SURGICAL TECHNOLOGY

PRINCIPLES AND PRACTICE

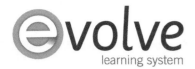
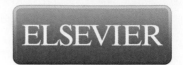
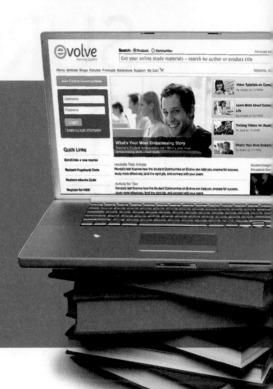

SURGICAL TECHNOLOGY
PRINCIPLES AND PRACTICE

SIXTH EDITION

Joanna Kotcher Fuller, BA, BSN, RN, RGN, MPH
Emergency Medical Coordinator
Medical Emergency Relief International, UK-Global

Consulting Editor:
Julie Armistead, CST, CRCST, BA
Surgical Technology Program Director
Virginia College
Macon, Georgia

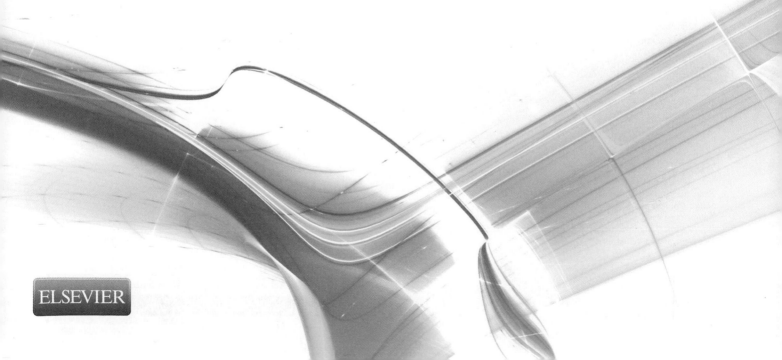

ELSEVIER

3251 Riverport Lane
St. Louis, Missouri 63043

SURGICAL TECHNOLOGY: PRINCIPLES AND PRACTICE, SIXTH EDITION   ISBN: 978-1-4557-2506-9

Notices

Knowledge and best practice in this field are constantly changing. As new research and experience broaden our understanding, changes in research methods, professional practices, or medical treatment may become necessary.

Practitioners and researchers must always rely on their own experience and knowledge in evaluating and using any information, methods, compounds, or experiments described herein. In using such information or methods they should be mindful of their own safety and the safety of others, including parties for whom they have a professional responsibility.

With respect to any drug or pharmaceutical products identified, readers are advised to check the most current information provided (i) on procedures featured or (ii) by the manufacturer of each product to be administered to verify the recommended dose or formula, the method and duration of administration, and contraindications. It is the responsibility of practitioners, relying on their own experience and knowledge of their patients, to make diagnoses, to determine dosages and the best treatment for each individual patient, and to take all appropriate safety precautions.

To the fullest extent of the law, neither the Publisher nor the authors, contributors, or editors, assume any liability for any injury and/or damage to persons or property as a matter of products liability, negligence or otherwise, or from any use or operation of any methods, products, instructions, or ideas contained in the material herein.

Library of Congress Cataloging-in-Publication Data

Fuller, Joanna Ruth.

  Surgical technology : principles and practice / Joanna Kotcher Fuller, Julie Armistead.—6th ed.

      p. ; cm.

  Includes bibliographical references and index.

  ISBN 978-1-4557-2506-9 (hardcover : alk. paper)

  I. Armistead, Julie.   II. Title.

  [DNLM: 1. Operating Room Nursing.   2. Operating Room Technicians.   WY 162]

  LC classification not assigned

  617′.0231–dc23

                                        2012014598

Vice President and Publisher: Andrew Allen
Executive Content Strategist: Jennifer Janson
Senior Content Development Specialist: Kelly Brinkman
Publishing Services Manager: Catherine Jackson
Senior Project Manager: Mary Pohlman
Designer: Jessica Williams

Printed in Canada
Last digit is the print number: 9 8 7 6 5 4 3 2 1

SURGICAL PROCEDURE REVIEW PANEL

BETH APPLEGATE-DEBO, CST
Crouse Hospital
Syracuse, New York

CALE BLAINE, CST
Doctors Hospital at Renaissance
Edinburg, Texas

TAMMY L. CAPESTRO, CST, EMT-B
SSM St. Clare Surgical Center
Fenton, Missouri

DAVE FREEMAN, CST
Renton Technical College
Seattle, Washington

DEON KULA, CST,CRCST, EMT-B
Elgin Community College
Chicago, Illinois

KIMBERLY MILLER, CST
Certified Surgical Technologist
Three Gables Surgical Hospital
Proctorville, Ohio

PAUL NICHOLS, CST
Surgical Technologist
SSM Health Care, St. Clare Health Center
St. Louis, Missouri

GWEN O'ROURKE, AS, CST
Surgical Technologist
Jacksonville, Florida

COLETTE RYERSON-FERRELL, RN
Bartlett Regional Hospital
Juneau, Alaska

MATTHEW C. SCHAAB, BS, CST
Instructor
Medical Careers Institute
Richmond, Virgina

GREG SCHAFER, RN
Wishard Hospital
Indianapolis, Indiana

JONI WIGGINS, CST III
Palo Alto Medical Foundation
Mountain View, California

CONTENT REVIEWERS

BECKY BRODIN, RN, MA, CNOR
Program Director, Surgical Technology
Saint Mary's University of Minnesota
Minneapolis, Minnesota

NICOLE CLAUSSEN, CST, MS, FAST
Program Director of Surgical Technology
Rolla Technical Center
Rolla, Missouri

LORI GROINUS, CST
Surgical Technologist Program Coordinator
Rasmussen College
St. Cloud, Minnesota

JESSIE A. HERNANDEZ, OTC, CST
Surgical Technologist/Trauma Service Technologist
William Beaumont Army Medical Center
Department of Defense/United States Army
El Paso, Texas

JULIA HINKLE, RN,MHS, CNOR
Professor/Program Chair Surgical Technology
Ivy Tech Community College
Evansville, Indiana

RUTH ANNE LETEXIER, CST, BSN, PHN
Surgical Technology Program Director
Northland Community & Technical College
East Grand Forks, Minnesota

KATHY PATNAUDE, CST, AOT, BS
Surgical Technology Program Director
Midlands Technical College
Columbia, South Carolina

KARIE M. TENNANT, AAS, CST
Program Director, Surgical Technology
Virginia College
Columbia, South Carolina

Shortly after the historical entry of operating room technician as a civilian allied health profession, *Surgical Technology: Principles and Practice* was introduced as the first and only textbook written by a certified surgical technologist and intended solely for the study of surgical technology. Since that time this textbook has been in continuous publication, with succeeding editions that paralleled the growth of the profession.

The sixth edition of *Surgical Technology: Principles and Practice* represents a long-term partnership between educators and students that spans more than 20 years. Throughout this period there have been striking advances in biotechnology and associated demands for professional development of the surgical technologist. The Association of Surgical Technologists was instrumental in creating structures for course accreditation through a number of collaborating agencies. *Surgical Technology: Principles and Practice* has been there to support students throughout the growth and development of the profession. It has kept pace with technological advances in the profession but also with a wider role in patient care. The surgical technologist today is not only a team player but also a decision maker, a role that requires greater demands on personal as well as technical skills. *Surgical Technology: Principles and Practice* continues to provide authoritative information in a manner that encourages students to think strategically and creatively as they face new professional challenges.

A number of new areas of study have been added to the surgical technology curriculum. This edition includes the most recent curriculum requirements with electronic resources for both students and instructors to make the transition smoother and to ensure that all material and references are authoritative and up to date.

Surgical technologists must be current in all aspects of government and professional standards related to safety. Patient and health worker safety has been a major focus in all editions of *Surgical Technology: Principles and Practice*. This edition provides the current standards, and includes the names and web addresses of the authoritative agencies and professional bodies that create the standards, so that students and instructors can be continually informed of any updates.

WHO WILL BENEFIT FROM THIS BOOK?

This textbook has been written primarily for surgical technology students. The book's comprehensive approach covers all core content required for instruction in surgical technology programs that are accredited by both the Commission on Accreditation of Allied Health Education Programs (CAAHEP) and the American Board of Health Education Schools (ABHES). Although primarily a student textbook, the progressive technical discussions and comprehensive approach make it a standard reference book for central processing staff, surgical nurses, medical students, and interns working or rotating through surgery.

WHY IS THIS BOOK IMPORTANT TO THE PROFESSION?

Surgical Technology: Principles and Practice is an important work, not only because it was the first textbook written for and by a surgical technologist, but because it is based in sound evidence-based practice and a high level of scholarship. Textbook standards must be soundly based in responsible scholarship. For students and instructors, this means that information—no matter what the form—must be thoroughly researched and include sources of the information.

Standards of practice are established by the coordinated efforts of the many peer-reviewed professional and governmental organizations involved in medicine, nursing, environment safety, infectious disease, and patient protection. These practices are evidence-based. *Surgical Technology: Principles and Practice* presents these standards as the basis of practice using language and terms widely recognized by the medical and nursing community. One of the important goals of *Surgical Technology: Principles and Practice* has been to present facts and material without pretention or jargon—to make it accessible to students so they can achieve their personal career goals. The sixth edition continues in these traditions.

NEW TO THIS EDITION

The sixth edition of *Surgical Technology: Principles and Practice* presents important new material required for the continuing growth of the profession. This edition contains all additions to the latest surgical technology curriculum. These topics have been integrated into existing chapters and include up-to-date references and resources for students and instructors.

New to this edition is a chapter on community disaster planning and response. This material was developed for surgical technologists as an accreditation requirement of CAAHEP. The chapter explains federal, state, and local disaster management structures and also presents an illustrative case study of a disaster. Internet-based resources are provided throughout the chapter so that students and instructors can easily access formal training programs in disaster response and also get more information on specific topics.

A new chapter on trauma surgery has also been added. This chapter synthesizes skills that students acquire in preparation for their work as surgical technologists, with new information on the methods and practices of trauma surgery. Most importantly, the chapter explains the principles that form the basis of trauma surgery and provides insight into how to apply previously learned skills into the trauma specialization.

LEARNING AIDS

A variety of pedagogical features are included in this text to aid learning:

Chapter Outlines, Learning Objectives, and Terminology, with glossary-style definitions at the beginning of each chapter, set the stage for student learning.

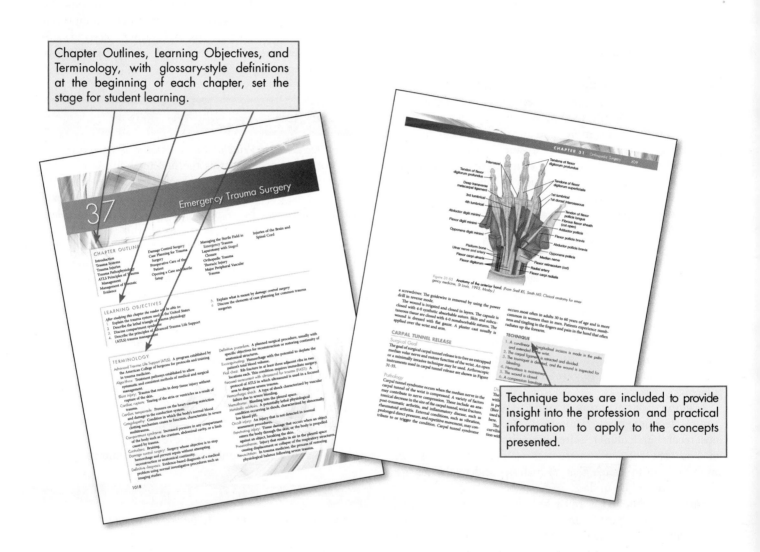

Technique boxes are included to provide insight into the profession and practical information to apply to the concepts presented.

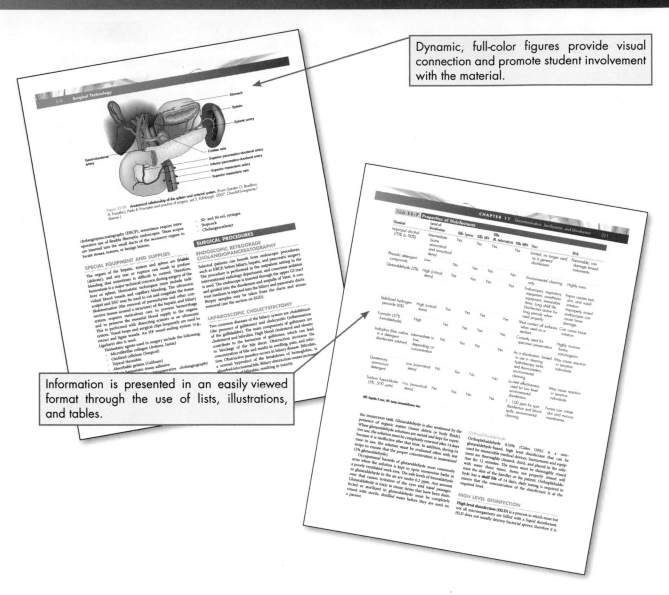

Dynamic, full-color figures provide visual connection and promote student involvement with the material.

Information is presented in an easily viewed format through the use of lists, illustrations, and tables.

ANCILLARIES

FOR THE INSTRUCTOR

Evolve

Surgical Technology: Principles and Practice offers several assets on Evolve to aid instructors:

- Test Bank: An Exam-View test bank of more than 1400 multiple choice questions that feature rationales, cognitive levels, and page number references to the text. This can be used as review in class or for test development.
- PowerPoint Presentations: One PowerPoint presentation has been developed for each chapter. These can be used as is or as a template to prepare chapter lectures.
- Image Collection: All of the images from the book are available as JPEGs and can be downloaded into PowerPoint presentations. These can be used during lecture to illustrate important concepts.

- Text Answer Key: All of the answers to the Review Questions from the text, along with talking points for the Case Studies.
- Workbook Answer Key: All of the answers to the Workbook exercises.
- TEACH Instructors Resource: Includes lesson plans, lecture outlines, and PowerPoint slides, all available via Evolve. The TEACH Instructors Resource provides instructors with customizable lesson plans and lecture outlines based on learning objectives. With these valuable resources, instructors will save valuable preparation time and create a learning environment that fully engages students in classroom participation. The lesson plans are keyed chapter by chapter and are divided into convenient lessons that break up the chapters logically. The Lesson Plans include a wide variety of classroom, online, and homework activities for students. In addition to the lesson plans, instructors will have unique lecture outlines in PowerPoint with talking

points, thought-provoking questions, and unique ideas for lectures.

FOR THE STUDENT

Student Workbook

The student workbook includes:

- Comprehensive review of terminology, anatomy, and chapter content that are reinforced by a variety of recall exercises.
- Application exercises that encourage students to put concepts into practice.
- Critical thinking exercises that take information to the next level and prepare students for the real world through patient case scenarios.

Evolve

Student resources on Evolve:

- Skills Videos that correspond to specific content covered in the text.
- A mock certification exam that prepares students for the exam by testing their knowledge on important concepts.
- Chapter activities that provide review of content covered in text for additional practice.
- Archie Animations that show various anatomy and procedure demonstrations discussed in the text.
- Flash cards to provide a quick review of terms found throughout the textbook.
- Content updates to keep the text current. And more!

Acknowledgments

Special thanks for this edition of *Surgical Technology* go to several key people who have been instrumental in the production of this edition. Jennifer Janson, Executive Content Strategist, has been associated with the text for many years and provided excellent oversight and major decision making. Kelly Brinkman, Senior Content Development Specialist, has been instrumental in managing the flow and organization of manuscript and artwork, and advising on content and organization. I would like to give special praise to Mary Pohlman, Senior Project Manager, for implementing the layout of the text. Her expert design has improved readability while maintaining visual appeal in the text, making it much easier for the reader to match the text with the images. Mary's editorial expertise has also been a great help in completing this edition of the book. I would also like to acknowledge the consultant work of Julie Armistead, who has updated the ancillaries and provided consultation on curriculum requirements.

Contents

PART II   SURGICAL TECHNOLOGY PRACTICE

CHAPTER OUTLINE

Introduction

Historical Evolution of the Profession

AST: The Association of Surgical Technologists

Affiliated Organizations

Training and Certification

The Role of the Surgical Technologist

Other Perioperative Responsibilities

Task Integration

Careers for Certified Surgical Technologists

Becoming a Health Care Professional

Personal Attributes for Success

LEARNING OBJECTIVES

After studying this chapter the reader will be able to:

1. Understand the development of the role of the surgical technologist, including the organizations that support the profession
2. Describe the process of training and certification for the surgical technologist
3. Discuss the role of the surgical technologist
4. Discuss career opportunities available to the surgical technologist
5. Describe the attributes of a professional
6. List the personal attributes needed for success as a surgical technologist

TERMINOLOGY

ABHES: Accrediting Bureau of Health Education Schools. Organization that offers accreditation to higher education institutions.

ACS: American College of Surgeons. A professional organization that establishes educational standards for surgeons and surgical residency programs.

Allied health profession: A profession that follows the principles of medicine and nursing but that focuses on an expertise set apart from those practices.

AORN: Association of periOperative Registered Nurses. The professional organization for surgical nurses; originally known as the Association of Operating Room Nurses.

AMA: American Medical Association. Association founded in 1847 made up of medical doctors whose mission is to promote healthy lifestyles across all patient populations.

ARC/STSA: Accreditation Review Council on Education in Surgical Technology and Surgical Assisting. The ARC/STSA establishes, maintains, and promotes quality standards for education programs in surgical technology and surgical first assisting.

ANSI: American National Standards Institute. Organization that creates business and health standards to serve as a baseline for assessment.

Assistant circulator: The surgical technologist in the nonsterile role of the surgical team responsible for monitoring conditions in the operating room as related to patient care, safety, documentation, distribution of sterile supplies and counts. A registered perioperative nurse in this role would be considered a circulator and will have additional responsibilities.

AST: Association of Surgical Technologists. The professional association for surgical technologists that strives to uphold and support the standards of patient care and the profession.

CAAHEP: Commission on Accreditation of Allied Health Education Programs. Accredits health science programs, including those for surgical technology.

Certification: Acknowledgment by a private agency that a person has achieved a minimum level of knowledge and skill. Certification usually is established by graduation from an accredited institution and passing a written examination. Certification does not confer legal status.

Continuing education: More formally called *professional development*. It demonstrates an ongoing learning process in an individual's profession. Continuing education (CE) credits are provided by a professional organization. Credits are earned by attending lectures and in-service presentations or by study and examination. Usually only peer-reviewed professional literature qualifies for CE credits.

CST: Certified surgical technologist. A surgical technologist who has successfully passed the certified examination given by the National Board of Surgical Technology and Surgical Assisting.

CST-CFA: Certified surgical technologist–certified first assistant. A surgical technologist with advanced training who has successfully passed the certification examination for surgical first assistants and is credentialed by the National Board of Surgical Technology and Surgical Assisting.

Licensure: Professional status, granted by state government, that defines the limits (scope) of practice and regulates those who hold a license.

National Certifying Examination for Surgical Technologists: A comprehensive written examination required for official certification by the Association of Surgical Technologists, developed by the NBSTSA.

NBSTSA: National Board of Surgical Technology and Surgical Assisting. The NBSTA (formerly the Liaison Council on Certification for the Surgical Technologist) is responsible for all decisions related to certification such as eligibility, renewal, and revocation, as well as developing the certification examination.

NCCT: National Center for Competency Testing. A nonprofit organization that provides a certification examination for nonaccredited programs and on the job training, and other trained surgical technologists whose programs are not recognized by the Association of Surgical Technologists.

Nonsterile team members: Surgical team members who handle only nonsterile equipment, supplies, and instruments. The circulator is the primary nonsterile team member.

ORT: Operating room technician. Former name for surgical technologists (name changed to *surgical technologist* in the early 1970s).

Professional attributes: Positive behaviors and traits of a professional, highly regarded by the public and professional peers. They include such traits as honesty, reliability, tact, diplomacy, and commitment to the profession.

Proprietary school: Private, for-profit school.

Scrub: Role and name commonly applied to the surgical technologist or licensed nurse in the sterile scrub role during surgery.

Sterile personnel: Members of the surgical team who have performed a surgical scrub or hand and arm antisepsis procedure. They don sterile gown and gloves and either perform the surgery or assist directly. Sterile personnel include the surgeon, assistant(s), and scrub. Other sterile personnel such as a scrub nurse, students, and preceptors may also be part of the sterile team.

Surgical conscience: In surgery, professional and personal honesty about one's actions, mistakes, and abilities.

INTRODUCTION

Surgical technology is an allied health profession. Professionals in allied health follow the principles of medicine and nursing in that they participate in the health and well-being of people through specific tasks and expertise. However, allied health professionals have distinct expertise that is both humanistic and technical. Allied health professionals are highly trained and must have a global view of health, as well as the education and capability to focus on highly technical aspects of health care delivery. Other allied health professions include emergency medical technologists, nuclear medicine technicians, and specialists in the fields of medical physics, hemodialysis, bioengineering, dentistry, and respiratory therapy. In the past 2 decades, the number of allied health professionals has increased enormously, as have their educational requirements. Advances in technology and the need for specialist training have resulted in the development of new allied health professions and expanded the roles of those already in existence. Surgical technology has also followed this trend.

Whether the surgical technologist is trained in an intensive military program or through rigorous study and practice in a civilian health facility, the profession offers a variety of challenges and opportunities.

HISTORICAL EVOLUTION OF THE PROFESSION

The profession of surgical technologist, as it is defined today, is developing as a result of rapid, monumental developments in technology in general. Advances in optics and digital technology especially have contributed to the highly complex equipment required for modern surgical procedures.

Surgeons have always needed skilled assistants, including those whose particular role was centered around surgical instrumentation. Beginning with the development of effective anesthesia and antisepsis in the late 19th century, the role of the nurse in surgery has been well documented. In the late 1800s, she prepared instruments for surgery, and in the early 1900s, she assisted in surgical procedures and in the administration of ether, called "etherizing." Her duties from about the 1920s to the 1940s were those of today's circulator. She also instructed student nurses in their surgical education. Often the operating room supervisor was the only graduate nurse in surgery, and it was her duty to oversee the student nurses as they completed their rotation in surgery.

The need for assistive personnel in surgery did not arise until World War II. During World War I, Army corpsmen worked on the battlefield to offer aid and comfort to the wounded, but they had no role in surgery. World War II dramatically changed that. With the development of antibiotics, such as penicillin and sulfa, war surgeons could operate on and save the lives of many more patients than previously was possible. Technological advances also created a need for trained personnel who could assist the surgeon.

The increase in battlefield survivors created a drastic shortage of nurses. In addition to the nurses needed to staff the field hospitals, many more were needed at base hospitals. At home, extra nurses were trained to attend to the wounded who returned from battle. To supply the field hospitals in the Pacific and European theaters, the Army began training corpsmen to assist in surgery, a role that previously had been filled only by nurses. By this time, however, corpsmen were expected to administer anesthesia and also assist the surgeon directly during surgery.

When nurses were not available, such as on combat ships, corpsmen worked under the direct supervision of the surgeon. In this way, a new profession was born, and the Army called these corpsmen operating room technicians (ORTs). From this time on, the military played a significant role in refining the position of the ORT. Each branch of the military provided specific training and job descriptions for the ORT, who received secondary training after becoming a medic.

After World War II, the Korean War caused a continued shortage of operating room nurses, and the need for fully trained nurses in the operating room was questioned. At this time, the operating room supervisors began to recruit former corpsmen to work in civilian surgery. Their primary function was that of a circulator. Registered nurses continued to fill the role of the scrub or "instrument nurse" until about 1965, when the roles were reversed. At this point, hospitals began training civilian ORTs.

In 1967, prompted by the need for guidelines and standards in the training of paramedical surgical personnel, the Association of Operating Room Nurses (AORN) published a book, *Teaching the Operating Room Technician*. In 1968 the AORN board of directors created the Association of Operating Room Technicians (AORT). Formal training for the civilian ORT began in proprietary schools across the United States.

Along with organizational independence came steps toward formalizing the technologist's education. The AORT created two new committees, the Liaison Council on Certification for the Surgical Technologist (LCC-ST) and the Joint Review Committee on Education. In 1970, the first certifying examination for operating room technicians was administered, and those who passed were given the title Certified Operating Room Technician (CORT). In 1973, the AORT became independent from the AORN, and the profession changed its title to Association of Surgical Technologists (AST). The certified technician became known as a certified surgical technologist (CST).

AST: THE ASSOCIATION OF SURGICAL TECHNOLOGISTS

The AST is the surgical technologist's professional organization. The association supports students and graduate surgical technologists through its many services and publications. State assemblies and local chapters of AST link surgical technologists with their national association and provide forums for learning, discussion, and advocacy. The association is actively involved in training and curriculum development. At the national level, AST provides the following support to student and graduate surgical technologists, the public, and teaching institutions:

1. Maintains Practice Standards, Code of Ethics, and Code of Conduct for surgical technologists
2. Publishes a professional journal, *The Surgical Technologist*, which provides news, legislative updates, and articles for professional development
3. Holds annual conferences for surgical technologists and educators
4. Maintains a membership registry
5. Provides opportunities for continuing education (professional development)
6. Provides leadership, standards, and direction for the profession through its Standing Committees
7. Represents surgical technologists and advocates for standards of patient care through state and federal legislative bodies and the general public

8. Coordinates with the Accreditation Review Council on Education in Surgical Technology and Surgical Assisting (ARC/STSA) to establish educational standards for surgical technologists
9. Maintains regional and local chapters of the Association of Surgical Technologists
10. Provides academic scholarships through its foundation

It is important for surgical technology students to become active members of the AST and to promote the standards of the profession. Participation in conferences and educational seminars ensures that the high standards set by the organization are maintained through a process of continuing education and public awareness. Also, association with peers in the profession provides opportunities to share experiences and maintain current practices.

The website of the Association of Surgical Technologists can be accessed at http://www.ast.org.

AFFILIATED ORGANIZATIONS

As a body of professionals, surgical technologists are supported by a number of key organizations and partners. Each has a designated role in promotion, certification, accreditation, and continuing education.

ACCREDITATION REVIEW COUNCIL ON EDUCATION IN SURGICAL TECHNOLOGY AND SURGICAL ASSISTING (ARC/STSA)

The ARC/STSA provides educational standards and recommendations required for accreditation of programs in surgical technology and surgical first assisting. The ARC/STSA collaborates with the Commission on Accreditation of Allied Health Education Programs (CAAHEP), which accredits programs on recommendation of the ARC/STSA. Accreditation is granted to a school only after a full on-site evaluation of the program and its facilities to ensure compliance with ARC/STSA standards This includes an evaluation of the courses that must adhere to an approved core curriculum.

The Accrediting Bureau of Health Education Schools (ABHES) is another nonprofit accrediting body. ABHES is recognized by the U.S. Department of Education as both an institutional and specialized accreditation body in health training and education. Its students may apply to take the AST certification examination.

The ARC/STSA website can be accessed at http://www.arcst.org.

NATIONAL BOARD OF SURGICAL TECHNOLOGY AND SURGICAL ASSISTING

The National Board of Surgical Technology and Surgical Assisting (NBSTSA) (formerly the LCC-ST) oversees certification and credentialing of surgical technologists and surgical technologist-first assistants. The organization is responsible for the eligibility, granting, revoking, and denial of certification.

Students who have graduated from schools accredited by the CAAHEP or by ABHES can sit for the AST certification examination. The organization's policies, procedures, and certification test information can be found at the NBSTSA website, http://www.nbstsa.org.

TRAINING AND CERTIFICATION

Surgical technologists are trained in 2-year colleges, the military, and proprietary (for-profit) certificate programs. The curriculum for surgical technologists is varied and intense. Certification through the Association of Surgical Technologists requires graduation from a CAAHEP-accredited school or one approved by the ABHES. The ABHES offers accreditation to higher education institutions approved by the U.S. Department of Education and includes hospital-based, Veterans Administration (VA), and federally sponsored Armed Forces programs.

CERTIFICATION

Certification by examination is available for qualified STs through the NBSTSA. Certification demonstrates a standard of knowledge and understanding of the principles of surgical technology. It is an important commitment to establishing and maintaining quality assurance in patient care throughout the surgical technologist's career. Certification is mandatory *in some states* for an individual to work in the profession. This requirement is the national trend because it provides a demonstrable standard of knowledge. Certification is not the same as state licensure, which is described in Chapter 4. The comprehensive examination covers the principles and basic practices of surgical technology, including basic sciences and patient care in the operating room. Students have the opportunity to take the examination before graduation. A passing grade on the examination confers the right to certification and the title Certified Surgical Technologist.

Eligibility

To be eligible to take the certification examination, the applicant must meet one of the following criteria:
- The individual must be a graduate of a surgical technology program accredited by CAAHEP (see earlier discussion) or by the ABHES.
- The individual must currently be or previously have been a CST.
- Graduates from accredited military programs and previously certified surgical technologists with lapsed membership are also eligible to sit for a certification examination.
- Students may apply to take the examination before graduation; however, the results of the examination are not released until proof of graduation is presented.

NATIONAL CENTER FOR COMPETENCY TESTING

The National Center for Competency Testing (NCCT) has developed certification examinations for surgical tech-

nologists; these examinations are separate from the AST certification process. The NCCT certification process is essential for trained medical military staff, whose educational programs are not recognized by the AST. For certification as a surgical technologist, the NCCT requires scrub experience from all applicants, with a minimum of 150 validated, documented surgical cases. The NCCT also requires applicants to have a high school diploma or equivalent, and they must meet any of the following eligibility requirements:
- Be a graduate of an operating room technician, surgical technician, or surgical technologist program offered by a school or college recognized by the U.S. Department of Education.
- Be a graduate of a formal operating room technician or surgical technology training program, with 1 year of validated work experience in the past 2 years or 2 years of work experience in the past 4 years.
- Have 7 years of validated scrub experience within the past 10 years.
- Be a medical doctor (MD), registered nurse (RN), licensed practical nurse (LPN), or licensed vocational nurse (LVN) with extensive, documented scrub experience.
- Applicants must pass the certification examination to receive the credential tech in surgery–certified, or TS-C (NCCT).
- The NCCT also requires individuals to maintain continuing education (CE) credits for certification. Those who pass the surgical assistant certification examination earn the credential assistant in surgery–certified, or AS-C (NCCT).

The NCCT website can be accessed at http://www.ncctinc.com.

CONTINUING EDUCATION

Continuing education provides an opportunity for professionals to improve their knowledge and competency. The AST provides resources for CE credits through its CE resources available directly from the AST, through online courses, or through *The Surgical Technologist*, the professional journal published by the AST.

CLINICAL LADDER PROGRAM

The Clinical Ladder program was established by the AST to provide incentives for surgical technologists to advance their clinical skills and competency in key areas. According to the AST, the proposed clinical ladder provides a "tool for measuring the ongoing progress of the surgical technologist from one level to another." The stated goals of the clinical ladder are primarily to:
- Improve patient care
- Encourage employer recognition of the surgical technologist
- Promote accountability
- Increase the visibility of the surgical technologist's role

Box **1-1** Proposed Clinical Ladder

Level 1: Entry Level

Entry-level surgical technologist (ST) is the first level after graduation from an accredited surgical technology program and includes the first year of practice. The technologist should have scrubbed in general surgery, orthopedics, obstetrics and gynecology, genitourinary surgery, and otorhinolaryngology procedures at several levels of complexity. He or she will be able to demonstrate practical use of anatomy and physiology, pharmacology, and medical terminology and will be able to assist in the care of the patient at a basic level. The entry-level technologist demonstrates sound understanding of aseptic (surgical) technique and applies this knowledge in practice. The ST is also expected to apply basic knowledge about electricity and other energy sources in the perioperative environment. He or she takes part in training programs and orientation to more advanced skills and techniques.

Level 2: Proficient

The certified surgical technologist at level 2 has at least 1 year of employment, demonstrates the skills necessary for routine scrub roles across the specialties, and can respond to emergency situations in surgery. At this level, the technologist assists in circulating duties and assumes greater responsibilities in patient care. The level 2 technologist participates in decision making with his or her peers and seeks educational experience to advance his or her practice skills.

Level 3: Expert

The expert-level role includes a proficiency in all expected tasks in surgery and includes advanced-level practice in surgical equipment and highly technical instrumentation. The expert technologist is capable of scrubbing complex cases across the specialties and takes an active role in their planning. He or she is a role model for other technologists and participates in teaching and mentoring programs for students. The expert technologist may be asked to become involved in acquiring new equipment for the operating room, which might include planning purchases or leases with vendors.

- Encourage experienced surgical technologists to collaborate with colleagues to allow for professional growth

The Clinical Ladder program defines specific levels of practice (I through III) and provides clinical and learning objectives for each level. The levels are characterized by increasing technical ability and responsibilities for tasks involving patient care and management (Box 1-1). The clinical ladder is not a requirement but a model for advancement. Because individuals are unique, no one system fits everyone. Many technologists enter the profession as highly critical thinkers, able to problem solve, and achieve some of the "higher" objectives while still in their first or second year of practice.

THE ROLE OF THE SURGICAL TECHNOLOGIST

Today's certified surgical technologist has a broad scope of practice and many career choices. The exact role on the job varies according to specialization and the type of institution in which the CST works. Chapter 21, Case Planning and Intraoperative Routines, provides technical discussions of the common duties and roles of a surgical technologist. Here we provide fundamental information about the roles a surgical technologist can fulfill. The full job description document as established by the AST is located at www.ast.org.

SCRUB ROLE

As a member of the **sterile team**, the technologist is a scrubbed, gowned, and gloved participant in surgery. In very simple terms, the sterile team, which also includes the surgeon and assistant(s), delivers direct surgical care by performing the surgery or by providing technical assistance to those who perform the surgery. In this position the technologist is often referred to as the *scrub*. This is the traditional role of the individual who prepares and passes instruments, medical supplies, medications, and equipment during the surgery. The scrub also assists the surgeon in specific, well-defined tasks as needed during the procedure. The term *scrub* has been used to describe this role for many years and predates the current profession of surgical technologist as it is practiced today. The name *scrub* remains in common use, because surgical traditions are highly regarded. Even though the role is highly evolved, the name remains as part of the tradition. The scrub role can be fulfilled by various professionals, including RNs and licensed vocational and practical nurses. The surgical technologist in the scrubbed role may also be referred to as STSR (surgical technologist scrub role), scrubbed ST, or simply ST. In this text the term *scrub* is used interchangeably with *scrubbed ST*. The *scrub* role is different from those of *surgical assistant* and *circulator*, which are discussed later.

Surgical procedures require a variety of instruments, supplies, and equipment. These range from a relatively small number of basic instruments to very large instrument "sets" that contain specialty instruments for a specific body system and its tissues. Complex procedures can involve more than one body system. These cases require hundreds of items to be immediately available for the surgeon's use. Some instruments require assembly "on the field" (the immediate sterile work area of the team), sutures must be prepared, and supplies such as sponges, medications, solutions, and electronic devices must be carefully delivered to the surgeon throughout the procedure. These are presented as needed at the moment they will be used.

The scrub must also protect the sterile field from contamination and communicate effectively with the surgeon to prevent errors, such as passing the wrong instrument or passing it in the wrong position. Errors consume valuable time and cause disruptions that are distracting to the surgeon and are not conducive to safe surgery. This means that the scrub must anticipate every step of the surgery and maintain the instrument tables in a neat and orderly way at all times. The scrub also communicates with the nonscrubbed circulator to receive other items needed during a surgical procedure. Scrubs learn the flow and events of different procedures within their specialty by study and practice. The AST lists *general* duties of the surgical technologist in the scrub role that can be found at www.ast.org. The scrubbed ST performs many other tasks requiring training and special skills.

CIRCULATOR

The surgical technologist in the circulator role is identified as an **assistant circulator,** ST circulator, or STCR—surgical technologist circulating role. In this text the term *ST circulator* is used most frequently, and it is understood to refer to the role in an assistant position.

Unlike the scrub, who is a "sterile" team member and remains at the sterile field throughout the surgery, the circulator is a "nonsterile" team member. Traditionally, the role was fulfilled by a registered perioperative nurse, LVN, or LPN. In the past decade, the surgical technologist's training has expanded to include specific tasks performed by the circulator. The surgical technologist shares some but not all of the responsibilities of the RN. The exact duties vary somewhat by state, region, and health facility. Each of the fundamental practices of the ST in the circulator role are described in this text. Students can then adapt their practice according to the facility and location in which they work.

The circulator role is quite different from that of the scrub. The circulator does not directly contact (touch) any sterile instruments, supplies, or equipment. Instead, he or she performs direct patient care, obtains, delivers, and prepares the nonsterile equipment or nonsterile *connections* of sterile equipment. The circulator also distributes and opens sterile instruments and other supplies to the sterile team members using a method that protects the instruments from contamination. The circulator is also responsible for positioning the patient for surgery, assisting the anesthesia care provider, receiving tissue and other types of specimens from the sterile field for their proper containment, identification, and transfer to the pathology department. These are just a few of the many responsibilities of the circulator.

The circulator ensures that the patient chart, including results of diagnostic procedures, permits, and preoperative checklist, accompanies the patient to surgery. Other possible duties of the circulator include performing the surgical skin prep and urinary catheterization. Refer to the AST website for a list of basic ST circulator duties as established by the AST. Note that some of these duties vary according to state practice acts and facility policy.

SECOND ASSISTANT

Most surgical procedures require one or more assistants to the surgeon. When two assistants are needed, the ST may step into the **second assistant** position. This role is separate from that of first assistant described later. The tasks of the second assistant include but are not limited to the following:
- Maintain retraction on tissues
- Maintain a "dry" surgical site by operating suction devices and appropriate use of surgical sponges
- Assist with hemostasis as directed by the surgeon

- Properly assemble and attach wound suction devices at the close of surgery
- Apply wound dressings at the close of surgery

These tasks and many others requiring direct assistance have traditionally been performed by the scrub but are now officially designated in the role by the Association of Surgical Technologists. Other tasks that may be required include:
- Steadying and maintaining the position of the insertion tube during endoscopic surgery
- Irrigating the surgical wound, especially in microsurgery
- Cutting sutures that have been placed by the surgeon

The scope of practice in this role is defined by state Practice Acts (discussed in Chapter 4) and health facility protocol. It is important for perioperative professionals to understand that no facility, organization, or individual can override state Practice Acts.

OTHER PERIOPERATIVE RESPONSIBILITIES

EMERGENCY DUTY

The surgical technologist working in a hospital or other facility that provides 24-hour care is usually required to be on "call". This means that the ST is available outside normal working hours to respond to emergency cases.

INSTRUMENTATION SPECIALIST

In the role of specialist in the preparation, handling, and use of instruments, surgical technologists put into practice their specific knowledge about instrumentation, including its preparation for surgery. The skills and knowledge required for this role are the processes of sterilization and disinfection, inspection and troubleshooting of equipment, and assembly of instrument sets.

PATIENT CARE

The surgical technologist is more than a technical adviser and manager of equipment. The technologist is also a care provider. A surgical patient is exposed to numerous risks. Some are directly related to the technology used to accomplish the surgical goals; others are inherent in the procedure itself. The direct care that the surgical technologist, nursing, and medical team provide helps mitigate or eliminate these risks. Psychosocial support is equally important to the patient's recovery and well-being. Surgical technologists interact directly with patients and contribute to the patient's psychological well-being, especially in the preoperative period.

LEADERSHIP AND MANAGEMENT

Unique opportunities in leadership and management are available to experienced surgical technologists. Specialty services such as orthopedics, ophthalmology, and neurosurgery need team leaders to facilitate and direct personnel and to manage equipment in specialty departments. Other leadership opportunities are available in facilitating safety and emergency protocols.

Surgical technologists may choose to pursue an advanced degree in hospital administration and management. At advanced levels, the integrated experience of both technology and patient care is an excellent springboard for a broader managerial career.

PRECEPTOR

Surgical technologists often are asked to act as preceptors, teaching others while scrubbed. Some people enjoy this role and are natural teachers. Others are uncomfortable with the responsibility or are disappointed that they can no longer scrub cases alone. Serving as preceptor requires patience and a willingness to share knowledge and experience.

TASK INTEGRATION

An important concept for surgical technology students and experienced professionals alike is task integration. Because the role is complex, it is easy to lose sight of the importance of connecting or integrating tasks and responsibilities. The work of the surgical technologist is never performed in isolation. Every task and responsibility is an integral part of a larger domain of medicine. A holistic perspective is required to understand the relationships among patient care, the use of technology, and technical assistance. All are related to patient safety and achievement of the surgical objectives.

The specific domain of surgical technology is patient care in the perioperative setting, focusing on the safe use of technology and the art of surgery to promote the patient's well-being.

This larger picture casts the surgical technologist's role as a combination of five main areas of health care and technology:
- Assistant in surgical procedures as part of the surgical team
- Specialist in the preparation, handling, and use of surgical devices, equipment, and instruments
- Patient care provider in the perioperative setting
- Participant in leadership and management
- Educator and preceptor

Clearly, the surgical technologist has many roles and performs many tasks, ranging from the basic to the complex.

CAREERS FOR CERTIFIED SURGICAL TECHNOLOGISTS

FACILITY-BASED SURGICAL TECHNOLOGIST

The unique combination of health care and technological expertise opens the door to a wide range of roles and responsibilities. Most surgical technologists work in hospitals as members of the surgical team; this is the role that entry-level CSTs are trained to fulfill. It is a complex job involving many disciplines, including:

- Basic patient care
- Organization, use, and care of surgical instruments and devices
- Team-building skills
- Principles and practice of sterile technique
- Surgical procedures

Surgical technologists may also work as agency personnel. In this position, they are not permanent employees of a particular hospital, but rather work under short-term contracts in different hospitals. This provides a variety of experiences in different locations.

MILITARY SERVICE

The military offers a surgical technology program for a specialized setting; this is referred to as the operating room specialist course. The educational program parallels civilian requirements, with additional training in combat and war surgery and in golden hour treatment (the golden hour is the first hour of treatment close to the front lines). The military program was the prototype for surgical technologists and remains dedicated to high standards, offering care to the war wounded and to other military personnel and civilians in combat areas where the armed forces are deployed. Opportunities in military surgery extend to more complex tasks associated with emergency settings and to licensure for operating room nursing.

SPECIALTY PRACTICE

The hospital-based surgical technologist may specialize in one or more surgical specialties, such as orthopedics, neurosurgery, cardiac surgery, obstetrics, or plastic surgery. CSTs at the midlevel and advanced stages of their career have the experience and knowledge to provide expert assistance in these specialties, and their work is in high demand.

Many surgical technologists work as private scrub assistants in the specialties in which they trained as hospital employees. These positions require middle- and advanced-level experience, as well as management and leadership skills. Surgical specialists may be required to provide preoperative education to patients in the office practice, and they may also fulfill that role in the hospital or health care facility.

Educational requirements for the role of specialist begin with certification in basic surgical technology. More advanced education in patient care and management may be required to provide care in the medical office.

CERTIFIED SURGICAL TECHNOLOGIST– CERTIFIED FIRST ASSISTANT

The Certified Surgical Technologist–Certified First Assistant (CST-CFA) assists in surgical procedures to retract tissue and aid in exposure, hemostasis (control hemorrhage), closing of tissue planes (suturing or stapling), and other intraoperative techniques while under supervision of the surgeon. Surgical technologists represent one among several professions that can attain professional status as a surgical assistant. Others include the Registered Nurse First Assistant, the Physician Assistant First Assistant, and the Surgical Assistant Nurse Practitioner. Expanded professional roles of the RN and physician's assistant usually involve greater responsibility because these individuals provide complex perioperative care to the surgical patient.

Preparation for the CST-CFA role includes certification in entry-level surgical technology, graduation from surgical assisting programs accredited through Accreditation Review Council on Education in Surgical Technology and Surgical Assisting (ARC/STSA), or a CST who completes 350 cases in the CFA role within the last 2 years. Proprietary (certificate) programs are available for surgical assistance.

> *The Association of Surgical Assistants (ASA) website can be accessed at http://www.surgicalassistant.org.*

EDUCATOR AND CLINICAL INSTRUCTOR

The preferred educational pathway for the surgical technologist is a 2-year college degree or certificate program. In the future, a 4-year Bachelor of Science (BS) degree may become the norm. In the field of education, certified surgical technologists currently work as formal instructors and as clinical department heads. They also design and develop the curriculum for their institutions and manage departments. These roles are becoming increasingly widespread, because the profession is growing and the need for quality instructors has greatly increased.

Entry-level certification and at least 2 years of experience in surgery are the minimum requirements for an educator position. Specific requirements depend on the type of institution (e.g., proprietary and state or community level).

MEDICAL INDUSTRY REPRESENTATIVE

An increasing number of CSTs with advanced training and experience work as representatives in the medical services and equipment industry. Service representatives are responsible for advising and training hospital and private clinical staff in the use of a company's products. They often travel to clinical sites in their designated area and are available on call to answer questions and provide on-site assistance during surgery that involves the equipment. In this role, they promote their company's equipment, but they also have the technical expertise to troubleshoot problems.

The educational requirements for the role of medical services representative include entry-level certification plus experience and additional training in management and service provision, which is provided by the company. More advanced positions in medical industry management might require a degree in business.

CENTRAL PROCESSING MANAGEMENT

Materials management or central sterile processing is the management of cleaning, assembly, and sterilization of medical instruments and equipment used in surgery. This field is growing in complexity and scope, requiring the expertise of instrument technology and a thorough knowledge of safety and health standards. The scope of duties and responsibilities includes disinfection and sterilization processes, assembly of surgical instrument sets, and management of complex instrument systems. It also may include managing and ordering other supplies used in surgery and maintaining accurate records of processing, use, and distribution. The surgical technologist may manage a materials processing department or function under the supervision of others.

The educational requirements for the role of materials management and processing are basic entry-level certification and at least 1 year of experience in operating room technology. Some hospitals may require certification as a Central Processing Technician. Management positions may also require supervisory experience or an advanced degree.

RESEARCH PRODUCT AND DEVELOPMENT

The surgical technologist is well prepared to work in research product and development in the area of surgical instruments, supplies, and devices. In this role, the technologist documents the results for new products and provides essential information for their further development and production. Basic entry-level certification and additional education in research methodology are required.

BECOMING A HEALTH CARE PROFESSIONAL

The journey from student to health care professional is a process in which you will learn new skills and acquire knowledge in many different areas of study. You will have "hands-on" practice for many of the technical skills and will also have the opportunity to connect classroom knowledge directly to your work. In addition to the practice and theory, you will begin to develop as a *professional*. This is just as important as all the other knowledge and skills you acquire as a surgical technologist.

WHAT IS A PROFESSIONAL?

We often think of a professional as someone who is highly trained and uses his or her skills in the public sector. But the term *professional* means much more than just practicing skills and knowledge. Professionals have particular attributes—attitudes and behavior—that reflect a high standard of accountability, ethics, honesty, and respect for people. All health care providers go through the process of becoming professional. It is a normal part of learning and maturing in a chosen field of work.

> *Many students are more concerned about demonstrating hands-on skills than professional attributes. However, behavior deficiencies such as difficulty with patient interaction, communication, and other professional attributes are more important causes of performance problems in the clinical area.[1]*

Health professionals are among the most highly regarded professionals in our society. A central value from which many others are developed is the **public trust**. This means that patients, their families, and others in the care environment maintain a high level of confidence in the professionals who care for them. In return, health professionals are ethically and morally bound to respect patients as feeling individuals with dignity and humanity. Violation of the public trust by one individual reflects on others who are collectively part of that profession. This gives a sense of urgency and gravity to any situation in which professionalism and public trust are violated.

THE FOUNDATIONS OF PROFESSIONALISM

- **Personal integrity:** This means to be trustworthy, reliable, and responsible, not only on the job, but at all times, in all areas of one's life. We also expect medical professionals to be honest and transparent in association with patients, colleagues, and the public. Professionals are expected to manage their personal affairs so they do not interfere with the duties of the work or education. This means being punctual and organized for work (or study) when required. Respecting schedules and the time constraints of others is essential to obtaining and maintaining a professional career.
- **Consistency in character and behavior:** Professionals maintain professional demeanor even under stress. This means controlling one's emotions (self-regulation).
- **Respect for rules, regulations, and law:** Because of the nature of their work, health care professionals are required to comply with many types of regulations and rules—including those of their institution (school or health facility) and state and federal laws. Professionals may disagree with regulations and rules and can challenge them at the appropriate time and place while maintaining respect for the institutions that created them.
- **Discretion and tact:** Health professionals work in many difficult situations requiring diplomacy and good judgment. Team conflict, patient and family crises, management disagreements, and many other stressful situations sometimes need to be handled on the spot to prevent escalation. Person-to-person difficulties require a high level of professional maturity. The health professional thinks before speaking and considers the consequences of actions and words. Discretion also means maintaining a healthy separation between personal life (and its problems) and work and maintaining patient confidentiality at all times.

DEVELOPING PROFESSIONALISM AND PERSONAL DEVELOPMENT

Throughout a career, people are guided by instructors, clinical mentors, and peers in the development of professionalism. There are many opportunities to increase professionalism through work experience and association with colleagues.

Many people believe that professionalism cannot be taught, but only acquired by observation and interaction with people. The process of developing professionalism is enhanced when colleagues, instructors, and our mentors give us feedback on our behavior and attitudes. Feedback may be expressed concretely through job evaluations, or more casually through conversation or body language of people in the work environment. Positive behaviors such as helping others with work or admitting an error may not be acknowledged publicly, but they are noticed by others. On the other hand, not owning up to a mistake, avoiding unpleasant but necessary tasks, or other negative traits are also noticed in the workplace. We can learn a lot about ourselves by observing others' reactions to our behavior and regulating our behavior accordingly.

PERSONAL ATTRIBUTES FOR SUCCESS

Whereas professionalism is the expression of attitudes and behaviors conducive to public trust and accountability, personal attributes are individual characteristics that are more related to ethics and attitudes toward others. Personal attributes can be learned or modified, and some are developed with time and experience.

The surgical technologist can achieve career goals in a variety of settings, whether it is a high-profile institution, a military post in a war zone, or a small, community-based setting. Everyone has unique talents to bring to the workplace. Some surgical technologists prefer a quiet workplace in which interpersonal relations are emphasized. Others prefer a highly technical, high-pressure environment in which many overtime hours are required and a wide variety of procedures are performed. Regardless of the setting, certain personal attributes contribute to or are necessary for professional success.

CARE AND EMPATHY

Health care professionals maintain an enduring interest in the health and safety of others. Caring for others is not a part-time job. It is a lifetime vocation.

A person who chooses to enter a health care profession usually has the qualities of care and empathy. However, once the professional begins working, these qualities can be enhanced through personal growth, or they can be lost through job stress or personal crisis. Providing care in the health domain requires a devotion to human beings, in all their states and predicaments. Empathy is a response to the emotional or physical experience of another human being. Having the desire to contribute to the patient's well-being is the most important personal attribute of any health care worker.

In addition to exhibiting care and empathy on the job, health care professionals may enhance these skills by getting involved in community service that assists various patient populations. For example, volunteers are often needed at nursing homes and children's hospitals. While volunteering, your technical skills likely won't be used, but your skills in care and empathy will be further developed.

ORGANIZATIONAL SKILLS

A surgical technologist is required to have good organizational skills. This is the ability to prioritize tasks and equipment in a logical and efficient manner. For example, the surgical technologist is required to prepare, assemble, and physically arrange instruments and equipment in the order in which they will be needed. This requires overall knowledge of the surgical process and all the steps needed to complete the task. Any one procedure may require the organization of hundreds of items. Instruments, sutures, sponges, needles, electrosurgical devices, solutions, and medications all must be immediately available. Materials must be organized in a logical and methodical way so that they are readily at hand when needed. This skill is developed with practice and time.

MANUAL DEXTERITY

The surgical technologist must work quickly and deftly, sometimes with complex or very small instruments. Equipment must be assembled and handled efficiently and without confusion. This requires manual skills and keen observation. Excellent hand-eye coordination is required to master the skills needed to prepare for and assist during surgery. Speed is not always the most important skill; in fact, if the surgical technologist tries to work too fast, organization can break down, instruments can be dropped, and injuries can occur.

ABILITY TO CONCENTRATE

Surgery requires constant, focused attention on both the operative site and the equipment. Although lulls in activity may occur, the surgical technologist is in motion during most of the procedure, preparing equipment or passing instruments in the correct spatial position. At the same time, the ST must anticipate the next step of the procedure. This requires moderate to intense levels of concentration. Lapses in focus can increase the risk to the patient and other team members. Many operative accidents, such as needlesticks, accidental cutting or burning, and loss of items in the surgical wound, are the result not of a lack of knowledge or skill but of a lack of attention. The short- and long-term problems that are the most common causes of lost concentration include fatigue or lack of sleep, stress, and substance abuse. Professionals have a public responsibility to be proactive in resolving personal and workplace situations that interfere with patient care.

PROBLEM-SOLVING SKILLS

The work of the surgical technologist is complex. Problems arise in every workday. Some problems require technical expertise, whereas others need a combination of "people skills" or environmental adjustments. A person with good problem-solving skills is able to:
- Identify and define problems
- Demonstrate genuine willingness to seek solutions to problems

- Use time wisely and anticipate problems
- Gather appropriate information to solve problems
- Identify solutions and select the best alternative to achieve positive results
- Analyze the result and accept feedback from others as part of the learning experience
- Assess his or her own abilities (e.g., asking oneself, "Do I have what I need to solve this problem myself? If not, who can best assist?")
- Demonstrate flexibility (e.g., asking oneself, "If the problem cannot be solved with the time and resources available, what alternatives do I have?")

PERSPECTIVE

The ability to put events in perspective and enjoy the lighter side of work and life is a great asset. Humor, when expressed appropriately, can ease tension and promote good practice. However, not all humor is appropriate. Humor that is sarcastic, mean-spirited, prejudicial, or crude may create tension and disdain among team members.

 Watch Section 1, Unit 1: Overview of the Surgical Technologist on the Evolve website. http://evolve.elsevier.com/Fuller/surgical.

KEY CONCEPTS

- The profession of surgical technologist developed out of a need for qualified personnel who were familiar with the technical aspects of surgery and could assist in intraoperative patient care.
- The U.S. military has trained surgical technologists since World War II and continues to do so today.
- The Association of Surgical Technologists is the professional organization for surgical technologists. It provides its members with opportunities for career planning, training materials, national conferences, and professional and legislative support.
- The National Center for Competency Testing provides certification by examination for surgical technologists with documented surgical experience and academic qualifications. This includes individuals trained in the armed forces.
- Surgical technology is one of the fastest growing professions in the United States. Many opportunities are available for career placement and advancement.
- Surgical technologists may be employed in a health care facility, hospital, or private clinic. Many develop expertise in specialty areas such as orthopedics, cardiac surgery, trauma, ophthalmic surgery, and plastic surgery.
- Other opportunities exist in education and marketing for surgical manufacturers and as central service managers (materials management).
- The surgical technologist assists in surgery as a member of the sterile team. In nonsterile roles, the surgical technologist assists in preparing the patient and the supplies and equipment needed for a surgical procedure.

- Surgical technologists are required to have the same professional attributes as any other health professional. Honesty, professionalism, respect for others, empathy for patients and other staff members, and the ability to work on a team are necessary.

REVIEW QUESTIONS

1. What would be the impact on the surgical technology community if certification became mandatory in all states?
2. What types of job opportunities are available for surgical technologists?
3. Why do you think the role and duties of the surgical technologist have expanded in recent years?
4. In your opinion, which professional attributes can be learned and which can be acquired through practice and observation?
5. What is meant by the phrase *scope of practice*?

CASE STUDIES

Case 1

A surgical technologist student has graduated, passed the certification examination, and is interviewing for a jobs in hospitals that are level 1 trauma centers (able to take critical trauma patients in all specializations) that offer exciting career possibilities in several specialties. The graduate is required to provide three sources of reference for the applications. The graduate asks his clinical instructor and two other health care workers where he trained to provide references. In two out of five job interviews the graduate is told that while his academic record is good, his absenteeism and lack of punctuality indicated on his student record is inconsistent with the responsibilities and professionalism required at their medical center. They are concerned that the individual may have other work habits that could create mistrust or safety problems.

- What are the possible causes for habitual lack of punctuality on the job? How does it affect colleagues in the operating room?
- How should this person proceed with the interview process at the other medical centers? What are his options?
- What are the ways in which a student can *prevent* being habitually late in student and professional life?
- Would you hire this individual if he applied to your team?

Case 2

Achieving a high level of professionalism is usually the result of experience in the profession, a desire to learn and achieve, and interaction with others who can act as role models. In a group setting, describe the personal qualities of someone you know who demonstrates a high level of professionalism in their work (any profession). What particular behaviors and attitudes does that person have that contribute to your opinion?

Case 3

Intensive student experiences, such as those in allied health, often change an individual's general outlook and reflection on one's accomplishments. In a group setting, discuss what changes you hope will occur (in addition to achieving technical expertise and acquiring knowledge in the profession) and those that seem highly challenging. What strategies can you take to overcome the difficult challenges?

REFERENCE

1. Freeman J, Rogers J: *A comparison of rank ordered professional attributes by clinical supervisors and allied health students*, Accessed July 7, 2011, at. http://ijahsp.nova.edu/articles/Vol8Num3/Freeman.htm.

BIBLIOGRAPHY

Accreditation Review Council on Education in Surgical Technology and Surgical Assisting (ARC/STSA): http://www.arcst.org.

Accreditation Review Council on Education in Surgical Technology and Surgical Assisting: *ARC/STSA communiqué*. Accessed October 17, 2007, at http://arcst.org/core_curriculum.htm.

Association of periOperative Registered Nurses (AORN): *Standards, recommended practices and guidelines, 2011 edition*, Denver, 2011, AORN.

Association of Surgical Technologists (AST): *Standards of practice*. Accessed October 22, 2011, at www.ast.org.

Association of Surgical Technologists: *Surgical technology: a growing career*. Accessed October 12, 2011, at http://www.ast.org.

National Board of Surgical Technology and Surgical Assisting (NBSTSA): http://www.nbstsa.org.

U.S. Army Medical Department Center and School Portal: *Operating room branch*. Accessed October 12, 2011, at http://www.cs.amedd.army.mil/new_arrival.aspx.

U.S. Department of Labor: *Occupational outlook: surgical technologists*. Accessed October 12, 2011, at http://www.bls.gov/oco/ocos106.htm.

Communication and Teamwork

CHAPTER OUTLINE

Introduction
Communication
Cultural Competence

Professional Communication
   Skills

Stressors in the Perioperative
   Environment
Teamwork

LEARNING OBJECTIVES

After studying this chapter the reader will be able to:

1. Describe the elements of communication, including the meaning of content and tone in communication
2. Demonstrate body language and describe its meaning
3. Discuss the significance of touch in communication
4. Explain the significance of netiquette and how it should be used
5. List and describe the qualities of good communication
6. Discuss barriers to communication and how to overcome them
7. Demonstrate professional communication techniques
8. Recognize forms of abuse in the operating room and how to handle each type
9. Discuss types of problem behavior and how to cope with them
10. Define sexual harassment and discuss how to confront it
11. Describe the qualities of good teamwork
12. Explain how poor teamwork results in poor patient care

TERMINOLOGY

Aggression: The exertion of power over others through intimidation, sarcasm, or bullying.

Assertiveness: Communicating one's personal and professional needs to others; protecting one's own rights while respecting those of others.

Body language: Communication through facial expressions, posture, and gestures.

Consensus: Agreement among members of a group.

Emoticons: Small images or acronyms used to convey emotion in email and SMS (text message) communication.

Facilitator: A group leader who coordinates the direction and flow of a group meeting without influencing the content of people's contributions. It is similar to an *enabling* position in which people are encouraged to express ideas without fear of judgment.

Feedback: The response to a message; a component of effective communication.

Groupthink: In sociology and group behavior theory, the conformity of a group to one way of thinking and behaving. Groupthink creates two factions, those who agree (in-group) and those who disagree (out-group). This generates resentment and conflict in the workplace.

Lateral abuse: Verbal abuse or sabotage of people of equal job or professional ranking.

Message: The idea, concept, thought, or feeling expressed during communication.

Norms: Behaviors that are accepted as part of the environment and culture of a group. Norms usually are established by custom and popular acceptance rather than by law, although the two may not be mutually exclusive.

Receiver: The person to whom a message is communicated by a sender.

Sender: The person who communicates a message to another.

Sexual harassment: An extreme abuse of power in which an individual uses sexualized language, gestures, or unwanted touch to coerce or intimidate another person.

Therapeutic touch: The purposeful touching of another person to convey empathy, care, and tenderness.

Verbal abuse: Deliberate attempts to devalue, intimidate, bully, or embarrass another person using loud, vulgar, sexualized, or intimidating language.

Win-lose solution: In conflict resolution, a solution that leaves one party satisfied but the other party dissatisfied.

Win-win solution: In conflict resolution, a solution that allows both parties in a conflict to gain.

INTRODUCTION

Communication and teamwork are two of the most important components of patient care. Information must be passed accurately, and often very precisely, in the health care setting. The ability to communicate well is highly valued in professional settings. It is a skill that is developed over time, often with the aid of mentors, through self-reflection.

Surgery is performed by *teams* of health professionals. Within the team, each person knows his or her tasks and roles and is guided by knowledge and experience. The ability to form a cohesive group quickly and efficiently—even among those who do not know each other—is one of the challenges of teamwork in surgery. Some teams in the perioperative setting are more or less permanent. Department committees, policy groups, and surgical specialty teams meet regularly to communicate policy, for scheduling, for training, or for social functions. Hundreds of models are available to help people form teams, get along, be productive, and enjoy the process. No matter what model (if any) is used, the process requires active participation and willingness to work with others toward a common goal. This is the definition of a team.

COMMUNICATION

WHY STUDY COMMUNICATION?

Communication is a two-way process with various goals in mind. One person (the **sender**) provides information or expresses ideas and feelings, and another person (the **receiver**) obtains the information, processes it and gives feedback. In patient care, effective communication is crucial to understanding the patient's needs, feelings, and experiences. Being aware of your audience is key. Clear communication among coworkers is equally important, because it produces cohesion, harmony, and efficiency in the workplace. It gives personnel the information needed to establish priorities and act on them. It also helps solidify roles so that everyone knows what is expected of them. Good communication clarifies relationships, solves problems, and helps establish professional and social boundaries. It increases teamwork and reinforces team goals. Good communication greatly increases the safety of the environment for the patient. Poor communication results in poor patient care, errors, conflict, and stress.

In the health care setting, the exchange of information is everyone's responsibility. We communicate information about patients to others involved in their care, and this triggers specific actions. Information about equipment and safety is transmitted throughout the workday. Many messages need an immediate and specific response. In these and many other situations, effective communication can be critical in preventing patient injury.

Good communication is not accidental. It requires skill and practice. Everyone wants to be understood and to have his or her ideas and feelings respected. Even under the best of circumstances, however, communication can be difficult. Many health care workers are surprised to find that the greatest challenge in their work is not the work itself but the interactions and social climate of the workplace. This chapter is intended to increase understanding of communication skills and the way communication affects interpersonal relationships and team building.

Among the most important reasons to improve communication skills is maintaining respect, trust, and empathy among coworkers and management. The operating room environment is usually busy, tense, and even brusque. In this atmosphere, people sometimes feel a loss of control over their work. When individuals are allowed to express their needs in the workplace and others are willing to listen and respond, conflicts and destabilizing events can be defused or prevented.

ELEMENTS OF COMMUNICATION

In this chapter we discuss the five components of communication:

- The sender
- The receiver
- The message
- Feedback
- Methods of communication

Communication requires both a sender and a receiver. No communication takes place without both. The **message** is the concept, thought, idea, or feeling that is being expressed. It is the actual information of the communication. Information can be perceived as negative ("You must work the next two weekends"), positive ("Everyone is getting raises next month"), or neutral ("Please, shut the door"). The message has an effect based on the content itself.

For communication to be considered effective, one additional item is required—feedback. **Feedback** is a response by the receiver acknowledging receipt of the message and its content. In relationships with people we know outside the workplace, feedback is not an essential part of communication. Feedback in the health care setting is critical to patient safety. It ensures that the message was conveyed and that the receiver understood the message.

The method used to communicate is almost as important as the content of the message. The *delivery* is the way the message is expressed; it includes verbal and nonverbal communication. We use deliberate methods to communicate, such as speaking and writing. We also communicate through facial expression, body movement, and tone of voice. Some of these actions are deliberate, and others are inadvertent, a result of our feelings and attitudes.

VERBAL COMMUNICATION

Verbal communication is spoken or written. This includes phone conversations as well as written and electronic communication. In health care, the ability to convey information is critical to patient care, group morale, and team cohesion. The words that we select in day-to-day communication can have a powerful effect on the listener's reaction. When we speak thoughtlessly, without considering how the message is interpreted, we can cause conflict and injury to others. When we speak as we would like to be spoken to, we are more likely

Box **2-1** **Guidelines for Verbal Communication**
1. Focus on the receiver.
2. Use concrete words. Avoid descriptions that are vague and require the listener to "fill in the blanks" or guess your meaning.
3. Do not assume that the receiver will respond in a particular way. Allow the person the freedom to express personal views and opinions.
4. Do not judge the receiver or others in your dialogue; this engenders mistrust.
5. Avoid using strong emotional words; these trigger emotional reactions in others.
6. When speaking with someone, make eye contact with the person and be alert to cues that the individual is not listening or wants to terminate the conversation. Such cues include looking away or from side to side, fidgeting, and backing up.
7. On the telephone, do not carry on a background conversation while speaking to the person on the phone. It disrupts the phone conversation and prolongs it unnecessarily. If someone interrupts you while you are on the phone, ask that person to wait until you are finished.

to produce an environment conducive to problem solving and collaboration.

Some situations in the operating room require communication of brief, accurate information with little or no dialogue. Even in these cases, it is important to use language and a tone that are respectful and polite. Box 2-1 lists important considerations for communicating verbally.

Tone is the manner or implied feelings behind the message, reflected in emphasis on certain words or pitch of the voice. Tone can reveal attitudes about the receiver or the content of the message. Most people are familiar with the effect that tone has on the message. For example:

"Please! Keep-the-doors-closed!"

"Would you mind keeping those doors closed?!"

"Please keep the doors closed-thanks!"

In the first example, the sender emphasizes words by volume and by measured delivery. This conveys impatience and frustration. In the second example, the sender uses a bit of sarcasm to emphasize annoyance. In the third example, the sender simply expresses a need to keep the doors closed and shows appreciation for compliance.

The following sentence can be stated in many different ways to convey additional information about the message:

"I'm scrubbing with you again today, Dr. X …" (Neutral information)

Although not spoken, the sender's *tone* might convey any of the following additional meanings:

"… and I'm dreading it." (Worry)

"… and I'm really glad, because things go so smoothly in your rooms." (Positive anticipation)

"… and if you start yelling today, I'm going to report it to administration." (Threatening)

As most people who frequently use the Internet have learned, tone is often lost in email communication. This is one of the causes of misunderstanding and miscommunication. **Emoticons**, which are the small pictures and letters used to represent facial expressions, are helpful but cannot accurately convey the nuances of human expression.

NONVERBAL COMMUNICATION

Body Language

The way we use posture, gestures, and expressions to convey ideas and messages is called **body language**. These cues can emphasize the message or convey a meaning that differs significantly from what was intended.

Even if a person does not want to express his or her true feelings about the message, those feelings probably will be conveyed by the individual's body language.

One of the qualities of good communication is genuineness. Watch your own body language. Does it express what you feel? How do you think others read your body language? For example, you can request assistance from a colleague in many ways. Your words may sound polite, but your body language may convey impatience.

Another example is the manner in which we receive job assignments for the day. Not everyone can be assigned the cases he or she wants. When assignments are made, most supervisors try to match the skills of the personnel with the tasks required while also considering a complicated schedule and staffing problems. When you receive an assignment, do you respect the need to consider these factors? What does your body language convey? If you were the supervisor, how would you react to the person who rolls his eyes, shakes his head, sighs, or turns away abruptly when given an assignment? Table 2-1 describes some common examples of body language observed in Western culture.

Touch

Touch can be both an expression of comfort and a way of controlling people. Deliberate touch is almost never neutral. It is a powerful means of communication that can soothe and comfort. It can also demonstrate dominance. People who want to show their power over others sometimes use touch in a condescending manner. For example, consider the team leader who lays his hand on a subordinate's shoulder and says, "I know you won't mind working overtime tonight, since you had last weekend off." The team leader may be using touch to establish authority, because a boundary is broken. On the other hand, we are often compelled to reach out spontaneously to someone who needs comfort. Touch is a very delicate issue for many people. Consider the following behaviors that occur in the workplace:

- Engaging in horseplay or jostling
- Making intimate gestures in view of others (jokingly or not)
- Surprising someone from behind by touching or grabbing them

To some people, these behaviors seem innocent and acceptable, whereas others find them repugnant and offensive. Very

Table 2-1	Body Language Observed in Western Culture
Element of Body Language	**What It Demonstrates**
Hands on hips	Authority or anger
Arms folded across the chest	Resentment or guarding
Eye contact	Attention and respect for the speaker, confidence
Lack of eye contact	Lack of social comfort (note that people of different cultural backgrounds may not hold eye contact with the speaker because of their culture or faith)
Eyes cast downward	Contemplation, embarrassment, or contrition
Backing up	Social distance that is too close or a desire to leave
Rigid posture	Restrained emotions or tension
Upright posture	Confidence or a sense of well-being
One eyebrow raised	Doubt or mistrust
Both eyebrows raised	Surprise
Mouth covered by hand	Shock or sudden grief; embarrassment

often, the person who finds the behaviors acceptable cannot understand why others will not "loosen up" and participate. People who lack respect for others' feelings, values, and experiences demonstrate this in many ways, and touch is one of them. Many people simply do not want to be touched.

No one has the absolute right to touch another person. It is a privilege earned by trust and limited by the boundaries of culture and social custom.

Therapeutic touch is purposeful touch that conveys empathy, tenderness, and care. Therapeutic touch is one of the health professional's roles. For many people, it is a natural response to another's suffering. Training in therapeutic touch is directed toward the development and awareness of how touch can have a positive effect on patient outcome.

Silence and Stillness

Silence and stillness communicate powerful messages. Silence can mean contemplation, shock, inability to speak, disagreement, or concentration. Many people misinterpret silence and stillness as "dead space" that must be filled. They are uncomfortable with silence. However, allowing others to think carefully before speaking shows respect and self-confidence. Some people are naturally quiet and still, even in a busy environment. Individuals with this trait sometimes cause others discomfort because they behave differently from the norm. All people have a right to express their individual personalities unless they harm or disrespect the rights of others.

Sometimes a person who is uncomfortable with silence feels the need to provide a running dialogue (or monologue) to avoid silence. In the operating room, speaking can spread airborne contaminants. However, the modern operating room is far from silent. Even here, team members may keep up a constant verbal dialogue.

NETIQUETTE

Email has revolutionized the way people communicate worldwide. It allows almost immediate access to people without being face to face with them. Most people are aware of the genuine advantages and some of the problems that email can create in business and even personal relationships. **Netiquette** (short for *network etiquette*) is a set of guidelines to help people use email and other types of Internet communication in a way that promotes personal security, respect, and clarity. The Internet community continues to define the language used in formal and informal communication. People who grew up using the Internet are usually very fluent in electronic language, but many who are starting a professional career may not be familiar with some of the rules of netiquette used in *workplace* communication. These guidelines are meant to protect individuals as much as create good communication. They do not apply to communication among friends and classmates with whom there is a casual and friendly relationship. They apply to emails written to professional colleagues, instructors, and managers:

- Always type in a subject heading so that the reader can identify the transmission. The heading should be short, clearly defining the purpose of the message.
- It is appropriate in business or professional transmissions to begin the email with a greeting, as in a letter, (i.e., Dear Dr. X …").
- Use short sentences. Keep to the point, and avoid emotional content.
- Do not forward an email or attachment to someone else without the author's permission. This demonstrates your professional integrity and respect for privacy.
- When one message is to be sent to more than four people, the names should be formatted as a group and the email sent to the name of the group. This protects the confidentiality of the group members.
- Compress large attachments before sending them. This only takes a moment and will be greatly appreciated by the recipient.
- Avoid sending attachments that contain information already stated in the body of the email.
- Flaming is never appropriate.
- Remember that an email can be a legal document. What you say in an email can be stored, retrieved, and used later. Try to keep emails concise and to the point. Most people do not read an entire email, especially if it is long. They read the first few lines and skim the rest.
- Take the time to spell-check your email and correct formatting errors before sending. SMS language is not used for professional communication.
- Include your name and contact information at the end of the email. Do not assume that the receiver knows who sent the email. Sometimes email correspondents have each other's contact information, but it is helpful to include it in

the email to encourage a reply and to make it easier for the other person to make contact.

Blogs

Blogs are a way for people to talk with others in their personal and professional community about topics that interest them. It is a way to share information and express views. Professional blog sites—those intended for members of a particular profession—are valuable for learning and sharing technical information, mentoring, and being mentored. Most people who join a chat group or Internet forum are aware of the rules. However, it is good to review them from time to time. The rules of blogging and online forums, especially in the professions, are those of common courtesy and legal and ethical behavior. Personal opinions expressed in strong emotional language may quickly attract the attention of others who do not share this point of view. Online arguments can ensue, resulting in negative, rapid-fire language. In these cases the blog or discussion administrator, who monitors all messages, can step in and halt the discussion online. However, individuals may have already been hurt or offended by what was said up to that point. Posts in a forum are, by definition, public statements. People form opinions and impressions about other bloggers based on what is said. Things said in the forum may remain as public documents for several years.

To research netiquette and keep up to date on the latest Internet language, search "netiquette" plus your or another state's university. These websites are excellent resources for learning more about Internet language and tools.

CULTURAL COMPETENCE

Cultural competence is the ability to communicate effectively with people of different cultures and subcultures within populations. The ways in which people interact are closely linked to their culture. This includes not only language but also ways of expressing emotion, body language, methods of coping with illness or conflict, gender value, and attitudes toward authority.

Communication with people of different cultures requires respect for all human beings. Most people have heard others criticize newcomers to the United States with comments such as, "They should act like we do" or "They should learn the way we do things"—or, worse, "If they can't do it like we do, they should go back where they came from." These statements show the speakers' disdain for others who are different from them and a lack of knowledge about how cultural behavior or **norms** are formed. Social and interpersonal norms are imbued in people from the time they are born. Cultural beliefs are based on tradition and value systems that cannot be switched off and on. All people esteem their cultural values and deserve to have them respected by others.

Health professionals are required to achieve a level of cultural competence because their patients' welfare depends on it. This is best done through course work and programs that teach health workers about important cultural communication skills. Many large health facilities, medical facilities,

and allied health organizations offer such training for their employees and members.

QUALITIES OF GOOD COMMUNICATION

Listening (Receiving Skills)

People find it easy to talk with those who have good listening skills. Good listeners are often placed in management positions because of their ability to communicate ideas in a concise, accurate, and nonjudgmental way. People seek them out for advice because they know they will be heard fairly and with respect.

Listening requires active participation. Passive listening frequently leads to inaccurate interpretation or inability to respond to the information. Parts of the message may be lost because the listener is distracted or impatient to speak.

Many people begin to formulate a response before they have heard everything the sender has to say. Their thoughts are focused on what they want to say, and they fail to receive the message. Box 2-2 presents positive listening skills.

Box 2-2 Positive Listening Skills

1. Focus on the sender. Avoid listening to background noise or other conversations.
2. Avoid listening for what you want to hear; you may misinterpret the message.
3. Do not judge the sender. If you are preoccupied with personal details about the sender, you cannot interpret the message accurately.
4. Watch for nonverbal cues, such as facial expressions and body language. These help clarify the sender's attitude about the message and help you understand important aspects of the information.
5. Ask for clarification!
6. Rephrase the sender's content so that both of you know the message is understood—for example, "You mean that. ..."
7. If the sender begins to get sidetracked from the topic, redirect the conversation. Ask questions about the original issue, or ask the sender to return to the topic.
8. If you find that your attention has drifted, ask the sender to repeat what was just said.
9. Do not assume background information unless you know it. If the message seems unreasonable, there may be circumstances of which you are unaware. Be open to the possibility that a much bigger picture is involved than the one you see.
10. If you find the sender's language or comments in bad taste or offensive, say so without judgment—for example, "I feel uncomfortable when you talk about Dr. X that way" or "I wish you wouldn't use that kind of language, it's offensive to me." When asking another to change his or her tone or language, be sure to state your own feelings about it—for example, "When you get angry with me in front of everyone, I feel very uncomfortable. Can we talk in your office instead?"

Assertiveness

Assertiveness is the ability to express one's own needs and rights while respecting the needs and rights of others. It is not aggression or confrontation. **Aggression** is the exertion of power over others by intimidation, loudness, or bullying; these traits ignore others' feelings or take advantage of another's vulnerabilities. The aggressive person puts his or her own needs and desires above those of everyone else. In contrast, the assertive person communicates self-worth without showing arrogance or "pulling rank." *Assertion* means communicating your own needs and advocating for them while respecting the needs of others.

The assertive person does not submit to the aggression of others, but rather states his or her needs clearly, without hesitation or self-effacement.

You can convey assertiveness through nonverbal or verbal language. To show assertiveness using *body language*:

- Maintain good posture.
- Use eye contact when speaking and listening. In maintaining relaxed eye contact, shift your gaze on the other person from one eye to the other. A fixed stare can convey emotional intensity.
- Stand still and do not fidget or shift your weight; this conveys ambivalence.
- Place your arms at your sides; this communicates acceptance and genuineness.
- Curb annoying actions, such as knuckle cracking and foot tapping, which can be distracting.

To express assertiveness through *verbal language*:

- Do not interrupt people. Patience shows respect.
- State your question, request, information, or comment without hesitation.
- State your message without blame or criticism.
- State your own needs or feelings in a straightforward manner.
- Accept the consequences of your message. Remain calm and deliberate in your speech.
- Remain open to the responses.
- Remain engaged and attentive during conversation.
- If you are emotionally upset, take time to calm down before speaking (unless the patient or a coworker is at risk for harm). Strong emotions cloud the ability to think and speak coherently.
- Never assume that, because the work environment is intense, your own intensity has no effect on others; it does. Consider the following examples.

EXAMPLE 1

Statement A: "I came to ask you for the weekend off. My brother's coming in from overseas. I really want to spend time with him before he leaves again."

Statement B: "Uh, oh, I was thinking about this weekend. I, well, I've been on call for the last two weekends. I mean, I know you are short-staffed, but I was wondering if, you know, I could have this weekend off. I don't know, maybe it'll throw your schedule off. I just thought I'd ask."

EXAMPLE 2

Statement A: "I want to report that Dr. X threw another bloody sponge across the room today. It hit the wall and barely missed the circulator. Please speak to him."

Statement B: "I was in a room with Dr. X. You know how he is. But, well, I think maybe someone might need to talk to him. Maybe he shouldn't throw sponges. I mean, he did it again today. I know he's chief of surgery, but, well, isn't it bad practice? I mean, couldn't someone get hepatitis or something?"

Statement C: "This operating room is so awful. I mean, to let someone like that get away with throwing bloody sponges all over the room. No wonder people get hepatitis. Why don't you do something? You make these policies, but no one ever does anything about them!"

These examples demonstrate several ways of communicating the same problem. In example 2, the sender is concerned about appropriateness and safety with regard to the behavior of Dr. X. In statement B of both examples, the sender is not confident about reporting. He or she has needs but is reluctant to express them directly. In statement A of both examples, the messages are polite, clear, and to the point. They state the problem clearly, show respect for the receiver, and deliver the message without hesitation. The receiver knows exactly what the request is and can make a decision. Statement C in example 2 communicates disrespect for the receiver and anger at the situation, without actually stating what the problem is or who is involved. This type of approach is aggressive, not assertive. Equally important, it does not provide information for problem solving.

Respect

Respect for others communicates the recognition of value, both our own and that of other people. It shows that although we may not agree with another's opinion or beliefs, we value that person's right to express and act on them, as long as the person does not cause harm to others.

People immediately sense when another person respects them. The person's actions and speech clearly show it.

We all know individuals who are always respectful and easy to talk to. We admire them because we can trust them.

The respectful person:

- Is nonjudgmental
- Does not gossip
- Is discreet—does not reveal personal or confidential information about others
- Practices active listening—speaks directly and listens attentively to others, while maintaining eye contact, when appropriate
- Responds with empathy and sensitivity to others
- Waits for others to finish speaking before talking
- Does not demand another's attention
- Values the views and ideas of others
- Never uses others to gain personal advantage
- Does not disparage another person to appear smarter, more skilled, or "better"

Respectful people are well liked because others feel accepted in their presence. This quality is developed from one's past experiences and one's own self-esteem. Sometimes people do not realize that their behavior shows a lack of respect. They do not see the cues or have never been told that their communication is offensive or hurtful. Others feel entitled to treat people in a disrespectful manner because they were treated this way at some time in their lives. This type of person is often self-centered and may be socially isolated. Such individuals seek out others who find their behavior acceptable. This tactic allows the disrespectful person to validate his or her negative behavior and avoid the criticism of others who recognize it as harmful.

Clarity

Clarity means that the important aspects of the message are delivered without ambiguity or unnecessary information. Consider the following examples:

EXAMPLE 1

"You know, I just went to get Dr. X's curettes; you know, the ones he always wants on his total knees. … But I can't find them on the ortho cart. I don't know why people can't schedule these cases better. I don't know what to do now. Maybe they're in another room or something. Listen, I've got to go and scrub and I just don't have time to look for them now. This schedule is crazy. Can you find them for me?

EXAMPLE 2

"Dr. X's curettes aren't on the ortho cart and didn't come down with the setup. Would you mind calling upstairs? I need to scrub."

When you report a problem, such as the one in the previous examples, give the right person the necessary information, as in example 2. In that example, the receiver knows exactly what and where the problem is. He or she also understands the level of urgency and can act on this information without further questioning.

Information in the perioperative setting often is communicated on a "need to know" basis. Economical communication is not the same as withholding information.

Feedback

As mentioned previously, feedback is the response to the sender's message. Effective communication includes clear feedback. Poor communication can occur when a message is delivered but the receiver does not acknowledge understanding. In this case, feedback is missing. This may happen when the receiver is distracted, in a hurry, or reluctant to seek clarification.

Look for cues that the receiver understands the message. When the message is understood, the receiver should seek additional information or indicate the appropriate action. Just as the sender has a responsibility to clarify the message, the receiver should give direct, specific feedback. In health care, feedback is critical in discussions or reporting of safety issues. In the previous examples, a request is made to solve a problem with missing instruments. The person who asks for help must not assume that the other person will follow through. He or she must determine whether the coworker really will be able to locate the needed instruments.

How do we give feedback? We do it by repeating the message or reporting our response to the sender. Feedback gives the sender confidence that the receiver understands the importance of the message and will act on it. Without feedback, some ambiguity may exist about the receiver's ability or intention to take the information on board and respond appropriately. Consider the following examples:

EXAMPLE 1

A: "I just talked to the ED, and there's a patient with a gunshot wound in the chest. I'm calling thoracic to see who's on call. Can you call the anesthetist on duty?"

B: "Well, okay, but I was just going to lunch."

EXAMPLE 2

A: "Can you tell Dr. X that his 2 o'clock has been cancelled because the patient refused to sign the permit? The patient's sitting in the holding area."

B: "I'll do that right now. I just saw him going into the locker room. Do you want me to let him know that the patient is still in the holding area?"

In example 1, the sender has given an urgent message. The receiver does not convey assurance that the message is important. The sender may even wonder whether the requested task will be carried out. He or she does not need to know that the receiver was just going to lunch, and it is not relevant to the situation, which requires immediate attention.

Example 2 is a clear response to the request and includes clarification. There is no doubt about this person's understanding or willingness to follow through.

Appropriate Person, Time, and Place

Effective communication results when the delivery is appropriate to the situation. Communication should take place with the right person, at the right time, in the right place.

The chain of command must be respected in communication. Ask yourself, "Does this person need to know this?" If the message is urgent, do not delay. However, do not rush to someone with a problem that is not under that person's control or that the individual cannot resolve. Think about the consequences of your communication.

BARRIERS TO COMMUNICATION

Communication between individuals or groups can fail for many reasons. The following are some of the most common:

- **Perceptions.** Our perceptions of the environment may not coincide with those of others. We make assumptions about what we see, hear, and understand based on our perception of the situation. For example, one person may perceive an unemotional patient as "stoic," a strong, brave person facing illness. Another person may see the same patient as extremely anxious and fearful, speechless, and unable to express emotion because of the intensity of his or her emotions.

- **Bias.** *Personal bias* is our preexisting opinions about people because of their affiliations, culture, economic status, and even their diseases. Bias is an effective communication stopper because it does not allow new ideas or opinions to develop or to be revealed. The biased receiver already "knows" all he or she wants to know and is firmly rooted in a point of view.

- **Lack of understanding.** Sometimes the receiver does not have sufficient knowledge to understand exactly what the sender is trying to communicate. This is why *clarification* is so important in communication. Both parties have a responsibility to ensure that the message is clear. If the communication requires action on the part of the receiver, the need for clarification is even more pressing.

- **Social and cultural influences.** How we perceive a problem, situation, or action sometimes depends on our social and cultural background as much as our knowledge. These affect the way we evaluate and comprehend what is being communicated. Communication in any form is integrated into what we already know and believe. In a sense, there is no "pure" communication; each of us has a unique point of view of ourselves and the environment.

- **Emotions.** How we feel at the time of communication can have a powerful effect on our ability to receive and send messages. Emotions can block communication through distraction or prejudice. Communication is extremely difficult when people are in a state of intense anger or resentment. These emotions not only distort the message, but also prevent concentration and mental imaging, which are necessary for good communication.

- **Environmental barriers.** Communication sometimes fails simply because the environment prevents reception. Hearing is a particular problem in the operating room. Masks can cause words to sound muffled, and background noises, such as suction, irrigation, power equipment, or loud music, can distort communication.

- **Lack of a desire to communicate.** To be successful in sending and receiving information, a person must *want* to communicate. The desire to communicate creates greater attention, focus, and concentration, which are necessary for clarity and understanding.

PROFESSIONAL COMMUNICATION SKILLS

Chapter 6 provides guidelines and examples of communication with patients. Here we discuss communication with their caregivers—the family or friends of the patient with whom the surgical technologist interacts in the health facility. Professionalism in the clinical workplace includes how we communicate with the public, who are in an unfamiliar environment. Communication with the patient combines clinical knowledge with care for the patient as an individual. Communication with the patient's family and friends has other qualities that require different skills.

THE PROFESSIONAL RELATIONSHIP

The relationship between the health professional and the public, in this case family and friends, has particular characteristics:

- **The public most often has great respect for the knowledge and skills of the professional.** Health professionals are generally highly respected and trusted by the public. This often imposes a level of formality during communication between the family and the professional.

- **The public looks to the professional for reassurance.** When the patient is removed from the company of family, *it is a significant separation.* The family is naturally concerned and often worried. Emotions are high. The health professional may be the only "emotionally neutral" person in the setting, and the family needs this neutrality for reassurance.

- **The family may believe that the health professional has privileged or undisclosed information that is hidden from them.** This is not the same as mistrust in professional. It is simply part of the relationship and must be considered during communication.

- **Family members may be self-conscious or embarrassed to show their emotions in front of the health professional.** When a health professional steps into an emotional setting, he or she does not need to be drawn into the emotion of the context. Setting these boundaries is very important.

- **The health professional may feel awkward about dealing with the family's emotions and relationship with the patient.** Health professionals, especially those who are starting their career, may feel inadequate or out of place in the company of the patient and his or her family. This uncomfortable feeling may result in poor or inappropriate comments during communication.

DEVELOPING PROFESSIONAL COMMUNICATION SKILLS

Development of a professional attitude and relationships is as much a goal as learning how to assist in surgery. It is a skill that is developed with experience, and it is based on a number of clear principles.

Professionals maintain appropriate social boundaries when speaking to the public. Close relationships such as those among family members or good friends are more open than those among casual acquaintances. The relationship between the health professional and the public should have clear boundaries. It is somewhat formal and mutually respectful. The professional has a duty and responsibility to keep his or her emotions in check. Comments and conversation should be restricted to the job at hand.

Health professionals should avoid communicating their opinions about their facility, work colleagues, or other professionals in the health care setting to the public. This shows *discretion.* The professional understands the difference between a professional opinion and a personal opinion. The professional opinion is based on experience, skills, and knowledge, whereas personal opinion is often influenced by emotion. Expressions of personal opinions are out of place when a professional is speaking to patients and the families of patients, with whom we have a more formal relationship.

- A professional's attire communicates a sense of responsibility and accountability. Today's workplaces are more casual than in previous decades. However, most people still appreciate a professional way of dressing and grooming, especially in the health care setting. The way a professional appears to the family can determine their level of trust in our ability to care for the patient. An appearance of self-care and neatness demonstrates that we care about how others view us. It shows respect for the public itself. On the other hand, sloppy, casual attire and poor grooming in the professional workplace often communicate a much different message in the public's eye, and even among professionals themselves. The public does not know your professional skills and abilities. A sloppy appearance may communicate that one's work is also sloppy, the opposite of what professionals want to convey.
- The professional understands that some aspects of patient care may be very foreign to the family. When explaining certain procedures to the family, use simple but professional language that shows you respect them and their level of understanding about the health care process. The professional is careful not to alarm the family by using terms or words that are highly charged or that the public may simply not understand in the way that they do. Developing cultural competence is also a key to helping families cope. People of many cultures and languages enter the health care system in America. Professionals need to give extra effort in helping the patient *and their family* understand and cope with the process.

Sometimes health professionals are very uncomfortable in social interaction with the public in the workplace. Having a role model for appropriate communication is important. The best role model is one who seems to put people at ease, and with whom there is obvious trust and mutual respect. Notice not only how this person communicates verbally, but also how his or her body language conveys assurance and capability to do what is needed at the time.

Having a mental idea of what is to occur before the situation can ease the pressure of difficult communication. If you are going to transport the patient, know in your mind the steps needed and what you want to convey while in the presence of the patient and family. There is no harm in a mental "rehearsal" of your communication and actions. This is especially helpful for students who are aware that they are being watched carefully as they perform their tasks.

STRESSORS IN THE PERIOPERATIVE ENVIRONMENT

Coping with problem behaviors in the workplace is always a challenge. Because the operating room is a unique environment that often involves an established hierarchy and intense

work, problem behaviors frequently are accepted as the norm. The following are some characteristics of operating room work that contribute to lack of communication and disrupt team cohesion:

- **The work is stressful.** The operating room requires its personnel to work at a high level of mental, physical, and emotional strength. Because of the demanding schedules, strong lines of authority, and wide diversity of behavior and personality types, excellent communication skills are vital.
- **Close teamwork is necessary.** This holds true even when team members have little knowledge of each other's work styles and personalities. It is especially true in a teaching hospital, where surgical residents and medical, nursing, and surgical technology students rotate through the department regularly. Even when communication is good among team members, working under intense conditions with new people can be challenging.
- **People and departments compete for time, space, materials, and personnel.** All operating rooms, whether in a large metropolitan area or in a small community, must meet the needs of the patients with fixed levels of staffing, equipment, and time. When the patient load requires more resources than are immediately available, the potential exists for conflict over available personnel, supplies, and space. Conflict arises when the needs of one person override those of the others.
- **The model for team relationships is in transition.** The social model for teams in the operating room traditionally has been authoritarian, hierarchical, and intended to put people "in their place." Many of these social traditions are no longer accepted by administrators and professional associations. Whenever a major change in a social structure occurs, a period of testing and adjustment also occurs.

Problem behaviors cause mistrust, frustration, and interpersonal conflict. The person with problem behaviors uses extreme defensive or aggressive tactics to achieve a level of social comfort. Supervisors cannot resolve every conflict that arises. Each person on the unit must make an effort to communicate effectively and assertively. When personal attempts to resolve conflict fail, then the issue must be referred to management.

When working with people with problem behaviors, one must remember to *focus on the behavior, not the person.* Difficult people relate poorly to each other, their environment, and themselves because they have not learned how to meet their own needs in socially acceptable ways. They have not learned to cope. This does not dismiss the frustration and even humiliation that others experience with them. However, attacking the person in an attempt to cope with the behavior is neither productive nor helpful. In fact, it usually increases defensive behavior and alienates the person even more.

VERBAL ABUSE

Verbal abuse is a significant problem in the operating room. Despite changing social norms and professional acknowledgement of the problem at all levels, it persists. It is among the leading causes of burnout among team members. Verbal abuse has a negative effect on patient care, because it causes staff members to become tense, upset, and distracted, and the result is an increase in errors. Verbal abuse also reduces productivity and increases staff turnover.

What Is Verbal Abuse?

Verbal abuse is one of several types of sabotage in which the perpetrator overpowers an individual by demeaning the person and devaluing him or her. This is done through deliberate and often aggressive (and loud) criticism, public embarrassment, vulgar language, and personal attack. Sometimes verbal abuse involves sexual innuendos or insults.

Verbal abuse includes but is not limited to the following behaviors:

- Vulgar remarks directed toward staff members
- Violent public criticism and demeaning of another person
- Loud and abrasive comments or demands
- Comments intended to deliberately embarrass or hurt another person
- Sexual remarks and innuendos directed toward others

Violent behavior may accompany verbal abuse. This includes throwing or deliberately destroying instruments and other items. Any staff member who threatens or throws a dangerous object at another person may be violating the law and certainly should be reported.

Perpetuation of Verbal Abuse and Violence

No excuse is possible for verbal abuse. However, research has shown that circumstances and beliefs perpetuate it.

Verbal abuse by surgeons increases when they are allowed to show favoritism toward particular staff members. Others who are obliged to work with these surgeons on emergency calls or under other circumstances often are the targets of severe verbal abuse because they lack the "inside knowledge" of the select group. This type of treatment leads to conflict and resentment among staff members and increases the scope of the problem. People in the select group who feel secure in their positions sometimes use their power to belittle and criticize others, especially students or new employees. This behavior damages self-esteem and inhibits the newcomer's ability to fit into the group.

Verbal abuse sometimes is built into the operating room culture. An administration that does not address and act on the problem in a serious manner gives implied permission to continue the behavior. Victims who cannot seek sympathy from or action by those who can affect policy are left with little recourse. They may leave the job or suffer the abuse silently as their stress level increases. Administrative support is very important to changing operating room culture.

Rude, vulgar, and offensive behavior is *not a natural reaction to stress*. There are few professions that would tolerate it. It is a choice made by those who perpetrate it. The job stress experienced by surgeons and other operating room personnel is no greater than that of people in many other professions, such as firefighters, rescue workers, and police officers. Yet in these groups, one finds increased cohesion and support rather than abuse among coworkers. A culture of verbal abuse and passive aggression does not flow naturally from the environment; it comes from individuals who use their authority to hurt others.

Remember, as a student it is important to inform your instructors if you are the target of verbal abuse and to allow them to help resolve the situation.

Coping with Verbal Abuse

Assertive behavior is one of the most effective ways to counteract verbal abuse. The following guidelines describe specific coping behaviors.

1. **Remain calm.** To deescalate rising tension and disarm the abuser, you must prepare yourself to address the person. This often is very difficult, especially when the outburst is extremely demeaning and loud and includes foul language.
2. **Remind yourself of the following facts:**
   - "I have the right to confront this person."
   - "I have the right not to take this abuse."
   - "There is no acceptable excuse for this behavior."
3. **Make an assertive statement.** Do not engage in sarcasm or personal attack; this usually escalates the situation. Instead, state what you feel and what you want:
   - "Dr. X, please don't speak to me like that. It is rude and demoralizing."
   - "Dr. X, it is not necessary to scream at me. When you do that, I can't work."
   - "Dr. X, if I make an error, tell me what the error is. It's not necessary to yell and curse at me."

   After you have made your statement, proceed with your work. If the abuser continues, it sometimes is helpful just to ignore the person. The abuser will soon realize that you are not listening. The important fact is that you have stated your rights and are in control of yourself. If the situation continues, restate your position calmly.
4. **"Sidestep" the behavior.** With this tactic, you simply change the direction of the communication. For example, in response to an aggressive remark about an instrument that is not working, you state, "I'll get a replacement for that instrument right now."
5. **Do not become aggressive.** When you act aggressively in the face of aggression, it escalates the conflict and may cause a major crisis. This creates a risk to the patient and is not acceptable. The patient must never bear the consequences of anyone's behavioral problems. If you cannot stop the behavior, wait until after surgery, and then confront the abuser or report it *in writing*.
6. **Stand up for your coworkers.** If you are in a room where your coworker is being abused, defend the person. Your silence is approval of the abuser's behavior.
7. **If the abuse becomes violent (objects are thrown or threats are made), call for the supervisor.** Do not allow the abuse or other disruptive behavior to continue. Do not be afraid to request the presence of others who are in an administratively stronger position to stop the abuser.
8. **Challenge authorities who allow abuse to continue.** Seek justification for allowing abuse to continue, and do not

allow yourself to feel personal defeat in the face of the administration's complacency.

When an abusive situation has occurred, it is natural to want to tell the first person you see what has happened. However, pick the correct time and place. The operating room corridor is not the appropriate place to vent your feelings. Patients can overhear talk and become frightened and insecure. File a complaint with the operating room supervisor. You can do this face to face or in a written report, stating when the abuse occurred, what was said, and who was in the room. If you choose to meet with your supervisor, make an appointment. Do not burst into the supervisor's office demanding that the person "do something about Dr. X." If you need to vent your anger, avoid lashing out at others. This only spreads the effects of the abuse and multiplies the abuser's power to demoralize people. If possible, take a break and write down your feelings. Vent your stress in physical activity or other appropriate ways.

If you work with the abuser again, continue to reinforce your position: that that person is the abuser, and you have the right to tell him or her to stop. Continue to file appropriate written reports of the abusive behavior.

Abuse and Threat of Job Loss

Many people are reluctant to report abuse in the workplace for fear of losing their job. This may be a valid cause of concern, especially in environments that have tolerated abuse in the workplace for many years, or where one person in high authority can dominate a department. In this case, the best tactic is to keep documenting every case in which abuse occurred. Make sure you include the dates, specific procedures, and circumstances. Do not include patient names. If you are not comfortable submitting the documentation, keep it until you feel secure in presenting your case. Go about the reporting in a professional manner and know what your plan of action will be for different outcomes.

LATERAL ABUSE

Lateral abuse takes place among staff members of equal rank and position. This type of abuse may be completely ignored by management because they consider it a private problem involving personal conflict. In reality, it often is not a matter of personal conflict but a form of sabotage. Some examples of vertical abuse include the following behaviors:
- Failure to share information
- Demeaning a person in front of others
- Open or covert discrimination
- Mocking another person
- Taking the credit for another's work or accomplishments
- Directly sabotaging another's work
- Falsely reporting another person to management or staff

The most effective management of this type of abuse is assertiveness and reporting in writing. Defend your colleagues by exposing the abuser. If you do not agree with what others are saying, let them know. *Silence shows agreement with the abuser.* Act as you would like others to act for you if you were the one being abused. Follow the same strategies applied to abuse by someone in authority.

PROBLEM BEHAVIORS

Complaining

Legitimate complaints about conditions in the workplace are important and should be addressed. Legitimate complaints often lead to creative solutions that produce a safer and more efficient operating room. However, when people complain without the intention of seeking solutions, they erode morale and sometimes cause conflict. Chronic complaining can be contagious. When it becomes part of the workplace culture, it spreads discontent and feelings of helplessness or despair. Habitual complaining usually is not about occasional incidents. Habitual complainers usually are unhappy about many aspects of their lives. They do not look for solutions; they simply want everyone to know how they feel and seek out others to hear and validate their many complaints. It is helpful for people to share their feelings about incidents. By sharing their thoughts and emotions, they find support and empathy. Chronic complainers, however, have little regard for or knowledge about the unhappiness that they spread in the work environment. The following guidelines can be used in dealing with chronic complainers:
- Do not become a complainer yourself. Often we are tempted to jump in and agree with a complainer. This only perpetuates the problem. Offer a solution or suggest how the person might solve the problem. If the complainer rejects the solution immediately or gives more examples of how bad things are, you know that the individual is not interested in seeking solutions but simply wants to state and restate the negative aspects of work or of his or her personal life.
- Just listen. Sometimes silence has a powerful effect on the complainer. Listen without emotion and then simply leave. This is not a satisfying response to the complainer, and the person may stop.
- Confront the complainer. Complainers often dominate locker room conversation or complain in front of patients. If you are in the presence of a patient, simply say, "Not now" or "This isn't the time." Speak to the complainer in private and tell the person how you feel about the complaining and the effect it has on the team. Ask the person to curb the behavior. It is not necessary to speak harshly or unkindly. The individual does not complain out of maliciousness. The complainer is unhappy and does not know how to cope with this unhappiness.
- If possible, remove yourself from the situation. If other solutions do not work, simply do not stay with the complainer. Understand that listening to the complainer regularly is frustrating and tiring. Do not allow this person to increase your stress.

Gossip and Rumors

Gossip is the telling and retelling of events about another's personal life, professional life, or physical condition. It is insidious behavior that hurts people, erodes teamwork, and damages group ethics. Gossip is not the same as the normal sharing of news or events that occur in people's lives. It is communication about another person or event that is confidential or personal.

The goal of gossip is to shock or evoke intrigue. As gossip spreads, the story may change slightly and facts may become blurred, so that the only importance of the story is its ability to entertain, at the expense of someone else.

A rumor is information whose validity is in question. The damaging effect of a rumor is that, after the story begins to circulate, people assume that it is true and react as if the rumor were fact. If the rumor is unpleasant news, conflicts arise, and people may become resentful, angry, or even fearful. Ironically, people who spread rumors often fail to validate the rumor. As with gossip, the value of the rumor lies in its effect on others during the telling and retelling, not in whether it is based on reality.

Adopt the following rules in coping with gossip and rumors:

- Do not perpetuate rumors or gossip about others. If you find yourself participating in rumors or gossip, ask yourself whether you would want others to discuss the details of your personal life or other private news in public.
- Call attention to the behavior. One very effective way to do this is to make a remark such as, "We shouldn't be talking about Dr. X. That's his personal business." (Note that it is important not to accuse the other person; that is, do not say, "*You* shouldn't. …") You might also say, "It's not fair to talk about someone when he can't defend himself." The point is to reinforce to the gossiper that you do not want to carry gossip.

Groupthink

Groupthink is collective behavior and thinking. It is based on peer pressure and occurs when members of a group are polarized in their opinions, ways of doing things, and means of expression. It produces two categories of people: those who are "in" and those who are "out." Whether the values of the group are positive or negative, people avoid becoming isolated and strive to become part of the in-group. They change their own values to fit those of the in-group. In this way, group culture is created and maintained.

Groupthink establishes unwritten, unspoken rules. Those who do not follow the rules may be criticized or ostracized by their peers. Standards of practice are deeply affected by groupthink. When the group sets high standards, groupthink is a positive force. However, when aseptic technique and other practices slide, the people in the out-group may be the only ones trying to uphold the high standard.

Groupthink usually is a negative force because it does not allow freedom of speech or action without the implied threat of isolation. A surgical technologist should be an independent and critical thinker, uphold high standards, and act in a professional manner in every situation.

Criticism

Criticism is a helpful tool in correcting work habits or raising awareness about harmful or unsafe situations. When offered appropriately, criticism is specific, nonjudgmental, and focused on the task, not on the person. When criticism is used to exercise power over others or boost one's own self-confidence, however, it can be very destructive. People who criticize usually are insecure in their own lives. They use criticism as a

way to soothe the anxiety they experience as a result of self-dissatisfaction. Nevertheless, this does not give them the right to demoralize or demean others. Some critics are expert at finding vulnerabilities in their coworkers and using these to demonstrate their superiority. Staff members must not tolerate this behavior.

Habitually critical people often are defensive and may become resentful when confronted with their behavior. However, it is important to point out when their criticism is causing conflict. When confronting the critical person, you should do the following:

- State that you find the person's behavior distressing rather than helpful.
- Tell the person that if he or she wishes to discuss your work, you will do so in private. This formalizes the critical process and removes its ability to cause embarrassment in front of others.
- Ask the person to be specific about the problem. Respond with a request for clarification or simply state without emotion or further discussion your reason for behaving as you did.

EXAMPLE 1

Person A: "The way you stacked these things, I can't find anything!"

Person B: "Tell me how you would like them to be arranged."

Person A: "I don't know—that's not my job."

Person B: "But I can't improve things unless you tell me what the problem is."

EXAMPLE 2

Person A: "Why can't you ever loosen up in surgery? You're so serious."

Person B: "What bothers you about it?"

Person A: "You never laugh at any of my jokes."

Person B: "I just don't find that kind of humor amusing, and I'm usually pretty quiet during surgery."

In both of these examples, person B deflected person A's comments by being assertive or asking for clarification.

SEXUAL HARASSMENT

Definition

Despite increased awareness and the enactment of laws and policies regarding sexual harassment, it continues to be a problem in the operating room. **Sexual harassment** is an extreme abuse of power in which a person engages in the following types of behavior:

- Expects sexual favors in exchange for personal or professional gain (sexual coercion)
- Directs sexually explicit comments toward another
- Makes *any* unwanted sexual or casual physical contact with another person
- Directs vulgar or sexual innuendo at another

The legal implications of and responses to sexual harassment are discussed in Chapter 3. Behavioral responses to aid in coping with this behavior are discussed in this chapter.

| Box **2-3** | **Protecting Yourself Against Sexual Harassment** |

- If the institution does not have policies covering reporting and discipline, request that the process of developing such policies be initiated.
- Do not engage in sexual jokes or conversation yourself. Walk away from the scene or simply change the subject. If you are scrubbed and cannot leave, confront the person later. If you are afraid to make the report, ask another person who was present to support you. Explain why.
- Inform your coworkers that you recognize a given behavior as sexual harassment. If they agree, ask them to participate in a confrontation. If you are not the subject of the harassment but are present, help others by confronting the perpetrator as your coworker's advocate, especially if the victim is so humiliated that he or she cannot respond.
- Report incidents of sexual harassment, even if you are not the victim. Show support for those who are.
- Stand up for your rights. If you feel victimized, others probably do, too. Seek others out for support in taking appropriate action.
- If your supervisor does not respond to repeated reports, write a letter or speak to the person at the administrative level directly above the supervisor.

Coping with Sexual Harassment

Sexual harassment is illegal. However, because the victims are humiliated and embarrassed, they often feel powerless to do anything; incidents go unreported and perpetrators continue the behavior. The perpetrator often considers sexual harassment to be innocent behavior. He or she may believe that acts of sexual harassment are open to interpretation (unless the sexual content is blatant). Consequently, the victim may feel that there are no grounds on which to make an incident report. Any act that evokes humiliation, shame, or guilt should be reported. Documentation of an incident is the best way to elicit disciplinary action by those in a position to enforce the law.

Although it sometimes is difficult, the victim should confront the perpetrator when sexual harassment occurs and afterward submit a written report. For example:

"Don't touch me again. I don't like it, and I won't tolerate it."

"Don't use those kinds of sexual references around me. Your comments are inappropriate."

"My personal life is not open for discussion."

Box 2-3 presents specific defenses that personnel can use, in addition to confrontation, to prevent and stand up to sexual harassment.

TEAMWORK

TYPES OF TEAMS

A team is a group of people who come together to reach a common goal or set of goals. The surgical team is only one type of team that plans and implements patient care in the operating room. In some large hospitals, certain personnel work within a surgical specialty, such as cardiology or orthopedics. In this type of structure, surgical technologists work with their peers to design instrument sets, order equipment, and update the surgeons' procedural changes. The team may or may not have a team leader.

The surgical technologist also may participate in other types of interdepartmental teams to improve care or produce information for surveillance and monitoring. Within a team, different personalities, work styles, values, and cultures are brought together. The team must identify and prioritize the steps of the process to reach the desired goal of a positive outcome for patient treatment.

The surgical team includes the surgeons, anesthesia provider, assistants, surgical technologist, and registered nurse. They all work together on a single procedure. Communication usually is focused, task oriented, and at times intense.

A *group* does not have a common goal, but the people in the group share common professions, task requirements, or other characteristics. Group work and teamwork are very similar. Interpersonal relationships and the ability to resolve differences are equally important in a team and in a group. When people work on the same shift in the operating room, they form a group. An understanding is formed among them that they will help each other with certain tasks and try to resolve work-related obstacles.

CHARACTERISTICS OF GOOD TEAMWORK

Good teamwork is the result of healthy relationships within the team. This does not mean that conflicts do not arise. Conflict in groups is normal, because people have different ideas, problem-solving skills, values, and beliefs. The qualities of a good team reflect how conflict is managed. Individuals must retain valued traits, such as genuineness, self-assertion, and empathy, yet at the same time be willing to discuss, yield, and accept change.

Many different social and professional models of team building and collaboration have been devised. There is no "best" model for every situation. People work in teams for immediate (emergency) results, long-term project goals, creative output, and many other reasons. The dynamics of team interaction always include common social and psychological behavior. An earlier business model developed in the 1960s by Bruce Tuckman was based on five group processes: "forming, storming, norming, performing, and adjourning." More modern models allow for greater integration of psychological, social, and cultural perception, more flexibility in the creative process, and an emphasis on conflict resolution.

Conflict cannot be managed unless people communicate about their problems. Discussion means that the group must admit that a problem exists. Identifying the problem requires sharing of experiences and interpretations of events without judgment. Members of successful groups do not accuse others of wrongdoing. They simply state the facts and relate the effect. Although people's perceptions of events, situations, or problems may be different, it is important to focus on the problem, not the people. Attacks on others in the group lead to defensive behavior, which works against creating solutions.

Yielding

Yielding in teamwork does not mean giving up one's values or beliefs. It means accepting the fact that others have valid points of view and conceding when one has made incorrect assumptions or conclusions. People who are able to yield are open-minded and retain a sense of fairness during team interaction. A team member who tries to gain control of all decisions and conversations is unable to yield to other people's right to express their views. Such individuals cannot imagine any way but their way and make little or no attempt to broaden their thinking.

Change

The ability to accept change is crucial to good teamwork. Many people experience change as a positive event, but others face it with dread. One of the purposes of a team is to adjust to a changing environment, such as unfolding events during a surgical procedure, a change in instrumentation, or new responsibilities. When teams are confronted with change, they must adjust their ways of working to accommodate the change. Team members must identify new tasks or procedures and implement them with as little disruption as possible. This requires personal flexibility, one of the positive character traits identified in the successful surgical technologist.

Politeness

Politeness concerns the manner in which people speak to and behave toward each other. The attributes of acceptable behavior include respect, gratitude, and acceptance. The operating room culture does not always promote these attributes. This does not mean that they are unimportant. On the contrary, teams that honor and practice these qualities have a pleasant work atmosphere, are efficient, and show a high level of professionalism. They experience fewer conflicts, and team members show high self-esteem. Unfortunately, groupthink and aggressive behavior often overcome civility in the operating room. The most powerful way to instill civility in a group is to model it.

Polite behavior is not complicated or difficult. Saying "Thank you" or "Please" makes people feel appreciated and respected. Offering to help another person even if you have not been asked and responding to requests for help without resentment create an atmosphere of cohesion and empathy among coworkers. Speaking with others in a calm manner without sarcasm promotes evenness and reduces stress.

Collaboration

Collaboration is working together for a common purpose. In the operating room, personnel contribute their skills, time, and energy to the care of the surgical patient. Collaboration requires that everyone solve problems and obstacles as a group. Cooperation and the ability to accept one another's individual personalities contribute to successful collaboration. Successful patient outcomes result when each team member recognizes the relationship of his or her own responsibilities to the tasks of the other members. Each person understands that his or her contribution is one of many and that problems or strengths in one area affect the entire collaborative effort.

TEAM CONFLICT

Interpersonal Conflict

Personality clashes, attempts to gain control of the group, and power plays are some causes of team conflict. When stress occurs between two or more people on a team, all team members feel the tension. Other members feel frustrated because they cannot solve the problem. Team cohesion disintegrates, and members worry about productivity, safety, and accountability. Resolving the conflict may require mediation if the individuals involved cannot resolve their differences. Particularly in health care, the overall goal (patient care) must not suffer because of individuals' inability to get along or resolve differences.

Conflict Between Team Goals and Personal Goals

On the surface, a team's goals might seem obvious. Although each person is aware of the final outcome (i.e., the surgery is completed), the manner in which each person contributes to the final outcome is affected by personal goals. For example, if a student is scrubbed with a surgical technologist, the role of the surgical technologist is to be a teacher (preceptor). The overall goal remains the same: completion of the surgery in a safe and efficient manner. The goals of the student, however, are to learn about the procedure and practice skills that will allow the student to work independently. The surgical technologist may not want to give up control of the case. The surgical technologist may be concerned that the surgeon will blame him or her if the surgery is slowed or errors are made. Perhaps the surgical technologist wants to show the student how much he or she knows rather than allow the student to participate actively. In such a case, the student becomes frustrated, because a conflict of goals has arisen. In this type of conflict, the needs of each person must be discussed. The most favorable outcome is for each person to recognize the overall priority of needs and to be willing to yield to these priorities.

Conflicting Priorities

Setting team priorities requires **consensus,** which is agreement on what the goals are and how they will be reached. Everyone may understand the goal, but people may disagree on how to reach it. For example, during surgery, the surgeon's goal is to work quickly without pauses in the flow of the procedure. The surgical technologist's goal is to remain ahead of the surgeon, anticipating what will happen next and what instruments and supplies will be needed, at the same time providing what is needed in the present. To do this, the surgical technologist must use every moment to prepare as well as work in the present.

Consider a scenario in which the surgeon places used instruments out of the surgical technologist's reach. Suction devices, hemostats, and needle holders soon pile up at the opposite end of the work area from the surgical technologist. The surgeon has created a situation in which the surgical technologist cannot do the work. The surgical technologist reminds the surgeon of the need to return instruments. This causes interruption. The surgeon is frustrated, because he or she must periodically retrieve the instruments, and the surgical technologist must spend time requesting the instruments and sorting them. Cooperation is lacking. The solution, of course, is for the surgeon to place the used instruments within the surgical technologist's reach immediately after using them, but this is not the surgeon's main priority. In this case, it would be helpful for the surgical technologist to point out that the procedure would go more quickly and more smoothly if the used instruments were placed within reach. The surgeon may be unaware of this need or may not have thought about the effect of his or her work habits on achievement of the overall goal.

Role Confusion

Role confusion is discussed in Chapter 4. However, it is reemphasized here in the context of team conflict. It occurs when individuals are uncertain of what is expected of them. The following comments are common expressions of role confusion:

"That's not *my* job." (Anger)

"I thought *you* were supposed to do that." (Surprise and confusion)

"What am *I* supposed to do about that?" (Anger)

"No one told *me* that was part of my job description." (Distress and anger)

Most role confusion is a result of poor communication. Conflict occurs when one person assigns a task to another who does not have the ability or time to complete the task. In cases of delegation, the person who delegates the job is responsible for evaluating the outcome and assisting if help is needed.

When a task is transferred from one person to another with the same qualifications, the person completing the task must have both the freedom to work independently and the authority to carry out the task. You should never assign a task to someone else just to get rid of it. Learn whether that person is qualified, is capable of doing the job, and has the time to do it. Always request a specific job description when beginning employment.

When working on a team, ask for clarification of what is expected of each person. Do not give up responsibility for a task after you have accepted it. If you cannot complete it, you must pass the task to someone else who agrees and is qualified to complete it.

Conflict Resolution

The goal of conflict resolution is to attempt to find a solution that is acceptable to all parties. This is called a **win-win solution.** Another type of resolution is a **win-lose solution,** in which one party is satisfied but the other is not. This is not a satisfactory resolution, because resentment and frustration will continue. In extreme cases, a lose-lose situation will occur, where neither party has a satisfactory resolution.

The goal of conflict resolution is to find a win-win solution. This requires behaviors such as a nonbiased approach, flexibility, willingness to yield, and the ability to focus on the problem, not the people. The following are some steps for resolving conflicts:

- When discussing the problem, try not to consider your personal opinion or bias about the situation. Consider the problem and the objective (e.g., to provide smoother turn-around between cases).
- Remain open-minded about solutions. Do not get stuck on a single fact or solution.
- Gather information about the problem before discussing it. Then assess the information and how it relates to the problem.
- View the problem as a team problem, not as *your* problem. Even interpersonal conflict is a team problem because it affects everyone.
- Brainstorm for solutions. Offer suggestions without deep analysis. Brainstorming allows people to suggest creative or different solutions without fear of judgment.
- Address any interpersonal conflicts in the team before other problems are solved. Tension in the team competes for energy needed for other types of problem solving.
- Formulate a plan for improvement that includes necessary behaviors and the rationale for changes.
- Try to reach a win-win solution. If such a solution is not reached, go back over the plan and evaluate whether concessions can be made to achieve a more satisfactory resolution.
- Seek mediation if the conflict cannot be resolved.

MANAGING TEAMS

Surgical technologists are increasingly becoming team managers. They may manage other technologists on a specialty team or serve as managers for projects or for situations requiring technical expertise. Few technologists have previous management training; therefore, they must learn how to develop those skills by doing the job. Management practices have changed significantly in the past decade. Professional teams are more participatory in decision making, and a completely top-down approach is reserved for emergency situations in which the team leader must make decisions that have immediate and serious consequences.

Management styles were first popularized in the 1970s, when businesses began to seek methods of training managers for increased production. Early texts identified these styles based on the behavior of the manager and the context. The following styles were described:

- *Authoritarian* or *autocratic:* With this method, the manager makes most decisions with little or no input from the team.
- *Democratic:* This style allows team members to provide input in the decision-making process, and extensive discussion is pursued to support the final decisions.
- *Laissez-faire:* With this method, the manager allows the team to make the decisions based on loosely organized communication and little or no management.

The modern team leader is a **facilitator** or enabler. Managers are trained to develop the ideas of individual team members, clarify their common goals, and help set a course that will accomplish the objectives. Good management or team leading reflects particular qualities. An effective team leader will follow these rules:

- Listen to everyone with equal attention and respect.
- Set realistic goals.
- Keep the team focused and interested in the goals.
- Be alert for friction among team members.
- Remain unemotional in team interactions.
- Enable every team member to participate in discussion and input.
- Recognize that new ideas can be brought to the team in many ways; integrate them into the objectives.
- Allow team members to make mistakes; allow them to be human.
- Remember to encourage team members frequently; point out accomplishments.
- Meetings should be short, well planned, and focused.
- Allow others to speak more frequently than you do.
- Do not become involved in department politics, and do not criticize management.
- Be generous with your knowledge and humble about your opinions.

THE SURGICAL TECHNOLOGIST PRECEPTOR

The experienced surgical technologist may be asked to become a preceptor to new employees or surgical technology students. In this role, the surgical technologist tutors the student and shares the duties of a scrubbed technologist. Those who enjoy teaching and sharing information find the role very satisfying. However, patience and a good sense of timing are important. A balance between allowing the student freedom and preventing serious errors or frustration on the part of other team members is crucial to the preceptor role. Box 2-4 outlines important guidelines for serving as a preceptor.

KEY CONCEPTS

- Effective communication skills are extremely important in the health care professions. Patient safety and teamwork are based on the ability to deliver and receive information in all forms.
- The elements of communication are a sender, a receiver, the message, the means of communication, and feedback about the message.
- Verbal communication is written and spoken. Our choice of words and tone of voice often can alter the meaning of a message, resulting in positive or negative reactions in those with whom we are communicating.
- Communication is influenced by culture, attitude, point of view, emotions, and the desire (or lack of desire) to communicate.
- The qualities of good communication include focused listening, assertiveness, respect, and clarity.

Box 2-4	**Guidelines for Serving as a Preceptor**

1. If you are a student now, notice the problems you encounter. Think of the preceptors from whom you have learned the most and consider why you learned from them.
2. Develop a plan with the person for whom you are serving as preceptor. Discuss with the learner what each of you will do and how it will be done. For example, as the preceptor, you might start the case and then allow the learner to step in and complete it. You might also have the student perform certain tasks while you do others.
3. Never try to perform the same task at the same time as your student. For example, if the learner is passing instruments, allow your student time to think and act. Silently point to the correct instrument, but do not reach for it; this would result in hand collisions on the Mayo stand and frustration for everyone.
4. If the learner is struggling, try to help by coaching quietly in the background. If this is insufficient, ask the learner whether you should take over for awhile. This allows the student to regain composure.
5. Never make a learner feel inadequate or foolish; this will only intensify the person's lack of confidence. Encouragement is much more productive than criticism. If you cannot contain negativity, ask to be excused from preceptor duties.
6. Always introduce the learner to the surgical team before beginning the procedure. This allows the learner to feel like part of the team and encourages confidence.
7. Respect the learner as a person. Remember that the learning phase is only one aspect of this person's life. You have a privileged job in helping the student achieve goals. You are also in a position to hurt the student's confidence. This is especially true of adult learners, who may not be accustomed to steep learning curves.
8. If the surgeon becomes irritated or anxious because of the learner's lack of experience, support the learner. If the situation becomes critical, ask the learner to wait until the critical situation has passed. Then invite the student back into the case after assessing whether the surgeon is tolerant.

- Stressors in the environment can block good communication and teamwork.
- Verbal abuse in the workplace deeply affects relationships and attitudes on a team.
- Verbal abuse used to be an accepted norm in the workplace. It is no longer acceptable behavior and requires action on the part of those involved, as well as by management.
- Skills to manage verbal abuse are learned. Ample resources for these skills are available through human resource departments and in professional literature.
- Sexual harassment is not acceptable in today's workplace. All staff members can learn how to recognize and stop sexual harassment.
- Characteristics of good teamwork include yielding, the ability to change, politeness, and collaboration.

- Team conflict often arises when the goals of the team conflict with the priorities of individuals.
- Role confusion is an important source of team conflict. Clarification of everyone's role on the team is of utmost importance.
- Conflict resolution is a learned skill that can benefit all health care professionals.
- Important goals of team management are to enable the team to reach its objectives and to do this in a way that fosters appreciation for individual contributions.

REVIEW QUESTIONS

1. Give three examples of groupthink that you have observed.
2. Define *sexual harassment*. Give three examples of sexual harassment in the workplace.
3. What is the purpose of having teams?
4. What are the characteristics of good communication?
5. Why does communication sometimes fail?
6. What does it mean to withhold information deliberately?
7. What are some constructive ways to work with chronic complainers?
8. What would you do if you believed a coworker was spreading rumors about you?
9. What are the causes of cultural discrimination?
10. How do you distinguish between true verbal abuse and indiscriminate rude comments?

CASE STUDIES

Case 1

You have repeatedly been the victim of verbal abuse by one member of the surgical team. You avoid working with this person, as does almost everyone else. When you are assigned to work with her, you are tense and upset even before the case begins. How can you prepare yourself to work with this difficult person?

Case 2

In the situation described in the previous example, you have made repeated complaints to the operating room supervisor, who tells you that she cannot really do anything about it. What steps will you take next?

Case 3

You are among six surgical technologists on an orthopedics team in a large hospital. The team leader is aggressive and rude to you. You feel that his technical expertise is lacking and that he was made team leader because of his relationships with the sales representatives. How will you handle your working relationship with this person? How can you reduce your own stress?

Case 4

You are a new employee in a large hospital operating room. You have been assigned a preceptor with whom you have difficulty working. You are not learning much, because she won't let you do anything except observe. When you tell her you would like to do more, she declares, "You're not ready to do anything; just watch." After several weeks, the situation has not changed. What will you do?

Case 5

You are a student scrubbing in with your preceptor. When draping begins, you reach for the drapes and he pushes you out of the way, saying, "Dr. X likes me to do this." What will you do?

BIBLIOGRAPHY

Buback D: Assertiveness training to prevent verbal abuse in the OR, *AORN Journal* 79:1, 2004.

Clancy C: Team STEPPS: Optimizing teamwork in the perioperative setting, *AORN Journal* 86:18, 2007.

Dunn H: Horizontal violence among nurses in the operating room, *AORN Journal* 78:6, 2003.

Grove C, Hallowell W: *The seven balancing acts of professional behavior in the United States, 2002.* Accessed July 22, 2011 at www.grovewell.com/pub-usa-professional.html.

Reina D, Rein M: *Trust and betrayal in the workplace*, San Francisco, 1999, Berrett-Koehler.

3

Law, Documentation, and Professional Ethics

CHAPTER OUTLINE

Introduction
Law and the Surgical
  Technologist
Institutional Standards and
  Policy

Professional Standards and
  Practices
Legal Doctrines
Negligence
Intentional Torts

Documentation
Risk Management
Ethics
Ethical Behavior in
  Health Care

Combined Ethical and Legal
  Concerns
Ethical Dilemmas
Professional Codes of Ethics
Patients' Rights

LEARNING OBJECTIVES

After studying this chapter the reader will be able to:
1. Differentiate among law, standards of practice, and codes of conduct
2. Apply evidence-based practice in all areas of clinical duty
3. Explain the difference between licensure, certification, and registration
4. Access resources related to legal doctrines in the perioperative environment
5. Define sentinel event
6. Identify common areas of negligence in perioperative practice

7. Discuss the importance of documentation in the perioperative setting
8. Explain informed consent
9. Describe how to write an incident report
10. List and describe types of advance care directives
11. Discuss ethics as they apply to the surgical technologist
12. Describe situations where both legal and ethical issues could be present
13. Define and discuss *ethical dilemma*

TERMINOLOGY

Abandonment: A health professional's failure to stay with a patient and provide care, especially when there is an implied contract to do so.

Accountability: Accepting responsibility for one's actions. In a professional context, this means that roles and actions accepted by an individual within the context of their occupation require the person to accept responsibility for the consequences of carrying out those tasks.

Administrative laws: Laws created by an agency or a department of the U.S. government.

Advance directive: A document in which a person gives instructions about his or her medical care in the event that the individual cannot speak for himself or herself. Examples are a living will and a medical power of attorney.

Damages: Money awarded in a civil lawsuit to compensate the injured party.

Defamation: A derogatory statement concerning another person's skill, character, or reputation.

Delegation: The assignment of one's duties to another person. In medicine, the person who delegates a duty retains accountability for the action of the person to whom it is delegated.

Deposition: The testimony of a witness given under oath and transcribed by a court reporter during the pretrial phase of a civil lawsuit.

Dilemma: A situation or personal conflict that arises from a need to make a decision when none of the choices are acceptable.

Ethical dilemmas: Situations in which ethical choices involve conflicting values.

Ethics: Core values that define one's relationship with others.

Evidence-based practice: Professional practices and their standards based on established scientific research rather than opinion or tradition.

Hospital policy: Rules or regulations that hospital employees are required to follow. They are created to protect patients and employees from harm and to ensure smooth operation of the hospital.

Incident report: A written description of any event that caused harm or presented the risk of harm to a patient or staff in the course of normal health care.

Informed consent: A process and a legal document that states the patient's surgical procedure and the risks, consequences, and benefits of that procedure.

Insurance: A contract in which the insurance company agrees to defend the policy holder if that individual is sued for acts covered by the policy.

Laws: Standards of conduct that apply to all people in a given society.

Liable: Legally responsible and accountable.

TERMINOLOGY (cont.)

Libel: Defamation in writing.

Living will: A legal document stating the patient's wishes regarding care in the event the patient is unable to speak for himself or herself.

Malpractice: Negligence (as defined by the law) committed by a professional. Malpractice may be committed if a person deliberately acts outside of his or her scope of practice or while impaired.

Medical ethics: A branch of ethics concerned with the practice of medicine.

Medical power of attorney: A legal document signed by a person who is giving another individual the power to make health care decisions for the first person if he or she becomes incompetent, unconscious, or unable to make decisions for himself or herself.

Negligence: Negligence as it applies to health professionals can occur in two ways: it can be a failure to do something that a reasonable person, guided by the ordinary professional considerations would do; or, it can be the act of doing something that a reasonable and prudent person would not do.

Perjury: The crime of intentionally lying or falsifying information during court testimony after a person has sworn to tell the truth.

Practice acts: State law that establish and regulate the conditions under which professionals may practice including licensure, registration, educational requirements, scope of duties, and functions.

Professional ethics: Ethical behavior established by authoritative peers of a particular profession, such as medicine or law.

Punitive: Actions intended to punish a person who has violated the law.

Retained foreign object: An item that is inadvertently left inside the patient during surgery.

Safe Medical Device Act: A federal regulation that requires the reporting of any incident causing death or injury that is suspected to be the result of a medical device.

Sentinel event: An unexpected incident resulting in serious physical injury, psychological harm, or death. The *near miss* of injury or harm is also considered a sentinel event.

Sexual harassment: Sexual coercion, sexual innuendoes, or unwanted sexual comments, gestures, or touch.

Slander: Spoken defamation.

Standards of conduct: A set of rules or guidelines an organization writes for its members. The rules pertain to how people behave and are based on the principles that the organization values, such as professionalism, and personal integrity.

Statutes: Laws passed by state legislative bodies.

Subpoena: A court order requiring its recipient to appear and testify at a trial or deposition. Medical records also can be the subject of subpoenas.

TIMEOUT: A procedure in which the surgical team affirms the identity of the patient, correct procedure, and location (side), verification of informed consent, and other documents necessary to proceed with the surgery—formally called the Universal Protocol. The procedure is mandated by the Joint Commission.

Tort: Legal wrongdoing that results in injury to a person or property.

Unretrieved device fragment: A portion of a medical device that has broken off or come apart in the body and is not detected or removed. Examples are fragments of a broken surgical needle and a hinge pin of a surgical instrument.

INTRODUCTION

Health professionals in all settings are guided in their practice by standards, laws, regulations, and policies. They also follow an ethical code, which is expected of people who are highly accountable to the public. **Laws** reflect society's rules, which have been created by the people and enforced by their government. Law in most societies is intended to protect individuals from harm and promote a peaceful society. Violation of the law has legal consequences. *Professional standards* are specific requirements that help promote and ensure safety and care. Professional standards are a way of setting a level for the quality of care practiced by individuals in that profession. **Ethics** is the values that are highly regarded by individuals and society. They direct people in everyday life and in critical decisions involving others. The health professions have particular ethics related to beneficence (caring for others), accountability, integrity, honesty, and trust. This chapter provides an overview of the laws and standards applicable to the surgical technologist both as students and practitioners. A discussion of ethics is also included to provide a basis of active discussion and debate, necessary for professionals to clarify their own beliefs and relate them to society's expectations.

LAW AND THE SURGICAL TECHNOLOGIST

Law is a rule or set of rules that governments make to regulate people's behavior. Laws enable society to be cohesive, ordered, and peaceful. They also protect individuals from harm. Whether a person agrees with the law or not, there is a consequence for violating it. This may be a fine, imprisonment, or other types of **punitive** action. Laws are made by the government at all levels. State laws are called **statutes**; the law is called *statutory law*. Federal laws are made at the national level. There are many different kinds of laws such as tax, corporate, criminal, and malpractice laws. The health professions are particularly guided by certain kinds of administrative law and state law. These are discussed next.

ADMINISTRATIVE LAW

Regulations (also called **administrative laws**) are created and enforced by *government agencies*. For example, OSHA (Occupational Safety and Health Agency) issues and enforces regulations that protect employees and patients against risks in the work environment. These include hazards such as those caused by chemicals and electrical devices and risks associated with blood-borne diseases. The EPA regulates the use of chemicals such that those used in disinfection, sterilization, and environmental cleaning. The U.S. Food and Drug Administration (FDA) establishes laws that govern the safety of medicines and protect the public from medical devices that might be defective, unsafe, or hazardous. An example of an FDA regulation is the **Safe Medical Device Act**, which requires hospitals to report any incident in which a medical device is believed to be the cause of an injury or death.

Hospitals and other health care institutions are required to follow government regulations and also ensure that employees know their responsibilities with regard to the regulations. Failure of a health facility to comply with federal regulations can result in disciplinary action by the agency.

STATE LAW AND PRACTICE ACTS

Under the U.S. Constitution, each state has the power to pass laws that define and regulate its health professions. These state laws are called **practice acts**. They are enacted by the state legislature and may be modified by further legal proceedings. The purpose of a practice act is to "protect and benefit the public" by defining the type and level of education and experience required, licensing, certification, or registration requirements, and the scope of professionals' practice (what they can do within the boundaries of their profession).

The current laws are more detailed than in the past. In many states, surgical technologists are specifically named in the statutes, whereas in the past they were not. Many states now have statutes that discuss the practice of surgical technology and provide some scope of tasks, as well as requirements for education and certification or registration.

Surgical technologist practice acts vary from state to state. For this reason, graduates and students should access their state laws to study the statutes. Surgical technologists can research their state practice acts online by searching *state legislature* plus the state plus *surgical technologist*. Other key words to replace *legislature* are *state register* and *statute*. Because of the varied roles of the surgical technologist, there is active debate about surgical technologists' range of tasks. Legislators (those who make the laws) must ensure a balance between reimbursement for state and federal medical services and the realities of an available workforce. Lobbyists (those who propose change in the law) are concerned with advocacy and protection of the profession and appropriate advancement leading to greater esteem and financial reward. Both groups are motivated to protect the public and provide a high standard of care. Surgical technologists can become involved in their state legislative activities by contacting their state assembly.

DELEGATION

Delegation is the transfer of responsibility for a task from one person to another. Delegation of tasks to the surgical technologist is sometimes but not always defined by state practice acts. Surgical technologists are routinely delegated tasks by the surgeon, so it is best to check the practice acts and professional standards for the medical profession as well as for surgical technologists. Some surgical technologists and surgical first assistants are eager to accept responsibilities, whereas others feel uncomfortable with some of the tasks they are asked to do. In either case, it is wise to know the law ahead of time.

The basic guidelines for accepting a delegated task can be summarized in the following points:

- The delegee (the person to whom the task is delegated) must be *legally allowed to* perform the task. The legality of a task may be determined by the state's practice acts and by hospital policy standards of practice. Legal accountability may rest with both the delegee and the person delegating the task. This is because it is assumed that both professionals know their scopes of tasks or practice.
- The delegee must have received the appropriate training to perform the task safely.
- The delegee must be competent and able at the time of delegation to perform the task.

Accountability is taking responsibility for ones actions, including professional duties. As surgical technologists take on a wider scope of tasks than in the past, they are obliged to accept the personal responsibility that goes along with it. When a surgical technologist proceeds with a delegated task, he or she must agree to be identified as having carried out the task in the formal documentation process. Otherwise, the technologist should not agree to perform the task. This is for the protection of both parties. It is both an ethical and legal consideration, because taking the responsibility for an act also includes accepting the consequences of one's actions. If any form of coercion is routinely used in the delegation of tasks for which the delegee feels uncomfortable, *for any reason,* this should be documented and taken to the supervisory level, all the way through the chain of command, if necessary. This helps protect and promote everyone's right to act legally and ethically.

INSTITUTIONAL STANDARDS AND POLICY

Hospitals and other health care facilities are accredited by the Joint Commission through a rigorous process of performance evaluation in key areas of patient care. To achieve and maintain accreditation, facilities must establish standards and policies that meet or exceed those expected by the Joint Commission. Accredited hospitals and other health care facilities are also required to provide orientation training for their employees and to supply documents that detail their policies. New employees and students must be familiar with the policies that affect their professional role and duties. Violation of **hospital policy** may result in disciplinary action by the facility (which may jeopardize one's job in the future). Forgetting a policy or not knowing a policy is usually not an acceptable reason for failure to comply. Policies are usually logical and are beneficial for a smooth-running workplace. They are created by specialists within the organization, in consultation with the Joint Commission, who advise on best practices based on risk analysis and specific research in the areas of safety that are affected by those practices.

The operating room *procedure manual* is distinct from the hospital policy. It describes the operating room protocols for specific practices such as disinfection and sterilization methods, room turnover procedures, and chemical and laser safety precautions. Separate policy manuals may be used to detail the safe and careful use of particular equipment, protocols for moving and handling patients, preparation of the patient for surgery, and other specific areas of care.

PROFESSIONAL STANDARDS AND PRACTICES

Medical, allied health, and professional nursing organizations such as the American Academy of Surgeons, the Association of Surgical Technologists, and the Association of periOperative Registered Nurses publish **standards of practice** (also called practice standards). These are specific technical standards that list and describe the practices of the profession. They represent the highest standard of care within that specialty and are based on evidence derived from recent peer-reviewed scientific data. This is what is known as **evidence-based practice**, which relies on science rather than opinion or tradition. Examples of the hundreds of topics covered are parameters for disinfection and sterilization, the correct procedure to use for the hand scrub or hand antisepsis, the use and precautions related to antiseptics that are safe to use as patient skin preps, safety practices in laser surgery, and many others.

Perioperative practice covers a wide range of topics and subspecialties. This means that some technical practices are common to a number of different professions that provide guidelines on the same topic. Sometimes there are discrepancies in technical standards among professional organizations, and questions arise as to which is correct. In this case, the *source* of the technical information must be validated Technical standards must always be accompanied by appropriate citations or references that provide evidence for the standard. New technology and research can cause standards to become quickly outdated or obsolete. Therefore, professional organizations normally review the literature frequently so that practices keep pace with current medical science. However, professional institutions do not rush to change a standard based on a single new study, especially if the study itself does not follow appropriate research standards or if there was a conflict of interest on the part of the researcher. Box 3-1 lists websites related to perioperative practice standards, including those of the Association of Surgical Technologists.

In addition to technical and professional standards, an organization may publish **position statements.** These are public declarations of the organization's collective *opinion* on important topics rather than evidence-based standards of practice. A position statement represents the organization's point of view on important issues but may not be used to overturn law, practice acts, or hospital policy. Instead, position statements are used for advocacy and to publicly state what the organization believes.

AST publishes position statements on its website, http://www.ast.org.

Box **3-1**	**Resources for Public and Private Agencies**

American College of Surgeons (ACS): www.facs.org
American Medical Association (AMA): www.ama-assn.org
American National Standards Institute (ANSI): www.ansi.org
American Society of Anesthesiologists (ASA): www.asahq.org
Association for Professionals in Infection Control and Epidemiology (APIC): www.apic.org
Association of periOperative Registered Nurses (AORN): www.aorn.org
Centers for Disease Control and Prevention (CDC): www.cdc.gov
The Emergency System for Advance Registration of Volunteer Health Professionals (ESAR-VHP): www.phe.gov/esarvhp/pages/about.aspx
Environmental Protection Agency (EPA): www.epa.gov
U. S. Food and Drug Administration (FDA): www.fda.gov
International Association of Healthcare Central Service Materiel Management (IAHCSMM): www.iahcsmm.org
The Joint Commissions (TJC): www.jointcommission.org
Medical Reserve Corps (MRC): www.medicalreservecorps.gov
National Disaster Life Support Foundation (NDLSF): www.ndlsf.org
National Fire Protection Association (NFPA): www.nfpa.org
National Institute of Occupational Safety and Health (NIOSH): www.cdc.gov/niosh
Occupational Safety and Health Administration (OSHA): www.osha.gov
World Health Organization (WHO): www.who.int/en

CODE OF CONDUCT

A code of conduct is an organization's rules or guidelines for the behavior of its members. The purpose of a code of conduct is to ensure that the actions of individuals in that profession or organization are consistent with its core values. These are not laws, and there is no legal consequence for violating the code of conduct unless a standard coincides with an existing law. However, violation of the professional code of conduct may result in disciplinary action by the organization. This might include revoking membership in the organization, certification, or privileges to practice in a particular institution. Ethical behavior as described in a professional code of conduct is separate from *moral* behavior, which is based on principles of "right and wrong" that are usually defined in terms of societal approval influenced by culture, religion, and other social entities.

CERTIFICATION, LICENSURE AND REGISTRATION

The right to practice a health profession is granted when the individual achieves the educational, practice (number of clinical or contact hours), and examination requirements established by law (where one exists) or other regulating body. *Certification* is verification that an individual has completed the requirements needed to achieve a designated standard of knowledge or performance. Surgical technologist certification is granted by examination following successful completion of an accredited educational program. It demonstrates publicly that a measurable level of achievement has been reached. Surgical technology certification in one state does not restrict someone from practicing in a state other than the one in which they were certified. Certification is required in some but not all states.

Licensure is a legal requirement of the state and is not voluntary. This means that each state requires that a person be licensed *in that state* in order to practice their profession there. Examples of licensed health professionals are medical doctors, registered nurses, respiratory therapists, and radiology technologists. Licensure allows states to monitor and regulate professionals to protect the public. Most states allow *reciprocity*, which means that a person licensed in one state may apply for licensure in a different state. If the conditions of licensure are different from those in which the person is licensed, additional testing, study, or internship can be undertaken to meet the new requirements.

Registration of health professionals is an administrative process of the state government in which the state maintains an official record of the health professional's vital statistics, address, and place of employment for public protection. Registration allows the state to accurately identify the health professional and is also related to public safety and protection.

LEGAL DOCTRINES

Legal doctrines are rulings or conclusions drawn from many similar legal cases. They are used by lawyers and judges in the legal process. Historically, these doctrines were printed in their Latin form, as part of legal tradition. Today, the Latin terms are rarely used except in the legal setting (court cases, documentation, and communication among law professionals). The following terms are the most common in the medical setting:

- *Respondeat superior*—"let the master respond": Historically, the surgeon or health care facility was held responsible for the acts of others on the surgical team through a doctrine called "borrowed servant." However, this doctrine is outdated and is seldom enforced in modern practice. With advanced medical and surgical technology, highly trained members of the surgical team are now required to make informed decisions based on their own professional judgment and knowledge. This means that individual professionals on the surgical team are accountable for their own acts whether they are unintentional, negligent, or delegated. The surgeon, employing agency, or health care facility may also be named in the same or another lawsuit, but only when they are also found negligent in their duties.
- *Res ipsa loquitur*—"the thing speaks for itself": The defendant is judged to be guilty of an act of negligence even though there is no direct evidence it. This is based on the fact that the act is so obvious that "the thing speaks for itself." An example is leaving an instrument or sponge in the patient, which is an obvious source of harm and needs no other evidence that it happened.
- *Primum non nocere*—"first, do no harm": Many medical organizations use this slogan to emphasize that professionals have a legal and ethical responsibility to ensure that their care does not cause injury or harm. This doctrine may seem obvious but is fairly often violated when a health professional injures a patient unintentionally through negligence during normal care.
- While there is no doctrine of forseeability, this concept is embodied in the laws regarding negligence. It is very clear that a health professional must be able to predict specific dangers that can injure a patient and protect the patient from harm. Areas included are electrosurgery, laser use, patient positioning, and other usual activities with inherent risk.

NEGLIGENCE

A civil wrong (called a **tort**) is an act committed against a person or their property. In the health care setting, we are mainly concerned with *unintentional acts* of harm called **negligence**. Intentional acts of harm are covered by criminal law and include theft and violence against another person or the person's property.

Negligence is the most common cause of injury in the health care setting. It is defined as "the commission of an act that a prudent person would not have done or the omission of a duty that a prudent person would have fulfilled, resulting in injury or harm to another person." In other words, the negligent person fails to act in a situation that he or she should have known about and acted on. Health professionals can protect themselves against liability for acts of negligence by purchasing **malpractice** insurance. In the past it was very rare for a surgical technologist to be named in a lawsuit. However, the trend is changing. This may be due to the higher profile of the profession, surgical technologists taking on highrisk roles, or shifts in accountability within the legal system. Certainly there is an increasing trend to shift responsibility from the surgeon to other members of the surgical team. Nevertheless, any individual on the surgical team (*personal liability*) and the health facility itself can be held liable (*corporate liability*).

There are two schools of thought about whether an individual should take out malpractice insurance. One is that if one does carry malpractice, one is more likely to be sued for **damages** and responsible for monetary compensation. The other is that it is wiser to prepare oneself in the event a lawsuit is brought and won. Both are valid arguments. It is wise to review the options and the liability protection available when making a decision.

A **sentinel event** is "any unexpected occurrence involving death or serious physical or psychological injury, or the risk thereof." The phrase "or the risk thereof" means actions or situations in which there is a significant *risk* of adverse outcome. Sentinel events require documentation and reporting to hospital administration, which uses the information for risk assessment and intervention. An important resource on patient safety and sentinel events for surgical technologists and other perioperative professionals is the ECRI Institute. The institute is a leading authority on patient safety, used by many different professional organizations. The Patient Safety Authority, which collects and analyzes national data on sentinel events, publishes reports and case studies.

The specific ECRI website on patient safety is https://www.ecri.org/Pages/default.aspx, and the Patient Safety Authority can be accessed at http://patientsafetyauthority.org/Pages/Default.aspx.

MALPRACTICE

Negligence is unintentional harm. Malpractice is negligence committed by a professional. There are four elements that must be proven in order to show negligence:

1. There is a duty to the patient that is initiated the moment the patient receives treatment or care from a hospital or physician.
2. The duty is breached when there is a failure to meet the standard of care.
3. The breach causes injury to the patient.
4. The breach of duty results in damage to the patient, known as *causation* or *proximate cause*.

The plaintiff must prove that negligence was committed, and if the plaintiff is successful may be awarded compensation, also called damages. There are three types of damage: *Direct* (current and future medical expenses and loss of wages), *indirect damage* (pain and suffering, and emotional distress), and *punitive damage* (intentional conduct or gross negligence which not usually awarded in medical malpractice).

The consequences of malpractice may include a lawsuit. In this case, legal representation is required for both the plaintiff and the defendant who is being sued. Certain terms are important to understand the basic process of a lawsuit. If negligence is suspected and a lawsuit is to be filed, the medical professional will receive a summons or **subpoena** which is an order to appear as a witness to an incident. A meeting will take place in where testimony is given, called the **deposition**. The deposition is recorded by a court reporter and all lawyers involved in the case are allowed to question the witness. If a surgical technologist is required to testify about an incident at the hospital, the individual should check with the hospital administration before doing so. In some cases the hospital (or its insurance carrier) may provide a lawyer to be present during the testimony. The person giving a deposition who is directly involved in the lawsuit will have an attorney present. Unless a settlement is made early in the case, a jury is called to hear the evidence and produce a verdict. Testimony given during a court trial is given under oath. Lying under oath is *perjury* which is punishable by law. Once the verdict is given, the judge decides on the amount and type of damages awarded to the plaintiff.

COMMON AREAS OF NEGLIGENCE

Unintended Retained Foreign Objects

A **retained foreign object** is an instrument, sponge, needle, or instrument fragment (**unretrieved device fragment**) unintentionally left in the patient as a result of surgery or other invasive procedure. A retained object can result in infection, tissue destruction, and hemorrhage. Delayed healing and unresolved pain are additional consequences. Accountability for a retained object lies with the entire operating team. The standard protocol for preventing retained objects is the sponge, sharps, and instrument count (commonly called the *count*). The scrub and the circulator are responsible for the surgical counts, which must be performed in an exact way at prescribed times during the surgery. This protocol is described fully in Chapter 21. Surgical counts are documented according to hospital policy, and extra precautions may be taken according to specific circumstances.

Burns

Burns are the most frequent cause of injury in the operating room. The most common injuries are the result of misuse or negligent operation of electrosurgical equipment, heating blankets, hot solutions, hot instruments, lasers, and chemicals. Every person who works with these devices and agents is responsible for learning about the risks and must be able to demonstrate their safe use. The following are examples of actual cases of burn injuries caused by negligence:

- During laser surgery of the upper respiratory tract, special precautions for a laser-safe endotracheal tube are neglected. The endotracheal tube bursts into flames, causing third-degree burns of the patient's face and throat.
- Sparking from the electrosurgical device ignites a wet alcohol prep solution and surgical drapes, resulting in third-degree burns of the peritoneal cavity and thorax.
- A warm air blanket that covers the patient's body is connected improperly. The warm air hose disconnects from the blanket undetected. The patient suffers extensive burns that are not discovered until the end of surgery when the drapes are removed.
- An improperly placed dispersive electrosurgical pad allows current to flow to electrocardiographic leads, resulting in serious burns under the leads.
- A stainless steel retractor is removed from the steam sterilizer and immediately placed in the patient. The abdominal contents are burned by the hot instrument.
- Skin prep solutions (antiseptics) are allowed to pool under the patient. After the procedure, the drapes are removed to reveal the patient's blistered skin.
- Irrigation solutions are kept in warmers at excessively high temperatures. The lining of the body cavity in which the irrigation solution is used is burned by the hot solution.
- A hot ultrasound coagulation/dissecting instrument is inadvertently placed on the patient's skin, causing a second-degree burn.

Falls

Patient falls are the *leading* cause of death in hospitalized people older than 65 years. Hospital employees are also at risk for falls, which contribute to injury, lost workdays, reduced patient care, and expense in worker compensation claims. The following are examples of common circumstances in which falls occur in the perioperative environment:

- The side rails on a stretcher are not kept raised, or a safety strap is not secured on the operating room table.
- Children are left unattended, enabling them to crawl out of cribs or beds.
- An insufficient number of staff members are available to transfer a patient to and from the operating table. The patient falls to the floor.
- A sedated or disoriented patient climbs over the side rails or becomes entangled between the rails.
- Unsafe transfer techniques are used to move a patient to and from a wheelchair, resulting in a fall.
- An obese patient requires the use of an extra-large operating table and mechanical lifting device for transfer to the operating table. Another team is using the equipment, which was not scheduled. The team attempts to move the patient manually. There is loss of control of the patient, who falls to the ground, suffering a cranial fracture and internal bleeding.
- Water is allowed to pool on the floors around scrub sinks and cleaning and decontamination areas, causing slippery conditions.

Injury as a Result of Incorrect Patient Positioning

The patient can be seriously and permanently injured as a result of improper positioning for the surgical procedure. Overextension of limbs, pressure on bony prominences, loss of circulation as a result of poor or improperly placed padding, and restricted ventilation are some consequences of improper positioning. The surgeon, anesthesiologist, nurse anesthetist, surgical assistant, and circulator work collaboratively while positioning the patient to ensure safety.

Operating on the Wrong Patient or Wrong Site

No excuse is acceptable for operating on the wrong patient or the wrong site, or doing the wrong procedure. The consequences of these errors are so grave that the Joint Commission requires surgical teams to comply with a specific protocol in which the entire team participates. The Universal Protocol or **TIMEOUT** is a verification procedure in which the team pauses just before surgery begins to acknowledge essential information about the operative site and side, patient identity, position, and other crucial information about the patient and procedure. Surgery may not proceed until the protocol is completed. A record of the TIMEOUT is included in the operative record or other permanent form in the patient's chart. The Universal Protocol is described fully in Chapter 21.

The source of the protocol can be viewed online at http:// www.jointcommission.org/standards_information/up.aspx.

Incorrect Identification or Loss of a Specimen

Any tissue or foreign object removed from the patient during surgery requires careful handling and documentation. If the specimen is removed to confirm or rule out malignancy, improper labeling or loss of the tissue can have disastrous consequences for the patient, including misdiagnosis or delay in appropriate treatment. All specimens must be identified by the hospital pathology department. Some are forensic evidence that will be used to prove innocence or guilt in a criminal case. One of the key responsibilities of the surgical technologist is to handle specimens properly and deliver them off the surgical field. The surgical team must identify, label, and ensure delivery of specimens to the pathology department or other area specified by hospital policy. This procedure is described in Chapter 21.

Medication Errors

Surgical technologists are required to transfer medicines to the surgical field, to mix solutions, and to prepare medicines for administration. They are also required to label medicines received on the sterile field. This is necessary when drugs are transferred from their original container into another container or delivery system for use in surgery.

Studies in the past decade have shown that labeling errors are among the most prevalent and serious errors occurring during surgery. This can result in the wrong drug being transferred or administered, or the wrong strength mixed at the sterile field. Other errors include miscalculation of the amount of drug administered, which can be related to intermittent administration such as during the use of local anesthetic. The complete procedure for handling medicines in the operating room is located in Chapter 13.

Abandonment

Abandonment is defined as neglecting a patient or leaving a patient unattended when the patient requires the presence of a health care professional. Abandonment can result in falls or injury related to rapid deterioration of the patient's condition such as aspiration (breathing in fluid), choking, cardiac arrest, or other life-threatening events. These can happen very quickly and may be irreversible by the time help arrives. The surgical patient is especially vulnerable during the postoperative period and may be unstable coming into surgery. Abandonment may also be defined as leaving a patient unattended without providing handover of care to another qualified person. Examples of abandonment follow:

- A patient is left unattended in the operating room suite.
- A staff member leaves the operating room at the change of shift once the patient is on the operating table, and no relief is available.
- A patient is being transported to the operating room by stretcher and is left unattended in a hallway.
- A staff member agrees to work overtime, then leaves without notifying anyone.
- A health professional delegates care of the patient to a colleague who is unqualified to provide safe care.

An inadequate ratio between patients and staff and miscommunication between staff members can also result in a charge of patient abandonment.

Failure to Communicate and Miscommunication

Failures in communication can occur when a member of the team neglects to pass on vital information that requires action. The information can be about the condition of the patient or some important aspect of a procedure. Communication is often difficult in the operating room environment because staff is required to carry out multiple tasks and to continually anticipate new ones. Distraction is a major cause of neglecting to carry out a task. Recent studies have also shown that the noise level related to devices and loud music played during surgery can contribute significantly to poor communication and decreased safety for patients.

Loss of or Damage to the Patient's Property

Patients sometimes arrive in surgery with dentures, jewelry, hearing aids, or glasses. Loss or damage of these items can be very stressful for the patient. Any personal property must be properly labeled with the patient's name and hospital number. Property is then transferred to a designated area for safekeeping, according to hospital policy.

WHISTLE BLOWING

Whistle blowing refers to a policy in which institutions encourage their employees to report acts of misconduct or negligence of others. The policy has gained momentum in the past few years as equal rights in the workplace have increased. Health care workers no longer take the blame for wrongdoing by those in a position of authority. Historically it was common for a nurse or technologist to remain silent in order to "protect" the surgeon or institution. However, more and more professionals are finding out that this may not be the best action and certainly is no longer expected of professionals working in the health care system.

INTENTIONAL TORTS

An intentional tort is civil wrongdoing that is deliberate rather than the result of negligence. Because these are civil rather than criminal acts, the consequences are usually an award of money to the person who was injured by the one held **liable** for the wrongdoing.

INVASION OF PRIVACY

The patient has a right to both physical and social privacy. One of the most common offenses against the patient is invasion of privacy. Discussions about patients in public areas of the hospital are common. These are a violation of ethical and legal codes. Vivid descriptions of the patient's surgery or disease, including the names of the attending physicians, are commonly heard in cafeterias, hallways, and elevators. Family or friends overhearing these discussions can be devastated by their content. Any conversation about a patient must take place only within the therapeutic environment and never in public. (See also the later discussion of HIPAA.)

DEFAMATION

Defamation means deliberate efforts to erode the reputation of another person. If the actions are verbal, it is **slander**. If the statement is written, it is **libel**. Medical personnel sometimes witness practices or acts that they consider incompetent or dangerous to the patient. Failure to report incompetence (or

impairment, such as intoxication) is negligent because the harm may continue and more patients may be injured. However, exposing these events publicly could be considered defamation unless the statements are legally proven to be correct. This does not mean that people cannot discuss the actions of others. However, making statements in public, in published writing, or electronically such as in a blog site can invite a case of slander. This is a particular caution in light of social networking, which is available to a large community of people.

SEXUAL HARASSMENT

Sexual harassment is unwanted sexual coercion, lewd comments, innuendoes, or touching perpetrated by one person on another. Sexual harassment is identified when a person speaks or acts in a sexually aggressive manner that causes discomfort, embarrassment, humiliation, or shame. It is illegal and unethical. Over the past 20 years, sexual harassment increasingly has been condemned in the workplace. Incidents that used to be accepted as the norm in team relationships are no longer tolerated by institutions or health care workers themselves. No one in any profession is obliged to tolerate implied or actual physical or verbal sexual aggression. Because sexual harassment is defined differently by different individuals, it is best to document and report every instance of harassment as it occurs. The person who is harassed should retain an exact duplicate of the report. If the perpetrator is a superior, the report should be made above his or her administrative level or up the chain of command. Sometimes victims of sexual harassment do not report the abuse because they are afraid of losing their job. Talking about the abuse to peers often reveals others with the same experience, and the collective documentation can force institutions to act.

CIVIL ASSAULT AND BATTERY

Civil assault is the threat or attempt to harm another person, regardless of whether the threat is carried out. This is a punishable civil crime, and the victim may sue for mental distress as well as damages resulting from the assault. *Battery* involves contact with intent to injure and applies even if no injury occurred. An example of battery is chemical and physical restraints such as sedatives and restraints used on disoriented older patients to prevent them from wandering in the ward. In this case, restraints become a method of managing a group of patients all in one place, possibly against their will. This type of case might also be considered *false imprisonment.*

DOCUMENTATION

Documentation is a requirement in all areas of medical practice. It is both a method for health care providers to communicate and a record of all the patient's encounters with the medical system. Medical records are protected by law. Losing or misplacing a record or part of a record is a serious event. The use of electronic documentation is now common in most facilities and requires all personnel to become familiar with specific operating systems. The Joint Commission sets specific standards for the type of information that must be documented during surgery. However, documentation varies among individual facilities. General documents that the surgical technologist is likely to encounter are discussed later in this section. Specific documents are described within their subject in the text—for example, specimen and pathology documentation is detailed in Chapter 21.

The *Health Insurance Portability and Accountability Act of 1996 (HIPAA)* protects patients' medical records and other health information through its Privacy Rule. The goal of the Privacy Rule is to ensure that the individual's health information (called *protected health information*) remains confidential. Identifiable health information is any information relating to the individual's past, present, or future physical or mental health or condition and information about payments for health care. The Privacy Rule applies to any transmission of information through any medium, including electronic, paper, or oral means. Box 3-2 specifies information that cannot be shared. All employees of the health care facility must sign a confidentiality statement in which they agree to abide by the HIPAA Privacy Rule.

Box **3-2** **Health Privacy Act Identifiers that May Not Be Shared**

Individual identifiers include but are not limited to the following:
- Name and address
- Birth date
- Social Security number
- Photographs
- Medical record numbers
- Fax numbers
- Email addresses
- Health plan beneficiary numbers
- Account numbers
- Certificate/license numbers
- Vehicle identifiers and serial numbers, including license plate numbers

---

The complete document can be accessed at http://www.hhs.gov/ocr/privacy/hipaa/understanding/srsummary.html.

GUIDELINES FOR DOCUMENTATION

Documentation is the means of making a permanent legal record of the patient's interaction with health care providers and services. It is a way for health professionals to communicate patient procedures, diagnoses, treatments, condition, and recommendations for care. Many health professionals will consult the patient's medical record, so it is necessarily done in a standardized manner. Separate forms are required for many different types of documentation, but the method of documentation is consistent among health care facilities. The importance of correct documentation cannot be overstated. A mistake in documentation can lead to serious medical errors. The Joint Commission has developed a list of abbreviations that must not be used in documentation because they can be misread or misinterpreted. These are mainly related to drug administration and are shown in Table 3-1. The list also appears in Chapter 13 for emphasis.

The following general guidelines should be followed for health care documentation:

1. Every document must contain the patient's unique identifiers, including patient name, hospital or Social Security number, and other information required specifically for that health facility.
2. The date must be accurate. Never predate or postdate a document. Always document the correct time.
3. If you make an error in handwritten documentation, make a single line through the part that is incorrect and write in the correct information. Initial the change. Never use opaque liquids or tapes to blank out the error—it must remain in the record.
4. If the documentation is performed in writing, make sure it is legible, using *black* ink only. Documents must be kept clean and dry to prevent smearing. It is good practice to document away from areas where spills or splashes can occur.

Table **3-1** **The Joint Commission List of *Do Not Use* Abbreviations**

Do Not Use	Potential Problem	Use Instead
U (unit)	Mistaken for "0" (zero), the number "4" (four) or "cc"	Write "unit"
IU (International Unit)	Mistaken for IV (intravenous) or the number 10 (ten)	Write "International Unit"
Q.D., QD, q.d., qd (daily) Q.E.D., QOD, q.o.d., qod (every other day)	Mistaken for each other	Write "daily" Write "every other day"
Trailing zero (X.0 mg)* Lack of leading zero (.X mg)	Decimal point is missed	Write X mg Write 0.X mg
MS MSO₄ and MgSO₄	Can mean morphine sulfate or magnesium sulfate Confused for one another	Write "morphine sulfate" Write "magnesium sulfate"

(From The Joint Commission at http://www.jointcommission.org/assets/1/18/official_do_not_use_list_6_111.pdf. Accessed on March 1, 2012.)
Applies to all orders and all medication-related documentation that are handwritten (including free-text computer entry) or on preprinted forms.
*Exception: A "trailing zero" may be used only where required to demonstrate the level of precision of the value being reported, such as for laboratory results, imaging studies that report size of lesions, or catheter/tube sizes. It may not be used in medication orders or other medication-related documentation

5. Use brief, exact wording when documenting. Documentation is a record of facts only.

6. Remember that your documentation will be read by many professionals. Use correct spelling and do not use SMS or Internet language.

7. Avoid abbreviations.

8. When performing computer-based documentation, remember to log off when finished. Do not allow someone else to use your password, and do not give your password to anyone else.

9. The person performing the documentation must be identified by a signature. Never sign another person's document or allow someone else to sign for you.

COMMON TYPES OF DOCUMENTATION

Patient Medical Record

The patient's medical record is the sum total of all encounters with the health care system, including reports, assessments and investigations, surgical procedure records, nursing notes, anesthesia records, and dates of admission and discharge. Medical records may be stored electronically or in paper form. If the record is in paper form, the record may contain more than one file which may be dated by year. The patient medical record "travels" with the patient whenever he or she is admitted to the hospital. While the patient may not physically carry it, it is present during all health care encounters so that records can be kept in real time. All records are kept in the medical records department of the hospital. This is discussed in Chapter 4.

Informed Consent

A patient's operative consent form, or **informed consent**, is part of a process in which the attending practitioner (the one who actually performs the procedure) explains the risks, benefits, and alternatives of the surgery to the patient. The informed consent fulfills the patient's right to know what the procedure involves, the alternatives, and possible outcomes. Its importance as a legal document and a rights document cannot be overemphasized. The patient must be prepared to discuss and sign the document (or have a representative sign). This means that certain conditions must be met with regard to the patient's level of consciousness, means of communication, and ability to understand the consent. The surgeon or surgeon's representative may make a note in the patient's chart verifying that the patient appeared to understand the consent and that it was not signed under coercion. The consent is dated and the time stated to show that it was signed before the start of surgery. The practitioner who performs the surgery or other medical procedure is responsible for the process, which is required for the procedure to take place. The purpose of the consent is to document the fact that the patient understands the intended procedure and its consequences, risks, and alternatives. It gives patients an opportunity to ask questions and participate in choices and decisions about their care. Informed consent must not be obtained by coercion or pressure, and the process is only finalized when the patient acknowledges his or her understanding of information. The patient, surgeon, and a witness must sign the consent. An example of what the consent form might look like is shown in Figure 3-1.

All invasive procedures require informed consent, including blood transfusion and administration of anesthesia. Anesthesia consent may be required as a separate process. Some facilities have specific consent forms for elective procedures that result in sterilization, and for implantation of medical devices.

For the consent to be legal and valid, the patient must be able to understand the information on which the decision for intervention is made. Patients who are not native speakers of English may require an interpreter to ensure comprehension. Those with hearing impairment must have a qualified interpreter present. In the event the patient is not mentally competent to understand the information, the patient's representative must be present. *Health literacy* is an important concept in informed consent. This is the patient's ability to understand certain medical terminology used in the media and in educational settings. Patients who do not understand medical terms that are used in everyday media will have difficulty in comprehending informed consent. The law mandates health facilities and primary care practitioners to provide an explanation of the procedure in language that the patient can understand. If the procedure is elective the surgical consent may be prepared in the surgeon's office and signed several days before the scheduled date of the surgery. In emergency situations, the consent is prepared as close to the time of surgery as possible. The consent is legal only when all elements and special considerations are included, such as those listed in Box 3-3.

The main elements of a surgical informed consent are:

- The name and type of surgery, which are communicated using words and language the patient understands
- The risks, benefits, and possible outcomes of the procedure
- Alternatives to the procedure
- An assessment of the patient's understanding of the information
- The patient's acceptance of the procedure

In an emergency situation, when the patient is incompetent or unconscious and has no representative, the decision to act in beneficence may override other considerations. This is a decision made by the attending physician. In some cases a court order may be required for medical or surgical intervention. The laws concerning this vary by state. Special cases determine who can provide consent (see Box 3-3).

Patients who agree to participate as subjects in experimental surgery or other types of research must be fully informed of the risks and possible outcomes. These are contained in a special informed consent document designed by the Institution Review Board according to FDA regulations. The terms of the consent vary according to the specific case.

WITNESSING THE CONSENT The surgical consent is signed by the surgeon, patient, and a witness. By law, any adult, such as a legal guardian, spouse, or agency representative, can witness the patient's signature. The witness is only attesting to the fact that he or she observed the signing by the physician and patient, not that the patient understood the information. However, hospital policy may state who may or may not act

	Patient name:
Date of procedure:_____	Date of birth:

I,_____ , request and give consent to _____
(Type or print patient name)   (Type or print doctor or practitioner name(s))

to perform the following procedure(s) _____
                                                          (Please list site and side if appropriate)

_____

The benefits, risks, complications, and alternatives to the above procedure(s) have been explained to me.

I understand that the procedure(s) will be performed at Christiana Care by and under supervision of my doctor or practitioner. My doctor or practitioner may use the services of other doctors or practitioners, or members of the resident staff as he or she deems necessary or advisable.

I authorize my doctor or practitioner and his or her associates and assistants to perform such additional procedures, which in their judgment are necessary and appropriate to carry out my diagnosis or treatment.

I authorize the hospital to retain, preserve and use for scientific, teaching purposes, or to make other dispositions of, at their convenience, any specimens, tissues, or parts taken from my body during the course of this operation.

I consent to observers in the procedure area in accordance with hospital policy. I consent to a healthcare industry representative being present during the procedure, if necessary, to provide technical assistance or to perform calibration of equipment. I consent to photography or video taping of my surgical procedure for educational purposes, provided my identity remains anonymous and confidential.

I agree to being given blood or blood products as deemed advisable during the course of my procedure. The risks, benefits, and alternatives to receiving blood or blood products have been explained to me.

I consent to the administration of sedation or analgesia during my procedure. The risks, benefits, and alternatives to receiving sedation or analgesia have been explained to me.

If anesthesia is required, I consent to the administration of anesthesia by members of the Department of Anesthesiology. I also consent to the use of non-invasive and invasive monitoring techniques as deemed necessary. I understand that anesthesia involves risks that are in addition to those resulting from the operation itself including, but not limited to, dental injury, hoarseness, vocal cord injury, infection, nerve injury, corneal abrasion, seizures, heart attack, stroke and even death.

If applicable, I consent to the use of fluoroscopy. I understand that prolonged exposure to fluoroscopy may result in skin reactions, such as redness, irritation or a burn.

Please initial one of the following statements (females and those within child bearing years only):

_____To the best of my knowledge I am not pregnant.   _____I believe I am not pregnant.

I certify that I have read and understand the above consent statements. In addition, I have been offered the opportunity to ask my doctor or practitioner any questions I have regarding the procedure(s) to be performed and they have been answered to my satisfaction. I acknowledge that I have been given no guarantee or assurance as to the results that may be obtained from the procedure(s).

Signature of patient or decision maker	Date	Time	Doctor or practitioner signature/title	Date	Time
Relationship to patient if decision maker			Doctor ID # or print name		
Witness signature	Date	Time	Practitioner print name		
Witness print name					

Telephone Consent:

Name of person consent obtained from			Relationship to patient if decision maker		
Witness signature	Date	Time	Witness signature	Date	Time
Witness print name			Witness print name		

Figure 3-1   Sample informed consent document. *(From Rothrock JC: Alexander's care of the patient in surgery, ed 14, St Louis, 2011, Mosby.)*

as a witness in the perioperative environment. The attending surgeon may not act as a witness to the consent because of conflict of interest. Many health care facilities do not allow other members of the care team, such as the surgical technologist, to witness the consent for the same ethical reasons.

Intraoperative Record

The *intraoperative record* is specific documentation about the surgical procedure and includes patient assessment; technical information about the equipment and devices, drains, and implants used during the procedure; and record of the

TIMEOUT (Universal Protocol). Implants require registration of type, manufacturer, identification number, size, and other identifiers. The patient position and prep site must be indicated, along with details about specimens and medications. The names of all perioperative personnel who participated in the procedure are listed, and those who participated in the counts must sign at the close of surgery. See Figure 3-2 for an example of an intraoperative record.

Anesthesia Record

The anesthesia record is a document of the intraoperative anesthesia process including type, drugs and solutions used, methods, and any complications that occurred during the surgery. It is also used to document values for physiological monitoring, any unexpected interventions performed, and the outcome of the procedure. There is a section on the record for drains, for fluid loss during surgery, and also for replacement fluids or blood products given during the procedure.

Patient Charges

Patient charges are documented in a variety of locations in the chart. Usually there is a dedicated form in the patient chart for stating the service or equipment and appropriate charge. The process for documenting charges is part of the operating room policy and is easily accessed through the department.

Birth and Death Certificates

Birth certificates are issued by the health facility after the mother or her representative provides the required information. This information may vary among states. Death certificates are provided by the attending physician or the coroner. Birth and death certificates are legal documents and are certified in the county in which they occur.

Specimen and Pathology Records

Documentation must accompany all tissue or other specimens obtained during surgery. A description of the tissue, its origin, time of recovery, and any special identifiers must be included.

Specimen identification is critical in prevention of medical errors. Incorrect or lost documentation may result in delays or even failure to assess the tissue. All health care facilities publish a manual that states specifically how to submit a specimen and what information is required. A complete discussion of the care of specimens and their documentation is included in Chapter 21.

RISK MANAGEMENT

Incident reports provide the basis for a larger process with goals to prevent patient and employee harm, and determine how to decrease the number and type of incidents that occur in the health care facility. The process called risk management includes reporting of actual and potential risks and creating policies and protocols to prevent or mitigate risk. Health care workers are encouraged to be proactive in reporting patient and employee risks in the workplace so that accidents and sentinel events can be prevented.

Following a sentinel event including near misses, the risk management department is notified and an investigation is initiated to assess the causes of the event, the injuries (if applicable), and the outcome. If the event involves an injury to a patient or staff member, the injury is treated immediately to prevent complications. A report of the event is made as soon as possible which will lead to an investigation.

The purposes of the investigation are to evaluate every aspect of the event so that steps can be taken to reduce or mitigate future events. A second goal is to assess the legal implications for the health care facility and employees. The reports are never placed in the patient's chart but a description of the event and any injury is placed in the progress notes. Employees who fail to fill out an incident report is typically in fear of one's professional reputation or that of a colleague. However, all accidents must be reported and treated, if necessary, right away to prevent more serious repercussions later on. This applies to both patients and employees. An annual review of policies and procedures helps to determine whether these need to be modified to further manage risk. If there is an immediate risk to patients and employees, these are addressed right away. Employees have the right to work in a safe environment. Problems that arise because of reduced staffing and its relationship to patient safety must be presented with evidence in order to initiate change.

Throughout this textbook you will find many references to accident prevention. These are intended to alert the reader to potential risks associated with surgical technology. These risk reduction measures are located according to the environment or practice most commonly associated with the risk.

INCIDENT OR SENTINEL EVENT REPORT

An **incident report** or sentinel event report is a document submitted to the operating room supervisor or other designated manager describing an incident or sentinel event—that is, an event that causes injury, harm, or death, or one in which there was a "near miss" of any of these events. Incidents may also be reported for cases of internal conflict on the team

Instruction:
To be completed by RN.   Page 1 of 3

CASE PARTICIPANTS	
Attending surgeon:	Resident:
Attending surgeon:	Resident:
Attending surgeon:	Resident:
Assistant:	Assistant:
Anesthesiologist:	Anesthetist:
Perfusionist:	Autotransfusionist:
X-Ray tech:	Laser operator:
Circulating nurse:	Scrub person:
Circ relief: Time in: Out:	Scrub relief: Time in: Out:
Circ relief: Time in: Out:	Scrub relief: Time in: Out:
Circ relief: Time in: Out:	Scrub relief: Time in: Out:
Other/observer:	Other/observer:

CASE TIMES

Patient in O.R.: _____ Anesthesia induction: _____ Incision/start: _____ Closure/end: _____ Patient out: _____

Recovery in O.R. Start: _____   Recovery in O.R. Stop: _____

ARRIVAL TO O.R.

Via: ☐ Ambulatory ☐ Stretcher ☐ Patient bed ☐ Other: _____   ☐ Personal items to O.R.: _____

Pre-op skin condition: ☐ Dry and intact ☐ Other: _____

Safety strap applied ☐ Abdomen ☐ Thighs ☐ Other: _____

PLAN OF CARE

☐ Allergies verified ☐ Perioperative history and assessment reviewed ☐ Standard plan of care implemented

Plan of care exceptions: ☐ Latex precautions ☐ Contact precautions ☐ Airborne precautions ☐ Droplet precautions

☐ Other: _____

PATIENT POSITIONING

Body position: ☐ Supine ☐ Prone ☐ Lithotomy ☐ Sitting ☐ Lateral right side up ☐ Lateral left side up

☐ Other: _____

LEFT arm: ☐ Board ☐ Side ☐ Chest ☐ Arm holder   RIGHT arm: ☐ Board ☐ Side ☐ Chest ☐ Arm holder

Traction weight _____ lbs. ☐ Positioned by self ☐ Positioned by (initial): _____

Positioning device/site:

☐ Andrews bed ☐ Axillary roll ☐ Donut ☐ Fracture table ☐ Gel pads ☐ Hall Relton frame ☐ Jackson table

☐ Mayfield headrest ☐ McGuire positioner ☐ LamiRolls ☐ Stirrups ☐ Stryker frame ☐ VacPac

☐ Other/Comments: _____

INTERMITTANT COMPRESSION DEVICES	☐ N/A

Serial #: _____ Setting: _____mmHg   ☐ To O.R. with compression device on

Device type: ☐ Calf ☐ Thigh ☐ Bilateral ☐ Left ☐ Right   Applied by (initial): _____

SKIN PREP	☐ N/A

Hair removal method: ☐ None ☐ Dry clip ☐ Dry shave ☐ Wet clip ☐ Wet shave   Hair removed by (initial): _____

In O.R. Pre-op scrub: ☐ Betadine scrub ☐ Chlorhexidine ☐ Other: _____

Prep agent: ☐ Betadine ☐ Chloraprep ☐ Other: _____

22280 S(15730)(0808)C

Figure 3-2 Sample intraoperative record. *(From Rothrock JC: Alexander's care of the patient in surgery, ed 14, St Louis, 2011, Mosby.)*

Page 2 of 3

CATHETERS, DRAINS, TUBES	☐ N/A

Catheter/drain description: _____ ☐ Straight catheter

Location: _____ Collection device: _____

Balloon fill amount: _____ Inserted by (initial): _____ Date: _____ Time: _____

Drainage description: _____

☐ Present on arrival ☐ Removed at end of case

ESU/OTHER EQUIPMENT	☐ N/A

Type: ☐ Monopolar ☐ Other: _____ Serial #: _____ Settings:_____ Cut _____ Coag

    Grounding pad site: _____ Applied by (initial):_____

    ☐ Bipolar ☐ Tripolar   Serial #: _____ Setting: _____ Coag

    ☐ Argon beam coagulator   Serial #: _____ Beam Setting: _____

TOURNIQUET #1	☐ N/A

Tourniquet side: ☐ Left ☐ Right   Site: ☐ Thigh ☐ Calf ☐ Upper arm ☐ Forearm ☐ Ankle

Pressure _____mmHg   Time inflated: _____ Deflated: _____ Time inflated: _____ Deflated: _____

Pressure _____mmHg   Time inflated: _____ Deflated: _____ Time inflated: _____ Deflated: _____

Applied by (initial): _____ Serial #: _____ ☐ Tourniquet applied but not inflated

TOURNIQUET #2	☐ N/A

Tourniquet side: ☐ Left ☐ Right   Site: ☐ Thigh ☐ Calf ☐ Upper arm ☐ Forearm ☐ Ankle

Pressure _____mmHg   Time inflated: _____ Deflated: _____ Time inflated: _____ Deflated: _____

Pressure _____mmHg   Time inflated: _____ Deflated: _____ Time inflated: _____ Deflated: _____

Applied by (initial): _____ Serial #: _____ ☐ Tourniquet applied but not inflated

EXPLANTS	☐ N/A

Explant description: _____

LASER DATA	☐ N/A

Laser type/model/serial #: _____ Laser time: _____ ☐ Standby

X-RAYS and IMAGES	☐ N/A

Type: ☐ Angiography ☐ Flat plate ☐ Fluoroscan/self image ☐ Fluoroscopy

CELLSAVER	☐ N/A

☐ Used

GENERAL CASE DATA

O.R.:_____ ☐ ASA class: _____ ☐ Return to O.R. ☐ See implant record

Pre-op diagnosis: _____

Post-op diagnosis: _____ ☐ Same as Pre-op

SURGICAL PROCEDURE

Procedure performed:_____

_____

_____

_____

Anesthesia type: ☐ General ☐ M.A.C. ☐ Spinal ☐ Block (type) _____ ☐ Epidural ☐ Local

Wound class: ☐ 1 ☐ 2 ☐ 3 ☐ 4

Figure 3-2, cont'd

Continued

MEDICATIONS   ☐ N/A

Medication	Dose	Route	Given by (Initial)	Date	Time

Hemostatic agents: _____

IRRIGATION   ☐ N/A

Irrigation	Additives	Estimated In	Estimated Out

FAMILY COMMUNICATION   ☐ N/A

☐ By Phone   ☐ In person   Communicated to: _____

Communicated by (initial): _____   Date: _____   Time: _____

SPECIMENS/CULTURES

Number of specimen: Tissue:_____ Frozen section:_____ Culture:_____ Fluid:_____ Foreign body:_____ ☐ None

Examined and disposed per Dr. (Print Name):_____

Skin/bone freezer: Description:_____

PACKING   ☐ N/A

Packing type:_____   Packing site: _____

DEPARTURE FROM O.R.

Post-op skin condition excluding operative site:☐ Dry and intact ☐ Unchanged ☐ Other, description:_____

Via: ☐ Ambulatory ☐ Bed ☐ Crib ☐ ICU bed ☐ Post-op chair ☐ Stretcher ☐ Surgilifter ☐ Other:_____

Destination: ☐ PACU ☐ PACU Phase I ☐ PACU Phase II ☐ Home ☐ Other: _____

Dressings:_____

COMMENTS

Abbreviations:
ASA–American Society of Anesthesiology   Coag–Coagulation   M.A.C–Monitored Anesthesia Care   O.R.–Operating Room
Circ–Circulator   ESU–Electrosurgical Unit   Op–Operative   PACU–Post Anesthesia Care Unit

Initial	Signature/Title	Print Name	Initial	Signature/Title	Print Name

Figure 3-2, cont'd

Box 3-4 Examples of Sentinel Events

- Surgery performed on the wrong side
- Failure to obtain informed consent
- Treatment or a procedure initiated on the wrong patient (patient misidentification)
- Medication error
- Documentation errors
- Cardiac or respiratory arrest
- Retention of an object after surgery *even if the object is subsequently retrieved*
- Incorrect count and steps taken to resolve the count
- Suspected intoxication of personnel
- Any injury to a patient while that person is in the care of the perioperative staff
- Equipment failure resulting in injury
- Break in sterile technique that causes harm to the patient
- Suspected malpractice
- Failure to recognize or act when a potentially critical event occurs in the operating room
- Extreme inappropriate behavior by physicians or other staff members
- Bullying
- Sexual harassment
- Battery of a patient (includes inappropriate touching or a procedure for which informed consent was not obtained)
- Any violation of the patient's rights by another
- Loss of patient property
- Death of a patient

NOTE: Other events may require reporting according to hospital policy.

during surgery, bullying, sexual harassment, and other forms of coercion. Remember that the purpose of the report is not to make a judgment about an event, only to report it. The report lists the date and time the incident occurred, who was there, and what happened, exactly as it occurred without emotion or embellishment. The main reasons for the report are for quality assurance or risk reduction and to provide details in case legal action is taken by any of the individuals involved.

How to Write an Incident Report

A report is required whenever an event occurs that has resulted or might result in death, injury, or harm. *Harm* includes psychological as well as physical injury.

A report must be filed after events involving either patients or employees. Box 3-4 gives examples of sentinel events that require an incident report. Other events require reporting according to hospital policy. If you are unsure whether an incident requires formal reporting, it is best to seek advice from the department manager, who can provide a definitive answer.

Incident reports are completed in writing on the hospital's designated form. The forms include a place to list the personnel involved and the date, location, and time of the incident. A section is included in which the incident must be described by the person making the report in his or her own words. The statement must include *who* was involved, *where* the incident

occurred, *when* it took place, and *how* it happened. A witness should also be present when the report is completed.

These guidelines can be followed in writing the narrative part of the report:

1. **Write and submit the form as soon as possible after the event.** If you are uncertain whether an incident report is needed, ask for help.
2. **State only the facts and do not give your opinion about the incident.** An example of a proper statement is, "Dr. X smelled strongly of alcohol. His speech was slurred" or "The needle count was found to be incorrect at the close of surgery. A radiograph was ordered, which did not reveal the needle, and the needle was not found outside the patient."
3. **Use professional and precise language whenever possible.** It is *more proper* to state, "Dr. X appeared agitated and angry. He denied us time for a sponge count and proceeded to throw surgical scissors off the sterile field onto the floor." Language such as the following should be *avoided*: "Dr. X was acting horrible. He wouldn't even take a sponge count, and he smashed the Metz across the room."
4. **Write in the first person.** For example, "When I arrived in operating room 4, I saw the patient lying on the floor" is better than "The patient was seen by the surgical tech (me) on the floor in room 4."
5. **Do not be intimidated by others who want to protect individuals.** In some circumstances, employees may wish to protect others who were involved. Always use good ethical judgment; keep the safety of the patient in mind.
6. **Take your time in writing the report.** Try to write the report in a location where you are undisturbed by others. Fill out the form carefully and thoughtfully.
7. **Submit the incident report directly to the operating room supervisor or other designated personnel.** Do not leave the report where others can find it. Do not place it in the patient's chart.
8. **Remember that the report may be subpoenaed for legal action.** After an incident report is submitted to the risk management or legal department, an informal investigation may be conducted, or the hospital's **insurance** company will be notified. Further action is then taken if needed.

ADVANCE HEALTH CARE DIRECTIVE

An **advance directive** is a document in which a patient gives instructions about his or her medical care in the event the individual cannot speak for himself or herself because of incapacity. If the patient is incompetent or a minor, a guardian or family member may sign the advance directive. Various forms of advance directives can be used, and states have different regulations and standards for the implementation of directives. For example, an individual may refuse mechanical ventilation but accept medication. If the patient is considered to be in a persistent vegetative state, the guardian may request withdrawal from mechanical support systems. In most institutions, the advance directive must be reactivated with each separate hospital admission. The following sections explain the different types of advance directives.

Do Not Resuscitate Order

A *do not resuscitate* (DNR) or *do not attempt resuscitation* (DNAR) orders specifies that cardiopulmonary resuscitation must not be initiated in the event of cardiac or pulmonary arrest. The patient's status is clearly indicated on the front of the chart. Because of the effects of anesthetic agents on the cardiovascular and respiratory systems, some hospitals suspend a DNR order for the duration of the surgical procedure. The order must be rewritten when the patient is in the postanesthesia care unit (PACU).

Organ Donation

Patients have the right to refuse the removal of their organs for transplantation after their death. A number of religions and cultures forbid or limit certain types of organ transfers. Others may not provide consent for organ donation based on fears that the organs might be removed before death is pronounced. Regardless of the reason, documentation of this directive should be included in the patient's chart. Organ transplantation itself requires extensive documentation consistent with the complex nature of the procedure.

Refusal of Blood or Tissue Products

Patients may refuse blood or tissue products because of their faith or personal beliefs. Simply stating that one belongs to a certain faith does not automatically restrict medical intervention. If the patient is unable to communicate his or her wishes, lifesaving measures may be initiated. An advance directive is needed if the normal process of patient care, including transfusion, is unwanted.

Living Will

A **living will** is a legal document that specifically states the type of medical intervention or treatment the patient does not want. Possible interventions include artificial feeding, transfusions, specific diagnostic tests, pulmonary maintenance on a ventilator, and the use of medications. Living wills can be created with help from the state bar association, state nursing association, state medical association, or hospital. A living will is not the same as a last will and testament, which is a legal document used for the distribution of a person's property after death.

Medical Power of Attorney

The patient may assign a specific person to act as his or her proxy with regard to medical treatment. After the **medical power of attorney** is prepared and signed, the proxy thereafter can speak on behalf of the patient regarding his or her medical treatment. The medical power of attorney does not give up legal authority in any area except medical treatment.

ETHICS

Ethics is a branch of philosophy that defines people's behavior in their relationships with others and their environment. The definition of ethics and whether morality is the same as ethics is the subject of many philosophical and scholarly debates. There is no correct answer. Morality, or morals, may be described as personal standards that often are influenced by culture, religion, or traditions. Morality usually attempts to define what is right or wrong behavior. Ethics tends to be less focused on right and wrong and more intent on finding out what is *beneficial to humanity* in the long term. It addresses specific circumstances of an act. In many ways, these concepts overlap. For example, most people agree that stealing another's property is wrong or immoral. However, ethics might argue that some situations allow stealing. For example, is it permissible to steal food to save a child from starvation?

For the purposes of this text, ethics is discussed as it applies to a health professional's conduct in the care of patients— **medical ethics.** The focus is on **standards of conduct** that have been established by the health professions for their own members and that promote accountability and responsible, compassionate care of others.

One of the best-known ethical standards is, *"Do no harm."* This standard was established by the medical profession but has been adopted by many others. This simple phrase includes many deeper concepts, including the promise to every patient that no matter what treatment or advice is given, the patient will not be injured *as a result* of the treatment. It is an implied contract between the patient and the health care professional and the basis of trust in this relationship. Conflict in ethical decision making arises when a standard of behavior creates a **dilemma** (choices or decisions, none of which is satisfactory). Perhaps the choice of actions conflicts with the rights of another person or might result in harm. Dilemmas are resolved by making decisions based on the best outcome even if it is not entirely acceptable.

ETHICAL BEHAVIOR IN HEALTH CARE

Most people understand what is acceptable in a society and what is considered unethical. **Professional ethics** comprises the standards that society expects from those who provide services to them. Medical ethics defines the conduct of those in the health professions.

Ethical behavior in health care is based on a few very powerful directives for the health professional. These directives have far-reaching implications:

- Respect human individuality and uniqueness
- Do no harm
- Act with beneficence
- Act with justice
- Respect all confidences entrusted to you
- Act with faithfulness to the patient and others
- Act with honesty
- Respect the free will of the patient
- Give the patient's welfare priority over all else

These behaviors might be applied to any situation in life. In the care of patients, they have special meaning.

RESPECT HUMAN INDIVIDUALITY AND UNIQUENESS

Each person is different from all others. Each individual has needs that are specific to his or her personality, medical condition, psychological state, emotions, social life, and culture. Respect for these qualities is demonstrated when health professionals treat the patient as a person with a name, a history, and a lifetime of experiences that probably are very different from their own. We must act without judgment or condemnation.

When we encounter a patient who acts or looks very different from what we consider "normal" or "mainstream," we sometimes feel off-guard or even offended. Our first impressions tell us that this person is different and therefore unpredictable or even threatening in some way. Health professionals learn to curb these feelings and transform them into therapeutic action. A person may behave outside the norm, but he or she is human, with all the needs and pain of any human being. It is these characteristics to which health professionals must respond, not the patient's lifestyle, appearance, or mannerisms.

ACT WITH BENEFICENCE

Beneficence implies empathy and commitment to healing. It requires health professionals to move beyond aspects of the patient's condition that offend their senses or make them emotionally uncomfortable and instead focus on the use of their professional and personal skills. Active care of a patient who has a purulent infection, shows self-neglect, or has a condition associated with a social stigma is an act of beneficence and compassion.

ACT WITH JUSTICE

All patients have the right to equal treatment regardless of age, physical attributes, mental state, ethnicity, or socioeconomic status. Advocating for justice may mean speaking out in the workplace when equal rights are violated. It also means monitoring and challenging our own beliefs and perhaps even our prejudices. Health professionals must be culturally and socially sensitive. To act without sensitivity is to act without justice.

RESPECT ALL CONFIDENCES ENTRUSTED TO YOU

Confidential information about the patient should not be shared with others outside the operating room. Confidence among coworkers is also an expected ethical behavior. Gossip is an insidious but common breach of confidentiality. It extracts enormous cost in emotional hurt and can affect the professional and personal lives of people in profound ways that we may never realize.

ACT WITH FAITHFULNESS

It is your responsibility to remain faithful to the patient as his or her advocate. At all times, you must respect the patient's personal and physical privacy and honor the patient's trust in you. It is important to have trust in the work you do and the people with whom you work.

ACT WITH HONESTY

If you make an error, it is crucial that you admit it. When you are unsure about a procedure, be sure to ask for help and accept that help without resentment or anger. Falsifying information or records is dishonest, as is embellishing or diminishing your actions or those of others.

RESPECT THE FREE WILL OF THE PATIENT

All patients have the right to refuse care and to participate in their care. They have the right to receive information about their condition from their physicians and nurses and to ask for advocacy. Patients lose almost all physical freedom when they enter the hospital. Although not physically restrained (except in certain extreme circumstances), they lose mobility, the freedom to work and care for other family members, and the ability to participate in a normal life. Health care workers are expected to respect and respond to patients' freedom to make choices and express needs and concerns.

PATIENT'S WELFARE—PRIORITY OVER ALL ELSE

Surgical technologists are presented with many responsibilities and decisions during the course of a workday. Some decisions, such as what equipment to prepare for a case or the ordering of supplies, are straightforward, without ethical dilemma. Others situations, such as reporting alleged malpractice committed by a colleague, are laden with more serious ethical consequences. Most responsibilities and duties in the perioperative environment have a consequence (large or small) for the patient. The technologist has a duty of care to always act in favor of the patient's welfare. The implied contract between patient and care worker always favors outcomes that protect the patient from harm. During professional development, surgical technologists learn to think "outside" immediate consequences when making decisions. They become increasingly aware of their patients' vulnerabilities. Patient protection and welfare is consciously or unconsciously factored into every action and task.

SURGICAL CONSCIENCE

Surgical conscience is a specific set of professional attributes that are associated with being on the surgical team. It includes the following concepts:

- **Accountability:** taking responsibility for ones actions at all times both on and off the job. It is includes admitting when one has made an error even though there may be difficult consequences. Accountability is similar to responsibility.
- **Responsibility:** closely aligned with accountability. However, responsibility implies that a person is made responsible for specific acts or status either because the person volunteered to be the responsible person, or because their circumstances place them in a role of responsibility. Accountability is admitting your actions as the responsible person.

- **Confidentiality:** maintaining patient confidentiality is a required component of being part of a surgical team. Confidentiality must be maintained according to all HIPAA regulations.
- **Honesty and willingness to admit mistakes:** admitting mistakes applies to all aspects of health care. It includes admitting potential drug errors or any other event which may cause harm and requires action. In these cases "conscience" is the same as "ethics" because someone with sound professional ethics would not allow such mistakes to be kept secret at the cost of another person's harm.
- **Commitment to cost containment in the health facility:** using materials and supplies wisely to prevent waste and as a measure to prevent exceeding the facility and department budget.

Some people may blame stress or lack of resources for a poor surgical conscience. There are no reasonable barriers to maintaining sound ethics in surgery. Choices are based on what is right, fair, honest, and professional, and these sound choices are made for all patients, regardless of gender, race, religion, etc. Anyone contemplating a career in health care must be able to combat stress with positive activities, rather than sliding values.

COMBINED ETHICAL AND LEGAL CONCERNS

IMPAIRMENT

An impaired team member is a major threat to the safety of the patient and others in the environment. It is illegal to care for others while impaired by drugs or alcohol. Health care workers have both a legal and an ethical responsibility to report suspected impairment of a coworker or, if needed, to seek treatment for themselves. Self-destructive behavior, such as drug or alcohol abuse, reveals not a weakness but an illness. In reporting these behaviors, team members protect not only everyone in the environment but also the abuser. Treatment programs are available for those who need help. The goal is to return the health care worker to a productive and satisfying role in the workplace and to enable the individual to resume a stable personal and social life.

REFUSAL TO PERFORM AN ASSIGNED TASK

The surgical technologist has the right to abstain from participation in certain types of cases that violate his or her ethical, moral, or religious values. The facility must be informed of this when the surgical technologist is hired. It is not ethical to suddenly refuse to follow a directive on moral grounds unless the case is one that could never have been anticipated by the staff member. When offered a position, the surgical technologist should submit, in writing, a list of cases in which he or she declines to participate.

Occasionally a team member refuses to work with another person based on a history of inappropriate behavior or abuse. The surgical technologist should document and report the behavior before he or she is required to work with that person. To suddenly refuse to scrub a case, or worse, to walk out in the middle of a case, could be interpreted as abandonment of the patient. If the reason for refusal is a personality clash, steps must be taken to resolve the problem, because they can ultimately lead to poor patient care (see Chapter 2).

ETHICAL DILEMMAS

An **ethical dilemma** is a personal conflict that arises from the need to make a decision based on choices that are not completely acceptable. A common example is the overloaded lifeboat. If everyone remains on the lifeboat, it will probably sink. To remove individuals and prevent the boat from sinking will result in the immediate death of those thrown overboard. Neither option is satisfactory from an ethical viewpoint. Society tries to resolve dilemmas in many areas of medical ethics through ethics committees, public debate, and even laws. Medical technology has exceeded our ability to cope with the many ethical dilemmas as they relate to health and society. There are no "answers" to these debates, but health professionals should be aware of them.

- **Right to die.** Should an individual have the right to die when and where he or she wishes? Should this include assisted suicide?
- **Stem cell research.** Is it ethical to use stem cells obtained from discarded human embryos for cell regeneration?
- **Human cloning.** Is it ethical to allow researchers to perform the replication of a human being?
- **Good Samaritan law.** Should a health professional be allowed to help someone in need of assistance outside the health care environment without threat of liability if things go wrong? (States allow this by law, but the issue is still debated.)
- **Abortion.** Is it ethical for a woman to terminate her pregnancy?
- **Elective sterilization.** Do individuals have the right to undergo elective sterilization? What about forced sterilization?
- **Genetic engineering.** Is the process ethical?
- **Human experimentation.** What are the moral and ethical problems associated with human experimentation?
- **Medicare fraud.** What are the ethical and moral issues involved?
- **In vitro fertilization.** Is it ethical?
- **Artificial insemination.** What are the ethical implications?
- **Gender reassignment.** Should insurance providers pay for gender reassessment?
- **Animal Experimentation.** With advancements in technology, should animals be used for medical experimentation?
- **Communicable diseases.** What are the ethical implications when treating patients with highly contagious diseases?
- **Refusal of treatment.** Can the family of an incapacitated individual decide to refuse treatment for that family member if they believe it will cause or prolong suffering?

- **Organ donation.** Is it ethical to remove vital organs from a patient who is brain dead but maintained on life support systems? Can the family make this decision if the patient cannot express his or her wishes? Is it ethical to donate a liver to a person who suffers from chronic alcoholism?

Many other ethical dilemmas occur in day-to-day clinical work, including the following:

- **Loyalty.** A loyalty dilemma requires that a person be loyal to one person while being disloyal to another. For example, you are asked to comment on an act of negligence committed by a coworker that you witnessed. Do you incriminate your coworker by telling the truth or try to defend her even though you know she was negligent?
- **Confidentiality.** Your patient informs you that she is pregnant, but she has not told her partner or the physician. She asks you not to tell anyone.
- **Spiritual values.** You have notified your employer that you decline to participate in abortion procedures. You are called in for an emergency. When you arrive at the hospital, you learn that you will serve as scrub on a case of an incomplete self-induced abortion. No one else is available to serve as scrub. The patient is hemorrhaging.
- **Honesty.** You have incorrectly reported the amount of a local anesthetic used during a procedure. The patient has a toxic reaction, but it is eventually resolved with a good outcome for the patient. No one knows that you miscalculated the dosage and caused the reaction. Do you report it anyway, knowing that it might cost you your job?

One method of resolving ethical conflict is to examine your own beliefs thoroughly and come to a resolution about how you will act in certain circumstances. Not every ethical dilemma is predictable, but surgical technologists frequently are confronted with ethical decisions both small and large. These issues deserve thoughtful consideration. Speaking with other health care professionals or a mentor can help one define their personal values and integrate them into professional ethics.

ETHICAL DECISION MAKING

Ethical decisions come from choices that we make in our lives, based on personal values rather than opinions. Professional values were discussed earlier under Ethical Behavior in Health Care. These can easily be extended to one's personal life. An initial professional code of ethics is reflected in the decisions they make in the workplace and in other environments. It is not possible to make ethical decisions without first having a personal or professional code of ethics to follow. It is logical that our decision making should be consistent with the ethics we claim to live and work by.

PROFESSIONAL CODES OF ETHICS

Professional organizations, such as the Association of Surgical Technologists (AST), the American Nurses Association, the American Hospital Association, and the American Medical Association, have created codes of ethics that reflect

| Box **3-5** | **Code of Ethics of the Association of Surgical Technologists** |

1. To maintain the highest standards of professional conduct and patient care.
2. To hold in confidence, with respect to the patient's beliefs, all personal matters.
3. To respect and protect the patient's legal and moral rights to quality patient care.
4. To not knowingly cause injury or any injustice to those entrusted to our care.
5. To work with fellow technologists and other professional health groups to promote harmony and unity for better patient care.
6. To follow principles of asepsis.
7. To maintain a high degree of efficiency through continuing education.
8. To maintain and practice surgical technology willingly, with pride and dignity.
9. To report any unethical conduct or practice to the proper authority.
10. To adhere to the Code of Ethics at all times with all members of the health care team.

From the Association of Surgical Technologists, http://www.ast.org.

expectations of those professionals as they make decisions involving ethical issues. By acting in accordance with these ethics, professional health care workers demonstrate their advocacy for human rights, patient protection, and the laws of society. In all situations, the health care worker is the patient's advocate; the health care worker is doing what the patient would do if he or she were able. The AST has adopted a Latin phrase to describe its ethos: *Aeger primo*, which means "the patient first." The AST code of ethics is presented in Box 3-5.

PATIENTS' RIGHTS

Government agencies and established laws are created to protect patients. Professional organizations for health care workers establish and publish codes of ethics. These codes outline the behaviors expected of any member of the health profession. A health professional thus is expected to act in a certain way and within the ethical standards of the profession and the laws of the state. Health professionals have an unspoken contract to maintain a particular kind of relationship with their patients. The American Hospital Association has developed guidelines to help patients understand their rights in the hospital setting. These can be found in Appendix A.

KEY CONCEPTS

- Laws concerning the practice of medicine, nursing, and allied health have been established to protect the public.
- The surgical technologist's scope of tasks is defined by state law.
- The medical and nurse practice acts of each state provide information about the roles and responsibilities of health care workers.

- Health care policy is established by professional organizations and by health care facilities.
- Delegation is an important legal and professional concept in medicine. It is the transfer of responsibility for a task from one person to another. The conditions of delegation must be determined to protect the patient from harm.
- Civil liability derives from an act committed against a person or property. Acts of negligence in health care are causes of civil liability.
- Negligence is "the commission of an act that a prudent person would not have done or the omission of a duty and a prudent person would have fulfilled, resulting in injury or harm to another person."[1]
- Negligence is the most common cause of patient injury and death in health care.
- Examples of negligence include patient burns, falls, medication errors, improper patient positioning, abandonment of a patient, and retained surgical items. Failure to care for a surgical specimen correctly and failure to communicate about a potentially dangerous situation are also considered negligence.
- The patient's record is a legal document. Laws regarding the use of patient information are strictly enforced.
- Documentation in the perioperative environment is necessary to protect the patient.
- A sentinel event is one in which there is potential or actual injury or death in the work environment. A report must be completed for any sentinel event.
- A legal action may be brought against any health professional when a negligent act results in harm.
- Ethics is a branch of philosophy that defines people's behavior in relation to others and the environment.
- An ethical dilemma is a situation in which no desirable outcome exists no matter which ethical choice is made.
- Ethical behavior in health care is established by culture, society, and professional organizations.
- Professionals are expected to act in an ethical manner.
- Ethics in medicine involves issues such as confidentiality, honesty, respect for others, beneficence, and respect for the law.

REVIEW QUESTIONS

1. Define the relationship between accountability and delegation.
2. Who may delegate a task? Under what circumstances can a task be delegated?
3. What is sexual harassment? Why do you think people tolerate it in the workplace?
4. Negligence is the most common cause of lawsuits in medical practice. Define negligence and give three examples of negligent acts or behavior.
5. What are state practice acts?
6. What are the causes of negligence in the operating room?
7. What is informed consent? Why is it necessary? Who can witness informed consent?
8. How do you decide what ethical decisions to make?
9. What is the difference between the law and ethics?
10. What is an ethical dilemma?
11. Many bioethical dilemmas have arisen in our society, such as abortion, stem cell research, savior siblings, and organ donation. List at least five bioethical dilemmas that you find particularly difficult.

CASE STUDIES

Case 1

You are assigned to scrub on a case, and you have just finished setting up the back table and instruments. The surgeons are gowned and gloved. The circulator is completing the skin prep using an alcohol-based antiseptic. As soon as she finishes, the surgeons ask for drapes. You see that the patient's skin is still quite wet with the prep solution, and you hesitate in starting the draping, knowing that the prep solution has not dried. You remark on this to the surgeon and he replies, "Come on— come on, let's get going on this." A few minutes later, the edge of the drape catches fire. The fire is quickly extinguished, revealing a second-degree burn of the patient's skin. Who do you believe is responsible? What documentation is needed? Who should be notified?

Case 2

Your patient is a 70-year-old man scheduled for a hernia repair. Your role is assistant circulator. The RN circulator asks you to go to the holding area to see whether the patient has arrived. When you arrive at the holding area, the patient is there with the surgeon. The patient's speech is slurred, and he appears to have difficulty hearing the surgeon. As the surgeon looks over the chart, he notices that the patient has not signed the operative permit. He asks you to witness the patient's signing. What will you do?

Case 3

While scrubbed on a case involving surgical treatment of carpal tunnel syndrome, you complete the instrument, sponge, and needle count. You are missing a needle. You tell the surgeon that the count is incorrect. He replies, "Oh, don't worry. The needle can't be in the wound, it's too small. I would be able to see it. Let's close." What will you do?

Case 4

While in the locker room, you notice that one of your coworkers is emptying the pockets of her scrub suit. There are two vials of injectable medications. You cannot see what they are. She puts them in her purse and leaves. What do you do?

Case 5

You have been called into the office of the hospital's attorney to answer questions about a case 2 months earlier in which you scrubbed. The case involves the retained needle in the patient undergoing carpal tunnel surgery (see case 3), who is suing the hospital and staff. Based on how you answered the question in case 3, what are your thoughts as you wait to see the hospital's attorney?

Case 6

You have been asked to help position an 80-year-old man for hip surgery. He is under general anesthesia and is intubated. After the surgery, the anesthesiologist discovers that the patient's right ulna is fractured. The surgeon says, "We'd better fix this ulna now." Think about the events in this procedure. Who is responsible for the fracture? Can the surgeon repair the ulna without a permit? What (if anything) is the appropriate action for you as a surgical technologist at this point?

Case 7

You are scrubbed on a cholecystectomy case. You have been given sterile saline, Hypaque (a contrast medium used during radiography to observe strictures inside the ducts of the gallbladder), and thrombin (a coagulant). You put these in separate medicine containers on your back table. The surgeon asks you to prepare a syringe of 50% Hypaque and 50% saline. Instead, you hand her thrombin. Just as she begins to inject the bile duct, you realize that you made an error. What do you do? Who will be responsible for any injury to the patient?

REFERENCES

1. *Mosby's pocket dictionary of medical, nursing, and allied health*, ed 6, St Louis, 2009, Mosby.
2. Department of Health and Human Services, Centers for Disease Control and Prevention, National Institute for Occupational Safety and Health, *Slips, trips, and fall prevention for health workers*, http://www.cdc.gov/niosh/docs/2011-123/pdfs/2011-123.pdf. Accessed July 18, 2011.

BIBLIOGRAPHY

American Hospital Association: *The patient care partnership: understanding expectations, rights, and responsibilities.* Accessed July 19, 2011, at www.aha.org/aha/issues/Communicating-With-Patients.

Association of periOperative Registered Nurses (AORN): Position statement on correct site surgery. In *Standards, recommended practices and guidelines, 2007 edition*, Denver, 2007, AORN.

Association of Surgical Technologists (AST): *Standards of practice.* Accessed July 18, 2011, at http://www.ast.org.

Association of Surgical Technologists (AST): *Code of ethics.* Accessed July 19, 2011, at http://www.ast.org.

United States Department of Health and Human Services, Office for Civil Rights: *Summary of the HIPAA privacy rule.* Accessed July 19, 2011, at http://www.hhs.gov/ocr/privacy/hipaa/understanding/summary/privacysummary.pdf.

University of Washington School of Medicine: *Informed consent: ethics in medicine.* Accessed July 18, 2011, at http://depts.washington.edu/bioethx.

Virginia Board of Health Professions, Virginia Department of Health Professions: *Study into the need to regulate surgical assistants & surgical technologists in the Commonwealth of Virginia*, July 2010. Accessed January 23, 2012, at http://www.dhp.virginia.gov/bhp/studies/SurgicalAssistant_TechnologistReportFinal.doc.

4

The Health Care Facility

LEARNING OBJECTIVES

After studying this chapter the reader will be able to:
1. Describe the principles of operating room design
2. Describe the purpose of traffic patterns in the operating room
3. Identify the common items found in the surgical suite
4. Explain temperature and humidity ranges used in the surgical suite and why they are important
5. Discuss the functions of various work areas in the surgical suite

6. List common hospital ancillary services and describe their functions
7. Define *health care insurance* and discuss the ways patients pay for care
8. Describe an organizational chart and explain its significance in an organization
9. Describe the purpose of an organizational chart
10. Define *chain of command*
11. Identify perioperative professionals and their roles

TERMINOLOGY

Accreditation (of a health care facility): The process by which a hospital or other health care facility is evaluated by an independent organization. Accredited facilities are those that meet the standards of the accreditation agency.

Administration: Individuals who manage an institution, plan its activities, and provide oversight for day-to-day operations and employees. The administration is also a liaison between the facility and the community, government, and media.

Air exchange: The exchange of air between areas separated by a physical boundary. Standards for air exchange are regulated by health and safety organizations.

Back table: A large stainless steel table on which most of the sterile surgical supplies and instruments are placed for use during surgery. Before surgery, the back table is covered with a sterile drape and sterile instruments and other equipment are opened onto its surface. Supplies needed for immediate use are transferred to the Mayo stand.

Biomedical engineering technician: Professional who specializes in the maintenance, repair, maintenance, and safe operation of devices used in medicine, including surgical equipment.

Case cart system: Organizational method of preparing equipment and instruments for a specific surgery. Equipment is prepared by the central services or supply department and sent to the operating room.

Central core: The restricted area of the operating room, where sterile supplies and flash sterilizers are located.

Chain of command: A hierarchy of personnel positions that establishes both vertical and horizontal relationships between positions.

Decontamination area: A room or department in which soiled instruments and equipment are cleaned of gross matter and decontaminated to remove microorganisms.

Efficiency: The economic use of time and energy to prevent unnecessary expenditure of work, materials, and time.

High-efficiency particulate air (HEPA) filters: Filters installed in the operating room ventilation system that remove 99.97% of particles equal to or larger than 0.3 micrometers.

Integrated operating room: A type of structural and engineering design in which digital and computerized components such as cameras, monitors, and environmental controls can be controlled from a central location in the room. Components such as endoscopic control units and monitors are built into the room structure rather than as separate portable units.

Job description: A document that specifies duties, responsibilities, location, pay, and management structure of a job.

Job title: The name of a job, such as "Certified Surgical Technologist" or "Chief of Surgery."

Laminar airflow (LAF) system: A ventilation system that moves a contained volume of air in layers at a continuous velocity, with 800 to 900 air exchanges per hour.

TERMINOLOGY (cont.)

Organizational chart (organigram): A graphic depiction of an organization's chain of command that shows the lines of vertical (higher and lower) and horizontal (equal) administrative authority.

Personnel policy: A policy that sets forth the health care facility's job descriptions, role delineations, requirements for employment, and rules of conduct for personnel.

Postanesthesia care unit (PACU): The critical care area where patients are taken after surgery for monitoring and evaluation as they emerge from anesthesia..

Restricted area: The area of the operating room where only personnel wearing surgical attire, including masks, shoe coverings, and head coverings, are allowed. Doors are kept closed, and the air pressure is greater than that in areas outside the restricted area.

Risk management: The process of tracking, evaluating, and studying accidents and incidents to protect patients and employees. Risk management produces change in policy or enforcement of policy if the risk reaches an unacceptable level.

Role confusion: Lack of clarity about one's job duties and requirements.

Semirestricted area: A designated area in which only personnel wearing scrub suits and hair caps that enclose all facial hair are allowed.

The Joint Commission: The accrediting organization for hospitals and other health care facilities in the United States.

Traffic patterns: The movement of people and equipment into, out of, and within the operating room.

Transitional area: An area in which surgical personnel or visitors prepare to enter the semirestricted and restricted areas. Transitional areas include the locker rooms and changing rooms.

Unrestricted area: An area that people dressed in street clothes may enter.

INTRODUCTION

The services provided in the health care setting require specific facilities and a staff capable of delivering those services. Neither of these elements of health care can exist without the other. The facility itself must provide a safe environment for patients, staff members, and visitors. It also must *enable* the work of health care personnel in a way that encourages efficiency of time, movement (work), and space. This is done through the administrative and management process.

This chapter is an introduction to the perioperative environment and to the health care facility as a whole. It gives the rationale for operating room design and standards. It also provides important information about the professionals who work in the facility–specifically, what their roles are and where those roles fit into the larger organizational structure. Environmental safety for patients and perioperative personnel includes the methods, guidelines, and standards related to operating room technology. This topic is crucial for patient care and occupational safety of everyone who works in the surgical environment. It is covered in detail in Chapter 8, Environmental Hazards in the Perioperative Environment, and in Chapter 18, Energy Sources in Surgery.

STANDARDS AND RECOMMENDATIONS

Technical standards and recommendations for the physical perioperative environment are set by a number of different agencies and regulatory bodies that are concerned with safety, including infection control, structural engineering, and safety in the workplace. Some of the agencies listed here will be seen in later chapters covering additional focal areas, especially in the area of environmental safety, which is covered in Chapter 8:

- **Association for Professionals in Infection Control and Epidemiology** (APIC) conducts research and establishes guidelines for infection control measures (http://www.apic.org).
- **Agency for Healthcare Research and Quality** (AHRQ) National Guideline Clearinghouse (searchable database) (http://www.guideline.gov/browse/by-topic.aspx).
- **American Institute of Architects** (AIA) sets the primary standards and for health care facility engineering (http://www.aia.org).
- **Environmental Protection Agency** (EPA) sets and enforces regulations related to safety in the environment, including hazardous chemicals and radiation (http://www.epa).
- **Occupational Safety and Health Administration** (OSHA) regulates occupational hazards and safety (http://www.osha.gov/index.html).

ACCREDITATION

Accreditation, as it pertains to health care institutions and facilities, is the process by which a team of professionals evaluates a health care institution's practices and policies and the outcomes of patient care. **The Joint Commission** is the primary accreditation organization for all health care facilities (http://www.jointcommission.org).

The facility is awarded accreditation when these standards are met. Accreditation is a voluntary process, but government agencies and insurers use accreditation to determine whether an institution qualifies for patient care reimbursement. Accreditation implies a high standard of care and a commitment to public safety and welfare.

To earn accreditation by the Joint Commission, the institution must meet or exceed the high standards set by the commission. The Joint Commission bases its own standards on those of professional and governmental agencies. The Joint Commission is governed by a board of commissioners, made up of members of the American College of Physicians, the American Society of Internal Medicine, the American College of Surgeons, the American Dental Association, the American Hospital Association, the American Medical Association, and selected professionals. The Joint Commission standards apply to every area of the health care facility and focus on patient safety, protection, and quality care.

PRINCIPLES OF OPERATING ROOM DESIGN

The surgical department is structured and engineered to provide a safe and efficient environment for patients and staff members. Many different designs can be used, but all must achieve the following objectives:

1. Infection control
2. Environmental safety
3. Efficient use of personnel, time, space, and material resources

INFECTION CONTROL

Infection control is a multidisciplinary process. It involves many different areas of expertise and practice. The physical design of the operating room is one focal area. It is based on two basic principles:

- Physical separation between the surgical environment and any source of contamination
- Containment of sources of infection

Clean and *contaminated* areas (those with the greatest potential sources of infection) are physically separated when possible. For example, the cleaning and decontamination area is separated from the *surgical suites* (individual rooms where surgery is performed) by walls and corridors. The **decontamination area** is where surgical instruments and equipment are disinfected after use. The surgical department itself is separated from hospital corridors and units by doors that remain closed at all times.

When complete physical separation is impossible, contaminated objects are *contained* or confined in a prescribed area or a barrier. For example, the air in the surgical suite cannot be completely separated from the air directly outside the suite; therefore, it is contained by keeping the doors closed and by maintaining air pressure in the suite higher than it is outside. Nonporous materials are used for floors so that soil, debris, and body fluids remain on the surface, where they can be easily removed with disinfectant and water.

ENVIRONMENTAL SAFETY

The surgical environment contains many potential sources of environmental hazard. Some of these are obvious, but others are not. For example, although explosive anesthetic gases are no longer permitted, high level energy sources such as laser and electrosurgical devices are used routinely. Strong chemicals including sterilants are used to prepare surgical instruments and cleanse environmental surfaces. Extremely hot temperatures are used in the decontamination of equipment. High pressure gas canisters are used to contain medical gases and oxygen, which supports combustion and fire. Environmental engineering in the operating room follows national medical engineering standards for electrical circuits, inline gases, lighting, and other utilities. Strict safety standards ensure that patients and staff members are protected from extreme hazards and accidents such as fire, explosion, and electrocution. Refer to Chapter 8 for an in-depth discussion of environmental safety in the operating room.

EFFICIENCY

Efficiency is the economical use of time and energy to save unnecessary work, material resources, and time. Efficient use of space influences the use of time and contributes to safety. Work in the operating room is strenuous. Intelligent design can reduce physical stress by reducing movement and creating work systems that minimize strain. Time-saving practices are implemented to increase the number of patients served, but also to make the best use of people's skills and abilities. In an emergency, time sometimes is the most important factor in achieving a good outcome. Proper storage of sterile supplies and efficient use of space protect the sterility of the items and enable staff members to find what they need quickly and retrieve it safely. For example, equipment that is stacked too high for safe retrieval or equipment that obstructs hallways creates a risk of injury for both patients and employees.

TRAFFIC PATTERNS

Traffic patterns are physical routes for people and equipment in the health care facility and are specifically designed to prevent the transmission of infection. The number and concentration of microorganisms is high in certain areas of any health care facility and also in environments outside the facility. When traffic patterns are enforced in the operating room, they include entry *into* the operating room and movement of people and equipment *within* the department itself. Traffic patterns create boundaries between areas that carry the highest potential sources of infection and those that are the cleanest (most *aseptic*). This is crucial because disease-causing microbes are carried into the operating room on street clothing and shoes, food, insects, objects, and equipment. Health facilities differ in design, which may limit their ability to strictly monitor traffic. The following guidelines are those recommended by infection control agencies and the Joint Commission:

1. The movement of people and equipment into the perioperative area is controlled. Personnel can enter the department only through monitored doors. Fire exits are equipped with alarms to prevent people from entering the department from the outside.
2. The department is separated into three distinct areas—unrestricted, semirestricted, and restricted. Each is defined by its level of asepsis. Transitional rooms or corridors may exist between each of the three areas.
3. People coming into the department from outside the building or operating room department must be properly attired in order to pass to semirestricted and restricted areas.
4. Signs that designate the department areas and direct visitors are posted in clear view.

5. Adherence to traffic patterns applies to everyone, including visitors and hospital staff who normally work in other departments outside the operating room.

6. Traffic patterns are controlled by secure doors and monitored transition areas so that visitors and others new to the department layout can be appropriately directed.

UNRESTRICTED AREA

People enter the operating room department directly into the **unrestricted area**. This is a central location where visitors can be monitored and directed to change into surgical attire in order to proceed to the other areas. Personnel in street clothes and any portable equipment that has not been disinfected are confined to the unrestricted area. Family waiting areas and outer reception areas are also unrestricted areas.

SEMIRESTRICTED AREA

Only personnel wearing surgical attire (a scrub suit and a hair cap that encloses facial hair) are allowed in the **semirestricted area**. The corridors between surgical rooms, the instrument and supply processing area, storage areas, and clean utility rooms within the surgical department are semirestricted areas.

Patients are brought into a designated semirestricted area while awaiting surgery. In this environment they can be monitored and are shielded from the sights and sounds of operating areas, which might be distressing.

STERILE OR RESTRICTED AREA

Only personnel in complete scrub attire, including hair cap, mask, and facial hair covering, are permitted in a **restricted area**. These locations include the surgical suites, procedure rooms, sterile corridor, substerile rooms between surgical suites, and those where sterile supplies are kept.

OPERATING ROOM FLOOR PLANS

Many different types of floor plans meet the goals of infection control, environmental safety, and efficiency. Figures 4-1 and 4-2 show two examples of floor plans. In Figure 4-1, the surgical suites are separated from the workroom by a corridor. The surgical suites are arranged around a continuous corridor. The transitional areas are located at one end so that traffic into the department can be controlled at one location. In Figure 4-2, the **central core** contains clean and sterile equipment and supplies. Contaminated instruments and equipment are processed outside the central core in another area. The primary goal of the floor plan is to create a clear separation between soiled and clean equipment.

THE SURGICAL SUITE

EQUIPMENT AND FURNITURE

Equipment, furniture, and supplies in the surgical suite are stored in a standardized way that is familiar to all personnel.

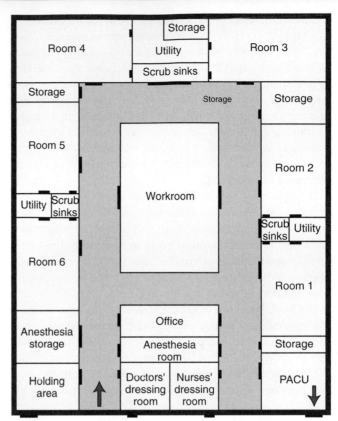

Figure 4-1 Racetrack-style operating room floor plan. *(Modified from Phillips N: Berry and Kohn's operating room technique, ed 11, St Louis, 2007, Mosby.)*

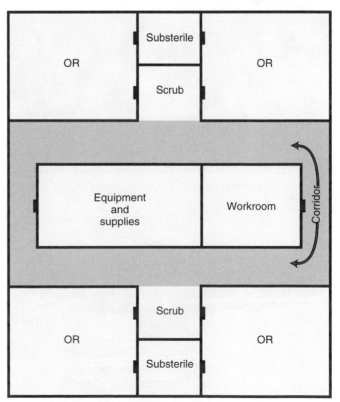

Figure 4-2 Operating room floor plan with a central core. *(Modified from Phillips N: Berry and Kohn's operating room technique, ed 11, St Louis, 2007, Mosby.)*

This facilitates efficient setup and ability to locate stored supplies rapidly. Every piece of equipment has a designated location. Basic components are standard to most surgical suites. Equipment needed during surgery includes the operating table, instrument tables, ring stands for solutions, computer station, digital imaging equipment, and electrosurgical unit. All rooms contain an anesthesia machine and physiological monitoring equipment. Sterile supplies are stored in recessed cabinets or in substerile rooms just outside the suite. Figure 4-3 shows a standard operating room with furniture and equipment in place.

The operating table is adjustable for height, degree of tilt in all directions, orientation in the room, articular breaks ("table breaks"), and length (Figure 4-4). This allows the patient to be positioned in any anatomical position to expose the surgical site fully and maintain safety. The table surface is covered with a firm removable pad. (The operating table is discussed in more detail in Chapter 19.)

The **back table** is a large, stainless steel table on which all instruments and supplies except those in immediate use are placed (Figure 4-5). For some procedures, more than one back table may be needed. Just before surgery, a sterile pack (cover with towels and drapes enclosed) is opened onto the table. This provides a sterile surface on which instruments and sterile supplies are distributed. After gowning and gloving, the scrubbed surgical technologist arranges all the equipment in an orderly manner.

Other small tables are used for skin prep kits, power equipment, and extra sterile supplies that may be too heavy or bulky to place on the back table during surgery.

The Mayo stand is a smaller table with one open end that can be raised or lowered (Figure 4-6). It also is covered with a sterile drape and used for instruments and supplies that are needed immediately during surgery. The Mayo stand is placed over or alongside the patient for quick access to instruments. As the case progresses, new instruments or supplies are added

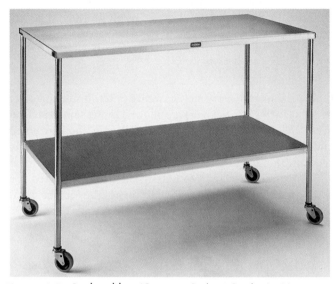

Figure 4-5 **Back table.** (Courtesy Pedigo Products, Vancouver, Wash.)

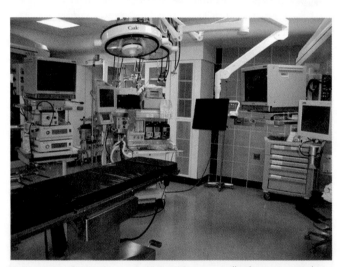

Figure 4-3 **Operating room suite.** (Courtesy Allegheny General Hospital, Pittsburgh, Pa.)

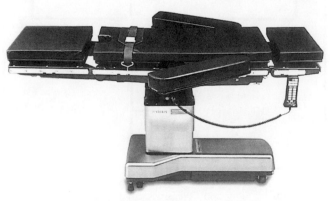

Figure 4-4 **Operating table.** (Courtesy STERIS, Mentor, Ohio.)

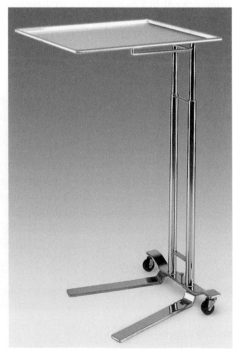

Figure 4-6 **Mayo stand.** (Courtesy Pedigo Products, Vancouver, Wash.)

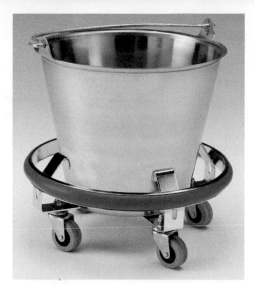

Figure 4-7 **Kick bucket.** *(Courtesy Pedigo Products, Vancouver, Wash.)*

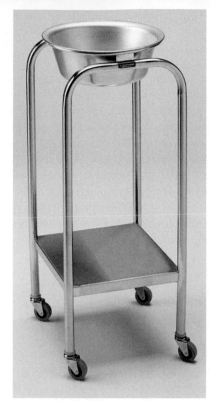

Figure 4-8 **Single ring stand.** *(Courtesy Pedigo Products, Vancouver, Wash.)*

to the Mayo stand and others placed in reserve on the back table.

The kick bucket is constructed of stainless steel and fitted into a wheeled frame (Figure 4-7). It has a specific use and is not a trash receptacle. The kick bucket is designated for soiled surgical sponges and other lightweight, nonsharp items that must be discarded during surgery and accounted for. During surgery, it is placed in a strategic location near the surgical field so that the scrub can drop items directly into it.

The ring stand is used to contain one or two stainless steel basins (Figure 4-8). The ring stand is designed to support the lip of the basin, which has been previously wrapped and sterilized. Before surgery, the wrapped basin is placed in the ring stand and the wrapper opened up to expose the basin. Sterile water or saline is poured into the basin for use during surgery.

SPECIAL PROCEDURE ROOM

Some types of surgical procedures require specialized rooms that contain the equipment and technology of that specialty. For example, transurethral (through the urethra) procedures of the genitourinary tract require continuous irrigation and a specialty operating table. A cystoscopy room is standard to all surgical departments. Other procedures, such as fluoroscopy-assisted cryosurgery, are performed in the interventional radiology or nuclear medicine department or the emergency department.

ENVIRONMENTAL CONTROLS AND SYSTEMS

AIRFLOW AND VENTILATION

Allowing airflow from unrestricted to restricted areas can increase the risk of infection. To reduce this risk, the air pressure in the surgical suite is maintained at a level 10% higher than the air pressure in adjacent semirestricted areas. The

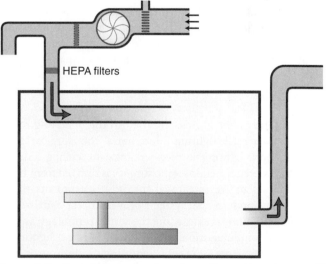

HEPA filters

Figure 4-9 **Operating room air system.** *(From Gruendemann BJ, Mangum SS: Infection prevention in surgical settings, Philadelphia, 2001, WB Saunders.)*

doors to the surgical suite must remain closed to maintain this positive pressure differential. When the door is opened, positive pressure from within the room pushes air out and prevents it from entering the suite from the semirestricted area outside. Fresh filtered air enters the operating room ceiling vents and is combined with existing air in the room (Figure 4-9). The standard for **air exchange** is a minimum of 15 and a maximum of 20 filtered air exchanges per hour.

High-efficiency particulate air (HEPA) filters are installed in the operating room ventilation system and remove particles equal to or larger than 0.3 μm. HEPA filters must be changed regularly to maintain their efficiency. Bacteria and molds can easily colonize heating and cooling vents and dirty filters, creating a major source of infection, especially in burn units.

A **laminar airflow (LAF) system** moves a contained volume of air in layers at a continuous velocity. HEPA-filtered exchanges range from 400 to 600 exchanges per hour. The function of a LAF system is to move large volumes of air containing particles and microorganisms out of the operating room suite. A LAF system is very expensive to implement and maintain. The use of LAF is currently being debated among infection control professionals as a cost-effective method of reducing surgical site infection, especially when compared to using strict aseptic techniques.

HUMIDITY AND TEMPERATURE

Air humidity is controlled to reduce the risk of infection and to minimize static electricity. When humidity is low, static electricity can create a fire hazard in the presence of flammable solutions and oxygen. High humidity may increase the risk of mold and bacterial growth on surfaces. The current standard for humidity in the operating room is 30% to 60%.

Temperature control is an important component of patient care and safety. The operating room is maintained at 68° to 73° F (20° to 23° C). This temperature range is less hospitable to the growth of microorganisms and maintains the temperature within the comfort range of patients and personnel. In extreme cases in which the patient's core temperature must be raised, such as for burn or pediatric patients, a warmer environment must be created to prevent hypothermia.

LIGHTING

Many different light sources are used in the operating room. Overhead surgical lighting illuminates the surgical field, whereas room lighting is recessed into the ceiling fixtures. Light that is used for endoscopic surgery is derived from fiber-optic cables that are integrated into the instruments themselves. Many modern light systems provide direct visualization on high-definition screens using the same technology as television and computer monitors. Modern surgical lighting is usually derived from LED (light-emitting diode) sources and halogen. LED is the newest generation of high-intensity light and is replacing halogen because of the relatively cool temperature and energy-saving features of LEDs. Halogen provides extremely intense light that is less fatiguing to the eyes than other types of light of equal intensity. Energy emitted by both halogen and LED lighting is given off as light rather than as heat, making it safe to use in surgery.

GASES

A number of different types of compressed gases are used as adjuncts to anesthesia and as power sources for pneumatic devices used during the surgical procedure. Oxygen, compressed air, nitrous oxide, and nitrogen are available through inline systems in most hospitals and outpatient surgical centers. Gas lines terminate at hoses that drop from an overhead panel in each surgical suite. Each hose is fitted with a safety valve to provide direct connections with anesthesia or surgical equipment. Facilities that do not have an inline supply of gases such as nitrogen and compressed air must use compressed gas cylinders that are stored in a designated room within the surgery department. Safety laws and procedures related to the storage and use of compressed gases are strictly monitored by the Joint Commission. A complete discussion for the use of compressed gas, including gauges, fittings, storage, and safety precautions, is found in Chapter 8.

Suction is needed during surgery to evacuate fluids, including blood from the surgical incision (wound), and to remove any fluids from the patient's airway during anesthesia. Like inline gas supply, suction is supplied through line systems that terminate at outlets or hoses fitted with safety valves. Suction tubing is fitted between collection units and safety valves. The strength of vacuum is measured in pounds per square inch (psi) and is adjustable.

ELECTRICITY

Electrical outlets in the operating room are necessary for a wide variety of equipment and medical devices. Because of the high risk associated with electrosurgical devices and electricity in general, there are numerous codes and standards related to electrical equipment and the types of outlets used. Perioperative personnel have many opportunities to learn about the safe use of electricity in surgery. Two chapters in this text are devoted to energy sources and associated hazards. Chapter 17, Physics and Information Technology, explains the nature of electricity, how it works, types of circuits, and important terms related to electricity. Chapter 18, Energy Sources in Surgery, discusses the actual use of electricity and other energies, how they are used in medical devices, and safety guidelines to protect patients and staff.

WORK AREAS

Surgical departments can vary widely in size, use of space, and types of work areas they contain. Regardless of the exact appropriation of space, every department strives to maintain the principles of asepsis—separating and confining contaminated areas to keep them apart from clean and sterile areas. The following are some examples of units in the surgical department.

SURGICAL OFFICES

A front office situated near the main entry doors serves as a central communication area for the department. General incoming calls may be received in and referred from this office. Because of its location, the office also is a monitoring point for personnel entering the department. Other offices include those of the operating room supervisor, head nurse, anesthesia director, and other department heads. Dictation rooms are set up for surgeons to make postsurgical reports and for general communication needs.

LOCKER ROOM/LOUNGE AREA

The locker room is a **transitional area** for those who need to change from street clothes to surgical attire. Clean scrub attire is located outside the locker room to protect it from contamination by fluids or soil inside the locker room. Locker and changing rooms for staff may be entered directly from outside the department using a key card or coded lock. A separate door leads into the semirestricted area, allowing staff to transition into the next level of environmental asepsis. Locker room facilities include showers and lavatories. Because the locker room itself is a transitional area, operating room attire must not be kept inside lockers along with street clothes, bags, and other personal items.

If the locker room leads directly into the lounge area, it is separated from the nonrestricted area. The areas are clearly delineated so that personnel dressed in street clothes do not frequent the lounge, offices, or other locations used by those who work in restricted zones. The lounge area often presents a problem for infection control, because personnel in street clothes may have easy access, and traffic control may be limited or even absent.

PATIENT PREOPERATIVE HOLDING AREA

Hospitalized surgical patients are transported to the preoperative holding area before being taken into the operating room. Outpatients (i.e., those coming from outside the hospital) may be escorted to a changing area and then to the holding area. Patients arrive via gurney or wheelchair and await surgery. The holding area is a check-in point where the surgeon, anesthesiologist, and circulating nurse can confirm that all laboratory and preoperative documentation is in order and the information on the preoperative checklist can be verified. In some health care facilities, emergency patients may be brought directly from the emergency department or other facility departments to the operating room suite without passing through the holding area.

SCRUB SINKS

Scrub sinks are located outside the surgical suites so that personnel can proceed directly to surgery immediately after hand antisepsis (Figure 4-10). Some operating room designs include closed areas for the scrub sinks, and these are restricted (masks are required). Scrub sink areas contain antiseptic hand rub, masks, face shields, protective eyewear, brushes, and surgical soap. The area around the scrub sink is kept clean and free of surface water.

SUBSTERILE ROOM

The substerile room is directly adjacent to the operating room suite and is entered through a common door between the two or more operating room suites. It is a restricted area, requiring

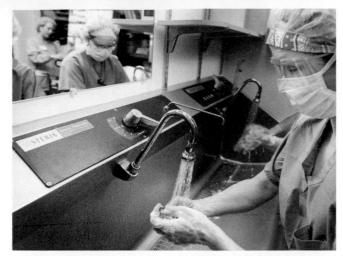

Figure 4-10   Scrub sink area. *(Courtesy STERIS, Mentor, Ohio.)*

complete surgical attire, including mask. The substerile room may contain large carts with specialty supplies such as dressings and suture, and there is usually direct access to a flash sterilizer so that unwrapped instruments can be transported directly from the sterilizer into the operating suite while remaining within the restricted areas.

STERILE INSTRUMENT ROOM

Sterile wrapped supplies are stored in designated restricted areas adjacent to the operating suites nearby. Specialty rooms, such as those used for orthopedics, genitourinary procedures, or cardiothoracic surgery, often have their own sterile supply rooms close by. Case cart systems are used in nearly all health facilities to decrease the number of instrument sets stored in the operating room itself.

EQUIPMENT STORAGE

Large equipment, such as the operating microscope, operating table attachments, and other heavy equipment, is kept in clean designated storerooms. Equipment must be arranged in a way that prevents damage during movement into and out of the room. Thousands of dollars of the operating room's yearly budget are spent on equipment repair as a result of poor storage systems in the operating room department. Many of these accidents occur when equipment is poorly stored in a space that is too small or in a manner that makes the equipment difficult to remove.

UTILITY WORKROOM AND DECONTAMINATION AREA

Soiled instruments and equipment are decontaminated and washed in a utility workroom or central processing area. Some operating rooms use a combination of systems, holding back certain specialty instruments for decontamination and sterilization in the utility workroom and sending the remainder to central processing. The workroom is located in an area convenient to the staff but well contained and away from all restricted areas to prevent cross-contamination of sterile and clean equipment and supplies.

When a **case cart system** is used, sterile supplies (e.g., wrapped instrument sets, single-use items, and drapes) are placed on a closed or open stainless steel cart by personnel in the central processing department. The case carts usually are prepared ahead of time (in many facilities the night before) and are sent to the operating room by central service personnel. As new cases are added to the schedule in the daytime, new case carts are assembled. After surgery, soiled instruments and equipment are placed on a cart and returned to the utility workroom and/or the central processing decontamination area where cart and instruments are decontaminated. The equipment then can be assembled in trays, wrapped, and resterilized. Special elevator systems are used to transport carts into and out of the operating room to central service.

CLEAN PROCESSING AREA

Any instruments that are not sent out of the department for decontamination and sterilization are brought to a clean processing room for assembly after decontamination. Items that are particularly delicate or that are used infrequently may be processed in this area. If an item must be reused in a later case and there is not enough time to send it to the central processing department, it may be cleaned and prepared in the clean processing room.

ANESTHESIA DEPARTMENT

The anesthesia workroom contains clean respiratory equipment, anesthetic agents, and adjunctive drugs. Tubes, hoses, valves, airways, and other equipment are stored in the workroom and organized neatly to avoid damage and to enable personnel to locate the items quickly. This semirestricted area also may have its own separate office. The anesthesia workroom may also be used to store clean physiological monitoring equipment. Sterile supplies and equipment used for intravenous access and for local and regional anesthesia are usually maintained in a separate sterile room in the anesthesia department.

POSTANESTHESIA CARE UNIT

A patient emerging from anesthesia faces many physiological risks. These include airway obstruction, cardiac arrest, hemorrhage, neurological dysfunction, hypothermia, and pain. Therefore, patients are taken directly from surgery to the **postanesthesia care unit (PACU)**. Critical care nurses in the PACU assist the patient in recovery from conscious sedation or general anesthesia. They assess, monitor, and document the patient's recovery from the time of arrival until the patient is discharged back to the hospital unit, other health care facility, or home. (Refer to Chapter 15 for a complete discussion of postanesthesia recovery.)

SURGERY WAITING AREA

The surgery waiting area for the patient's family is located outside traffic areas leading into the operating room but near the department. This waiting area allows families to be close to the operating room in a quiet environment. This is an unrestricted area where the surgeon and other surgical staff may communicate directly with family members. Some facilities also have side rooms where the surgeon may consult with the family in a secluded area.

INTEGRATED OPERATING ROOM SYSTEMS

The **integrated operating room** provides centralized control of surgical devices and equipment through a sterile remote- or voice-activated system. This enables the surgeon to activate endoscopic controls, imaging components, operating lights, table adjustments, insufflators, environmental controls, and many other devices that previously were managed individually. Integrated systems allow the surgical team to view patient monitoring output, as well as diagnostic imaging, on the central monitor or "inside" the image seen by the endoscopic camera. A nonsterile work station in the system provides secondary control of equipment and a standard computer for intraoperative documentation and access to patient records. Integrated operating room systems allow for advances in technology through software design that can be updated periodically.

SECTION II: HEALTH CARE FACILITY DEPARTMENTS AND FUNCTIONS

TEAM APPROACH TO PATIENT CARE

Perioperative staff members work in coordination with many different professionals and departments in the health care facility. The operating room often seems isolated and independent from other departments of the hospital. Physical barriers and procedures necessary to maintain strict asepsis seem to foster an atmosphere of independence. In fact, the operating room could not function without the collaborative efforts of departments outside the operating room. The efforts of many departments and caring staff members contribute to a safe surgery and uneventful recovery. Perioperative staff members must communicate effectively with those outside the operating room and help facilitate a cohesive team approach. Knowledge about the roles of other departments and the activities they perform contributes to this team approach.

Sometimes departments face multiple demands that may exceed their limits of available personnel and time. Patience, respect, and professionalism build good interdepartmental relationships, help reduce stress, and improve patient care.

Departments in the health care facility are distinguished by function (what they do) or by **administration** (the sector in which they are managed, such as nursing administrator or medical director). Every hospital has multiple departments and services. Box 4-1 lists the hospital departments found in most facilities.

Box 4-1 Hospital Departments

Patient Medical Services

Diagnostic Services
- Radiology
- Clinical laboratory/pathology
- Other diagnostic services (e.g., computed tomography, magnetic resonance imaging)

Patient Care Units
- Cardiovascular
- Labor and delivery
- Medical/surgical
- Neonatal
- Neurological
- Orthopedic
- Pediatric
- Trauma
- Psychiatric
- Renal dialysis

Intensive and Critical Care Units (ICUs)
- Cardiac telemetry
- Cardiac (CICU)
- Medical (MICU)
- Neonatal (NICU)
- Neurological
- Operating room
- Postanesthesia care (PACU)
- Trauma (TICU)
- Pediatric (PICU)

Anesthesia and Pain Management

Blood Bank

Outpatient or Ambulatory Surgery

Emergency Department (ED or ER)

Rehabilitation

Physical Therapy

Outpatient Medical Clinics

Nuclear Medicine

Food and Nutrition Services
- Dietitian
- Outpatient nutrition services

Psychosocial and Outreach Services

Patient Education

Community Health Services

Home Health Services

Hospice

Adult Day Care Services

Hospital Chaplaincy

Occupational Therapy

Employee and Administrative Services

Human Resources

Employee Education

Employee Health Services and Insurance

Accounting

Patient Accounts

Reimbursement

Managed Care

Auditor

Payroll

Environmental Services

Infection Control

Maintenance

Bioengineering (Clinical Engineering)

Housekeeping

Materials Management

Central Supply

Distribution

Communications

Switchboard

Paging System

Telecommunications

Mobile Radio Communications

Electronic Communications

Safety

Risk Management

Security

Records and Clerical Services

Medical Records

Admissions

PATHOLOGY

The pathology department receives all tissue samples and other specimens from surgery. A *pathologist* is a specialist medical doctor who examines specimens to determine the type of tissue or other material, to identify disease within the tissue, and to create a permanent legal record. If the surgeon requires an immediate tissue evaluation, as in the case of a suspected malignancy, the pathologist is available to perform a frozen section analysis. The specimen is frozen with liquid nitrogen and sliced into sections for microscopic examination. Immediate tissue analysis provides the information needed to make decisions about the need for more extensive surgery during the same procedure.

NUCLEAR MEDICINE AND INTERVENTIONAL RADIOLOGY

Nuclear medicine involves the use of radioactive materials or radiopharmaceuticals to diagnose and treat disease. These special procedures are performed in a designated nuclear medicine department, which has the technical capability to perform a variety of different procedures following the strict regulations needed to ensure patient and staff safety.

Interventional radiology uses radiography, magnetic resonance imaging (MRI), computed tomography (CT), ultrasound, and other imaging techniques to guide instruments into vessels and organs. Surgical technologists may be required to assist in interventional radiology because sterile technique is required. Examples of interventional radiology procedures are angiography, angioplasty, insertion of a gastrostomy tube, needle biopsy, and stereotactic procedures.

INFECTION CONTROL

Infection control personnel are specialists in the prevention and control of hospital-acquired infection. The health care environment is a potential source for the spread of many types of infection. Whenever people are in close proximity, especially people who are already ill or are debilitated by surgery, nutritional problems, stress, or trauma, the potential for infection is high. The infection control department develops policy based on the standards and recommendations of the Joint Commission, the Centers for Disease Control and Prevention (CDC), APIC, OSHA, and the National Institute for Occupational Safety and Health (NIOSH).

The objectives of infection control are to reduce the number of infections by prevention and to study the causes of infection within the facility. Infection prevention policies affect every department of the hospital. Important goals in infection control include educating staff members and patients, tracking policy compliance, and investigating the sources of infection.

BIOMEDICAL ENGINEERING

Biomedical engineering technicians (BMET, also called *biological engineers*) maintain the safety and operating condition of many of the hospital's medical devices, including those used in surgery. The complexity of sophisticated devices requires technicians who are specially trained in biomedical engineering. The biomedical engineering department is usually a separate department, but there may be an office dedicated to surgical equipment near the surgery department. Technicians may be called to the operating room in the event of equipment failure during surgery.

MATERIALS MANAGEMENT

The materials management department of a health care facility is the purchasing and logistics center for goods and supplies needed for the delivery of health care. It is also responsible for ordering new supplies and for implementing tracking systems to maintain the supply chain.

CENTRAL SUPPLY

Disposable items, linens, and equipment are distributed to hospital departments by the central supply department. Items usually are tracked by computer, and distribution is carefully managed to control hospital costs. In some health care facilities, this department may be responsible for receiving soiled equipment used in surgery. In this case, wrapping and sterilization are performed in separate areas of the department. Items may be purchased from this department or from a separate purchasing department.

PHARMACY

The pharmacy distributes medications to patient care units in the hospital. Medications and anesthetic agents used in the operating room are received from the pharmacy, either by regular delivery or by special requisition. Many modern surgical departments have their own pharmacy, which is stocked from the central pharmacy or directly from the vendors. Anesthetic agents usually are stored in the anesthesia department or pharmacy located in the surgical department.

LABORATORY

Diagnostic tests are performed in the hospital laboratory, where clinical laboratory personnel examine and analyze body fluids, tissues, and cells. Laboratory personnel perform chemical, biological, hematological, immunological, microscopic, and bacteriological tests. They also perform blood typing procedures. The data and results obtained in the laboratory are returned to the physician to aid evaluation and treatment of the patient.

BLOOD BANK

The blood bank provides blood products for transfusion in the surgical, postanesthesia care, and medical units of the hospital. Because of the stringent protocols regulating blood product transfusion, strict methods are followed for their handling, storage, transport, and identification. The surgical technologist may interact with blood bank personnel and should be familiar with the institution's policy regarding ordering and transporting blood products.

RISK MANAGEMENT DEPARTMENT

Because of the many environmental risks and the possibility for errors and omissions by personnel, surveillance is required to track the number and exact nature of adverse or sentinel events in a given time period. The cause of each event is studied, and policies are enacted to prevent future incidents of the same type. For example, if the incidence of chemical burns among staff members were increasing, the **risk management** team would investigate the circumstances, time of day, personnel involved (e.g., housekeeping, nursing), and other important aspects to identify the cause. The team then would develop a plan to reduce the number of incidents. The team might change existing policy regulating the use of chemicals or give personnel intensive training. After the plan is implemented, an evaluation is performed to determine whether the measures taken actually did reduce the number of chemical burns. Incident reports (see Chapter 3) are very important to risk management because they contain the information needed to analyze incidents and develop a plan of intervention.

COMMUNICATION SYSTEMS

The central communication point of a health care facility is designed to redirect calls to specific individuals or departments. With new voice and communication technology, staff can receive and transmit information through many different types of systems that reduce the need for hospital-wide intercom paging. Wireless, voice-controlled communication using smart phones and voice badges allow facility staff to communicate instantly with each other without the delay common in older pager systems. Modern intercom systems are designed for hands-off use and can be integrated for use inside and outside the health care facility. The operating room intercom system can be set up for voice control communication so that the surgeon can communicate directly with other departments such as pathology without stepping away from the surgical field. Messaging systems can now utilize smart phones to provide pages, text messages, and alerts sent through a web-based console. Web-based and satellite-based systems also allow teaching and telemedicine during surgical procedures.

MEDICAL RECORDS

The medical records department is responsible for receiving, maintaining, and transferring all patient records. Because patient records are legal documents, strict protocols determine when signatures are required, who may make entries, what must be included, and where the patient's documents are stored. Many, but not all, health care facilities use electronic record systems. When an electronic system is in use, patient records are accessed through a strictly monitored password system.

FACILITIES MAINTENANCE

The facilities maintenance department is responsible for environmental systems in the hospital. These systems include the hospital's power source (regular and emergency), ventilation, inline gases, suction, electricity, water, light, heat, cooling, and humidity control. Standards for environmental control and safety are established by the Joint Commission and government agencies. Perioperative personnel should never ignore or try to repair a system that malfunctions. Maintenance personnel are available at all times to respond to environmental emergencies.

ENVIRONMENTAL SERVICES

Environmental services personnel perform essential cleaning and decontamination services for all departments of the hospital. In the operating room, they maintain a clean environment and decontaminate the floors, furniture, and other surfaces between cases. They work with other team members to ensure rapid turnover from one case to the next.

SECURITY

Security services are provided in large and medium-sized health care facilities. Security officers are responsible for monitoring public activities in the facility, including traffic and staff identity. They respond to public disorder within the boundaries of the facility and are in direct communication with local enforcement authorities. Security personnel are not members of the police department. Their role is to reduce the level of security incidents and to implement training programs for security personnel.

NUTRITIONAL SERVICES

Nutritionists are licensed health care professionals who advise and perform care related to the nutritional status of patients. Nutritionists consult with medical and nursing personnel to provide a plan of care for a patient whose medical condition either contributes to or is caused by a diet that is harmful. They are also consulted for patients with particularly dietary needs such as those with kidney disease or patients who have undergone gastric procedures for obesity control. In addition to advising in special cases, they may also coordinate with dietary services in planning meals for the general patient population.

SECTION III: HEALTH CARE ADMINISTRATION

HEALTH CARE PROVIDERS

Most large health care organizations provide primary health care, inpatient and outpatient, diagnosis, and outpatient rehabilitation services. Primary or secondary (preventive) medical care is provided in a fixed location, such as the community hospital. The community hospital, whether privately or publicly owned, brings together people with different professional skills to provide coordinated services. Larger hospitals or medical centers also operate satellite facilities in rural or urban areas away from the central facility. Satellite facilities deliver various types of care or treatments. Services may include but are not limited to ambulatory surgery centers, clinics, urgent care centers, laboratory and radiology centers, physicians' offices, extended care, and rehabilitation facilities.

Surgery is performed in many different settings, including hospitals, community health centers, and freestanding clinics that may be privately owned or operated by nonprofit organizations.

Ambulatory surgical centers perform minor surgery that does not require postoperative hospital recovery. Ambulatory surgery and outpatient surgery departments in hospitals also are becoming increasingly popular. In addition, some types of surgery are being performed in surgeons' offices.

Surgery that requires general anesthesia, conscious sedation, or complex local anesthesia is performed in a hospital facility, where perioperative services are coordinated with the services of other departments. This setting provides continuity of care and ensures that emergency services are immediately available. This chapter focuses on the hospital-based surgical department. However, the principles of administration, organization, and physical layout are similar for all settings.

HEALTH CARE FINANCING

Health care financing in the United States is divided mainly among government structures, employer contributions, and private insurance.

GOVERNMENT ASSISTANCE

Government-assisted health care systems are managed by state and federal agencies. The *Medicaid system* assists in medical care for specific low-income families and individuals with special needs, including disability. The program is jointly funded by the state and federal government. Eligibility is dependent on both economic and health qualifications.

The *Medicare system* operates like an insurance plan in which individuals pay into a fund through their employment taxes and can later draw on the fund after age 65 for certain medical costs. The plan includes hospital and medical insurance and is also administered to people with specific types of permanent disability. Individuals or their spouses who paid into the Medicare system through their taxes generally do not pay for hospital insurance. Certain medical and prescription drug insurance is partly covered under a monthly premium paid by the individual through Social Security taxes.

PRIVATE INSURANCE

Private medical insurance programs require regular payments by an individual or group of individuals, who in turn receive partial or total payment for specific types of medical care. Insurance companies may contract specific health organizations to provide services at a reduced rate for their beneficiaries. These organizations are referred to as *preferred provider organizations* or PPOs. The *health maintenance organization* (HMO) is another system of health care delivery utilized by insurance companies. The HMO contracts with specific health care providers to deliver services using techniques and standards that are designed to be economical and efficient. The HMO sets the guidelines for care that must be followed by the contracted health care providers.

PAYMENT SYSTEMS

The specific payment systems in the insurance industry use standardized codes for a diagnosis and treatment modalities. The *diagnosis-related group* (DRG) is a list of services or "products" that hospitals deliver. For example, a surgical procedure is one type of product. The system of DRGs is used by Medicare and insurance companies to determine the amount of money the system pays out for its beneficiaries.

The International Classification of Diseases (*ICD*) code is an assigned number for specific medical conditions. The ICD code is used in combination with the DRG to determine the amount of money that the insurance company or Medicare provides for its beneficiaries. Another system used by medical providers is the Current Procedural Terminology (CPT) code, which is created and maintained by the American Medical Association to provide consistent terminology for medical procedures.

MANAGEMENT STRUCTURE

Hospital management and operational staff members usually are organized into separate bodies or groups of people whose joint functions and roles enable patient and community services. The board of directors or trustees is responsible for hiring the chief executive officer. It determines the hospital's administrative and development policies and mission statement, and it reviews the procedures for safe, ethical patient care.

The administrative sector designs and implements personnel procedures, policies, and financial systems. It communicates with the public and handles overall institutional issues, such as public relations and quality assurance.

The medical and other professional staff deliver services according to the privileges granted them by license and state codes. Management within these sectors usually is organized by departments and profession. Medical staff members usually are managed by the chief or head physician of the department. Professional nurses are managed by the nursing department. Allied health staff members are managed by their own department heads, or they may be administered by the nursing department. The management structure can be horizontal (many people sharing the same level of management) or vertical (fewer people at the management level).

ORGANIZATIONAL CHART (ORGANIGRAM)

An **organizational chart (organigram)** is a graphic representation of the management chain of command (Figure 4-11). The significance of the organizational chart is that it depicts each manager's areas of responsibility and accountability. It eliminates ambiguity about who is in charge of what and the level of responsibility. It is important to note that there is no standard organizational system, and different hospitals use various titles for their administrative and management staff. The terms *supervisor, manager,* and *director* are interchangeable in the general sense. All staff members have a responsibility to understand the management structure of the institution and in particular their department.

CHAIN OF COMMAND

The **chain of command** defines the relationship between management and staff members. An employee reports (is responsible to) the person directly *upward* on the organizational chart. Vertical alignment of positions indicates the authority that one position has over another. Horizontal alignment indicates equal authority. The fact that some positions are lower vertically than other positions does not necessarily mean that all the lower positions are under the authority of a given higher level person. For example, the chief medical engineer does not have administrative authority over the surgical technologist, even though that vertical position is higher.

Chain of command is important for several reasons. Management systems rely on the flow of information *from* specific people in particular positions *to* other specific positions. Certain information is critical to the outcome of work. For example, a safety warning about equipment is directed to all staff members who use that equipment. The direct link between the staff members and their immediate manager may be the most important source of that information. In another

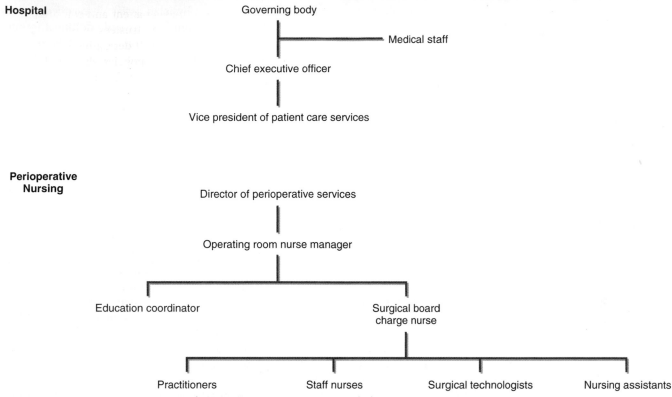

Hospital

Governing body

Medical staff

Chief executive officer

Vice president of patient care services

Perioperative Nursing

Director of perioperative services

Operating room nurse manager

Education coordinator

Surgical board charge nurse

Practitioners

Staff nurses

Surgical technologists

Nursing assistants

Figure 4-11 **Sample operating room organizational chart.** *(Modified from Phillips N: Berry and Kohn's operating room technique, ed 10, St Louis, 2004, Mosby.)*

example, an incident in surgery must be reported to the individual positioned to act on the consequences of that incident. This includes not only immediate action on health and safety, but also the process of analysis and risk management. Certain people in the chain of command are responsible for these tasks. Following the chain of command puts the person (or position) previously designated as the most appropriate in charge of the response.

The types and volume of responsibility required of managers in today's hospitals are much greater than ever before. Chain of command defines the domains and specific areas of focus for each manager. It allows managers to focus their attention where it is intended. This creates a more smoothly running department and better patient outcomes.

Chain of command is important for resolution of policy and protocol questions. Each staff member has a line manager whose tasks include resolving issues or directing them to another appropriate source. For example, if a staff member experiences abusive treatment in the operating room, that staff member must present the situation to his or her line manager. The line manager must be made aware of staff relations in the department and is best placed to counsel the individual and refer the situation to other authority if necessary. Except in unusual circumstances it is almost always unwise to skip the chain of command when reporting incidents or seeking information as this may be interpreted as a lack of respect for one's direct line manager or lack of faith in that person's ability to manage. This reflects badly on the manager to his or her own manager and peers.

STAFF ROLES

PERSONNEL POLICY

The responsibilities and functions of all employees in the surgical department are clearly defined in writing in the hospital manual covering its **personnel policy**. These policies are written to clarify job descriptions and to establish the accountability of each employee. They include topics such as employee safety, how to respond in emergency situations, insurance issues, and ethical conduct. These policies comply with state and federal laws and ensure that the hospital meets the minimum standards set by the Joint Commission. Policies must be strictly followed, because they define the practices necessary for the safe and efficient operation of the department. Employees are required to read these policies and often must sign a form stating that they understand the policies in order for the hospital to enforce compliance.

Each member of the hospital staff has defined duties and responsibilities. These are often referred to as a job description. A job description for each position is necessary to ensure that every person knows what is expected of him or her. The **job description** is a management tool to ensure that all tasks have been assigned appropriately. It is equally important for the individual to know exactly what his or her role is. **Role confusion** is a common cause of conflict in the workplace. This occurs when delegation or assignments are not clear or when an employee is not sure who is responsible for what. Assumptions that *someone else* is responsible for completion of a task can lead to *no one* doing it. This presents risks for patient safety, because many tasks have *shared* responsibility. Responsibility and accountability must be specifically handed over to ensure safety. Staff members are required to read their job description at the time of hiring to prevent confusion and conflict later on. The job description includes a **job title**, which identifies the position by name. This is another method of clarifying roles and responsibilities.

Many different professional personnel make up the modern perioperative team. Some roles overlap, whereas others are specific to a particular job according to professional standards, policy, training, and individual capability.

PERIOPERATIVE PROFESSIONALS

Surgeon

The surgeon is the patient's primary physician in the operating room and is responsible for guiding the surgical procedure. The surgeon operates under the prescribed policies of the hospital in which he or she works and is licensed under the medical practice acts in his or her state. The surgeon may be qualified as a medical doctor (MD), doctor of dental surgery (DDS), doctor of dental medicine (DDM), doctor of osteopathic medicine (DO), or doctor of podiatry (DPM).

Assistant Surgeon

The assistant surgeon is a medical doctor licensed to perform and assist in surgery. The assistant provides direct care to the patient according to the delegation of the surgeon and the needs of the patient. The assistant surgeon is qualified to deliver emergency care during a procedure and must be able to take charge of the surgical case in the event the primary surgeon is unable to.

Anesthesia Care Provider

The anesthesia care provider is an MD, DO, or Certified Registered Nurse Anesthetist (CRNA) and is a specialist in anesthesia and pain management. The anesthesia care provider is responsible for the meticulous assessment, monitoring, and adjustment of the patient's physiological status during surgery. He or she consults with the surgeon on the patient's specific physiological and medical condition before surgery and follows this care through the postsurgical recovery period.

Perioperative Registered Nurse

The perioperative registered nurse holds a current license in nursing (RN) and also may have advanced certification in perioperative nursing (certified nurse–operating room [CNOR]). The perioperative nurse functions as a circulating nurse (circulator) or as a scrub. Additional training permits a registered nurse to become a registered nurse–first assistant (RNFA). Refer to Chapter 21 for a complete description of the circulator role of the perioperative registered nurse.

Physician Assistant

A physician assistant (PA) is a medical professional who practices medicine under the supervision of a physician. A PA is required to pass a national certification examination and earn the title of a physician assistant–certified (PA-C). A PA in the operating room has received additional training in surgery. The PA may perform first-assistant tasks under the direct supervision of the surgeon and according to hospital policy.

Licensed Practical Nurse

The licensed practical nurse (LPN) (or licensed vocational nurse [LVN] in some states) has completed a 1- to 2-year program in a college, vocational, or technical school. After completing a state-approved practical nursing program, an LPN or LVN becomes licensed after passing the National Council Licensure Examination for Licensed Practical Nurses (NCLEX-LPN), which is the national qualifying examination for LPNs. In the operating room, the LPN or LVN usually functions in the role of scrub.

Certified Surgical Technologist

The role and of the certified surgical technologist is discussed throughout this text and the duties as a member of the surgical team are listed and described fully in Chapter 21. The certified surgical technologist (CST) prepares equipment and instruments before surgery, ensuring that all devices are safe and operative. Surgical technologists also assist in preparation of the patient immediately before surgery. They help position the patient, perform the antiseptic skin prep, and assist the surgeon in applying sterile drapes to protect the surgical site from contamination. They arrange the equipment, maintain it during surgery, and pass instruments to the surgeons. They also are responsible for setting up and maintaining instruments during the procedure and for safely handling and transporting soiled instruments for reprocessing. In addition, the CST may also function as the assistant circulator. This role is described in detail in Chapter 1.

Certified Surgical Technologist–Certified First Assistant

The certified surgical technologist-certified first assistant (CST-CFA) is a certified surgical technologist who has completed an educational program for assisting the surgeon during a procedure. For the purposes of patient reimbursement through Medicare, he or she is a "nonphysician surgical assistant." Certification requirements are established by the National Board of Surgical Technology and Surgical Assisting (NBSTSA). The CST-CFA practices as a surgical assistant by providing aid in exposure (retraction), hemostasis (controlling bleeding in the surgical wound), suturing, suctioning fluids from the wound, and other tasks as directed by the surgeon. The CST-CFA may be hired by a specialist surgeon or health care facility to perform in a role specific to that specialty, such as ophthalmic surgery, ear, nose, and throat (ENT) surgery, or orthopedic surgery.

Certified Surgical Assistant or Nonphysician Surgical Assistant

The certified surgical assistant (CSA) or nonphysician surgical assistant is an allied health qualification achieved by certification through the National Surgical Assistant Association. Qualifications for certification include graduation from an accredited surgical assistance school, military training, or a foreign medical degree. Physician assistants and registered nurses may also apply for qualification, which is recognized by the Accreditation Review Council on Education in Surgical Technology and Surgical Assisting (ARC/STSA) and approved by the Commission on Accreditation of Allied Health Education Programs (CAAHEP). There are also other credentialed surgical assistants (i.e., SA-C).

Certified Anesthesia Technologist

The certified anesthesia technologist is a member of the anesthesia patient care team and department. Anesthesia technologists directly assist the anesthesiologist, residents, and nurse anesthetist. They prepare and maintain equipment and supplies needed for administration of anesthetics and calibrate monitoring devices used during surgery. They assist with laboratory tests and obtain blood products and pharmaceuticals. Depending on their expertise, they may also perform technical and support roles in procedures involving anesthesia.

Operating Room Educator

The operating room nurse educator may be a registered nurse or certified surgical technologist with extensive operating room experience. This individual develops and implements educational programs, seminars, and in-services (informational training on new products or techniques) within the department. Not all surgical departments have a designated educator; some provide training on a more informal basis. The surgical technologist instructor is designated by the health care facility to orient and teach newly recruited surgical technologists or those in a specialty.

Independent surgical technology instructors are affiliated with their educational institution, not with the health care institution in which students have internships. The instructor upholds the policies of the health care institution and supervises students in compliance with these standards. The students also interact with health care facility staff members who may delegate individual tasks in accordance with the goals and objectives of the educational program. Cooperation and good communication between the surgical technology instructor and operating room staff ensure that students complete their educational requirements while following the policies of the health care institution in which they are learning.

Surgical Orderly or Aide

The surgical orderly participates in many types of patient care services, including transportation of the patient to and from the surgical department. The orderly also may participate in "turnover" (preparation of the surgical suite for the next patient). Orderlies often assist in the preparation of supplies and instruments for decontamination and sterilization. The work is demanding, because many members of the surgery department make many requests for their attention.

Central Sterile Processing Technician

The central processing or sterile processing technician is responsible for the safe management and sterilization of equipment in preparation for and after its use in surgery and other care units. Technicians are knowledgeable about the process of sterilization and decontamination, asepsis, and standard precautions. They assemble instruments and safely process them according to hospital standards. They also keep hospital and operating room inventories of instruments and equipment and may be responsible for ordering supplies.

Patient Care Technician

The patient care technician (PCT) is a multidisciplinary nursing assistant. He or she provides direct patient care in activities of daily living (ADL). These include patient mobility, dressing, eating, and toileting. The certified PCT may also perform phlebotomy (venipuncture), electrocardiography, and other technical roles.

ANCILLARY TECHNICAL STAFF

Radiology

Medical and technical radiology professionals may be involved in the perioperative setting before, during, and after surgery. The radiologist MD is responsible for the medical interpretation of diagnostic images produced by CT, fluoroscopy, MRI, and other complex imaging. Radiology technicians perform imaging procedures in the interventional radiology department or as on-call personnel who perform imaging in other departments of the health care facility, including surgery.

Electroencephalogram Technician

The electroencephalogram (EEG) technician is a specialist in measuring the brain's activities through a variety of procedures and tests, usually in a special department of the health care facility. The EEG technician may also perform brain activity monitoring duties during specific surgical procedures.

Medical Industry Representative

The medical industry representative is employed by surgical equipment and instrument companies to provide guidance and training on the company's products. The industry representative may be present in the operating room during procedures in which their products such as orthopedic implants are being used. Their role is to train members of the surgical team on the proper use of the products.

Cardiovascular Perfusionist

The role of the cardiovascular perfusionist is to provide extracorporeal (outside the body) oxygenation of the blood during cardiac bypass procedures in which the heart is placed in standstill. The perfusionist is responsible for setting up all equipment and for its safe operation during surgery.

Administrative Personnel

Health care managers and other administrative personnel are needed to provide oversight and development of the facility's goals and operations.

Health Care Facility Management

The chief executive officer (CEO) of the health care facility is responsible for the overall operational planning and implementation of the facility's strategic plan. This role may be shared with the chief operational officer (COO), who is expected to assume the role of CEO in that individual's absence. Additional roles of the CEO are ensuring that the facility complies with regulatory requirements and developing good communication among departments within the facility. The executive officer provides leadership within the facility and in the community.

Chief Operational Officer

The COO is responsible for oversight of the health care facility with a particular focus on the functioning of the medical services, personnel, and fiscal areas. This individual works with all levels of operations, developing strategic plans for operation and implementing them. The operational department covers a broad range of areas, including workforce recruitment and safety, information technology, communications, liaison with educational institutions, and research. The COO is a manager who troubleshoots problems in the actual day-to-day operations from a global perspective.

Director of Surgical Services/Operating Room Supervisor

The director of surgical services (also known in some areas as the operating room supervisor) is responsible for overseeing all clinical and professional activities in the department. Using evidence-based standards, he or she creates and implements policies about clinical and professional practices in the operating room. The operating room supervisor may represent the department at supervisory meetings, where he or she helps coordinate activities in other departments with those of the operating room.

Perioperative Nurse Manager

A perioperative nurse manager may assist the operating room director with his or her duties or may have separate responsibilities. If the director is absent from the department, the nurse manager may assume the role of supervisor if necessary. The nurse manager is responsible for the day-to-day activities of the operating room, although the individual may or may not participate in surgical procedures. The nurse manager usually is an RN with a Bachelor of Science in Nursing (BSN) and a master's degree in management. Responsibilities may include ordering and management of devices and materials, environmental safety, education, infection control, staff scheduling, and resolving staffing problems. The nurse manager often is responsible for organizing triage and emergency responses in the operating room.

Unit Clerk/Secretary

The surgical unit clerk or secretary receives scheduling requests from the surgeons or their representatives. The secretary also must answer the telephone and relay messages within and out of the surgical department. In the event of emergency, the secretary must assist the manager in rescheduling any cases that have been canceled and notify all personnel involved in these cases. The unit clerk maintains an orderly schedule and coordinates the scheduling needs of many different surgeons. The individual is knowledgeable about medical and surgical terminology, has excellent communication skills, and is able to cope with a variety of stressful situations.

KEY CONCEPTS

- The operating room is designed and engineered to provide infection control; environmental safety; and efficient use of personnel, time, space, and resources.
- The layout of the surgical department is based primarily on the principles of infection control—confining and containing areas and sources of contamination.
- Traffic patterns in the surgical department contribute to infection control and are strictly enforced.
- Operating room equipment and furniture are managed in a way that promotes safety and efficiency.
- The physical environment of the operating room, such as lighting, air exchange, temperature, and humidity, is strictly controlled. Standards for these elements are enforced by accreditation and safety organizations.
- Basic equipment and furniture needed for surgery are kept in each surgical suite. Special procedure rooms include supplies and equipment for surgical specialties such as genitourinary surgery, orthopedics, and plastic surgery.
- Designated areas of the surgical department include the surgical suites, substerile rooms, instrument storage areas, anesthesia workroom, and scrub sink areas. These are restricted areas.
- The health care facility has many different departments that interact with each other to provide patient care. Coordination among departments is essential for smooth teamwork.
- Perioperative personnel rely on departments such as interventional radiology, materials management, pharmacy, and the blood bank for day-to-day activities in surgery.
- All health care facilities have a mission statement and community goals on which they base their policies, procedures, and activities.
- Hospital policies are established in consultation with accreditation and safety organizations. Every employee must be familiar with personnel, health, and safety policies. They are also required to understand the policies of the department they work in.
- An organizational chart establishes the relationships between management and staff. These are ranked by chain of command.
- All personnel are required to have a job description so that they know what is expected of them.
- The surgical department employs many different types of professional and nonprofessional staff. Everyone has a responsibility to coordinate their work with others and to become familiar with each other's roles in the work place.

REVIEW QUESTIONS

1. How is the floor plan of the operating room related to patient safety?
2. What is a restricted area in the operating room?
3. How does the environmental air pressure in the operating room relate to the spread of infection?
4. Why is the operating room maintained at a specific humidity?
5. What is an integrated operating room?
6. What is the purpose of hospital accreditation?
7. What types of problems might employees experience if they are not familiar with the policies of their employer?
8. An organizational chart outlines, in graphic form, the levels of responsibility within an organization. Why do you think it is important to delineate management responsibilities?
9. What is the purpose of a chain of command?
10. In many health care facilities, employees are asked to sign or initial their job description, showing that they have read it. Why is this important?

CASE STUDIES

Case 1

The floor plan of the surgical department is one of the main strategies for infection control. Working in a group, design a floor plan that meets the criteria discussed in this chapter without duplicating the designs already shown.

Case 2

The concept of *chain of command* was introduced in this chapter. The importance of this concept is often overlooked as simply a paper exercise that only concerns management. However, in actual practice, it is extremely important. Analyze the following situation and discuss how chain of command affects the outcome:

A single mother employee is experiencing difficulty in the workplace due to difficulties balancing care of her children with the work schedule. If she could change her work schedule to coincide with the hours she needs to be home, it will solve the problem. She sends an email to someone in human resources who she believes might be more sympathetic than her line manager—after all, it is a human resources problem. What effect will this have on resolution of the problem? What reaction do you feel the line manager might have? What about the person in human resources?

Case 3

An employee's job description is an important document for clarification of roles, responsibility, and accountability. What is the effect of a job description that is extremely vague? What is the relationship between a job description and chain of command?

BIBLIOGRAPHY

ASHRAE Standing Standard Project Committee 170 (SSPC 170): *ANSI/ASHRAE/ASHE Standard 170, Ventilation of Health Care Facilities.* Accessed July 11, 2011, at http://sspc170.ashraepcs.org.

Association of Surgical Technologists: *Job description: surgical assistant.* Accessed July 11, 2011, at http://www.ast.org.

Association of Surgical Technologists: *Job description: surgical technologist.* Accessed July 21, 2011, at http://www.ast.org.

Ninomura P, Rousseau C, Bartley J: Updated guidelines for design and construction of hospital and health care facilities. Accessed July 11, 2011, at http://www.newcomb-boyd.com/pdf/ASHRAE%20 rousseau%20et%20al.pdf.

U.S. Department of Labor, Occupational Safety and Health Administration: *Surgical suite module.* Accessed July 21, 2011, at http://www.osha.gov/SLTC/etools/hospital/surgical/surgical.html.

CHAPTER OUTLINE

LEARNING OBJECTIVES

After studying this chapter the reader will be able to:

1. Discuss different types of disasters
2. Discuss the common features of a disaster
3. Explain the role of government agencies during
   a disaster
4. Define NIMS and explain its relationship to the state
   emergency response
5. Define the four phases of the disaster cycle
6. Locate documents useful for making a home disaster plan

7. Describe the main components and strategy used by
   communities to prepare their local disaster plan
8. Define Incident Command System and explain how it works
9. Describe basic human needs in a disaster
10. List the primary components of a health care facility disaster
    plan
11. Discuss ethical dilemmas that accompany disasters
12. Explain the possible roles of the surgical technologist during
    a disaster

TERMINOLOGY

Agency for Healthcare Research and Quality (AHRQ): Agency
that provides disaster-related research, resources, training, and
recommendations for health care facilities, communities, and
individuals.

All-hazards approach: An integrated strategy for disaster
management that focuses on the common features of all
disasters, regardless of the cause or origin.

American Red Cross: National organization that provides
humanitarian assistance and technical support during disasters
and emergencies.

Bioterrorism: The intentional release of biological agents (e.g.,
bacteria, viruses, mycotoxins) to create illness and death in
humans, animals, and the environment. Modes of
transmission include air, water, and food.

Declared state of emergency: A status conferred on a
disaster by the state governor or the president (for a
federal declaration). An official declaration of emergency
entitles the state in which the disaster occurs to receive
federal aid through the Federal Emergency Management
Agency (FEMA).

Disaster: A catastrophic event that affects a large portion of the
population and poses significant risk to human life and
property. A disaster overwhelms local resources and requires
outside assistance.

Disaster recovery: A phase of the disaster cycle in which
the community returns to a functional level after a
disaster. Recovery has no defined interval and may
take years.

Emergency: A more geographically isolated event than a disaster
that can be handled by local emergency services, such as
ambulances, the fire department, or paramedics.

Federal Emergency Management Agency (FEMA): Federal agency
responsible for all aspects of coordination, management, and
response for nationally declared disasters. It also provides
extensive training programs in disaster preparedness
management and response for professionals and members of
the community.

Logistics supply chain: The event-related process of handling
material goods from the point of procurement to the point of
delivery to the end user.

Mass casualty event (MCE): An emergency in which the number
of victims overwhelms the human and material capacity of
available health care services. An MCE usually is associated
with a geographically isolated event (e.g., transportation
accident, industrial accident).

Medical Reserve Corps (MRC): Medical volunteer agency that is
committed to supporting public health and emergency
response in the community.

Mitigation: A process or intervention intended to reduce the level
of injury or harm. For example, mitigation against the effects
of a hurricane includes early warning systems that may predict
the strength and location of the storm.

National Disaster Medical System (NDMS): Agency that
maintains a database of trained on-call medical, paramedical,
and allied health personnel for emergency deployment during
a disaster.

TERMINOLOGY (cont.)

Natural disaster: Widespread damage and risk of injury caused by forces of nature, such as a hurricane, a tornado, an earthquake, floods, and extreme heat or cold.

National Disaster Life Support Education Consortium (NDLSEC): Organization of health professionals committed to providing education, standards, and guidelines for volunteers so that the needs of the public are met during a disaster or emergency situation.

National Fire Protection Association (NFPA): Organization that develops and distributes codes and standards that aim to lessen the threat of fire and hazards, as well as their potential impact in the community.

Pandemic: A public health emergency in which an infectious disease spreads throughout a large population, often across international boundaries.

Shelter-in-place: During a disaster, individuals may be required (or may choose) to shelter-in-place rather than evacuate the hazardous areas. This means that people remain where they are until the environment is safe or until rescue workers can reach the site.

Surge capacity: The number of patients a health care facility can manage in an emergency.

Vulnerability: Exposure to the risk of harm. In disaster management, vulnerable populations are those with a higher than normal risk. This may be related to their age, mobility, inaccessibility, or other condition that hinders or prevents aid.

INTRODUCTION

In recent years, disasters such as the 9/11 terrorist attacks, Hurricane Katrina, Asian tsunamis, wildfires in Australia, and the threat of a flu pandemic have revealed a need for increased disaster preparedness among all sectors of the community, including health care. As a result, government, social, and professional groups have increased funding for research, training, and implementation of disaster programs designed to inform the public, create new systems, and train professionals in disaster preparedness. The World Health Organization (WHO), the Centers for Disease Control and Prevention (CDC), and many academic institutions and national health organizations now provide training at all levels of disaster management. Recognition that different types of disasters require common response strategies, training for disaster is based on an **all-hazards approach** in which communities and disaster specialists learn basic management and responses that can be applied with some modification to many different types of emergencies.

Disaster preparedness training is required for the health professions, including allied health. The Commission on Accreditation of Allied Health Education Programs (CAAHEP), has added emergency preparedness to its accreditation standards. The organization has stated that allied health students "must have an understanding of their specific role in an emergency environment, both as citizens and health professionals."

Disaster preparedness training and management is a broad interdisciplinary process that involves many agencies and individuals. This chapter is intended to introduce the surgical technologist to disaster terminology, core principles, and the disaster environment. It is not intended to train people in management or other roles specific to disasters. These roles depend on the emergency plan of the health care facility and may require more extensive training. There are many courses on all-hazard preparedness available including those for health professionals. For a list of agencies that provide all-hazard courses, refer to the last section of this chapter, Resources for Students and Instructors.

ACRONYMS

Government and international institutions often use a variety of acronyms to define documents, agencies, and doctrines. These are usually familiar to those who work in those sectors, but are confusing for others. Acronyms used in this chapter are necessary for studying federal government documents and processes. A list is provided here for reference:

AHRQ	Agency for Healthcare Research and Quality
CDC	Centers for Disease Control and Prevention
DHHS	Department of Health and Human Services
DHS	Department of Homeland Security
DHSES	Division of Homeland Security and Emergency Services
DMAT	Disaster Medical Assistance Team
EMA	Emergency management agency
EOP	Emergency operations center
FCC	Federal Communications Commission
FEMA	Federal Emergency Management Agency
HazMat	Hazardous materials
HICS	Hospital incident command system
HRSA	Health Resources and Services Administration
MCE	Mass casualty event
NDMS	National Disaster Medical System
NIMS	National Incident Management System
NRF	National Response Framework
NWS	National Weather Service
START	Simple triage and rapid treatment
WHO	World Health Organization

TRAINING

Although currently no standardized curriculum exists for disaster preparedness for health care professionals, the need for such a curriculum has been nationally recognized. Individual professional organizations are responding to this need by creating objectives and guidance statements. While this work is in progress, allied health and other professionals can increase their capacity to respond to disaster and mass casualty events by taking specific courses in disaster management.

| Box **5-1** | **Proposed Health Care Worker Competencies for Disaster Training** |

1. Recognize a potential critical event and implement initial actions.
2. Apply the principles of critical event management.
3. Demonstrate critical event safety principles.
4. Understand the institution's emergency operations plan.
5. Demonstrate effective critical event communications.
6. Understand the incident command system and the health care worker's role in it.
7. Demonstrate the knowledge and skills needed to fulfill the health care worker's role during a critical event.

Hsu E, Thomas T, Bass E, et al: Health care worker competencies for disaster training, *BMC Medical Education* 6:19, 2006.

This chapter is an introduction to the disaster environment in accordance with the academic requirements of CAAHEP.

A number of governmental agencies and academic institutions offer excellent disaster preparedness courses (see resources at the end of this chapter), and many of them are free, available as podcasts or live broadcasts. A wealth of federal, state, and community disaster training is available at all levels, including advanced academic degrees for disaster managers. These are intended for students and instructors. Advanced courses are also available in specific topics, such as bioterrorism, public health, and infectious disease. Basic competencies for disaster training are shown in Box 5-1.

CLASSIFICATION AND DEFINITION OF DISASTERS

A **disaster** is a catastrophic event that poses a large-scale risk to human life and property. Most important, a disaster *overwhelms local resources and requires outside assistance*. Disasters often are associated with human tragedy and widespread environmental devastation.

It is important to distinguish between a disaster and an emergency. A disaster causes widespread disruption in the social order, as well as injury and loss of property. In other words, disasters have far-reaching *social* consequences. An **emergency** is a more geographically isolated event that can be handled by local emergency services, such as ambulances, the fire department, or paramedics. For example, a motor vehicle accident or house fire can have tragic implications for those directly involved; however, unlike a disaster, these emergencies do not threaten the entire community.

A **mass casualty event (MCE)** is a localized emergency, such as a transportation accident (e.g., major air crash), explosion, or structural collapse, in which the number of victims overwhelms local health care services. A mass casualty event may overwhelm local health care services, but it does not usually constitute a large-scale disaster requiring federal assistance.

TYPES OF DISASTERS

Disasters and emergencies are classified by type and cause. The type of disaster can influence the response and may have implications for federal or state funding and reimbursement for property loss.

Traditionally, disasters were classified simply as "human-made" or "natural." However, today's global and regional disasters do not fit easily into these categories. Although we sometimes use these terms for broad discussion, root causes such as globalization, climate conditions, and widespread environmental degradation have blurred the categories. It is easy to see how the definitions lose meaning when we discuss whether a flood was caused by a torrential storm, loss of topsoil and vegetation related to farming practices, or poor engineering of levees on a flood plain. The current nomenclature for hazards used by the Federal Emergency Management Agency is *Natural*, *Technological/Accidental*, *Pandemic*, and *Terrorist*.

We then define the disaster specifically according to probable causes (Table 5-1). A classification of disasters informs the level of response needed:

- Level I: Local emergency teams are able to manage the immediate consequences and aftermath of the event.
- Level II: Requires regional assistance from surrounding communities
- Level III: Statewide and federal assistance is required because the effects of the disaster have overwhelmed local and regional resources.

Natural Disasters

A **natural disaster** is one that arises from a force of nature, such as a hurricane, a tornado, an earthquake, floods, and extreme heat or cold. Natural disasters are often complicated by other environmental factors, including those caused by populations. Overcrowding in communities, failure to meet building codes or lack of building codes, and even inequitable health care systems can place vulnerable populations at even higher risk when a disaster occurs. The more we study the effects of population growth, land use, and other social and technological pressures, the more apparent it is that human presence and activities may be the root cause of many disasters described as "natural." For example, mud slides and flooding may be initiated by excessive rainfall, but the root cause often is deforestation and urbanization of natural flood plains, which alter the geography. The following are considered to be natural disasters:

- **Blizzard:** A winter storm characterized by high wind and blowing snow resulting in low or no visibility. Blizzard conditions are often extremely cold. High winds can also pick up fallen snow, causing blizzard conditions.
- **Ice storm:** Freezing rain falls during an ice storm, covering all exposed areas with a thick, slippery, glasslike layer of ice. The weight of the ice causes the collapse of roofs, power lines, trees, and other solid structures. Transportation is halted because of dangerous road conditions, and power outages are widespread.
- **Extreme heat:** Temperatures that exceed the body's ability to regulate itself result in death unless the body can be externally cooled. During a heat wave, power grids may fail because of overload from urban use of air conditioners. People who do not have the means to cool the body are most vulnerable, including older adults, poor, and

Table 5-1 Natural and Human-Made Disasters, Health Risks, and Mitigation

Type of Disaster	Health Risks/Effects	Mitigation/Response
Climatic		
Flood	Drowning Overflow of sanitation collection sites Driving through or into water Contamination of drinking water	Early warning Environmental surveillance Structural preparation Land use planning and preparation
Hurricane	Drowning Injury from debris Massive property damage	Surveillance Early warning Evacuation
Tornado	Injury from debris Structural collapse Massive property damage	Surveillance Early warning Safety shelter Evacuation
Winter storm	Vehicle accidents Hypothermia Carbon monoxide poisoning Structural collapse from ice and snow Ice jams Flooding	Identification of shelters Establishment of shelter-in-place plan Adequate supplies of sand, salt, heavy equipment Distribution of weather radios Extra food stocks in communities
Extreme heat	Heat cramps Heat exhaustion Heat stroke Fatal hyperthermia	Identification of vulnerable groups Surveillance
Earthquake	Injury and death from structural collapse Risk of tsunami	Strategies for rescue Building and retrofitting for structural soundness (to prevent structural collapse)
Wildfire	Smoke inhalation Carbon monoxide poisoning Burns Injury from falling structures Heat stress (especially for responders) Electrical hazard	Evacuation plan Management of hazardous fuel in wild lands and forests Community awareness and education Build backfires Create fire breaks
Tsunami	Drowning Injury from structural collapse and high-velocity debris	Earthquake surveillance and early warning systems Evacuation
Volcano	Asphyxiation from toxic gas and ash Inundation by mud and lava	Early warning Evacuation
Landslides, avalanches, and mudslides	Drowning, inundation by mud and debris Injury related to high-velocity debris and water Electrical risks Disrupted roadways/lack of access to health care	Land use and urban planning Environmental surveillance Early warning Community education
Infectious Disease		
Pandemic, emerging infectious diseases, epidemic	Flu viruses	Adequate stockpile of vaccine Adequate stockpile of medical supplies and drugs Community education Surveillance
Unintentional and Technical Disaster		
Transportation accident (train, air disaster, motor vehicle, marine)	Traumatic injuries Burns Drowning	Response includes search and rescue. Federal agencies may become involved in investigations.
Explosion	Burns Head and other traumatic injury Ear injury	Following safety standards in the workplace Workplace training in safety and first aid

Continued

Table **5-1** **Natural and Human-Made Disasters, Health Risks, and Mitigation—cont'd**

Type of Disaster	Health Risks/Effects	Mitigation/Response
Hazardous material spill	Burns Lung injury Nerve damage Systemic poisoning	Early detection of the agent Early identification of the agent Protective measures according to type of agent Decontamination areas may be needed for victims and hazardous materials crews that work on the front line
Radiation	Nuclear accident	Protection from radioactive fallout Protection from contamination in the area Safe use of food and water Monitoring and treatment of victims of radiation exposure
Intentional Violence/Terrorism		
Bioterrorism	Anthrax Botulism Plague Smallpox Tularemia Viral hemorrhagic fevers	Enhanced diagnosis capacity Surveillance Establishment of case definitions Training and education Preparation of health care facilities Establishment of safe areas
Chemical	Caustic agents Pulmonary Explosives Flammable gas and liquid Blistering agents Nerve agents Blood agents Dioxins Oxidizers Incapacitating agents Respiratory (pulmonary) agents Metals Vomiting agents Toxic alcohols	Early detection of the chemical Early identification of the agent Rapid surveillance and reporting systems Specific training for primary health workers Personal protective equipment (PPE) for workers and civilians Availability of specialists in rapid removal Provision of shelter-in-place Case definitions of adverse effects Preparatory training before an incident occurs
Radiation	Dirty bombs Nuclear blast Radiation poisoning	Protection from radioactive fallout Protection from contamination in the area Safe use of food and water Monitoring and treatment of victims of radiation exposure
Explosion or bombing	Blast injury Burns Injury from high-velocity debris	Community education about disaster plans Health care facilities prepared for mass casualty

homeless. More people die from heat waves in the United States than any other weather-related disaster.

- **Drought:** A climate condition that features lack of rain (precipitation) is called a drought. Drought conditions result in failed crops and low water levels in reservoirs used for human use. The most famous drought in recent history was during the 1930s in the central region of the country (the Dust Bowl). In severe drought conditions such as occurred during the Depression, thousands of families were forced to leave their land and homes to seek food and work.
- **Earthquake:** Movement of earth's tectonic plates that causes them to move past each other results in pressure on the boundary. When the pressure reaches a critical level, an earthquake occurs. Earthquake disaster can cause massive loss of life and property from collapsed structures. Water and power lines are often affected, and logistic systems for bringing in aid may be crippled for weeks (Figure 5-1).
- **Flood:** Floods are usually related to both weather and land use. Poor drainage, lack of engineered waterways, and construction in flood plains with a known history of previous mass flooding contributes to loss of life and property during a flood. The risks for populations are often related to inability or refusal to evacuate the flood area as warnings are issued.
- **Forest fire:** Forest fires occur every year in the United States as a result of lightning strikes and more commonly from human activity near large forest lands. As urban

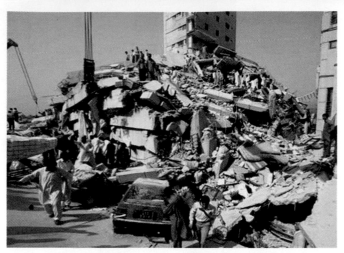

Figure 5-1 Earthquake in Bam, Pakistan. *(From Marx J: Rosen's emergency medicine, concepts and clinical practice, ed 7, St Louis, 2010, Mosby.)*

communities continue to encroach on wild forest lands, fires become increasingly common.

- **Hurricane:** A combination of conditions including warm oceans, moisture, light winds, and a weather disturbance can lead to a hurricane. Most hurricanes do not reach land but remain over the ocean. However, as the conditions build, the hurricane can move quickly, reaching coastal and urban communities very fast. Hurricane categories are based on the Saffir-Simpson scale. A category 3 or higher is a major event with sustained winds of 74 mph or higher.

- **Tornado:** This is a narrow rotating column of air that forms during a thunderstorm. The column or "funnel" extends from the base of the thunderstorm to the ground, moving rapidly across the land while rotating extremely fast. Although the energy released during a tornado is very destructive, the actual footprint may be small (perhaps only 100 or 200 yards) in comparison to a hurricane.

- **Tsunami:** An earthquake or volcano generated on the ocean floor can create very long, powerful waves on the ocean surface. Such a wave is called a tsunami or tidal wave. On the open ocean, the wave can be very shallow. However, as it reaches shallow land near shore, the height of the wave increases. Waves of enormous speed and force can completely destroy structures in their path. Just before reaching the shore, water on the coastline retracts quickly, often below the lowest tidal point. Once on shore, the tsunami crosses the shoreline, going far inland, and then pulls back, taking with it most of the debris created by the wave.

- **Snow avalanche:** Snow avalanches are familiar to most people who ski or live in mountainous areas. Avalanches are large swaths of snow, ice, and rock that fall along slip planes that are weakened by warming weather or water. The avalanche may take trees, boulders, and buildings in its path.

- **Mudslide:** Similar to an avalanche, a mudslide is the release of thousands of tons of mud from an incline. The cause is usually unstable slippage planes that may be natural (related to the type of soil) and made active by loss of topsoil and vegetation. Mudslides commonly occur in regions that have

been cleared for forestry activity or urbanization. Particular types of soil are prone to slides, and houses or whole communities built in these areas are at high risk. A mudslide can be fast moving and very destructive, carrying debris, trees, buildings, and boulders in its path.

Technological Disasters

Technological or industrial disasters are *unintentional* events caused by human activity, compounded by error or negligence. They can be caused by the release and spread of toxic substances involved in manufacturing, transportation, building, and extraction of natural resources such as oil and minerals. In many of these disasters, specific methods are used to contain and neutralize toxic materials. Technological disaster can be particularly frightening for communities because many of the dangers are hidden and represent an unknown. The effects of these disasters are often experienced for decades, as we have seen in Chernobyl and in the 1984 Bhopal disaster in India. At Bhopal, an accident at the Union Carbide plant released a pesticide component into the air, immediately killing at least 4,000 people and causing lifelong disability in an estimated 400,000 others. The following disasters are technological disasters:

- **Explosion:** Large-scale explosions can occur where flammable materials are used in manufacturing or in large storage facilities, including oil refineries, chemical plants, and manufacturing facilities. Victims at the site of the disaster suffer severe injury from the blast and fire. Communities are affected if chemicals are released into the environment. This can have short-term or long-term health implications.

- **Hazardous material accident:** Hazardous material accidents occur in conditions similar to those for explosions, with greater risk in refineries and other locations where large amounts of hazardous materials are stored or manufactured. Disaster response in this type of situation depends on identification of the hazardous material and the ability to contain the material or to mitigate the effects. HazMat specialists are needed to manage and advise on the response.

The federal government's Agency for Toxic Substances and Disease Registry provides HazMat Emergency Preparedness Training and Tools for Responders, including a dictionary of hazardous materials, on their website: http://www.atsdr.cdc.gov/hazmat-emergency-preparedness.html or search for "ATSDR HazMat."

- **Radiation accident:** Radiation accidents such as the Fukushima nuclear crisis and Chernobyl are uncommon but devastating to communities. The unpredictable outcome of a radiation disaster can create fear and anxiety for many decades after the event. During the disaster, containment of the leak and evacuation of the population are the two main features of community and technical responses. Specialists in radiation technology are needed on site to help manage the disaster and evacuate victims to appropriate treatment centers in the region.

- **Transportation accident:** Large-scale aviation, vehicle, and train accidents often result in mass casualty events. If the accident is caused by environmental conditions such as snow, fog, or ice storm, these can complicate rescue efforts and prevent emergency crews from reaching health care facilities. Air accidents that occur over urban areas multiply the effects many times. In all mass casualty situations, triage and treatment begin at the site of the accident unless it is unsafe to remain in the area.

Pandemic

A **pandemic** is a wide-scale, rapidly contagious infectious disease, whereas an epidemic is localized to a specific population. In recent years, human immunodeficiency virus/acquired immunodeficiency syndrome (HIV/AIDS) and flu have been the major causes of worldwide pandemics. Community response to pandemics and epidemics includes prevention through public health practices such as immunization, health education, and testing. At the clinical level, containment of the infectious agent requires isolation, strict hand washing, disinfection, and sterilization of patient care items. Although clinics are often very busy with flu patients during the winter season, there are few occasions when all services are overwhelmed, and these are usually temporary.

Acts of Terrorism

Current community and public health attention to all-hazards approach began with the events of 9/11 and other terrorist threats that followed. Extensive education, planning, and preventive measures have been put in place to enable a response to a variety of terrorist threats and actual events.

- **Bioterrorism**: This the intentional release of harmful biological agents (disease-causing bacteria or viruses) into the environment. A specific group of biological agents is associated with bioterrorism for their properties. They are easy to disseminate into the environment on a warhead or other means, they are rapidly fatal with high public health impact, and they require specific treatment and complex methods to mitigate their effects. The most common agents associated with bioterrorism are anthrax, botulism, plague, smallpox, tularemia, and viral hemorrhagic fevers. Some emerging infectious diseases such as hantavirus are also being considered as possible threats.
- **Chemical terrorism:** This is the use of chemical agents for intentional harm in the population. Chemicals include blistering and caustic agents that enter the respiratory system and the nerve gas groups that cause paralysis. Flammable chemicals such as napalm used during the Vietnam War are also in this group. Disaster planning for biological and biochemical terrorism is complex and highly technical. Special procedures for detection, analysis, and protection against individual chemicals and biotoxins are a specialty in disaster preparedness. HazMat training is provided by the CDC and other government agencies.
- **Bombing/direct attack:** A direct terrorist attack, as occurred on 9/11 and in the Oklahoma City bombing, creates a mass casualty event in which all disaster preparedness systems for rescue, triage, evacuation, and national security are immediately put in place (Figure 5-2). In addition to the health emergency services, civil and national defense alerts are also activated. These may involve military presence at the site of the disaster. Chain

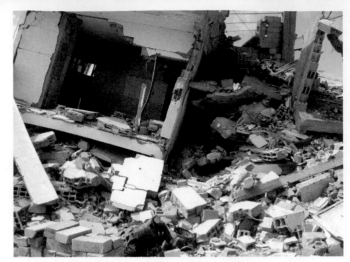

Figure 5-2 Bombing in Gaza, 2010. *(Photo by J. Kotcher.)*

of command may change according to the priority set by government agencies such as Homeland Security. State and national responders may be rapidly deployed to the area of the bombing.

DISASTER MANAGEMENT AND GOVERNMENT STRUCTURES

Disaster management is the strategy used in preparedness and response at different levels of government (federal, state, and local) and by communities themselves. A primary feature of disaster management is rapid, decisive, effective action. This requires a somewhat hierarchical management structure. Because all disaster plans involve government agencies, each level of governance (federal, regional or state, community) *flows from the one above it.* For example, the state disaster plan is based on the procedures and protocols of the federal agencies. Facility plans (including those for health care facilities) must be in accordance with state and federal systems such as those directed by OSHA and DHHS.

Disaster plans and protocols are consolidated at each government level through that level's emergency system following the *chain of command.* At the community and facility level, each has its own protocols for the disaster plan that are compatible with state and federal regulations. This means that doctors, nurses, or allied health professionals do not have to know the detailed points of the federal government disaster plan (discussed later), but they must understand and be able to practice the disaster plan for their community and for the health care facility and the department in which they work. On the other hand, *disaster managers* (specialists in the management aspects of disaster) must be familiar with all levels of the disaster plan.

FEDERAL LEVEL: AGENCIES AND ROLES

Governmental and nongovernmental agencies contribute to management and coordination during a disaster. The type of agency and the level of involvement depend on the nature of the disaster, the size of the affected population, and the location and extent of the affected area. The federal framework for

<table>
<tr><td>

Box **5-2** **Key Principles of the National Response Framework**

1. Engaged partnership
2. Tiered response
3. Scalable, flexible, and adaptable operational capabilities
4. Unity of effort through unified command
5. Readiness to act

</td></tr>
</table>

disasters management is implemented by the **Department of Homeland Security (DHS)**, which ensures that the disaster response is consistent with the country's doctrines and laws (especially constitutional law). This is especially important during a terrorist attack of any kind. The key policy document of the DHS is called the **National Response Framework (NRF)**. The information and guidance of the framework contains the following sections:

- Roles and responsibilities (of disaster managers)
- Actions (policy and procedure)
- Organization (how the nation is organized in a disaster)
- Planning
- Resources

The *principles (doctrine)* of the framework are listed in Box 5-2.

> The National Response Framework document can be accessed at http://www.fema.gov/pdf/emergency/nrf/nrf-core.pdf, or search for "FEMA National Response Framework."

Federal Emergency Management Agency

The **Federal Emergency Management Agency (FEMA)** is responsible for the coordination, management, and response for nationally **declared disasters**. It also conducts training programs in disaster preparedness, management, and response for professionals and nonprofessionals. FEMA assistance is only available in disasters that have been "declared" a **state of emergency** by the governor of the state where the disaster occurred. Once the governor has declared a disaster, a formal request is made to the federal government. This results in a federal declaration of the disaster that releases federal funding and other resources to help out with the disaster.

FEMA collaborates with many different partners, including community-based organizations, to implement disaster response. Its four federal partners are:

1. Federal Communications Commission (FCC)
2. National Weather Service (NWS)
3. National Disaster Medical System
4. Department of Health and Human Services

National Incident Management System (NIMS)

FEMA uses the **National Incident Management System (NIMS)** to implement its work. NIMS defines the management structure, objectives, chain of command, and procedures necessary for disaster coordination and response. NIMS is intended for use by all levels of government, nongovernmental organizations, and also the private sector. There are five main components and many subsections in the system. The five are:

- Preparedness
- Communications and Information Management

- Resource Management
- Command and Management
- Ongoing Management and Maintenance

Training for NIMS is available through FEMA, which maintains a large database of resources and references. NIMS courses can be taken on site, and individuals can access online training (see later links) through the agency's Center for Domestic Preparedness and Emergency Management Institute.

Health Resources and Services Administration

HRSA, an agency of the Department of Health and Human Services, oversees two primary agencies that are involved in the medical (health) response to disaster management:

- **Agency for Healthcare Research and Quality (AHRQ).** This agency provides disaster-related research, resources, training, and recommendations for health care facilities, communities, and individuals.
- **National Disaster Medical System (NDMS).** This agency maintains a database of trained on-call medical, paramedical, and allied health personnel for emergency deployment during a disaster. It also trains first responders. NDMS response teams are established in each state, and trained professionals are recruited as needed to maintain a full team. Specialist teams include:
  - DMAT (Disaster Medical Assistance Team)
  - DMORT (Disaster Mortuary Operations Response Team)
  - NVRT (National Veterinary Response Team)
  - NNRT (National Nurse Response Team)
  - NPRT (National Pharmacy Response Team)

Disaster Medical Assistance Team

Disaster Medical Assistance Team (DMAT) is the on-call volunteer health assistance team for FEMA. Individuals on DMAT teams are deployed in their usual roles as health care professionals and also perform associated tasks. Individuals on the DMAT teams must be available for rapid deployment and able to work in resource-poor disaster environments. Health professionals with specific skills such as radiation, chemical, or other types of trauma are needed in special circumstances. Health care professionals, including surgical technologists, who are interested in applying can make application to their state or local DMAT organization. For information on state DMAT teams, go to http://www.demat.org or search for "DMAT FEMA." Community members may also join their local Community Emergency Response Team (CERT). See http://www.citizencorps.gov/cert. Further opportunities for volunteering are with the Emergency System for the Advance Registration of Volunteer Health Professionals (ESAR-VHP).

Centers for Disease Control and Prevention

Among its many programs and mandates, the CDC is a key information, training, and research organization for disasters and emergencies. Through local partners, it provides public health education to inform people about existing and emerging threats to the population. It provides research and strategic guidelines for all types of health problems including those resulting from bioterrorism, environmental and technical disaster, infectious disease outbreak, and other public health issues. The CDC Coordinating Office for Terrorism Preparedness and Emergency Response (COTPER) is a federally supported agency that funds technical assistance and stockpiles the drugs, antidotes, vaccines, and medical supplies needed during a disaster. Its Emergency Operations Center monitors threats so that disaster response can be more efficiently and effectively coordinated. The agency also provides extensive disaster training for health care providers and the public.

STATE AND LOCAL: AGENCIES AND ROLES

Disaster planning, management, and coordination at the state level are implemented through each state's emergency management agency or EMA (e.g., the Alabama Emergency Management Agency, the Colorado Office of Emergency Management, and the Florida Division of Emergency Management). State EMAs coordinate closely with FEMA and local emergency management agencies (LEMAs).

> A list of the state EMAs can be found on the FEMA website: www.fema.gov/about/contact/statedr.shtm.

Governmental and nongovernmental agencies are involved in disaster coordination and response at the local level. Local governments are responsible for management, using protocols and guidelines established by the EMA and FEMA. Individual agencies provide services according to their capacity and expertise. Their local knowledge is particularly helpful in coordinating with state and federal disaster managers. The **American Red Cross** and other nongovernmental agencies provide humanitarian assistance and technical support during disasters and emergencies. Local chapters of the Red Cross also provide courses and training for health care professionals and the community. Individuals who wish to volunteer to help in community disaster response can register with the Red Cross through their state EMA. (Further information is available at the organization's website, http://www.redcross.org.) Local communities plan for disasters with the help of FEMA guidelines and disaster specialists.

THE DISASTER CYCLE

Up to this point, we have discussed types of disasters and the government structures that are involved in setting guidelines, structures, documents, and chain of command for a disaster. From here, we move to the community level, the facility, and the actual events of the disaster. The *disaster cycle* (Figure 5-3) is a framework for action from the start of planning until communities are able to function again following a disaster. The disaster cycle is a convenient structure for planning and implementation. This framework is used in mainstream disaster planning at all levels and can be changed as needs arise. One or more of the phases may take place at different times or at the same time. The important fact to take away is that the disaster cycle provides grouping of the complex action points of all hazard preparedness.

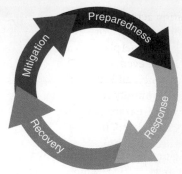

Figure 5-3   The disaster cycle—planning and implementation model.

I.   PREPAREDNESS

The preparedness phase is the first step in planning for a disaster. It encompasses numerous complex activities that have a common goal. This is to ensure that individuals, communities, and government sectors are able to respond effectively to different types of disasters. Planning is carried out using the guidelines, procedures, and recommendations provided by governmental agencies (e.g., FEMA), health agencies (e.g., the CDC), and research and academic institutions experienced in disaster management. When a disaster occurs in a hospital, medical office, or stand-alone surgery center, an executable plan must be in place to prevent wasted resources, both human and material. Without adequate planning, the disaster environment can rapidly deteriorate, increasing loss of life and property.

Local Team Building

Local team building for disaster planning is derived from the community. Experts from the community form the basis of the team, which has the capacity to discuss important issues and create a working plan. Representatives or lead coordinators from important sectors include the following:

- Law enforcement
- Fire service
- Public works, water, and sanitation
- Public health
- Emergency medical services
- Emergency paramedical services
- Search and rescue
- Ambulance service
- Social and children's services
- Mental health practitioners
- Public health specialists
- Water and sanitation engineers
- Veterinary service
- Structural specialists
- Health care facility management

Other groups such as utility companies, community service organizations, and transportation authorities can provide support input to the planning process.

Risk Analysis and Mitigation Strategy

Once the team is formed, a risk analysis is carried out to target the most likely hazards in that particular community. Even though the overall approach is "all hazards," there are certain mitigation activities that must be carried out according to areas of vulnerability. For example, an area may be near chemical, nuclear, or fuel plants that might create a community-wide disaster in the event of an accident. Natural risks such as flooding, hurricane, and tsunami may also be potential hazards. Each community considers its risks and plans accordingly within the all-hazard framework. Once the risk assessment has been completed, the risk reduction plan is designed. This is where specific technical recommendations are made to protect people and property.

Resource Assessment

No plan can be implemented without the resources to do it. At this point, communities must assess their capacity to fulfill the disaster plan. This includes available communication services, logistical capacity, and human resources.

The Response Plan

The response plan is developed with consideration of the assessment of resources, risk evaluation, and input from specific community interest and service groups. The plan addresses the process of activation, what will be done and how, who is involved, and the criteria for triggering the response. It includes the sequence of different responses, levels of action, and the actual organization of the response. There is no single plan that fits all communities. A list of general components for an emergency plan is shown in Table 5-2.

In addition to the main disaster preparedness plan, states require specific plans to meet health and safety codes. Examples of these are:

- Plan for Hazardous Materials Incident Response (HazMat Plan)
- Risk Management Plan for toxic flammable explosive substances that includes management of oil spills and other chemicals released into the waters or air
- Dam Failure Emergency Action Plan for mitigation and response to dam failure
- Crowd Control Plan used for mitigation of crowd disasters involving venues with a capacity of more than 5,000 people
- Radiological Emergency Response Plan, specific to commercial nuclear power plants and hazards associated with nuclear disaster

- School Safety Plan developed to protect school children in event of disaster
- Hospital Disaster Plan, specific to health care facilities, employees, and patients
- Nursing Home Disaster plan to provide mitigation and response to patients and staff
- Adult Health Care Facility Disaster Emergency Plan for protection of residences and shelters of adults in the community
- Long-Term Care Facility for the Mentally Retarded Emergency Plan for care and protection of residents and staff
- Electric Utility Storm Plan designed to protect the population and restore power in an emergency or disaster
- Airport Emergency Plan to mitigate and plan for hazards associated with airports and their use in disaster

The Local Incident Command System

The local incident command system (ICS) is the on-site (local) disaster management process used during all disasters. The system is designed during the preparation phase and implemented during the response. Many operational sectors in the community such as health care facilities, law enforcement, public works, and schools are integrated into the system, in which one or several commanders take the lead, and various sector leaders work under the commanders' line management (Figure 5-4). Horizontal and vertical communication within the ICS promotes coordination, information gathering, appropriate response, and analysis during an ongoing disaster. This top-down approach is necessary so that decisions affecting people's lives and property can be made quickly by experienced disaster managers. Individual sectors within the ICS include planning, logistics, health, communications, operations, finance, and others.

The ICS is used to overcome coordination problems common to disasters and emergencies, such as:

- Competing goals or standards among agencies
- Many responders with no specific tasks or objectives
- Poor communication among responders and agencies
- Lack of clarity about what is to be done and how
- No clear chain of command
- No overall plan or the responders are unaware of the plan

Table 5-2 Primary Objectives of a Local Disaster Plan

Objective	Explanation
1. Activation of emergency response personnel	Based on which organizations have been identified in planning phase. The level of activation depends on the predetermined threshold or trigger.
2. Command post operations center	Responding personnel need a place to meet. This may correspond with the emergency operations center (EOP).
3. Public announcements, hazard and service information	People in the community need to receive updated information about the emergency. The plan must include methods for information dissemination.
4. Management of resources	During a disaster, resources can be depleted or used inefficiently. The plan includes a resource management team that coordinates private and government sources of all types of resources.
5. Restoration of vital services	Critical services such as power, fuel, sewer, and roadways are essential to aiding victims and preventing additional emergency situations. A strategy for restoration of vital services is addressed at the planning stage.

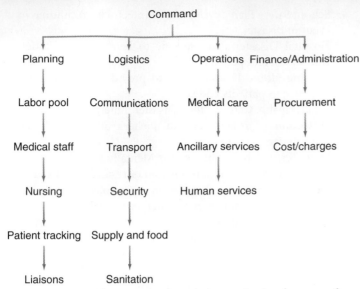

Figure 5-4 Incident command system—organizational structure for management. *(From Townsend CM: Sabiston's textbook of surgery, ed 18, Philadelphia, 2008, Saunders.)*

The ICS may be implemented locally for a single facility, such as a hospital, or it may be strategically based to provide management for the entire community or state. A more complex command system may include *incident commanders* who are heads of organizations involved in the disaster. This system is then called incident command. When implemented for an individual health facility such as a hospital, it is called an *HICS* (hospital incident command system). The ICS mandate must follow the NIMS structure and protocols for consistency and efficient use of resources during an emergency. The operational goals of an ICS are:

- To meet the needs of the incident
- To provide a system under which different agencies can rapidly become operational
- To provide logistic and administrative support to operational staff
- To prevent duplication of efforts

Coordination

Coordination is the process by which the efforts and activities of groups and individuals are organized to make the most efficient use of resources. Disaster planning coordination prevents duplication of efforts and gaps in service and takes place throughout the disaster cycle. The coordinating body may be a specially trained team or individuals who manage a particular sector, such as health, logistics, or administrative duties. Coordinators are responsible for meshing the activities of service providers or front-line responders and ensuring that they are in compliance with the disaster plan, standards, and recommendations. Uncoordinated groups actually may become a burden or a risk during the response phase. Coordination requires a clear, concise plan; a means of communication during the disaster; and trained individuals to oversee the coordination. Good coordination requires an overall plan that is both strategic and realistic. All health care facilities coordinate efforts to put their disaster plan in order. They coordinate with other local agencies and service providers and meet regularly to review their plan.

Logistics and Supply Chains

During a disaster, normal supply chains and locations of goods, including food, often are disrupted. Disaster preparedness, therefore, includes extensive logistical planning for emergency procurement, storage, and distribution of supplies and equipment. Categories of supplies and materials needed in a disaster include shelter materials, medical supplies, food and water, nonfood items (e.g., blankets, tarpaulins, soap), and communications equipment. The **logistics supply chain,** the stages of supply from procurement to end user, may require predisaster placement or stockpiling. Local disaster agencies ensure that all responders are familiar with the regional plan so that the supply chain can be activated quickly and smoothly. Points of distribution (PODs) of supplies are preplanned along with alternative sites. The federal government's *Strategic National Stockpile* of drugs and medical supplies, maintained by the CDC, is available in the event of terrorist attack, disease outbreak, or other public health emergency. Antibiotics, emergency medicines, airway equipment, intravenous fluids, and dressing materials are included in "push packs" for immediate distribution in an emergency.

For more information on this program, see http://www.cdc.gov/phpr/stockpile/stockpile.htm.

Emergency Exercises

Exercises in which disaster responders do a "dry run" of a disaster are an essential part of disaster preparedness. Hospitals and other types of health care facilities are required by the Joint Commission to implement a facility exercise at least once a year. However, it also is important that local or regional agencies and responders perform emergency exercises that include all those who would be involved in the event of a disaster. Predisaster exercises are valuable for revealing gaps and weaknesses in overall plans, which can be resolved before a disaster occurs. Analysis of lessons learned from large emergencies or previous disasters also is important in strategic planning before a disaster or mass casualty event occurs.

Personal and Family Preparedness

National and state agencies encourage individuals and families to prepare for a disaster or local emergency in specific ways to mitigate the effects of the disaster on personal health, safety, and communication. A model plan includes logistical problems that might arise such as inability to access drinking water, failure of usual communication systems (phone, Internet), and evacuation. Methods of evacuation and designated meeting places for families are also included in the model plan.

Shelter in disasters is crucial for health and safety. Any plan for disaster or emergency includes a strategy for sheltering in place. This requires preplanning to maintain a supply of food, water, and other necessities at home or work site, including pet care. Prolonged sheltering may be necessary in emergencies where it is impossible to move people or when a group of people have no alternative but to stay where they are. Examples of this are groups that have been moved to large sports stadiums or other public facilities until individual homes or shelters can be provided.

A model plan includes an evacuation kit containing a 3-day supply of personal and "survival" items. This type of simple "go bag" is also important for health care providers who may be called out to assist in an emergency. It should include your wallet, copies of personal identification cards or passport and contact information.

Excellent resources for developing personal and family all-hazard preparedness plans are available from the Centers for Disease Control and from FEMA. Refer to http://www.bt.cdc.gov/preparedness or http://www.fema.gov/pdf/areyouready/areyouready_full.pdf. An additional resource on animals in emergency can be accessed at http://www.fema.gov/individual/animals.shtm.

II. MITIGATION

Mitigation, or risk reduction, is a process or activity that minimizes the impact of an event. In general, when a disaster cannot be averted or avoided, mitigation is used to reduce the disaster's effects on people, the infrastructure, property, and the environment. Mitigation is sometimes placed first on the disaster cycle or in association with preparedness. It might also occur as part of the response.

Many types and levels of mitigation can be used, depending on the type of disaster and the environment in which it occurs. For example, structural mitigation may involve changing planning and building codes or actually rebuilding structures so that they can withstand the forces of an earthquake. The engineering and construction of structures, such as dams, seawalls, and defensible spaces, are mitigation activities. Construction of an elaborate communications (i.e., with LEMA) and technological infrastructure, such as early warning and detection systems, also is part of the mitigation process, as is isolating patients with contagious disease.

III. RESPONSE

The process of disaster response is complex and often very difficult. The environment is stressful and often disturbing, and the work is demanding. Even the best preparation and coordination plans can be quickly overwhelmed by the unpredictable events and conditions of a disaster. The work of preparation is over; now is the time to implement the plan. You hope for the best but understand that not every detail can be accounted for in the planning stage. Things can go wrong—but you do your best and remember your ethical mandates to do no harm. Remain cooperative and keep your head, even under great psychological pressure. Keep track of your own mental and physical health status.

Community Disaster Response

Although specific types of disasters create particular needs in a population, many scenarios are common, especially in natural disasters in which significant human needs and damage to the infrastructure result. Some common scenarios are:

- Loss of shelter (buildings or other means of escaping environmental hazards)
- Sudden requirement to shelter large numbers of people
- Disruption or alteration of communications, including access to electronic information
- Disruption, alteration, or destruction of the usual methods of transport
- Sudden need for large-scale health care services
- Sudden need for relocation of patients and newly injured
- Disproportionate effects on vulnerable sectors of society (older adults, impoverished, chronically ill, homeless, and others)
- Diversion of logistical support normally available for health needs
- Loss of infrastructure (systems and structures)
- Shortage of human resources
- Disruption, alteration, or destruction of power sources
- Disruption or destruction of water supply lines
- Possible contamination of drinking water
- Rapid depletion of medical supplies
- Scarcity of food
- Diversion of human resources and changes in roles

It is not possible to predict all the effects of all disasters. However, part of disaster planning and management is to assess the life-threatening effects of the disaster, prioritize needs, and analyze the best use of resources.

Human Needs in a Disaster

Many disaster response activities are implemented to provide basic, immediate human needs: shelter, sanitation, food and water, and medical assistance.

EVACUATION AND SHELTER Shelter protects people from environmental conditions, including extreme weather. It also offers an element of safety and a sense of security. Shelter may be a single building or a group of buildings away from the disaster area, or it may be temporary structures, such as tents. Shelter also offers protection from injury or further harm. In a disaster, shelter or protection may be the most immediate human need. Naturally, food and water are essential for life, but people's first instinct is to escape harm, and this often equates with shelter or evacuation. Evacuation is a way of moving people away from a disaster to protect them from catastrophic morbidity and mortality. Once an order has been made for evacuation, messages are sent out through local radio and other media still accessible. It is often part of the disaster scenario. People are assisted with transportation during an organized evacuation. Evacuation teams composed of community responders such as fire and other emergency personnel are identified in the predisaster planning stage. Vulnerable individuals in the population must be identified during the disaster planning phase. Some people cannot evacuate because of illness, physical incapacity, or lack of understanding of the risks. Others choose not to evacuate because they do not want to leave their home or pets. This may increase their risk of injury and often poses additional hazards for rescuers, who must come in to assist late in the disaster. Gaps in these services can create a separate type of humanitarian crisis in which people are left homeless and dependent on agencies for long periods.

The alternative to evacuation is **shelter-in-place**, in which people remain where they are, usually in a building or other structure, in a relatively safe location within the structure. A safe room or location sometimes can be fitted to resist debris impact or to prevent contamination by outside air. The decision to shelter-in-place is based on risk analysis and usually is communicated to the population through the media. An example of a disaster that might require shelter-in-place is a tornado or other extreme weather event in which people remain below ground until the disaster is declared over. A chemical disaster or bioterrorism is another type of event in which remaining inside to avoid toxic fumes or vapor may be the safest course of action.

MEDICAL AID Medical aid in a disaster is carried out in existing health care facilities or mobile clinics. During the planning phase of disaster management, all facilities that are equipped to take patients are involved in medical aid. Stand alone offices and smaller facilities are assigned roles according to their capacity. The type of aid needed depends on the nature of the disaster. For example, earthquakes that cause buildings to collapse result in a high rate of orthopedic and other crush injuries. Chemical disasters result in toxicity and may include large numbers of burn victims. Transporting victims who need medical aid is a difficult problem when roads are blocked by collapsed structures or flooded with water.

INFECTION CONTROL Prevention of disease transmission is one of the primary objectives during a disaster. Infection control applies to evacuation facilities (shelters and camps) health care facilities, and community health. Important operational needs related to disease prevention in the disaster setting include but are not limited to the following:

- Control of infectious disease in evacuation centers
- Safe water
- Sanitation
- Health messages to the community
- Safe disposal of medical waste
- Collection and destruction of garbage
- Control of animal and insect pests in congested areas
- Shelter from harsh environments

Infection control procedures during a disaster must be followed as closely as possible. This includes wearing personal protective equipment (e.g., hand protection and masks) when handling body fluids and rigorous hand washing. When hand washing facilities are not available, bottled water or an alcohol-based hand rub is used to prevent cross infection. If the disaster itself is caused by an infectious agent, such as during a bioterrorism attack, community volunteers and HazMat teams will distribute appropriate protective clothing, respirators, and eye protection to those people closest to the focal point of the disaster. Decontamination procedures must be set up at a health care facility where appropriate equipment and supplies are available.

FOOD Food security often is threatened during a disaster, because the normal means of procuring and transporting food are interrupted or destroyed. Food shortages also create panic in an unstable environment. Problems with the food pipeline sometimes emerge days rather than hours after the onset of a disaster, because supply lines may be destroyed or the disaster environment prevents a sufficient flow of food into the logistics pipeline.

MENTAL HEALTH NEEDS Social and psychological assistance is needed in every disaster. People are best able to use their innate coping strategies when the social structure is maintained. Disaster response, therefore, includes measures to reunite families and maintain social cohesiveness. Although critical incident counseling during a disaster is controversial, immediate psychological aid can assist some individuals traumatized by the effects of a disaster. Mental health providers are among those who are needed in the immediate and short-term disaster response.

PROTECTION Protection from criminal threat may be necessary during a disaster or emergency, especially when resources are scarce and the usual protection measures are diminished or absent. In large disasters, local law enforcement agencies often divert personnel to lifesaving and rescue efforts. Curfews may be enforced during a disaster to help prevent violence and loss of property.

VULNERABLE POPULATIONS The term **vulnerability** (exposure to risk) often is discussed in association with disasters and emergencies. Vulnerable populations are those with a particularly high risk of injury or harm as a result of the disaster. People living in a flood plain, those living in substandard housing, people with learning and physical disabilities, and older adults are particularly vulnerable in disasters. They may not fully appreciate the danger of the situation or may not be able to respond to evacuation orders. Poorly constructed housing and physical isolation also contribute to vulnerability. Disaster planning at the community level includes the ability to locate and assist special needs populations and those living in difficult physical circumstances.

REUNIFICATION Often in disasters, family members are separated and there may be no way for them to contact each other. The Red Cross has a mandate to assist families in reunification during disaster. There are different methods and means for providing reunification, which depends on collecting names and other information and funneling it through one or two sources. Electronic reunification is sometimes the best method of keeping a database, and local radio stations can assist in making announcements. It may be necessary for families to have more than one designated person to be the center point of communication in case that person loses contact with the others for some reason. The local Red Cross agency is almost always the best way to begin the process, because they have many years of experience in reunification.

Health Care Facility Disaster Response

The following is a mass casualty disaster scenario with events as they might occur in a health care facility. Not all services are represented in this short scenario, but these examples may be helpful in understanding the disaster environment and for tabletop analysis.

Local community members and the media report that an explosion and fire have taken place at 2:00 AM in a large local furniture factory located in a semiurban area in which there is also forestry activity. The fire is being fueled by the structure itself, its contents, and a large chemical warehouse where flammable materials are stored. The fire is spreading rapidly, and there are many injuries from the explosion and collapse of the building. The families living near the factory are low-income factory workers, and their houses are low-quality structures mainly made of chip wood. The community has one hospital with a helipad. The nearest large health care facility is 100 miles away.

1. Within minutes of the explosion, the first victims arrive at the 100-bed health care facility by private car from surrounding neighborhoods. News arrives that hundreds of severely wounded people will follow shortly.

2. The emergency department staff rushes to evacuate all existing nonurgent patients from the department.

3. The hospital incident command system has been activated, and hospital staff are called in according to the facility emergency plan. The command center is put in place at the security desk.

4. The hospital administrator contacts other county and state emergency managers to notify them of the disaster and possible need for assistance.

5. Department heads report to the command center and call as many of their employees as possible. All incoming staff report to the command center before going to their units. Job sheets are filled out for special assignments according to need and urgency.

6. ICU and nursing management begin to discharge patients who do not need essential medical care. Local taxi and volunteer vehicles are found to take patients who are able to leave the hospital home from the facility in order to make room for emergency cases.

7. Emergency communication systems are in place, but there are not enough handheld VHF radios. The mobile network system is overloaded. The primary communications system in the emergency department is used to make radio calls.

8. The emergency services—ambulance, fire, and other rescue vehicles—have all been deployed, and victims are being brought in by emergency crews. Triage has been performed by doctors and nurses in the emergency vehicles and near the hospital entrance. All patients are identified using numbered disaster tags.

9. A runner is sent to all departments to inform them of the type and approximate number of victims they can expect.

10. A triage area is established outside the emergency department, but people from the community arrive and enter the area looking for loved ones. There are two hospital security officers who recruit three other hospital staff to help with crowd control. A visitor control center is then set up in the lobby and manned by two social services staff. A third is on the way.

11. A temporary morgue has been set up, but it is far from the emergency department, requiring travel outside the building to avoid patients and the public.

12. The hospital administrator contacts the county emergency office to request RACES (Radio Amateur Civil Emergency Service) personnel to assist in providing radio communications.

13. Perioperative personnel have arrived and start setting up rooms for emergency surgery. The operating room supervisor contacts purchasing to request extra supplies. A runner is assigned to transport the needed supplies.

14. Clinical staff has arrived and are already on duty in the treatment areas (e.g., surgery, radiology, blood bank). Technical staff is deployed to the operating room to help with instrument processing and transportation of patients.

15. Police and other law enforcement professionals arrive to help with crowd control and communications.

16. Members of the maintenance department lock all outside doors except those for employees, the emergency department, and the front lobby.

17. A headquarters for members of the media is set up in the hospital cafe.

18. Housekeeping staff bring additional beds from the supply room and create additional ward areas.

19. There are 35 burn victims who need airway care. They are triaged by two emergency department doctors. Eight of the victims need immediate intubation. The anesthesia technologist and two respiratory therapists are brought in to assist in intubation of the victims.

20. A phone line in the medical records department is designated for receiving outside calls and communication with relatives.

21. The incident command system, which includes bringing in regional actors to assist in the emergency, is partially effective. However, there are not enough managers to direct and coordinate the efforts.

22. Triage is notified when operating rooms and recovery areas are ready to take additional patients.

23. As the initial wave of victims is cared for at the hospital level, community organizations are setting up shelter accommodation in the town. Emergency vehicles arrive from other state regions to take victims to other facilities for care.

24. The hospital's helicopter is joined by an additional flight crew and helicopter to assist.

25. Emergency cases continue to be seen well into the next day, and evacuation of residents from the fire area is ongoing. The fire is still burning but moving away from the town center. The emergency services will be working for another 6 days to care for victims and place people in temporary shelters.

In the fictional scene just described, we can see activation of many different types of emergency services that require preplanning.

However, even with the best planning, there is no way to predict exactly how the health care facility or community will cope with the needs of people during a specific disaster event. The health care needs of populations in disaster or emergency events vary widely according to the type of event, the location, and population density. Some disasters result in high morbidity but low mortality, whereas in others such as earthquakes, fewer people are injured than killed. In the early days of a disaster, the focus is on survival and rescue. After the initial burden of victims has been handled, other needs emerge, including management of patients who were not urgent at the time of the disaster but who nevertheless need care. Chronic-disease, reproductive, and mental health needs can become critical when patients do not have access to health care services.

OPERATIONAL CONSIDERATIONS DURING THE RESPONSE

Communication A disaster or large-scale emergency may result in loss of usual methods of communication, or existing networks may be overwhelmed as people try to connect with relatives, friends, and service providers. A major health care facility has the ability to communicate using satellite or high-frequency radio. Health and safety messages to the community are more difficult but can be achieved by radio transmission. Local radio stations are particularly effective in transferring health messages and also providing links between individuals and families. Staff will be oriented to disaster communications during drills and training sessions. At least three different communication systems will be activated for backup. All hospital employees are normally oriented to emergency alert signals (fire and patient emergency codes) during the first week of employment. The usual emergency alert systems for the hospital may be suspended during a community disaster.

Medical Facility Evacuation Evacuation of a medical facility may sometimes be necessary because of structural hazards or immediate threat from fire, chemical, or bioterrorism. The decision to evacuate patients is difficult because in the midst of a disaster, managers must evaluate the risks of moving people as compared to the dangers of staying in place. In general, a structural evaluation must be made by qualified personnel such as facility engineers. Medical personnel must ensure that care of the patients can be continued and that the evacuation destination is safer than the one being evacuated. Naturally, when there is an immediate undeniable threat, such as a structural fire that is out of control, the objectives are to move people as quickly as possible away from harm. Planning before a disaster occurs can help set thresholds for threats that require evacuation. Evacuation may be partial (moving to another part of the building or outside) or complete (moving to another facility). The procedures and protocols for a facility evacuation can be located in the disaster guidelines for that facility. Patient evacuation is carried out by trained first responders.

Surge Capacity **Surge capacity** is the ability of a health care facility to quickly increase its capability to receive and treat patients. In disasters that have a high burden of injuries, this becomes a critical issue. A system for transferring patients from one facility to another may not be functional (e.g., flooded roads or building debris may block access). Health care facilities can determine the maximum number of casualties they can receive, but the environment of the disaster may not permit the movement of patients to other locations. Strategies to increase surge capacity include discharge of elective cases, not admitting nonemergency cases, and conversion of nonpatient areas into makeshift wards. Calling in staff from other health care facilities is often necessary to reach surge capacity, but space to work in, supplies, drugs, and medical equipment are also needed.

Staff Assignments One of the first events to occur in health care facility disaster management is activation of the emergency plan, including the deployment of all facility staff. Disaster plans for all health care facilities include a protocol for callout of staff. In most cases, staff is called in by a member of the facility incident command system. Individuals report to their incident command station and then their usual duty area, or they might be assigned tasks at another location. Facility departments are assigned roles during development of the disaster response plan or by the incident commander at the time of the event. Roles are assigned using a *job action sheet* (JAS). This is a tool used to define a person's functional role during an emergency. The JAS is completed by the unit leader or section leader for that professional. The important data include the position (which may not be the person's usual role), whom to report to, the purpose of the role, and tasks to be completed and in what order. The disaster plan must designate the exact reporting or assembly area for staff and the names of those who are assigned. The role of the surgical technologist during disaster response is most likely his or her usual role in the operating room, which might include helping with instrument and equipment reprocessing. The surgical technologist may be required to assist outside his or her scope of practice.

A set of job action sheets for the California Emergency Services Authority can be accessed online at http// www.emsa.ca.gov/hics/job.asp, or search for "California Emergency Job Sheets." This website provides good examples of typical job sheets used in many different kinds of disasters.

Note that the ICS is enacted at the management level, not the operational level. The "hands on" roles and responsibilities are delegated by the facility ICS manager according to the disaster plan for that facility.

Triage Triage is a process in which casualties are given emergency medical treatment according to the probability of their survival. The surgical technologist is expected to support the role of triage as needed. Triage is a necessary procedure when the number of people needing medical attention overwhelms the services available. The process requires rapid, clear, decisive thinking and action by medical personnel. No standard scoring system is used in triage. However, a common practice is to differentiate patients by the following parameters:

- Those not needing emergency care
- Those with the greatest chance of survival with medical care
- Those for whom medical intervention will aid survival
- Those whose chance of survival would not increase with medical intervention

Triage is performed at the disaster or mass casualty site, in transit to a health care facility by emergency vehicle, or in the health care facility itself. People with minor injuries and their

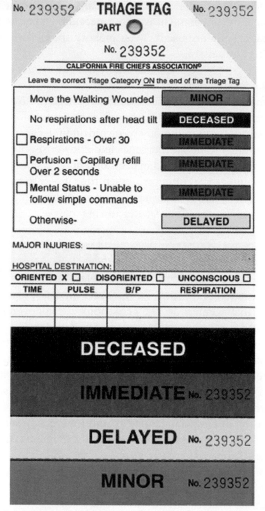

Figure 5-5 Triage system tag used to identify victims according to survival chances. *(From Marx J: Rosen's emergency medicine, concepts and clinical practice, ed 7, St Louis, 2010, Mosby.)*

families often crowd to a medical facility for reassurance during a disaster. However, an attempt must be made to triage each person to ensure that a seriously injured or ill person is not overlooked. Triaged individuals are assigned a category and tagged using a color or other code tag that can be identified by other health care workers (Figure 5-5).

In very large disasters where there are mass casualties, such as 9/11, a rapid triage system is used by emergency medical personnel. The START (simple triage and rapid treatment) system is used when the number of casualties overwhelms the capacity to fully assess victims. The system uses basic metabolic signs: respiration, perfusion, and mental status. Training in the START system is available at health care facilities and as part of overall disaster training in the community.

Advanced first aid courses, including first responder techniques, are available for communities and through disaster training management groups. To access these courses, refer to the list of resources at the end of this chapter.

Supplies and Drugs Supplies are managed during an emergency by the procurement officer and his or her staff. Accounting must be kept for all supplies, even if the system is

streamlined for emergency purposes. This is necessary so that as supplies are depleted, an immediate rough inventory and request for a regional stockpile can be made. In some events, a request for medical supplies is made at the beginning of the disaster, with knowledge of what supplies are likely to run out.

Drugs are managed by the pharmacy department with runners actively assisting in distribution of drugs following orders. Orders must be recorded and dispensed in a way that allows tracking.

Items that require refrigeration can be kept cold using the facility's emergency generator or cold packs that are prepacked and ready for use in emergency.

Morgue A facility morgue is set up near the back of the hospital if overflow room is needed. The location should be selected to prevent casual or accidental viewing of bodies by visitors. The morgue is usually an assigned task of the pathology department. Someone from the department stays on duty at all times, and bodies are removed from the premises as soon as feasible. Disaster tags are necessary for all bodies, and all forms must be filled out at the time the body is delivered to the morgue area.

PROTECTION OF FACILITY RECORDS Protection of medical records during disasters is a topic that is currently being debated by disaster managers and health care facilities. Unless the facility keeps electronic records off site or in multiple sites, there is no easy way to solve the problem of lost or damaged records. In large disasters, patients may travel far from their usual health care facility for treatment or may be relocated for extended periods of time without their records, unless they keep updated documents with them. There are also questions about the security of all electronic medical records.

IV. RECOVERY

The recovery phase of a disaster is not defined by a particular event or activity. **Disaster recovery** is a complex process in which the risk of morbidity and mortality is reduced or mitigated to a level at which the community can cope. This does not mean that losses are reverted to predisaster levels. Complete "recovery" from a major disaster may take many years.

Recovery activities and objectives are targeted at all components of society. This includes not only repair and reconstruction of physical structures, but also recovery from the economic, social, and psychological effects of the disaster. This means that disaster recovery is built into the planning and response phase. Available resources (human and material) are first targeted toward survival and then toward regaining an acceptable level of normality within the community.

Within the health care facility, one area is converted to a communications room for internal and external use. Communication generated from the health care facility is limited to essential transmissions only. A media representative is also needed to work from the communications area. This is necessary because people's need for information may override the need for accuracy in reporting, resulting in a worsening situation of public anxiety.

Humanitarian Aid and Professionals

International aid workers usually are sent to an emergency or disaster by individual United Nations or nongovernmental organizations. International responders are professionals, specially trained in international humanitarian response. Most have at least a bachelor-level education in their profession, with additional training or experience in the international context. In the health sector, doctors, nurses, anesthesiologists, midwives, and nurse practitioners are needed to fulfill the roles and responsibilities created by complex emergencies such as conflict and disaster.

Surgical technologists may enter the field of international aid. Because few people are deployed for a given disaster, all aid professionals are required to have extensive experience, professional training, or both. One person may be required to do the job of three people, with cross-cutting responsibilities within the team. Top coordinators in the specific sectors (e.g., medical, logistics, shelter, nutrition) usually are master's level trained with additional certification in security, team management, and other sectors according to their role.

The minimum entry degree for health responders is the bachelor of nursing with certifications in tropical medicine and/or public health in disaster. Health professionals are managed by the agencies that contract with them for a disaster.

> Further information on international relief resources and career opportunities is available at the website http://reliefweb.int. This is the designated website for the United Nations Office for Coordination of Humanitarian Affairs. A mirror site can be accessed by searching for "Relief web."

ETHICAL DILEMMAS IN DISASTER

We observe the best and worst in human behavior during a disaster. Communities all around the world pull together when there is a common threat. People are often surprised at the level of personal sacrifice and courage seen in emergency situations. In fact, it is very common for people to empathize with others and to offer comfort, shelter, and sustenance. But there is another side of disaster that reveals the tragedy of choice, perceived need, and perceived loss. Here are some examples of situations in which these issues become very real:

1. Marginalized populations such as those living in poverty, older adults, physically and mentally challenged, and chronically ill are often invisible during a disaster. Their needs have not been preplanned. They cannot advocate for themselves and rely on others to advocate for them. If the social and political will is not there, they may be forgotten in a crisis.
2. People who have immediate access to disaster assistance are helped first. If disaster assistance is unable to reach all the people who need aid, those who can travel are better able to travel to the assistance.
3. Individuals' perceived needs are often very different from each other. The perception of what is essential for survival or even comfort may be far above or below what the reality of the situation can provide or that agencies should provide.
4. Disaster assistance agencies and managers must make choices during mass disaster. Who should be rescued first? What criteria are used? What priority should be given to aiding animals?
5. Should people be compensated by the government for loss that occurred during a disaster?
6. In multiple disasters within a state or region, how can we decide where to place resources?

These questions and many more are often debated publicly by community leaders, emergency and disaster specialists, and ethicists. Students involved in disaster response should debate the legal and ethical implications of these issues to explore or provide clarity about one's personal convictions and to understand those of others.

RESOURCES FOR STUDENTS AND INSTRUCTORS

In appreciation of the need for resources on disaster plans and disaster management in the classroom, the following list is provided to assist surgical technologist students, instructors, and others who need quick access to essential, trustworthy information, including online training courses. In most cases the title of the document describes the content. Where it is not clear, a brief explanation is provided. Each website has been assessed for relevance to the CAAHEP requirements:

- Division of Homeland Security and Emergency Services
  Provides federal and state planning documents, training, and other resources.
  http://www.dhses.ny.gov/planning
- FEMA Emergency Management Institute
  Training courses online and on site
  http://training.fema.gov/EMIWeb/IS/is100HCb.asp
- FEMA Introduction to the Incident Command System for Healthcare/Hospitals
  Training course online
  http://emilms.fema.gov/IS100hcb/index.htm
- Institute for Disaster and Emergency Preparedness
  All-hazards courses online
  https://nova.edu/idep/indix.html
- National Incident Management System
  Training Program, September 2011
  http://www.fema.gov/pdf/emergency/nims/nims_training_program.pdf
- FEMA National Preparedness Directorate
  Online course catalogue
  http://www.fema.gov/pdf/emergency/nims/nims_training_program.pdf
- FEMA, developing and maintaining emergency operations plans
  Comprehensive Preparedness Guide (CGP) 101 version 2.0 September 2010
  http://www.fema.gov/pdf/about/divisions/npd/CPG_101_V2.pd
- FEMA, Emergency Management Institute
  Independent Study Program
  http://training.fema.gov/IS/isfaqdetails.asp?id=2&cat=General

- Department of Homeland Security, National Response Framework, 2008
  The federal document for all disasters
  http://www.fema.gov/pdf/emergency/nrf/nrf-core.pdf
- Centers for Disease Control and Prevention, Preparing and Responding to Specific Hazards
  http://www.bt.cdc.gov/hazards-specific.asp
- NOVA Institute for Disaster and Emergency Preparedness
  Provides courses, education, and training for groups. Works with all major disaster agencies.
  http://www.nova.edu/idep/index.html
- U.S. Department of Health and Human Services, CDC, Public Health Emergency Response Guide for State, Local, and Tribal Public Health Directors. Version 2.0, April 2011
  Explains local preparedness and planning in detail
  http://www.bt.cdc.gov/planning/pdf/cdcresponseguide.pdf
- FEMA, Incident Command System (ICS)
  http://www.fema.gov/emergency/nims/IncidentCommand System.shtm#item2
- The International Disaster Database, Centre for Research on the Epidemiology of Disasters (CRED)
  Epidemiology of past disasters, including disaster profiles, lists, and trends
  http://www.emdat.be/result-disaster-profiles?period =1900%242011&disgroup=group&dis_type='Complex +Disasters'%24Complex+Disasters&Submit=Display+ Disaster+Profile

KEY CONCEPTS

- Disasters overwhelm local resources and require outside assistance.
- An important factor that distinguishes a disaster from an emergency is that an emergency is a geographically isolated event that can be handled by local health and emergency services.
- A mass casualty event is a localized emergency, such as a transportation accident (e.g., major air crash), explosion, or structural collapse, in which the number of victims overwhelms local health care services.
- The two main categories of disasters are natural disasters and human-made disasters.
- Natural disasters are caused by forces of nature, such as a hurricane, a tornado, an earthquake, floods, and extreme heat or cold.
- Human-made disasters are the result of intentional or unintentional human action, such as technical accidents (e.g., chemical or radiation disasters) and terrorist and conflict-related disasters.
- Although many different types of disasters can occur, they often have common characteristics because they affect individuals and the community in general.
- Vulnerable populations are those with a particularly high risk for injury or harm as a result of a disaster.
- Federal and local agencies are responsible for the management of a disaster. The Federal Emergency Management Agency is responsible for overall coordination and management of nationally declared disasters.
- Only a disaster that is a declared state of emergency by the governor of the state where the disaster occurred qualifies for FEMA assistance.
- The National Incident Management System is a set of guidelines that defines the management structure, objectives, and chain of command during a disaster.
- At the state level, disasters are managed by that state's emergency management agency.
- The all-hazards approach is a disaster management strategy that emphasizes the common elements of all types of disasters. It is defined by four phases: mitigation, preparedness, response, and recovery.
- Mitigation or risk reduction is a process or activity that minimizes the impact of a disaster.
- The preparation phase of a disaster includes numerous coordinated activities with the common goal of ensuring that individuals, communities, and government sectors can respond effectively to a variety of different types of disasters.
- The objective of disaster response is to prevent injuries and loss of life and to protect against property loss.
- Evacuation is a way of moving people away from a disaster to prevent catastrophic morbidity and mortality.
- The alternative to evacuation is shelter-in-place, in which people remain where they are (usually in a building or other structure) in a relatively safe location within the structure.
- Currently, no national standard exists for training health care professionals in the all-hazards approach to disaster preparedness. Allied health and other professionals can increase their ability to respond to disaster and mass casualty events by taking specific courses in disaster management.
- Primary care and allied health professionals usually assist in a disaster by performing their normal role and occasionally by performing tasks that are outside their usual job description but not outside their scope of practice.
- Surgical technologists are trained in a variety of professional skills that are needed during a disaster. The specific role of the surgical technologist may be determined at the time of the disaster.
- International disasters include all the elements of a disaster in developed countries, as well as other constraints and complexities, such as conflict, war, and an unstable or failed government.
- In the health sector, doctors, nurses, anesthesiologists, midwives, and nurse practitioners are needed to fulfill the roles and duties created by complex emergencies, such as conflict and natural disaster.

REVIEW QUESTIONS

1. What are some of the differences between a disaster and an emergency?
2. Differentiate between a natural disaster and a human-made disaster.
3. Define *state of emergency*. What government official declares a state of emergency, and why is this done?

4. What is the all-hazards approach to disaster preparedness and management?
5. Define *mitigation*. Give several examples of mitigation in natural disaster management.
6. What is an incident command system? Why is this used during a disaster?

CASE STUDY

Case 1

An earthquake has occurred with the epicenter approximately 50 miles from your workplace. You hear on the radio that all primary health care and allied health care employees should be on standby for immediate duty. You receive a call to come into the facility and remain on duty there for an "indefinite period of time." You will be staying at the hospital until the first phase of the disaster has passed. How will you prepare yourself mentally for this assignment? Can you predict what coping mechanisms you will use to respond to the coming days of work, which will bring an unusual level of fatigue and stress?

Case 2

One of the important issues to consider in disaster planning is "altered care." Currently, a debate is going on among disaster professionals and health care workers about the reality of health and care standards in the disaster environment. The Agency for Healthcare Research and Quality has stated that to save as many people as possible during a disaster, compromises in health care delivery are necessary; this is called "altered care." The AHRQ points out that this may mean restricting medical supplies to certain types of patients or using ventilators only for surgical patients. It also might mean compromise in normal isolation techniques. In some disasters, two or more surgical patients might be operated on side-by-side in the same operating room. If you were asked to discuss this topic among your peers, what would you add to the discussion? This is both an ethical and a technical discussion. What is your opinion about what surgical practices could be altered during a disaster?

Extensive research on this topic is available at http://www.ahrq.gov/research/altstand/altstand2.htm.

Case 3

Discuss the significance of having an incident command system structure during a disaster or mass casualty event. Top-down management has advantages and disadvantages. Discuss these in detail. Apply any previous experience you have had with management in analyzing a possible disaster scenario in which all major decisions come from one central location. What would happen if you overrode the system and ignored a few directives (even though you believe it to be in the best interest of the patients)?

Case 4

You are employed by a busy medical center as a certified surgical technologist and team manager for orthopedics. Your supervisor notifies you that you must attend 2-day training on disaster preparedness. Your colleagues, who must also attend, do not want to "waste" the time and feel that the information is too far removed from day-to-day practice. What response in favor of disaster preparedness will you give them? How would you encourage others to become more engaged in the training?

BIBLIOGRAPHY

Agency for Health Care Research and Quality (AHRQ): *Mass medical care with scarce resources: a community planning guide.* AHRQ Pub. No. 07-0001, February 2007. Accessed September 26, 2011, at http://www.ahrq.gov/research/mce.

American Medical Association/American Public Health Association (AMA/APHA): *Improving health system preparedness for terrorism and mass casualty events.* Accessed September 26, 2011, at http://www.ama-assn.org/resources/doc/cphpdr/final_summit_report.pdf

American Nurses Association: *Adapting standards of care under extreme conditions: guidance for professionals during disasters, pandemics, and other extreme emergencies,* Columbia School of Nursing, New York, 2008, American Nurses Association.

Association of periOperative Registered Nurses (AORN): AORN guidance statement: mass casualty, triage, and evacuation, *AORN Journal* 85:792–800, 2011.

Centers for Disease Control and Prevention: *Public health preparedness: strengthening CDC's emergency response: a CDC report on terrorism preparedness and emergency response (TPER)-funded activities.* Accessed September 26, 2011, at http://emergency.cdc.gov/publications/jan09phprep/index.asp.

Columbia University Mailman School of Public Health: Available at http://www.ncdp.mailman.columbia.edu/index.html

Coppola D: *Introduction to international disaster management,* Oxford, 2007, Butterworth-Heinemann.

Department of Homeland Security: *National response framework, 2008.* Accessed September 26, 2011, at http://www.fema.gov/pdf/emergency/nrf/nrf-core.pdf.

Health Systems Research: *Altered standards of care in mass casualty events.* AHRQ Pub. No. 05-0043. April 2005. Accessed September 27, 2011, at http://www.facs.org/trauma/disaster/pdf/standards_care.pdf.

Hsu E, Thomas T, Bass E, et al: Health care worker competencies for disaster training, *BMC Medical Education* 6:19, 2006.

New York State Emergency Management Office: *Emergency planning guide for community officials, 2008.* Available at http://www.dhses.ny.gov/oem/planning/documents/Planning-Guide.pdf.

Markenson D, DiMaggio C, Redliner I: Preparing health professions students for terrorism, disaster, and public health emergencies: core competencies, *Academic Medicine* June, 2005. Available at http://www.proteusfund.org/files/pdfs/Terrorism%20Or%20All-Hazards.pdf.

Occupational Safety and Health Administration: *OSHA disaster site worker training program.* Available at http://www.osha.gov/SLTC/emergencypreparedness/index.html.

U.S. Department of Health and Human Services, CDC: *Public health emergency response guide for state, local, and tribal public health directors.* Version 2.0, April 2011. Available at http://www.bt.cdc.gov/planning/pdf/cdcresponseguide.pdf.

6

The Patient

CHAPTER OUTLINE

Introduction
Fundamental Human
  Needs—Maslow

Therapeutic Communication
Cultural Competence

Spiritual Needs of the Patient
Special Patient Populations

LEARNING OBJECTIVES

After studying this chapter the reader will be able to:

1. Define patient-centered and outcome-oriented care
2. List and discuss human needs as described in Maslow's hierarchy
3. Describe human basic physiological needs
4. Discuss common psychological needs of the surgical patient and family

5. Demonstrate appropriate communication with the surgical patient
6. Define cultural competence and discuss its importance in ethics and health care
7. Define spirituality as it applies to patient care
8. Identify special patient populations and needs

TERMINOLOGY

Body image: The way an individual perceives himself or herself physically in the eyes of others.

Cultural competence: The ability to communicate with people of other cultures and belief systems. Health institutions are required to provide access to resources for achieving and promoting cultural competence.

Elimination: The physiological process of removing cellular and chemical waste products from the body.

Maslow's hierarchy of human needs: A model of human achievement and self-actualization developed by psychologist Abraham Maslow.

Mobility: The ability of an organism to move. As a protective mechanism, mobility allows an organism to move away from harmful stimuli.

Nutrition: Usually refers to the intake of food by an organism.

Patient-centered care: Therapeutic care, communication, and intervention provided according to the unique needs of the patient and centered on those needs.

Physiological: Refers to the biochemical and metabolic processes of an organism.

Reflection: Communication with the patient that helps the individual connect his or her current feelings with events in the environment.

Therapeutic communication: A purposeful method of communication in which the caregiver responds to explicit or implicit needs of the patient.

INTRODUCTION

As a member of the patient care team in the operating room, the surgical technologist directly contributes to the patient's physical and psychological well-being. Patients undergoing surgery are often fearful and worried, not only about the outcome of the surgery, but also about the process that they cannot control during the perioperative period. Patients undergoing general anesthesia are more likely to feel anxiety than those having a local anesthetic. The surgical technologist has many opportunities to help the patient through this difficult process during the preoperative period, transport, circulating duties, and outpatient care.

Understanding and empathy for the patient evolve from knowledge of the patient's physical and psychological needs. Every patient is unique, and a positive surgical outcome depends on patient-centered care that is holistic—that is, takes into account many different dimensions of care. In **patient-centered care**, the surgical team bases its assessments, planning, and interventions on the patient as an individual. These unique needs are revealed through information from others, the patient's records, astute observation, and good communication with patients themselves.

FUNDAMENTAL HUMAN NEEDS—MASLOW

In the 1970s, psychologist Abraham Maslow developed a theory about human needs. His model, known as **Maslow's hierarchy of human needs**, is depicted as a triangular hierarchy in which the critical needs to preserve life are at the base levels (Figure 6-1) and other needs that create emotional, social, and spiritual fulfillment flow upward. This model is still used to describe fundamental human needs. The most basic of human needs are **physiological**—that is, they involve the biochemical, mechanical, and physical processes of life (Table 6-1). According to Maslow's model, the most basic requirements for life must be fulfilled in order for the higher levels to be achieved. Maslow's model provides an excellent guide for patient care and a method of prioritizing the patient's needs.

PHYSIOLOGICAL DOMAINS

Physiological needs, also called *life functions*, are those that sustain life. In the patient care environment, enabling life functions takes priority over all other needs. Life functions are:

- **Respiration:** The act of breathing and taking in oxygen. Without the exchange of oxygen for carbon dioxide, cells and tissue cannot survive.
- **Nutrition:** This is the process of taking in food for energy, growth, and repair. It includes the intake of essential electrolytes to maintain cellular function.
- **Transport:** The body must be able to transport substances to tissues and cells. This is accomplished by the circulatory system. We can see the result of lack of transport in ischemic disease, where inability of the vessels to carry oxygen results in tissue necrosis. In diabetes, absence of insulin, which regulates the transport of glucose to cells, results in serious metabolic disturbances.

- **Excretion:** Waste products are produced as a result of normal metabolism. These must be shunted from the tissues that produce them out of the body. Without excretion, the buildup of metabolic wastes results in severe toxicity. This is seen in kidney disease, in which the body's normal filtering and excretion system is unable to remove toxic cellular waste materials which may lead to death. Carbon dioxide is a waste product that is excreted through exhaled breaths. Retention of carbon dioxide results in hypercapnia, which can be life-threatening.
- **Reproduction:** This applies not only to the species, but also to cellular reproduction, which is necessary for tissue growth and repair.
- **Growth:** This includes the normal growth and development from infancy to adulthood and also the growth of cells and body systems. Growth is also repair of tissues following disease or tissue trauma, including the tissue trauma of a surgical procedure.
- **Repair:** Repair is the process that occurs following illness and trauma. Unless the body is overwhelmed by the disease or trauma, new tissues develop to replace those that have been damaged, and the body's immune system provides the chemical processes needed to initiate recovery.
- **Movement:** The body must be able to react to harmful conditions in the environment. This is apparent when we approach a hot surface or perceive irritating fumes in the air. We immediately withdraw from the source. Patients

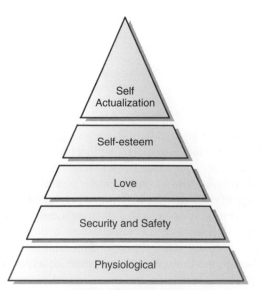

Figure 6-1 Maslow's hierarchy of human needs.

Table 6-1	Basic Physiological Needs of the Patient
Type of Need	**How Needs Are Met in the Perioperative Environment**
Nutrition, water	Administration of intravenous replacement fluids and nutritive or electrolyte fluids
Shelter	Control of temperature through cloth blankets, air heating, or cooling blankets
Air and oxygen	Maintenance of an open airway
	Provision of the proper mix of oxygen with anesthetic or room air
	Attention to signs of oxygen deficit
Rest and sleep	Protection from environmental stress such as noise, light, or cold
Elimination	Catheterization or opportunity to void as needed
	Medical attention to conditions that prevent elimination
Movement	Freedom from restraint and assistance with movement when patient is unable to move on his or her own
	Protecting the patient from harm
Freedom from pain	Observation of the patient for signs of pain
	Administration of pain medication
	Exercise of care when moving the patient

undergoing general anesthesia are unable to withdraw from pain. This is why meticulous care is required in patient positioning and in the use of medical devices such as warm air blankets or a pneumatic tourniquet, which can cause serious injury during surgery.

SECURITY

Security is the absence of perceived and real physical or psychological harm. In the physical realm, people need to be safe from any threat to their well-being. Threatening psychological events can contribute to illness and anxiety and can diminish the ability to make decisions, have relationships with others, and care for one's self. Surgical patients need to trust in those who care for them, not only for comfort and a sense of well-being, but also to reduce stress that can prolong recovery after surgery. High levels of anxiety before surgery contribute to alterations in physiological processes, including to anesthesia and adjunct drugs. It has been demonstrated that patients experiencing extreme anxiety in the preoperative period are more likely to have problems such as delirium as they emerge from general anesthesia. Anxiety is also linked to increased requirements for postoperative analgesia and contributes to poor communication between patient and caregiver.

Fear of surgery can be complex, involving previous social and emotional experiences. Many patients approach their surgery with anxiety and fear. Even though a patient may understand the objectives of the surgery, emotions can overwhelm this understanding.

Reassurance and open acknowledgment of the patient's fears are good methods of communicating empathy. The patient feels greater security when team members explain, honestly and professionally, what is occurring and why, in a way that is not overly technical or dismissive of the patient's fears. For example, the patient safety strap is secured as soon as the patient is transferred to the operating table. Rather than saying jokingly, "I'm putting this strap on so you don't get away" it is better to use reassuring statements, such as, "The operating bed is very narrow. I'm putting this strap over your legs to remind you to stay centered on the bed." This statement acknowledges that a safety issue exists and it is being addressed.

Common Patient Fears

Patients share many common fears:

- **Anesthesia:** Many patients fear that they will not awaken from the anesthetic or that they will feel pain while remaining paralyzed (called *anesthesia awareness*). Although this condition is real, it has been given a great deal of attention by the media and depicted in fictional broadcasts. This has created a public fear that is unwarranted. The anesthesia care provider normally explains the process during the anesthesia history and physical and can anticipate fears of anesthesia awareness, even if the patient does not ask about it directly. An empathetic anesthetist or anesthesiologist can relieve many of the patient's anxieties related to the anesthetic agents, physiological care during anesthesia, and the experience of emergence from general anesthesia.

- **Death:** Fear of death during or after surgery is common among patients. This fear often is greater in a patient who is about to receive a general anesthetic. The concept of being held unconscious and in another's control increases feelings of impending death.

- **Pain:** Fear of pain is a normal protective mechanism. However, surgical patients sometimes have extreme fear of postoperative pain. They might not have sufficient information about their postoperative care, or they may have experienced severe pain in the past.

- **Disfigurement:** Patients undergoing radical or reconstructive surgery have realistic fears about disfigurement. Body image is a very important psychological consideration. People identify themselves with the way they perceive their looks, which often influences their ability to relate to others. Disfigurement is attached to social stigma and rejection, which are powerful triggers for fear and anxiety. Patients undergoing radical cosmetic surgery or reconstructive procedures of the face can be particularly fearful of disfigurement. Adolescents are also very concerned about body image and the physical changes brought about by surgery.

- **Loss of control:** When patients enter the health care system, they often feel a loss of personal rights and control. For the surgical patient, these feelings are intensified with the anesthesia experience. The patient may also anticipate immobilization as a result of pain or loss of function. Whereas some patients are quite stoic about their surgery, others may act regressive, exhibiting childlike behaviors including helplessness.

- **Physical exposure:** The fear of physical exposure of the body is quite strong in many patients, especially adolescents. This fear can be eased by maintaining the patient's dignity at all times, covering the body unless absolutely necessary for a procedure.

- **Loss of privacy:** Many patients are afraid that information about their health may not be held in confidence. They fear that the information may result in loss of employment or that it will injure their relationships with others. The ethical responsibility to hold all patient information in strict confidence cannot be overemphasized. (Refer to Chapter 3 for a more complete discussion of patient privacy.)

SOCIAL DOMAINS

Love, Belonging, and Acceptance

Love and belonging are powerful needs. They determine our sense of well-being through others' acceptance and nurturing. Love and belonging affirm our humanity and provide emotional fulfillment. Social and medical science research has demonstrated that a sense of belonging has a dramatic effect on physical and emotional health. People who are actively involved in their community and family experience a sense of connectedness that is demonstrated in good health and even longevity. Social and personal support seems to have a positive effect on the immune system and seems to decrease stress, which is a determinant of many diseases.

Family support of the patient is extremely important during illness. The surgical patient is often accompanied in the preoperative period by family members and partners, who wait for them during the procedure and postoperative recovery period. The support and care of family and friends is reassuring and healing. Family members may accompany the patient as he or she is taken to the operating room. The moment of separation can be very emotional. A professional, caring attitude toward both patients and family is important for all.

Feelings of acceptance or being accepted contribute to a healthy ego and the ability to pursue goals and objectives in life. Illness can result in loss of employment or an unexpected change in vocation, resulting in a lower income. Western media focuses on social acceptance based on youth and appearance. Surgery that is disfiguring or results in disability can threaten the patient's sense of acceptance by their family and community. Even undergoing surgery to create a more youthful or aesthetic appearance can create preoperative anxiety related to uncertainty about the outcome.

Self-Esteem and Self-Image

Maslow's model includes self-esteem and self-image, because our perception of ourselves influences motivation and relationships, both social and personal. The restrictions imposed by illness and recovery on the patient's ability to pursue self-defining activities can be a great source of anxiety. Self-image is closely associated with body image. **Body image** is the way we perceive ourselves physically in the eyes of others. When we are comfortable with our body image, we feel good about ourselves. When a person's body image is altered suddenly or is perceived to be altered, feelings of embarrassment, rejection, and isolation can arise. Patients who need counseling to adjust to sudden changes in their appearance can be guided to support groups or trained specialists.

Self-image is dependent not only on physical appearance but also on people's normal roles within their family and community. Patients may view their roles of responsibility as severely threatened or changed by their inability to carry out certain physical or mental functions as a result of illness and surgery. The parental role, care of the household, and reproductive role may become difficult or blurred by illness. People also identify with groups that give them a sense of belonging and of being needed. Sports activities, clubs, or even solitary pursuits that are important to the patient may suddenly become unavailable to them because of illness. The needs of a patient in a health care facility cannot be met in the same way the patient might be accustomed to in day-to-day life. This can be very distressing to the patient.

Self-Actualization

Self-actualization is the highest level of Maslow's model. It is the individual's ability to plan and achieve his or her life goals based on the physical, social, and psychological freedom to pursue those achievements. Personal goals are whatever that person defines as a goal or an achievement. They are unique and usually highly valued by each individual. The frustration and grief many patients feel during illness is related to their actual or perceived inability to achieve goals because of their

illness. Surgical patients are vulnerable to this risk because of the added psychological burden of altered body image or loss of function. This can be related to the surgery itself or to the illness that requires the surgery. Perioperative caregivers can help their patients through this difficult situation by understanding the meaning of individual loss.

COPING WITH ILLNESS AND SURGERY

The patient's personal experiences through illness and surgery are unique to the individual. Patients' reactions to illness and therapeutic interventions depend on previous experiences with illness, cultural factors, age (or more specifically, developmental stage in life), knowledge about their condition, and resilience to stress. An important role of all health care providers is assisting patients to cope with their illness. Surgical technologists in different health care settings have varying levels of social and professional contact with patients. In some settings the surgical technologist may have only brief encounters with patients, whereas in others, contact is extensive. Regardless of how brief or extended the professional relationship is, the surgical technologist can anticipate the patient's immediate needs through verbal and nonverbal cues.

Preparation for patient support includes exploring one's own attitudes and beliefs that might interfere with support (therapeutic) communication. Professional development in this area can be transforming for the health professional. Some of the more important attitudes that need to be explored are:

- What are my own beliefs about how to cope with stress?
- What are my beliefs about disability?
- How do I normally act around older adults in the community?
- What are my personal opinions about morbidly obese individuals?
- Do I like children? Do I like being around them?
- What are my assumptions about blind people? Do I assume they need my help in the community?
- What do I know about people who are traumatized? How much of this knowledge is based on what I've seen in the popular media (e.g., TV, movies)?
- Do I know how I would cope if faced with a life-threatening disease?
- What is my attitude toward immigrants, illegal or otherwise?
- What are my core beliefs about faith and spirituality?

It is difficult for anyone to step outside their own beliefs and attitudes and walk in the other's shoes. But in health care, this is required. Professionals explore their own attitudes in order to monitor themselves—to learn about the realities of others in society so they can avoid stereotyping and prejudice. It is a process that requires continual attention if we truly want to be health professionals.

THERAPEUTIC COMMUNICATION

Today's health care system often requires surgical facilities to perform as many procedures as possible in a 24-hour period. The surgical patient is in the center of a storm of activity, in a very busy environment that is frightening and authoritative. Patients have little or no control over what is happening and are handed from one person to the next, often with no knowledge about the roles of the people involved in their care.

Perioperative personnel can alleviate some of the patient's fears and concerns by using **therapeutic communication**. This is a specific way of relating to a patient that encourages him or her to express any concerns, and responds to those concerns with empathy and support.

- Even if the encounter is brief, using therapeutic communication skills will contribute to a positive surgical outcome by helping the patient through the perioperative experience.
- Listen to the patient attentively. Show your interest by making eye contact (unless this is culturally inappropriate; e.g., in traditional Islamic cultures, women do not make direct eye contact with men).
- Explain what you are doing in plain, simple language. Look for cues that the patient understands. Do not assume that because the message was given, it was also received and comprehended.
- Continual questioning can make a person feel uncomfortable. Therapeutic communication allows patients to express needs and concerns at their own pace.
- Do not talk about yourself. It is inappropriate for team members to share personal information with the patient or with coworkers in the presence of the patient.
- Joking and offensive language can have serious effects on the patient's sense of security. Although it is not meant to offend the patient, it is not only disconcerting but also unprofessional. Would you want to hear the details of someone's date while waiting to have abdominal surgery for cancer?
- Refer questions when you do not know the answers. Be honest about what you do not know. Patients often are unaware of the professional roles of their caretakers. If you are asked a medical question or one that requires assessment or other specialized skills, refer the question to licensed personnel. Ask the patient if he or she has discussed the issue with the physician. It is better to delay an answer than to mislead or give information that is outside the scope of one's role.

TECHNIQUES IN THERAPEUTIC COMMUNICATION

- **Active listening:** Make eye contact (as appropriate within the patient's culture) and listen attentively. Do not allow yourself to be distracted while communicating with the patient. If your attention is split, you may convey a lack of concern.
- **Providing information:** Although some patients do not want to know the details of their surgery, most are eager to understand what is occurring around them. Look and listen for cues that the patient needs information. He or she may not ask specific questions, but instead show concern or worry about some aspect of the environment.
  Example: "I'm here to escort you to surgery. I'll also be assisting during the procedure."

- **Focusing:** The health care provider stays on point. He or she focuses on crucial communication that can affect the outcome of care.
  Example: "I see on your chart that you didn't want to remove your wedding ring. Is it difficult to remove, or is it important that you keep it even during surgery?
- **Paraphrasing and restatement:** This is restating what the patient has said, using different wording.
  Example: "When you say that no one is at home to help you, you mean that no preparations have been made to help you with daily activities like preparing meals after your surgery?"
- **Clarifying:** The health care professional needs to clearly understand what the patient is saying or implying.
  Example: "Does your aunt plan to wait for you here, or should I show her where the surgical waiting area is?"
- **Reflection:** Patients may comment on their surroundings to communicate uneasiness or fear. Sometimes an abrupt comment requires the caregiver to reflect on what the problem might be. In the following example, the patient is trying to express discomfort and perhaps fear. A skilled caregiver understands that the patient is not only cold but also angry about being helpless in this situation and unable to meet his or her own environmental needs. The caregiver acknowledges the patient's frustration and responds appropriately.
  Example: Patient: "It's always so cold in these places. With all the money these hospitals make, the least they could do is turn up the heat."
  Response: "The temperature is low for safety reasons. I'll get you a warm blanket."

CULTURAL COMPETENCE

Cultural competence is the ability to communicate and interact with people of different cultures and beliefs. Health care providers were among the first professionals to recognize the need for cultural competence. Meeting a patient's needs depends on good communication, trust, and respect for the other's values. Culture is not only a difference of ethnicities, language, and faith systems. It also includes subcultures related to specific developmental stages (particularly within adolescent populations) and sectors of society that are marginalized because of poverty, disability, addiction, and homelessness.

Knowledge about the different cultures in one's community is the beginning of study in cultural competence, but it does not cover all situations. Appreciation of diversity does not necessarily lead to cultural competence. Lists of cultural beliefs might not be valid for all people in that cultural group. This type of information can be helpful, but we risk stereotyping by relying on such lists. There are other ways that health professionals can develop cultural competence, starting with communication skills.

Communication between health care professionals and patients touches on the rights of people to be treated equally, regardless of their beliefs, economic situation, age, or physical or psychological state. The Joint Commission has initiated a program of patient-centered communication that requires all accredited hospitals to provide the means of communication to all patients, including those who speak languages other than English. Those health care facilities that fail to institute patient-centered communication access will risk losing accreditation after January 2012. The standards address the implications of patient safety, basic ethical and legal rights to understand their condition and treatment, and further marginalization of groups that cannot communicate easily because of language, disability, mental, or physical status.

Cultural competence is proactive. It establishes real methods to help patients access the care they need and exercise their right to knowledge, understanding, and participation in decisions that affect their health. The three components are attitudes, knowledge, and skills. Whereas diversity training that instills appreciation and respect for people of different cultures has been available for many years, cultural competence is less familiar as a form of study in which people not only are sensitized to the rights of diverse populations, but also acquire skills and methods to ensure quality health care across diverse groups. Students and employees can and should advocate for training in this area. Box 6-1 lists resources for instructors and students who want to pursue training in this important area of patient care.

SPIRITUAL NEEDS OF THE PATIENT

Spirituality is a sense or understanding of something more profound than humanity that is not perceived by the physical senses. Spirituality is not necessarily the same as religion, although they often are expressed as one entity. It is an awareness or belief in an energy or power greater than humankind. This power may be referred to as creator, spirit, or God, or the patient may have no name for it. In the religious setting, spiritual life is integrated into rituals (practices that have special meaning) and ceremonies common to those who practice a particular faith. Patients often express their religious faith in the health care setting through prayer or other rituals that are sacred in their faith. Ritual defines life-changing events and is important to physical and mental healing. For many it *is* the healing force. Many health professionals avoid becoming involved in the spiritual needs of the patient because they are uncomfortable or perhaps have not faced this dimension of

care in the past. With today's short-stay practices, patients can come into the health care facility and leave the same day, even after complex procedures. In this environment, caregivers do not have the opportunity to become familiar with spiritual practices and enable patients to express themselves in the health care setting.

Patients may bring religious items into the health care setting that reinforce their faith and provide a source of strength. These may be items that assist in prayer, icons, religious jewelry, and prayer books. It is very important to safeguard these items to prevent their loss. Jewelry may not be worn in surgery in which electrosurgery will be used. If a patient is reluctant to remove an item, the caregiver explains carefully what the risks are. Whenever possible, a family member can take care of the jewelry until the patient returns from surgery.

All operating room staff should learn where prayer areas are in their facility and how to contact the facility's chaplain in the event that spiritual support is requested.

The disposition of body parts is very important in many faiths, which require the special burial of any tissue removed from the body. Hospital policy usually prevents tissue from being released to the public for reasons of public health. It is best to check with hospital policy on this issue.

Practicing Jehovah's Witnesses do not allow administration of blood or blood products or storage of their own blood for later transfusion. Most members of the church are familiar with the problems that can arise with caring for minors who require blood transfusion. This is a dual legal and medical problem with which church spokespersons and doctors are very familiar. Adults do have the right to refuse blood products, and this is respected by the medical community.

SPECIAL PATIENT POPULATIONS

THE PEDIATRIC PATIENT

The pediatric patient presents particular challenges in both communication and the physiological response to surgery. Pediatric patient groups are defined according to approximate chronological age ranges. The age group reflects the developmental stage, as shown in Table 6-2.

Physiological Considerations

In pediatric patients, the size of anatomical structures, the relative fragility of the body, and the ratio of surface area to

Box **6-1**	Resources for Teaching and Learning Cultural Competence in Health Care

- *Diversity, improving health care for a diverse world.* Available at http://www.diversityrx.org.
- American Medical Association: *Ethical force program.* Available at http://www.ethicalforce.org.
- Gilbert M, ed: *Principles and recommended standards for cultural competence education of health care professionals.* Prepared for the California Endowment. Available at http://www.calendow.org/uploadedFiles/principles_standards_cultural_competence.pdf.
- Cultural Competence 101, in *Diversityrx.org.* Available at http://www.diversityrx.org/topic-areas/cultural-competence-101.

Table **6-2**	Pediatric Age Groups
Development Stage	**Age Range**
Infant	Birth to 18 months
Toddler	19 months to 3 years
Preschool	4 to 6 years
School age	7 to 12 years
Adolescent	13 to 16 years

volume present particular risks for surgery. Loss of even a small amount of blood or fluid is severe in the pediatric patient. The large surface area compared to mass predisposes the patient to hypothermia or hyperthermia during surgery. This can result in excess fluid loss or hypoglycemia, especially in infants.

Developmental Stages

Children of different developmental stages have predictable fears, responses, and reactions to hospitalization and the process of surgery. Knowledge of these stages can help the surgical technologist understand the behaviors exhibited by children in the operating room.

Infants need to be physically close to their caretakers. They should be held as much as possible until the procedure begins. Stress is high in infant patients. They have been separated from the familiar feel, smell, and sight of their primary caregiver, and feedings have been stopped before surgery. For these reasons, they are difficult to comfort and may cry continually.

Toddlers suffer frustration and loss of autonomy, as well as extreme anxiety, when separated from their primary caretaker. The operating room environment can be terrifying to a toddler, who expresses this by crying and screaming or through aggression and regression (acting younger than his or her actual age group). Toddlers are especially difficult to restrain. They require patience and understanding from their caregivers. Stronger restraint (or more restrainers) usually causes more terror and increased resistance. Taking the time to instill calm is the humane way to provide medical intervention. When this is unsuccessful, rapid sedation may be required.

Preschoolers also suffer extreme fear in the operating room environment. These patients commonly view the hospital and surgical experience as a type of punishment or as deliberate abandonment. Prone to fantasy, they may imagine extreme mutilation as a result of surgery. Because they are unable to understand what the inside of the body actually looks like, they interpret descriptions of surgery literally. They are concrete thinkers and understand words such as cut, bleed, and stick in extreme, literal, and often exaggerated forms.

School-age children are more compliant and cooperative with health care personnel, but many tend to withdraw from their caregivers. They are curious about their bodies and often insist on "helping" with their own care. They are very sensitive about body exposure, which can be extremely stressful. For school-age children, receiving information is a way of coping with their fears. They welcome explanations and descriptions of how things work and how devices and equipment in the environment relate to their own bodies.

Adolescents are very sensitive about body image and changes in the body. They resent any intrusion on their privacy and bodily exposure. They also fear loss of control. At times stoic and curious, they are grateful for concrete information about the surgical environment and the procedure itself. Among their many concerns, potential loss of presence with their peers and fear of being "left out" because of illness or deformity are very important. A more extensive discussion on the needs of the pediatric patient can be found in Chapter 35.

THE OLDER PATIENT

The life expectancy of people living in the United States is expected to steadily increase over the next 10 years. The health care system has seen noticeable transformations in the quality and number of services for the older patient. These indicators demonstrate that older people themselves seek improved quality of life that is available to them with improved medications, surgical technology, and healthier lifestyles than in the past. Healthy aging is now an important part of all medical curricula in the United States.

The older patient approaching surgery has a number of important challenges that must be investigated before the final decision is made. These are both physiological and social. A successful surgical outcome depends on the patient's care after surgery as much as on the technical expertise employed during the procedure.

Social Considerations

Unless the surgery is an emergency procedure and the patient will remain in care for some time, an important consideration is whether the patient has help at home following the hospital stay. Will the patient be able to carry out routine daily activities called ADLs or *activities of daily living*? These include dressing, toileting, bathing, possibly cooking, and other simple, necessary tasks in the household. If the patient needs assistance in ADLs, this will be considered as part of the surgical plan. The preoperative assessment will also determine whether family or community members are available to assist the patient in the longer postoperative period. This is important both from a health and safety standpoint and also in resocialization of the patient in the community.

MOBILITY Older patients are carefully assessed for their level of **mobility**, both before surgery and the level to be expected after the procedure. Mobility can affect the risk of falls and the patient's access to emergency help if needed. This is part of the ADL evaluation but includes any history of sensory alterations, which increase the risk of falls.

NUTRITIONAL STATUS Older patients often have lost an acute sense of taste and smell, which is reflected in body weight. The patient may be undernourished or malnourished because of sensory problems or related to access to food. Many older people who are unable to use public transportation and lack community assistance simply do not get out of their homes to buy needed food. This is an increasing problem in communities in which older people are afraid to go outside because of local crime. Loss of essential nutrients leads to many different illnesses that further debilitate the older person.

COGNITIVE IMPAIRMENT Cognitive impairment can often be related to poor nutrition (lack of certain essential minerals), language barriers, anxiety, or true organic brain disease. A psychological assessment of the patient is performed to establish the nature of the impairment and to assess the risk of general anesthesia, which in some cases can cause prolonged impairment. Older patients who are cognitively impaired need special care to ensure that they understand the choices and decisions that must be made when surgery is planned. If they are unable to speak for themselves, the family or an appointed representative takes the responsibility. It is also important to distinguish between cognitive impairment and sensory impairment, which may affect the patient's ability to understand and communicate effectively.

The older patient may face many physical challenges in surgery. These are related to coexisting disease, nutritional status, metabolic balance, and risks associated with certain types of surgery (e.g., procedures involving major blood vessels, abdominal and thoracic conditions). Surgery that involves significant blood loss (e.g., hip replacement or repair) can also be high risk for the older patient.

The normal physiological alterations of aging (Table 6-3) often affect the decision on whether surgery should be performed. Some of the important areas of preoperative evaluation are listed below:

- The cardiovascular system loses elasticity, and circulation is often decreased, particularly to vital organs such as the kidneys and heart.
- The lung tissue loses elasticity. This can lead to postoperative pneumonia, which is among the most common hospital-acquired infections. Accessory muscles of the respiratory system may be atrophied, and spinal curvature can restrict movement.
- Decreased functioning of the digestive system and poor appetite can lead to low nutritional status both before and after surgery. Peristalsis is reduced in the gastrointestinal system, leading to slow stomach emptying and intestinal blockage. Absorption of nutrients is delayed or impaired.
- Kidney function may be significantly decreased in older patients. This can lead to electrolyte and fluid imbalance. Loss of sphincter control leads to urinary incontinence.
- Older patients are often very sensitive to anesthetic agents and other drugs, which must be carefully dosed to avoid adverse effects.

Chronic illness and stress can weaken the immune system necessary for a successful recovery from surgery. Older patients are at risk for skin, joint, muscle, and bone injury, especially during transfer and positioning. During the aging process, soft connective tissue loses tone, mass, and elasticity. This increases the risk of skeletal injury. The older patient's skin often is dry and extremely fragile. Decreased body fat increases the patient's risk for hypothermia. Decreased range of motion is accentuated in the older patient, and joints must be manipulated carefully during moving, handling, and positioning. These fragile conditions require increased vigilance and care in the perioperative environment. Transportation, transfer, and positioning are performed slowly under the direction of the anesthesia care provider or surgeon. The patient's core temperature must be maintained at all times before, during, and after surgery, and blood loss and urinary output must be monitored carefully.

Communicating with Older Patients

Recent recognition of negative communication practices among health care providers treating older patients has

Table 6-3	Physical Changes that Occur with Age
Body System	**Changes**
Respiratory	Chest diameter decreases from front to back (anterior to posterior). Blood oxygen level decreases. Lungs become more rigid and less elastic. Recoil of alveoli diminishes.
Gastrointestinal	Peristalsis diminishes. Liver loses storage capacity. Motility of stomach muscles decreases. Gag reflex diminishes.
Cardiovascular	Capillary walls thicken. Systolic blood pressure increases. Cardiac output decreases.
Musculoskeletal	Muscle strength decreases. Range of motion decreases. Cartilage decreases. Bone mass decreases.
Sensory perception	Progressive hearing loss occurs. Sense of smell diminishes. Pain threshold increases. Night vision decreases. Sensitivity to glare increases. Sense of body position in space (proprioception) can decrease.
Genitourinary	Bladder capacity diminishes. Stress incontinence in women occurs. Kidney filtration rate decreases. Reproductive changes occur in women: Vaginal secretions decrease. Estrogen levels decrease. Reproductive organs atrophy. Breast tissue decreases. Reproductive changes occur in men: Testosterone production decreases. Testicular size decreases. Sperm count decreases.
Skin	Skin loses turgor (elasticity). Sebaceous glands become less active. Skin becomes thin and delicate. Pigment changes occur.
Endocrine	Cortisol production decreases. Blood glucose level increases. Pancreas releases insulin at a slower rate.

brought needed attention to better care for the aging population. Along with an awareness of the need for more knowledge about the aging process, there is also more emphasis on the dignity of the older patient—teaching caregivers not to stereotype or make assumptions about their patients. One of the most important shifts in attitude involves *infantilizing* the adult—"treating the patient as a small child." This includes speech patterns that use short sentences with simple grammatical structures spoken in a high-pitched voice by the care provider. Research in this area has shown poor medical outcomes for patients who are exposed to this type of communication. Instead, health care providers are encouraged to speak to the older patient as they would to any adult and to clarify communication when necessary.

The following tips can be helpful when communicating with an older patient:

- Do not use clichés. Do not reach for the first available, easiest response. For example, if the patient says that she is a burden to others in her illness, do not respond with, "Oh, I'm sure you're no bother." Instead, support the patient in her feelings—for example, "It must be very difficult for you to have surgery right now."
- Do not refer to the patient by diminutives such as "sweetie" or "honey." These names are offensive to many patients. They convey a lack of respect for the patient as an adult with a lifetime of accomplishments and knowledge. Always address the patient by his or her proper name.
- Do not assume that the older patient is cognitively impaired. The normal aging process does not include dementia. Some patients are slightly disoriented in the hospital. Perioperative caregivers can help orient the patient by explaining procedures and identifying personnel in the environment.

THE PATIENT WITH A SENSORY DEFICIT

Sensory deficit is an alteration in one or more of the body's senses such as hearing, sight, touch, and smell that may result in the patient's inability to interpret the environment. The operating room environment can seem overwhelming to many patients and can be especially confusing to one with a sensory deficit. Hearing- and sight-impaired patients are often well adjusted to their usual environment but may experience anxiety in the operating room, which is often bright, busy, and noisy.

It is always a good idea to check the patient's chart before making assumptions about the level of impairment. Good communication also includes involving patients in their care by asking which side to approach them on, which is their better ear, and other environmental aids.

Hearing Impaired

Different types of hearing loss are associated with specific parts of the auditory system. There are three basic types—sensorineural, conductive, and mixed hearing loss. Each causes different kinds of deficits, which may include dizziness and poor balance. These are important physiological conditions that health professionals should be aware of in order to deliver safe care. The severity of the loss is described on a scale ranging from slight to profound. *Sensorineural* loss occurs with damage to the inner ear or nerves that conduct signals to the brain. In this type of loss, sounds are perceived as very faint even when the actual level of sound is high. Voices sound muffled or unclear. Sensorineural hearing loss is most common in the aging process but may also be caused by head trauma, malformation of the inner ear, or toxic drugs. *Conductive* hearing loss is the result of sound not being conducted through the outer ear, canal, eardrum, and ossicles. Common causes are infection, fluid in the middle ear, perforated eardrum, a foreign body in the ear, and absence or malformation of segments of the auditory system. In some auditory problems,

certain frequencies are blocked while others can be heard more clearly. Older patients often suffer from loss of upper frequencies, which makes communication difficult because speech is heard at these frequencies.

Caring for the patient with hearing deficit requires specific techniques. It is important to try and decrease ambient noise when communicating with the patient. Blocking out unnecessary environmental sounds increases the patient's ability to understand speech. Speak in a normal pitch and ask which is the good ear. Face the patient when speaking, and do not wear a surgical mask in areas that do not require one. Speak slowly and distinctly, and get the patient's attention before starting to speak. For patients who are profoundly deaf, an interpreter must be present. Writing is another method of communication, but it is best to find out ahead of time which method the patient prefers. Always allow hearing-impaired patients to keep their assistive devices as long as possible when they are being transported to the operating room. The anesthesia care provider may advise on this and ensure that hearing aids are kept secure and returned to the patient after surgery.

Sight Impaired

Visual impairment can take many forms, with specific associated problems. Clarity of vision is only one of the symptoms of sight deficit, which most people are familiar with—farsightedness and near-sightedness. Other conditions cause high sensitivity to glare and bright light, or darkness in portions of the field of vision. Peripheral vision may be lost so that only a small portion of the field of vision is seen, as if through a small hole. Glaucoma causes this type of deficit. In macular degeneration, the field of vision appears with a darkened or gray smudge that blots out images at the center of the field. Cataracts result in loss of visual sharpness, with images appearing as they might be seen through a lens coated with petroleum jelly. Diabetic retinopathy produces prominent areas of complete darkness in varying shapes and sizes in the vision. Retinitis pigmentosa results in a very small area of vision located in a mostly black field of sight.

Patients who have long-standing visual deficits have usually acclimated to their normal environments using visual aids, or even a guide dog for those with complete blindness. However, when a patient is challenged with a new environment, or if he or she has other sensory problems, the inability to see can be stressful. When assisting patients with sight deficit, orient the patient as much as possible. Explain the sounds and feel of the preoperative environment in simple but direct terms. When transferring the patient to the operating table, take the patient's hand gently and guide it to the operating table so he or she can feel the surface and direction of the move. Never put patients on a lateral transfer device without explaining to them what to expect or helping them feel the device. When prepping the patient for a local anesthetic, warn him or her ahead of time about the feel of the liquid and the extent of the prep area. Using common sense, empathy, and active communication with the patient usually results in a positive outcome.

As with hearing-impaired patients, allow the sight-impaired patient to keep eyeglasses as long as possible in the preoperative period. You can also offer the option of keeping their eyeglasses (according to facility policy), reassuring them that they will have their glasses as soon as possible after surgery.

THE MALNOURISHED PATIENT

A malnourished patient lacks the necessary nutritional reserves to support the process of healing. The postoperative period requires high metabolic activity during the healing process. Protein and carbohydrates are in particularly high demand by the body to rebuild tissue and meet the physiological demands of organ systems. The patient who enters surgery undernourished (without enough food intake to support health) or malnourished (lacking the right kinds of food to support body functions) is at high risk. Cancer, alcoholism, metabolic disease, neglect, and advanced age are a few conditions that often result in malnutrition or undernutrition.

The malnourished patient is susceptible to injury during moving and handling and requires extra attention during surgical positioning. Supportive connective tissues that normally help protect the patient are decreased in size and strength in the malnourished person. Tissues do not have the resilience needed for support of the skeletal system. Nerves and blood vessels are very close to the surface, where they can be easily bruised or injured.

Anesthesia tolerance is another problem in malnourished individuals. The body's normal metabolic processes are affected by lack of essential elements and poor **elimination** of waste products. Poor electrolyte balance can also affect the body's ability to metabolize anesthetic agents and has a direct effect on the electrical activity of the heart.

THE BARIATRIC PATIENT

As the prevalence of morbidly obese or bariatric patients continues to increase in the United States and worldwide, it has become necessary for health care professionals to learn how to mitigate specific risks for this population. The National Center for Health Statistics states that more than 60% of adults in the United States are overweight or obese, and a sizeable number are morbidly obese. Weight categories are defined by the National Institutes of Health using the body mass index or BMI. This is the relationship between height and weight. The formulas used are:

$$BMI = \frac{\text{Weight in kilograms}}{\text{Height in meters squared}}$$

or

$$BMI = \frac{\text{Weight in pounds} \times 703}{\text{Height in inches squared}}$$

The National Institute of Health defines obesity as a BMI of 30 or more and morbid obesity as a BMI of 40 or greater. This figure represents a clinical extreme and presents specific surgical risks that must be considered during their medical care. These complications also are present for the moderately and severely obese patient who may also be classified as high risk based on their BMI and associated (comorbid) disorders.

Certain types of diseases that are associated with obesity can be life-threatening. Surgery can compound the risks, and great care is taken to prepare for adverse events related to anesthesia and surgery itself.

Airway obstruction is a high risk for obese and morbidly obese patients. Extra tissue in the neck and around the trachea can make intubation difficult. Many obese individuals suffer from a collapsed airway during sleep (sleep apnea) under normal conditions. Administration of general anesthesia complicates this risk even more.

Hemodynamic function (movement of blood through the body and blood pressure) can be greatly altered in the bariatric patient. The heart must work harder to move blood around the body, and severe blood pressure changes can occur rapidly during the positioning and movement required for surgery. The extra work required by the heart results in an enlarged heart and inability to shunt the blood in and out. This often leads to congestive heart failure and hypertension. Kidney disease is a common result of severe hypertension and inability to rid the body of waste products such as urea, nitrogen, and excess salts. Fluid balance is therefore critical in these patients.

Venous stasis is an additional problem of the vascular system that results in edema of the lower extremities and high risk for deep vein thrombosis or thromboembolism. A blood clot that forms in the venous system during surgery may break loose in the postoperative period, causing stroke or pulmonary embolism.

Respiratory problems including difficulty breathing are common in bariatric patients. The extra effort needed to move air through the lungs is related to increased tissue in the thorax and shortness of breath due to overexertion of the heart muscle, which cannot keep up with the oxygen needs of the tissues.

Moving and Handling the Bariatric Patient

The bariatric patient is at high risk for injury during moving, handling, and positioning for surgery. Mechanical devices are available for lateral transfer to the operating table; however, neurological injury, blood pressure shifts, and musculoskeletal complications can occur during positioning (see Chapter 19). Specialty equipment such as a bariatric operating table, positioning aids, and long safety straps must be prepared before the patient is brought into the operating room.

THE PATIENT WITH DIABETES

Diabetes mellitus is an endocrine disease that disrupts the metabolism of carbohydrates, fats, and proteins. When diabetes is not controlled, severe damage to vascular and neurological tissues results. The risks associated with surgery in diabetic patients are complex. They arise from impairments in the healing properties of the vascular system and in the efficient use of glucose for tissue metabolism. Because many diabetic patients have a compromised vascular system, their risk of infection at the surgical site is higher than for other groups. They also are subject to prolonged wound healing, hypertension, and peripheral edema.

Diabetes mellitus is a common disease in the obese individual. Two types of diabetes are prevalent. Both types can be life-threatening. In diabetes, the required amount of insulin needed for the metabolism of carbohydrates, protein, and fat does not match the insulin available. Metabolic fuels, especially glucose, are necessary for cells to function. Insulin is the key to making the fuels available to all tissues in the body. In *type 1 diabetes*, which is often diagnosed in childhood, the insulin-producing beta cells of the pancreas are destroyed through an autoimmune process. The severity of the disease depends on the level of beta cell destruction. *Type 2 diabetes* is caused by obesity and advanced age. In this case, there is impaired insulin secretion and insulin resistance at the cellular level. Without insulin to carry glucose into the cell, glucose remains in the blood, with severe consequences. Surgery puts extra stress on the body, which translates into a need for extracellular fuel. Other diabetic complications are related to ischemic vascular disease, in which the blood vessels themselves are abnormal, causing delayed healing. Postoperative cardiac arrest may be more common in diabetics, and slower wound healing means a greater risk of infection and longer hospital stay.

THE IMMUNOSUPPRESSED PATIENT

The patient whose immune system is compromised or suppressed faces the threats of postoperative infection and delayed healing. The body requires a healthy immune system to respond to the trauma of surgery and to defend it against potentially infectious microorganisms in the environment. Immunosuppression is a result of certain diseases such as human immunodeficiency virus/acquired immunodeficiency syndrome (HIV/AIDS) and also antineoplastic agents used for the treatment of cancer. Patients undergoing organ transplantation or who have had an organ transplant in the past receive immunosuppressants. Corticosteroids used in the treatment of autoimmune disorders are also immunosuppressants.

Surgery of the immunosuppressed patient is performed only when necessary to avoid exposing the patient to complications common to this patient population. These include poor healing related to the depressed immune system and metabolic problems related to specific diseases that require immunosuppression. Other complications are specific to comorbid conditions.

HIV patients no longer present the extremely high risks seen before the advent of advanced antiretroviral drug therapy in the mid-1990s. HIV-positive patients who required surgery before this time were usually deferred or treated using non-surgical interventions. Because HIV is now considered a chronic disease rather than a fatal condition, the decision to perform surgery on the HIV patient now is dependent on extensive preoperative investigations that measure the immune system's strength, and also on the patient's general medical condition. With the use of preoperative antibiotics and close observation postoperatively, HIV patients are now undergoing orthopedic surgery, gastric banding, and even kidney transplantation. Problems related to HIV transmission during surgery are a different matter, and strict adherence to universal precautions is imperative.

THE TRAUMA PATIENT

Incidents of personal violence such as gunshot or knife wounds, automobile crashes, industrial accidents, falls, and automobile or pedestrian accidents are some of the more common causes of trauma. In older adults, falls account for 40% of trauma, whereas in younger populations the main cause is assault and motor vehicle accidents (MVAs). MVAs are also the second most common cause of trauma in older adults. Many accidents, especially MVAs, are avoidable, and the cost in human suffering is enormous. Federal and state agencies are working hard to develop programs to teach the public and encourage compliance with the use of seat belts, abstaining from drugs and alcohol before driving, and child safety in vehicles.

Trauma hospitals are those that are staffed and equipped to handle trauma cases on emergency. These are designated by levels I, II, and so on, according to their capacity to handle a variety of types of trauma. This mainly relates to the types of specialist surgeons immediately available. Rural areas are the least served by trauma centers. However, air ambulance services are available for most rural areas. The problem is one of time. The most important factor in saving lives is action within the first hour following the trauma, called the golden hour.

The patient who is admitted emergently for trauma surgery is normally stabilized to some degree in the emergency department before coming into the operating room. Insertion of chest tubes, intubation, fluid resuscitation, the start of blood transfusion, and other lifesaving measures can be performed in a well-staffed emergency department.

From the point of arrival at the trauma center to transport into the operating room, the attending surgeons will obtain as much information on the patient's past and present medical history as possible. The patient's family and friends are vital in providing information that can assist in surgical decision making. If no one is available to provide a history, the risks may increase. Witnesses to the trauma can also supply important information about the nature of the event, which aids diagnosis. Injuries may be undetected, especially if the patient cannot answer questions. The trauma patient may arrive in surgery in a precarious physiological state, with extensive blood loss, severe shock, and fluid-electrolyte imbalance. Intoxication from alcohol or drugs can alter the physiological response to surgery and complicate the process and method of anesthesia. During this time, family and friends are notified, if they are not already on site at the hospital. Nursing staff and the attending doctors will provide psychosocial care and try to give as much information as possible to help the family cope with the events.

As soon as the patient is stable enough, surgery commences quickly. Trauma cases often require more than one team operating on different areas of the body. This is particularly true for motor vehicle accidents in which there are multiple areas of trauma such as head, pelvis, and extremity injuries. During surgery, physiological monitoring is very important, and metabolic tests such as blood gas levels, blood pH, and total blood cell count, especially platelets, may be carried out frequently during treatment. Autotransfusion is often used, especially in crush injuries and abdominal or thoracic trauma. Patients in critical or serious condition are transferred to intensive care or another designated specialty unit following surgery.

Psychosocial support of the patient and family can be extremely delicate in trauma cases. Families want and deserve to know the condition of their loved one. However, there may be no way to summarize the condition of an unstable patient. Surgery in complex trauma cases can last many hours, and there may be no way to predict the actual duration. As soon as a patient is transferred from one department to another, it is important to let the family know exactly where the patient has been taken and whom to speak to about the patient's medical condition. Patients who retain consciousness and cognitive ability are understandably frightened about their condition and are often focused on pain levels. Unable to interpret the flurry of activity in their environment, they can feel isolated, even when the activity is focused on them. A gentle touch on the patient's hand or shoulder can make a strong statement of caring and empathy. Orienting patients by telling them where they are and describing the environment in simple terms, using a soothing tone, is usually very comforting.

THE PATIENT WITH A DEVELOPMENTAL DISABILITY

Developmental disabilities refer to a large group of diseases or conditions that affect movement, posture, cognitive ability, behavior, and other mental processes. The following conditions are included in but not limited to this category:

- Cerebral palsy
- Cognitive disability (including genetic or chromosomal syndromes)
- Learning disabilities
- Asperger disorder
- Autistic spectrum disorders

The developmentally delayed patient may also have comorbid psychiatric disabilities. There is a very large spectrum of diseases that can regarded as developmental and learning disabilities. For the purposes of this discussion, it is important to understand that the syndromes are complex. Although many exhibit common features, each patient expresses the condition according to his or her personality, environment, previous experience in the health care system, and complex emotional factors.

The Person Is Not the Disease

In caring for patients with developmental delay and in communication with others on the care team, it is important to use terms that respect the individual and that apply to that patient. For example, Down syndrome is only one of many chromosomal defects resulting in development and learning disability. Its proper name is *Down*, not *Down's* syndrome. When speaking about a patient with family members, friends, and colleagues, use "people-first" language. A person with a disability *has* the disability. He or she is not a "victim" of Down syndrome or "afflicted by cerebral palsy." These language cues indicate that the patient has only one dimension—the disease.

This is simply not the case. Some guidelines for people-first language are:

- Name the person first, not the disability:
  A person with a disability, not a disabled person
  An adult with autism, not an autistic adult
- Use neutral expressions:
  A child *with* cerebral palsy, not *afflicted with* cerebral palsy
  An individual who had a stroke, not a stroke *victim*
- Use preferred language:
  Use *cognitive disability*, not *mentally retarded*
  Accessible parking instead of *handicap parking*

The perioperative experience for patients with learning or developmental disability may not require special techniques outside of empathetic, safety-conscious care. In cases in which patients are physically difficult to manage because of agitation, the anesthesia care provider will provide guidance in order to prevent injury to the patient or others on the team.

Positioning the patient may present difficulties because many developmental syndromes are accompanied by skeletal malformations that affect the patient's range of motion and ability to lie in certain positions. Here, the patient's chart, especially the recent medical history and preoperative physical examination, can provide essential information to prevent injury. Positioning may require some creative means of providing support to vulnerable nerves, blood vessels, and bony prominences while also allowing adequate surgical exposure. Special physiological needs and airway precautions are of primary importance in some types of developmental syndromes.

THE PATIENT WITH A HISTORY OF PSYCHOLOGICAL TRAUMA

Severe psychological trauma can result in a number of different syndromes and physical symptoms that the perioperative staff may encounter. Not all patients with psychological trauma are diagnosed with post-traumatic stress disorder (PTSD). This is only one of many syndromes identified in the DSM— the *Diagnostic and Statistical Manual of Mental Disorders*, in which psychological disorders are classified and identified by symptoms.

Patient populations with trauma disorders come from all parts of society, and there are many causes. Veterans from recent and past wars are among the largest group. Others include rescue workers, medical workers in humanitarian aid, and those who have experienced sexual assault and other violent crime.

When caring for patients with PTSD or any other trauma-related syndrome, it is important to understand some of the symptoms that are common among most such patients:

1. The person reexperiences the trauma emotionally through the senses when triggered by specific cues in the environment. For example, a torture victim seeing or hearing an electrical device in use may suddenly begin to relive the torture experience, including the pain response. A woman who was raped and is undergoing a gynecological examination may suddenly believe and feel that she is being raped again.

2. The patient with a trauma syndrome experiences vivid nightmares and may not be able to sleep more than a few minutes at a time throughout the night. These patients are continually exhausted and sleep deprived.

3. Flashbacks of the traumatic event occur as sensory (smell, taste, feeling) events that can recur daily or many times a day.

4. The patient with severe trauma symptoms—especially those arising from sexual torture, criminal assault, or political torture—may not be able to withstand touch by another person or objects that trigger the patient.

5. Individuals with a severe trauma history have a heightened startle reflex. Sudden noise, approaching them from behind, or sudden touch can cause rapid withdrawal or protective actions such as covering the head or seeking cover. This is particularly acute in veterans and others who have spent time in war zones.

6. The trauma experience may result in severe depression, which is a comorbidity with the trauma syndrome.

Patients with severe trauma symptoms may avoid seeking care for medical problems because of the need for exposure to a busy, brightly lit environment in which they will be required to be examined (touched) and possibly have tests or procedures that trigger an episode of terror and dread. Such patients must be allowed to control their care, refuse certain parts of an examination or test, and thus protect themselves from further psychological trauma. Many who have been raped prefer to have gynecological examinations under general anesthesia.

Patients with a trauma diagnosis are often debilitated by their symptoms but are not necessarily permanently ill. Now that the medical profession accepts and understands the consequences of trauma, effective medication and other types of therapy are available. Symptoms can arise decades after the trauma, and individuals, especially those traumatized in previous wars, are now able to receive the care they need.

THE PREGNANT PATIENT

The pregnant patient may be scheduled for certain kinds of urgent surgery that are not related to the pregnancy. Minimally invasive surgery allows procedures on the gallbladder and other upper abdominal procedures that were not attempted in the past. Lower abdominal procedures are not performed as frequently because of the obvious risks to the fetus. The safest period for surgery is during the second trimester.

Appendicitis is the most common cause of acute surgical problem during pregnancy. Delay can lead to perforation, preterm labor, and death of the fetus in about 35% of cases.[1] The decision to operate rests with the patient care team—including the gynecologist or obstetrician, operating surgeon, and anesthesiologist. Fetal monitoring is necessary throughout the perioperative period in order to quickly detect any changes in fetal circulation and danger to the fetus. Gallbladder and biliary tract disease is the second most common nongynecological condition that requires surgery in pregnancy. Only those cases that cannot be treated medically are presented for surgery.

Aside from the mechanical danger to the fetus, surgery during pregnancy has other risks related to anesthesia, gas exchange, hemodynamics, and electrolyte balance. These are all considered carefully before the final decision is made.

Preparation for the patient follows normal protocols for safe perioperative care, with particular attention to the patient's position, and additional obstetrical and gynecology staff are on hand to assist in fetal monitoring and consultation during the procedure. The patient must be placed in a left side-lying position. This decreases pressure on the inferior vena cava that would compromise fetal circulation. Antiembolic stockings or a sequential compression device is used to prevent deep vein thrombosis. Aspiration precautions are used because the pregnant patient has lower than normal esophageal sphincter pressure and delayed emptying of the stomach. Many other physiological processes are used to protect both the patient and fetus. A more complete discussion of the pregnant patient is found in Chapter 25.

THE SUBSTANCE ABUSE PATIENT

Substance abuse patients are patients that are impaired by a legal or illegal substance. The substance may be drugs, alcohol, or any other substance that impairs decision making. When a patient comes to the operating room for surgery who may be impaired, there are many aspects that can alter a planned procedure. Aspiration and blood loss are common conditions that can occur with a patient under the influence of a substance.

THE ISOLATION PATIENT

A patient who is resistant to any organism is considered to be an isolation patient. Prior to surgery, healthcare workers should take the normal precautions of gloving, gowning, and working within the sterile field. Circulating personnel should wear gloves and an isolation gown. Patients being transported go directly into the operating room and the patient's chart is placed in a bag. Patients recover in the operating room or return directly to their floor.

KEY CONCEPTS

- The needs of humans have been summarized in a theory known as Maslow's hierarchy of human needs. This theory, which is commonly used to identify areas of focus for patient care, includes physiological needs, protection, and relational and personal needs.
- Direct patient care prioritizes the physiological and emotional needs of the patient.
- Communication with the patient establishes the basis of all care.
- Therapeutic communication is a learned skill that all health care professionals can develop.
- Cultural competence is the ability to interact with all people regardless of their culture or belief.
- Cultural competence cannot be learned by reading or studying cultures. It is developed through training and experience with people.

- Health care workers must examine their own beliefs and prejudices to become truly culturally competent.
- Cultural competence includes respect for and acknowledgment of another's faith or spiritual beliefs.
- Special patient populations have particular physiological and psychological needs.
- Patients with a severe hearing deficit or language barrier require an interpreter to ensure their understanding of the surgical procedure and its consequences.
- The pregnant patient may undergo certain surgical procedures unrelated to her pregnancy, but only after consultation with the medical care team.
- Patients who are fearful or anxious about their surgery may exhibit regressive behavior.
- Pediatric patients, especially adolescents, are particularly sensitive about body exposure and self-image.
- The older patient is given a very complete preoperative evaluation to reduce the risk of metabolic, structural, and physiological problems that can complicate recovery.
- Developmental disabilities are a large group of diseases or conditions that affect movement, posture, cognitive ability, behavior, and learning processes.
- Special populations include pediatric and older patients, those with sensory deficits, and those who are immunosuppressed. Trauma patients and those with chronic diseases also have special needs that must be considered in their care.

REVIEW QUESTIONS

1. Define *patient-centered care*.
2. Discuss the domains of Maslow's hierarchy.
3. What is body image? In what ways does body image influence a patient's anxieties about surgery?
4. What methods would you use in therapeutic communication?
5. Define *cultural competence*. Why is cultural competence important in health care? What is the difference between cultural competence and diversity awareness?
6. What is developmental disability? Research some medical conditions that result in developmental disability.
7. What would you do to communicate with a patient who does not speak English? What if no interpreter is available?
8. Why might the patient with a sensory deficit particularly anxious in surgery?

CASE STUDIES

Case 1

Your patient is an 85-year-old woman. As the team begins to move her to the operating table, she cries out and begins crying. What do you think could be the possible causes of her extreme distress?

Case 2

You are preparing equipment for a cardiac procedure. The patient has been brought into surgery and is lying on the operating table. He says to you, "How long do you think this will take?" How will you respond? What possible concerns does this patient have? Is he expressing these concerns to you through his question?

Case 3

You are assisting the circulator with a 3-year-old patient about to have a tonsillectomy. The patient is screaming and kicking. He is crying and saying he wants his mommy. The circulator calls for more help to restrain the child. When you attempt to soothe him, he kicks you. What will you do? What is this patient experiencing? What can you provide for this patient?

Case 4

The patient is a 20-year-old brought to the operating room for an emergency cesarean section. She is crying. She says to you, "I hope I don't lose the baby. When will my doctor be here?" What is your response?

Case 5

The patient is a 40-year-old woman from Southeast Asia. She does not speak English. You overhear a coworker mimicking her attempts to speak to staff members. The patient overhears this, too, and begins to cry silently. How will you respond to her? Will you respond to your coworker?

REFERENCE

1. Gabbe SG, Niebyl JR, Simpson JL, editors: *Obstetrics: normal and problem pregnancies*, ed 5, New York, 2007, Churchill Livingstone.

BIBLIOGRAPHY

Dreger V, Tremback T: Management of preoperative anxiety in children, *AORN Journal* 84:5, 2006.
National Center for Cultural Competence and the Center for Child and Human Development: *A definition of linguistic competence.* Accessed November 12, 2007, at http://gucchd.georgetown.edu/nccc.
National Center for Cultural Competence and the Center for Child and Human Development: *Cultural competence: definition and conceptual framework.* Accessed November 11, 2007, at http://gucchd.georgetown.edu/nccc.
Rosén S, Svensson M, Nilsson U: Calm or not calm: the question of anxiety in the perianesthesia patient, *Journal of Perianesthesia Nursing* 23(4):237, 2008.
Wood B: Caring for a limited-English-proficient patient, *AORN Journal* 75:2, 2002.

Diagnostic and Assessment Procedures

7

CHAPTER OUTLINE

LEARNING OBJECTIVES

After studying this chapter the reader will be able to:

1. Describe the proper procedure for taking the patient's vital signs
2. Accurately document vital sign measurements
3. Describe the use of an electrocardiograph
4. List and define commonly used imaging studies
5. Discuss basic blood and urine chemistry tests
6. Describe different methods of tissue biopsy
7. Describe the effects of malignancy on the body
8. Discuss cancer screening

TERMINOLOGY

ABO blood group: Inherited antigens are found on the surface of an individual's red blood cells. These antigens identify the blood group (i.e., type A blood has type A antigens). Also known as blood type.

Acute illness: Sudden onset of disease or trauma or disease of short duration, usually 3 weeks or less.

Benign: A term used to characterize a tumor that does not have the capability to spread to other parts of the body and usually is composed of tissue similar to its tissue of origin.

Chronic illness: An illness that has continued for months, weeks, or years.

Complete blood count (CBC): A blood test that measures specific components, including the hemoglobin, hematocrit, red blood cells, and white blood cells.

Computed tomography (CT): An imaging technique that allows physicians to obtain cross-sectional x-ray views of the patient. The result is a CT scan.

Contrast medium: A radiopaque fluid used in radiation studies to determine the shape and density of the anatomy.

Diastolic pressure: The pressure exerted on the walls of the blood vessels during the resting phase of cardiac contraction.

Differential count: A test that determines the number of each type of white blood cells in a specimen of blood.

Doppler studies: A technique that uses ultrasonic waves to measure blood flow in a vessel.

Electrocardiography: A noninvasive assessment of the heart's electrical activity displayed on a graph, the electrocardiogram. In the United States, *electrocardiogram* is abbreviated correctly as ECG. EKG is the European abbreviation.

Endoscopic procedures: Medical assessment of body cavities using a fiberoptic instrument (endoscope).

Fluoroscopy: A radiological technique that provides real-time images of an anatomical region.

Hematocrit (Hct): The ratio of red blood cells to plasma.

Hemoglobin (Hgb): The oxygen-carrying molecule found in red blood cells.

Imaging studies: Diagnostic tests that produce a picture or image.

Invasive procedure: A medical or nursing procedure in which the skin is broken or a body cavity is entered.

Magnetic resonance imaging (MRI): A diagnostic technique that uses radiofrequency signals and magnetic energy to produce images.

Malignant: A term used to characterize tissue that shows disorganized, uncontrolled growth (cancer). Malignant tissue has the potential to spread locally or to distant areas of the body. It is then termed *metastatic*.

Mean arterial pressure (MAP): The average amount of pressure exerted throughout the cardiac cycle.

Metastasis: The spread of malignant or cancerous cells to a local or distant area of the body.

Neoplasm: A tumor, which may be benign or malignant.

Nuclear medicine: Medical procedures that use radioactive particles to track target tissues in the body.

Orthostatic (postural) blood pressure: Refers to a technique used to check the patient's blood pressure in the upright and recumbent positions.

Palpating: Assessing a part of the body by feeling the outline, density, movement, or other attributes.

Partial thromboplastin time (PTT): A test of blood coagulation used in patients receiving heparin to determine the correct level of anticoagulation.

Positron emission tomography (PET): A type of medical imaging that measures specific metabolic activity in the target tissue.

Prothrombin time (PT): A measurement of the time required for blood to clot.

Pulse pressure: A measurement of the difference between the systolic pressure and diastolic pressure. This can be a significant sign of metabolic disturbance.

TERMINOLOGY (cont.)

Radioactive seeds: Small "seeds" of radioactive material implanted in tissue for cancer treatment.

Radionuclides or isotopes: In nuclear medicine, radioactive particles are directed at the nucleus of a selected element to create energy. These special elements are referred to as *radionuclides* or *isotopes*.

Radiopaque: A substance that is impenetrable by x-rays (gamma radiation).

Sphygmomanometer: An instrument used to measure blood pressure.

Staging: An international method of classifying tissue to determine the level of metastasis in cancer.

Systolic pressure: The pressure exerted by blood on the walls of vessels during the contraction phase of the cardiac cycle.

TNM classification system: An international system for determining the extent of metastasis and the level of cell differentiation, two important factors in treatment and prognosis of cancer.

Transcutaneous: Literally "through the skin"; it refers to a procedure in which a needle or other medical device is inserted from the outside of the body to the inside through the skin.

Tumor marker: An antigen present on the tumor cell, or a substance (protein, hormone, or other chemical) released by cancer cells into the blood.

Vital signs: Cardinal signs of well-being: pain, temperature, pulse, respiration, and blood pressure. These are measured to assess a patient's basic metabolic status.

INTRODUCTION

The first step in medical and surgical decision making is assessment, which provides clues and information about the nature of the patient's illness and the possible causes. Selection of the tests and procedures used to evaluate the patient's condition begins with a general assessment, which can lead to more complex investigations. The assessment begins with a baseline history (described in detail in Chapter 14) and physical examination.

Diagnostic procedures and tests often are performed as part of an assessment to confirm or rule out a diagnosis. In some cases invasive tests are required. An **invasive procedure** involves breaking intact skin or mucous membrane or inserting a medical device into a body cavity. Noninvasive procedures are limited to skin contact or no direct contact with the body. Interventional radiology procedures combine technologies such as x-ray or other imaging tools with invasive techniques.

The surgical technologist participates in selected invasive diagnostic and interventional procedures. These are performed in the surgical suite or in a designated specialty department. Routine tests such as blood analysis, urinalysis, and other *chemistry* studies are performed in the laboratory by technologists trained in that specialty. Conclusions about the result of a test or series of tests contribute to the diagnosis. Primary health care providers such as doctors and nurses use advanced skills in patient assessment, interpretation of tests, and the disease process to make strategic decisions about treatment.

This chapter is an orientation to commonly performed tests and diagnostic procedures. Surgical technologists participate in a variety of invasive diagnostic procedures described in this chapter and throughout the book. **Endoscopic procedures**, in which a fiberoptic instrument is passed through a body cavity for examination and biopsy, are described in Chapter 24 and in each procedural chapter according to specialty. Bacteriological and other tests required for investigation of infectious diseases are described in Chapter 9. Diagnostic tests associated with a particular medical specialty are described in the chapter associated with that specialty.

CONCEPTS RELATED TO PATHOLOGY

Pathology is the study of disease and can also refer to specific illness. Illness can be caused by a number of different environmental and physiological conditions, or one single factor. The term *etiology* refers to one or more causes. For example, you might see "etiology unknown" written in the patient's chart. This simply means that the cause is unknown at the time of examination. Primary health care providers use the word *idiopathic* to mean that the condition arose suddenly or spontaneously without apparent cause such as "idiopathic hypertension" meaning the patient developed high blood pressure. The terms *morbidity* (rate of illness in the population) and *mortality* (rate of death in the population) are used in the field of epidemiology, which focuses on population health. For example, "Syndactaly virus is associated with high morbidity and low mortality in most populations."

When a patient is being assessed, specific terms are used to describe a disease process and outcome. When discussing the disease itself, we usually refer to its *course*. For example, "the patient experienced abdominal pain throughout the course of the infection." A more formal term referring to the origin and development of the disease is *pathogenesis*. During the patient assessment, the primary health care provider differentiates between objective (measureable) *signs* of the condition (e.g. rash, fever, injury, loss of function) and *symptoms*. Whereas signs are objective (they can be observed independently of the patient's experience), symptoms are subjective. Symptoms are what the patient reports. For example, "The patient reports gradual loss of vision in the left eye over 5 days." This is a symptom. On the other hand "There is marked swelling of the lower lid, with serosanginous drainage at the medial punctum." These are signs of disease.

Events related to the disease state are also qualified using specific terms. A *complication* of disease is separate from the primary problem, but occurs at the same time or as a consequence of the main problem. A complication usually causes the main problem to be more serious or complex. For example "The non union fracture was caused by postoperative infection, complicated by poor nutritional intake. Sometimes the term *exacerbation* is used to mean worsen or become more serious. A *syndrome* is a unique group of signs associated with a specific disease.

The course of the disease is defined by specific terms. The *prognosis* is a prediction of the outcome of a condition or medical intervention. This is usually expressed with general terms such as excellent, good, or poor. If the disease subsides (goes into *remission*) and then returns again, it is a *relapse*. An illness that results in death is said to be *terminal.*

The treatment of disease also uses special vocabulary. *Curative* refers to treatment that is meant to resolve the medical problem. However *palliative* care is intended to make the condition more tolerable, without actually curing it.

VITAL SIGNS

Taking a patient's **vital signs** allows an overall evaluation of the person's well-being. This is the most basic form of clinical assessment. In some facilities, the surgical technologist may measure the patient's vital signs. These are documented and reported to the registered nurse or surgeon. The surgical technologist is not expected to interpret the measurements or make a diagnosis based on the results. However, *accurate measurement* is always required. The vital signs include:

- Temperature
- Pulse
- Respiration
- Blood pressure

A change in the vital signs can be an early warning of an **acute illness** (one that comes on suddenly) or a sign of a **chronic illness** (long-term disease). Vital signs are measured whenever a patient requires medical assessment. During general anesthesia or deep sedation, vital signs are measured with complex biomedical devices. In simple procedures performed with a local anesthetic, noninvasive techniques are used. The person measuring the vital signs must report immediately any variation from the *baseline values* (i.e., those taken at the beginning of an assessment period). The baseline values may vary from "normal" limits. Upward or downward trends and deviations from the baseline values are an indication of important changes in the patient's condition. The methods used to measure the patient's vital signs in a clinical or outpatient setting are less exacting than those used by the anesthesia care provider during general anesthesia. The anesthesia care provider often uses internally placed devices, whereas external devices are used in cases only requiring local or regional anesthetic.

TEMPERATURE

The body requires a core (internal) temperature of approximately 99° F (37.2° C) to maintain physiological functions. The core temperature is regulated by the hypothalamus through a complex feedback system that balances the core temperature with environmental factors. However, when environmental factors or disease exceed the body's ability to adjust, vital functions deteriorate, and this can result in serious tissue injury or death.

Temperature is recorded and documented in degrees Celsius. The formula for conversion from the two systems is:

$$\text{Fahrenheit} \rightarrow \text{Celsius} \quad °C = \tfrac{5}{9}\,(°F - 32)$$

$$\text{Celsius} \rightarrow \text{Fahrenheit} \quad °F = \tfrac{9}{5}\,°C + 32$$

Methods of Measuring Temperature

The site where the temperature is measured affects the reading that results.

- The oral temperature is measured under the tongue (*sublingually*). The tongue is highly vascular and accurately reflects the core temperature. The normal oral temperature in a person at rest is 98.6° F (37° C). The range is 96.4° to 99.1° F (35.8° to 37.3° C).
- Temporal artery temperature measured with a temporal artery thermometer (TAT) is approximately 0.8° F (0.4° C) higher than oral temperature.
- The *tympanic* temperature accurately assesses core temperature through the external auditory canal.
- The *rectal* temperature varies from 0.7° to 1° F (0.4° to 0.5° C) higher than the oral value.
- The *axillary* temperature is measured at the axilla. Readings are 0.5° to 1° F (0.3° to 0.6° C) lower than the oral value.
- The forehead, or *skin*, temperature varies with environmental changes.

Use of Thermometers

Always wear gloves when taking the patient's temperature. Probe and tympanic thermometers can harbor an infectious biofilm that may not be visible. Even though only the probe cover comes in contact with patient tissue, the units are often heavily laden with bacteria.

The TAT has replaced many other types of patient thermometers in the clinic setting. The thermometer probe is noninvasive and accurate when used properly. It can be used on patients of all ages. After disinfection with an alcohol wipe, the probe is gently swiped in a straight line from the center of the forehead laterally to cross the temporal artery, lifted from the skin and placed briefly behind the ear lobe. It is not placed at the temple, which is a common user error. The device can be calibrated to provide an output reading as oral temperature. The *electronic probe thermometer* consists of a sensing probe connected to a handheld reader with a light-emitting diode (LED) or liquid crystal display (LCD) format. This type of thermometer is used primarily for oral and axillary measurements. Only a designated rectal probe thermometer is used for measuring the rectal temperature.

A clean probe cover must be used on each patient to prevent the spread of infection. The measurement is displayed after about 30 seconds.

To use the electronic thermometer, make sure the batteries are charged and the unit is clean. Insert the tip into a new disposable probe cover and press gently. This attaches the cover to the probe. Then proceed as follows:

- *Oral temperature:* Gently insert the probe under the patient's tongue.
- *Axillary temperature:* When the thermometer is used in the axilla, make sure the tip of the probe does not extend

outside the body. In children, it is best to hold the upper arm in contact with the body to ensure an accurate reading. Stabilize the probe until the reading is obtained.

- *Rectal temperature:* Rectal temperature readings are seldom performed or required because safer and more accurate technologies have been developed. Have the patient lie on his or her side with the uppermost knee flexed. The probe tip should be lubricated after the probe cover is applied. Spread the buttocks with one hand and gently insert the probe approximately 1½ inches (3.75 cm). If stool is encountered during insertion, remove the probe, replace the cover, and begin again. Stabilize the probe until the reading is completed. The risk of puncturing the rectal mucosa and musculature exists when a rectal probe is used. This method is used *only when no other method is available.* The tympanic or temporal method is preferred over the rectal method. Remove the probe and dispose of the cover in a hazardous waste container. Wash your hands thoroughly and record the measurement.

- *Tympanic membrane thermometer:* This may be used on conscious or unconscious patients. It is the preferred method of temperature assessment in the clinical setting. The tympanic thermometer receives infrared signals from the eardrum. It provides an accurate reading of core temperature, because the tympanic membrane shares its blood supply with the carotid artery. The instrument is shaped like an otoscope, and single-use probe covers are used to prevent cross-contamination among patients. To use the thermometer, clean the probe using a soft alcohol wipe. Place a disposable probe cover over the tip. Direct the tip into the external ear canal. Rotate the thermometer slightly to seat it into the ear canal and retract the skin in front of the ear to seat the tip. Release the skin before taking the reading. Remember that the infrared beam must "see" the tympanic membrane for an accurate reading. Press the activate button and wait for an audible beep from the thermometer. Remove the earpiece gently and dispose of the cover. Record the measurement.

Glass thermometers, which contain a colored solution, have been replaced by electronic or digital instruments. Mercury is no longer used in the manufacture of glass thermometers because of concerns with environmental safety. Health care workers occasionally may be required to use a glass thermometer, which first must be briskly shaken to lower the liquid column.

MEASURING THE PULSE

The pulse is a reflection of the stroke volume (amount of blood pumped through the heart) of each beat. The pulse is felt in the artery as it expands with each heartbeat. The normal heart rate varies according to age, condition, and metabolic level. Disease or injury alters the metabolic level and affects the heart rate, rhythm, and strength. Table 7-1 lists normal resting pulse rates by age. The normal pulse rate for an adult is 60 to 100 beats per minute.

The heart rhythm normally is regular. However, in younger adults and children, the rate may decrease with respiratory inspiration (inhaling). The *strength* of the peripheral pulse can

Table **7-1**	Normal Pulse and Respiratory Rates by Age*	
Age (Years)	**Normal Pulse Rate (Range) (Beats per Minute)**	**Normal Respiration (Breaths per Minute)**
0	120 (70-190)	30-40
1	120 (80-190)	21-40
2	110 (80-130)	25-32
4	110 (80-120)	23-30
6	100 (75-115)	21-26
8	100 (70-110)	21-26
10	90 (70-110)	21-26
12	90 (70-110)	18-22
14	85 (65-105)	18-22
16	85 (60-100)	16-20
18	75 (55-95)	12-20
Adult	75 (60-100)	10-20
Athlete	50-60 (50-100)	10-20

*Male children may have slightly lower values.

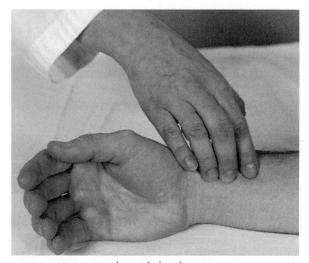

Figure 7-1   **Measuring the radial pulse.** *(From Jarvis C: Physical examination and health assessment, ed 5, Philadelphia, 2008, WB Saunders.)*

vary with changes in metabolism, disease, or injury. A normal pulse feels elastic and has moderate strength. A "bounding" pulse is one that feels exceptionally strong, whereas a weak pulse may be barely palpable or "thready." A three-point or four-point scale is used to report the strength of the pulse:

- Bounding: 3+
- Normal: 2+
- Weak 1+
- Absent: 0

The pulse is measured by **palpating** (feeling) an artery. In a routine assessment, the radial artery is used. This is located along the radius on the inner side of the wrist (Figure 7-1). You may need to position your fingers in several locations to find the pulse. Always use the pads of your first three fingers to measure the pulse, because the thumb has its own pulse, which may be confused with the patient's pulse. Also, applying

Box **7-1**	**Location and Method of Palpating Major Arteries**

- The temporal artery is located between the ear and outer eye in the depression above the cheek bone.
- The carotid artery is located in the depression between the sternocleidomastoid muscle and the trachea, at the side of the neck midway between the clavicle and the jaw.
- The brachial artery can be felt in the groove that runs along the side of the biceps muscle on the inside (medial aspect) of the upper arm. To locate this artery, flex the biceps to locate the groove and then relax the muscle to palpate. This pulse can also be felt in the antecubital fossa behind the elbow. This is the artery used to measure the patient's blood pressure.
- The radial artery is most often used to assess a patient's pulse in the clinical setting because it is easily accessible. Palpate this artery by placing the fingers on the radial bone and sliding them slightly toward the inner wrist so that they rest in the groove next to the bone.
- The femoral artery is very important in surgery. This artery is most often used to cannulate the larger vessels of the trunk for an angiogram (arteriography) and for placement of stents. To palpate the artery, place your fingers in the deepest furrow of the groin where the upper leg joins the pelvis. You may have to press firmly, because the femoral artery lies deep in the fascia and muscle.
- The popliteal artery is an extension of the femoral artery. It can be felt at the back of the knee in the depression at the top of the tibia, behind the patella.
- The dorsalis pedis branches from the popliteal artery and is located over the front of the foot in the depression between the great and second toes.
- The posterior tibial artery lies in the furrow between the Achilles tendon and the tibial process (ankle bone).

excessive pressure depresses the artery and stops circulation. Although the radial artery normally is used to measure the patient's pulse, any other artery can be used. Box 7-1 describes the location and method of palpating major arteries.

When you have located the pulse, count the number of beats in 30 seconds and multiply by 2 to get the beats per minute. The baseline reading (the first taken) should be counted for a full minute. Also, if at any time the pulse is irregular, you must count for 60 full seconds. Keep in mind that an irregular pulse or a missed beat may result in a difference of 4 or 5 beats per minute in the measurement.

RESPIRATION

The respiratory rate is an objective assessment of the number of breaths per minute. The respiratory rate is altered by exertion, metabolic stress, strong emotion, and the effect of specific drugs, which can depress or stimulate the autonomic nervous system.

The respiratory rate is measured by observing the patient's thorax and abdomen and recording the breaths per minute. It

is measured when the patient is unaware, because people often alter their breathing pattern when under observation. The respiratory rate can be counted while the pulse rate is obtained. To measure the respiratory rate, count the number of breaths in 30 seconds and multiply by 2. Normal respiratory rates are listed in Table 7-1.

NOTE: *Medical assessment of breath sounds, such as tone, pitch, pattern, and rhythm, is required for complex assessment of respiratory disease.*

BLOOD PRESSURE

Blood pressure is the force exerted on the vessels walls by the blood as it is pumped through the body. Vascular pressure changes during the cardiac cycle (filling of the heart chambers and shunting of blood through the heart). When the blood is forcefully pumped through the left ventricle, pressure is at its greatest. This is called the **systolic pressure**. As the heart muscle relaxes between contractions, blood pressure is lowered. This is called the **diastolic pressure**. The **mean arterial pressure (MAP)** is the average amount of pressure exerted throughout the cardiac cycle. When blood pressure is assessed, the difference between the diastolic and systolic pressures can be a significant sign. This is called the **pulse pressure**. Figure 7-2 shows changes in pressure that occur throughout the cardiac cycle. Many diseases cause changes in blood pressure. It also is important to understand how normal physiological processes can affect blood pressure.

Factors that Affect Blood Pressure

Normal blood pressure for an adult is 120/80 mm Hg. Pressure varies by age and is affected by various other normal physiological conditions, including:

- Weight
- Exertion
- Stress
- Strong emotion

Gender is another factor; blood pressure tends to be lower in adult women than in men. Important normal physiological factors that influence blood pressure include:

- *Cardiac output:* The total amount of blood pumped through the heart in 1 minute.
- *Stroke volume:* The amount of blood pumped during ventricular contraction. Total blood volume alters cardiac output.
- *Peripheral vascular resistance:* The static pressure of the blood vessels against the flow of blood. As blood vessels contract and relax, peripheral vascular resistance changes. Vessel obstruction also increases vascular resistance.
- *Resilience of the cardiac and vascular systems:* The elasticity of the vessels and heart muscle directly affects vascular pressure.

Procedure for Taking Blood Pressure

A simple blood pressure assessment requires both the diastolic and systolic measurements.

Blood pressure is measured with an electronic (digital) or manual **sphygmomanometer**, which requires the use of a

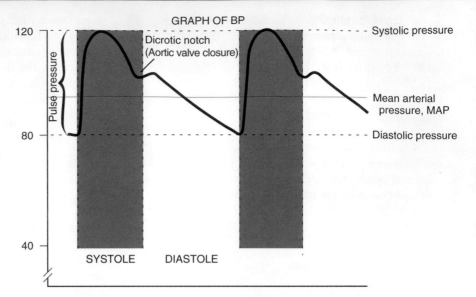

GRAPH OF BP

Figure 7-2 Graph of the cardiac cycle. *(From Jarvis C: Physical examination and health assessment, ed 5, Philadelphia, 2008, WB Saunders.)*

stethoscope. The stethoscope method provides a more thorough assessment.

The method used to take the blood pressure is critical to obtaining a correct reading. Table 7-2 lists common errors in blood pressure measurement. A sphygmomanometer has three components: the cuff, the pump, and the gauge. A manual blood pressure apparatus has a round gauge with numerical values and a pointer. Electronic blood pressure devices display the measurement on an LED or LCD panel attached to the control unit. The blood pressure cuff is an inflatable bladder covered with fabric that is secured to the patient's limb with Velcro.

Blood pressure can be measured in several locations on an arm or a leg. For adults, the most common location is the upper arm (i.e., the brachial artery). The cuff should be no larger than 40% of the circumference of the person's upper arm. Cuffs are available in many sizes, from pediatric to extra large. An incorrectly sized cuff is a common error in blood pressure measurement (see Table 7-2). This can lead to a falsely high or low reading.

The patient should be sitting or lying in a relaxed position. The arm must be at the level of the heart, and it should be supported on a surface. The person taking the reading may also support the arm, but it must be at heart level. Wrap the cuff around the patient's upper arm so that the air tubes are in line with the inner arm and brachial artery (Figure 7-3).

How to Use a Manual Sphygmomanometer

1. Before taking a reading, you must locate the general systolic pressure. Palpate the brachial artery, which is just above the antecubital fossa. Center the cuff above the fossa. Do not allow the cuff to slide down, because this obscures the measurement.
2. With your fingers over the brachial artery, inflate the cuff until the arterial pulse is no longer palpable. Continue to inflate another 25 to 30 mm above this point.
3. Release the cuff and wait 10 to 15 seconds. This allows blood to return to the artery.

Table **7-2**	Common Errors in Blood Pressure Measurement
Result of Measurement	**Cause of Inaccuracy**
False high systolic and diastolic pressures	• Blood pressure taken when patient is upset or anxious • Measurement taken after exertion • Wrong size cuff (too narrow) • Cuff too loose or unevenly wrapped • Arm below heart level
False low systolic and diastolic pressures	• Arm above heart level • Failure to inflate cuff sufficiently
False low systolic pressure	• Failure to inflate cuff sufficiently • Cuff deflated too quickly
False low diastolic pressure	• Stethoscope pressed too hard on artery
False high diastolic pressure	• Cuff deflated too slowly • Stopping deflation and reinflating • Failing to wait longer than 2 minutes between readings
Any type of error	• Working too fast • Faulty technique • Defective equipment

4. Place the bell end of the stethoscope over the artery and inflate the cuff to the level you previously measured.
5. Slowly deflate the cuff and listen for the first sound of the pulse. Observe the correct level on the gauge or liquid column. *This is the systolic reading.*
6. Continue to deflate until you hear a muffled pulse and then the disappearance of the pulse. The diastolic measurement is *the point where the pulse was no longer audible.*
7. If the difference between the muffled sound and no sound is greater than 10 mm Hg, you must document all three measurements. In some facilities, the middle sound is always documented.

8. To document the blood pressure, write the systolic pressure over the diastolic pressure (e.g., 140/70). If you document the middle sound, it is written between the diastolic and systolic pressures (e.g., 140/97/70). Documentation also includes identification of the artery used for measurement, and the side. Figure 7-4 shows the relationship between auscultatory sounds and pressure.

If the patient is to be assessed for **orthostatic (postural) blood pressure**, the pulse and blood pressure are measured with the patient in the recumbent position and again while the individual is sitting or standing. The patient's posture for each reading must be indicated in the documentation.

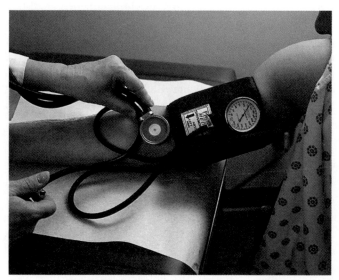

Figure 7-3 **Correct positioning of the blood pressure cuff.** *(From Jarvis C: Physical examination and health assessment, ed 5, Philadelphia, 2008, WB Saunders.)*

NOTE: *A simple digital (automatic) sphygmomanometer provides the pulse rate, systolic pressure, diastolic pressure, and MAP. However, it does not measure important anomalies in the auscultatory sounds, and readings may be inaccurate, depending on the quality of the instrument and its maintenance.*

ELECTROCARDIOGRAPHY

Electrocardiography measures the electrical activity of the heart and displays it on a graph, known as an **electrocardiogram (ECG)**, for evaluation. To obtain the readings, electrodes are placed at strategic locations on the chest wall and extremities. These coincide with the heart's conductivity pattern. A 12-lead ECG is used for a complete assessment; a simple assessment can be made with a three-lead ECG (Figure 7-5). ECG monitoring is a routine procedure for any patient undergoing general anesthesia or sedation, in the postoperative period, and for selected high-risk patients.

The ECG machine has a console with a roll of paper that feeds automatically when the leads are in place and the machine is activated. Electrical activity through the heart is graphed by time and strength of impulse. This produces characteristic patterns indicating normal or abnormal conduction, which are recognizable to trained personnel.

As a diagnostic tool, an ECG provides detailed information about heart conduction. Each phase of the cardiac conduction system is represented on the graph. The waveforms correspond to the impulses that stimulate heart action, which pushes the blood through the chambers and valves. One complete heart cycle is represented by a series of waves, which have characteristic peaks, troughs, and duration. This is called a *QRS wave*. A normal QRS wave form in shown in Figure 7-6. Certain kinds of patterns and variations indicate disturbances

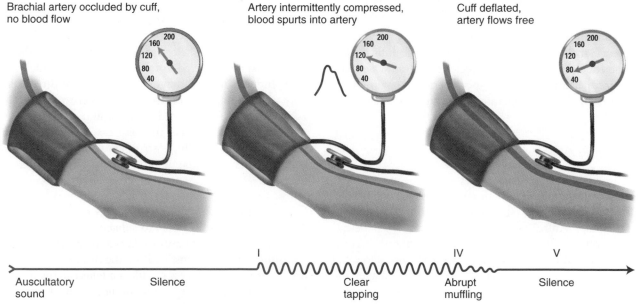

Brachial artery occluded by cuff, no blood flow

Artery intermittently compressed, blood spurts into artery

Cuff deflated, artery flows free

Auscultatory sound — Silence — I Clear tapping — IV Abrupt muffling — V Silence

Figure 7-4 **Korotkoff sounds and blood pressure.** Taking the blood pressure with a sphygmomanometer and stethoscope provides a detailed assessment of the sounds. *(From Jarvis C: Physical examination and health assessment, ed 5, Philadelphia, 2008, WB Saunders.)*

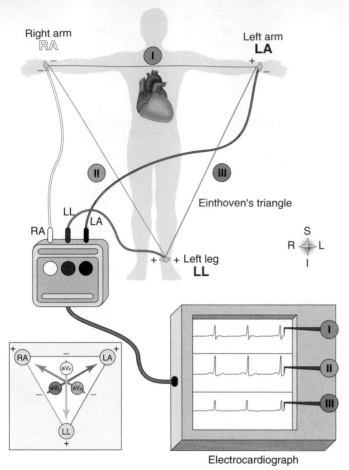

Figure 7-5 **Three-lead electrocardiogram (ECG).** *(From Thibodeau G, Patton K: Anatomy and physiology, ed 6, St Louis, 2007, Mosby.)*

NOTE: *Because radiographs use gamma radiation, all personnel must wear protective attire that prevents the penetration of radiation. (Safety precautions and protection against gamma radiation in the perioperative environment are discussed in detail in Chapter 8.)*

The images formed by x-rays display contrasts in density. An extremely dense substance produces a white image, whereas air produces a black image. Contours and outlines of organs, systems, and tissue are displayed as a combination of white, black, and grays. Images are taken from different angles and positions in order to visualize the structures from all sides and aid in assessment. These are interpreted by the radiologist, who reports to the surgeon or other physician ordering the tests. Diagnostic x-rays are often used to confirm a condition or to provide baseline studies for comparison following a surgical procedure. Baseline x-rays are taken in the radiology department as part of the preoperative preparation of the patient. Many different forms of x-ray imaging are used in modern diagnostic medicine. Radiography is also used in combination with other imaging techniques such as computed tomography and fluoroscopy.

Standard Radiography

The standard x-ray film is obtained with a fixed or portable x-ray machine. Both types are used in modern operating rooms. The portable machine is transported to the operating room on an on call basis so that images can be obtained during surgery as needed. Many types of x-ray procedures can be done intraoperatively. They are most commonly used during orthopedic surgery, biliary procedures, and vascular surgery. An x-ray film might also be taken when a surgical count cannot be resolved and the risk exists that an item was left in the patient.

Intraoperative anterior-posterior x-ray films are obtained with the use of a Bucky platform. This is a Plexiglas or carbon platform mounted on the operating bed frame. The technician slides the film into the platform from the head or foot of the table. When done properly, this does not risk contamination of the sterile field. However, the target of the radiograph must be protected from contamination by the overhead tube. The machine is brought into position at the sterile field only after the area is protected with sterile drapes (Figure 7-9). A draped, portable radiographic film stand is used when other views are required. In these cases, the scrub protects the sterile field, including instrument tables and other draped equipment, from contamination by the overhead radiograph machine.

Contrast Radiography

The term **radiopaque** refers to substances that x-rays cannot penetrate. In diagnostic medicine, a drug called a **contrast medium** is injected, instilled, or ingested to outline hollow organs or vessels before x-ray films are taken. The liquid contrast medium produces a solid white field in the area of the medium. Crevices, deviations, and the shape of a hollow structure can be clearly viewed on x-ray films or by fluoroscopy. (Contrast media are discussed in Chapter 13.)

in the conduction system which may be caused by disease, physiological disorder, and certain drugs.

IMAGING PROCEDURES

As the name implies, **imaging studies** involve a "picture" of the patient's anatomy. Imaging studies provide information about the function and shape of regional anatomy. Selected studies are performed in the perioperative environment during surgery or in a separate department of the facility (Figure 7-7).

RADIOLOGY

X-rays are electromagnetic particles with a relatively short wavelength. A radiographic (x-ray) image is created when radiation passes through structures and strikes a medium (e.g., radiographic film) positioned in line with the penetrating rays. X-rays penetrate body tissue at different rates according to density. Some materials and tissue do not allow full penetration of the x-rays (Figure 7-8). X-ray images are recorded, and the output is available as electronic data or film. Historically all radiographs were recorded onto film. This method has been replaced by digital images, which can be stored on discs and transferred electronically.

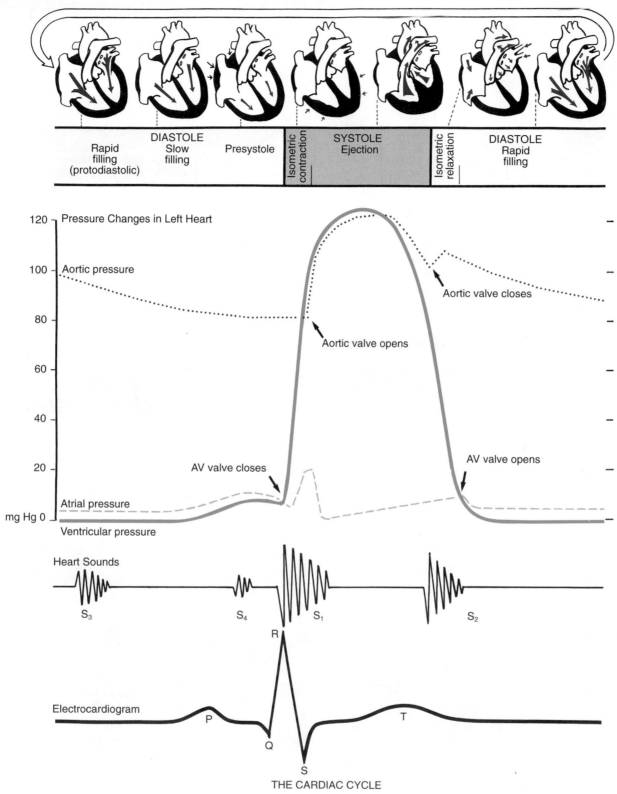

Figure 7-6 **Cardiac cycle QRS wave.** AV, Atrioventricular. *(From Jarvis C: Physical examination and health assessment, ed 5, Philadelphia, 2008, WB Saunders.)*

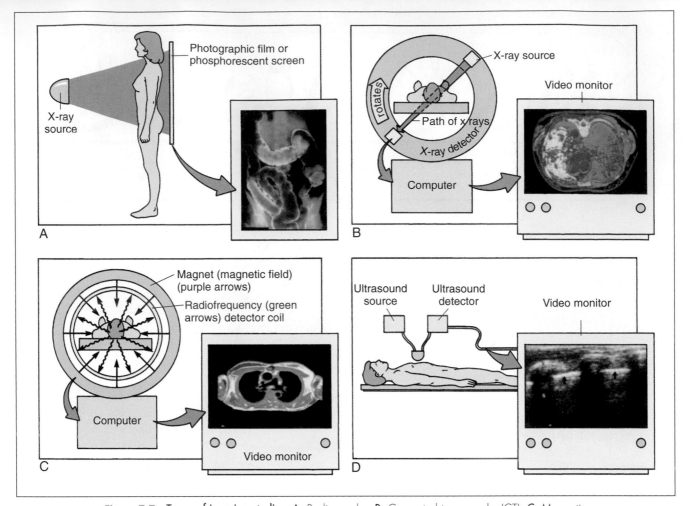

Figure 7-7 **Types of imaging studies. A,** Radiography. **B,** Computed tomography (CT). **C,** Magnetic resonance imaging (MRI). **D,** Ultrasonography (US). *(From Thibodeau G, Patton K:* Anatomy and physiology, *ed 6, St Louis, 2007, Mosby.)*

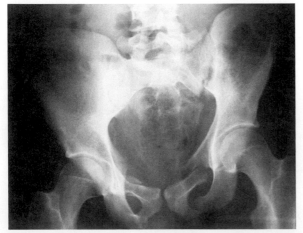

Figure 7-8 Flat radiograph of the pelvis showing dislocation of the left hip. *(From Garden O, Bradbury A, Forsythe J, Parks R:* Principles and practice of surgery, *ed 5, Edinburgh, 2007, Churchill Livingstone.)*

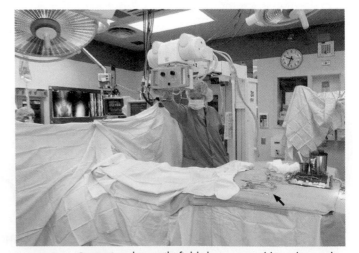

Figure 7-9 Protecting the sterile field during portable radiography. *(From Ballinger PW, Fra ED:* Merrill's atlas of radiographic positions and radiologic procedures, *vol 3, ed 10, St Louis, 2003, Mosby.)*

Contrast radiography carries a risk of allergy to the radiopaque medium, especially when the agent is injected. A careful patient history is used to determine whether the patient has had any previous reaction to contrast media. Allergy to iodine or agents containing iodophor may indicate sensitivity to contrast media. There is no evidence that allergy to shellfish indicates sensitivity or allergy to contrast media.

Specific details for intraoperative contrast studies are described in the surgical procedure chapter for that specialty.

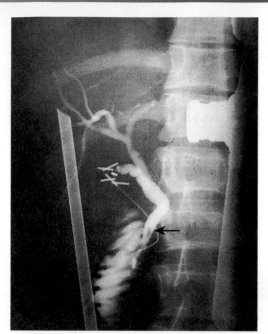

Figure 7-10 Endoscopic retrograde cholangiography showing the biliary tree *(arrow)*. Note the surgical staples and endoscopic ports on the left. *(From Garden O, Bradbury A, Forsythe J, Parks R: Principles and practice of surgery, ed 5, Edinburgh, 2007, Churchill Livingstone.)*

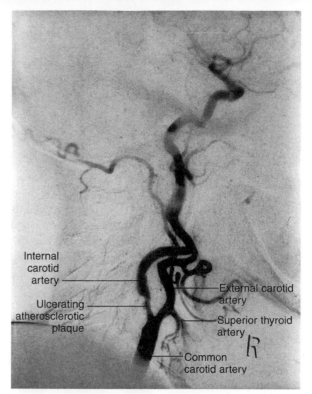

Figure 7-11 Carotid angiography using a contrast medium injected intravenously. *(From Garden O, Bradbury A, Forsythe J, Parks R: Principles and practice of surgery, ed 5, Edinburgh, 2007, Churchill Livingstone.)*

Contrast studies are used in nearly every medical specialty. The most commonly performed are:

- *Cholangiography:* A contrast medium is injected into the biliary tree. This outlines the ducts of the biliary system for suspected stones, tumor, or dilation (Figure 7-10).
- *Angiography:* A contrast medium is injected into the cardiovascular system to determine areas of stricture or other anomalies of blood flow in vessels (Figure 7-11).
- *Myelography:* A contrast medium is injected into the subarachnoid space for visualization of the spinal cord and nerve roots.
- *Retrograde pyelography:* A contrast medium is instilled into the urinary tract for visualization of the bladder, ureters, and kidney. This procedure is used to identify stones, strictures, tumor, or other anomalies of the urinary system.
- *Gastrointestinal studies:* In studies of the gastrointestinal system, barium, a radiopaque element, is used to fill and outline the structures. An upper gastrointestinal study is used to identify problems in the esophagus, stomach, and small intestine. For a study of the large intestine, barium is instilled into the distal colon and rectum (Figure 7-12).

FLUOROSCOPY

Fluoroscopy combines radiography with an image intensifier that is visible in normal lighting. A digital monitor allows the moving images to be seen in real time. Fluoroscopy is used diagnostically and intraoperatively during procedures using contrast media or during implantation of a biomedical device.

Mobile C-Arm

The mobile C-arm fluoroscope is used in surgery for real-time imaging (Figure 7-13). The head of the fluoroscope is directed through the body onto an image intensifier on the underside

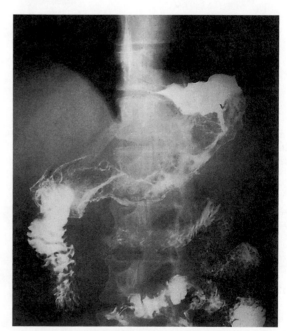

Figure 7-12 Barium study of the stomach showing extensive gastric carcinoma. *(From Garden O, Bradbury A, Forsythe J, Parks R: Principles and practice of surgery, ed 5, Edinburgh, 2007, Churchill Livingstone.)*

of the C. The C-arm can be moved into place so that the operating bed is centered between the tube and the intensifier. Multiple images can be taken by moving the machine along the axis of the operating table. The C-arm is draped before positioning to allow freedom of movement along the sterile field and has replaced portable x-ray machines in many hospitals.

COMPUTED TOMOGRAPHY

In **computed tomography (CT)**, x-ray and computer technologies are combined to produce high-contrast cross-sectional images. This technique allows precise tissue differentiation and determination of the dimensions of anatomical structures. CT is enhanced with contrast media to assess structures such as ducts, blood vessels, and the gastrointestinal system.

MAGNETIC RESONANCE IMAGING

Magnetic resonance imaging (MRI) uses radiofrequency signals and multiple magnetic fields to produce a high-definition image (Figure 7-14). In this process, the patient is exposed to electromagnetic energy, which is emitted inside a closed body tube or an open platform. MRI produces two- or

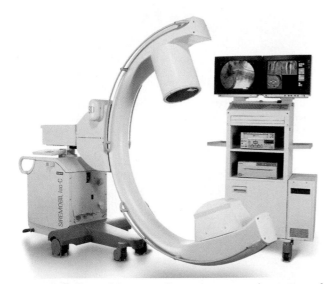

Figure 7-13   The mobile C-arm fluoroscope is used in surgery for real-time imaging. *(From Ballinger PW, Frank ED: Merrill's atlas of radiographic positions and radiologic procedures, vol 3, ed 10, St Louis, 2003, Mosby.)*

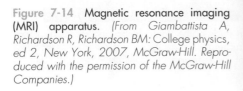

Figure 7-14   Magnetic resonance imaging (MRI) apparatus. *(From Giambattista A, Richardson R, Richardson BM: College physics, ed 2, New York, 2007, McGraw-Hill. Reproduced with the permission of the McGraw-Hill Companies.)*

three-dimensional digital images in cross section and is used mainly to detect structural abnormalities, including tumors (Figure 7-15). Because the process involves a high level of electromagnetic energy, any metal in range of the device may be drawn toward the source of emission. This poses a genuine risk for injury to the patient and personnel working in the area. Images can also be distorted by the presence of metallic substances in the tissue. These include biomedical devices such as a pacemaker, vascular clips, and certain kinds of tattoos containing metal-based dye. MRI is performed in the interventional medicine or radiology department and occasionally intraoperatively in facilities that have a dedicated surgical suite.

POSITRON EMISSION TOMOGRAPHY

Positron emission tomography (PET) uses the combined technologies of computed tomography and radioactive scanning. PET is performed to produce an image not of a structure, but rather of a metabolic process. In this technique, a biological substance to be followed in the body is "labeled" with radioactive atoms. The labeling is performed by injection. During PET, the radioactive particles emitted by the atoms are traced and computed to provide an image of the physiology and biochemical properties of tissue. These are displayed in three-dimensional color representations of the structure, such as the brain or heart.

ULTRASOUND

Ultrasound energy is generated by high-frequency sound waves. As a diagnostic tool, the sound waves are directed at tissue, which reflects the waves back to produce a real-time image. The images are digitalized for viewing, storage, and reproduction. Ultrasonic waves can be clearly traced through liquid or semiliquid substances. When the ultrasound probe is applied to skin or mucous membrane for deep tissue assessment, a gel coating is used as an interface because the high-frequency waves cannot be precisely tracked through air.

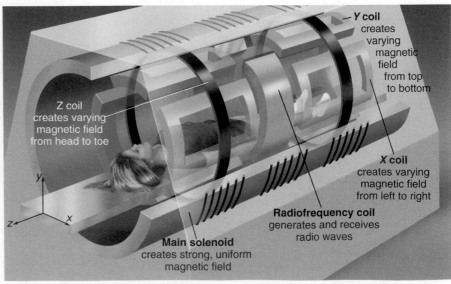

Y coil creates varying magnetic field from top to bottom

Z coil creates varying magnetic field from head to toe

X coil creates varying magnetic field from left to right

Radiofrequency coil generates and receives radio waves

Main solenoid creates strong, uniform magnetic field

Ultrasound has many applications, both intraoperatively and outside surgery. It is commonly used to obtain images of abdominal viscera and for pregnancy assessment. Images represent tissue density. The outline and internal density are identified by shades of black, white, or gray. When combined with the Doppler technique, ultrasound is used vascular surgery to track the movement of blood and provide a screen image of velocity and viscosity. An intraoperative ultrasound probe is used to assess vascular structures and tissue density. Echocardiography is used in the same way to demonstrate motion of the heart.

Doppler studies use ultrasound for specific measurement of vascular flow. The Doppler probe, or transducer, provides **transcutaneous** (through the skin) measurement of vascular obstruction. The sounds reproduced by the Doppler technique differ in pitch and quality and correspond to the movement of blood through a vessel. Doppler sounds can be directly interpreted, or they may be transmitted as wave signals and digitally displayed on a screen for interpretation.

BLOOD TESTS

Blood tests routinely are done to assess the blood's chemistry, function, structure, and composition. The structure and type of blood cells present are also important assessment findings. Many hundreds of blood tests can be done and are routinely performed in the health care setting. The most basic tests are the complete blood count, tests for coagulation, overall blood chemistry, and verification of blood type. The arterial blood gas (ABG) test usually is performed in critical care situations.

COMPLETE BLOOD COUNT

The **complete blood count (CBC)** is a basic test used to evaluate the type and percentage of normal components in the blood (Table 7-3). A blood sample is drawn from the vein and centrifuged. This separates it into cellular and liquid components for evaluation. The CBC is a basic blood test used for screening medical, infectious, and other types of diseases. When formulating a diagnosis, physicians always consider variations in normal blood values along with other signs and symptoms; they are never considered in isolation.

The blood components measured are:

- **Hemoglobin (Hgb):** The oxygen-carrying protein attached to red blood cells (erythrocytes).
- *Red blood cell count:* Erythrocytes make up most of the volume in peripheral blood. They are produced in red bone marrow and live for about 120 days. Their main function is to deliver oxygen to cells.
- **Hematocrit (Hct):** The percentage of red blood cells in the blood (by volume).
- *Platelet count:* Platelets have important functions in the blood clotting mechanism, including clot retraction and activation of coagulation factor.
- *Differential leukocyte count:* White blood cells (leukocytes) are essential to the immune process. The **differential count** measures the number of each type of leukocyte by volume of blood. These are *monocytes, macrophages, band neutrophils, eosinophils, basophils,* and *lymphocytes.*

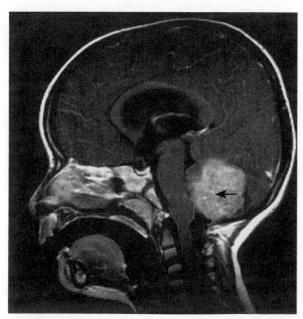

Figure 7-15 Magnetic resonance imaging of a tumor filling the fourth ventricle *(arrow).* MRI uses radiofrequency signals and magnetic energy to produce high-resolution images. *(From Garden O, Bradbury A, Forsythe J, Parks R: Principles and practice of surgery, ed 5, Edinburgh, 2007, Churchill Livingstone.)*

Table **7-3**	**Components of the Complete Blood Count**
Component	**Normal Values**
Hematocrit (Hct)	Men 45% (38%-51%)
	Women 40% (36%-47%)
Hemoglobin (Hgb)	Men 14-17 g/dL
	Women 12-16 g/dL
	Children 12-14 g/dL
Erythrocytes	Men 5.0 (4.5-6.0) million
	Women 4.5-5.5 million
Reticulocytes	1.0%
Leukocytes, total (WBC)	5,000-10,000 (100%)
Differential White Blood Cells	
Segmented neutrophils	2,500-6,000 (7%-40%)
Band neutrophils	0-500 (0%-5%)
Eosinophils	50-300 (1%-3%)
Basophils	0-100 (0%-1%)
Monocytes	200-800 (4%-8%)
Lymphocytes	1,000-4,000 (7%-40%)
Platelets	200,000-500,000

METABOLIC PANEL

The metabolic panel includes a number of tests to determine serum levels of substances that are crucial for metabolism. Many types of metabolic panels can be done. The *basic metabolic panel* includes blood glucose, carbon dioxide, creatinine, urea nitrogen, bicarbonate, and several important electrolytes. The exact tests included in any metabolic panel are determined by health care regulatory agencies and may change with reimbursement regulations.

COAGULATION TESTS

A number of blood studies may be performed to determine coagulation, which is a critical factor for the surgical patient. The tests are used to assess disease states and to monitor patients who are receiving antiplatelet drugs for a clotting disorder.

The mechanism of blood clotting is an extremely complex physiological activity that is divided into two processes, the *intrinsic pathway* and the *extrinsic pathway.* The extrinsic pathway occurs at the tissue level, and the intrinsic pathway occurs in the vascular system. Both systems activate a chemical called *factor X* and the formation of *fibrin* for clotting. The chain reaction of physiological events in the coagulation process is controlled by many chemicals, called *factors,* which are identified by Roman numerals. These are released in specific order, and if one is missing, the clotting mechanism is altered.

The prothrombin time (PT) and partial thromboplastin time (PTT) are determined to evaluate the extrinsic coagulation system. They are also used for screening congenital deficiencies of factors II, V, VII, and X.

The **prothrombin time (PT)** is a measurement of coagulation time. The PT generally is used to monitor the patient on long-term anticoagulant therapy.

The **partial thromboplastin time (PTT)** or activated partial thromboplastin time (APTT) is commonly performed to assess the functional ability of the coagulation sequence. In this test, partial prothrombin is added to coagulated blood. The test is most commonly used to determine the effects of heparin therapy or to screen for clotting disorders.

ARTERIAL BLOOD GASES

Blood pH is regulated by an increase or decrease in specific ions (acid and base). A measurement of these ions (bicarbonate [HCO_3^-] and carbonic acid [H_2CO_3]) provides a snapshot of this balancing mechanism. The partial pressures of carbon dioxide (CO_2) and oxygen (O_2) are also measured and provide an assessment of the patient's ventilatory capacity. Oxygen saturation (O_2Sat) is the amount of oxygen attached to hemoglobin and available to the cells. Blood drawn for ABG testing is usually taken from the radial artery and must be kept cold during transport, because temperature affects the accuracy of the results.

ABO GROUPS

A person's blood type, or **ABO blood group**, is based on inherited antigens found on the surface of an individual's red blood cells. The *Rh type* refers to whether a specific antigen called *Rh* is present. An individual is typed as Rh positive or Rh negative according to whether this antigen is present.

The four significant ABO antigens are A, B, O, and AB. Individuals who lack A and B antigens are typed as *O*. Those who have type A antigens are typed as *A*. Those with B antigens are typed as *B*, and those with both A and B are typed as *AB*.

An individual develops antibodies to the antigen he or she does not have. For example, a person with type A antigens develops antibodies to type B antigens. In the case of a transfusion, the antigen reaction is predictable when the ABO group is known.

The significance of the ABO grouping is that a transfusion of blood containing antibodies to the specific antigens of the blood group can cause a transfusion reaction. This can be a mild allergic reaction or a life-threatening condition. Blood incompatibility can lead to a hemolytic reaction in which the recipient's blood cells are destroyed. For this reason, any patient receiving blood products must be tested for blood grouping before transfusion is performed.

ELECTROLYTES

Body fluids contain both organic and inorganic substances. These substances are essential for homeostasis. Molecules of inorganic substances are capable of splitting to yield a charged particle or substance, called an *electrolyte*. Positively charged electrolytes are called *cations,* and those that are negatively charged are called *anions* (Table 7-4). Cations function mainly in the transmission of nerve impulses to muscles. The highest percentage of positive ions is found in the blood, the cells, intercellular spaces, and the gastrointestinal tract. Electrolyte imbalance can result in severe physiological disturbances. The cations potassium, sodium, calcium, and magnesium are routinely measured in blood. Several anions are measured directly (e.g., ion gap). For more complex information on this topic, a blood chemistry or pathophysiology text should be consulted.

Potassium

Potassium is found mainly in the cells. It is necessary for the transmission of nerve impulses to skeletal, smooth, and cardiac muscle. It also functions in the conversion of carbohydrates for cellular energy and is critical in maintaining osmolality in the cells. *Hypokalemia* (decreased serum potassium) can result from persistent and severe vomiting and diarrhea, extensive tissue trauma, or shock. Certain drugs can also cause a drop in potassium.

Table **7-4** **Electrolytes**

Cations	Anions
Sodium (Na^+)	Chloride (Cl^-)
Potassium (K^+)	Phosphate (PO_4^{3-})
Magnesium (Mg^{2+})	Bicarbonate (HCO_3^-)
Calcium (Ca^{2+})	Sulfate (SO_4^{2-})

Sodium

Sodium is the most plentiful electrolyte found outside the cell. It is responsible for regulation of body and cellular fluids and plays a critical role in the transport of substances into and out of the cell. It binds with specific negatively charged electrolytes to maintain the blood pH. *Hyponatremia* (low sodium) is caused by prolonged vomiting and diarrhea, use of certain diuretics, and surgery.

Calcium

Calcium is found in the cells and also in the extracellular fluid. It is most important in promoting myocardial contraction and in the conversion of thrombin to prothrombin, which is part of the blood-clotting mechanism. Calcium contributes to cell permeability and is necessary for the development and maintenance of bone tissue. *Hypocalcemia* can result from parathyroid disease, vitamin D deficiency, and specific drugs such as corticosteroids and some diuretics.

Magnesium

Magnesium is important in the neurotransmission of all muscles but especially the myocardium. Like calcium, it contributes to cell permeability and also protein and carbohydrate metabolism. Magnesium is necessary for the transport of sodium and potassium through the cell membrane. Hypomagnesemia can be caused by drugs such as corticosteroids, laxatives, and some diuretics.

URINALYSIS

Standard urinalysis is performed to assess the body's overall health, with particular focus on the urinary tract. Simple screening is performed with a dipstick coated with reagents that register the levels of different substances in the urine. These substances are:

- Albumin
- Bilirubin
- Glucose
- Ketones
- Leukocytes
- Blood nitrite
- Urobilinogen

The pH and specific gravity are also assessed. The color, clarity, and odor of the urine are interpreted in the overall assessment. The sample is centrifuged to create sediment, which is examined for microorganisms, crystals, cells, and casts. Urine culture is performed to determine the exact organism associated with a urinary tract infection.

MICROBIOLOGICAL STUDIES

Tissue specimens and fluid suspected of being infected are analyzed to determine the presence and type of microorganisms. Samples that are suspected or known to be contaminated are taken intraoperatively in selected procedures. This is based on evidence of pus, inflammation, or devitalized tissue. A sample confirms the diagnosis and aids treatment decisions. One of the tests used to detect infection is the culture and sensitivity (C & S) test. In this test, a sample is allowed to incubate on a culture medium. After colonization, a number of tests are performed on the colonies to identify the exact microorganism. The sensitivity test exposes the cultured microorganisms to a variety of antibiotic substances during incubation. This determines which of the antibiotics interferes with growth.

PATHOLOGICAL EXAMINATION OF TISSUE

Pathology is the study of diseases. Tissue pathology is the examination of tissue for the presence of disease. In surgery, pathology specimens are routinely obtained and sent to the pathology department for analysis. Each type of tissue requires special care to ensure that the cells are not damaged.

TISSUE BIOPSY

Biopsy is the removal of tissue for analysis and diagnosis. Protocols for tissue preservation vary according to the type of tissue, whether it will be examined immediately, and how it is to be analyzed. The protocol for handling specimens is developed by the facility's pathology department and is available for all perioperative personnel to study. (Chapter 21 presents information on the handling of specimens.) Biopsy specimens can be obtained in a number of ways:

- *Excision:* The surgical removal of a small portion of tissue. Excision usually refers to removal by cutting (also called *excisional biopsy*).
- *Needle* or *trocar biopsy:* The removal of tissue with a hollow needle or trocar, which is inserted into the tissue. A core sample of the tissue is removed in one or more locations of the suspected area. The needle can be inserted through the skin (percutaneously) or into tissue exposed during surgery. A hollow trocar may be used to remove a large core of tissue such as bone marrow.
- *Brush biopsy:* A biopsy brush, a very small cylindrical brush, is used to sweep a hollow lumen or cavity for cells. This technique is commonly used in diagnostic procedures of the throat structures and bronchi. The procedure removes only superficial cells and does not cut into the tissue. After biopsy, the brush is withdrawn and immediately swished in liquid preservative or saline to prevent drying.
- *Aspiration biopsy:* Fluid for pathological examination may be removed from semisolid tissue by aspirating the fluid (removal with a syringe). The term *centesis* refers to aspiration of fluid.
- *Smear:* A smear is obtained by passing a swab or small brush over superficial tissue. The swab is passed over a glass microscope slide, which is sprayed with a cell fixative. The specimen can then be examined microscopically by the pathologist.
- *Frozen section:* Immediate microscopic and gross (without aid of the microscope) examination of suspect tissue is performed by *frozen section*. In this procedure, the tissue is removed and immediately placed in liquid nitrogen. This freezes the sample. It is then sliced into single-cell sections and analyzed microscopically. A surgical procedure is purposefully scheduled with a frozen section to determine the need for radical or more extensive excision of a tumor. A

permanent section fixes the tissue slices on slides for preservation. (Chapter 21 presents a complete discussion of the intraoperative care of frozen section tissue.)

CANCER TERMS AND CONCEPTS

Surgery commonly is performed to diagnose or treat cancer. Terms related to cancer treatment, classification, and diagnosis are used in the perioperative setting. A basic understanding of these terms and their origin is an important aspect of surgical practice.

DEFINITIONS

A **neoplasm**, or tumor, is an abnormal growth. A tumor is classified as malignant or benign. A **malignant** tumor is composed of disorganized tissue that exhibits uncontrolled growth. Malignant tissue has the potential to spread from the original site (called the *primary tumor*) to other parts of the body. A **benign** growth is composed of cells belonging to a single tissue type and does not spread to distant regions of the body. Any word with the ending *-oma* refers to a tumor (e.g., osteoma, leiomyoma, lymphoma).

COMPARISON OF MALIGNANT AND BENIGN TUMORS

A benign tumor often resembles the tissue in which it originates. It does not undergo histological change (changes in the tissue type) but remains consistent during growth. These tumors usually are encapsulated or confined and do not infiltrate the tissue bed. A benign tumor may continue to grow but does not take over the functions of the original tissue. In contrast, a malignant tumor develops a disorganized vascular system and usually contains different types of cells or tissue. It invades the tissue of origin and captures its nutrients and often its blood flow. Malignant cells release toxins that kill normal cells, and the tumor grows quickly and invasively. Cells from the malignancy break off and enter the lymph system, where they are transported to other areas of the body. New tumors may develop from these seed cells; this is called **metastasis**. Eventually the tumor disrupts or halts the normal function of vital organs. Malignancy usually results in death unless it is treated early.

A benign tumor may impinge on nearby tissue or organs. This can interrupt blood supply, cause pain, or alter the function of healthy tissue. However, the tumor grows slowly compared to malignant tissue, and the benign tissue does not invade the healthy tissue or deplete its nutrients.

EFFECTS OF MALIGNANCY ON THE BODY

Malignancy causes specific injury to the body:

- The risk of thrombosis (blood clot) is increased as a result of inappropriate production of clotting factors by the tumor itself. The tumor may also block blood vessels, resulting in clotting.
- Pain is caused by direct injury to tissue or by pain mediators released by the tumor. As the tumor impinges on healthy tissue, the tissue dies, resulting in severe pain.
- Cachexia (tissue and body wasting) is characteristic of malignancy. As the tumor destroys tissue, the patient's metabolism is altered. Nutrients normally received by healthy tissue for growth and repair are captured by the malignant tissue, which continues to grow and spread.
- Anemia occurs as a result of internal bleeding and the body's inability to replace red blood cells.
- As the malignancy spreads, changes occur in the function of the target tissue. This results in many different disease conditions, depending on the organ or tissue function.

DIAGNOSTIC METHODS

Several tests commonly are performed to screen for suspected cancer. The exact type of test depends on the affected tissue.

Tumor Markers

A **tumor marker** is an antigen present on the tumor cell or other substance (protein, hormone, or other chemical) released by the cells into the blood. Some markers are specific for certain types of cancer cells. Markers are not always reliable for diagnosing malignancy, because some benign tumors can also release markers. Tests for tumor markers are most useful in patients undergoing treatment when a comparison provides information during the course of therapy. An assessment tool for the detection of prostate cancer is measurement of the tumor marker prostate-specific antigen (PSA). Another common assessment marker is CA-125, which is present in some types of ovarian cancer.

Biopsy

A tissue biopsy is a sample of tissue, cells, or fluid that is removed from the body and examined for suspected disease. A tissue biopsy can be a small segment of the suspected tissue, a cell washing, a smear, or a blood sample. The Pap smear (Papanicolaou test) is a familiar type of routine biopsy for cervical cancer. The frozen section specimen described previously is another type of biopsy.

Tumor Staging

Two methods are used to classify malignant tumors; this is called **staging**. One is by analysis of the cellular characteristics; the other is by the spread of cancer (i.e., the metastatic pattern). Staging provides a basis on which to select the most beneficial treatment. It also indicates the progress of treatment and the outcome, or *prognosis*. The staging process is an internationally used system called the **TNM classification system** (Box 7-2). *T* refers to the extent of the tumor, *N* refers to lymph node involvement, and *M* is the extent of metastasis. Tumors are also graded according to the level of cellular differentiation. Grades I through IV indicate decreasing levels of differentiation. Grade I cells show the most differentiation. Decreased differentiation indicates more serious disease; thus, grade IV has greater risk of lethality than grade I.

Box **7-2**	**Tumor-Node-Metastasis (TNM) Classification System**

Tumor

Tx	The tumor cannot be assessed.
T0	No evidence of a primary tumor.
Tis	Carcinoma in situ.
T1-T4	Increasing tumor size or involvement of healthy tissue.

Nodes

Nx	Lymph nodes cannot be assessed.
N0	No evidence of lymph node involvement.
N1-3	Increasing involvement of regional lymph nodes.

Metastasis

Mx	Metastasis not assessed.
M10	No evidence of distant metastasis.
M1	Distant metastasis confirmed and site indicated.

CANCER PREVENTION AND SCREENING

Many forms of cancer can be treated in the early stages of the disease. Public health promotion and screening procedures enable people to learn about cancer and protect themselves against some cancers.

An updated review of screening recommendations can be found on the National Cancer Institute's website at http://www.cancer.gov.

NUCLEAR MEDICINE

Nuclear medicine involves the use of radioactive particles, which are directed at the nucleus of a selected element to create energy. These special elements are referred to as **radionuclides or isotopes**. Radionuclides emit gamma radiation and can be used for diagnosis and treatment. Administered intravenously, orally, or by direct deposition, they can be traced to reveal the structure and function of an organ, a system, a cavity, or a tissue.

RADIATION THERAPY

Tissue destruction by ionizing radiation is used in the treatment of a neoplasm. The delivery and implantation systems for radiation therapy include needles, seeds, and capsulated implants. Radiation therapy procedures are carried out in designated areas of the hospital or health care facility by specially trained personnel. In addition to implantation procedures, intraoperative radiation therapy is used to deliver a single dose of radiation to a specific area of the body.

In needle delivery systems, cesium-137, a radioactive isotope, is enclosed in dose units and contained in special hollow needles for insertion into tissue. The needles are placed around the borders of the tumor. These are connected by heavy sutures and secured to the patient's skin. The needles remain in place up to 7 days.

Radioactive seeds can be implanted directly into the tumor mass and may be left in the patient indefinitely. Cesium-137,

iodine-125, and iridium-192 are used in this procedure. Seeds generally are used in tumors that cannot be removed by surgical resection because of precarious location or size. The procedure may be performed intraoperatively or in the interventional radiology department.

Short-acting radiotherapy in high doses can be delivered through *brachytherapy*. In this procedure, a capsule containing high-dose radiation is implanted using a special catheter. Radioactive pellets are inserted into the implanted catheter for several days and then removed. This treatment is used in breast and prostate cancer.

Historical Highlights

For many years it was thought that an allergy to shellfish meant that a patient was also allergic to injectable iodinated contrast media. There were never any clinical data to support this, but the misinformation continued to be widespread. The theory was formally debunked in the early 2000s. Allergic reactions to injectable contrast media do exist in about 3% of cases, but these are unrelated to shellfish.

For more information see the U.S. Department of Health and Human Services, Agency for Healthcare Research and Quality, Reaction to Dye, available at http://www.webmm.ahrq.gov/case.aspx?caseID=75, or search on "AHRQ dye."

KEY CONCEPTS

- The first step in medical and surgical decision making is assessment of the problem.
- An invasive procedure involves breaking intact skin or mucous membrane or inserting a medical device into a body cavity. Noninvasive procedures are limited to skin contact or no direct contact with the body.
- The vital signs include temperature, pulse, respiratory rate, and blood pressure, and in the health care setting, a measurement of the patient's level of pain.
- Filling of the heart chambers and shunting of blood through the heart is called the systolic pressure. As the heart relaxes between contractions, the pressure decreases. This is called the diastolic pressure.
- An ECG machine measures the electrical activity of the heart.
- The images formed by x-rays display contrasts in density. An extremely dense substance produces a white image, whereas air produces a black image.
- The term *radiopaque* refers to substances that x-rays cannot penetrate.
- In surgery, the mobile C-arm fluoroscope is used for real-time imaging.
- In computed tomography, x-ray and computer technologies are combined to produce high-contrast cross-sectional images.
- Magnetic resonance imaging uses radiofrequency signals and magnetic energy to produce images.
- Positron emission tomography uses the combined technologies of CT and radioactive scanning.

- During ultrasound imaging, high-frequency sound waves are directed at tissue. These are reflected back to produce an image of the tissue.
- Doppler studies use ultrasound to measure vascular flow. The reflected sound waves can be interpreted directly or transmitted as waveforms on a digital output monitor.
- The complete blood count is a basic test used to evaluate the type and percentage of normal components in the blood.
- The prothrombin time is a measurement of coagulation time.
- The ABO blood groups, also known as blood types, are categorizations based on inherited antigens found on the surface of an individual's red blood cells.
- Electrolytes are vital for homeostasis and are responsible for nerve impulses, fluid balance, transport of substances into and out of the cell, and balancing of the blood pH.
- Biopsy is the removal of tissue for analysis and diagnosis.
- Excision is the surgical removal of a small portion of tissue. Excision usually refers to removal by cutting (also called excisional biopsy).
- Brush biopsy is performed with a very small cylindrical brush used to sweep a hollow lumen or cavity for cells.
- In an aspiration biopsy, fluid for pathological examination is removed from semisolid tissue by aspirating fluid (removal with a syringe).
- A smear is obtained by passing a swab or small brush over superficial tissue. The swab then is passed over a glass microscope slide and sprayed with a cell fixative.
- A frozen section is removal of tissue for immediate pathological assessment. The tissue specimen is frozen and passed through a device that produces single-cell sections for examination.
- A neoplasm, or tumor, is excessive, disorganized growth of tissue.
- A malignant neoplasm consists of nondifferentiated cells that have the potential to break loose from the original site and spread to other parts of the body.
- Tissue destruction by ionizing radiation is used in the treatment of a neoplasm. The delivery and implantation systems for radiation therapy include needles, seeds, and capsulated implants.

REVIEW QUESTIONS

1. Describe the factors that can increase core temperature in the clinical setting.
2. Which methods of temperature assessment accurately reflect core temperature?
3. How do you correctly document the patient's vital signs? Give examples and explain what they mean.
4. What are the causes of a falsely high blood pressure reading?
5. What is "postural" blood pressure?
6. The peaks and troughs on the ECG reading correspond to what?
7. What is the purpose of a contrast medium?
8. What is the differential leukocyte count?
9. Compare the main differences between a malignant and a benign tumor.
10. What is a tumor marker?
11. Why do you think people do not take advantage of screening procedures for cancer?

CASE STUDIES

Case 1

While assisting the circulator during outpatient surgery under local anesthesia, you are asked to take the patient's vital signs for the duration of the case. Explain the following:

1. You do not know what the patient's *normal* vital signs are. Do you need to know this in order to carry out this role?
2. You cannot find an available digital blood pressure apparatus so you must use a stethoscope and manual sphygmomanometer. Is this important to the documentation?
3. The circulator asks you to record all three elements of blood pressure. What does he mean and how do you measure it?
4. You are required to take vital signs every 15 minutes. You have missed one blood pressure reading. The next diastolic reading you get is elevated by 20 points. The pulse rate is elevated by 15. Should you report this immediately or repeat the measurement?

Case 2

During emergency surgery, you are assisting the circulator. You are asked to rush to the laboratory and pick up 2 units of blood for the patient. You arrive at the lab and are handed 2 bags of blood. When you return to the operating room you discover that the patient's name as documented with the blood is incorrect. How should this have been prevented?

Case 3

According to your knowledge of arterial blood gases, why would getting blood gases be an emergency procedure? Why do you think the blood must be arterial rather then venous blood?

BIBLIOGRAPHY

Chernecky C, Berger B: *Laboratory tests and diagnostic procedures*, ed 2, St Louis, 2008, Mosby.

McPhee S, Papadakis M, Tierney L: *Current medical diagnosis and treatment*, ed 46, New York, 2007, McGraw-Hill.

Porth C: *Pathophysiology concepts of altered health states*, ed 6, Philadelphia, 2007, Lippincott Williams & Wilkins.

Environmental Hazards

8

CHAPTER OUTLINE

Introduction
Risk and Safety

Technical Risks
Chemical Risks

Biological Risks
Musculoskeletal Risks

LEARNING OBJECTIVES

After studying this chapter the reader will be able to:

1. Identify the types of risks that are present in the operating room
2. Explain the importance of the fire triangle
3. Discuss fuels and sources of ignition commonly found in the operating room
4. Describe how to respond appropriately to a patient fire
5. Identify methods associated with preventing fires in the operating room
6. Describe measures to safely store, transport, and use compressed gas cylinders
7. Discuss the principles of electricity in the operating room
8. Identify precautions to prevent exposure to ionizing radiation

9. Describe methods to avoid chemical injury
10. Describe toxic substances in smoke plume
11. Identify the practice of Standard Precautions
12. Discuss various techniques to prevent sharps injuries
13. Identify the practice for transmission-based precautions
14. Identify methods of properly handling and disposing of hazardous waste in the operating room
15. Describe the symptoms of true latex allergy
16. Identify necessary precautions to prevent latex reaction in allergic patients
17. Describe proper body mechanics for lifting, pulling, and pushing objects

TERMINOLOGY

Airborne transmission precautions: Precautions that prevent airborne transfer of disease organisms in the environment.

Blood-borne pathogens: Harmful microorganisms that may be present in and transmitted through human blood and body fluids.

Electrocution: Severe burns, cardiac disturbances, or death as a result of electrical current discharged into the body.

Electrosurgical unit (ESU): Medical device commonly used in surgery to coagulate blood vessels and cut tissue.

Eschar: Burned tissue fragments that can accumulate on the electrosurgical tip during surgery; eschar can cause sparking and become a source of ignition.

Flammable: Capable of burning.

Grounding: A path for electrical current to flow unimpeded through a material and disperse back to the source or disperse into the ground.

Hypersensitivity: A cell-mediated immune response to a substance in the body.

Impedance (resistance): The ability of a substance to stop or alter the flow of electrons through a conductive material.

Latex: A naturally occurring sap obtained from rubber trees that is used in the manufacture of medical devices, supplies, and patient care items.

Neutral zone (no-hands) technique: A method of transferring sharp instruments on the surgical field without hand-to-hand

contact. A neutral zone is identified, and sharps are exchanged in this zone.

Occupational exposure: Exposure to hazards in the workplace; for example, exposure to hazardous chemicals or contact with potentially infected blood and body fluids.

Oxidizers: Agents or substances capable of supporting fire.

Oxygen-enriched atmosphere (OEA): An environment that contains a high percentage of oxygen and therefore presents a high risk for fire.

Personal protective equipment (PPE): Clothing or equipment that protects the wearer from direct contact with hazardous chemicals or potentially infectious body fluids.

Postexposure prophylaxis (PEP): Recommended procedures to help prevent the development of blood-borne diseases after an exposure incident such as a needlestick injury.

Risk: The statistical probability of a given event based on the number of such events that have already occurred in a defined population.

Sharps: Any objects that can penetrate the skin and have the potential to cause injury and infection. Sharps include but are not limited to needles, scalpels, broken glass, broken capillary tubes, and exposed ends of dental wires.

Smoke plume: Smoke created during the use of an electrosurgical unit (ESU) or laser. This smoke contains toxic chemicals, vapors, blood fragments, and viruses.

TERMINOLOGY (cont.)

Standard Precautions: Guidelines issued by the Centers for Disease Control and Prevention (CDC) to reduce the risk of transmission of blood-borne and other pathogens.

Transmission-based precautions: Standards and precautions to prevent the spread of infectious disease by patients known to be infected.

Underwriters Laboratories (UL): A nonprofit agency that tests and certifies electrical equipment in the United States.

Volatile: A substance with a low boiling point such as alcohol that converts to a vapor at low temperature.

INTRODUCTION

The potential for accident and injury in the operating room is one of the highest in the health care setting. High-voltage equipment, chemicals, exposure to blood and body fluids, and stress injury are some of the risks that perioperative personnel encounter daily.

Management of environmental risks requires knowledge of the risk, a plan of action, and continuous monitoring. A successful injury reduction plan considers both the human factor and the technological aspects. Education, awareness, and compliance with recommendations and safety protocols are equally important. This chapter discusses hazards in the operating room environment and provides a basis for knowledge and understanding of the hazards for patients and personnel.

RISK AND SAFETY

Risk is the statistical probability of a harmful event; it is defined as the number of harmful events that occur in a given population over a stated period. In other words, risk represents the number of times an event actually occurs under specified conditions in a specific environment. For example, the risk of contracting human immunodeficiency virus (HIV) as a result of working in the health care environment is based on the number of people who have contracted HIV through **occupational exposure** in the past (based on yearly statistics). Risk and probability are not difficult to measure when sentinel event reporting is performed each time there is an accident or injury in the workplace. Statistics are collected and analyzed so that risk can be measured and policies put in place to prevent future accidents. People often ignore risk factors because they believe themselves immune from harm, or they believe they will somehow escape the danger. They know that risk exists, but not for themselves. Taking risks means trying to beat the odds, but it does not change the probability that a given event will occur.

In the health care setting, taking a risk for oneself often means risking the safety of the patient and other staff members.

Most of the discussions in this chapter focus on the technical aspects of accident and injury. However, human factors also contribute to risk. Some of the human causes of injury include:

- Fatigue in the workplace
- A work culture focused on completion of tasks rather than the methods used to complete the tasks safely

- Rushing through tasks to get the work done
- Lack of knowledge about the risks involved
- Emotional strain and stress, which may influence work habits

A culture of safety is crucial to injury reduction in the workplace. This means that staff members must have *awareness* of the risk, *accept* the responsibility for harm reduction, and *act* on prevention measures.

The risks discussed in this chapter focus on the three types of potential injury that represent the most common sources of accidents:

- *Technical risk factors:* Hazards related to medical devices and energy sources
- *Chemical risk factors:* Hazards related primarily to liquid, gas, and solid chemicals in the perioperative environment
- *Biological risk factors:* Hazards related to the transmission of infectious disease

SAFETY STANDARDS AND RECOMMENDATIONS

A number of private, professional, and government organizations create standards and recommendations aimed at reducing injury in the health care setting:

- *ECRI Institute:* A nonprofit research organization designated as an evidence-based practice center by the U.S. Agency for Healthcare Research and Quality and a collaborating agency of the World Health Organization. Note that ECRI is not an acronym. The initials ECRI have a historical origin. http://www.ecri.org
- *Association for Professionals in Infection Control and Epidemiology (APIC):* http://www.apic.org
- *Centers for Disease Control and Prevention (CDC):* An agency of the federal government and the central authority on infectious diseases. http://www.cdc.gov
- *U.S. Environmental Protection Agency (EPA):* http://www.epa.gov
- *U.S. Food and Drug Administration (FDA):* http://www.fda.gov
- *The Joint Commission:* http://www.jointcommission.org
- *Occupational Safety and Health Administration (OSHA):* http://www.osha.gov

These organizations can be contacted for further information on patient and occupational risks in surgery. Standards are periodically updated and renewed. The surgical technologist should remain current, because hazards and risks change as new technologies develop.

TECHNICAL RISKS

Technical risks related to medical devices remain high in spite of increased awareness and safety programs in health care facilities. The expanded role of surgical technologists places them in an important position to influence safety practices in the surgical department. In the future, surgical technologists may have even greater responsibilities for the departmental management of devices in surgery. As medical and surgical technology becomes increasingly complex, the demand for safety and awareness also increases.

FIRE

Fire in the operating room historically has been a great risk. In the past, many fires were associated with flammable anesthetics and unregulated combustible materials. Although these are no longer used, fire is still a real risk. All accredited health care facilities have a responsibility and mandate to orient employees and students to fire safety practices, including the use of fire extinguishers and facility evacuation procedures.

Fire Triangle

Fire requires three components:
- *Oxygen* (available in the air or as a pure gas)
- *Fuel* (a combustible material)
- *Source of ignition* (usually in the form of heat)

These components are commonly present in the operating room (Figure 8-1).

OXYGEN Normal air contains about 21% oxygen. An environment that contains a greater concentration of oxygen is called an **oxygen-enriched atmosphere (OEA)**. The operating room is an OEA because oxygen is used in conjunction with general anesthetics and in patient care. Consequently, the risk of fire is high. Oxygen is heavier than air, so it settles under drapes and in confined areas, such as body cavities, where it remains trapped. Also, oxygen molecules are produced when nitrous oxide, used in anesthesia, decomposes in the presence of heat, and this adds to the accumulated level of oxygen.

As the concentration of oxygen increases in the environment, so does the *speed* of ignition, *duration* of the fire, and the *temperature* of the flames. Items that normally would not burn in atmospheric air are highly flammable in the presence of oxygen. Oxygen and nitrous oxide are called **oxidizers**, because they are capable of supporting fire.

FUEL Any material capable of burning is potential fuel for a fire. Materials and substances that burn are called *flammable*. Note that the words *flammable* and *inflammable* have the same meaning; both indicate combustibility. Sources of fuel commonly found at the surgical site are listed in Table 8-1. Although many items used in the surgical setting are considered "flame resistant" or "flame retardant," they may easily catch fire and continue to burn when ignition occurs in an OEA.

Flammable Chemicals

Alcohol is now commonly used in skin prep solutions and is a high risk source of fuel in surgical fires. An alcohol concentration greater than 20% is flammable and highly **volatile** (i.e., vaporizes at a low temperature). Most skin prep solutions contain 70% alcohol.

Vapor from alcohol can be trapped under drapes. When the vapor is ignited, the fire is hidden from view. Second- or

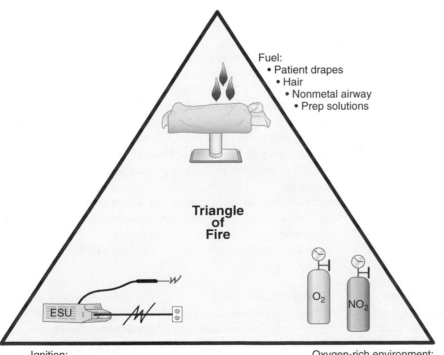

Figure 8-1   The triangle of fire.

Fuel:
- Patient drapes
- Hair
- Nonmetal airway
- Prep solutions

Triangle of Fire

ESU

O₂   NO₂

Ignition:
- Electrosurgical unit
- Laser
- Faulty electrical equipment

Oxygen-rich environment:
- Oxygen
- Nitrogen

Table 8-1 Fuel Sources at the Surgical Site

Fuel Source	Fire Prevention
Oxygen-rich environment (OEA)	Tent drapes away from the patient's head during surgery.
Dry sponges and drapes	Place the tip of the electrosurgical unit (ESU) in a holder.
	Use wet towels, wet sponges, or nonflammable drapes at the operative site.
Endotracheal tube and other flammable anesthesia equipment	Use only laser-approved airways and endotracheal tubes.
	Use a reflective shield between the patient's head and the surgical field.
Volatile prep solutions	Drape the patient only after all prepping solutions are dry.
	Tent drapes to allow the escape of vapors when an alcohol-based prep is used.
	Always check for solutions pooling under the patient before draping.
Lanugo (fine body hair on the patient)	Use a water-based gel on lanugo near laser or ESU sites.
Petroleum-based products	Do not use around laser or ESU sites.
Suction catheter and other peripheral venous catheter (PVC) devices	Do not use around ESU or laser sites.
Smoke plume evacuator tip	Use noncombustible evacuator tip.
	Use moist sponges around laser area.
Gastrointestinal gas	Use suction to remove gases at operative site.

third-degree burns can occur within moments of ignition. Most fires arising from alcohol prep solutions occur in combination with an electrosurgical spark (ignition). Although alcohol is highly volatile, it is widely used because it is inexpensive, readily available, and effective.

Chemicals such as cyanoacrylates (fibrin glue), used as tissue glue and for taking tissue grafts, and methylmethacrylate (bone cement) are volatile and flammable. Petroleum products, such as ointments, also can ignite.

Medical Devices

Rubber, plastic, Silastic, and vinyl materials are flammable. Medical devices made of these materials are common in surgery. Disposable anesthesia equipment, such as endotracheal tubes, airways, masks, cannulas, and corrugated tubing, is a hazardous source of fuel.

Endotracheal tubes, except those made especially for laser surgery, are frequently the cause of patient fires during laser surgery of the head, neck, and face. An endotracheal fire can begin as an explosion, causing extensive burns within seconds. The fire moves quickly along the oxygen path and spreads to the lungs, face, hair, and drapes.

Drapes and Gowns

Surgical drapes and gowns are flame resistant. However, in an OEA they can ignite easily. The operating table mattress and positioning devices made of foam and liquid gels also are potential fuel. As these items burn, they release toxic gases that are an additional source of injury.

Intestinal Gases

The intestine normally produces hydrogen, oxygen, nitrogen, carbon dioxide, and methane. Some gases are produced by normal bacteria in the gastrointestinal tract, and others are ingested with food. Forty percent of these gases are contained in the large bowel. Hydrogen and methane are present in sufficient quantities and concentration to be an important risk. Methane is explosive at concentrations of 5% to 15%.

SOURCES OF IGNITION Any heat-producing device has the potential to cause a fire. The more intense the heat, the more rapidly oxidation and ignition are likely to occur. Many potential sources of ignition can be found in the operating room.

Laser

Approximately 13% of surgical fires involve lasers.[1] Laser surgery of the trachea and adjacent structures is performed in an OEA close to flammable material. During laser surgery of the neck and throat, a nonflammable endotracheal tube and aluminum-coated drapes are used. In spite of these precautions, laser energy remains a potent source of ignition in an OEA during surgery.

Electrosurgical unit

The **electrosurgical unit (ESU)** uses electrical energy to coagulate and cut tissue. The active electrode can reach 1,292° F (700° C), hot enough to ignite surgical drapes and other supplies. The tip of the active electrode can become coated with **eschar** (oxidized tissue residue), which holds heat in much the same way as charcoal. Eschar causes sparking and ignition. Small bits of eschar can be released into the wound as burning embers (e.g., into the throat during neck surgery).

Sparking can occur when the active electrode comes in contact with metal. Sparks can ignite volatile gases, liquids, drapes, and sponges, especially in an OEA. (Chapter 18 presents a complete discussion of the hazards associated with the ESU.)

High-Speed Instruments

Other, less obvious devices can ignite combustible materials in surgery. These include power instruments, burrs, drill bits, saws, and the harmonic scalpel, which uses high-frequency sound waves to cut and coagulate tissue. When high-speed drills are used, the active tip is irrigated to prevent the buildup of heat created by friction between the metal tip and the bone.

Hot drill bits, saw blades, and other metal tips should never be placed in contact with drapes or other combustible materials.

High-Intensity Light

Light sources used in surgery are intense and bright. Although modern surgical light is cooler than in the past, these light sources are still a risk. Fiberoptic light, used in endoscopic instruments, is particularly intense. The light source is delivered through a fiberoptic cable. When the cable is detached from the endoscope, light emitted from the cable can easily ignite drapes, cloth, or other materials. (The safe use of fiberoptic light is fully described in Chapter 24.)

Electrical Malfunction

An electrical short or other malfunction can cause sparking (electrical arcing), which can ignite combustible materials on the surgical field. If an electrical device malfunctions during surgery, it must be removed from service immediately and sent out of the department for repair by the bioengineering department or manufacturer. Perioperative staff should never attempt to repair malfunctioning electrical equipment.

Fire in the Operating Room

PATIENT FIRE Patient fire is a devastating event. Approximately 21% of patient fires occur in the airway, 44% on the face, 8% inside the patient, and 26% on the skin.[2] It takes only moments for a flash fire to engulf the patient. To stop the progression of the fire, *the triangle of fire must be broken*. This means that one or more components (fuel, oxygen, or source of ignition) must be removed from the fire.

During a patient fire, time is critical. Three steps are immediately taken to protect the patient and stop the fire:
1. Shut off the flow of all gases to the patient's airway.
2. Remove any burning objects from the surgical site.
3. Assess the patient for injury and respond appropriately.

The anesthesia care provider reduces the flow of oxygen in the event of fire around the airway. At the same time, burning objects are removed from the field as safely as possible. The surgical technologist must stand by for direction from the surgeon and other staff members in the room. Patient fires usually can be contained when one of the elements of the fire has been removed. The next phase of the emergency focuses on the patient's injuries.

Structural Fire

If the fire extends beyond the immediate patient area, the surgical team must activate the hospital evacuation plan. This plan is based on four immediate actions, which are easily remembered by the acronym *RACE*:

Rescue patients in the immediate area of the fire.

Alert other people to the fire so that they can assist in patient removal and response. Activate the fire alert system.

Contain the fire. Shut all doors to slow the spread of smoke and flame. Always shut off the zone valves controlling inline gases to the room.

Evacuate personnel in the areas around the fire.

If the fire is limited to a small area, appropriate extinguishing agents may be used to put it out. Personnel should never let a fire get between them and the exit.

FIRE DRILLS AND EXTINGUISHERS Fire drills are held regularly in all health care facilities. Staff training on fire includes emergency response, the location of fire extinguishers and fire escape routes, and how to activate the fire alert system. Most fire extinguishers used in the operating room are water-based, carbon dioxide, or dry powder. Carbon dioxide is the preferred type for operating room fires.

During fire extinguisher training, employees and students are asked to remember the acronym *PASS*:

Pull the ring from the handle.

Aim the nozzle at the base of the fire.

Squeeze the handle.

Sweep the fire with tank contents.

Fire Prevention

- Fire prevention is the responsibility of everyone working in the operating room. Risk reduction strategies have been developed by the Joint Commission, ECRI, AORN, and other professional organizations concerned with the protection of patients and staff members. The following strategies are the focus of risk management:
- Participation in fire drills
- Demonstration of the use of firefighting equipment
- Developing methods for rescue operation
- Gas shutoff procedures
- Location of ventilation and electrical systems
- Review of code "red" (fire alert) policies
- Review of fire department procedures
- Developing a safety culture

Risk Management

AORN has established fire risk management strategies based on current recommendations for perioperative personnel. These are shown in Tables 8-2 and 8-3.

COMPRESSED GAS CYLINDERS

Gases such as oxygen, nitrous oxide, argon, and nitrogen are compressed into metal tanks, called *cylinders* for medical use:

- *Oxygen* is contained in portable tanks and is used when inline systems are not available or when patients are transported.
- *Compressed* nitrogen and air are used as a power source for instruments such as drills, saws, and other high-speed power tools.
- *Argon* is used during laser surgery.
- *Nitrous oxide* is an anesthetic gas.
- *Carbon dioxide* is used for insufflation of the abdominal cavity during laparoscopy or pelviscopy.

Cylinder Components and Specifications

A compressed gas cylinder is made of heavy steel, able to withstand the high pressure of the gas and to resist puncture or breakage. The wall of a large cylinder is approximately ¼

Table 8-2 Fire Management Strategies: Ignition

Risk	Management
Electrosurgical unit (ESU)	• Use the lowest possible power setting. • Place the patient return electrode on a large muscle mass close to the surgical site. • Large reusable return electrodes should be used according to the manufacturer's instructions. • Always use a safety holster. • Do not coil active electrode cords. • Inspect the active electrode to ensure its integrity. • Do not use the ESU in the presence of flammable solutions. • Ensure that electrical cords and plugs are not frayed or broken. • Do not place fluids on top of the ESU control unit. • Do not use the ESU near oxygen or nitrous oxide. • Ensure that the ESU active electrode tip fits securely into the active electrode handpiece. • Ensure that any connections and adaptors used are intended to connect to the ESU and fit securely. • Do not bypass ESU safety features. • Ensure that the alarm tone is always audible. • Remove any contaminated or unused active accessories from the sterile field. • Keep the active electrode tip clean. • Use wet sponges or towels to help retard fire potential. • Never alter a medical device. • Do not use rubber catheters or protective covers as insulators on the active electrode tip. • Use *Cut* or *Blend* instead of *Coagulation* when possible. • Do not open the circuit to activate the ESU. • Make sure the active electrode is not activated near another metal object that could conduct heat or cause arcing. • After prepping, allow the prep solution to dry and the fumes to dissipate. Wet prep and fumes trapped beneath drapes can ignite. • Provide multidisciplinary in-service programs on the safe use of ESUs based on the manufacturer's instructions
Argon beam coagulator	• Argon beam coagulators combine the ESU spark with argon gas to concentrate and focus the ESU spark. Argon gas is inert and nonflammable, but because it is used with an ESU, the same precautions as with an ESU should be taken. • Always use a safety holster. • Make sure the active electrode is not activated near another metal object that could conduct heat or cause arcing.
Laser	• Use a laser-specific endotracheal tube (i.e., a tube that has laser-resistant coating or contains no material that will ignite) if head, neck, lung, or airway surgery is anticipated. • Wet sponges around the tube cuffs may provide extra protection to help retard fire potential. Moist towels around the surgical site also may retard fires. • Keep towels moist and away from the edge of the surgical site to retard fires. • Do not use liquids or ointments that may be combustible. • Inflate cuffed tube bladders with tinted saline so that inadvertent rupture may be detected during chest or upper airway surgery. • Do not use uncuffed, standard endotracheal tubes in the presence of a laser or the ESU. • If an endotracheal tube fire occurs, oxygen administration should be stopped and all burning or melted tubes should be removed from the patient immediately. • Prevent pooling of skin prep solutions. • Have water and the correct type of fire extinguisher available in case of a laser fire. • Ensure that the alarm tone is always audible.
Fiberoptic light sources and cables	• Ensure that the light source is in good working order. • Place the light source in standby or turn it off when the cable is not connected. • Place the light source away from items that are flammable. • Do not place a light cable that is connected to a light source on drapes, sponges, or anything else that is flammable. • Do not allow cables that are connected to hang over the side of the sterile field if the light source is on. • Make sure light cables are in good working order and do not have broken light fibers.

Table 8-2 **Fire Management Strategies: Ignition—cont'd**	
Risk	**Management**
Power tools, drills, and burrs	• Instruments and equipment that move rapidly during use generate heat. Always make sure they are in good working order. • A slow drip of saline on a moving drill or burr helps reduce heat buildup. • Do not place drills, burrs, or saws on the patient when they are not in use. • Remove instruments and equipment from the sterile field when not in use.
Defibrillator paddles	• Select paddles that are the correct size for the patient (e.g., pediatric paddles on a child). • Ensure that the gel recommended by the paddle manufacturer is used. • Adhere to appropriate site selection for paddle placement. • Contact between the paddles and the patient should be optimal, and no gaps should be present before the defibrillator is activated.
Electrical equipment	• Ensure that all equipment is inspected periodically by biomedical personnel for proper function. • Check the biomedical inspection stickers on the equipment; they should be current. • Do not use equipment with frayed or damaged cords or plugs. • Remove any equipment that emits smoke during use.

Modified from the Association of periOperative Registered Nurses (AORN): Fire prevention in the operating room. In *Standards, recommendations, practices and guidelines, 2007 edition*, Denver, 2007, AORN.

Table 8-3 **Management Strategies: Fuel and Oxidizers**	
Fire Risk—Fuel	
Fuel Sources	**Management Strategies**
Bed linens Caps, hats Drapes Dressings Gowns Lap pads Shoe covers Sponges Tapes Towels	• Assess the flammability of all materials used in, on, or around the patient. Linens and drapes are made of synthetic or natural fibers. They may burn or melt, depending on the fiber content. • Do not allow drapes or linens to come in contact with activated ignition sources (e.g., laser, electrosurgical unit [ESU], light sources). • Do not trap volatile chemicals or chemical fumes beneath drapes. • Moisten drapes, towels, and sponges that will be near ignition sources. • Ensure that oxygen does not accumulate beneath drapes. • If drapes or linens ignite, smother small fires with a wet sponge or towel. Remove burning material from the patient. • Extinguish any burning material with the appropriate fire extinguisher or with water, if appropriate.
Prep solutions	• Use flammable prep solutions with extreme caution. • Do not allow prep solutions to pool on, around, or beneath the patient. • After prepping, allow the prep solution to dry and the fumes to dissipate. • Do not activate ignition sources in the presence of flammable prep solutions. • Do not allow drapes that will remain in contact with the patient to absorb flammable prep solutions.
Skin degreasers	• Skin degreasers may be used before skin prep to degrease or clean the skin or as part of the dressing. These products may contain chemicals that are flammable. Allow all fumes to dissipate before beginning surgery. The laser or ESU should not be used after the dressing is in place.
Body tissue and patient hair	• The patient's own body can be a fuel source. Coat any body hair that is near an ignition source with a water-based jelly to retard ignition. • Ensure that surgical smoke from burning patient tissue is properly evacuated. Surgical smoke can support combustion if allowed to accumulate in a small or enclosed space (e.g., the back of the throat).
Intestinal gases	• The patient's intestinal gases are flammable. The ESU or laser should be used with caution whenever intestinal gases are present. Do not open the bowel with the laser or ESU when gas appears to be present. • Use suction during rectal surgery to remove any intestinal gases that may be present.

Continued

Table **8-3**	Management Strategies: Fuel and Oxidizers—cont'd

Fire Risk—Oxidizers

Oxidizers	Management Strategies
Oxygen	• Oxygen should be used with caution in the presence of ignition sources. Oxygen is an oxidizer and is capable of supporting combustion. • Ensure that anesthesia circuits are free of leaks. • Pack wet sponges around the back of the throat to help retard oxygen leaks. • Inflate cuffed tube bladders with tinted saline so that inadvertent ruptures can be detected. • Use suction to help evacuate any accumulation of oxygen in body cavities such as the mouth or chest cavity. • Do not use the laser or ESU near sites where oxygen is flowing. • Use a pulse oximeter to determine the patient's oxygenation level and the need for oxygen. • Allow oxygen fumes to dissipate before using the laser or ESU. • Oxygen should not be directed at the surgical site. • Ensure that drapes are configured to help prevent oxygen accumulation when mask or nasal oxygen is used. • With a large fire, turn off the gases; with an airway or tracheal fire, disconnect the breathing circuit and remove the endotracheal tube. • Stop supplemental oxygen for 1 min before using electrocautery or laser for head, neck, or upper chest procedures.
Nitrous oxide	• The strategies to manage oxygen also should be used to manage risks associated with nitrous oxide.

From the Association of periOperative Registered Nurses (AORN): Fire prevention in the operating room. In *Standards, recommendations, practices and guidelines, 2011 edition,* Denver, 2011, AORN.

inch (0.63 cm) thick, and the gas is pressurized to 2,200 pounds per square inch (psi). A regulator is fitted into the cylinder stem valve by a threaded connection. The regulator contains two gauges; one displays the flow of gas from the regulator to the equipment being used, and the other shows the amount of gas in the tank (in psi). The regulator is activated by a valve handle. A valve stem or hand wheel is fitted into the top of the tank. Gas flows through the regulator when the tank valve is opened.

The contents of gas cylinders are identified by a stamp or stencil on the tank itself or by a cylinder tag. *Do not* identify medical gases contents by the color of the cylinder. Tank colors vary from vendor to vendor, and there is no international standard for tank color. Using the wrong gas can result in accident or severe injury. Safety guidelines mandated by OSHA and the Compressed Gas Association (CGA) advise that only the cylinder tag or stamp/stencil located on the cylinder itself should be used to identify the gas.

Hazards

Two types of hazards are associated with compressed gas cylinders: physical hazards, which are related to the high pressure in the cylinder, and chemical hazards, which are related to the flammability oxidative qualities, toxicity, or other properties of the gas.

Any compressed gas cylinder can explode or rupture, because the gas is under extremely high pressure. If the gas is also flammable or supports combustion (e.g., oxygen and nitrous oxide), the risk increases significantly. Cylinders must be handled with caution. A leak in a tank or separation of the valve from the tank can propel the tank with the force of a missile, sending it through walls and into objects and people. A cylinder explosion sends high-speed metal particles from the fragmented cylinder into the environment in the same way as a bomb causes injury from shrapnel. All perioperative personnel must be familiar with the proper handling of gas cylinders (Figure 8-2).

Handling of Gas Cylinders

Many modern operating rooms have inline gas outlets that dispense oxygen, nitrogen, and air. Even so, gas cylinders, especially oxygen and nitrogen, are common in the hospital environment. The surgical technologist should be familiar with the following procedures for opening, adjusting, and connecting the cylinder to a hose for use in pneumatic powered surgical instruments:

1. The gas cylinder has two valves. One opens the cylinder and allows gas to flow to the regulator. This valve is located on top of the cylinder. Cylinders have either a hand wheel or stem valve with no turn wheel. The stem valve is operated using a valve *spindle key*, which remains with the cylinder at all times while it is in use. Do not use a wrench or other tool to operate the stem valve, because this can result in damage to the valve stem. Only tools that are provided with the cylinder should be used to operate the valve.

2. The second valve is located on the regulator. This valve controls the flow from the regulator to the tubing connected to the user end. It must be adjusted according to the specific requirements of the instrument or device that uses the gas.

3. The right-hand gauge displays the pressure in the cylinder. The left-hand gauge displays the pressure in the power hose connected to the instrument.

4. If the regulator is already attached to the cylinder, *slowly* turn the valve to "crack" it open. Then turn the

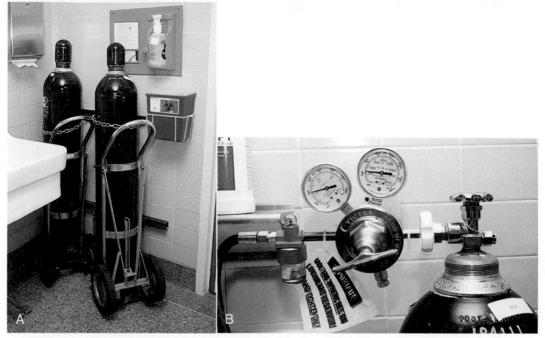

Figure 8-2 Handling of compressed gas cylinders. **A,** Proper storage of gas cylinders. **B,** Close-up of valves. *(From Ignatavicius DD, Workman L: Medical-surgical nursing: critical thinking for collaborative care, ed 4, Philadelphia, 2002, WB Saunders.)*

valve to full open position. With the valve in this position, the tank pressure is displayed on the right-hand pressure gauge.

5. Do not use the tank if the pressure is less than 500 psi. This means there is insufficient gas remaining in the tank. A small amount of residual gas (and pressure) in the tank prevents debris (e.g., rust, dust) from entering the hose. Particles entering the hose can damage the equipment or cause injury. Therefore it is unsafe to run the tank dry.

6. Attach the connector hose securely to the regulator outlet. Most connectors can be attached by pushing and turning firmly.

7. Turn the regulator wheel handle to set the pressure at the correct level. The required pressure level depends on the instrument manufacturer's specifications. Some instruments must be running to set the correct pressure. Make sure the correct pressure is maintained throughout use.

8. After use, turn off the tank pressure valve. Then bleed the gas remaining in the air hose by activating the instrument.

9. Close the regulator valve by rotating the regulator dial. The pressure should now read zero.

10. Do not return a tank to storage if the pressure is below 500 psi. The tank must be replaced.

11. *Regulators are gas-specific and are not interchangeable.* Do not attempt to modify a regulator gauge to fit the gas you are using.

STORAGE AND TRANSPORT All personnel should be familiar with safety precautions used for the storage and transport of gas cylinders. These are described in Box 8-1.

ELECTRICITY

Risk

Electrical malfunctions are a leading cause of hospital fires in the United States. Accredited hospitals are required to install explosion-proof outlets and to comply with building and environmental codes enacted to prevent electrical fire. However, electrical equipment also must be maintained. The probability of malfunction increases as devices become technologically more sophisticated and have greater requirements for repair and maintenance.

Characteristics of Electrical Energy

The nature and mechanics of electrical energy are described fully in Chapters 17 and 18. A few points are extracted here for the sake of discussion. The characteristics of electricity (the flow of electrons) are current, voltage, impedance (resistance), and grounding.

- *Current* is the rate of electrical (electron) flow. Direct current (DC) is low voltage and originates from a battery. Alternating current (AC) is transmitted by a 220- or 110-V line, such as that normally found in wall outlets. The available power is much higher with AC than with DC.
- *Voltage* is the driving force behind the moving electrons.
- **Impedance (resistance)** describes the ability of a substance to stop the flow of electrons (electricity). Electricity follows the path of least resistance. Nonresistant materials include metal, water, and the human body. When electricity enters the body and is not directed back to the source, severe burns and cardiac arrest can result. This is commonly referred to as **electrocution**.

| Box **8-1** | **Guidelines for Storage and Transport of Gas Cylinders** |

1. Label storage areas with the names of the gases stored there.
2. Never use a gas cylinder that is not labeled properly.
3. A gas cylinder must be secured at a point approximately two thirds of its height at all times. Each cylinder should be secured individually with a chain, wire cable, or cylinder strap.
4. Store cylinders so that the valve is accessible at all times.
5. Never store oxygen cylinders in the same area as flammable gases.
6. Cylinders must never be stored in public hallways or other unprotected areas.
7. Never use grease or oily materials on oxygen cylinders or store them near these cylinders.
8. Always secure a gas cylinder before transporting it. Use a caged rack, chain, or other secure device designed to prevent the cylinder from falling or tipping over.
9. Do not store cylinders of different gases together or allow one to strike another.
10. Never store gas tanks near heat or where they might come in contact with sources of electricity.
11. Never roll, drag, or slide a gas cylinder. Always use a hand cart to transport a tank.
12. Do not tamper with tank safety devices.
13. Always read the identification label of any gas cylinder. Do not rely on the color for identification.
14. Do not attempt to repair a cylinder or valve yourself. The tank must be returned to the bioengineering department or regulator supplier for repair.
15. Never use pliers to open a cylinder valve. Cylinders are equipped with a wheel or stem valve to initiate the flow. Operation of stem valves requires a key, which must remain with the cylinder at all times.
16. Make sure all compressed gas storage areas have adequate ventilation.

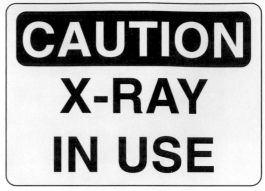

Figure 8-3   Hazard warning that radiographic equipment is in use.

- All switches must be protected from moisture.
- Only devices intended for use around fluids should be used.
- All equipment must be properly grounded.
- Any instrument or device must be switched to the off position before the power plug is removed.
- All equipment used in the operating room must be inspected and must be approved by **Underwriters Laboratories (UL)**. This agency develops and maintains standards of safety for consumer electrical products. Electrical items that do not have a UL approval rating must not be used.

The most common source of electrical injury to the surgical patient is the ESU.

Chapter 18 presents a complete discussion of the risks and proper use of the electrosurgical unit and other power equipment.

IONIZING RADIATION

Risk

Radiograph machines, fluoroscopes, and unshielded radioactive implants produce ionizing radiation in amounts high enough to damage tissue. Exposure occurs when workers are not protected during procedures that use radiography or fluoroscopy. Hazard warnings should be posted whenever radiographic or fluoroscopic studies are in progress (Figure 8-3).

The extent of tissue damage depends on the duration of exposure, the distance from the source of radiation, and the tissue exposed. Repeated exposures have cumulative effects. Among the risks of overexposure to radiation are genetic mutation, cancer, cataract, burns, and spontaneous abortion. Certain areas of the body are more vulnerable than others. These are the areas in which cell reproduction is the most rapid, including the ovaries, testes, lymphatic tissue, thyroid, and bone marrow.

Injury Prevention

Radiography and fluoroscopy are frequently used in diagnostic areas and in the operating room. Lead shields are the most effective method of blocking radiation. The distance from the radiation source, the duration of exposure, and the quality of

- **Grounding** is the discharge of electrical current from the source to ground, where it is dispersed and rendered harmless. As long as electrical current can travel unhindered through the body and is directed back to its source, electrocution does not occur. An improperly grounded electrical device can send electricity through the patient but does not control its dispersal to the ground. Normal grounding is established by the use of a three-prong plug. Two of the prongs send the current through the device. The ground wire, or third prong, connects the device to the ground. If no ground wire is used, current can leak into other conductors and will follow a nonresistant path.

Preventing Electrical Malfunction

- Equipment with frayed cords or devices with exposed wires must never be used.
- Cords must not be spliced or threaded through solid obstacles.

the shielding are the most important parameters determining risk and protection.

Safety Precautions During Use of Ionizing Radiation

- Although lead aprons are uncomfortable and heavy, team members should wear them under their sterile gowns during any procedure that requires radiation. Many lead aprons shield only the front of the body; therefore, workers should face the radiation source during exposure.
- A lead apron must be worn during fluoroscopy to prevent exposure to scatter radiation.
- Lead aprons must be stored flat or hung in a manner that prevents bending of the material.
- Remember that a lead apron protects only the areas of the body that are covered by the apron. The eyes and hands are not protected.
- Lead glasses should be worn during exposure to a fluoroscope.
- Neck shields are available to protect the thyroid, which is sensitive to radiation, during fluoroscopy.
- Nonsterile workers should step outside the range of exposure, either behind a lead screen or outside the room. Those who must remain in the room during exposure must maintain a distance of at least 6 feet (1.8 m) from the patient. The safest place to stand is at a right angle to the beam on the side of the radiograph machine or origin of the radiation beam.
- In the radiology department, the walls are lined with lead to protect workers when diagnostic studies are performed. In this circumstance, personnel may be able to step behind the lead wall while the equipment is in operation.
- Whenever possible, a mechanical holding device should be used to support radiograph cassettes to prevent exposure of the hands.
- Lead-impregnated gloves must be worn any time the hands are directly exposed to the radiation beam, such as during fluoroscopy or when radioactive implants or dyes are handled.
- Dosimeters are available to measure the cumulative radiation dose for those who are often exposed to radiation.
- Perioperative staff members should rotate through cases involving ionizing radiation. This prevents overexposure of the same staff members.

MAGNETIC RESONANCE IMAGING

Risk

Perioperative staff members may assist during magnetic resonance imaging (MRI) procedures. MRI provides a three-dimensional view of the patient's anatomy using radiofrequency. Whenever MRI is used, the primary risk is the presence of metal, which can be drawn from its source and into the path of the powerful magnetic field. For this reason, absolutely no metal objects are permitted in the environment during this process. Also, a substantial risk of injury exists from certain types of metal implants in the patient or staff members and

personal items, such as scissors or jewelry. Only plastic and titanium objects are safe to use during MRI procedures.

CHEMICAL RISKS

TOXIC CHEMICALS

Risk

Perioperative staff are exposed to many different types of chemicals. The majority of these are hazardous and can produce serious long-term effects, such as respiratory or skin problems, genetic changes, and fetal injury. It is important to remember that although exposure to a particular chemical may be brief, constant exposure to chemicals in a variety of work situations has a cumulative effect. For example, in a given day a surgical technologist might be exposed to glutaraldehyde disinfectant, vapor from methylmethacrylate cement, formaldehyde used as a specimen preserver, a phenolic agent used during environmental cleaning, and peracetic acid used as a sterilizing agent. Although the effects of any single exposure may be limited, the cumulative and synergistic effects can be much greater.

Standards and guidelines for handling chemicals are designed to reduce the risk of occupational exposure and associated injuries. All hazardous chemicals approved for use in the United States are issued a *Material Safety Data Sheet* (MSDS). The MSDS describes the chemical, precautions for handling the chemical, hazards associated with the chemical, and firefighting techniques and first aid for exposure. Each department in the health facility is required to maintain an MSDS for chemicals used in that department, and employees must have access to these.

Exposure

Toxic chemicals can enter the body through the respiratory tract, by direct skin contact, by splash contact, or by ingestion. **Personal protective equipment (PPE)** protects personnel against high concentrations of chemicals. Exposure to an airborne chemical (vapor) is measured by concentration, in parts per million (ppm) or milligrams of substance per cubic meter of air (mg/m^3). Every chemical used in the health care setting has a safe limit of exposure, which is determined by government agencies.

Prevention

Chemicals used in the health care setting must carry a label containing information about the chemical, including its intended safe use, toxicity, and postexposure measures. All personnel must be familiar with chemical labels and know how to interpret them (Box 8-2). When working with any chemical, you must know and use the appropriate concentration and the proper procedure (e.g., glutaraldehyde must be used under a hood to prevent respiratory irritation). Hazard warning labels are posted on the container and in storage areas (Figure 8-4). Chemicals transferred from larger containers to smaller ones must be labeled with the exact information found

Box 8-2 | Reading a Chemical Label

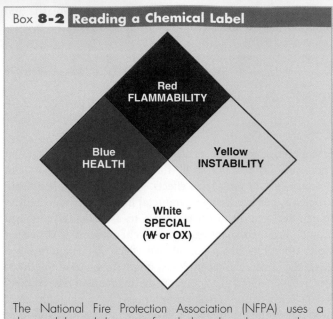

The National Fire Protection Association (NFPA) uses a diamond-shaped diagram of symbols and numbers to indicate the hazards associated with a particular chemical.

Blue   Health hazard
Red   Flammability
Yellow   Reactivity
White   Other hazards

Each category is given a score that corresponds to the hazard level:

4   Extreme
3   Serious
2   Moderate
1   Slight
0   Minimal

on the original container. Table 8-4 lists the chemicals commonly found in the operating room environment.

SMOKE PLUME

A **smoke plume** is created during laser surgery and electrosurgery. Smoke plumes contain harmful toxins that must be removed from the immediate surgical environment because they are known to contain benzene, hydrogen cyanide, formaldehyde, blood fragments, and viruses—potentially harmful when inhaled. All safety organizations including the National Institute for Occupational Safety and Health (NIOSH) recommend an efficient evacuation and filtering system. A suction tip at the exact site where smoke is generated filters the smoke and absorbs minute toxic particles. This equipment must be used according to the manufacturer's instructions. Filters are

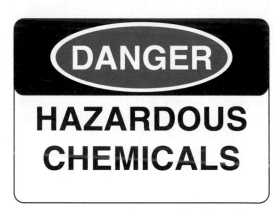

Figure 8-4   Hazard warning for chemicals.

Table 8-4 | Hazardous Chemicals Commonly Used in the Operating Room Environment

Substance	Use	Precaution
Anesthetic gases	General anesthesia	Must be scavenged by anesthesia machine. Be wary of possible fetal injury.
Ethylene oxide	Sterilization	Objects must be aerated in chamber. Personnel should wear dosimeters to measure exposure. Do not handle objects until aeration is complete.
Peracetic acid	Sterilization	Use goggles, face shield, and gloves when operating sterilizer.
Glutaraldehyde	Disinfection	Use only under hood. Wear gloves, mask, and goggles.
Phenolic compounds	Decontamination (environmental)	Use proper dilution. Wear gloves and goggles.
Sodium hypochlorite (1 ppm)	Decontamination (environmental)	Use proper dilution. Wear gloves and goggles.
Formaldehyde	Tissue preservative	Wear masks, gloves, and goggles.
Methylmethacrylate	Bone cement	Do not wear soft contact lenses around this substance; it causes corneal burns and melts contact lenses. Wear mask, gloves, and goggles.
Fibrin glue	Tissue glue	Wear goggles, gloves, and mask.

considered toxic waste and are handled according to institutional and government policy. (The details of smoke plume control and risks are discussed in Chapter 18.)

BIOLOGICAL RISKS

DISEASE TRANSMISSION IN THE PERIOPERATIVE ENVIRONMENT

Sources of infection and the ways diseases are spread from one person to another are discussed in Chapter 9. In this section, transmission precautions and recommendations are linked with activities in the perioperative environment.

The primary focus of disease control in the health care environment is on preventing contact with blood and body fluids.

STANDARD PRECAUTIONS

At the start of the HIV/acquired immunodeficiency syndrome (AIDS) crisis, the CDC and other agencies involved in public health safety became concerned about the possibility that health care workers might contract or transmit blood-borne disease in the course of their work. The response to this problem was a set of practices for handling blood and body fluids called *Universal Precautions*. Initially these guidelines applied only to body fluids capable of transmitting blood-borne viruses, particularly HIV. Later the concept was expanded to include contact with all body fluids capable of harboring any pathogenic microorganism. The new guidelines, published in 1996, were called **Standard Precautions**.

In 2007, the 1996 Standard Precautions were modified and updated. This is the standard now used in all medical settings (Box 8-3). The objective of Standard Precautions is to prevent the transmission of any infectious agent in the health care setting. The assumption is that *any person* may harbor potentially infectious microorganisms. Therefore, the practices of the standard apply to all patients and all contact with blood and body fluids.

The practices focus on the following points:

- Personal protective equipment (PPE) that provides an efficient barrier between the health care worker and body fluids
- Hand hygiene and asepsis using an effective technique
- The special handling of biological waste and linens (e.g., surgical drapes, towels, sheets) used in patient care
- Special handling procedures for sharp items, especially hypodermic needles, scalpel blades, and sharp instruments
- Specific procedures when a health care worker is injured by a contaminated needle or other sharp
- Disinfection (decontamination) of all inanimate surfaces in the medical environment
- Decontamination of all medical devices and instruments between patients
- Encouraging single-use medical supplies and equipment when possible

---

Box **8-3** **Recommended Practices for Preventing Transmissible Infections in the Perioperative Setting**

1. Health care workers should use Standard Precautions when caring for all patients in the perioperative setting.
2. Hand hygiene should be performed before and after each patient contact.
3. Protective barriers must be used to reduce the risk of skin and mucous membrane exposure to potentially infectious material.
4. Health care practitioners should double-glove during invasive procedures.
5. Contact precautions should be used in providing care for patients who are known or suspected to be infected or colonized with microorganisms that are transmitted by direct or indirect contact with patients or items and surfaces in patients' environments.
6. Droplet precautions should be used when caring for patients who are known or suspected to be infected with microorganisms that can be transmitted by infectious large-particle droplets that generally travel short distances (i.e., 3 feet [0.9 m] or less); diseases caused by such microorganisms include diphtheria, pertussis, influenza, mumps, and pneumonic plague.
7. Airborne precautions should be used when caring for patients who are known or suspected to be infected with microorganisms that can be transmitted by the airborne route; diseases caused by such microorganisms include rubella, varicella, tuberculosis, and smallpox.
8. Health care workers should be immunized against epidemiologically important agents according to the regulations of the Centers for Disease Control and Prevention (CDC).
9. Work practices must be designed to minimize the risk of exposure to pathogens.
10. Personnel must take precautions to prevent injuries caused by needles, scalpels, and other sharp instruments.
11. The activities of personnel with infections, exudative lesions, nonintact skin, and/or blood-borne diseases should be restricted when these activities pose a risk of transmission of infection to patients and other health care workers.
12. Policies and procedures that address responses to threats of intentionally released pathogens should be written, reviewed periodically, and readily available within the practice setting.
13. Policies and procedures that address responses to epidemic or pandemic pathogens should be written, reviewed periodically, and readily available within the practice setting.
14. Personnel should demonstrate competence in the prevention of transmissible infections.

Modified from the Association of periOperative Registered Nurses (AORN): Transmission of transmissible infections. In *Standards, recommended practices and guidelines*, 2007 edition, Denver, 2007, AORN.

Hand Washing

Hand washing is the most important method of preventing disease transmission in the health care setting.

- Wash your hands after touching blood, body fluids, secretions, excretions, and contaminated items, *regardless of whether gloves are worn*. Wash your hands immediately after removing your gloves between patient contacts. You may need to wash your hands between tasks and procedures on the same patient to prevent cross-contamination of different body sites.

- Wear gloves when touching blood, body fluids, secretions, excretions, and contaminated items. Put on clean gloves just before touching mucous membranes and nonintact skin. Change gloves between tasks and procedures on the same patient after contact with material that may contain a high concentration of microorganisms. Remove your gloves immediately after use, before touching uncontaminated surfaces, and before going to another patient.

Personal Protective Equipment

- Wear a mask and eye protection or a face shield to protect against splash contamination. Prescription eyeglasses are not considered adequate because they do not shield the sides of the eyes.

- A clean, nonsterile cover jacket should be worn to protect the skin and prevent soiling of clothing during procedures and patient care activities likely to generate splashes or sprays of blood, body fluids, secretions, or excretions.

- Remove a soiled gown as promptly as possible and wash your hands to prevent the transfer of microorganisms to other patients or environments.

Patient Care Equipment and Linens

- Patient care equipment and linens must be handled in a way that prevents contact with skin and clothing.

- Handle soiled linens with gloved hands only.

- Hold soiled linen away from your body and place it in a biohazard laundry bag for disposal. Always wear gloves when handling patient care items.

- All contaminated single-use (disposable) items must be placed in biohazard bags for disposal.

- Sharps for disposal are contained in a special puncture-proof container and disposed of as contaminated waste.

- Multiple-use items must be decontaminated between patients.

SHARPS INJURY

The most common means of transmission of **blood-borne pathogens** to health care workers is sharps injuries. **Sharps** are such a threat to health care personnel that OSHA has issued the Blood-Borne Pathogen Rule, a special set of regulations for handling and disposing of sharps.

More information on the OSHA standards is available at http://www.osha.gov/pls/oshaweb/owadisp. show_document?p_table=STANDARDS&p_id=10051.

Sources of Injury

- Hypodermic needles
- Suture needles
- Scalpel blades
- Needle-point electrosurgical tips
- Trocars, such as those used to perform endoscopic surgery or to place wound drains
- Sharp instruments, such as skin hooks, rakes, and scissors
- Metal guide wires and stylets
- Orthopedic drill bits, screws, pins, wires, and cutting tips, such as saw blades and burrs

Certain tasks are associated with a high risk of sharps injury:

- Passing and receiving a scalpel
- Preparing and passing sutures
- Collision of two individuals' hands when they reach for the same sharp instrument
- Mounting or removing a scalpel blade from the handle
- Manually retracting tissue
- Suturing

The risk of sharps injury can be reduced by following recommended guidelines and standards. This means performing tasks in a specific way. All health care workers are responsible for their own safety and the safety of others on the team. Therefore, compliance with guidelines is a combined ethical and safety issue.

Risk Reduction

- Whenever possible, retractable or self-sheathing needles and scalpels should be used.

- Blunt suture needles are now recommended over sharp needles.

- If hollow-bore hypodermic needles are used, they must never be recapped by hand. The cap is replaced by grasping it with an instrument. Removable needles must be handled only with an instrument, never by hand. Self-sheathing needles have nonremovable parts.

- Scalpel blades must be mounted and removed with an instrument.

- Used disposable syringes and needles, scalpel blades, and other sharp items should be placed in appropriate puncture-resistant containers located as close as practical to the area where the items were used. The container must be removed and replaced at frequent intervals to prevent overflow, another common source of sharps injury.

- During surgery, sharps are contained on a magnetic board or in a special holder that can be contained and disposed of properly.

- All health care employees should be immunized against the hepatitis B virus (HBV).

Neutral Zone (No-Hands) Technique

The **neutral zone (no-hands) technique** during surgery was developed because the evidence shows that most sharps injuries in surgery occur when instruments are passed and received. OSHA, the CDC, AORN, and the Association of Surgical Technologists (AST) now strongly recommend that the neutral zone technique be adopted in surgical settings whenever possible. The technique uses a hands-free space (e.g., a designated receptacle) on the sterile field where sharps can be placed and picked up so that the surgical technologist and surgeon do not hand instruments to each other directly. (This technique is described in Chapter 21.)

HUMAN FACTOR

Although the nature of blood-borne disease, its transmission, and prevention methods are known, the human factor must be included in the planning and implementation of any risk reduction program. The following are some reasons people have difficulty with risk reduction:

- Working too quickly.
- Distraction from the task at hand.
- Failure to comply with precautions and standards ("It can't happen to me").
- Extreme fatigue.
- Distraction related to environmental noise, including loud music and conversation. Recent studies have shown that loud music playing during surgery contributes to medical errors because it prevents clear communication.
- Lack of support in designing and maintaining a prevention program.
- Difficulty abandoning old and valued methods of working.
- Difficulty adapting to newer, safer medical devices.

POSTEXPOSURE PROPHYLAXIS

Postexposure prophylaxis (PEP) is a risk reduction strategy that is used after exposure to blood or other body fluids. It involves the administration of drugs and testing. PEP is voluntary; no health care worker should be coerced into receiving it. However, the decision must be made quickly, because the preventive drugs are most effective when given within 24 hours after exposure.

Components of Postexposure Prophylaxis

Individuals exposed to HBV should be tested for HBV surface antigen, and an immunization series should be initiated. Health care workers who have not been previously vaccinated should be given hepatitis B immune globulin (HBIG) if the incident involved mucous membrane exposure or penetrating exposure to a patient's blood or other body fluids.

PEP for HIV consists of a regimen of antiviral drugs followed by regular testing. PEP must be initiated soon after exposure and has a limited effect, and additional health risks are associated with the medications used. Because PEP must be initiated within a brief period after exposure, it is vital that health care workers be evaluated rapidly and that the patient be screened for HIV before leaving the health care setting.

Antibodies generally take 25 days to 3 months to appear on standard HIV tests. The attending physician assesses the patient's HIV exposure risks. PEP includes the use of two or three antiretroviral agents to prevent the virus from attacking the immune system. These drugs are administered orally, and the regimen usually lasts for 1 month. These antiretroviral agents have a number of side effects that must be considered before PEP is initiated.

TRANSMISSION-BASED PRECAUTIONS

Transmission-based precautions are implemented when a patient is known or suspected to have a highly infectious disease and Standard Precautions are insufficient to prevent transmission to others. These guidelines are used in addition to Standard Precautions.

Airborne Transmission

Airborne transmission precautions reduce the risk of transmission of airborne agents by droplet nuclei up to 5 micrometers in size (see Chapter 9). Because of their small size, such droplets remain suspended in the air and disperse widely in the environment.

A patient with a disease that can be spread by airborne transmission must wear a surgical mask during transport. Health care personnel must wear respiratory protection when within 3 feet (0.9 m) of such a patient. Masks must pass NIOSH-approved high-efficiency particulate air (HEPA) standards to be completely effective.

Airborne transmission precautions must be taken for the following diseases:

- Measles
- Varicella (including disseminated herpes zoster)
- Tuberculosis

NOTE: More detailed information on tuberculosis can be obtained from the CDC publication Guidelines for Preventing the Transmission of Tuberculosis in Health Care Facilities.[3]

Droplet Precautions

Droplet precautions are implemented to reduce the risk of infectious disease transmission by large, moist aerosol droplets. These are spread from the mouth, nose, oropharynx, and trachea to a susceptible host. The traveling distance of droplets is 3 feet (0.9 m) or less, and they do not remain suspended in the air. Patients with any of the diseases that can be transmitted in this way must be separated from other patients by at least 3 feet (0.9 m), and health care workers must wear a mask when within 3 feet (0.9 m) of the patient.

A partial list of the infections for which droplet precautions should be implemented includes:

- Invasive infection with *Haemophilus influenzae* type B
- Invasive infection with *Neisseria meningitidis*
- Streptococcal pharyngitis
- Rubella

Contact Precautions

Contact precautions are used with patients known or suspected to harbor an infection transmitted by direct contact. In addition to Standard Precautions, the following steps are required:

- Gloves must be worn and hands must be washed before and after contact with the patient.
- Health care personnel must wear protective gowns.
- All items that come in contact with the patient must be disinfected or sterilized.

Contagious conditions for which implementation of contact precautions is required include:
- Infection with the herpes simplex virus
- Impetigo
- Noncontained abscesses, cellulitis, or decubitus ulcers
- Disseminated herpes zoster
- Infection with *Clostridium difficile*
- Infection with any multidrug-resistant bacterium

HAZARDOUS WASTE

Definition

The EPA defines medical waste as any solid waste generated in the diagnosis, treatment, or immunization of humans or animals, in research that involves people or animals, or in the production or testing of biologicals. This includes, for example:
- Soiled or blood-soaked bandages
- Culture dishes and other glassware
- Discarded surgical gloves after surgery
- Discarded surgical instruments and scalpels
- Needles used to give injections or draw blood
- Cultures, stocks, and swabs used to inoculate cultures
- Removed body organs (e.g., tonsils, appendices, limbs)

Besides the EPA, the federal agencies associated with the regulation of various aspects of medical waste include the FDA, OSHA, and the Nuclear Regulatory Commission (NRC). Medical waste disposal also is regulated at the state level, and each state has laws that apply specifically to medical waste.

Waste Handling

Infectious waste is separated from all other waste and placed in red biohazard disposal bags. (The common term for medical waste is *red bag waste*.) The biohazard symbol (Figure 8-5) may or may not appear on the bag. The bag color and biohazard symbol are a form of hazard communication to anyone who later handles the waste material. Any person handling infectious waste, from the point of generation until its destruction, must wear PPE. Gloves must be worn at all times. Face shields and protective gowns protect the handler from splash hazards.

Guidelines for the handling and disposal of waste in the operating room environment include the following:
- Always wear gloves when handling any object contaminated with blood or body fluids.
- Red waste bags for infectious material must be available during case cleanup.
- Do not place noninfectious waste in red waste bags. The cost of processing is 10 times higher for infectious waste than for noninfectious waste.
- Place all sharps in an impenetrable sharps container.
- Do not overload sharps containers. Container overflow is one of the major causes of blood-borne disease transmission among health care workers.
- If it is necessary to examine items in a refuse bag, separate the items carefully by spreading them on an impermeable sheet or drape. Never handle waste material unless you can see what is contained in the refuse bag. Sharps may be present among trash and cause serious injury.
- Handle suction canisters and other blood containers with extreme caution. The practice of opening suction canisters used during surgery and pouring the contents into an open hopper puts workers at extremely high risk for disease transmission. Blood and fluid solidifiers are available. After fluids are solidified, they can be placed in tear-resistant plastic bags.
- Bags must not be loaded beyond their tensile strength. Double bagging may be necessary.
- Separate soiled reusable linen from disposable paper products and unsoiled items at the point of use.
- Keep all contaminated (soiled) or potentially contaminated waste separate from uncontaminated goods.
- Do not compact waste contained in plastic bags. Pack loosely and secure the open end.
- When transporting medical waste, do not use trash chutes or dumbwaiters. Use a transport cart.

A designated area of the operating room is reserved for the disposal of infectious waste. This must be completely separated from restricted and semirestricted areas of the department. Biohazard signs should be posted in areas of waste disposal.

LATEX ALLERGY

Sensitivity and true allergy to latex rubber are risks to both patients and personnel. True allergy is differentiated from other types of immune responses. True allergic response, which is mediated by the immune system, is described in Chapter 9. Table 8-5 lists three types of skin reactions to latex.

Allergy and Sensitivity

Latex is a naturally occurring sap obtained from rubber trees. It is used commercially in the manufacture of many products, including medical devices, supplies, and patient care items. True allergy is an abnormal immune response to a substance. Previous exposure and sensitization are required for the body to initiate the formation of antibodies against the allergen.

Latex allergy is a local or systemic reaction mediated by the body's immune system. The reaction causes the release of

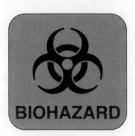

Figure 8-5 Biohazard warning label.

Table 8-5 Allergic and Nonallergic Skin Reactions

Type of Reaction	Symptoms/Signs	Cause	Prevention/Management
Contact dermatitis (nonallergic)	Scaling, drying, cracks in skin. Bumps and sores, especially on the dorsal side of the hand, caused by gloves.	Skin irritation caused by gloves, powder, soaps, and detergents. Incomplete rinsing after hand washing and surgical scrub. Incomplete hand drying.	Use alternative products. Rinse hands thoroughly after exposure to detergents and antiseptics. Dry hands completely before donning gloves.
Allergic contact dermatitis (delayed hypersensitivity or allergic contact sensitivity)	Blistering, itching, crusts, similar to a poison ivy reaction. Cracks that occur on hands or arms after skin exposure, caused by gloves.	Chemicals used in latex processing, including accelerators (thiurams, carbamates, and benzothiazoles).	Correctly identify cause. Use gloves that do not contain these chemicals.
Natural rubber latex (NRL) allergy (IgE/histamine mediated) (type I immediate hypersensitivity)	Hives in the area of contact with NRL. Generalized redness, nasal irritation, wheezing, swelling of the mouth, and shortness of breath. Can progress to anaphylactic shock.	Direct contact with or breathing of natural latex proteins, including those contained in glove powder or found in the environment.	Eliminate or drastically reduce exposure to NRL protein. Use nonlatex, powder-free gloves.

histamines, which occur normally in the body. This causes edema (swelling) and redness. When histamines are released in massive amounts, the reaction can be life-threatening. The extent of the reaction depends on the exact location and nature of the contact. Allergies are a response to proteins within a substance.

Hypersensitivity is a cell-mediated response. It is a type of delayed reaction that causes dermatitis on contact with the object. In the case of latex gloves, supplies, and medical devices, this reaction generally is related to chemicals in the latex product rather than the latex itself.

Nonallergic dermatitis (skin inflammation) is caused by many irritants found in the operating room environment. Chemicals, antiseptic residue from surgical scrub or hand washing, and glove powder are known to cause irritation in some sensitive individuals.

All health facilities have a latex-safe cart available for patients known to be allergic to latex. The cart contains supplies needed for management of the patient with latex sensitivity. Latex cannot be eliminated from the medical environment completely, but risk reduction is an important factor in preventing injury.

Exposure and Symptoms

Patients and perioperative personnel can be exposed to latex through the skin, circulatory system, respiratory system, and mucous membranes. Gloves and glove powder containing latex molecules are a major concern, but many other medical devices contain latex as well.

Latex can cause skin reactions, including sores, skin cracks, lumps, and itching. Latex can come in contact with the circulatory system through intravenous catheters, tubing, and other intravascular devices. If the latex reaches the bloodstream, large amounts of chemical mediators are released. These can

cause severe bronchial obstruction, pulmonary edema, and death.

Individuals at Risk

- People who have had repeated surgeries or frequent contact with medical devices, especially in early childhood
- Individuals who have a positive reaction to a serum latex antibody test
- Anyone with a history of asthma or allergies to particular foods
- Individuals with a history of undiagnosed allergic symptoms after contact with medical devices

Sources of Latex in the Operating Room

The operating room environment has many potential sources of latex. The most common concern among surgical personnel is latex gloves. Most surgical and examination gloves contain latex because of its strength and resilience. However, nonlatex gloves are available. Box 8-4 lists common sources of latex.

Prevention and Risk Reduction

Prevention of latex injury requires identification of those at risk and avoiding contact with devices that contain latex. A supply area containing latex-free devices should be maintained for patients known to be allergic to latex. If the patient is known to be latex sensitive, a warning sticker is placed on the person's chart. The information also is included in the patient information.

Workers who believe they are sensitive or allergic to latex should be tested. The use of low-allergen latex and powder-free gloves is recommended by NIOSH and other organizations concerned with the health risks of latex in the health care setting.

MUSCULOSKELETAL RISKS

CAUSES OF MUSCULOSKELETAL INJURY

Musculoskeletal injury is a risk to all personnel working in the operating room. The lumbosacral area, wrist, shoulder, and neck are particularly vulnerable. The causes of musculoskeletal injury are classified according to the types of movement and the workload involved.

Exertion is the amount of physical effort needed to perform a task, such as moving an object. The amount of exertion required for a task varies with the duration and nature of the task; it also can be modified by changing one's posture or grip.

Posture is a critical component of musculoskeletal stress. Twisting or turning the body disrupts normal balance. Other high-risk positions include bending, kneeling, reaching overhead, and holding a fixed position for a long time.

Repetitive motion places stress on tendons and muscles. Factors that affect the risk are the speed of the movement, the required exertion, and the number of muscles needed to complete the action.

Contact stress is excessive direct pressure against a sharp edge or hard surface. Increasing the pressure increases the risk of damage to nerves, tendons, and blood vessels.

MECHANICAL INJURY PREVENTION IN THE ENVIRONMENT

In the operating room, musculoskeletal injuries most often occur as a result of the following:

- Lifting, positioning, transporting, and transferring the patient (see Chapter 19)
- Retrieving and shelving heavy instrument trays overhead or near the floor
- Moving heavy equipment (e.g., the operating table, operating microscope, imaging equipment)
- Catching items that are falling
- Tripping over tubing or electrical cords
- Balancing a heavy instrument tray in the hand while distributing it onto the sterile field
- Attaching cords to wall sockets or overhead inline connectors
- Climbing over operating room clutter or trying to retrieve a heavy item from a cluttered environment

Prevention of musculoskeletal injuries involves creating a safe work environment and using good body mechanics.

Supporting the Body

Fatigue and stress affect muscle control, which can lead to injury. Standing and walking for long periods put extra stress on muscles, tendons, and joints.

Perioperative personnel can reduce muscle fatigue while standing by placing the feet shoulder width apart. If a lift (raised platform) is used, it should accommodate a wide stance. Two lifts may be needed so that the scrubbed technologist is not required to step up and down while working between the instrument table and the patient.

Shifting the weight back and forth on a level surface can reduce muscle strain. Standing on one foot for long periods, however, increases stress and puts the body off balance. Elevating the feet during breaks helps increase circulation to the legs.

Support stockings and leggings significantly reduce muscle ache. These can be purchased in medical supply stores. Supportive shoes distribute pressure on the foot to prevent heel spurs and arch problems.

Storage Systems

Heavy items such as large instrument trays must be stored at elbow height, never above the head or at floor level. If they must be stored at floor level, attention to good body mechanics in retrieving these items helps prevent lower back injury. The appropriate way to shelve equipment is to place the heaviest items even with the elbows and smaller items on shelves above and below this height.

Clutter

When the surgical suite is crowded with equipment, workers are inclined to shift their weight off balance to move around. Tubing and power cords are added risks. Reducing clutter usually requires planning. Extra space may not be available for the equipment needed, but clutter can be consolidated. Bring in only what is needed for immediate use. Avoid draping cords over furniture and equipment. Consolidate extra supplies on a designated cart, which can be placed away from traffic areas.

Safe Body Mechanics

Developing good body mechanics is a conscious activity. Students and new employees should learn these methods before entering the clinical area for work. If you are injured on the job, obtain medical care as soon as possible.

LIFTING When lifting an object, keep it close to your body. This reduces the force of exertion. Figure 8-6 demonstrates

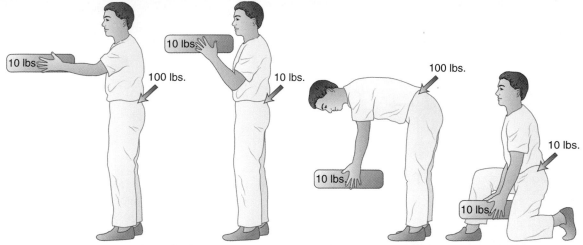

Figure 8-6 Weight on the back in various lifting positions. *(Redrawn from Saunders DH, Saunders R: Evaluation, treatment, and prevention of musculoskeletal disorders, vol 1, ed 3, Chaska, Minn, 1995, Saunders Group.)*

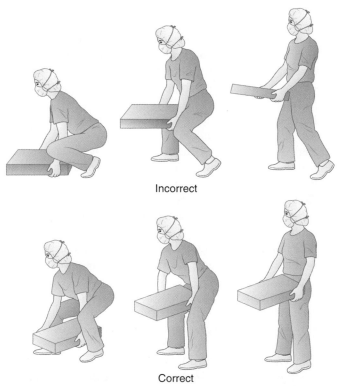

Incorrect

Correct

Figure 8-7 Body mechanics: Correct and incorrect lifting techniques. *(Redrawn from Saunders DH, Saunders R: Evaluation, treatment, and prevention of musculoskeletal disorders, vol 1, ed 3, Chaska, Minn, 1995, Saunders Group.)*

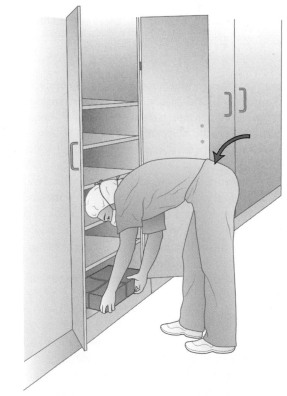

Figure 8-8 Unsafe body mechanics: Locking the knees creates the potential for back injury.

force exerted on the back in various lifting positions. Figure 8-7 illustrates safe and unsafe lifting techniques.

• Always bend at the knees when raising or lowering a heavy object. This takes pressure off the lower back and uses the body's heaviest muscles to do the work. Remember to keep your back straight and legs wide apart with both feet flat on the floor for balance.

• Never lock the knees and bend over to pick up an object (Figure 8-8). This puts stress on the lower back and does not permit use of the thigh muscles to help lift the body.

PUSHING AND PULLING When pushing a cart ahead of you from a standstill, place one foot behind the other. The back foot should be braced comfortably (Figure 8-9). Use the back foot to push off while transferring your weight to the front foot. Pushing is the preferred method of transporting objects

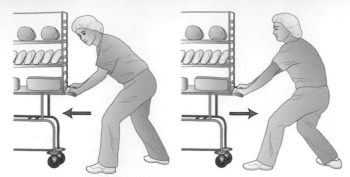

Figure 8-9   Safe methods of pushing and pulling a cart. Note the position of the brace foot.

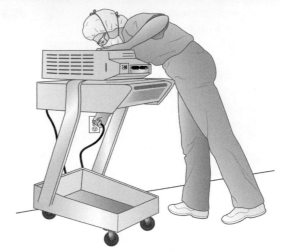

Figure 8-10   Bending and twisting at the same time creates the risk of back injury. Avoid putting weight on one foot, which decreases balance.

rather than pulling. Make sure you can see any obstacles in your path.

- When pulling a cart toward you, use the same stance as in pushing. Use your front leg to exert backward pull while the back foot maintains balance and support.
- When performing a horizontal transfer (straight across from one surface to another), use abdominal and arm muscles actively. Do not simply lean back and pull.

BENDING

- When you must bend or reach upward to connect an electrical outlet or inline gas connection, never twist your body or balance on one foot (Figure 8-10). This combination not only places the body off balance, but it also increases the risk of back injury, because the standing leg is locked in position.
- To lift or transfer a patient, use your abdominal muscles to hold the weight of your upper body. When the abdominal muscles are not engaged in exertion, the back muscles, especially those in the sacral and lumbar region, must support the entire trunk; this is a common cause of back injury. Tighten your abdominal muscles as you lift and notice that your back feels much more supported.

KEY CONCEPTS

- The potential for accident and injury in the operating room is one of the highest in the health care setting.
- Management of environmental risks requires a knowledge of the risks, a plan of action, and monitoring.
- Risk is the statistical probability of a harmful event and is defined as the number of harmful events that occur in a given population over a stated period.
- A work culture of safety is critical to injury reduction.
- Fire requires three components: oxygen, fuel, and a source of ignition.
- The operating room is an oxygen-enriched environment that supports combustion and fire.
- As the concentration of oxygen increases in the environment, so do the speed of ignition, duration, and temperature of a fire.
- Medical devices made of flammable materials are common in surgery.

- Any heat-producing device has the potential to cause a fire.
- Sparking can occur when an active electrode comes in contact with metal. Sparks can ignite volatile gases, liquids, drapes, and sponges, especially in the presence of oxygen.
- During a fire, the most important priority is protecting the patient.
- Immediate action during a fire is described by the acronym RACE: rescue patients in the immediate area of the fire; alert other people to the fire so that they can assist in patient removal and response; contain the fire; evacuate personnel in the areas around the fire.
- Compressed gases in steel cylinders are associated with serious accidents and fatalities related to explosion or rupture of the tank.
- A ruptured gas cylinder can become a projectile capable of penetrating walls. Safe handling techniques can prevent rupture.
- The most common source of electrical injury to the surgical patient is the electrosurgical unit (ESU). (Chapter 18 presents a complete discussion of the risks and proper use of electrosurgical equipment.)
- Ionizing radiation used in the operating room and interventional radiology departments can cause tissue damage. The most important method of reducing risk is to prevent exposure by using lead shields, aprons, and other protective devices.
- Magnetic resonance imaging uses radiofrequencies to provide a three-dimensional view of the patient's anatomy. Metal can be drawn into the magnetic field, causing severe injury or death.
- Dangerous chemicals are used in the perioperative environment for disinfection, sterilization, specimen preservation, and preparation of surgical implants.
- All staff members must have access to information about specific chemicals in their work environment. Precautions, hazards, and safety information are contained in the Material Safety Data Sheet (MSDS).

- A smoke plume is created whenever tissue is burned, such as during electrosurgery and laser surgery. Smoke plumes are known to contain toxins and therefore must be removed from the immediate surgical environment.
- Transmission of blood-borne disease organisms is a primary risk to personnel working in the surgical environment.
- The risk of disease transmission is significantly reduced when personnel follow Standard Precautions.
- All patients are considered potential sources of disease transmission. For this reason, Standard Precautions are used at all times and with all patients.
- The most common source of transmission of blood-borne pathogens to health care workers is sharps injuries. To reduce the risk of blood-borne disease transmission by sharps injuries, OSHA has established a set of rules pertaining to their handling and disposal, the *Blood-Borne Pathogen Rule*.
- A neutral zone technique prevents injury from sharps on the surgical field. With this method, no sharps are passed from one person to another by hand. Instead, a no-hands zone is established in which the surgeons and scrub pass and retrieve sharp items.
- Postexposure prophylaxis (PEP) is used after injury with a contaminated instrument. PEP includes a regimen of antiviral drugs and testing for hepatitis B.
- Transmission-based precautions are implemented when a patient is known to have or suspected of having a highly infectious disease and Standard Precautions are insufficient to prevent transmission to others.
- Hazardous waste is specifically defined by the Environmental Protection Agency (EPA). Disposal of medical waste is highly regulated by state laws. Medical personnel must handle medical waste according to facility policies, which are based on state regulations.
- Latex allergy is an immune response to latex rubber and can result in serious injury or death. Previous exposure and sensitization are needed for the body to initiate formation of antibodies to the allergen.
- Many medical and surgical devices contain latex. Prevention of latex injury requires identification of those at risk and avoidance of contact with devices containing latex.
- Musculoskeletal injury is a risk to all personnel working in the operating room. The lumbosacral area, wrist, shoulder, and neck are particularly vulnerable.
- The primary causes of musculoskeletal injury are stress, lack of balance, overexertion, and repetitive motion.
- Proper body mechanics prevents musculoskeletal injury. However, staff members often neglect good mechanics because of personnel shortages, rushing, or fatigue.

REVIEW QUESTIONS

1. What is the definition of risk? What is meant by risk management?
2. Under what circumstances might perioperative personnel bypass safety precautions?
3. Describe the elements of the fire triangle.
4. What characteristics of oxygen make it particularly dangerous in the perioperative environment?
5. What is an endotracheal fire?
6. Define the RACE procedure during a fire.
7. What are the elements of the PASS procedure for the use of fire extinguishers?
8. What is the rationale behind Standard Precautions?
9. Why were Standard Precautions developed?
10. Describe postexposure prophylaxis.
11. Define *hazardous waste*.
12. What is the minimum safe distance from a source of ionizing radiation during radiography?
13. What is a Material Safety Data Sheet?
14. What is the safest way to lift a heavy object from floor level?
15. How can you protect against musculoskeletal stress when standing for long periods?

CASE STUDIES

Case 1

You are scrubbed on a tonsillectomy. The patient is fully covered by drapes, and the case has started. The surgeon is using electrosurgery to coagulate a bleeding vessel in the throat. Suddenly there is an arc of fire emanating from the patient's throat, igniting the head drape. What are your initial responses as a surgical technologist?

Case 2

In the preceding case, there is a *mouth gag* (a type of retractor that attaches to the Mayo stand and holds the patient's mouth open) firmly in place. Does this change your response?

Case 3

You have been asked to retrieve a nitrous oxide tank from the storeroom and bring it to the surgical suite. You load the tank on a transportation cart. While in transit through the hallway, the tank falls to the floor and you suddenly hear a loud hissing sound from the top of the tank. What is your response?

Case 4

You have finished a busy day at work and are passing through one of the hospital wards to see a friend. As you walk past a utility room, you see that a small fire has started near the linen cart. What do you do?

Case 5

After a case in outpatient surgery, you are hurrying to clean up so that you can scrub on the next case. You suddenly cut your hand on a sharp retractor that has been soaking in an instrument basin. You decide not to tell anyone because you are sure there won't be any consequences, and you don't have time to fill out an incident report or go the emergency department. Two weeks later you regret your decision and are worried about the incident. You may face disciplinary action for not reporting the injury, but you are extremely worried. What would you do?

REFERENCES

1. ECRI Institute: *A clinician's guide to surgical fires: how they occur, how to prevent them, how to put them out.* Accessed September 8, 2011, at http://psnet.ahrq.gov/resource.aspx?resourceID=1427.
2. Eagan J: *Fire prevention and safety during surgical procedures* in Covidien energy-based professional education. Accessed February 29, 2012, at http://www.valleylabeducation.org/fire/pages/fire-disclose.html
3 Shuster L, Chinn RYW: Guidelines for preventing the transmission of tuberculosis in health care facilities, *Morbidity and Mortality Weekly Report.* Atlanta, June 6, 2003, The Centers for Disease Control and Prevention.

BIBLIOGRAPHY

Association of periOperative Registered Nurses: Fire safety in perioperative settings, *AORN Journal* 86(Suppl 1):S141, 2007.

Association of periOperative Registered Nurses: *Standards recommendations, practices and guidelines, 2007 edition,* Denver, 2007, AORN.

Bruley ME: *Surgical fires: perioperative communication is essential to prevent this rare but devastating complication.* Accessed September 8, 2011, at http://www.ncbi.nlm.nih.gov/pmc/articles/PMC1743921/pdf/v013p00467.pdf.

Centers for Disease Control and Prevention: *Implementing and evaluating a sharps injury prevention program.* Accessed September 8, 2011 at http://www.premierinc.com/safety/topics/needlestick/downloads/sharps-workbook-2008-high.pdf.

ECRI: A clinician's guide to surgical fires: how they occur, how to prevent them, how to put them out, *Health Devices 2003* 32(1):5, 2003.

Graling P: Fighting fire with fire safety, *AORN Journal* 84(4):561, 2006.

Groah L: Is there a relationship between workplace and patient safety? *AORN Journal* 84(4):653, 2006.

Joint Commission: *Preventing surgical fires,* Issue 29. Accessed September 8, 2011, at http://www.jointcommission.org/assets/1/18/SEA_29.pdf.

Joint Commission on Accreditation of Healthcare Organizations: Special report: 2005 Joint Commission National Patient Safety Goals. *Joint Commission Perspectives on Patient Safety.* September 2004. Available at http://www.jcrinc.com.

Lyczko E: Anesthesia and medical gas systems safety, *AORN Journal* 84(5):746, 2006.

McCarthy P, Gaucher K: Fire in the OR—developing a fire safety plan, *AORN Journal* 79(3):588, 2004.

Occupational Safety and Health Administration: *Revision to OSHA's bloodborne pathogens standard: technical background and summary,* Accessed April 11, 2012 at http://www.osha.gov/needlesticks/needlefact.html.

Occupational Safety and Health Administration: *Hazard recognition.* Accessed January 15, 2008, at http://www.osha.gov/SLTC/bloodbornepathogens/recognition.html.

Occupational Safety and Health Administration: *Bloodborne pathogens—OSHA's bloodborne pathogens standard.* OSHA Fact Sheet, January 2011. Accessed September 8, 2011, at http://www.osha.gov/SLTC/bloodbornepathogens/index.html#standards.

Salmon L: Fire in the OR: prevention and preparedness, *AORN Journal* 80:42, 2004.

Smith C: Surgical fires: learn not to burn, *AORN Journal* 80:24, 2004.

Microbes and the Process of Infection

CHAPTER OUTLINE

Introduction

Classification of Organisms

The Cell and Its Components

Tools for Identifying Microbes

The Process of Infection

Disease Prevention

Microorganisms and the
Diseases They Cause

Immunity

LEARNING OBJECTIVES

After studying this chapter the reader will be able to:

1. Explain the different classification of organisms and the binomial system
2. Describe components of the cell and cell transport
3. Discuss methods of identifying microbes
4. Identify the basic components of a biological microscope and describe their function
5. Relate the study of microbiology and the process of infection to surgical practice
6. Describe blood-borne pathogens
7. Describe the phases of types of infections
8. List and describe types of bacteria and the diseases they cause

9. Explain the significance of multidrug-resistant organisms
10. List and describe types of viruses and the diseases they cause
11. List and describe types of fungi and the diseases they cause
12. List and describe types of protozoa and the diseases they cause
13. Describe the body's defense mechanisms against infection
14. List the ways a person acquires immunity to pathogenic organisms
15. Relate a good surgical outcome to the patient's immune response

TERMINOLOGY

Aerobes: Organisms that favor an environment with oxygen. Strict aerobes cannot live without oxygen.

Aerosol droplets: Droplets of moisture small enough to remain suspended in the air; such a droplet can carry microorganisms within it.

Anaerobes: Organisms that prefer an oxygen-poor environment. Strict anaerobes cannot survive in the presence of oxygen.

Bioburden: A measure of the number of bacterial colonies on a surface.

Contaminated: A surface, substance, or tissue that is not completely free of microorganisms.

Cross-contamination: The spread of infection from one person to another or from an object to a person.

Culture: The process of growing a microbe in a laboratory setting so that it can be studied and tested.

Diffusion: Uniform dispersal of particles in a solution or across a membrane.

Direct transmission: The transfer of microbes by direct physical contact with the microbes.

Droplet nuclei: Dried remnants of previously moist secretions containing microorganisms. Droplet nuclei are an important source of disease transmission.

Endospore: The dormant stage of some bacteria that allows them to survive in extreme environmental conditions, including heat, cold, and exposure to many disinfectants. Endospores are commonly referred to as spores.

Entry site: In microbial transmission, the sites where microorganisms enter the body.

Fomite: An intermediate inanimate source in the process of disease transmission. An object, such as a contaminated surgical instrument or medical device, can become a fomite in disease transmission.

Infection: The state or condition in which pathogenic microorganisms invade and colonize in the body or body tissues.

Inflammation: The body's nonspecific reaction to injury or infection that results in redness, heat, swelling, and pain.

Necrosis: Tissue death.

Nosocomial infection: Another term for hospital-acquired infection (HAI) or health care–acquired infection; an infection acquired as a result of being in a health care facility.

Opportunistic infection: Infection in a weakened individual, or as the result specific drugs, usually by colonization of a bacterium that does not usually cause disease. The host may be debilitated by another disease or the immune system may be compromised.

Pathogen: A disease-causing (pathogenic) microorganism.

Prion: An infectious protein substance that is resistant to common sterilization methods.

Resident microorganisms: The microorganisms that normally colonize certain tissues of the body, usually without harm to the host.

TERMINOLOGY (cont.)

Sterile: Completely free of all microorganisms.

Suppurative: Having developed pus and fluid.

Vector: A living intermediate carrier of microorganisms from one host to another. An example is the transmission of the bubonic plague. The vector is a flea, and the bacterium is transmitted to the human through a bite from an infected flea.

Virion: A complete virus particle.

Virulence: The degree to which a microorganism is capable of causing disease.

INTRODUCTION

Microbiology is the study of microscopic organisms called microbes or microorganisms. In the operating room, we are particularly concerned with preventing infections caused by bacteria and viruses transmitted by instruments, equipment, and personnel. To understand how disease is transmitted and prevented, we first need to study the organisms themselves and the diseases they cause. This chapter in particular explains the relationship between microbes and infection. Box 9-1 presents a short summary of important events in the history of microbiology.

Microbiology is a highly complex field with many subspecialties. *Medical microbiology* is the study of infectious diseases caused by microorganisms. Subspecialties of medical microbiology are concerned with specific species (e.g., virology, bacteriology, parasitology).

Pathology is the study of disease mechanisms, diagnosis, and treatment. Nonmedical microbiology includes the study of microbes in the environment or those used in commercial products. Plant microbiology is an important field of study for understanding habitats in the environment and preservation of species. The study of microbial diseases in plants often focuses on the development and protection of food crops.

Epidemiology is the study of disease or event (e.g., trauma) patterns. Epidemiology specifically focuses on the incidence (number of *new* cases or events in a given time period, who is affected (what populations), and the existing burden of the disease (total number of cases per population at a given time).

A new field of study related to infectious disease is called *emerging diseases*. This is related to new diseases or known diseases that have not previously been a public health problem but are becoming a threat.

CLASSIFICATION OF ORGANISMS

A simple definition of an organism is a living thing or system, capable of reproduction, reaction to stimuli, growth, and maintenance or metabolism. There are many different types of organisms. A mammal is an organism, and so are one-celled bacteria.

Science uses several different methods to classify organisms. The oldest method was developed 300 years ago by Carolus Linnaeus, and his system is called the *Linnaean system*. The Linnaean system classifies living things as either plant or animal according to evolutionary descent. Of course, since Linnaeus's work, classification (taxonomy) has become much more sophisticated and complex. A commonly used system in biology has seven categories or classifications, listed here from smallest to largest:

- Species
- Genus
- Family
- Order
- Class
- Phylum
- Kingdom
- Domain

BINOMIAL SYSTEM

The *binomial system* is a method of naming organisms. Each organism is named specifically according to its genus and species, which are Latin or Greek words. For example, human beings are classified as genus *Homo* and species *sapiens*. The disease typhoid is caused by the bacterium *Salmonella typhi*. When the scientific name of an organism is typed, the genus is capitalized (*Salmonella*) and both the genus and species are italicized (*Salmonella enterica*); when the scientific name is

---

Box **9-1**	**Important Events in the History of Microbiology**

1677: Anton van Leeuwenhoek develops the light microscope and observes "little animals" under magnification.

1796: Edward Jenner develops the first smallpox vaccination.

1850: Ignaz Semmelweis discovers the association between hand washing and a decrease in puerperal infection.

1861: Louis Pasteur disproves the theory of spontaneous generation and develops the germ theory of infection.

1867: Joseph Lister first practices surgery using antiseptic practices.

1876: Robert Koch offers the first proof of the germ theory using *Bacillus anthracis*.

1882: Robert Koch develops the Koch postulates. Paul Ehrlich develops the acid-fast stain.

1884: Christian Gram develops the Gram stain.

1885: Louis Pasteur develops the first rabies vaccine.

1892: Dmitri Iosifovich Ivanovski discovers the virus.

1900: Walter Reed proves that mosquitoes carry yellow fever.

1910: Paul Ehrlich discovers a cure for syphilis.

1928: Alexander Fleming discovers penicillin.

1995: The first microbe genome sequence (for *Haemophilus influenzae*) is published.

written out, the capitalization stays the same and the name (both parts) is underlined.

THE CELL AND ITS COMPONENTS

Cell theory was developed in the 1600s, shortly after the invention of the microscope. This theory is the basis of modern biology and states that:

1. The cell is the fundamental unit of all living things.
2. All living things are composed of cells.
3. All cells are derived from other cells.

The cell is the basic unit of a living organism. Cellular organisms are divided into two types, prokaryotes and eukaryotes, each descended from different groups. Figure 9-1 shows both types of cells.

CELLS OF EUKARYOTES (COMPLEX ORGANISMS)

Plants, animals, and single-celled organisms are composed of many types of cells. This basic type of cell in a complex organism such as a mammal is called a *eukaryotic cell*. All cells that make up the human body are eukaryotic. Different tissues are composed of variations of the eukaryotic cell. For example, a muscle cell has features that distinguish it from a nerve cell (neuron). However, both are eukaryotic. The cells of a fish or a fungus are also eukaryotic cells.

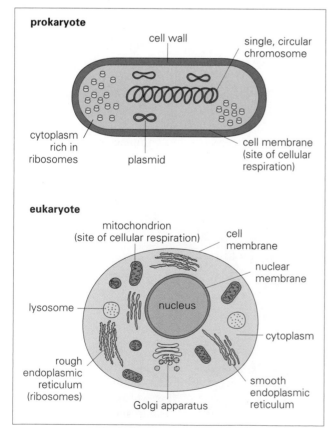

Figure 9-1   Eukaryote and prokaryote cells. Only bacteria and the Archaea groups are prokaryotes. *(From Goering R, Dockrell H, Wakelin D, et al: Mim's medical microbiology, ed 4, St Louis, 2008, Mosby.)*

The eukaryotic cell is the basic cell that makes up multicellular organisms and some types of single-celled organisms. There are many different kinds of eukaryotic cells, but all have the same basic structure, which includes a cell membrane and many specialized structures inside the cell.

- *Cell membrane:* A eukaryotic cell is surrounded by a double-layered membrane. The inside of the cell contains a semiclear liquid, called *cytosol,* and small bodies called *organelles,* which perform the cell's metabolic functions.

Organelles

A eukaryotic cell has many types of smaller interior organs called organelles (Figure 9-2):

- *Nucleus, chromatin, chromosomes:* The *nucleus* is the largest organelle. It is surrounded by a complex membrane that forms interconnected folds called the *endoplasmic reticulum.* The nucleus contains a protein substance called *chromatin* that contains the cell's deoxyribonucleic acid (DNA). This enables the cell to replicate. During reproduction, the chromatin forms double strands called *chromosomes.*
- *Nucleolus:* The nucleus also contains a *nucleolus,* which has proteins and ribonucleic acid (RNA), which is also necessary for cell reproduction. RNA transfers the cell's genetic information from the DNA in the nucleus to the ribosomes along the folds of the endoplasmic reticulum. These small organelles are the site of protein synthesis for cell reproduction.
- *Inner membranes and their vacuoles and Golgi apparatus:* The cell has a complex network of membranes that form compartments for the organelles. This system is called the *endomembrane system.* The endomembrane can "pinch off" to form new closed compartments as needed; these are called *vacuoles.* They may store molecules or transfer waste out of the cell. They also wall off any harmful substances inside the cell. Smaller sacs called vesicles store substances and transport waste. The *Golgi apparatus* is another extension of the endomembrane. This organelle stores and modifies large molecules and transports them inside the cell.
- *Mitochondria:* The *mitochondria* are composed of an outer membrane and many inner compartments. Mitochondria synthesize *adenosine triphosphate (ATP),* which provides energy for cell metabolism.

CELLS OF PROKARYOTES (MICROBES)

A *prokaryote* is one of a group of single-celled microbes that includes only bacteria and a smaller, primitive group of single-celled organisms called *Archaea.* In medicine, we are mainly concerned with the bacteria, because they cause disease.

- *Genetic material:* A prokaryotic cell (bacterium) does not develop into a complex organism with tissue differentiation. It remains as a single cell but multiples into colonies. One of the main differences between a prokaryote and a eukaryote is that the prokaryote has no nucleus. The genetic material for the prokaryote cell is coiled in an area called the nucleoid. This structure contains chromosomes, but DNA may also lie outside this region in a small circular

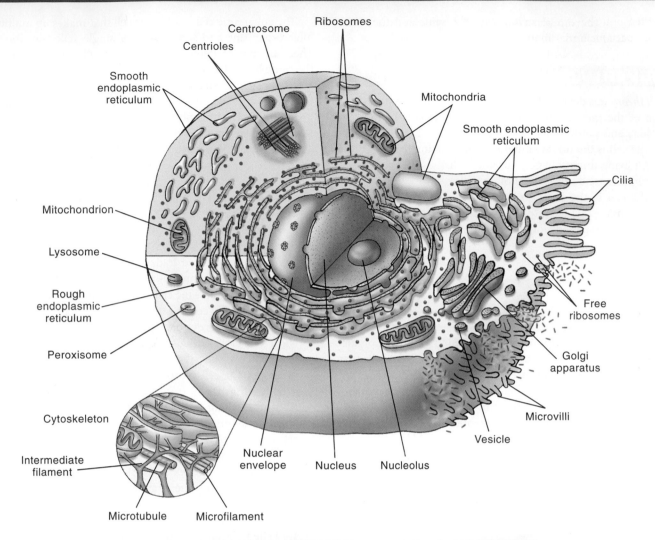

Centrosome
Centrioles
Ribosomes
Smooth endoplasmic reticulum
Mitochondria
Smooth endoplasmic reticulum
Cilia
Mitochondrion
Lysosome
Rough endoplasmic reticulum
Peroxisome
Free ribosomes
Golgi apparatus
Microvilli
Vesicle
Cytoskeleton
Intermediate filament
Nuclear envelope
Nucleus
Nucleolus
Microtubule
Microfilament

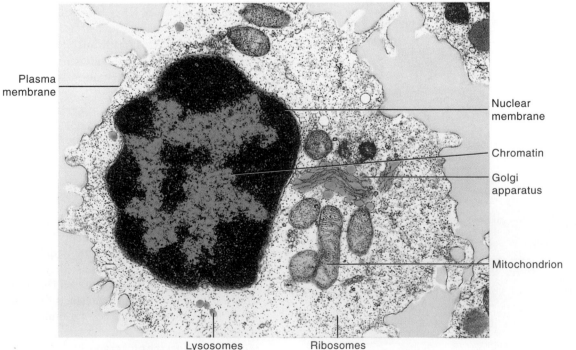

Plasma membrane
Nuclear membrane
Chromatin
Golgi apparatus
Mitochondrion
Lysosomes
Ribosomes

Figure 9-2 Eukaryotic cell demonstrating organelles, which are units of metabolic function within the cell. *(From Thibodeau G, Patton K: Anatomy and physiology, ed 6, St Louis, 2007, Mosby.)*

molecule called a plasmid. The only true organelle of the prokaryote is the ribosome, which synthesizes protein.

- *Cell membrane:* All prokaryotes are surrounded by a cell membrane, and some have a rigid *cell wall.* The cell wall is very important in the classification of bacteria.
- *Flagellum and pili:* A long filament extends from the surface of the cell. This structure may occur as a single strand (*flagellum*) or in small "tufts" (*flagella*). The flagella are used for movement. *Pili* are another type of surface extension on bacterial cells. A single *pilus* attaches to another bacterium as a means of infusing its cytoplasm and genetic material. Some bacteria can attach their pili to human tissue and can alter the body's immune response to the bacteria.
- *Capsule or slime layer:* Some bacteria have a *capsule,* or *slime layer.* This protects the cell from drying and also provides resistance to chemicals and invasion by viruses.

CELL TRANSPORT AND ABSORPTION

Cells absorb molecules and other substances across their outside membranes and synthesize others from substances inside the cell. The movement of substances occurs by two different methods, called *passive transport* and *active transport.* Active transport requires energy (chemical or electrochemical), whereas passive transport does not.

Passive Transport

This is the simple movement of particles in a solution. An example of passive transport is **diffusion**. When salt is added to water, the salt crystals simply disperse in the water. No energy is needed for this to occur. When the particles cross a permeable membrane, such as that of a cell, it is called *osmosis* (Figure 9-3).

The cell membrane is selective and allows only certain substances to cross. Water tends to move from the side with fewer particles to the side with more particles, which dilutes the side with more particles. Water continues to move until the concentration and water pressure are equal on both sides of the membrane (Figure 9-4).

Active Transport

In order to function, cells require some substances to be unequal in their distribution between the outside and inside of the cell. The cell does this by "pumping" the substance across the membrane rather than simply allowing it to disperse as in passive transport. The pumping is accomplished by chemical or electrochemical action that requires cellular energy.

ENDOCYTOSIS This is a type of active transport in which the cell carries a substance into the interior by engulfing it. In *pinocytosis,* the cell takes in water and small particles by

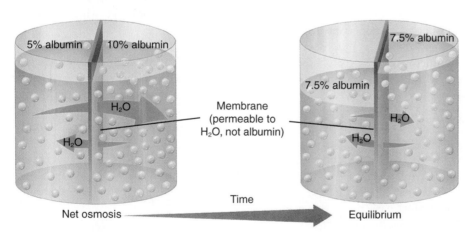

Figure 9-3 The process of osmosis, which is the passage of water through a *selectively permeable* membrane. On the left, the container holds two concentrations of albumin. On the right, the membrane has allowed water, but not albumin, to pass through, creating equilibrium. (*From Thibodeau G, Patton K: Anatomy and physiology, ed 6, St Louis, 2007, Mosby.*)

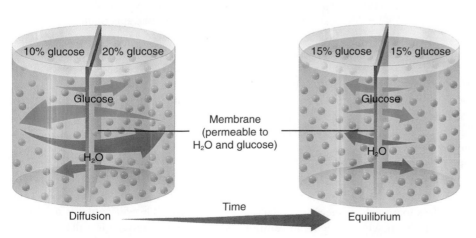

Figure 9-4 Diffusion across a membrane. The container on the left shows two separate concentrations of glucose. The membrane allows glucose to pass through until the two sides are equal in concentration. (*From Thibodeau G, Patton K: Anatomy and physiology, ed 6, St Louis, 2007, Mosby.*)

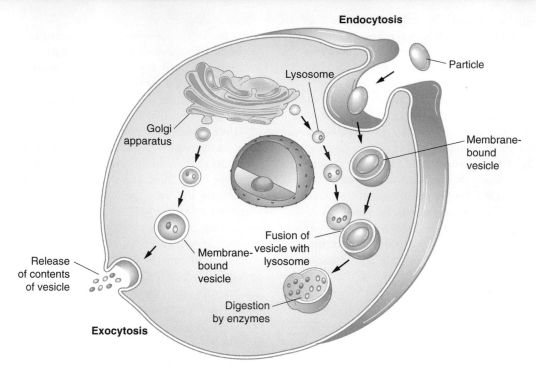

Figure 9-5 **Endocytosis and exocytosis.** Materials are transported into and out of a cell by means of a vesicle. Fusion of the vesicle with the lysosome causes the material to break down. The contents of the vesicle are released by exocytosis. *(From Thibodeau G, Patton K: Anatomy and physiology, ed 6, St Louis, 2007, Mosby.)*

surrounding them with a membrane-covered blister or vesicle. The material is completely enclosed by the membrane and moved to the interior of the cell, where it is transported to the needed location or outside the cell.

In *phagocytosis,* large particles such as microbes are engulfed and digested by a cell structure called a *lysosome.* The digested substances are then released from the cell by a process called *exocytosis* (Figure 9-5).

TOOLS FOR IDENTIFYING MICROBES

The study of microbes in medicine includes identifying them and testing their sensitivity to antimicrobial agents. This requires special laboratory procedures and tools. Most basic laboratory procedures focus on the bacteria, because this group of microbes causes most infectious diseases, and accurate identification often is critical for treatment and prevention.

CULTURE

In order to identify a specific type of bacteria, a sample must allowed to grow (colonize) outside the body. This is called a bacterial **culture**. After a sample of tissue or fluid is obtained, a very small amount of the sample is applied to a special plate or test tube that contains a semisolid or liquid medium conducive to microbial growth. Many different types of culture media are used to grow colonies of bacteria. After the bacteria are inoculated into the culture medium, the plate or test tube is placed in a warm culturing oven for several days to a week to allow the bacteria to proliferate. Samples of the newly

cultured microbes are then ready for testing and identification. Figure 9-6 shows bacterial colonies growing on culture media.

Bacteria are routinely tested for their sensitivity to antimicrobials (commonly called antibiotics). This is done by inoculating a culture plate with the microbe and placing small paper discs impregnated with various antibacterial agents on the sample. The procedure is called *culture and sensitivity testing.* The antimicrobial agents that prevent microbial growth of the particular bacteria show no cultures in that region of the culture plate. The microbe is said to be *sensitive* to that chemical. The antimicrobial discs that are *not* effective in halting microbial growth show a proliferation of colonies in the region of that agent (Figure 9-7).

STAINING

Staining is used to prepare a microbial specimen for examination under the microscope. A large variety of colored stains are available to perform specific tests. Staining takes place after the microbe has been applied to a glass slide. Many staining techniques require multiple steps, which include several "baths" with different solutions and meticulous care of the specimen. Bacteria commonly require staining, but fungi also may be stained for microscope viewing.

Gram Staining

Gram staining is routinely performed to differentiate bacteria into two primary groups called gram-positive and gram-negative bacteria. The bacterial cell wall contains a layer of sugars and amino acids. In some bacteria, this wall is very thin,

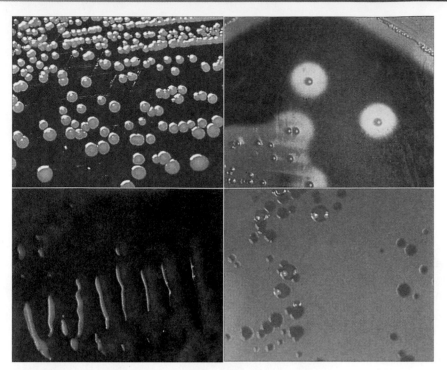

Figure 9-6 Bacterial colonies cultured in the laboratory using a Petri dish and culture media. *(From Goering R, Dockrell H, Wakelin D, et al: Mim's medical microbiology, ed 4, St Louis, 2008, Mosby.)*

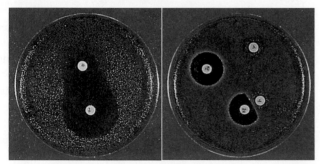

Figure 9-7 **Testing for culture and sensitivity.** This is a common method of determining which antibiotics are effective against a specific bacterium or fungus. Various types of antibiotic agents impregnated on paper are positioned in the culture medium, which has been inoculated with the microorganism. Note the areas of no colonization around some of the squares. *(From Goering R, Dockrell H, Wakelin D, et al: Mim's medical microbiology, ed 4, St Louis, 2008, Mosby.)*

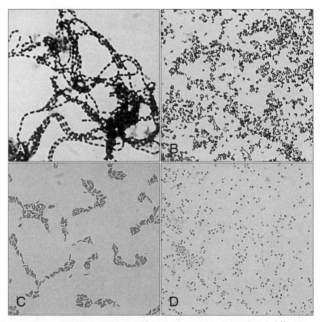

Figure 9-8 **Gram staining.** This technique is used to differentiate between gram-positive and gram-negative bacterial types for identification. **A** and **B,** Gram-positive bacteria stain dark purple, revealing a thick cell wall. **C** and **D,** Gram-negative bacteria stain pink due to the absence of a cell wall. *(From Goering R, Dockrell H, Wakelin D, et al: Mim's medical microbiology, ed 4, St Louis, 2008, Mosby.)*

> See the tables on the Evolve website that review staining techniques and culturing techniques. http://evolve.elsevier.com/Fuller/surgical.

whereas in others it is thick. Gram staining reveals the thicker wall; these bacteria are gram positive. The bacteria with the thinner wall do not absorb the stain and are gram negative. Under the microscope, gram-positive bacteria appear dark purple, whereas gram-negative bacteria stain pink (Figure 9-8).

Acid-Fast Staining

The acid-fast staining technique is used primarily for identification of *Mycobacterium* organisms, especially *Mycobacterium tuberculosis*. In this procedure, the bacteria are exposed to an acidic stain, which is taken up by the cell wall. The Ziehl-Neelsen test is most commonly used. This test uses the stain carbolfuchsin or methylene blue, which colors the cell wall pink, leaving a blue background. Another form of acid staining uses a fluorescent stain, which requires fluorescence microscopy for identification.

BIOCHEMICAL TESTING

Identification of the shape and size of bacteria is insufficient to establish the exact species. Tests that analyze the cell's biochemical activity are performed to differentiate bacteria. All metabolic functions are mediated by enzymes, which act on a substrate or base substance. Different biochemical tests reveal the substrates involved in metabolism and the end products. This information is used to identify specific bacteria or other microbes.

MICROSCOPY

The laboratory microscope is one of the most important tools used to identify and study microbes. The microscope magnifies specimens for identification of shape, size, staining properties, and other important attributes. Following is a discussion of the use of the microscope. The two main types of microscopes are the *optical microscope* and the *scanning probe microscope*. The optical microscope uses a series of lenses to focus light on the object being viewed. The light waves provide contrast, which can be enhanced by stains and other substances. The *electron microscope* is a type of optical microscope that uses electrons rather than light waves to provide contrast.

The *scanning probe microscope* uses a physical probe that tracks the contours and surfaces of the object and creates an image based on the findings. This type of microscope can view the object at a molecular level and is used in extremely fine examinations for industrial, biochemical, and medical purposes.

The *optical microscope* is commonly used in medical microbiology for routine identification and study of tissue, cells, and microorganisms. A simple optical microscope is pictured in Figure 9-9. Many different types of optical microscopes use an exterior or interior light source to illuminate the subject.

Parts of a Microscope

A biological microscope has one or two eyepieces, a series of lenses, a light source, focus adjustment, and a strong base that stabilizes the microscope. Modern microscopes use an electric light source contained inside the body or located at the bottom under the stage, where the specimen slide is placed for viewing. The following parts make up the microscope.

1. *Ocular (eyepiece):* One or two oculars are located at the top of the microscope. The viewer looks into the eyepieces, through which the image of the object is viewed. The eyepieces are directly in line with the series of lenses that focus the light and bring the image into clear view. A monocular microscope has only one eyepiece, and a binocular microscope has an eyepiece for each eye. Binocular microscopes allow adjustment of each eyepiece to accommodate the viewer's visual acuity and the distance between each eye. The eyepiece lenses are located near the top of the eyepiece.
2. *Tube:* The tube, or viewing tube, connects the eyepiece to the objective lens, which is located directly over the stage.
3. *Arm:* The arm connects the viewing tube to the base and balances the microscope. It also is used for carrying the microscope; one hand is placed on the base and the other around the arm.
4. *Objective lens:* This set of lenses is located at the bottom of the tube. The lens powers, or magnification, differ among microscopes. The common laboratory microscope has 10×, 40×, and 100× lenses. These are in line with the eyepiece lens, which is usually 10×. Thus the collective magnification is 10 times the power of the objective lens. Objective lenses are color-coded for easy identification.
5. *Focus adjustment knobs:* Two focus adjustment knobs are located near the arm. These provide fine and coarse focus

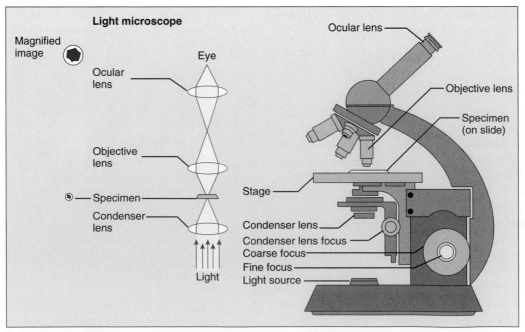

Figure 9-9 Light microscope showing the lens system and parts. *(From Erlandsen SL, Magney JE: Color atlas of histology, St Louis, 1992, Mosby, p 27.)*

by moving the serial lenses vertically. Because the focus adjustment moves the objective lenses directly over the subject, the danger exists of direct contact (and damage) to the objective lens. Some microscopes have a rack stop to prevent this.

6. *Rack stop:* This is a vertical adjustment that prevents direct contact between the objective lens and the specimen. The rack stop is common on student microscopes to prevent damage to the objective lens (and slide).

7. *Nosepiece:* This is a round fitting for the objective lenses. The nosepiece revolves to place one of the objective lenses directly over the subject being viewed.

8. *Stage:* This is the flat area just under the objective lenses where the specimen slide is placed. The stage can be moved with knobs so that the specimen can be scanned from side to side or up and down. The slide is secured on the stage by a clip mechanism.

9. *Illuminator (light source):* Intense, evenly distributed light is needed to view the specimen. This is provided by the light source, which is located under the base of the microscope directly under the condenser. Tungsten or quartz halogen light bulbs are commonly used in the laboratory microscope.

10. *Condenser:* This mechanism is located under the stage and contains two sets of lenses that focus light on the subject. The condenser has a diaphragm, or iris, that can be adjusted to allow more or less light into the viewing area. The condenser is operated with a diaphragm lever located just under the stage.

How to Use a Microscope

Using a microscope properly requires "hands-on" instruction and practice. The microscope itself is a delicate and expensive instrument with numerous components. In addition, the specimen itself requires preparation. If the slide is prepared improperly, the specimen will be damaged or obscured.

Guidelines for caring for the microscope include the following:

1. Always carry the microscope by the arm and the base, using both hands.

2. Use only laboratory-grade, lint-free lens paper to clean the objective lenses. The lenses are very delicate and can be easily scratched with coarse paper. Lint from cleaning materials can obscure the lenses.

3. Provide a clutter-free surface for the microscope during use.

4. Always store the microscope with the objective lenses in their highest position to prevent damage.

5. Never attempt to insert a slide with the objective lenses lowered.

6. Store the microscope in a dust-free environment with a cover.

The microscope requires some setting up and adjustments in the illumination system before use. Once these are accomplished, a simple specimen can be used to practice with the microscope. Follow these steps to prepare a simple specimen for viewing under the microscope:

1. Prepare the specimen using a glass slide and cover slip. (Slides that have been commercially prepared beforehand are best for learning in the beginning.)

2. Make sure the lowest power objective is in position over the stage. It should be placed in its closest position over the specimen.

3. Position the slide specimen on the stage and secure the spring clip. The stage should be centered under the objective.

4. Observe the specimen through the eyepiece. Slowly raise the objective using the coarse adjustment knob. Use the fine focus adjustment to clarify the image.

5. Use the condenser diaphragm to adjust the amount of light, which is critical for a clear view.

6. View the specimen on the next highest power by turning the nosepiece. Do not move the specimen.

7. Use the fine focus adjustment to clarify the image.

8. Immersion oil is required to view images with the red-coded objective lens. This further focuses the light.

THE PROCESS OF INFECTION

Biological advances have led to a new understanding of how microorganisms interact with the environment and the human body to cause disease. Historically, we simply identified an organism as beneficial, neutral, or harmful. We now understand that the microbe-host relationship changes according to the environment (including the environment of the body) or differences in the microbe itself.

It is important to note that specific microbes (mainly bacteria) can infect and cause disease in many different body systems and tissues, depending on the condition of the host, the portal of entry of the microbe, and complex biochemical conditions in the cell environment. Some bacteria prefer specific organ systems, whereas others are capable of crossing body systems and causing **infection** in different areas of the body via the bloodstream, lymphatic system, or natural pathways such as ducts and other tubular structures.

MICROBES IN THE ENVIRONMENT

Commensalism

In *commensalism,* one organism uses another to meet its physiological needs but causes no harm to the host. For example, the normal human intestinal tract contains many different types of bacteria, such as *Escherichia coli,* that are essential for metabolism. The bacteria survive in balance with the body as long as they remain in the intestine. However, if *E. coli* escape the intestine and enter the sterile tissues of the body, such as when the bowel is perforated by trauma or disease, the result can be fatal. The presence of *E. coli* bacteria in the bloodstream can result in destruction of vital organs and can cause death very quickly.

During bowel surgery, special techniques are used to prevent the bowel contents from contacting the sterile abdominal cavity. The surgical technologist has an important role in this process, which is called *bowel technique.*

Mutualism

In mutualism, each of the organisms benefits from their relationship in the environment. For example, *Staphylococcus aureus* inhabits normal, healthy skin. These bacteria proliferate in this environment, and they protect the skin from other invading organisms. However, the stress of disease, a break in the skin, and other conditions cause the bacteria to multiply rapidly and create infection.

Parasitism

A *parasite* is an organism that lives on or within another organism (the host) and gains an advantage at the expense of that organism. Infectious disease is the result of a parasitic relationship between the host and the invading organism.

Organisms that cause infectious disease are called *pathogenic* organisms.

Opportunistic Organisms

Only about 3% to 5% of all microbes are pathogenic. However, nonpathogenic microbes (those that do not usually cause disease) that live in and on the body can become pathogenic under certain conditions. When this occurs, the microbe is described as opportunistic. An **opportunistic infection** is one that occurs when the host is weakened in some way and its usual defenses are inadequate to prevent the microbe from causing disease. This occurs in human immunodeficiency virus/acquired immunodeficiency syndrome (HIV/AIDS) and can also occur in surgical patients who are weakened by the surgical process.

REQUIREMENTS FOR INFECTION

Not every contact with a **pathogen** results in infection. Certain conditions must be favorable for the pathogen to gain entry into the body and proliferate:

1. *The microbe must have an **entry site** and an exit site.* Microbes often are environmentally suited to a specific body system, and their entry site and exit site are often the same.
2. *Microbes must be present in sufficient numbers.* The number of invading microbes is called the *dose.* An infection or disease can be established only if a sufficient number of disease organisms are present. The number of microbe colonies on a surface is referred to as the **bioburden.**
3. *The environment must be well suited to the pathogen.* Once the pathogen gains entry into the body, the conditions for nutrition, oxygen requirements, pH, and temperature must be conducive to bacterial colonization and proliferation.
4. *The host must be unable to overcome the harmful mechanisms of the pathogen.* Infection develops only if the host's natural or artificial immunity cannot prevent microbial proliferation.

DISEASE TRANSMISSION

Diseases can be transmitted through a number of different pathways (Figure 9-10).

Direct Contact

Microorganisms are transferred from a host through direct contact or an intermediate source. The source can be nonliving (**fomite**) or living (**vector**). In the operating room, only sterile supplies and instruments are used. **Sterile** means completely free of all microorganisms.

A nonsterile (**contaminated**) surgical instrument can become a fomite by transmitting microorganisms into sterile tissue. Instruments and medical devices can harbor pathogenic bacteria encased in dried blood and body tissue that was not removed during the cleaning process. Other common fomites in the hospital are bed linens, wound dressings, and contaminated urinary catheters. Insects or rodents carry pathogens from one surface to another or between hosts. Food attracts vectors and therefore is not permitted in the operating room.

Airborne Transmission

Water droplets carry organisms from one surface to another. They can also enter the body directly through the respiratory tract or another entry site. Water droplets are forcefully expelled during talking, coughing, or sneezing. Another example of contamination by water droplets occurs in the processing of instruments and equipment in the surgical department. Cleaning always takes place away from restricted and semirestricted areas to prevent contamination by droplets released from contaminated wash water.

Airborne transmission also occurs via **droplet nuclei** (dried remnants of previously moist secretions containing microorganisms). Droplet nuclei or **aerosol droplets** can remain suspended in the air because of their small size (usually 1 to 5 micrometers). They are infective for long periods and transmit disease when individuals breathe in the particles. Aerosol droplets can settle on surfaces and transmit disease by direct contact.

Transmission by Body Fluids

Blood-borne pathogens are a risk to hospitalized patients and health care personnel, who may acquire disease through contact with blood and body fluids. Strict protocols for isolating and handling medical waste, body fluids, specimens, and soiled equipment in the hospital environment have been established to prevent infection. These protocols are called *Standard Precautions.* Exposure to blood-borne pathogens in the workplace requires immediate attention. The Centers for Disease Control and Prevention (CDC) has established guidelines for the management of exposure based on the type of pathogen and the nature of the exposure. Immediate care is available to all health care workers.

Oral Transmission (Ingestion)

Oral transmission occurs when a pathogen is ingested in food or through fecal-oral transmission. Fecal-oral transmission occurs when the infectious agent is shed by the infected host and acquired by the susceptible host through the ingestion of contaminated material. Poor hygiene among patients and hospital staff contributes to the spread of pathogens in this way. Frequent hand washing in the health care setting is very important to the prevention of oral disease transmission.

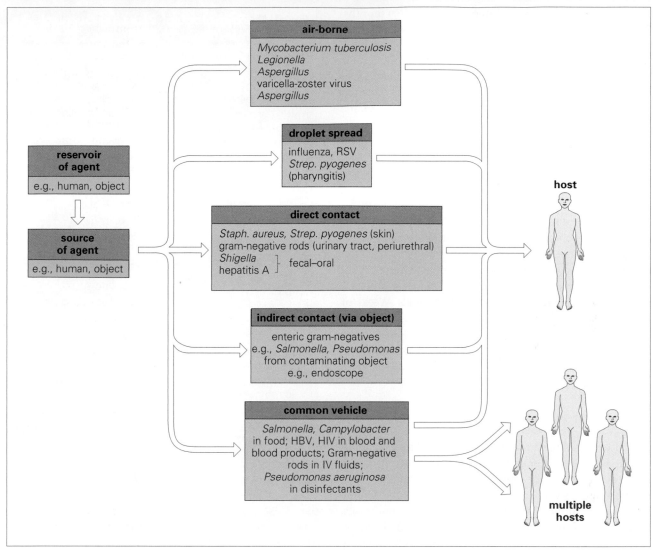

Figure 9-10 **Methods of disease transmission.** Microorganisms leave or gain entry into the body through one of these routes and may colonize unless the body is able to overcome and destroy the microbes. *HBV*, Hepatitis B virus; *IV*, intravenous; *RSV*, respiratory syncytial virus. *(From Goering R, Dockrell H, Wakelin D, et al: Mim's medical microbiology, ed 4, St Louis, 2008, Mosby.)*

Portal of Entry

To proliferate and cause disease, infectious organisms must gain entry to the body. The following are common means of entry.

- *Urogenital infection* almost always results from an outside source, usually the urethral orifice. The female urogenital tract is especially vulnerable to infection, because it is very short. Bacteria enter the urethral orifice and proliferate in the bladder, causing cystitis (infection of the bladder). The most common cause of urinary tract infection in females is *E. coli,* which is present in the large intestine and shed with feces.
- *Skin penetration* can result in local, regional, or systemic infection. The skin normally is a very efficient barrier against bacterial infection. However, when the skin is broken, bacteria can invade less protected tissues and cause local infection. If not resolved, a local infection can enter the vascular system and cause systemic disease.

- *Sexually transmitted diseases (STDs)* are spread when the mucous membrane of an infected person comes in contact with the mucous membrane of an uninfected person, usually during sexual contact. The intact mucous membrane can help defend the body against disease transmission by secreting mucus, which cleanses the membrane. However, sexually transmitted diseases are prevented only with the use of condoms or abstinence.
- *Mother to infant transmission,* or vertical transmission, occurs from one generation to another through breast milk.
- *Ingestion of particular microbes* by mouth may result in gastrointestinal infection.

PHASES OF INFECTION

The course of an infection follows a pattern of distinct phases.
1. *Incubation:* In this phase the pathogens actively replicate, but the host shows no symptoms. This may be a short

period (hours), or it may continue for days or even months. The incubation period is affected by the physical status of the host, the port of entry, and the number of infectious organisms present in the body.

2. *Prodromal phase:* In this phase symptoms begin to appear. They may be very mild or vague at the start of the infection or may include certain clinically important signs of the disease.

3. *Acute phase:* In this phase the organism is at its most potent, and symptoms are very apparent. Cellular damage and destruction of tissue are characteristic of many diseases at this stage.

4. *Convalescence:* During this phase proliferation of the infectious organism slows and symptoms subside. Tissue begins to heal, and the body starts to regain strength and normal function.

These stages apply to diseases that resolve with treatment or by natural course. However, not all diseases resolve. A *chronic infection* may develop in some individuals. Weeks or months may be required for resolution, when all the disease organisms are eliminated from the body. Also, a person may harbor disease organisms but show no signs or symptoms; this person is referred to as a *carrier.*

HOSPITAL-ACQUIRED INFECTION

A hospital-acquired infection (HAI), also called a **nosocomial infection,** is an infection acquired while the patient is in a health care institution. The most common HAI is urinary tract infection in patients who have been catheterized. In the United States, about 2 million patients a year develop infections, including surgical site infections, as a result of hospitalization. Seventy percent of the bacteria that cause these infections are resistant to at least one of the drugs commonly used to treat that infection. The spread of a hospital-acquired infection from person to person is called **cross-contamination**. Introduction of an infection from one part of the body to another is called *self-infection* or autoinfection.

SURGICAL SITE INFECTION

Surgical site infection begins when a pathogenic or nonpathogenic microorganism colonizes sterile tissues. This can be caused by:

- Contamination of the tissues before surgery, such as a ruptured bowel or a traumatic wound caused by a foreign object.
- Contamination during surgery due to poor aseptic technique (discussed in Chapter 10).
- Contamination of the incision after surgery.

Some wound infections are minor, involving only the skin, whereas others occur in deep tissue or body cavities. The infection may remain localized or spread throughout the body. The patient's general condition at the time of surgery is a predictor of risk. Certain surgical patients have a high physiological risk of infection (Box 9-2).

Box 9-2 Physiological Risks for Surgical Site Infection

- *Age:* The immune system of an older patient is less responsive than that of a younger patient. Tissues heal more slowly, and innate body defenses are less effective. Older patients are often undernourished.
- *Undernourishment or malnourishment:* Essential proteins required for tissue healing and body defenses against infection often are missing in the diet of these patients. Low body fat predisposes the patient to lowered body temperature, which increases physiological stress.
- *Diabetes mellitus:* The diabetic patient is at extremely high risk of infection because of problems with the circulatory system, which must be properly functioning to support a healthy immune system. Poor peripheral and visceral circulation prevents the flow of nutrients and oxygen to traumatized tissue, which increases the overgrowth of both resident and disease-producing microorganisms.
- *Substance or alcohol abuse:* These patients are often malnourished. Liver damage related to substance abuse and alcohol abuse leads to poor conversion of glycogen to glucose, which is necessary for cellular metabolism. Immune function often is depressed.
- *Immune suppression:* Patients with acquired immunodeficiency syndrome (AIDS) or other immune diseases, those undergoing cancer therapy, and those who have been prescribed high doses of corticosteroids have impaired immune function.
- *Long preoperative stay in the hospital:* A prolonged preoperative stay allows the body to incubate and colonize bacteria and other microorganisms commonly found in the hospital environment, especially antibiotic-resistant forms.
- *Surgical wound classification:* Contaminated wounds are associated with a higher risk of infection in the postoperative patient.
- *Long operative procedure:* Long procedures put the patient at higher risk for exposure to airborne pathogens and direct contact with contaminated medical devices and instruments.

The severity of the infection is influenced by the type, **virulence,** and number of invading bacteria, as well as the organism's sensitivity to antibiotic treatment.

The infection usually is treated at the first signs. A culture specimen is taken if there is exudate present. Antibiotic treatment may be initiated immediately. The wound is observed for further signs of infection and the patient monitored closely.

A small, localized area of infection sometimes develops at the wound site. This type of *abscess* is easily treated. However, a surgical site infection that spreads and becomes systemic can cause serious disease or death. In moderate to severe infection, the patient's temperature becomes elevated soon after surgery. The patient may experience pain at the incisional site or deep within the wound.

Exudate (an accumulation of pus, drainage, dead cells, and serum) may appear around the incision. The wound then is described as **suppurative**. The site becomes extremely tender or painful. If the infection is localized, antimicrobial therapy may be initiated and the infection eradicated. Deep infections, however, may lead to widespread areas of tissue death (**necrosis**), accumulation of pus, and breakdown of the sutured tissue layers.

Infection occurring at the surgical site can cause other problems such as breakdown of the incision layers. As suture materials degrade in the presence of bacteria, the wound may split open, a condition known as *dehiscence.*

A large accumulation of pus leads to the spread of infection into adjacent tissues. An uncontrolled infection in a body cavity results in inflammation of the lining of that cavity (e.g., peritonitis in the abdomen). This can be rapidly fatal as vital organs are infected and fail.

Treatment

A superficial surgical site infection usually is treated at the first signs. A culture specimen is taken. This is a sample of the wound exudate that is incubated and allowed to proliferate for testing. The wound is observed for further signs of infection and the patient monitored closely. Deep infection may not be diagnosed until days after the surgery and is often accompanied with pain and fever. Antibiotic treatment is started immediately. If the symptoms do not resolve, the wound may be incised again so that pus, necrotic tissue, and devitalized tissue can be removed. This procedure is called an *incision and drainage* (I & D). Advanced treatment includes intravenous (IV) antibiotic therapy and continuous wound drainage. If the infection remains localized, the prognosis for resolution is good. However, systemic infection can result when bacteria migrate into the vascular system, causing septicemia and widespread organ damage.

When infection is present, the wound cannot be sutured, because infected tissues cannot withstand the tension of sutures and bacterial toxins rapidly break most suture material. Instead, the wound is packed with gauze dressings and allowed to heal from the bottom to the exterior.

Isolation

Certain diseases and infections require the patient to be isolated from others in the environment. Patients with highly resistant bacterial infections are treated in the hospital using isolation procedures in which equipment and supplies needed for patient care are contained in the patient's room. Nurses and other care providers must put on gowns, face masks, and gloves while handling any contaminated medical supplies and must discard protective equipment in the patient's room before leaving.

Patients with highly contagious infections that are transmitted primarily through droplet transmission are almost never brought into the operating room for treatment. Within the health facility, those caring for them must wear a mask, gown, and gloves. (See Chapter 6 for additional information on the isolation patient.)

DISEASE PREVENTION

The most important reason for studying certain aspects of microbiology is *disease prevention.* No other area of health care has a greater impact on populations, including patients undergoing surgery. Important methods of disease prevention in the health care facility include the following:

- Hand washing
- Learning and practicing Standard Precautions and isolation precautions
- Learning and practicing aseptic technique
- Good personal hygiene practices
- Strict disinfection and environmental cleaning in the facility
- Proper use of antiseptics and chemical disinfectants
- Isolation of infected patients according to standard guidelines

Note that hand washing is the most important and effective method of disease prevention in the health care facility and in the community.

Standard and isolation precautions are standards established by the CDC that establish special techniques to stop the spread of infection in the health facility environment. Standard Precautions are discussed thoroughly in Chapter 8. Isolation precautions are carried out when a patient is infected with a highly transmissible disease. This type of patient is unlikely to be a candidate for surgery. However, all health professionals should be aware of the standards and know when to apply them.

> The most recent version of the standards is available in the following CDC document: 2007 Guideline for Isolation Precautions: Preventing Transmission of Infectious Agents in the Healthcare Settings, available at http://www.cdc.gov/hicpac/pdf/isolation/isolation.pdf.

MICROORGANISMS AND THE DISEASES THEY CAUSE

BACTERIA

Bacteria are prokaryotic organisms. They represent a very large population of microbes in the environment and affect animals, humans, and plants. Most live without causing harm to other organisms. However, a few species cause serious disease. Bacteria that cause infection are called *pyogenic.* This group includes streptococcal, staphylococcal, meningococcal, pneumococcal, and gonococcal organisms and the coliform (intestinal) bacilli. These organisms typically cause suppuration (pus) and tissue destruction that can lead to systemic involvement and ultimately death.

Structure

Bacteria represent the largest variety of infectious microorganisms and cause the greatest number of postoperative infections and other HAIs. Bacteria exist in a variety of shapes, sizes, and forms, which are created by the cell wall. Bacteria can exist singly or in groups, called colonies. Figure 9-11 shows a generalized bacterium.

Identification of specific bacteria is an important goal in the diagnosis of infectious diseases. Many tests can be performed on bacterial cells to identify their exact classification

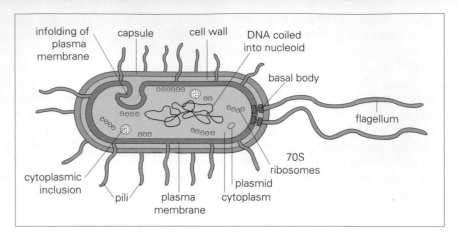

Figure 9-11 Generalized bacterial cell. Note both the cell wall and the plasma membrane, which differentiate the prokaryote from most eukaryotic cells. A wide variation in morphology is seen among bacteria types. *(From Goering R, Dockrell H, Wakelin D et al: Mim's medical microbiology, ed 4, St Louis, 2008, Mosby.)*

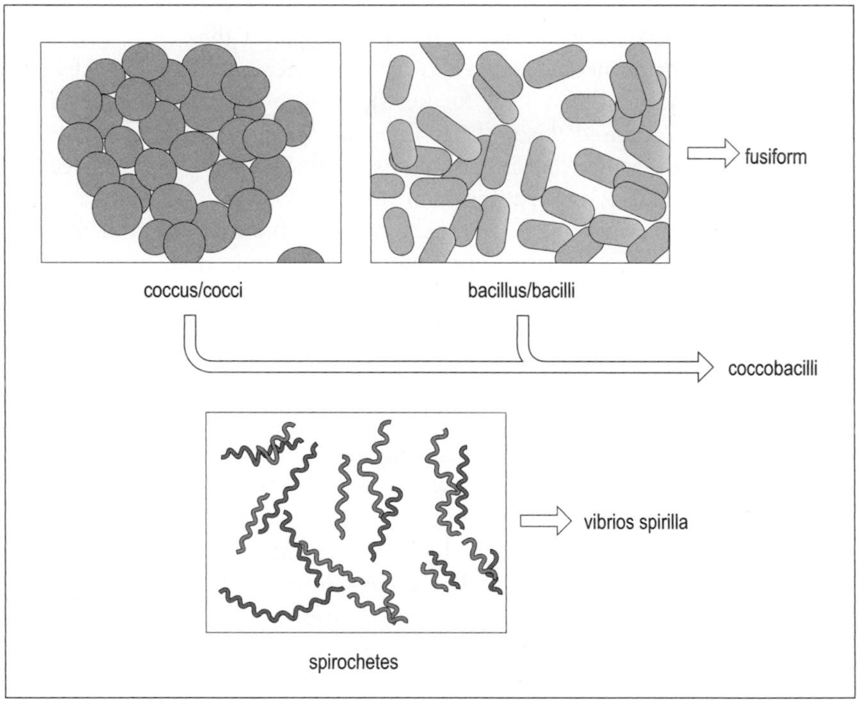

Figure 9-12 The three basic shapes of bacteria. *(From Goering R, Dockrell H, Wakelin D et al: Mim's medical microbiology, ed 4, St Louis, 2008, Mosby.)*

and disease potential. Other tests are performed to determine the organism's susceptibility to antibacterial drugs.

Bacteria are partially classified according to their shape (Figure 9-12). This can be determined by staining the bacteria and observing them under the microscope. Bacteria take the following basic shapes:

- Rod-shaped bacteria are *bacilli,* which occur singly or in pairs, chains, or filaments. Rods can be slightly curved or straight.
- Curved or spiral-shaped bacteria are *spirochetes,* which may be coiled or loosely curved.
- Spherical bacteria are *cocci,* which occur singly (micrococci), in chains (streptococci), in pairs (diplococci), or in clusters (staphylococci).
- Other shapes sometimes seen are square and tetrahedral, but these are less common.

Motility

Bacteria move using a number of different kinds of mechanisms. The flagella and pili described earlier are the most common methods. The flagella rotate and propel the cell in different directions. Pili also create motility by anchoring to a surface and retracting, which allows the pili to move the cell along. Some bacteria move by using the host's cytoskeleton, a network of filaments within the cytoplasm.

Environmental and Nutrient Requirements

Important environmental parameters for all microorganisms include temperature, oxygen, pH, moisture, and atmospheric pressure. Bacteria are found everywhere in the natural world, living under a wide variety of conditions. Those that infect humans require moderate conditions.

Bacteria that produce spores can live in temperature ranges of −4° to 194° F (−20° to 90° C). Oxygen requirements for bacteria vary widely. Some require oxygen to live and grow (strict **aerobes**). Others cannot live in the presence of oxygen; these are called strict **anaerobes.** Anaerobes are important in the process of infection, because they can proliferate in deep traumatic or surgical wounds. *Facultative* bacteria can live with or without oxygen.

Bacteria have evolved to withstand extremes of the pH spectrum. For example, the normal pH of blood is 7.35 to 7.45. *Helicobacter pylori* can invade the gastric mucosa and reproduce at a pH of 2. The normal pH in the body prevents most pathogenic organisms from proliferating, but a change in pH can destroy the normal "resident" bacteria and allow pathogens to invade the body.

Bacteria that are significant in infectious disease prefer a moist environment. One method of destroying bacteria is *desiccation* (drying). Resistance to drying makes bacteria such as mycobacteria, which cause tuberculosis, a public health problem, because the bacteria can spread through dried sputum.

Bacteria obtain nutrient substances from their immediate environment. Some bacteria can synthesize many nutrients from substances available within the cell. Others require a more complex variety of organic compounds, which they take in from their environment. Most bacteria require basic elemental nutrients:

- Carbon
- Oxygen
- Nitrogen
- Hydrogen
- Phosphorus
- Sulfur
- Potassium

Reproduction

Bacterial cells reproduce by asexual fission into two new cells. In this process, the genetic material is replicated and moves to separate areas of the cell. A septal membrane develops, splitting the mother cell into two halves, which separate into daughter cells.

Some bacteria are capable of producing a vegetative reproductive form called an **endospore** (commonly referred to as a *spore*). This is a dormant phase in the reproductive cycle in which the bacteria form a thick, multilayered protein wall around their genetic material. The wall resists extreme environmental conditions such as boiling, drying, chemical destruction, and high pressure. When environmental conditions are favorable, the spore becomes active and reproduction (colonization) begins. Two important spore-forming bacteria are *Clostridium tetani* (tetanus) and *Bacillus anthracis* (anthrax).

Bacterial Growth

Bacteria grow at a rate that corresponds to their environment and nutritional status. A favorable environment, one that meets the bacteria's essential requirements, results in more rapid colonization than an environment in which the bacteria must compete for resources. In the laboratory, bacteria can be provided with essential environmental and nutritive requirements. In this way, their growth patterns can be studied.

Bacteria show four characteristic phases of growth:

1. *Lag phase:* This period occurs immediately after the growth medium is inoculated with the sample bacteria. During this phase, the bacteria do not divide, but they may be processing or synthesizing components of the growth medium in preparation for cell division. This is a period of increased metabolism for the bacteria as they adjust to the environment.

2. *Exponential (log) phase:* This phase is characterized by active and sometimes rapid cell division. The rate usually is constant, depending on the growth medium. This rate often is referred to as the *doubling time* or *generation time* of the bacteria.

3. *Stationary phase:* In this phase, the bacteria have used up their available nutrition in the growth medium and the amount of space available for growth. The by-products of reproduction have accumulated, and these inhibit further growth. During this phase, cell division stops.

4. *Death phase:* In the restricted culture medium, the death phase follows the stationary phase. The bacteria can no longer survive and the colony dies out, usually at the same rate as the growth phase.

Pathogenicity

Bacteria cause disease by gaining entry into the host and colonizing tissue. Bacteria have many different mechanisms for adhering to host cells and evading the immune system. They can overcome and destroy the body's defensive white blood cells. Some are capable of hemolysis, the destruction of red blood cells. One of the most potent pathogenic mechanisms of bacteria is the release of toxins by the bacterial cell.

Endotoxins are chemicals contained within the cell wall of bacteria. When the bacterial cell ruptures, endotoxins are released into the bloodstream and spread to different organ systems. The toxic effects of these substances include fever, diarrhea, shock, extreme weakness, and sometimes death.

Exotoxins are proteins produced as a result of bacterial metabolism. Exotoxins break down surrounding tissue, which allows the pathogen to spread and colonize freely. Exotoxins enter specific body cells and disrupt the cell's chemical and physical structure. For example, *Clostridium botulinum* produces a highly concentrated toxin that damages the nerve-muscle mechanism and causes paralysis in the host. Exotoxins released by bacteria and other microbes are listed in Table 9-1.

Important Bacterial Pathogens

GRAM-POSITIVE COCCI Gram-positive cocci are responsible for about one third of all bacterial infections in humans. Many are responsible for surgical site infections. They produce pus, and some are resistant to antibiotic therapy.

The streptococci are further classified by their ability to reduce the levels of iron in hemoglobin through hemolysis. Two groups of hemolytic streptococci are the *alpha-hemolytic* streptococci and the *beta-hemolytic* streptococci.

STAPHYLOCOCCUS AUREUS *Staphylococcus aureus* is the most widespread cause of surgical site infections. It normally resides in healthy skin, but when transmitted to the surgical wound by direct or indirect contact, it can cause an infection. From 30% to 70% of people are skin carriers of *S. aureus*. When confined to the surgical wound itself, it produces copious amounts of pus, which spreads and erodes tissues. The organism also causes endocarditis (infection of the lining of the heart) when it colonizes heart valves. Invasion of the bone causes osteomyelitis.

STAPHYLOCOCCUS EPIDERMIDIS *Staphylococcus epidermidis* is a normal resident of the skin. However, it can cause infection

Table **9-1** Bacterial Toxins and Diseases

Bacteria	Exotoxin	Tissue Damaged	Mechanism	Disease
Clostridium tetani	Tetanospasmin	Neurons	Spastic paralysis	Tetanus
Clostridium perfringens	Alpha toxin	Erythrocytes, platelets, leukocytes, endothelium	Cell lysis	Gas gangrene
Clostridium botulinum	Neurotoxin	Nerve-muscle junction	Flaccid paralysis	Botulism
Corynebacterium diphtheriae	Diphtheria toxin	Throat, heart, peripheral nerve	Inhibits protein synthesis	Diphtheria
Shigella dysenteriae	Enterotoxin	Intestinal mucosa	Fluid loss from intestinal cells	Dysentery
Escherichia coli	Enterotoxin	Intestinal epithelium	Fluid loss from intestinal cells	Gastroenteritis
Vibrio cholerae	Enterotoxin	Intestinal epithelium	Fluid loss from intestinal cells	Cholera
Staphylococcus aureus	Alpha toxin	Red and white cells (via cytokines)	Hemolysis	Abscesses
	Hemolysin	Red and white cells (via cytokines)	Hemolysis	Abscesses
	Leukocidin	Leukocytes	Destroys leukocytes	Abscesses
	Enterotoxin	Intestinal cells	Induces vomiting, diarrhea	Food poisoning
	TSST1	—	Release of cytotoxins	Toxic shock syndrome
	Epidermolytic	Epidermis	Cell lysis	Scalded skin syndrome
Streptococcus pyogenes	Streptolysin O and S	Red and white cells	Hemolysis	Hemolysis, pyogenic lesion
	Erythrogenic	Skin capillaries	Inflammation	Scarlet fever
Bacillus anthracis	Cytotoxin	Lung	Pulmonary edema	Anthrax
Bordetella pertussis	Pertussis toxin	Trachea	Destruction of epithelium	Whooping cough
Legionella pneumophila	Numerous	Neutrophils	Cell lysis	Legionnaire's disease
Listeria monocytogenes	Hemolysin	Leukocytes, monocytes	Cell lysis	Listeriosis
Pseudomonas aeruginosa	Exotoxin A	Cell lysis	Cell lysis	Various infections

in other parts of the body when spread by medical devices such as catheters, prosthetic valves, and orthopedic implants.

STREPTOCOCCUS PYOGENES Many HAIs are caused by *Streptococcus pyogenes* (a group A beta-hemolytic streptococcus). This potentially lethal pathogen causes surgical site infection; it spreads via the lymphatic system to other sites in the body, causing anaerobic infection and tissue death. Burn patients are particularly vulnerable to streptococcal infection. Surgical site infection is most commonly caused by **direct transmission** from a contaminated surface.

STREPTOCOCCUS PNEUMONIAE *Streptococcus pneumoniae* is the primary cause of pneumonia and otitis media (middle ear infection). The pathogen is spread mainly through the respiratory tract. It colonizes the nose and nasopharynx and then spreads to the lungs and middle ear. The bacteria are coated with a thick capsule and cell wall, which prevent its destruction by the body's white blood cells. Because of this resistance mechanism, respiratory disease caused by *S. pneumoniae* can be fatal in children and older adults.

Gram-Negative Rods and Cocci (Aerobic)

PSEUDOMONAS AERUGINOSA *Pseudomonas aeruginosa* is found in the normal gastrointestinal tract and in sewage, dirt, and water. It has emerged as an increasingly important pathogen in hospitalized patients. It can infect nearly all body systems. *P. aeruginosa* infection is especially prevalent in burn patients who lack healthy skin as a barrier against airborne bacteria. *P. aeruginosa* can cause septicemia (systemic vascular infection), osteomyelitis, urinary tract infection, and endocarditis. It is highly resistant to antimicrobial agents.

NEISSERIA GONORRHOEAE Gonorrhea is a sexually transmitted disease spread from person to person by direct contact with *Neisseria gonorrhoeae*. The infection usually remains localized in the reproductive tract but may become systemic. The bacteria can cause blindness in the newborn of an infected mother; however, this can be prevented by instilling antibiotic drops into the newborn's eyes. If the disease is not treated, it may lead to sterility and endocarditis.

NEISSERIA MENINGITIDES Bacterial meningitis is a highly contagious infection of the meninges that cover the brain and spinal cord. Two forms of the disease are caused by *Neisseria meningitidis*, one that is transient and resolves spontaneously and a more serious form that can result in seizures, respiratory arrest, and coma.

BORDETELLA PERTUSSIS *Bordetella pertussis* is a bacterium that causes whooping cough, a life-threatening disease in children. Vaccination against *B. pertussis* has reduced the mortality rate significantly. Before the vaccine was developed, whooping cough was a major killer of children.

ENTERIC BACTERIA The enteric bacteria are also gram-negative rods; however, they are facultative anaerobes and can grow in an oxygen-poor environment. This group of pathogens inhabits the intestinal tracts of humans both in a disease state and as resident (normal) bacteria.

ESCHERICHIA COLI *E. coli* organisms are resident bacteria of the gastrointestinal tract. Postoperative infection caused by this bacterium occurs when the organisms are transmitted via a contaminated object such as an endoscope or catheter. Direct transmission occurs when the gastrointestinal tract is perforated and bowel contents spill into the sterile peritoneal cavity. *E. coli* is the most common cause of urinary tract infections. In the bloodstream, *E. coli* can spread to other organs and cause severe tissue destruction or death.

SALMONELLA ENTERICA *Salmonella enterica* is a common cause of food poisoning (acute gastroenteritis). The bacterial infection is spread from person to person by contaminated food and fecal contact. The disease causes diarrhea, vomiting, and fever, which usually resolve without treatment.

SALMONELLA TYPHI As mentioned previously, the bacteria *S. typhi* causes the disease typhoid. The infection is spread via contaminated water and food. In communities where sewage treatment is lacking, the bacteria can contaminate local drinking water and cause widespread infection. Bacterial colonies can persist in the intestine long after antibiotic treatment, and a disease carrier may continue to infect others while showing no symptoms.

When ingested, the bacteria penetrate the intestinal wall and enter the mesenteric lymph nodes. They release a powerful endotoxin that enters the bloodstream and causes septicemia, cardiovascular infection, and death. Several types of typhoid vaccine are available, but the vaccine usually is given only to individuals at risk, such as those traveling or working in an area where sanitation is poor.

Spore-Forming Bacteria

The spore-forming bacteria are significant because of their ability to resist destruction. They are extremely important in the health care setting. In the perioperative environment, any process of sterilization is defined by its ability to destroy not only all microbes but also bacterial spores.

CLOSTRIDIUM PERFRINGENS *Clostridium perfringens* is an anaerobic bacterium that causes rapid tissue death in deep wounds deprived of oxygen. This is a relatively rare infection, but it does occur in health care settings. Historically, it has been a common infection of deep, penetrating combat wounds. In true gas gangrene, the tissue is destroyed by the toxins of the *C. perfringens* bacilli. *Clostridium novyi* bacilli, another type of clostridia, invade the necrotic tissue and release toxic gases. Systemic absorption of these gases is fatal. The disease is transmitted directly from a contaminated source to an open or penetrating wound.

CLOSTRIDIUM TETANI *Clostridium tetani* is the causative bacteria of tetanus, a disease of the nervous system. *C. tetani* bacterium is an anaerobic organism commonly found in soil and intestinal tracts of humans and other mammals. The toxins released by the bacilli travel along the peripheral nerve pathways, eventually reaching the central nervous system. Severe muscle spasms, convulsions, and eventual paralysis of the respiratory system lead to death from asphyxia. Transmission is through direct contact with the bacilli, usually through an open or penetrating wound.

CLOSTRIDIUM DIFFICILE *Clostridium difficile* is a spore-forming bacterium that causes severe diarrhea. It is easily spread among patients who are immunocompromised, and the infection can be rapidly fatal. Strict attention to asepsis, especially hand washing, is needed to control its spread in the health care setting.

Mycobacterial Infections

As mentioned previously, the bacillus *Mycobacterium tuberculosis* causes the disease tuberculosis (TB). The human strain of the bacterium causes dense nodules or tubercles to form in localized areas of the body, including the lungs, liver, spleen, and bone marrow.

Tuberculosis is a serious concern in areas where people live or work in crowded conditions. Multidrug-resistant strains of *M. tuberculosis* are increasingly common throughout the world. TB kills about 3 million people and infects about 9 million every year worldwide. The organism primarily causes respiratory disease, but it also can infect other areas of the body, including vital organs. The infection is spread by inhalation of the bacteria in droplets or dust containing dried mycobacteria. The infection can be introduced into the body via medical equipment such as respiratory, diagnostic, or anesthesia equipment.

After the bacteria have entered the respiratory system, they are engulfed by white blood cell components. The mycobacteria that are not destroyed by the body become encased in granular "tubercles," which remain in the lungs. These become calcified and fibrotic. If the infected person's immune system becomes weakened, the bacteria can again become proliferative.

RICKETTSIAE Rickettsiae are a type of bacteria carried by specific species of ticks, mites, and fleas. The insect transmits the bacteria to its host through a skin bite. Once the bacteria enter the host's body, they move through the bloodstream and attach to the inner lining of the blood vessels (endothelium). The cell then ingests the bacteria, which continue to multiply and enter other host cells. Rickettsiae are identified by staining, using the same techniques as those for bacteria in general.

Diseases caused by rickettsiae include typhus, Q fever, and Rocky Mountain spotted fever. Rickettsial disease can persist in the body for long periods. Prevention of disease involves avoiding exposure to ticks, fleas, and mites that carry the bacteria.

Important bacterial diseases are listed in Table 9-2.

Multidrug-Resistant Pathogenic Bacteria

Certain strains of bacterial pathogens have evolved to be partly or completely resistant to the most powerful antimicrobial agents available. Certain strains of bacteria are of grave concern, because they are easily transmitted, colonize rapidly, and can be lethal. The symptoms of these infections are the same as with the original nonresistant strains. However, treatment becomes problematic, because resistance leads to spread of the infection and severe debilitation and/or death.

Treatment with antimicrobial agents destroys some pathogens, but the more resistant microbes survive and are

Table 9-2 Important Bacterial Infections

Gram-Positive Cocci

Organism	Major Infection	Less Common Infection	Vaccine Preventable
Staphylococci			
S. epidermidis	Bacteremia in immunocompromised individuals	Most often associated with indwelling devices	No
S. saprophyticus	Urinary tract infections	—	No
S. aureus	Boils, impetigo, wound infections, osteomyelitis, septicemia	Pneumonia, endocarditis, toxic shock syndrome, food poisoning	No
Streptococci			
Beta-Hemolytic			
S. pyogenes (group A)	Tonsillitis, impetigo, cellulitis, scarlet fever (rheumatic fever, glomerulonephritis)	Puerperal sepsis, erysipelas, septicemia	No
Alpha-Hemolytic			
S. pneumoniae	Pneumonia, otitis media	Meningitis, septicemia	Yes (some serotypes)
S. viridans	Dental caries	Subacute bacterial endocarditis	No
Group D Streptococci			
S. faecalis (enterococci) (Enterococcus faecalis)	Urinary tract infections, wound infections, intra-abdominal abscess	Bacteremia, endocarditis	No

Gram-Negative Cocci and Coccobacilli

Organism	Major Infection	Less Common Infection	Vaccine Preventable
Neisseria			
N. meningitidis	Meningitis, septicemia	Arthritis	Yes (serogroups A/C)
N. gonorrhoeae	Gonorrhea, pelvic inflammatory disease	Arthritis, conjunctivitis	No

Aerobic Gram-Positive Bacilli

Organism	Major Infection	Less Common Infection	Vaccine Preventable
Spore-Forming			
Bacillus			
B. anthracis	Anthrax	—	Yes
Non–Spore-Forming			
Listeria			
L. monocytogenes	Neonatal sepsis, meningitis	Septicemia in immunocompromised individuals	No
Corynebacterium			
C. diphtheriae	Diphtheria	Skin infections	Yes
C. urealyticum	Cystitis	—	No
C. jeikeium	Infection associated with prosthetic devices and intravenous or cerebrospinal fluid (CSF) catheters		No

Modified from Hart T, Shears P: *Color atlas of medical microbiology*, London, 2000, Mosby.

transmitted to other hosts. The resistance is passed to succeeding generations of microbes through simple replication or via plasmid exchange, which carries the genes of the resistant strain to other microbes. Resistance occurs when the antibiotic used only partly destroys the pathogen or when antibiotic treatment is stopped before the microbes are destroyed.

Natural selection of resistant strains has been hastened by a combination of microbe strength and the indiscriminate and improper use of antibiotics. *Antibiotic-resistant* bacterial infection is a primary focus of public and clinical health researchers. Unfortunately, as new and more powerful drugs are developed, resistant strains also develop. The incidence of multidrug-resistant organisms (MDROs) in the United States has increased steadily in the past few decades.

Strict isolation protocols are used for patients with an MDRO. The surgical technologist must be knowledgeable about these protocols, which are established by the health institution in which the technologist works. In addition to following all protocols, all health care workers must carefully practice hand washing procedures. These are discussed in detail in the next chapter.

METHICILLIN-RESISTANT STAPHYLOCOCCUS AUREUS AND EPIDERMIS Methicillin-resistant *Staphylococcus aureus* (MRSA) is a virulent form of *Staphylococcus* that is transmitted mainly by direct contact with the hands, equipment, and supplies. Health care workers who carry the bacteria in their respiratory systems may become carriers of the disease. They do not become ill but can transmit the pathogens to others in their environment. MRSA can occur in surgical incisions, in burns, and on urinary catheters, chest tubes, and other common devices used in the health care setting.

Recently MRSA has been discovered in the community, outside the health care setting. The infection can be fatal and is particularly serious in debilitated patients. Vancomycin traditionally has been used to treat MRSA. However, a new strain has developed—vancomycin-resistant *Staphylococcus aureus*. Methicillin-resistant *staphylococcus epidermis* is another MDRO found in the clinical setting and implicated as a source of wound infection.

VANCOMYCIN-RESISTANT AND VANCOMYCIN-INTERMEDIATE RESISTANT STAPHYLOCOCCUS AUREUS Infection with vancomycin-resistant *S. aureus* (VRSA) was first diagnosed in the United States in 1997. Since then, the incidence of the infection has increased steadily, and a new strain has also emerged, vancomycin-intermediate resistant *S. aureus* (VISA). These strains can be treated with other antibiotics. However, the infection can be fatal in severely debilitated patients.

VANCOMYCIN-RESISTANT ENTEROCOCCI Vancomycin-resistant enterococci (VRE) infection is transmitted by direct contact or through intermediate sources, including furniture, equipment, and the hands of health care workers. Enterococci inhabit the intestine and female genital tracts of healthy individuals. However, patients previously treated with vancomycin, surgical patients, and those who are debilitated or have a suppressed immune system are at particular risk for VRE

infection. The bacteria are transmitted through contact with stool, urine, or blood and by the hands of health care workers. The bacteria cause urinary tract infection, septicemia (blood infection), and wound infection.

MULTIDRUG-RESISTANT TUBERCULOSIS Multidrug-resistant tuberculosis (MDR TB) has emerged in the past few decades as a serious public health risk worldwide, including in the United States. It also is a risk for all health care workers. Transmission is the same as for nonresistant TB. However, MDR TB continues to increase in virulence and is fatal without treatment. A newer strain, called extensively drug-resistant TB (XDR TB), is rare but has a greater risk of mortality. This strain is resistant to both the first- and second-line drugs normally used to treat TB. All strains of TB are transmitted by airborne particles and droplets, direct contact with inanimate objects, and direct contact with an infected individual.

MISCELLANEOUS BACTERIAL PATHOGENS
Haemophilus influenza—Meningitis
Klebsiella pneumonia—Pneumonia
Porphyromonas gngivalis—Peridontal disease and intestinal infection
Streptococcus mutans—Dental caries
Moraxella catarrhalis—upper respiratory infection
Acinobacter—wound and systemic infection especially in immunocompromised patients
Treponema palladium—syphilis
Streptococcus agalactiae—one of the group B stretococcal bacteria found normally in the vagina but may infect the newborn during birth.
Mycobacterium leprae—leprosy
Chlamydia trachomatis—genital and reproductive system infection
Gardnerella vaginalis—genital infection
Mycoplasma hominis—may be related to pelvic infection
Proteus miribalis—urinary tract infection
Bartonella—opportunistic bacterial infection

VIRUSES

A **virus** is a nonliving infectious agent that ranges in size from 10 to 300 nm. A virus is not a cell. It is referred to as a virus particle. A complete virus particle is called a **virion**. These agents cause some of the most lethal infections known. Although they can be extremely pathogenic, they are unable to metabolize outside the host cell. While inside the host's cells, they are unable to infect another individual. Viruses are transmitted by inhalation, in food or water, and by direct transmission from an infected host via blood or body fluids. Some viruses may also be transmitted by insects. Viruses are found throughout the living environment and cause disease in many different organisms.

Classification

Viruses are classified by a number of complex systems and categories, such as by morphology (shape and structure), chemical composition, and method of replication.

Morphology

A virion consists of a double or single strand of either DNA or RNA. This genetic material is surrounded by a protein coating (capsid). The total structure is called a *nucleocapsid*. Depending on the type of virus, the nucleocapsid can take on many different complex geometric shapes. Some virions are enclosed in a membrane, or envelope, derived from the host cell (Figure 9-13). A virion has no organelles.

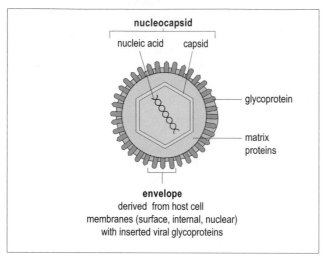

Figure 9-13   Construction of the virus, showing the envelope and nucleocapsid. *(From Goering R, Dockrell H, Wakelin D et al: Mim's medical microbiology, ed 4, St Louis, 2008, Mosby.)*

Replication and Transmission

Although viruses contain genetic material, they cannot replicate without a host cell. To replicate, they inject their DNA or RNA into another cell and dissolve its genetic material. The virus uses the host cell's physiological mechanisms to replicate its own genetic material. The virus then synthesizes new capsids, assembles new virions, and ruptures the cell to release them. The cycle of replication and lysis (bursting) of the host cell is called *lysogenesis*.

Some types of viruses remain inside the host cell in latent form. In this state the virus is not infective, but it continues to replicate. Under certain favorable conditions, the virus begins to replicate more actively and produces disease symptoms, perhaps years later. Examples of viruses that follow this cycle are the herpes simplex virus and the poliovirus.

A virus that invades bacterial cells is called a *bacteriophage* (Figure 9-14). Bacteriophages are widely dispersed throughout living organisms and may display a parasitic, commensal, or symbiotic relationship with their bacterial host. Bacteriophages can replicate and spread or remain inside the bacterial cell. Bacteriophages are currently being tested for use in medicine and food production as a way to destroy harmful bacteria.

Viruses are also capable of transforming normal cells into cancerous cells, which lose their original functional and metabolic characteristics through genetic changes. These cells divide rapidly and develop into tumor tissue. Specific cancer-inducing viruses include the hepatitis A virus and certain types of the human papilloma virus.

Figure 9-14   Life cycle of the viral bacteriophage. The bacteriophage is a bacterial virus that can survive outside or inside the bacterium and reproduce using the bacterial cell. *(From Goering R, Dockrell H, Wakelin D et al: Mim's medical microbiology, ed 4, St Louis, 2008, Mosby.)*

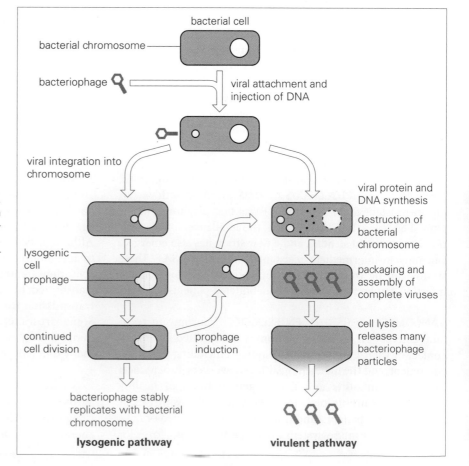

Pathogenicity

Pathogenicity is defined less clearly in viruses than in bacteria. We know some of the mechanisms that create and sustain viral disease in certain strains. These include the following:

- *Ability to enter a healthy cell:* The virus enters the host cell by attaching to its membrane or wall, where it is absorbed by phagocytosis.
- *Ability to develop:* The virus is able to redirect the cell's genetic material to viral replication rather than cell reproduction.
- *Ability to resist the host's defense mechanisms:* The virus may be recognized by the body's immune system, which attacks its own cell, killing it.
- *Cell transformation:* The virus's ability to mutate the cell can result in the formation of cancer growth in some cells.
- *Ability to synthesize substances not normally produced by the host cell.*
- *Ability to initiate structural changes in the host cell:* These changes lead to cell death or to abnormalities that alter the cell's functions.

Pathogenic Viruses

HUMAN IMMUNODEFICIENCY VIRUS/ACQUIRED IMMUNODEFICIENCY SYNDROME Infection with HIV is pandemic (a worldwide epidemic). Approximately 33.4 million cases of HIV have been reported worldwide.[1] The global effect of AIDS has changed practices and procedures in health care dramatically.

HIV is transmitted via blood-to-blood contact, sexual contact, and contact with certain body fluids. The body fluids known to transmit HIV are:

- Blood
- Semen
- Vaginal secretions
- Breast milk
- Cerebrospinal fluid
- Synovial fluid
- Amniotic fluid
- Any body fluid containing blood

HIV may be transmitted when the body fluids of an infected person are deposited on the mucous membranes or into the vascular system of another person. Sexual contact and use of contaminated needles are primary modes of transmission in the general public. The risk of transmission during sexual contact increases when partners also are infected with another sexually transmitted disease. HIV can be transmitted to the fetus in utero and to the infant who receives breast milk from an infected mother. A neonate also may be infected during delivery.

Casual contact with an infected person does not transmit the virus. Although HIV has been found in saliva, tears, and sweat, the number of pathogens found in these body fluids has been very small. Contact with these fluids has not been shown to result in the transmission of HIV. Occupational risk to health care workers is highest in needlestick and other sharps injuries. There is little evidence of a risk of transmission from an infected health care worker to a patient.

A person infected with HIV may show no symptoms yet still transmit the disease to others. This is because early in the disease process, the body's immune system is able to attack the virus. As long as such individuals are not tested, they may continue to transmit the disease to others without realizing that they are infected. Weeks after the initial infection, mild illness occurs, followed by increasingly serious disease manifestations. Years may pass before symptoms of AIDS begin to appear. The conversion from HIV infection to AIDS-related complex to AIDS is poorly understood. HIV infection is confirmed by the presence of specific antibodies.

AIDS is not a separate disease organism but a syndrome that results from infection with the HIV virus. Patients with AIDS lack normal immune response, and certain diseases are common in these individuals. A true diagnosis of AIDS is made when the presence of one or more of these diseases is confirmed (Box 9-3). Currently, AIDS has no cure. However, the disease now can be controlled with drug therapy.

Extensive information about AIDS and its treatment can be found on websites for the CDC and the United Nations Committee on HIV/AIDS.[1]

Box 9-3 Opportunistic Infections and Tumors in Acquired Immunodeficiency Syndrome (AIDS)

Viruses
Disseminated cytomegalovirus (lungs, retina, brain)
Herpes simplex virus (HSV-1 and HSV-2) (lungs, gastrointestinal tract, central nervous system [CNS], skin)
JC papovavirus (brain: progressive multifocal leukoencephalopathy)
Epstein-Barr virus (EBV)

Bacteria*
Mycobacteria (e.g., *Mycoplasma avium*, *Mycobacterium tuberculosis*: disseminated, extrapulmonary)
Salmonella (recurrent, disseminated; septicemia)

Protozoa
Toxoplasma gondii (disseminated, including the CNS)
Cryptosporidium (gastrointestinal tract: chronic diarrhea)
Isospora (gastrointestinal tract: diarrhea persisting longer than 1 month)

Fungi
Pneumocystis jiroveci (lungs: pneumonia)
Candida albicans (esophagus, lung)
Cryptococcus neoformans (CNS)
Histoplasma capsulatum (disseminated, extrapulmonary)
Coccidioides (disseminated, extrapulmonary)

Tumors
Kaposi sarcoma[†]
B cell lymphoma (e.g., brain; some are EBV induced)

Other
Human immunodeficiency virus (HIV) encephalopathy (AIDS dementia complex)

Data from Goering R, Dockrell H, Zuckerman M, et al: *Mims' medical microbiology*, ed 2, London, 1998, Mosby.

*Also pyogenic bacteria (e.g., *Haemophilus*, *Streptococcus*, *Pneumococcus* spp.), which cause septicemia, pneumonia, meningitis, osteomyelitis, arthritis, abscesses, and other diseases; multiple or recurrent infections, especially in children.

[†]Associated with human herpes virus 8, an independently transmitted agent; 300 times more common in AIDS than in other immunodeficiency conditions.

VIRAL HEPATITIS Viral hepatitis is a disease of the liver that is caused by one of five significant viruses. The hepatitis B, C, and D viruses are blood-borne pathogens, which are transmitted when blood from an infected person enters the body of another person (a transmission similar to that for HIV). Hepatitis A and hepatitis E are transmitted through contaminated food or water.

The hepatitis A virus (HAV) is transmitted by ingestion and by close contact with an infected person. Fecal and oral routes are the common modes of transmission. This virus cannot be cultured, but hepatitis can be diagnosed through a serological test that shows the presence of antibodies to HAV. Hepatitis A is rarely fatal, and one infection results in permanent immunity to the disease.

Infection with the hepatitis B virus (HBV) causes chronic hepatitis, cirrhosis, massive liver necrosis, and death. Like HIV, HBV is transmitted through blood and body fluids. The virus is 100 more times infective than HIV. It can be spread through sexual contact and is found in most body secretions. Infected mothers also pass it to infants in 70% to 90% of births. Infected infants have a 90% chance of becoming chronic (long-term) carriers.

The incubation period of HBV is 10 to 12 weeks, during which time the virus can be detected through serological testing. The disease causes general weakness, arthralgia, myalgia, and severe anorexia. Fever and upper abdominal pain also may be present. Some patients develop cirrhosis and liver cancer as a complication of the disease. There is no cure for the disease, so only the symptoms are treated. However, a safe, effective vaccine is available, and all health care workers and those coming in contact with blood products or body fluids should be vaccinated.

Hepatitis C virus (HCV) is transmitted by blood transfusions and blood products. The virus also is found in saliva, urine, and semen. Health care workers, those who receive blood transfusions, intravenous drug abusers, organ transplant recipients, and hemodialysis patients are at high risk for the disease. The symptoms are similar to but milder than those of hepatitis B. About 50% of patients develop chronic hepatitis and cirrhosis and may require liver transplantation. The highest rates of infection are found in transfusion recipients and intravenous drug abusers. HCV is a causal agent of liver cancer.

Hepatitis D virus (HDV) is associated with HBV as a coinfection. It is a blood-borne virus that is acquired as a secondary infection with HBV or as a result of HBV. When the two infections occur together, they result in more rapid liver destruction and more severe clinical manifestations than HBV alone.

Hepatitis E is caused by the hepatitis E virus. It causes serious acute liver disease and is transmitted by contaminated water. The disease is does not develop into chronic form.

HUMAN PAPILLOMA VIRUS The human papilloma virus (HPV) is a potentially cancer-producing virus that occurs in about 15% of the population. Approximately 40 types of HPV exist, although only a few of them are oncogenic. The virus is found throughout the animal population but is species specific. It is transmitted through sexual contact and therefore is a significant public health concern. Both men and women can be affected. Chronic HPV infection may develop into cervical cancer in women and noninvasive penile and anal cancer in men. The virus types are divided into two groups: high risk and low risk (for cancer association). Some of the low risk types cause genital warts (condylomata), which can be removed. However, the virus may persist in the body after removal of the lesions.

HPV may cause no symptoms and can lie dormant for many years. Predictors for HPV in women include:

- Women younger than 25 years of age
- Multiple sex partners
- Early onset of sexual activity (younger than 16 years old)
- Male partner with a history of multiple partners

Predictors in men include multiple partners. Disease rates are higher in the males having sex with males (MSM) population.

A vaccine for HPV is available for girls and young women. No evidence supports the effectiveness of the vaccine for men. A routine Papanicolaou (Pap) test is one of the best methods of detecting cervical cancer in women. The Pap test detects changes in the cervical endothelium caused by the HPV virus.

MISCELLANEOUS PATHOGENIC VIRUSES This group of viruses and the diseases they cause are of public health concern but not necessarily related to surgery.

Rubella

Varicella zoster—chicken pox

Variola—German measles

Morbillivirus—measles

Entervirus—polio

Lyssavirus—rabies

Information on HPV from the CDC can be found at http://www.cdc.gov/STD/Hpv/hpv-clinicians-brochure.htm.

PRIONS

The **prion** (a proteinaceous infectious particle) is a unique pathogenic substance. It is a protein particle that contains no nucleic acid. It is believed to be a modified form of normal cellular protein that arises through mutation. It then is transmitted by ingestion or direct contact, especially during medical or surgical procedures. Prions are resistant to all forms of disinfection and sterilization normally used in the medical setting. They cannot be cultured in the laboratory, and the immune system does not react to them. Only a few prion diseases affect human beings. The most important is Creutzfeldt-Jakob disease (CJD) and the newly emergent variant of CJD.

CJD is a rare transmissible disease of the nervous system that is progressive and always fatal. The disease may have an incubation period of up to 20 years. Although CJD is not contagious, it is transmissible. The mechanism of transmission currently is unknown. CJD represents a threat in the health care setting because it is known to be transmitted by contaminated electrodes during neurosurgical stereotactic surgery, corneal grafts, and direct contact with neurosurgical instruments that have been used on patients with CJD. For these reasons, current infection control standards require the use of disposable instruments for these types of surgical procedures or specialized decontamination procedures. Protocols for CJD have been established to help prevent transmission.

FUNGI

Fungi are found worldwide on living organic substances, in water, and in soil. More than 70,000 species of fungi exist, but only 300 are pathogenic. They are composed of eukaryotes classified into two groups, molds and yeasts.

Characteristics

Yeasts are unicellular, and molds are multicellular. Like the bacterial endospore, fungal spores are resistant to heat, cold, and drying. They have a cell wall and obtain their nutrients through absorption. Fungi are distinct from plants and animals. They occur as a single cell or as filaments called hyphae. These occur as a complex mass called a mycelium. The mycelium is divided into compartments, each containing a nucleus. Many fungi are visible without a microscope, and colonies may be grown in the laboratory for identification and drug sensitivity testing.

Identification

Fungi can be identified in the laboratory by direct observation of their form after culture. A specimen of the fungus is allowed to grow in a suitable medium and then observed for the shape, pattern, and color of the fungal colony. Further testing can be done by staining the cells and observing them under the microscope.

Reproduction

Fungi are capable of sexual or asexual reproduction, depending on the species and environment. Sexual reproduction takes place in the mycelium, which contains the sex cells needed for meiosis (reproductive cell division). Spores are released through sexual reproduction, and these may go on to produce a new colony. Fragmentation of the mycelium may also initiate the growth of a new colony.

Transmission to Humans

Fungal diseases occur as superficial or deep mycoses. Superficial fungi, which affect the skin, hair, nails, mouth, and vagina, are transmitted by direct contact with the source and cause mild disease symptoms. The yeast *Candida albicans* normally is established in the oral cavity of the newborn and persists as a commensal organism throughout life. At times of immune stress or disease, oral *Candida* can proliferate. Deep fungi enter the body through the respiratory tract or through breaks in the skin or mucous membranes. Medical devices, such as catheters and intravenous cannulas, also can infect a healthy individual. In the health care setting, fungi can survive in the heating and cooling ducts of the ventilation system, releasing spores into the environment from which patients and workers can become infected.

Pathogenicity

Deep or disseminated fungal infections can be fatal. Patients who are immunosuppressed or who are weakened by metabolic disorders, infectious diseases, or trauma are at high risk for serious *mycotic* (fungal) disease. Healthy individuals are rarely infected with deep mycosis. Pathogenic fungi are described in Table 9-3.

Pathogenic Fungi

ASPERGILLUS FUMIGATUS *Aspergillus fumigatus* is a significant fungal pathogen. It is an opportunistic infection in immunosuppressed patients. This fungus invades the body through the lungs and blood vessels and can cause vascular thrombosis and partial blockage of the airways. In a severely compromised patient, invasive *Aspergillus* infection often is fatal.

CANDIDA ALBICANS *Candida albicans* is a common cause of opportunistic infection. It is a normal resident of the mouth, vagina, and intestine. However, it can proliferate in individuals who are immunosuppressed or weakened by disease and in patients taking antibiotics. When localized in the oral cavity or vagina, the infection usually can be treated successfully with antifungal drugs. Systemic or disseminated infection can spread to any location in the body, including the heart, kidneys, and other vital organs.

Table 9-3 Medically Important Fungal Infections			
Type of Fungus	**Location**	**Disease**	**Causative Organism**
Superficial	Keratin layer of skin, hair shaft	Tinea nigra, pityriasis versicolor	*Trichosporon Malassezia Eosinophilia*
Cutaneous	Epidermis, hair, nails	Tinea (ringworm)	*Microsporum Trichophyton Epidermophyton*
Systemic	Internal organs	Coccidiomycosis	*Cryptococcus*
		Histoplasmosis	*Candida*
		Blastomycosis	*Aspergillus*
		Paracoccidioidomycosis	*Pneumocystis*

Modified from Goering R, Dockrell H, Zuckerman M, et al: *Mim's medical microbiology*, ed 4, St Louis, 2008, Mosby.

PNEUMOCYSTIS JIROVECI Infection with *Pneumocystis jiroveci* (formerly known as *Pneumocystis carinii*) is widespread in the general population but usually produces only mild symptoms. *Pneumocystis* pneumonia (PCP) is a common respiratory disease among patients with AIDS. Patients who are immunosuppressed, including those receiving immunosuppressive drugs for organ transplantation, are at high risk for the disease. The infection is difficult to diagnose because the symptoms are nonspecific and the fungus cannot be isolated from the patient's sputum through normal methods.

CUTANEOUS MYCOSES Superficial fungal infections invade the superficial layers of the skin. The filaments of the fungus spread into dead (keratinized) skin, hair, and nails. These cause irritation and oozing and may encourage the development of a superficial bacterial infection.

PROTOZOA

Characteristics

Protozoa are a group of single-celled eukaryotic organisms. Protozoa are free-living in a variety of freshwater and marine habitats. Approximately 65,000 different species have been identified (compared to 4,500 species of bacteria). A large number of protozoa are parasitic in animals, including human beings. Most have complex life cycles with intermediate hosts that facilitate their transmission and reproduction. Single-celled protozoa reproduce by binary fission. They can infect any tissue or organ of the body. The organisms usually enter through an insect bite or by ingestion. Once in the body, they selectively reproduce in particular anatomical structures, such as the intestine, skin, blood, liver, or central nervous system. Protozoa feed on a wide variety of substances in the environment, including algae and bacteria. These are absorbed through the cell membrane.

The structure of protozoa varies widely by species, which allows identification by microscopic examination. Most protozoa have a well-defined shape and cell membrane, or envelope. They range in size from 1 to 300 micrometers. Many have an outer layer, called an *ectoplasm,* which contains the organelles used for feeding, locomotion, and defense. The cytoplasm contains organelles usually found in eukaryotic cells (described previously).

Mobility

Protozoa move through their watery environment by a variety of mechanisms. These are used to classify the protozoa. *Ciliates* are protozoa that move by multiple projections (cilia), which extend as hairlike fibers around the periphery of the ectoplasm. The cilia move in waves, providing locomotion. *Flagellates* have a single flagellum ("tail") or multiple flagella, which propel them in different directions. *Amoebae* move by using a pseudopod (false foot), which extends and pulls the cell along. Amoebae are attracted or repelled by concentration gradients in their environment, and they feed by absorption through the pseudopod.

Pathogenicity

Protozoa cause a wide variety of diseases in animals and human beings. These diseases often are characterized by destruction of the host cells by ingestion. Protozoa are able to resist or avoid many of the body's defenses by changing the antigens on their surface or by ingesting the immune complement of the cell, thereby disabling it. Widespread cell destruction results in the disease characteristics of different protozoal species and of the tissue they invade.

Gastrointestinal disease is characterized by simple diarrhea or dysentery. Protozoa feed on the mucosa and red blood cells of the host. This can result in severe dehydration, anemia, perforation of the intestine, and proliferation in other organs.

Protozoal diseases of the central nervous system (CNS) can result in severe destruction of nerve cell tissue or blood vessels. This leads to encephalitis and death. Malaria is the most significant protozoal disease of the CNS and a major killer of children in Africa and Asia. Protozoa that infect blood and organs destroy blood cells and tissue, including the liver, kidneys, heart, and lymph system. Important pathogenic protozoa are described in Table 9-4.

ALGAE

Algae are eukaryotes that belong to the plant kingdom; they include sponges and seaweed. They are classified as microbes but have no pathogenic effect on human beings. Structurally they vary widely, from single-celled organisms to colonies and large plants that can reach several hundred feet in length. They occur in freshwater and saltwater sources globally. Widespread commercial harvesting of algae for food products, manufacturing, and agriculture threatens these species, which are important in the food chain and in the ecology of wetlands and water-borne animals.

IMMUNITY

The immune system defends the body against harmful substances, including disease microorganisms. *Immunity* is the body's ability to accept substances that are part of the body ("self") and eliminate those that are not ("nonself"). The study of immunity and the immune system often is difficult, because it involves many terms and complex concepts.

The body has two general types of immunity, innate and adaptive:

- *Innate immunity* (also called *nonspecific immunity*) exists from the time of birth. This type of protection is not targeted at a specific substance but occurs as a physiological reaction whenever an injury occurs or foreign substances are present in the body.
- *Adaptive immunity* is conferred through exposure to a specific substance or microbe called an *antigen*. When exposure occurs, the immune system develops *antibodies,* which are specific proteins that can stay in the system and trigger it to launch its defenses during subsequent exposure to the microbe or substance

Table **9-4** Important Protozoal Parasites			
Anatomical Location	**Species**	**Disease**	**Method of Transmission**
Intestine	*Entamoeba histolytica*	Amebiasis	Ingestion of parasite cysts in water or food
	Giardia intestinalis	Giardiasis	
	Cryptosporidium spp.	Cryptosporidiosis	
	Microsporidia	Microsporidiosis	
Urogenital tract	*Trichomonas vaginalis*	Trichomoniasis	Sexual contact
Blood and tissue	*Trypanosoma* spp.	Trypanosomiasis Sleeping sickness Chagas' disease	Reduviid bug Tsetse fly
	Leishmania spp.	Visceral leishmaniasis (kala-azar) Cutaneous leishmaniasis	Sand fly
	Plasmodium spp. (*P. vivax, P. ovale, P. malariae*)	Malaria	*Anopheles* mosquito
	Toxoplasma gondii	Toxoplasmosis	Ingestion of cysts in raw meat; contact with infected cat feces

Modified from Goering R, Dockrell H, Zuckerman M et al: *Mim's medical microbiology*, ed 4, St Louis, 2008, Mosby.

INNATE IMMUNITY

Chemical and Mechanical Body Defenses

The body has many different chemical and mechanical defenses against infection. These are sometimes called "first-line" defenses against infection.

- Intact skin, including the mucous membranes, serves as an excellent barrier against the transmission and spread of infection. The normal flora of the skin, fatty acids derived from perspiration, excretions of sebaceous glands, and the rapid growth of keratin prevent bacterial entry into deeper tissues. Specific skin tissues are specialized in their ability to defend the body against infection. For example, skin appendages such as the eyelashes and nasal and ear hair prevent contamination by dust and droplets.
- The respiratory system has many different defense mechanisms. Microscopic cilia that line the respiratory tract continually sweep particles from the surface of the tract. The action of the cilia moves material toward the mouth and nose and prevents it from settling in the lower respiratory tract. Mucus in the respiratory system traps particles and bacteria, which are forced out through the cough reflex.
- Bacteriostatic chemicals in saliva, low pH in the stomach, and resident flora in the intestine prevent infection. Gastrointestinal transmission occurs by ingestion (eating or drinking food or water contaminated with infectious microorganisms). We ingest many different types of foreign material and bacteria each day. Despite the body's defenses, virulent disease organisms can quickly invade the tissues of the intestine and proliferate.
- **Resident microorganisms** compete with invading microbes for the environment. Shortly after birth, an infant's body begins to acquire a wide variety of bacterial colonies in certain tissues of the body. Resident microorganisms are found in areas of the body that communicate with or are exposed to the outside environment (Figure 9-15). The gastrointestinal system has a complex environment that includes different resident bacteria that can be harmful outside of the gastrointestinal system. All other tissues in the body are normally sterile. The resident microbes help prevent invading, potentially disease-causing microorganisms from colonizing in tissue.
- The inflammatory response is the body's innate immune response to injury. The four classic signs of **inflammation** are heat, redness, swelling (edema), and pain.
Almost immediately after tissue injury, blood vessels temporarily constrict at the site of injury. Constriction of capillaries helps reduce bleeding and restricts the movement of any microbial toxins present. This is rapidly followed by localized arterial and venous dilation. As a result, the injured area becomes red and warm. Local capillaries become more permeable, which allows plasma to escape into the surrounding tissue. The plasma dilutes any toxins in these tissues; it also increases the thickness (viscosity) of the local blood supply and encourages clotting. These processes result in swelling, pain, and impaired function of the affected part.
- When microorganisms invade the body, a cellular response is initiated. Specialized white blood cells (leukocytes) rush to the site and surround and engulf them. This process, called phagocytosis, is an immune response triggered by the process of inflammation. Once the microorganism is inside the leukocyte, the leukocyte's lysosomes fuse with the microorganism and digest it. Nonliving remnants of the microorganism are then released from the leukocyte. Two types of "digesting cells", called phagocytes, are involved in this process. *Neutrophils* are carried to the site of infection within 90 minutes. Within about 5 to 48 hours, *macrophages* arrive and continue to engulf and digest large amounts of bacteria. Regional lymph nodes collect cellular

debris and act as centers for more intensive phagocytic activity. Pus at the site of an infection is composed of dead cells, lymphocytes, and living and dead pathogens.

ADAPTIVE IMMUNE SYSTEM

The *adaptive immune system* is triggered by exposure to a specific potentially harmful substance, such as a disease microorganism in the environment or through a vaccination. This protein substance is referred to an *antigen*. When exposed to an antigen, the body forms antibodies, which attach to the cells and remain there temporarily or throughout life.

- Antigens are *nonself* substances that trigger the immune system to launch a defense.
- Antibodies are *self* substances that provide protection to the body.

ACTIVE IMMUNITY

Active immunity develops when the body is stimulated to form its own antibodies against specific disease antigens. This type of immunity usually is permanent. The best immunity is formed from a live antigen.

Active immunity can occur after vaccination or exposure to the disease. In this process, T and B lymphocytes are activated to bring about the production of antibodies (proteins that remain in the immune system memory). When the body is exposed to the disease pathogen again, the antibodies are activated and quickly destroy the organisms. Immunity can last for years or a lifetime.

A person can develop active immunity in two ways:
1. By getting the disease.
2. By vaccination, which is an injection containing a small amount of disease antigen. The antigen is modified to prevent the recipient from developing the disease, but it is effective in stimulating the formation of antibodies.

PASSIVE IMMUNITY

Passive immunity develops when the body receives the specific disease antibodies from an outside source. This eliminates the need for the body to synthesize them. Passive immunity, which is temporary, occurs when:
1. The fetus receives antibodies in utero from the mother's immune system or breast milk (natural immunity).
2. A person receives a specific antibody for a specific antigen, created in equine or human tissue. The antibody usually is given by injection. Tetanus antitoxin is an example of an injectable antibody.

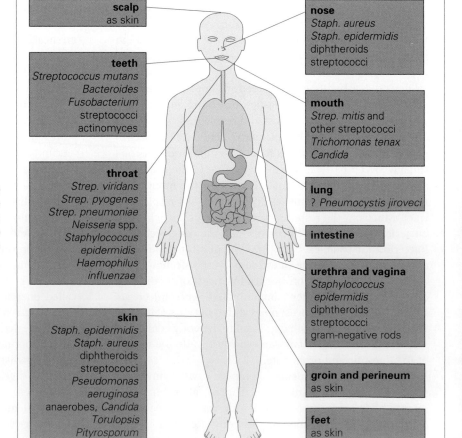

Figure 9-15 A, Normal body flora (resident bacteria). Normal flora protect the body against infection by competing successfully for resources (e.g., nutrition, moisture). They are well adapted to the body and also aid in body functions, such as digestion.

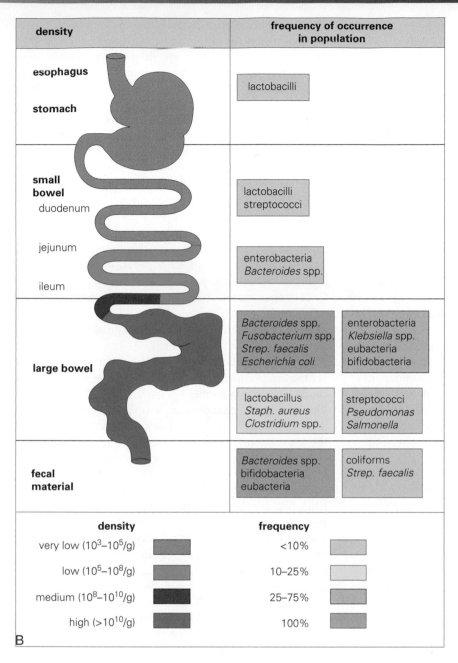

density	frequency of occurrence in population
esophagus **stomach**	lactobacilli
small bowel duodenum jejunum ileum	lactobacilli streptococci enterobacteria *Bacteroides* spp.
large bowel	*Bacteroides* spp. enterobacteria *Fusobacterium* spp. *Klebsiella* spp. *Strep. faecalis* eubacteria *Escherichia coli* bifidobacteria lactobacillus streptococci *Staph. aureus* *Pseudomonas* *Clostridium* spp. *Salmonella*
fecal material	*Bacteroides* spp. coliforms bifidobacteria *Strep. faecalis* eubacteria

density		frequency	
very low (10^3–10^5/g)		<10%	
low (10^5–10^8/g)		10–25%	
medium (10^8–10^{10}/g)		25–75%	
high (>10^{10}/g)		100%	

B

Figure 9-15, cont'd **B,** Normal flora of the gastrointestinal system and their frequency. *(From Goering R, Dockrell H, Wakelin D et al: Mim's medical microbiology, ed 4, St Louis, 2008, Mosby.)*

VACCINES

Vaccination provides a form of adaptive immunity. Vaccines are modified forms of disease organisms that create immunological memory in the body. They produce the same immunological response as the disease itself, without the risks involved in the disease process. Vaccination provides artificial immunity against specific organisms.

Vaccines are classified into two main types and their subtypes:

1. Live attenuated vaccines
   - Viruses
   - Bacteria
2. Inactivated vaccines
   - Whole
   - Fractional

Live attenuated vaccines contain modified disease organisms, either viruses or bacteria. Modification of the organism prevents the recipient of the vaccine from experiencing the effects of the disease, but immunity is still conferred. Examples of attenuated vaccines licensed in the United States are polio, measles, mumps, varicella, and rubella.

Inactivated vaccines contain whole viruses or bacteria, or fractional components of the organisms. Protein-based fractional vaccines are called toxoids. These are inactivated bacterial toxins.

HYPERSENSITIVITY

Immune response to a substance is referred to as hypersensitivity. Hypersensitivity occurs only in individuals who have previous exposure and sensitivity to the substance. A hypersensitivity reaction may be mild, producing a rash, mild respiratory distress leading to asthma, or gastrointestinal symptoms. The reaction can be immediate or delayed up to 12 hours after exposure. A severe immediate reaction is referred to as *anaphylactic shock,* which can be quickly fatal.

ALLERGY

True allergy is a process mediated by the immune system. A substance that causes a hypersensitivity reaction is called an allergen. Allergens gain entry into the body by many routes. In the perioperative environment, it is very important to know the patient's allergies. These may include medications and latex rubber, which is contained in many medical devices, including surgical gloves.

Immediate and Delayed Reaction

The two types of true allergic reactions are immediate and delayed. Delayed reactions are mediated by T lymphocytes. Immediate reactions are mediated by antibodies. Allergic reactions are divided into four categories:

- *Type I:* These reactions are characterized by inflammation of tissues, which is caused by the release of *histamine* in the body. This causes increased permeability of blood vessels and constriction of bronchioles, leading to difficulty breathing. The most extreme form of sensitivity is anaphylactic shock, which can lead to death.
- *Type II:* A type II reaction is called a *cytotoxic reaction.* It causes the onset of powerful immune defense mechanisms, which can result in injury or death. Mismatched blood transfusion and hemolytic disease in newborns are type II reactions.
- *Type III:* Type III reactions are caused by antigen-antibody complexes, which produce tissue damage when they trigger an immune response. An example of a type III reaction is allergy to antibiotics. Symptoms include itching, rash, severe tissue swelling, and fever. This usually resolves in several days.
- *Type IV:* Type IV reactions are cell-mediated reactions (not related to antibodies) that occur 24 to 72 hours after exposure to the agent. An example of this delayed hypersensitivity is a positive reaction to the tuberculin skin test, in which a small amount of killed *M. tuberculosis* is injected into the skin.

Autoimmunity

In certain diseases, the body does not recognize "self". Consequently, it mounts a mild to severe immune response to its own tissues, causing fever, swelling, and tissue destruction. Examples of autoimmune diseases are rheumatoid arthritis, systemic lupus erythematosus, and ulcerative colitis (single organ autoimmune disease).

KEY CONCEPTS

- Microbiology is the study of microorganisms and their relationship to the environment.
- The Linnaean system of classification is used in biology to distinguish specific groups of organisms.
- Living cellular organisms are divided into two groups, eukaryotes and prokaryotes.
- Eukaryotes are the cells of complex organisms such as mammals.
- Bacteria belong to the prokaryote class of cells.
- Microbes are identified by their morphology, staining tendencies, and reactions to biochemical tests. Gram staining is a basic test performed for differentiation.
- Chemical tests can be performed on bacteria only if they are grown in a laboratory environment (culturing). After culturing, the bacteria are tested for sensitivity to antimicrobial drugs (culture and sensitivity).
- Microbes are classified by types according to the Linnaean system. The major groups are bacteria, viruses, fungi, protozoa, rickettsiae, and prions.
- Cells contain various types of organelles, which aid in the cell's metabolism.
- Substances move into the cell mainly by diffusion, osmosis, active transport, and pinocytosis.
- The relationship between a microbe and its host depends on the environment, the condition of the host, and the condition of the microbe.
- The biological relationship between organisms living together is called *symbiosis.* If neither organism is harmed, the association is called *commensalism;* if the association benefits both, it is *mutualism* and, if one is harmed and the other benefits, it is *parasitism.*
- Bacteria are the most important group of microbes in medicine, because they cause most diseases.
- Bacteria vary in their environmental and physiological needs. These include nutrition, oxygen requirements, pH, and temperature. Oxygen requirements are particularly important in wound management. Aerobic bacteria require oxygen, and anaerobic bacteria do not. Anaerobic bacteria produce powerful toxins that can be fatal in the host.
- Bacterial toxins are produced by living bacteria as products of metabolism (exotoxin), or the toxins are released after the bacteria die (endotoxin).
- Specific types of bacteria live normally in human tissues. These are called *resident flora,* and they aid in digestion and defense against disease.
- Prions and viruses are nonliving but able to cause disease.
- Creutzfeldt-Jakob disease and variant CJD are fatal, transmissible diseases of the nervous system. They are important in surgery because although rare, the prion responsible for the diseases cannot be destroyed by normal sterilization methods.
- Hepatitis and HIV/AIDS are the most important infectious diseases caused by viruses. The hepatitis B virus and HIV are blood-borne microbes transmitted through contact with body fluids.
- Disease transmission occurs only when certain conditions are met. These include a method of transmission, a portal of entry into the body, a sufficient dose of microbes, a suitable environment for microbe reproduction, and insufficient resistance in the host.

- Infectious disease is transmitted by direct contact, airborne droplets, oral transmission, and ingestion of microbes.
- Urinary catheterization causes the greatest number of hospital-acquired infections in the United States. Surgical site infection is the second most frequent HAI.
- Multidrug-resistant organisms have evolved because of the overuse and misuse of antimicrobial agents worldwide.
- The immune system defends the body against infection by innate immunity and adaptive immunity. Innate immunity is present at birth, and adaptive immunity is conferred by previous exposure to the disease-causing organism, either naturally or by immunization.
- Hypersensitivity to a substance in the environment is also mediated by the immune system and can result in serious illness or death.

REVIEW QUESTIONS

1. How is the environment of a pathogen related to the disease it causes?
2. In what ways are viral and bacterial diseases transmitted?
3. List the body fluids that can transmit HIV.
4. What particular protection does the bacterial spore provide in prolonging the life of bacteria?
5. Why are antibiotics not effective against viral infections?
6. What is a resident bacterium? What protection does it provide?
7. How do viruses replicate?
8. How is hepatitis B transmitted?
9. What characteristics make CJD such a risk?
10. Define these terms: *antibody, antigen, passive immunity,* and *active immunity.*
11. What is the most important method of preventing disease transmission in the health care setting?

CASE STUDIES

Case 1

Direct contact with pathogenic microorganisms is the most common cause of hospital acquired infection. How might a dermal (skin) staphylococcus infection of a staff member result in a urinary traction infection of a patient? Describe a possible pathway of contamination during a normal workday.

Case 2

Surgical patients are at risk for opportunistic infection. Describe what this means and give specific examples of why the surgical patient is at risk.

Case 3

The study of microbiology and infectious disease transmission are the basis of the more advanced practice of aseptic technique which is the method used to prevent infection. How do these topics relate to *surgical conscience* introduced in Chapter 1?

REFERENCE

1. Joint United Nations Committee on HIV/AIDS and the World Health Organization (UNAIDS/WHO): *AIDS epidemic update 2009*. Accessed April 12, 2012, at http://www.who.int/hiv/pub/epidemiology/epidemic/en/index.html.

BIBLIOGRAPHY

American Social Health Association: *Fact sheet on HPV*. Accessed July 23, 2011, at http://www.ashastd.org/pdfs/hpv/hpv_learn_patfactsheet.cfm.

Atkinson W, Hamborsky J, McIntyre L, Wolfe S, editors: *Epidemiology and prevention of vaccine-preventable diseases*, ed 12, Washington, DC, 2011, Public Health Foundation. Accessed July 23, 2011, at http://www.cdc.gov/vaccines/pubs/pinkbook/default.htm.

Centers for Disease Control and Prevention: *Prion diseases: about prion diseases*. Accessed July 24, 2011, at http://www.cdc.gov/incidoc/dvrd/prions.

Centers for Disease Control and Prevention: *Healthcare-associated infections (HAIs)*. Accessed July 24, 2011, at http://www.cdc.gov/hai/index.html.

Centers for Disease Control and Prevention: *Human papillomavirus: HPV information for clinicians*. Accessed July 24, 2011, at http://www.cdc.gov/std/Hpv/hpv-/common-clinicans/ClinicianBro-fp.pdf.

Control Practices Advisory Committee: *2007 guidelines for isolation precautions: preventing transmission of infectious agents in healthcare settings*. Accessed May 25, 2008, at http://www.cdc.gov/ncidod/dhqp/pdf/isolation2007.pdf.

Edwards J, Peterson K, Mu Y, et al: *National Healthcare Safety Network report: data summary for 2006 through 2008, issued December 2009*. Accessed July 24, 2011, at http://www.cdc.gov/nhsn/PDFs/dataStat/2009NHSNReport.pdf.

Goering R, Dockrell H, Zuckerman M, et al: *Mim's medical microbiology*, St Louis, 2008, Mosby.

Klevens M, Morrison M, Nadle J, et al: Invasive methicillin-resistant *Staphylococcus aureus* infections in the United States, *Journal of the American Medical Association* 298:15, 2007.

Seigel J, Rhinehart E, Jackson M, et al: *Management of multi drug-resistant organisms in healthcare settings*, 2006. Accessed November 5, 2007, at http://www.cdc.gov/ncidod/dhqp/ar.html.

World Health Organization: *WHO guidelines on hand hygiene in health care*. Accessed July 23, 2011, at http://shqlibdoc.sho.int/publications/2009/97892415906_eng.pdf.

10

The Principles and Practice of Aseptic Technique

CHAPTER OUTLINE

LEARNING OBJECTIVES

After studying this chapter the reader will be able to:
1. Review the standards and recommendations related to aseptic technique
2. Clearly define terms related to aseptic technique and the principles of asepsis
3. Explain the concepts of barriers and containment
4. Explain surgical conscience
5. List and describe the principles of aseptic technique
6. Explain the relationship between personal hygiene and asepsis
7. Describe and explain the importance of surgical attire
8. Practice hand washing, the surgical handrub, and the surgical scrub using the correct methods
9. Demonstrate proper gowning and gloving techniques
10. Explain how to open a sterile tray of instruments
11. Define and give examples of evidence-based practice

TERMINOLOGY

Antiseptics: Chemical agents approved for use on the skin that inhibit the growth and reproduction of microorganisms.

Asepsis: The absence of pathogenic microorganisms on an animate surface or on body tissue. Literally, *asepsis* means "without infection", whereas *sepsis* literally means "with infection". In surgery, asepsis is a state of minimal or zero pathogens. Asepsis is the goal of many surgical practices.

Aseptic technique: Methods or practices in health care that reduce infection.

Chemical barrier: The barrier formed by the action of an antiseptic; it not only reduces the number of microorganisms on a surface, but also prevents recolonization (regrowth) for a limited period.

Contamination: The consequence of physical contact between a sterile surface and a nonsterile surface in surgery resulting in the potential or actual transfer of microbes from one surface to another.

Containment and confinement: A foundation concept of aseptic technique in which sterile and nonsterile surfaces are separated by physical barriers or distance (space).

Double gloving: Wearing two pairs of gloves, one over the other, to reduce the risk of contamination as a result of glove failure or puncture.

Gross contamination: Contamination of a large area of tissue by a highly infective source.

Hand washing: A specific technique used to remove soil, debris, and dead cells from the hands. Hand washing with an antiseptic also reduces the number of microorganisms on the skin.

Nonsterile personnel: In surgery, team members who remain outside the boundary of the sterile field and do not come in direct contact with sterile equipment, sterile areas, or the surgical wound. The circulator, anesthesia care provider, and radiographic technician are examples of nonsterile team members.

Physical barrier: In surgery, a barrier that separates a sterile surface from a nonsterile surface. Examples are sterile surgical gloves, gowns, and drapes. A physical barrier, such as a clean surgical cap, prevents a bacteria-laden surface, such as the hair, from shedding microorganisms.

Resident flora: Microorganisms are normally present in specific tissues. Resident flora are necessary to the regular function of these tissues or structures. Also called *normal flora*.

Scrub: The scrubbed surgical technologist or nurse assisting in surgery. Also refers to the surgical hand scrub performed before surgery.

Scrubbed personnel: In surgery, members of the surgical team who work within the sterile field. Also called *sterile personnel*.

Sharps: Any objects that can penetrate the skin and have the potential to cause injury and infection, including but not limited to needles, scalpels, broken glass, and exposed ends of dental wires.

Sterile field: An area that includes the draped patient, all sterile tables, and sterile equipment in the immediate area of the patient. The patient is the center of the sterile field.

TERMINOLOGY (cont.)

Sterile item: Any item or medical device that has been exposed to a process that destroys all microbes, including spores.

Sterility: A state in which an inanimate or animate surface harbors absolutely no viable microorganisms.

Strike-through contamination: An event in which fluid from a nonsterile surface penetrates the protective wrapper of a sterile item, causing it to become contaminated.

Surgical conscience: In surgery, the ethical motivation to practice excellent aseptic technique to protect the patient from infection. Surgical conscience implies that the professional practices excellent technique regardless of whether others are observing.

Surgical handrub: The systematic application of antiseptic foam or gel on the hands before gowning and gloving for a sterile procedure. The surgical handrub may be used as an alternative to the traditional hand scrub under certain conditions.

Surgical hand scrub: A specific technique for washing the hands before donning a surgical gown and gloves before surgery. The scrub is performed with timed or counted strokes using detergent-based antiseptic. The surgical hand scrub is designed to remove dirt, oils, and transient microorganisms and reduce the number of resident microorganisms.

Surgical wound: The superficial and deep tissue layers of the surgical incision. This is the center of the surgical field.

Surgical site infection (SSI): Postoperative infection of the surgical wound. The goal of surgical skin preparation is to prevent postoperative wound infection.

Transient flora: Microorganisms that do not normally reside in the tissue of an individual. Transient microorganisms are acquired through skin contact with an animate or inanimate source colonized by microbes. Transient flora may be removed by routine methods of skin cleaning.

INTRODUCTION

Aseptic technique is a set of practices that are used to create and maintain the sterile field and prevent **surgical site infection (SSI)**. Surgical site infection is often the result of contamination of the tissues by microorganisms during the intraoperative period. The infectious microorganisms can be *endogenous*—caused by bacteria from the patient's own skin or mucous membranes, or *exogenous*—bacterial contamination by sources outside the patient's body. Exogenous microorganisms originate from health care personnel; from contaminated instruments, supplies, and equipment; and from the environment, including airborne droplets and particles. Aseptic technique is among the most important areas of study for surgical personnel.

When students first begin to learn aseptic technique, with its many rules and precautions, they often feel awkward and afraid of making errors. This is a normal reaction to a completely new way of performing what was previously a simple task, such as pouring liquid from a bottle or putting on gloves. It is important to understand that the learning process always feels uncomfortable, especially when others are watching. However, the learning environment is where mistakes are made and corrected. There is no easy way to assimilate new ways of doing things except by practice. Repeated practice develops the confidence necessary for learning.

The practices of aseptic technique are derived from many sources. A particular practice is established by close evaluation of research data through a process of peer review (study by professionals who hold the same or higher degree as the researchers). References for the practices and guidelines defined in this textbook are cited so that instructors, students, and organizations can access and evaluate them. Where there is no established guideline or there has not been enough reliable information to establish a guideline, this is stated also. An introduction to evidence-based practice was presented in Chapter 3. In this chapter the topic is expanded so that students can learn how to apply critical thinking skills to standards and practices of aseptic technique, which are always based on scientific evidence and never on opinion or tradition.

STANDARDS AND RECOMMENDATIONS

Standards for aseptic technique are established by specific agencies that study and research infection control. Some research studies have been performed by individual academic institutions and then evaluated for their validity by standards agencies. Professional organizations set guidelines by examining all the previously validated work. The following standards agencies are actively involved in infection control research and publication of authoritative documents (in alphabetical order):

- Agency for Healthcare Research and Quality (AHRQ), National Guideline Clearinghouse (searchable database): http://www.guideline.gov/browse/by-topic.aspx
- Centers for Disease Control and Prevention (CDC) Hospital Infection Control Practices Advisory Committee (HICPAC): http://www.cdc.gov/hicpac/pubs.html
- Evidence-Based Practice Network: http://www.nursing center.com/evidencebasedpracticenetwork/JournalArticle. aspx?Article_ID=1136019
- Occupational Safety and Health Administration (OSHA): http://www.osha.gov/index.html
- Morbidity and Mortality Weekly Report (MMWR), Recommendations and Reports: http://www.cdc.gov/mmwr/ mmwr_rr/rr_cvol.html
- Society for Healthcare Epidemiology of America (SHEA): http://www.shea-online.org See also *Guidelines and Re sources:* http://www.shea-online.org/GuidelinesResources. aspx
- Professional Organizations, Association of periOperative Registered Nurses (AORN): http://www.aorn.org
- Association of Surgical Technologists (AST): http:// www.ast.org

CONCEPTS AND DEFINITIONS

STERILITY

When an object is sterile, it is *completely free* of all living microorganisms including microbial spores. All nonsterile surfaces are considered *potentially* contaminated with pathogenic microorganisms. All body tissues, except those that communicate directly with the environment outside the body, are normally free of microorganisms. The introduction of microbes into tissue can result in an infection. Microbes can be transmitted or introduced into tissues by direct contact, by air droplets, and by airborne particles.

Sterility is absolute. Something is either sterile or not sterile—there is no "partial sterility."

Surgery is performed under sterile conditions. All instruments, medical devices, supplies, and materials used in a surgical procedure are sterile. Sterile drapes are placed around the surgical incision site extending over the patient's body, and members of the scrubbed team wear sterile gown and gloves. The draped patient, instrument tables with equipment and supplies, and the scrubbed, gowned, and gloved sterile team form the **sterile field**. During surgery, this area is tightly controlled and has defined boundaries. The superficial and deep tissues of the surgical incision are collectively called the **surgical wound**. *This is the center of the sterile field.*

CONTAMINATION

Contamination is the contact between a sterile surface or object and a nonsterile item, substance, or entity.

Contaminated + sterile = contaminated.

The term *contaminated* is used in several ways:

- It defines an item or surface that was previously sterile but comes in contact with a contaminant, such as a sterile instrument that falls to the floor. The instrument is contaminated. The surgeon's gloved hand accidentally touches the nonsterile edge of the surgical drape. His glove is contaminated. The scrubbed surgical technologist accidentally punctures her glove with a suture needle. The *needle* is contaminated (remember that skin is not sterile).
- It is an *event* in which a **sterile item** or surface has come in contact with a nonsterile item or surface—for example, an infected appendix has ruptured, spilling pus into the abdominal cavity. Gross contamination of the peritoneal cavity has occurred.

Gross contamination is the contamination of the surgical wound or sterile field by a highly infective source such as in the example just given. Gross contamination can lead to systemic infection because of the number and type of microorganisms that enter the body. Even in the presence of gross contamination, aseptic technique is maintained, because wound contamination with one type or strain of microorganism does not eliminate the pathogenic potential of others in the environment.

THE CONCEPT OF BARRIERS

One of the foundation principles of aseptic technique is based on the concept of creating a barrier between the sources of contamination and a sterile surface. To better understand and practice aseptic technique, consider the concept of **containment and confinement**. A **physical barrier** prevents a nonsterile surface from touching a sterile surface. In other words, it contains (encloses) or separates a source of contamination.

Hair caps and masks are barriers that contain sources of contamination (hair, dander, exhaled air). A sterile table cover provides a barrier between the nonsterile surface of the table and sterile equipment placed on the cover. A **chemical barrier** is produced by the residual effect of **antiseptics** used during patient skin preparation and the surgical scrub or handrub.

Distance is another type of barrier. As the distance between a sterile surface and a nonsterile surface increases, the risk of contamination decreases. As you are learning aseptic technique, visualize an imaginary space around sterile objects and the sterile field. This space is perceived, first consciously and then unconsciously, as off limits to nonsterile objects and personnel. Over time, surgical personnel develop a sense of intrusion when nonsterile objects are too close to the field. Nonsterile items and personnel must remain at least 12 inches (30 cm) from a sterile field.

SURGICAL CONSCIENCE

Aseptic technique is based on **surgical conscience**—that is, the ethical and professional motivation that regulates a professional's behaviors regarding disease transmission. All members of the surgical team are jointly responsible for reporting and responding to breaks in aseptic technique so that steps can be taken to mitigate the risk of infection. In the case of gross contamination, this may mean starting the patient on intravenous antibiotics. If the gloved hand is contaminated, the glove is changed as soon as possible. A contaminated instrument is passed off the sterile field. If irrigation fluids are contaminated, they are discarded and new sterile basins and fluids are obtained. Admitting and reporting any break in technique demonstrates a high level of professional maturity and surgical conscience. If a sterile team member contaminates the field without knowing, others may quickly report the break—"Dr. X, your glove touched the anesthesia screen." One of the important roles of the scrubbed surgical technologist is to protect the field; this includes watching for breaks in technique and reporting them quickly.

THE PRINCIPLES OF ASEPTIC TECHNIQUE

Aseptic technique encompasses the practices used to create, protect, and maintain the surgical field.

The objectives of the technique are *containment, confinement, reduction,* and *elimination of microorganisms* to prevent contamination of the sterile field. Techniques are based on the central principle that microorganisms transmit disease from objects, surfaces, air, and dust to patients and personnel.

Aseptic technique is a method of "doing and thinking" used during the entire surgical process.

The concepts described in this chapter form the foundation of surgical technique. Developing good aseptic technique takes time and practice, and everyone makes mistakes. Minor breaks in aseptic technique usually can be corrected. Postoperative infections, or a high rate of postoperative infections in a health care facility, are usually due to a combination of many small breaks (errors) in aseptic technique rather than one single break.

The **sterile field** is the physical area starting with the surgical incision at the center and extending to include the patient drapes, sterile instrument tables, and any draped equipment such as the operating microscope. It also includes scrubbed team members. The sterile field is *created* using specific rules and standards. The following practices pertain to any situation in which a sterile field exists:

1. **Sterile surfaces contact only sterile surfaces; nonsterile surfaces contact only nonsterile surfaces.**

   Contamination of a sterile surface occurs when a nonsterile surface touches a sterile surface (e.g., the circulator's bare hand accidentally touches the surgical technologist's glove while delivering sterile items to sterile personnel).

2. **A sterile item is considered sterile only after it has been processed using methods that have been proven effective and that yield measurable results.**

   Before any sterile item is distributed to the sterile field, the wrapper must be inspected for tears, holes, and signs of water damage. The chemical sterility indicator must also be inspected. Biological indicators are placed in batches of sterile goods to verify the correct functioning of a sterilizing system. Although an item has been through the process of sterilization, it might not be sterile. Many conditions and events can alter the sterility of the item, including puncture holes or tears in the wrapper, moisture, or failure of the sterilizer system.

3. **Sterile drapes, gowns, gloves, and table covers are barriers between a nonsterile surface and a sterile surface.**

   Materials used as barriers against contamination are chosen for their density, strength, ability to resist moisture, and ease of use. Materials that do not meet minimum standards for patient safety are not be used.

4. **The edge of any sterile drape, wrapper, or covering is considered nonsterile.**

   When a sterile item is opened, the edge of its wrapper must not touch the item. Maintaining a wide margin between the sterile item and the edge prevents possible contamination of the item as it is delivered to the field. A 1-inch (2.5-cm) margin from the perimeter of a sterile wrapper is considered not sterile. When sterile items are opened and distributed, the nonsterile hand is protected under the wrapper. A specific technique is used to open and distribute sterile goods.

5. **Sterile liquids in bottles with an edge (lip) that is protected with a sealed sterile cap may be delivered directly from the bottle into a sterile container on the field.**

   Medication vials often are sealed with aluminum caps. When the metal cap is pried open, the edge of the vial is considered contaminated, because the top cannot be removed without dragging the nonsterile cap across the lip of the vial. When you begin to pour sterile solution into a container, do not stop pouring until the container is empty. Pull the container away from the sterile field so that no residual liquid can drip down the nonsterile side of the container into the sterile receptacle below. Sterile fluids are distributed from a single bottle all at one time.

6. **If any doubt exists about the sterility of an item, consider it contaminated.**

   Before opening the wrapper of any sterile item, inspect it for signs of contamination. Tears, holes, wear marks, or water spots on any wrapper are signs of questionable sterility. When in doubt, do not use the item.

7. **The draped patient is the center of the sterile field during surgery.**

   Draped items and sterile personnel form the periphery of the field. Sterile drapes create a barrier between a nonsterile surface and the working area of the sterile field. For example, the operating microscope, ring basin, and back table are draped. Equipment that is not draped must remain outside the sterile field, with at least 12 inches (30 cm) allowed between the sterile and nonsterile surfaces.

8. **Sterile gowns are considered sterile only in front from midchest to table level.**

   Sterile personnel should not drop their forearms or hands below waist level nor raise them above the midchest. The axilla itself is considered nonsterile even though protected by a gown because it is an area of friction.

9. **Sterile personnel must pass other sterile personnel back to back or front to front.**

   Even though wraparound gowns are used in most surgical settings, the sterility of the back cannot be guaranteed because the person wearing it cannot observe it, this is called surgically clean. Sterile personnel never turn their back to the sterile field.

10. **Sterile tables are considered sterile only at table height.**

    The top of a sterile table is the only surface considered sterile. Suture ends must not hang over the table edge. Table drapes must not be repositioned once they have been placed, because this changes the level of the sterile area. Tubing, cords, and hoses that are secured to the patient drape must not be pulled up to create additional slack. This brings the nonsterile portion of the tubing up to the sterile field. The scrub is responsible for measuring and allowing for necessary slack before securing these items in place when they are first brought onto the sterile field. The Mayo tray that extends over the patient is sterile because it is continually monitored and is completely covered using a continuously sterile tubal drape.

11. **Sterile personnel remain within the immediate area of the sterile field.**

Scrubbed personnel must not move away from the sterile field. Sterile personnel are sometimes required to move around the periphery of the field to perform their tasks. However, moving outside the immediate sterile area compromises aseptic technique. Sterile personnel should not leave the room to retrieve items from another area, even if that area is restricted (e.g., the sterile core where supplies are flash-sterilized).

12. **Nonsterile team members never lean over or reach over a sterile surface to distribute sterile goods to the field. They do not pass between two sterile surfaces.**

When sterile packages are opened, the opener must hand items to personnel or deposit them on sterile surfaces in such a way as to avoid reaching over previously opened goods. Many commercially prepared surgical items are packaged so that they can be flipped onto the sterile field from a safe distance. If the wrapper does not permit this technique to be used, **nonsterile personnel** must pass the item directly to scrubbed personnel.

13. **Movement is kept to a minimum during surgery**.

Team members should move around the operating suite as little as possible. This applies to both scrubbed and nonsterile personnel. Traffic into and out of the surgical suite creates air currents that sweep contaminated particles into the operating room. Doors to the operating room suite should remain closed when sterile supplies are opened and when surgery is in progress.

14. **Drapes and linens should be handled as little as possible and with a minimum of movement.**

This prevents the release of lint and dust particles, which create a vehicle for transmission of airborne bacteria. When draping a surface, always unfold the drapes; never shake a drape to loosen or unfold it. At the close of surgery, fold or roll soiled drapes toward the center, taking care to contain the contaminants. Never drag a soiled drape from a surface and bundle it up against your body, even if you are wearing protective attire. This spreads contaminated particles into the environment.

15. **Talking is kept to a minimum during surgery.**

The mouth is a major reservoir for bacteria. Talking forces the breath into the air and immediate environment. Masks worn to prevent the release of bacteria-laden moisture are not 100% effective and, when improperly worn, provide little protection against the dissemination of aerosol droplets containing microorganisms.

16. **Moisture carries bacteria from a nonsterile surface to a sterile surface.**

When water comes in contact with a sterile drape or gown, it can cause **strike-through contamination**. This occurs when moisture from either side of the drape serves as a vehicle for bacteria to infiltrate the drape from the nonsterile surface. Most disposable drapes are tightly woven to prevent strike-through. With continuous contact, blood and fluids can penetrate gowns and drapes. Woven (reusable) drapes are treated with a chemical that resists moisture, but they are not completely impervious. When copious amount of fluid are anticipated during a case, impervious drapes must be used.

17. **The sterile field is created as close as possible to the time of surgery and is monitored throughout the procedure.**

When sterile supplies have been opened, the sterile setup is vulnerable to contamination. Sterile supplies should be opened as close to the time of surgery as possible. In reality, however, cases may be delayed or even canceled. Currently no data are available to suggest that leaving a sterile setup exposed increases the risk of a surgical site infection. After a room is opened, it must be constantly monitored for contamination. A sterile setup must not be covered as there is no way to remove the drape without risking contamination.

HEALTH AND HYGIENE

Perioperative personnel must be particularly meticulous in practicing good hygiene in order to prevent potentially pathogenic microbes from being introduced into the surgical environment. Personnel must be free of any contagious illness or infection that might be transmitted to the patient and others in the operating room. Bacterial shedding from the nasopharynx and skin is a particular risk. Open sores or even small skin wounds shed bacteria, which can be transmitted by direct contact on the hands. Individuals with persistent skin conditions resulting in inflammation and infection may be a significant source of microbial transmission to patients, equipment, and other staff members. Sebum produced normally by the skin protects and maintains suppleness. However, an overproduction of sebum or obstruction of the glands creates a medium for bacterial proliferation. Daily bathing removes excess sebum and bacteria. Perfumes should not be used in the operating room. Particular attention is given to the hands and nails, which are kept short and neat. Bacteria proliferate under the nails, which represent a significant source of transmission. This is discussed in greater detail later.

SURGICAL ATTIRE

Surgical attire, including scrub suit, head covering, mask, shoes, and jacket, is worn in the restricted and semirestricted areas of the surgical environment and other areas of the facility where invasive procedures are performed. Scrub suits and cover jackets are manufactured from fabrics that shed little or no lint to prevent bacterial transmission by airborne particles. The selection of surgical scrub attire purchased from commercial vendors is the responsibility of the surgical supervisor or manager, in collaboration with the facility's infection control and purchasing departments. Appropriate guidelines are related to the density and composition of cloth used in the manufacture of surgical scrub suits; these are considered to ensure barrier protection, comfort, and safety.

A trend in homemade surgical caps and staff returning home wearing scrub suits worn during the workday has created increased debate about the need to use only a health care–accredited laundering facility. Also, it has been shown that some facilities have actually promoted home laundering as a cost-cutting measure.

Home laundering of surgical attire is not specifically sanctioned by any standards agency or organization. This is because home facilities do not achieve washing and drying parameters needed to meet disinfection requirements. All standards agencies require that scrub attire that is contaminated with blood and other body fluids must be removed immediately and laundered by the facility or a commercial laundry. The required standard for donning (putting on) freshly laundered surgical attire implies that these items are provided by the facility and never stored in contact with personal belongings, which carry a high bioburden. The practice of keeping home-laundered caps and cover jackets in personal lockers and wearing them for several days between cleanings does not meet any accepted standard of **asepsis**.* Health care personnel who leave the facility and enter the community wearing surgical attire risk spreading infection to others in public and at home.

CURRENT STANDARDS ON HOME LAUNDERING

- *AORN:* "All individuals who enter the semirestricted and restricted areas should wear freshly laundered surgical attire that is laundered at a health care–accredited laundry facility or disposable attire provided by the facility and intended for use within the perioperative setting."[†]

- *ARHQ:* "No recommendations on how or where to launder scrub suits, restricting use of scrub suits to the operating suite or for covering scrub suits when out of the operating suite. Home laundering of visibly soiled surgical attire is not recommended."[‡]

- *AST:* "Home laundering of OR attire to include scrub suits, cloth warm-up jackets, and cloth hats is not recommended".[§]

- *CDC and HICPAC:* "Although OSHA regulations prohibit home laundering of items that are considered personal protective apparel or equipment (e.g., laboratory coats), experts disagree about whether this regulation extends to uniforms and scrub suits that are not contaminated with blood or other potentially infectious material. Health-care facility policies on this matter vary and may be inconsistent with recommendations of professional organizations."[§]

JEWELRY

Jewelry of any kind is a potential source of pathogens. Microorganisms proliferate freely under rings and bracelets. Necklaces and earrings that are not confined under scrub attire pose a risk of falling onto the surgical field or even into the surgical wound. Exposed necklaces or earrings may become contaminated with blood or other aerosolized particles that can spread infection. Rings and watches that are not removed prevent effective asepsis during routine hand washing because they trap bacteria between the jewelry and skin.

The recommended standard issued by all agencies is to remove all jewelry or completely confine it inside scrub clothes.* Body piercing jewelry should be confined or removed. Piercings may contain a bacterial count up to 21 times greater under the jewelry than on the metal itself. A draining or inflamed piercing track is considered an open infection.[†]

Identification badges are necessary in the professional environment and can be worn securely on the scrub top. Many facilities require badges to be placed at the waist, rather than on the shoulder. Badges attached to cloth or chain lanyards can carry a high bioburden and can be a source of bacterial shedding unless routinely disinfected.

There is no evidence that a *healed* tattoo presents a source of contamination. However, fresh tattoos on exposed skin can be considered an open wound that would prevent an employee from working in surgery. Hospital policy determines whether any healed tattoos not covered by uniforms or scrub attire are permitted. Fashion accessories such as false eyelashes should not be worn.

SCRUB SUIT

The scrub suit is worn by both sterile and nonsterile surgical personnel in the perioperative environment. The suit is designed to prevent the shedding of skin particles and hair into the environment and to protect the wearer from contact with soil and body fluids. Perspiration and normal exudate from sebaceous glands in the skin contain large colonies of bacteria, which are shed with friction and movement. The scrub suit helps prevent the release of these substances but is not considered personal protective equipment.

The scrub suit consists of a shirt and pants (Figure 10-1). It is made of lint-free material and should fit closely to the body. The suit should not be so tight as to produce chafing,

---

*Guidelines for Environmental Infection Control in Health-care Facilities: Recommendations of CDC and the Healthcare Infection Control Practices Advisory Committee (HICPAC) 2003.

[†]AORN, *Surgical Attire* in Perioperative Standards and Recommended Practices, 2011 ed, Denver, 2011.

[‡]U.S. Dept of Health and Human Services, Agency for Healthcare Research and Quality, Prevention of surgical site infections. Accessed February 27, 2012 at http://www.guideline.gov/content.aspx?id=12921.

[§]AST, AST recommended standards of practice for wearing the lab coat, cover gown, or other appropriate apparel effective 2008), in Standards of Practice. Accessed February 24, 2012 at http://www.ast.org/educators/standards_table_of_contents.aspx.

[§]Sehulster L, Chinn R: Control Guidelines for Environmental Infection Control in Health-care Facilities: Recommendations of CDC and the Healthcare Infection Control Practices Advisory Committee (HICPAC) *MMWR,* 52(RR10):1-42, 2003.

---

*AST guideline states "AST recommends that no jewelry be worn by surgical team members in the restricted area." http://www.ast.org/educators/standards_table_of_contents.aspx

AORN 2011 guidelines state "Jewelry including earrings, necklaces, watches, and bracelets that cannot be contained of confined within the surgical attire should not be worn. Jewelry that cannot be confined within the surgical attire should be removed before entry into the semirestricted and restricted areas." From AORN Perioperative Standards and Recommended Practices, 2011 Edition. Denver, 2011.

[†]Bartlette GE, Pollard TC, Bowker KE, Bannister CC. Effect of jewellery on surface bacterial counts of operating theatres. *J Hosp Infect.* 2002;52(1):68-72.

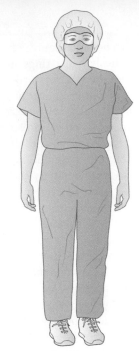

Figure 10-1 Correct attire for perioperative personnel working in restricted areas.

which increases the release of skin and hair particles laden with bacteria. The top should be secured at the waist, tucked into the pants, or fit close to the body to prevent contact with sterile surfaces. The drawstring ties should be tucked into the pants.

A clean scrub suit is donned whenever personnel enter the restricted or semirestricted area of the operating room. Before donning the pullover scrub top, the hair should be covered with a clean head cap. This prevents shedding hair and dander onto the scrub top.

- When a scrub suit has been soiled by blood or body fluids, surgical personnel must remove it in such a way as to prevent skin contact with the soiled area. Grossly soiled scrub suits are placed in a biohazard laundry receptacle so that they do not spread contaminants.
- Personnel should change into street clothes before leaving the health care facility or when traveling between buildings according to health facility policy.
- Personnel such as maintenance engineers or law enforcement entering the semirestricted or restricted area for a short time must don a single-use jumpsuit or freshly laundered scrub suit. Head and facial hair must be completely covered by a surgical cap, hood, or bonnet.

USE OF COVER GOWNS AND LAB COATS

Historically, a cover gown (nonsterile surgical gown) or lab coat was worn any time surgical staff left the department temporarily. This standard was enforced because of a single study claiming that the practice reduced contamination of the scrub suit and therefore decreased the risk of surgical site infection. However, the study was later declared flawed. Since that time, no studies have been able to validate the use of cover gowns or lab coats for the purpose of lowering infection rate. The practice is now dependent on facility policy, which may be related to public image (the perception of surgical personnel by patients and families) and on tradition. Because it is not an evidence-based practice, professional infection control organizations are unable to validate it.

Current Guidelines

- *AORN:* "Wearing cover apparel over surgical attire outside of the perioperative suite may be required for some health care personnel in some health care organizations for a variety of reasons . . . The use of cover apparel has been found to have little or no effect on reducing contamination of the surgical attire. Health care personnel should change into street clothes whenever they leave the health care facility or when traveling between buildings located on separate campuses."[*]
- *AHRQ:* "No recommendations on ... restricting use of scrub suits to the operating suite or for covering scrub suits when out of the operating suite."[†]
- *AST:* "Covering scrub attire may eliminate the need for a fresh pair of scrubs when reentering the surgical department and consequently decrease costs. ... Cover apparel such as a lab coat, cover gown, or other appropriate clothing should be worn when exiting the surgery department."[‡]

NONSTERILE COVER JACKET

Long-sleeved cover jackets (also called warm-up jackets) are often worn by nonsterile perioperative personnel, especially circulators, for comfort and to prevent contamination of the surgical field through bacterial shedding from the arms. Cover jackets are worn in the restricted and semirestricted areas of the operating room. OSHA recommends that jackets be buttoned or snapped closed during use. Previously worn jackets should never be kept in lockers and then reused because they can be a potential source of contamination rather than a barrier. Ideally, jackets should be freshly laundered by the health care facility. Cotton fleece jackets are also not recommended because they release large amounts of lint particles carrying dust, skin squames, and bacteria into the environment.

---

*Association of periOperative Registered Nurses (AORN): Recommended practices for surgical attire in *Standards, recommended practices and guidelines,* 2011 edition, Denver, CO.
†U.S. Dept of Health and Human Services, Agency for Healthcare Research and Quality, *Prevention of surgical site infections* accessed February 27, 2012 at http://www.guideline.gov/content.aspx?id=12921.
‡AST recommended standards of practice for wearing the lab coat, cover gown, or other appropriate apparel effective 2008, in Standards of Practice, accessed February 24, 2012 at http://www.ast.org/educators/standards_table_of_contents.aspx.

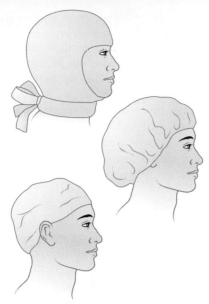

Figure 10-2 Approved head covers. All hair must be completely covered.

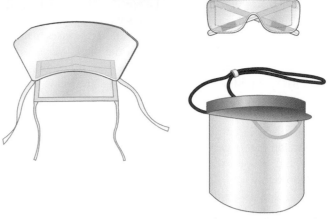

Figure 10-3 Protective eyewear required for surgical personnel.

HEAD COVERING

Disposable head caps, bouffant bonnets, or hoods are worn to reduce contamination of the surgical field by loose hair and dandruff from the scalp. Caps are meant to contain all hair and to cover the scalp line, nape of the neck, and sideburns completely (Figure 10-2). Males with facial hair should wear a cap that is specifically designed to cover this hair. The cap is put on before the scrub suit to prevent shedding of hair onto the clean scrub top.

The use of cloth (home-laundered) caps is not recommended, but may be subject to the policy of the individual institution. Homemade cloth caps worn as fashion accessories and reused day after day are a potential source of contamination. The scalp and hair are a rich source of *Staphylococcus aureus* and other bacteria, which proliferate under surgical caps. All infection control agencies validate the donning of freshly laundered scrub attire at the start of the work shift and whenever scrub attire is soiled.

PROTECTIVE EYEWEAR AND FACE SHIELD

OSHA mandates the use of protective eyewear or face shields as part of its blood-borne pathogen standard to protect workers exposed to splashing by blood and other potentially infectious materials (OPIM). Protective goggles, masks, or face shields are required during any procedure, including endoscopic surgery, in which there is a risk that blood, other body fluids, or particles of tissue could splash on the face*(Figure 10-3). The policy is reinforced by all professional organizations and safety standards agencies.

*Occupational and Safety and Health Administration, "Bloodborne pathogens" in *Code of Federal Regulations (CFR) 29: Part 1910.1030*

Specific criteria are as follows:
- Eyewear must extend from the brow to the top of the surgical mask and over the temples. This protects the eyes from the front and sides. Regular eyeglasses are not approved for safety use unless they have solid side shields.
- Impervious face shields offer increased protection. These extend from brow to chin.

MASK

Masks are worn to protect the intraoperative environment from contamination by aerosol droplets generated by the mouth, oropharynx, nose, and nasopharynx. Talking, coughing, and sneezing forcefully spread droplets onto the sterile field and surrounding environment. Masks are worn in the restricted areas of the operating room and in locations where sterile instruments and supplies are stored. In some facilities, masks may also be required in semirestricted areas. When used properly, masks block droplets and filter air. They also protect the wearer's nose and mouth from contact with particles of tissue and body fluids, especially during drilling, sawing, cutting, and tissue liquefaction. They provide a barrier against infectious microorganisms from patient respiratory secretions, blood, and other body fluids. Masks are made of lint-free synthetic material that is woven loosely enough to allow the breath to pass through effectively but tightly enough to filter 99% of particles of 5 μm or larger.

To protect the patient and the wearer, masks must be worn properly:
- The mask must cover both the nose and the mouth. Any pliable insert over the nose bridge of the mask should be molded over the nose to fit snugly.
- Ties must be secured at the top of the head and around the neck. Ties should not be crossed at the back of the head because this allows the sides of the mask to tent, allowing breath to bypass the mask and escape from the sides.
- Double masking is not recommended. When two masks are worn, the open spaces of the material are doubled, requiring the wearer to exert more respiratory force during inhalation and exhalation. This causes air to be forced in and out of the sides and defeats the filtering process.

- The wearer must remove and dispose of the mask immediately on leaving any restricted or semirestricted area. Even after a short time, bacterial colonization increases to a very high level on the inside surface of the mask. Masks are to be changed between surgical procedures. When masks are worn around the neck, they present a significant source of contamination.
- To remove the mask properly, the wearer should untie the top strings, then the bottom strings, without handling the portion that covers the face. The mask should be discarded in the proper waste receptacle and the hands washed thoroughly.
- Fresh masks are to be worn for each surgical procedure.
- Masks should either be *left on or left off*; they should never be worn around the neck with the ties dangling. Perioperative professionals can advocate for a policy of mask removal by encouraging vendors not to advertise surgical products using photos that depict individuals with masks left hanging over scrub attire or around the neck.
- Specialized masks are worn during laser procedures. These masks are designed to filter out particles that are smaller than those filtered by standard surgical masks; these smaller particles are created when cells are destroyed by laser energy.

SHOES AND COVERS

Shoes worn in the operating room must be dedicated for that use and should not be worn outside. Perioperative personnel should wear shoes that are comfortable and easy to keep clean and that protect the wearer against foot injury. Shoes with perforations over the top, side, and back do not protect the wearer from contamination with blood and body fluids and may be a source of cross-contamination. When selecting shoes for use in the operating room, it is important to consider injury from slips, falls, and penetration by instruments such as scalpels that may be accidentally dropped from the field. Backless shoes are a hazard in case of patient or facility emergency when staff must move quickly. From a health point of view, shoes can cause arch and back problems if they do not offer good support. This may not be apparent in the first few years of employment, but can become apparent later in a career. Cushioning for the foot is also important to prevent inflammation of the fascia that covers the bottom of the foot, including the arch. Shoes that have evenly distributed insole cushioning can help to prevent this problem.

Shoe covers protect shoes from contamination by blood and body fluids and should be worn when splashes or spills can reasonably be expected to occur. No evidence indicates that the use of shoe covers reduces the risk of surgical site infection; the primary purpose of shoe covers is to protect the wearer and prevent the tracking of blood and other body fluids outside the surgical suite. Shoe covers must be changed if they become wet or soiled. Clean shoe covers must be changed or removed before the staff member leaves the department. If gross contamination or pooling of blood, body fluids, or other liquids is possible, such as during some orthopedic or obstetrical cases, impervious shoe covers that extend to the knee can be worn.

PERSONAL AND PATIENT CARE ITEMS

Personal and patient care items brought into the operating room environment from outside can be a significant source of bacterial contamination. Stethoscopes should not be worn around the neck and must be disinfected between patient uses. Fabric stethoscope covers also harbor a high bioburden and should not be used. Belt packs (fanny packs or backpacks) are laden with dust containing lint, hair, fibers, and other contaminants and must not be worn in the operating room.

 Watch Section 2 Unit 2: Surgical Attire on the Evolve website. http://evolve.elsevier.com/Fuller/surgical

HAND HYGIENE

OVERVIEW

Hand hygiene is the most important tool for preventing infection in the health care setting. Organic debris, soil, and microorganisms can exist on the hands without any visible evidence, and as staff move from one task to another, touching patients and equipment, they can easily transmit microbes by direct contact.

Skin contains both **transient flora** and **resident flora** (resident microbiota). Transient microbes compete with resident flora for colonization by adapting to or changing existing resources needed for reproduction. Colonization signals the start of infection when the bioburden is high. Resident flora are protective through the consumption of existing nutrients in the skin environment. Even if colonization of transient microbes is not successful in one individual, their numbers can be sufficiently high for transmission to other surfaces and individuals whose normal resistance is low because of disease, physiological stress, or injury. Resident flora remain in the deeper skin tissues, whereas transient microbes accumulate on the epidermis, where they can be removed or destroyed by washing and the use of antimicrobial substances.

Hand hygiene is such a critical topic in the spread of disease that the World Health Organization (WHO) has launched an international campaign to promote hand hygiene practices to reduce hospital-acquired infection, including postoperative wound infection. WHO has published its research in a comprehensive document that reviews hand hygiene practices, existing data on the types of infections related to poor hand hygiene, and recommendations for effective preventive practices, including a review of preparations used in hand hygiene.

HISTORICAL BACKGROUND OF CURRENT RECOMMENDATIONS

In the surgical setting, three types of hand hygiene are used according to specific situations. These are the routine hand wash, the handrub with antiseptic, and the traditional surgical scrub. The traditional surgical scrub in which the sterile team used hard bristle brushes and antiseptic soap was used until 2002 as the exclusive technique for hand antisepsis before surgery. In that year, the CDC published a guideline advising against artificial nails and nail polish and advocating the use of alcohol-based handrub for all health care workers to prevent hospital-acquired infection. It was also found that harsh scrubbing of hands and arms resulted in abrasion and dermatitis, which actually encouraged the growth of microorganisms in the skin. The guideline recommended that the traditional 10-minute scrub be replaced with either an alcohol-based handrub *or* a scrub using a soft brush or sponge and antiseptic soap for 2 to 6 minutes.

The 2002 CDC ruling had widespread effects, including new research studies involving comparisons between the alcohol-based handrub and the traditional scrub. The conclusions drawn from these studies led to the current recommendations for hand hygiene in the operating room.

FINGERNAILS

To prepare the hands for all types of patient care, including surgery, a consensus on standards has been reached by professional organizations and health standards agencies including WHO:

- *The fingernails must be no longer than $\frac{1}{4}$ inch.* Nail tips should be level with the fleshy tip of the finger. The subungual (under the fingernails) area hosts a greater number of bacterial colonies than any other area of the hand. Long fingernails easily puncture gloves and make handling of equipment more difficult. Long nails can also scratch or dig into the patient's skin during transfer and positioning.
- *Nail polish must not be worn by surgical personnel.* Nail polish itself has not been proven to be a source of microbial proliferation. However, chipped or flaking polish is known to support bacterial growth.
- *Artificial nails must not be worn in the surgical environment.* Artificial nails harbor pathogenic bacteria (particularly gram-negative bacteria) and fungi between the real and synthetic nails, especially when the artificial nail is chipped or cracked. Bacterial counts remain high even after scrubbing of artificial nails with antiseptic solution.
- *Before performing any hand hygiene procedure, inspect the hands for visible soil, and remove all jewelry, including watches and rings.* Bacteria and fungi proliferate underneath rings and watches, creating a source of contamination.

Criteria for selecting a hand hygiene procedure depend partly on the condition of the hands. Inspecting the hands ensures that the proper method is used. Whenever there is visible soil, the hands must be scrubbed until all traces of soil are removed. Antiseptic handrubs are not effective on soil. The subungual area should be routinely cleaned using a disposable plastic nail cleaner. A nail cleaner is preferred over a nail brush, which can cause small abrasions that can harbor microbes under the nail. This should always be done during the first hand wash of the day and before the surgical scrub. Surgery personnel who have been involved in gardening or another activity that causes gross soiling should remove all visible traces of soil from the hands and under fingernails before entering the surgical environment.

Before performing hand antisepsis (traditional scrub or handrub) for a surgical procedure, the surgical technologist or

scrub nurse opens the sterile gown, towel, and gloves onto a small table on which no other sterile supplies have been opened. Never don gown and gloves directly from a surgically draped surface, and do not allow anyone else entering the sterile field to do so. This is to prevent the contamination of sterile instruments, table covers, and other equipment by water dripping from the hands and arms onto the sterile items.

ROUTINE HAND WASHING

Routine **hand washing** is an *event-related* practice (performed before and after a specific task or event). It requires a specific method with individual steps (Figure 10-4).

Antiseptic liquid soap is used in the health care setting for routine hand washing. Plain soap, without antiseptic, is effective in removing soluble fatty acids, soil, and debris from the skin surface. Plain bar soap is not used in the clinical environment because it can spread bacteria from one user to the next. Containers that dispense plain soap can also become contaminated with bacteria and fungi that colonize and proliferate. Topping up a dispenser without draining and cleaning it increases the risk of microbial proliferation in the reservoir. Dispensers that are refilled with individual vacuum-sealed bags are preferred over dispenser reservoirs refilled from a bulk container. Specific antiseptic agents are used for routine hand washing and surgical scrub (Table 10-1). They reduce the number of bacterial colonies and provide barrier protection that inhibits the growth of bacteria over time.

When to Perform Routine Hand Wash

Hand washing should be performed at the following times:

- At the beginning and end of each workday
- Before and after patient contact
- After any surgical case
- Between contacts with potentially contaminated areas of the same patient
- Before contact with sterile packages
- Whenever hands are visibly soiled
- After removing gloves
- Before performing the surgical handrub
- Immediately after contact with blood or body fluids, regardless of whether gloves were worn at the time of contact
- Before and after eating
- After personal hygiene care
- After toileting

Technique

The hand washing procedure should take 15 to 60 seconds or more if hands are very soiled. Gather all supplies needed prior to hand washing.

1. Remove *all* jewelry from hands and forearms.
2. Wet the hands 2″ above wrists thoroughly under running water.
3. Apply sufficient liquid antiseptic soap to cover all hand and 2″ above wrist surfaces. Rub the hands together, palm to palm in a circular motion.
4. With right palm over left dorsum (back of the left hand), interlace the fingers and rub vigorously. Repeat with the

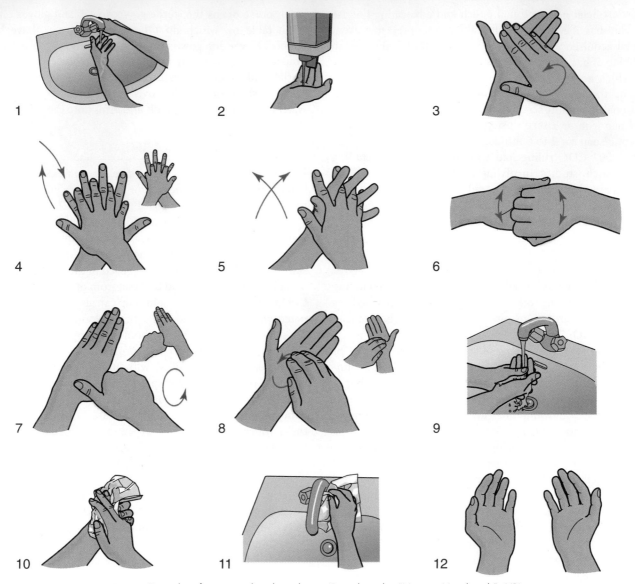

Figure 10-4   Procedure for routine hand washing. *(Based on the "How to Handwash", URL: http://www.who.int/gpsc/5may/How_To_HandWash_Poster.pdf © World Health Organization 2009. All rights reserved.)*

opposite hand. To ensure that the spaces between the fingers are adequately washed, spread the fingers and weave the two hands together, rubbing continuously.

5. While clasping the fingers of one hand into the cupped fingers of the opposite hand, wash the backs of all the fingers by rubbing them in a horizontal direction back and forth.

6. Clean the web space between thumb and first finger by clasping the thumb of one hand into the opposite palm. Reverse for the opposite hand.

7. Rub the fingers of one hand into the opposite palm using a circular motion. Repeat on the opposite hand.

8. In a back and forth motion, rub soap 2″ above the wrist.

9. Rinse hands under running water, keep fingers pointed downward / hands lower than elbows. making sure that all traces of soap are removed. Do not shake water from hands.

10. Dry hands using a single-use towel from fingers to wrist and turn off the faucet with towel. Do not shake water from hands.

11. Avoid contact with non-sterile surfaces during the hand wash. If you come in contact with a non-sterile surface, you must repeat the steps over. Be sure to check and follow the policy on hand washing at your healthcare facility.

TRADITIONAL SURGICAL SCRUB

The purpose of the surgical scrub is to remove soil and reduce the number of resident and transient microbes on the hands and arms to an absolute minimum. The surgical scrub is performed immediately before gowning and gloving for a surgical or invasive procedure (Figure 10-5). The surgical scrub does not sterilize the skin. However, the use of approved antiseptics along with standardized scrub technique reduces the

| Table **10-1** | **Surgical Hand Scrub Agents** | | | | |

| Agent | Residual Protection | Bactericidal Activity | | Toxicity | Comments |
		Gram-Negative Organisms	Gram-Positive Organisms		
Povidone-iodine (iodophors)	Minimal	Moderately good	Moderately good	Possible irritation, allergy, and toxicity. Can be absorbed through skin.	Commonly used. Effective against mycobacteria, fungi, and viruses. Effective in the presence of organic substances. Must be rinsed thoroughly from skin. *Caution:* Care must be taken not to allow iodophor detergents to splash into the eyes.
Chlorhexidine gluconate (alcohol-detergent based)	Good with repeated use	Good	Good	Nonirritating to skin. Highly ototoxic; causes severe eye damage on contact with cornea.	Not absorbed by the skin. Not effective in the presence of organic debris except in a detergent base.
Alcohol-based skin cleaners	None	Excellent	Excellent	Damaging to mucous membranes and eyes. Nontoxic on skin. Can be very drying.	Contain skin emollients to prevent drying. If used as a surgical hand cleaner, should be preceded by thorough mechanical cleaning.
Triclosan	Moderate with repeated use	Inhibits growth	Inhibits growth	Nontoxic on skin. Absorbed through skin.	Not fungicidal. Viricidal activity unknown. Effective against *Mycobacterium tuberculosis.* Least effective of surgical hand scrubs. Use only when personnel cannot use other skin scrub agents.

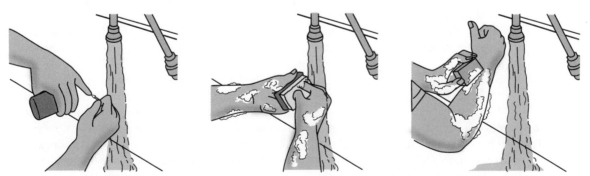

Figure 10-5 Procedure for surgical hand scrub. *(Redrawn from Rothrock: Alexander's care of the patient in surgery, ed 14, 2012, Elsevier.)*

number of microbes on the skin and provides continuous antimicrobial action. This is important, because bacteria can proliferate quickly in the moist environment between gloves and skin.

The surgical scrub is performed with a disposable sterile sponge brush combination. These are available at scrub stations along with other supplies such as soap, masks, face shields, nail cleaners, and antiseptic handrub products. The disposable prewrapped scrub sponge is impregnated with antiseptic soap. The surgical scrub is performed before donning gown and gloves, before use of handrubs when the hands are visibly soiled, and after direct exposure (skin contact) with blood or other body fluids. There are two acceptable methods. One is the timed scrub and the other is to count the number of sponge brush strokes used on each part of the hand and arm.

During the scrub, avoid splashing water on the front of the scrub suit, as this can result in contamination of the sterile gown. Turn off the tap using knee or foot control when not needed; this conserves water. The tap can be turned on for the final rinse at the end of the scrub. Always remember to discard used sponge brushes in the appropriate receptacle at the end of the scrub.

Technique

Prepare for the surgical scrub by ensuring that the scrub suit top is tucked into the scrub pants or is the proper fit so that it remains dry. Remember to adjust the surgical mask, face shield, or eyewear before starting the scrub. If you are using the timed method, allow 3 to 5 minutes total for the scrub or according to the soap manufacturer's directions. More time should be allowed if the hands or arms are very soiled. The scrub techniques for both methods (timed and counted) proceed as follows: one hand to the same arm, the opposite hand and arm. One sponge brush is used for both hands and arms. While performing the scrub, you may not return to an area that you have already scrubbed. Do not allow the scrubbed hand or arm to contact any part of the sink, faucet, or scrub suit. If any part of the hand or arm touches these, add 1 minute extra scrubbing time to that area. Avoid splashing water on the scrub suit, because this can cause contamination of the surgical gown by wicking bacteria from the nonsterile scrub suit to the sterile gown. Gather all supplies prior to surgical scrub, including choosing an appropriate hand scrub agent such as Povidone, Iodine, Chlorhexidine, alcohol based skin cleaners, or Triclosan (see Table 10-1). Open gown and gloves on a surface on which no other sterile supplies have been exposed. Don all PPE before beginning the surgical scrub.

1. Remove all jewelry and check the integrity of the skin and nails.
2. Perform routine hand washing and include the forearms, using antiseptic soap. Rinse the hands and arms thoroughly by passing the arms through the running water from hand to elbow.
3. Keep the hands and forearms above the elbow to allow water and soap to drain from the elbow, not toward the hands.
4. Unwrap a sterile scrub brush packet and remove the nail cleaner. Hold the brush in one hand while carefully cleaning the subungual area on each finger, using a nail cleaner under running water. Discard the nail cleaner in the proper receptacle.
5. Begin timing or counting strokes at this point.
6. Hold the sponge under the running water and squeeze to release soap. The scrub begins with the nails. Pass the nails back and forth across the sponge.
   Counted method: Nails—30 strokes per hand
   Timed: 2 minutes for the entire hand
7. Each finger has four sides. Scrub each side of each finger individually, between the fingers in the web spaces.
   Counted method: 10 strokes for each side of each finger and thumb
   Timed: Continuation of 2 minutes for the entire hand

8. The dorsal and palm side of the hand are scrubbed.
   Counted method: 30 strokes for each side of the hand
   Timed: 1 minute for each hand
9. The forearm has four planes. Scrub each plane separately in a circular motion to 2″ above the elbow.
   Counted method: 10 strokes for each of the four planes
   Timed: 1 minute for each arm, 2″ above the elbow covering all four planes
10. Remember to scrub one hand and arm before moving to the opposite hand and arm. At the end of the scrub, which terminates at 2″ above the elbow of the second hand and arm, drop the sponge brush into the appropriate waste receptacle.
11. Keep the hands higher than the elbows at all times, with upper arms well away from the body. When the scrub is complete, rinse the hands and arms by passing first the hand and then the arm under running water, keeping the elbows flexed. Do not move the arms back and forth through the water.
12. Avoid contact with non-sterile surfaces during the surgical scrub. If you come in contact with a non-sterile surface, You must re-scrub that area.
13. Proceed to the operating room, continuing to hold hands above the elbows and the arms away from the scrub suit. Enter by pushing the door open with your back, keeping the elbows flexed. Proceed to drying, gowning, and gloving. Make sure to dry the hands well, to facilitate smooth gloving.

SURGICAL HANDRUB

An approved, alcohol-based handrub can be used in place of the traditional surgical scrub unless mandated differently by the health care facility. Because the application of handrub products does not remove debris, the hands—including the subungual area—and arms must be thoroughly washed and dried before the product is applied. Many studies have demonstrated that, when done properly, the antiseptic hand and arm rub is as effective as the traditional surgical scrub just described, unless hands or arms are grossly soiled. In order to be completely effective, all surfaces of the hands and arms must be wet with the antiseptic product. The cidal effect of the product is dependent on the amount of time it is left on the skin, as stated by the manufacturer's guidelines. A period of 2 to 3 minutes is standard. Alcohol rub products are not dried off with a towel, but allowed to air dry.

Accumulation of the skin emollients contained in handrub products can create a sticky residue on the skin. This is uncomfortable and makes gloving more difficult. Skin residue can be removed by a thorough wash or hand scrub with no decrease in the efficacy of subsequent uses of the product. Lotions used by operating room personnel can interfere with the effect of alcohol- and even water-based disinfectants used in hand hygiene. It is very important to select a lotion that is water-soluble and does not contain petroleum products, which can interfere with the barrier properties of latex gloves. Perfumed lotions must not be used, because they can increase or cause nausea in patients.

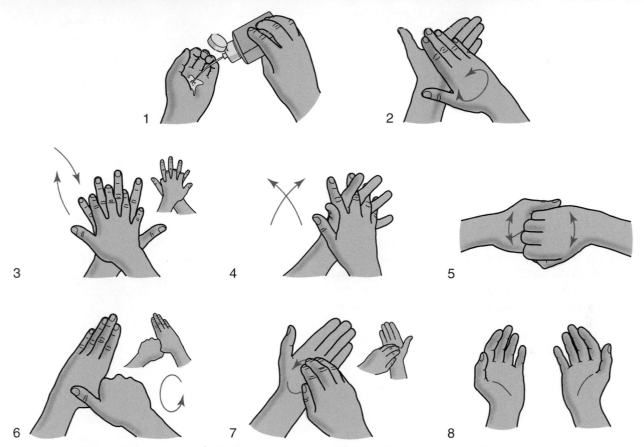

Figure 10-6 Procedure for hand and arm rub. (Based on the "How to Handwash", URL: http://www.who.int/gpsc/5may/How_To_HandWash_Poster.pdf © World Health Organization 2009. All rights reserved.)

Technique

Open gown and gloves on a surface on which no other sterile supplies have been exposed. Don mask and face shield before beginning the **surgical handrub**.

1. Following manufacturer's guidelines, dispense the appropriate amount of antiseptic liquid into the palm of one hand, using your elbow to activate the dispenser.
2. With fingers of the one hand together, dip the fingertips into the antiseptic held by the other hand. Use a circular motion several times to expose the fingernails and tips to antiseptic (5 seconds).
3. Spread antiseptic to the entire hand, including individual digits, wrist, forearm, and elbow area, covering all surfaces. Use circular movements to spread the chemical to every surface of the arm (10 to 15 seconds). Make sure there is sufficient gel to keep the skin wet.
4. Repeat the process on the opposite hand and arm. Repeat the procedure for covering fingertips, hand, wrist, and arms.
5. Finally, dispense 2 to 5 mL of rub into the palm of one hand to thoroughly cleanse the hands again. Cover all surfaces, including webs, backs, and palms. The backs of the fingers are covered by interlocking cupped hands together with a back-and-forth movement.
6. Apply rub to the web of the thumb and palm by interlocking them.

7. When hands are dry, proceed to the operating suite with forearms flexed above the elbows, ready to don sterile gown and gloves.

The handrub procedure is illustrated in Figure 10-6.

SUMMARY OF HAND HYGIENE PROCEDURES

The following is a summary of when to use each of the hand hygiene procedures. Health care facility policy may determine their use:

- Use *routine hand washing* frequently during the workday and specifically between patient contact and to remove visible soil before and following certain events that were listed earlier.
- The *traditional surgical scrub* using a sponge brush, antiseptic soap, and water is performed in place of the handrub in case of visible soil on the hand or arms following contamination of the hands or arms by potentially infectious body fluids.
- The *surgical handrub* is performed in place of a traditional surgical scrub except when the hands and arms are grossly soiled or have come in contact with body fluids. The first handrub of the day should be preceded by routine hand wash and drying with disposable towel.

GOWNING AND GLOVING

Sterile gowning and gloving occur immediately after preparation of the hands and arms for a surgical procedure. Following the surgical scrub or handrub, proceed directly to the operating suite. With your back to the door, enter the suite while still holding the arms and hands at a right angle to the body to prevent water from dripping toward the hands (following a wet scrub). This position also ensures that the hands and arms do not brush against the scrub suit, which would contaminate them. The following is the proper technique for drying the hands and arms following the **surgical hand scrub** with water and antiseptic soap (Figure 10-7):

1. After entering the operating room from the scrub sink area, proceed to the gowning and gloving table.
2. Remove the towel by grasping only the edge and lift it up and away from the sterile gown and gloves. Do not hesitate, because water may drip from the hands onto the sterile gown and gloves, which would contaminate them. If hands are dry, skip this procedure and gown directly.
3. Allow the towel to unfold so that the long edge hangs down between your two hands. Bend forward slightly at the waist so the sterile towel does not touch the scrub suit. Use one end of the towel for one hand and arm and the other end for the other hand and arm.
4. Blot the skin, working from hand to wrist to arm, without moving back over a previously dried area.
5. Keep the towel out in front of you where you can see it. After drying one hand and arm with one end of the towel, begin drying the other hand by placing the wet hand at the other end of the towel while confining it to its own side.
6. Dry the second hand and arm using the same blotting technique. Never rub the skin back and forth—always use a blotting motion, moving from hand to arm without returning to the area already dried. When you are finished, drop the towel into the appropriate receptacle. Proceed immediately to gowning.

GOWNING YOURSELF

Surgical gowns are worn by all sterile personnel. The gown is donned immediately before the start of surgery and may be changed during surgery if it is contaminated or penetrated by blood or other fluids. Most single-use gowns, particularly those used in orthopedic surgery, have a moisture-proof barrier that is laminated to the gown from the axillary line to the hips. The gown is a wrap-around type, which covers both the front and back of the wearer. However, the back is still considered nonsterile because it cannot be monitored by the wearer.

The surgical technologist or scrub nurse dons a sterile gown immediately after drying the hands (Figure 10-8).

When gowning, consider the gown as having two surfaces: an inside surface that will contact the nonsterile scrub suit and bare skin of the hands and arms, and an outside surface that will be considered sterile only from the waist to the axillary line and from the hands to the elbows.

Surgical gowns are folded inside-out before packaging. This allows scrubbed personnel to grasp the presenting surface of the gown with bare hands to put it on, because that surface

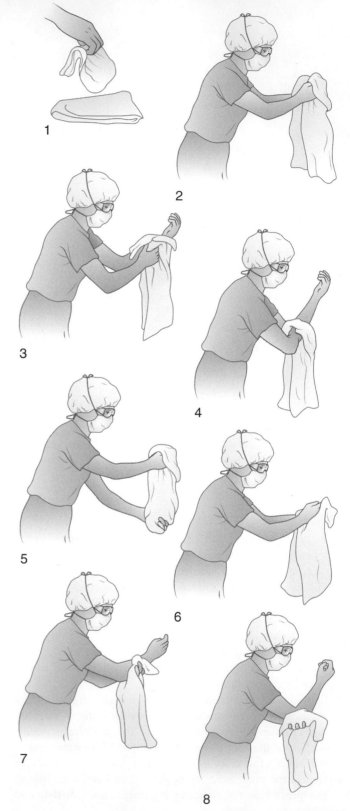

Figure 10-7 Procedure for drying the hands after the surgical scrub.

will be the nonsterile side. Care must be taken not to grasp the gown at the neckline, because the sterile (outer) section of the gown may become contaminated.

1. After drying the hands and arms, grasp the gown just below the neckline and lift it up and away from the table, without

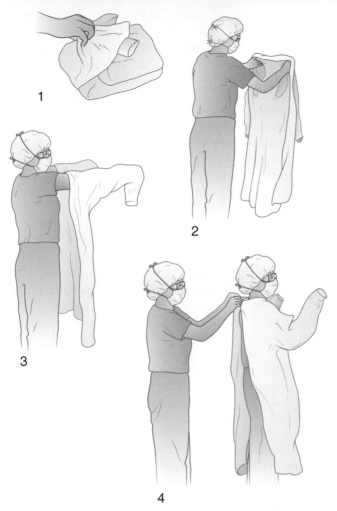

Figure 10-8 Procedure for gowning oneself.

the circulator holds the tab, he or she will pull the wrap around the back of the gown At this point it is necessary to release the gown tie from the tab. The gowned person pulls the tie sharply to release it from the tab, which is still held by the circulator. The ties can now be secured at the side of the gown.

GLOVING

Many types of surgical gloves are commercially available. The common considerations in choosing gloves are the glove material, tensile strength, thickness, and economy. Tactile sensation is important, especially in surgical specialties that require the use of fine instruments and in which delicate tissues are encountered. Thicker gloves are more appropriate for repeated contact with heavy instruments or if copious bleeding is likely, such as during orthopedic surgery.

Double gloving (wearing two pairs of surgical gloves) has been demonstrated to reduce the risk of glove failure, which increases with surgical time and prolonged handling of tissues and supplies. Glove punctures are associated with the transmission of blood-borne pathogens to health care workers and microbial contamination of the surgical site. The CDC recommends double gloving on all invasive procedures. No set rule governs glove sizes when double gloving. The outer glove can be one size larger or smaller or the same size. Using colored gloves as the first pair may make it easier to detect a puncture in the top glove. However, if there is any doubt, gloves must be changed.

Historical Highlight

Before the development of the surgical glove, surgeons operated bare-handed and disinfected the hands by dipping them into 5% hypochlorite solution (household bleach). Early surgical gloves were made of thick rubber and were washed and sterilized after each case by the instrument nurses.

Closed Gloving

Closed gloving is performed immediately after gowning. It is the most effective method for preventing contact between the skin and the outside of the sterile glove. When you are learning the closed gloving technique, think of the glove as having two surfaces or planes, the inside and the outside. Before the gloves are touched, the entire glove is sterile, inside and outside. As soon as gloving is initiated, however, the *inside* surface is considered nonsterile.

The technique for gloving is among the most difficult skills for students to learn. One of the best ways is to have an experienced person glove while you are also gloving in a practice session or dry run. Follow each step as the other person gloves. The experienced person must move slowly so that the student can follow these actions. The actions will need to be repeated in order to firmly establish correct technique. Always stand next to (not across) from the demonstrator to avoid confusion about which way the hand and glove are oriented. Take your time when learning to glove. It is better to be methodical and slow at first. Speed and efficiency will follow with practice. Students are often nervous when learning to glove. In practice sessions without a patient, the hands can be dusted with

touching anything else with bare hands. Remember, the inside surface of the gown faces inward, toward you.

2. Step away from the table and allow the gown to unfold in front of you. Do not touch the (outside) surface facing away from you.

3. Being careful not to lower the gown, look for the armholes and place your hands and arms inside the sleeves. Advance your hands, pushing them through to within about 1 inch (2.5 cm) of the knitted cuff edge. Do not allow the fingertips to extend beyond the knitted cuff and sleeve. Avoid raising your arms as you push them through the sleeves. At this point the circulator may secure the neck and inside ties. The circulator assists in securing the gown's back wrap (discussed next). Keep hands well inside the gown cuff and proceed to glove using the *closed* technique (see later discussion).

Securing the Gown Wrap

After gloving, the circulator will assist in securing the surgical gown wrap. Wraparound gowns have a paper tab attached to the front tie. The tab is used to pull the tie and wrap around the back of the gown at the side. Pass the tab carefully to the circulator. Remember to maintain sterility by not allowing your gloved hand to touch the circulator's hand. As

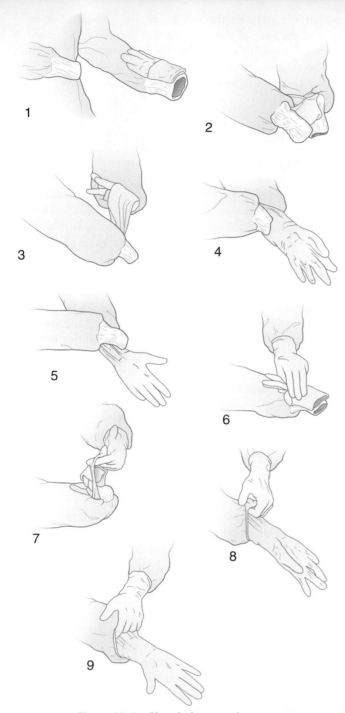

1

2

3

4

5

6

7

8

9

Figure 10-9   Closed gloving technique.

wrapper with the fingers up and the cuffed (wrist) part at the bottom edge of the wrapper. The upper and lower edges of the wrapper are folded inward. To open the wrapper, grasp the two center edges and open them outward to expose the gloves. To keep the edges from closing up again, evert them slightly; this will remove some of the memory in the folds.

3. Position the left hand with the palm facing upward, as if you are about to receive an object in your hand. Pick up the glove with your right hand shielded by the gown and place the glove, palm to palm and cuff to cuff, over the left hand. The glove is oriented correctly if the glove fingers point to your elbow.

4. Working inside the gown cuff, grasp the under edge of the glove cuff between your left thumb and fingers. Using your protected right hand, grasp the upper edge of the glove cuff. The palm of the glove should still be oriented to your palm. If it is not, you will have difficulty sliding the hand into the glove, a common problem at this point. To correct misalignment of the glove, grasp it at the cuff and realign it correctly, *palm to palm.*

5. Keep the hidden fingers within 1 inch (2.5 cm) of the outside edge of the knitted cuff, and make sure your thumb is well inside the seam of the cuff. This prevents another common obstacle, which occurs when the left hand slips back into the gown sleeve.

6. Pull the glove on. Grasp the left glove cuff and advance your left hand into the glove.

7. Repeat with the other hand. After gloving, check both hands for any sign of punctures or tears. If a defect is apparent, the circulator removes the glove, and gloving is repeated on that hand.

Open Gloving

Open gloving is used during sterile procedures that do not require a sterile gown, such as preoperative skin preparation of the patient, assisting in minor skin procedures, catheterization, and when a scrubbed member changes a glove without changing his or her gown.

When gloving, consider the two surfaces of the glove, the outside and the inside. The glove has a cuff that exposes the *inside* of the glove. This inner surface is considered the nonsterile surface, even though it is sterile until touched with the bare hand. The outside remains sterile. The wrapper is considered sterile to within 1 inch (2.5 cm) of the edges.

The following are the steps in the technique for open gloving (Figure 10-10). In this description, the right hand is gloved first.

1. Open the outer nonsterile wrapper and deliver the inner sterile wrapped gloves onto a clean, dry surface.

2. Grasp the edges of the glove wrapper with bare hands and expose the gloves. Before releasing the glove wrapper, make sure that it will stay open. The palms of the gloves should be facing upward, thumbs to the outside.

3. Using your left hand, grasp the uppermost side of the right glove cuff. Do not touch the wrapper underneath or the outside of the glove. Pick up the glove and slide your right hand into it, keeping your hand palm up, oriented to the

cornstarch, which dries the skin and helps gloves slide onto the hand more easily.

Use the following technique to perform closed gloving. In this description the left hand is gloved first, but the right hand can also be gloved first (Figure 10-9):

1. Begin closed gloving after donning a sterile gown. Do not allow your fingers to protrude outside the knitted cuff of the gown. You will maneuver sterile gloves onto your hands with your hands hidden from view under the gown's cuffs.

2. The glove wrapper is folded so that the side edges come together at the middle. The gloves are oriented in the

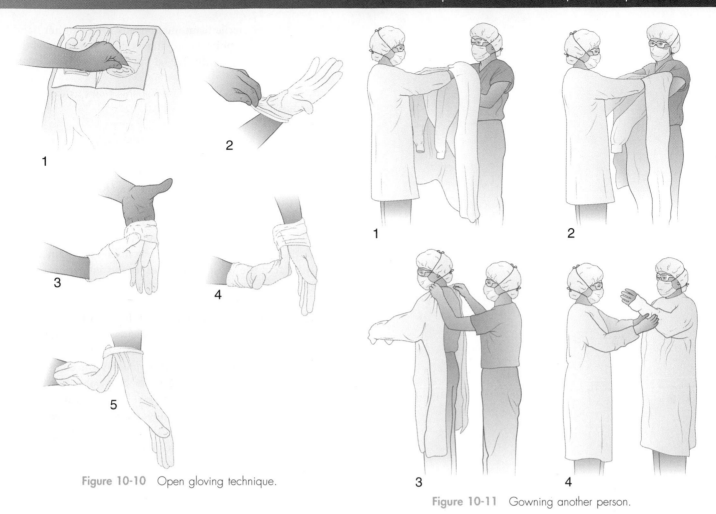

Figure 10-10 Open gloving technique.

Figure 10-11 Gowning another person.

palm of the glove. Leave the cuff turned down until you glove the other hand.

4. To glove the left hand, slide the fingers of your sterile gloved hand under the cuff. This positions your gloved hand (sterile) in contact with the outside (sterile) surface of the other glove. Keep the palm up as you slide your bare hand into the glove. You may unroll the cuff carefully, but do not allow the gloved hand to touch any bare skin.

When learning to glove, students sometimes experience difficulty removing the glove from the open sterile wrapper. Very thin or short-cuffed gloves are difficult to put on without contaminating the sterile side of the glove or the glove wrapper. Remember that as long as you do not touch the sterile surface with your nonsterile fingers, you have not contaminated either one.

GOWNING AND GLOVING OTHER TEAM MEMBERS

After the surgical technologist has set up sterile supplies and instruments, the other members of the surgical team enter from the scrub sink area. Gowning and gloving of the other team members precede all other activities and are as much a social tradition as a necessary part of the surgical routine. During gowning and gloving, the surgeon greets the scrub,

circulator, and anesthesiologist and may introduce other members of the team. This time allows formal acknowledgment of the team members and what is to be done before the actual start of surgery. The surgeon also may clarify the need for special instruments or equipment at this time. Interaction among team members during the process of gowning and gloving often sets the tone for the entire surgery.

When the sterile team members enter the operating room, the scrub hands an unfolded towel to the surgical team leader (lead surgeon) and then to the other members of the team.

Gowning Other Team Members

The following technique is used to gown other team members (Figure 10-11):

1. When the team member reaches out for a towel for drying, pass the sterile towel over the team member's hand so that the long edge of the towel falls between the person's two hands.
2. Grasp the folded gown, step away from any nonsterile surface, and allow the gown to unfold. Create a cuff over your gloved hands by placing them below the neckline and shoulders (away from the top edge) as shown in Figure 10-11. Position the gown so that the person you are gowning can easily insert his or her hands into the armholes as shown.

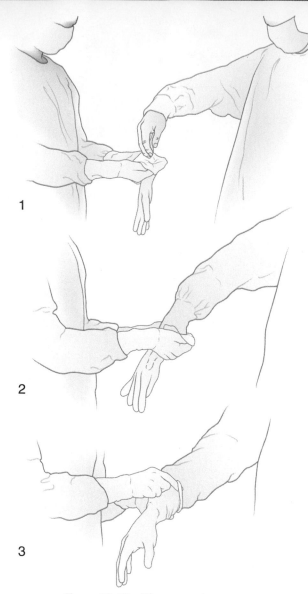

1

2

3

Figure 10-12   Gloving another person.

3. After the team member has stepped forward and placed his or her arms into the sleeves, the circulator will pull the gown up by grasping the neckline or inside of the shoulder seams. Once the gown is fitted over the shoulders, pull the sleeves up to expose the person's hands and proceed to gloving immediately. The circulator will secure the back of the gown.

Gloving a Gowned Team Member

The following technique is used to glove a gowned team member (Figure 10-12):

1. Open the glove wrapper and place the gloves and wrapper near you on the sterile table.
2. Grasp the glove under the cuff and spread the opening with your thumbs held well away from the glove or tucked securely under the cuff.
3. Orient the glove so that the palm of the glove faces the person you are gloving. Offer the right glove first, then the left.

4. Make sure the sterile team member inserts his or her hand into the glove by pointing all fingers downward. Allow the cuff edge to recoil gently. Repeat the process with the other glove.
5. The gown wrap can be secured at this point as described previously.

CONTAMINATION OF GLOVE OR GOWN

Gowns are considered sterile from the chest to the level of the sterile field and 2 inches above the elbows to the cuffs. Cuffs are contaminated when the hands extend beyond them within the glove. Therefore, the cuff must not be exposed. This can occur when the sleeves are pulled up inadvertently during a procedure. The cuff edge of the gown must remain at or slightly beyond the wrist at all times to prevent exposure.

Contaminated Glove

Contact between the sterile glove and a nonsterile surface results in contamination of the glove, which must be replaced with a new sterile glove. Note the following:

- *The sterile team member is double-gloved*: If the contamination is a puncture, both the inner and outer gloves are changed. If contamination occurred by direct contact with a nonsterile surface, only the upper glove is changed.
- *The sterile team member is single-gloved*: The glove is changed as soon as possible. If this is not practical, a sterile glove may be placed over the contaminated glove, using open technique until the gloves can be changed.* The following steps should be followed when replacing a contaminated glove:

1. The sterile team member presents the contaminated gloved hand to the circulator palm upward (Figure 10-13).
2. The circulator, wearing nonsterile gloves, grasps the contaminated glove below the wrist and removes it.
3. The preferred method of replacing a single glove is to ask another sterile team member to glove the hand using closed technique (assisted gloving) as described earlier. If this is not possible, open glove technique is used.
4. If only the top glove is contaminated, the glove can be replaced using open-gloving technique.

Contaminated Gown

If the gown is contaminated during surgery, both the gown and gloves must be changed:

- The contaminated team member steps away from the sterile field to allow the circulator access to the gown. The circulator pulls the gown forward off the shoulders, bundling it inward to contain the front, which has been exposed to blood and body fluids.
- Another team member may regown the person, or he or she can gown and glove themselves using closed technique as described earlier.

*AORN: Perioperative standards and recommended practices, 2011 edition, Denver, 2011, AORN.

Contaminated Sleeve

Many health care facilities allow the use of sterile sleeves that can be fitted over a contaminated sleeve. The replacement sleeve must be manufactured to the same standards of quality and impermeability as the gown. There are no established standards for this as long as the sleeve can be donned without a break in aseptic technique. Another person can assist by cuffing the top of the sleeve while the arm is inserted. If this is not possible, one can don the new sleeve by maintaining a wide cuff for one hand while slipping the sleeve over the contaminated arm. The top of the sleeve must be released in a way that prevents the gloved hand from touching the contaminated sleeve more than 2 inches above the elbow.

REMOVING STERILE ATTIRE

When removing sterile attire, always remove the gown first and then remove the gloves (Figure 10-14):

1. To remove a disposable gown, grasp the gown at the shoulders and pull downward and forward, away from the body, turning the sleeves inside out. This releases or breaks the closures. Roll the gown inside out as it slides over your arms and gloved hands. Try not to rip the gown off forcefully, as this can release contaminated particles into the environment. Cloth gowns must be untied at the neck and back by the circulator.
2. Roll the gown so that the contaminated outside surface is contained inward.
3. Dispose of the gown in a biohazard bag.

Gloves are removed after the gown (Figure 10-15):

1. Grasp one glove at the inner wrist, using the opposite gloved hand. Pinch the cuff with the opposite hand.
2. Pull the glove off. It will turn inside out as you remove it.
3. Place bare fingers inside the cuff of the opposite hand without touching the soiled glove and roll it off your hand.
4. Dispose of both gloves in a biohazard receptacle without touching the outside of the gloves.

Watch Section 2 Unit 4: Scrubbing, Gowning and Gloving on the Evolve website. http://evolve.elsevier.com/Fuller/surgical

Remember—glove to glove, bare skin to bare skin when removing a soiled glove.

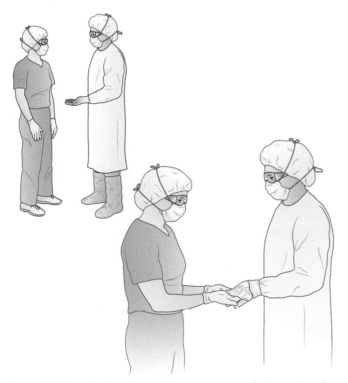

Figure 10-13 Circulator removing a contaminated glove. Note that the circulator does not touch the scrub's glove with bare hands.

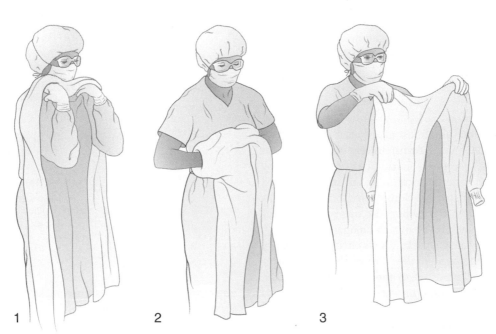

1   2   3

Figure 10-14 Removing the gown using aseptic technique. Note that the gown is immediately turned inside out to contain the contaminated side.

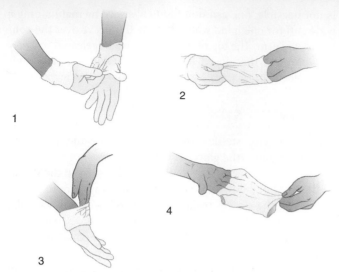

Figure 10-15 Procedure for removing contaminated gloves. Note that the bare hand does not touch the outside of the glove.

OPENING A CASE

Opening a case means to prepare the surgical suite for a procedure and open sterile items. All equipment and furniture are arranged, and sterile supplies are brought into the room.

Depending on the complexity of the surgery, the amount of equipment to be prepared, and the degree of emergency, the scrub and circulator open the case about 15 to 20 minutes before the start of surgery. In extremely large cases, more time may be needed for opening supplies and setting up.

After the case is opened, the sterile items should be monitored constantly. The ideal technique is to have someone physically in the room to observe the sterile setup. Covering the setup with a sterile drape is not recommended because of the risk of contamination when the cover is removed. Leaving a room vacant and posting a sign on the door advising staff members that the case is open also is not an acceptable practice.

LINEN PACK

Linen packs are included in almost all surgical setups. These include linen or nonwoven gowns, towels, and other soft items. Preassembled case packs can be custom-designed by the institution to include surgical supplies routinely used during specific types of surgery. Some commonly preassembled packs include abdominal, orthopedic, and minor surgery packs. The large case pack is the first to be opened.

Before opening any sterile pack, always check the integrity of the outside of the package and the external chemical indicators for verification of exposure to the sterilization process. Any packages with tears, holes, or water marks are contaminated and should be removed from the room for reprocessing and replaced with new packs.

The large pack is opened on the back table, because that is the center of the scrub's work area. After the large pack is

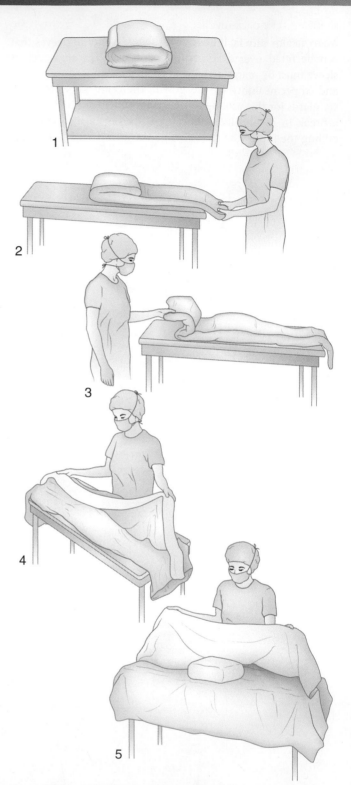

Figure 10-16 Procedure for opening a linen pack on the back table. The linen pack usually is opened first to provide a sterile surface on which other items can be distributed.

unwrapped, instruments, suture packs, and other sterile items are opened onto the draped surface and later organized and set up in logical order.

The following technique is used to open the large pack on the back table (Figure 10-16):

1. Center the pack on the table and orient it so that the long ends of the outside drape line up with the long end of the table.
2. If the pack is very large and has been square-wrapped, the recommended practice is to move around the package rather than reaching across it. In this case, grasp the folded edge of the top fold with both hands and pull the edges toward you.
3. Move to the other side of the table and repeat this process on the opposite top fold. Allow 1 inch (2.5 cm) of margin between the edge of the drape and your nonsterile hand. Remember not to lean over the table while opening the pack.
4. Do not readjust the table drape after it has been opened.

INSTRUMENT TRAYS

The following technique is used by nonsterile personnel to open an instrument tray properly (Figure 10-17):

1. When opening large instrument trays or other heavy equipment, set the tray on a small table and open it in place.
2. A nonsterile person opening a sterile pack should position themselves in a way that allows opening the wrap without stretching the arm or hand over it. Never lean over the sterile pack or tray to open the far side of the wrap. Reaching over a sterile surface violates a basic principle of aseptic technique.
3. Open each side flap individually.
4. Drape small tables in the same manner. Place the drape on the table. Grasp only the edges of the drape to unfold the drape. Flaps must be opened in such a way that the nonsterile arm and hand do not reach across the sterile surface. Move around the table if necessary, always bringing the edge of the drape toward you.
5. As sterile items are opened, use more tables if necessary.
6. Do not stack heavy sterile instruments precariously high or in such a way that they might be dropped.

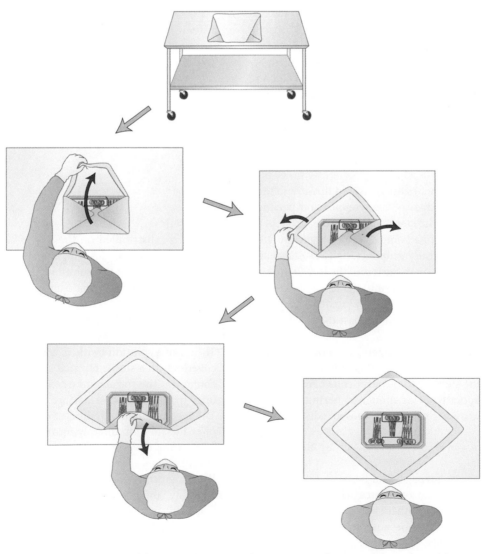

Figure 10-17 Method used by nonsterile personnel to open a small instrument tray on a table. Note the order in which each flap is folded back to prevent contamination by the hand and arm.

7. Avoid holding a heavy instrument tray in one hand and removing the wrapper with the other. This puts excessive strain on the wrist, and you may drop the tray. Instead, use additional small tables.

BASINS

Basin sets are placed on a ring stand and opened in the same manner as large instrument trays. Do not reach over the basin to open it. It is better technique to move around the sterile package and pull the flaps toward you.

If water is found in a basin when the sterile wrapper is opened, the basin is considered contaminated. This is caused by a problem in steam sterilization, and the central service department must be notified. The load in which the basin was sterilized will be located, and those items will be removed from service.

DELIVERING STERILE GOODS ASEPTICALLY

When items are opened during the setup and the scrub is sterile, the circulator opens these items and delivers them aseptically. The circulator opens envelope-wrapped trays or other small items by grasping the top flap and peeling it back and down. Side flaps are opened next, followed by the near flap. As the flaps are peeled back from the sterile item, they cover the circulator's nonsterile hand so that the item can be passed safely to the scrub. The scrub may take the item directly (Figure 10-18), or the circulator may carefully set the item on a sterile surface without allowing contamination of the object (e.g., tray, instrument) or the sterile surface.

Peel Pouches

Items wrapped in sealed pouches are delivered directly to the scrub by grasping the top edges of the wrapper and peeling the wrapper apart to reveal the sterile item (Figure 10-19, *A*). Suture packets also can be flipped onto the field (Figure 10-19, *B*). This is done by opening the peel pouch halfway and then quickly popping the wrapper open the rest of the way to propel the contents out of the package and onto the sterile field. Do not reach over the sterile surface when flipping items onto the field. Take care to avoid flipping the item past the sterile field and onto the floor.

When opening peel pouch wrappers, do not allow the item to slide out of the package; this contaminates it, because the edge of the sterile pack is never considered sterile. Instead, peel the wrapper back far enough to permit the item to drop out cleanly, away from the exposed edges of the wrapper.

Sharps

Scalpel blades and other **sharps** should be passed directly to the scrub or unwrapped in an open area where they are in plain view. Blades, trocars, and other sharps should not to be opened into instrument trays, because the sharps can be hidden by other instruments. If a sharp item is accidentally covered during opening, warn the scrubbed team of its location to prevent injury during the setup.

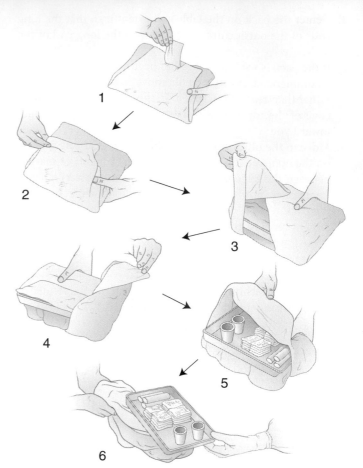

Figure 10-18 Procedure for distributing wrapped items. Note that the nonsterile (outside) of the wrapper does not touch the sterile inner surfaces.

Solutions

Solutions are distributed on the sterile field so that the fluid does not come in contact with the side of the bottle or any area below the sterile lip. Solutions are manufactured so that the cap can be removed aseptically, preserving the inner lip of the container.

The recommended practice for distributing solutions is as follows:

1. The lip of a solution bottle is considered sterile only if it is covered with a sterile top that extends over the edge of the container. The top must be removed by pulling it straight up, which protects the sterility of the inner lip.
2. The recommended method of distributing a solution is to pour the solution directly into a container set close to the edge of the table or held in the hand of the scrub (Figure 10-20).
3. When pouring sterile liquids, empty the entire container and move the downturned container away from the sterile field. This prevents any liquid from running over the edge of the container and contaminating the field. *After the bottle has been opened and its contents poured, the lip of the bottle is no longer considered sterile. All of the solution must be distributed at one time.*

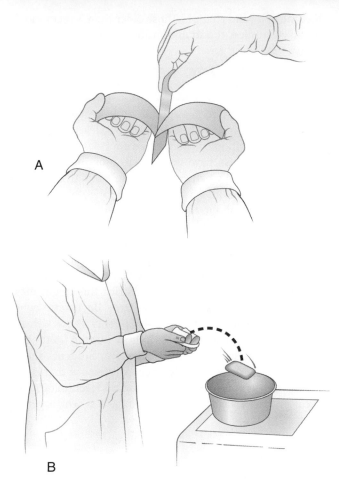

Figure 10-19 **A,** Distributing suture contained in a peel pouch wrapper. **B,** Suture packs may be flipped onto the sterile field. *(Redrawn from Phillips N: Berry and Kohn's operating room technique, ed 10, St Louis, 2004, Mosby.)*

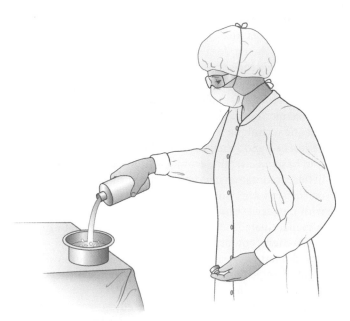

Figure 10-20 Distributing sterile liquids to a sterile container. Note that the bottle is not suspended directly over the sterile bowl. *(Redrawn from Phillips N: Berry and Kohn's operating room technique, ed 10, St Louis, 2004, Mosby.)*

4. Never remove the cap of a medicine vial using an instrument and then pouring out the contents. The lip of the vial is potentially contaminated by the instrument. (Chapter 13 presents a complete discussion of the sterile distribution of drugs.)

CONTAMINATION DURING SURGERY

When an item or surface becomes contaminated during surgery, it must be isolated or removed from the sterile field. Contamination events must be treated on a case by case basis. Instruments and other small items can be passed off to the circulator without handling the contaminated end. Scrubbed team members need to reglove or regown in the event of their contamination.

When draped equipment or the sterile field becomes contaminated, all items in the area of the contamination must be passed off to the circulator. The contaminated surface is then contained with a *nonpermeable* drape. If the boundaries of the contamination are not clear, a wide area of containment or covering is necessary.

REALITY VERSUS STANDARDS

As surgical personnel develop experience, they clarify their own practices and compare them with those of the people around them. Even after acquiring excellent technique, people may consciously (or unconsciously) disregard certain practices because of lack of peer or administrative support, lack of professional motivation, or simple apathy. Some professionals become very discouraged when others in the department do not support efforts to maintain high standards. Standards vary slightly according to the practice setting and the policies of individual institutions. Surgical personnel can and should discuss the aseptic technique practices of their team, department, or institution as long as they have *evidence* to demonstrate that these practices are below the normal safety standard. Always remember, however, that criticism of those in your internship facility will probably not be welcomed. Each individual must try to practice the highest standards possible, even if colleagues are not supportive.

EVIDENCE-BASED PRACTICE IN ASEPTIC TECHNIQUE

Aseptic technique is an area of perioperative practice that is frequently and often enthusiastically debated among health professionals, organizations, and infection control specialists. Today, there are many good studies that cover the most important areas of infection control in the operating room.

USING EVIDENCE-BASED PRACTICE

Evidence-based practice does not rely on *past* practices to define *current* ones. It relies on science and evidence rather than opinion or tradition. Evidence-based practice considers only best practices based on current research.

Evidence-based practices are rooted in the following questions:

- Why is this technique used in this situation?
- What is the rationale (logical, reasoned basis) behind a particular practice or procedure?
- Is this the *best* (e.g., beneficial, scientifically based, most effective) way to accomplish this? What is the evidence that this works?

Evidence-based practice provides rationales for all the standards and recommendations made by professional organizations in disease transmission, biotechnology, patient safety, and advances in surgical practice. Throughout this text, you will see sections titled Standards and Recommendations. These sections list the professional bodies that have been established as authoritative sources of information for that area of practice. No professional organization would attempt to set a standard without first carrying out the scientific studies or research required to support that standard. When we follow a directive in the operating room, we always have the right to ask, "What is the rationale for this and what is it based on?" If there is no evidence-based rationale, the practice may not be valid.

EXAMPLES OF EVIDENCE-BASED PRACTICE

The following are just a few examples of evidence-based practice.

1. *Double gloving.* In the past, double gloving (wearing two pairs of sterile surgical gloves) was practiced only in orthopedic cases in which heavy cutting instruments were used. Glove splitting and tearing are common in traditional orthopedic surgery. The current practice is for all scrubbed personnel to double glove, regardless of the type of surgery. This is based on numerous studies arising from the risk of blood-borne diseases and rates of contamination arising from glove tear or puncture.

2. *Surgical hand scrub.* Historically, the 10-minute scrub was a symbol of excellent aseptic technique. Use of a stiff brush and strong antiseptic was considered the only method adequate for preparing the hands before every surgical procedure. Raw skin and dermatitis were common among scrub personnel. Studies now show that vigorous scrubbing breaks down the skin, reducing its natural barrier against microorganisms and inviting infection. The surgical handrub, using an approved alcohol-based antiseptic, has been shown to be at least as effective as the hand scrub, as long as visible dirt is removed. Without evidence based on valid testing procedures the handrub would not have been acceptable in the past because of the highly regarded tradition of the 10-minute hand and arm scrub.

3. *Annotated research.* All professional journals and textbooks have an ethical responsibility to publish information that is based on research and evidence. Recommendations for techniques and standards must be backed up by a reference to the evidence. This may be in the form of a citation, a bibliography, or a list of references that states a *recent* (usually within the past 5 years) source of the information that is established as an authority. Five years is the usual lifetime of a valid citation. Those older than 5 years should be suspect unless the source has been revalidated.

LEARNING HOW TO RESEARCH: PRACTICES AND STANDARDS

Students should begin to incorporate evidence-based practice into their profession from the day they being learning. Curiosity and academic inquiry should lead to a desire to validate the learning. You also have the right to look up these references and determine whether they are authoritative.

The Internet provides a vast amount of information for students to learn about their chosen profession. However, students should seek evidence that the website is authoritative and presents evidence-based information. Just because something is on a website or in print does not mean it is true. If there are no references, or the references are outdated and do not seem to be based on authority, this might mean that the author bypassed this standard. Be careful when using websites that are edited by the public. These websites do not validate the qualifications of those putting up the data or the methods used to reach conclusions. Students should always check the dates of a reference. A reference that is 8 or 10 years old is questionable for today's technology and medical practices. If it is worth learning, it is worth getting it right.

KEY CONCEPTS

- Evidence-based practice is a way of making decisions and acting on proven methods. It uses rational decision making rather than opinion or past practice. Methods derived through evidence-based practice can be traced to accepted authority (peer review) and the highest level of professional inquiry.
- Professional surgical technologists are engaged in health care practices that use evidence-based knowledge and methods. The modern surgical technologist must be familiar with evidence-based thinking and acting.
- Aseptic technique is a method of preventing contamination of instruments, supplies, and equipment used in critical and semicritical areas of the body.
- Aseptic technique is based on a set of principles that must be learned and practiced until they are intuitive.
- The basis of aseptic technique is the concept of barriers between contaminated and sterile surfaces. Sterile objects or surfaces are contained or confined to prevent contact with nonsterile objects.
- A contaminated surface is one that has potentially or actually come in contact with a nonsterile object.
- The domains of aseptic technique include surgical attire, hand hygiene, gowning and gloving, surgical drapes, and techniques for handling sterile equipment.
- Perioperative personnel are required to wear scrub suit attire that has been freshly laundered and not previously worn.
- A surgical cap is worn to cover all hair, which can be a source of bacterial contamination in the environment.

- During surgery, a sterile gown and gloves are worn as barriers between nonsterile skin and clothing and the surgical wound and sterile equipment.
- The sterile field is the area covered by sterile drapes. It includes scrubbed personnel who are gowned and gloved. The draped patient is the center of the sterile field.
- The rules of asepsis include methods of moving around the sterile field, the distribution of sterile supplies and equipment, and methods of preserving sterility.
- Surgical conscience is the practice of aseptic technique, reporting when sterility has been broken, and taking measures to reestablish sterility when necessary. In cases of gross contamination of the surgical wound, medical therapy may be initiated to prevent infection.

REVIEW QUESTIONS

1. What is the purpose of aseptic technique?
2. How do standards agencies decide on rules of aseptic technique?
3. What strategy would you advise for another student who is extremely nervous about gowning and gloving?
4. As a student, would you let the surgeon know if he contaminated his glove during surgery?
5. How would you go about researching a question related to aseptic technique? Would you use Wikipedia?
6. Transient microorganisms are found on the uppermost layer of the skin. Where are resident microbes found?
7. While putting on sterile gloves, you touch the glove wrapper with your finger. Is the wrapper still sterile?
8. What is the sterile field?

CASE STUDIES

Case 1

After you have performed the hand scrub, you enter the surgery suite and proceed to the area where your gown and gloves are located. As you are removing the towel, you notice that some water from your hand has dripped onto your sterile gown. What will you do?

Case 2

During surgery, you notice that the surgeon has a hole in his glove. You notify him of this. He replies, "Don't worry about it." How will you respond?

Case 3

During surgery, you are moving a heavy instrument tray from one area of the sterile table to another. As you pick up the tray, the corner of the instrument tray accidentally rips the sterile sheet covering the entire back table. What will you do?

Case 4

When you open your sterile basins while setting up a case, you notice moisture on the inside of one of the basins. What is the significance of this?

Case 5

After gowning, you are donning your sterile gloves when you puncture the glove, creating a large hole. What should you do? What is the proper technique for correcting this problem?

Case 6

After gowning the surgeon, you notice a large tear in the sleeve of the surgeon's gown. What should you do? What is the proper technique for correcting this problem?

BIBLIOGRAPHY

Association of periOperative Registered Nurses (AORN): *Standards, recommended practices and guidelines, 2011 edition*, Denver, 2011, AORN.

Association of Surgical Technologists (AST): *Standards of practice*. Accessed July 3, 2012, at http://www.ast.org.

Centers for Disease Control and Prevention: *Airborne precautions*. Accessed August 23, 2011, at http://www.cdc.gov/hicpac/2007ip /2007isolationprecautions.html.

Centers for Disease Control and Prevention: *Contact precautions*. Accessed August 23, 2011, at http://www.cdc.gov/ncidod/dhqp/ gl_isolation_contact.html.

Occupational and Safety and Health Administration: Bloodborne pathogens. In *Code of Federal Regulations* 29 CFR 1910.1030. Accessed April 12, 2012 at http://cfr.vlex.com/ vid/1910-1030-bloodborne-pathogens-19686796

Sehulster L, Chinn R: Control Guidelines for Environmental Infection Control in Health-care Facilities: Recommendations of CDC and the Healthcare Infection Control Practices Advisory Committee (HICPAC), *MMWR* 52(RR10):1–42, 2003.

World Health Organization: WHO guidelines on hand hygiene in health care, Geneva, 2009, World Health Organization. Accessed August 23, 2011, at whqlibdoc.who.int/ publications/2009/9789241597906_eng.

11

Decontamination, Sterilization, and Disinfection

LEARNING OBJECTIVES

After studying this chapter the reader will be able to:

1. Review the standards and recommendations related to aseptic technique
2. Correctly use terms related to disinfection and sterilization
3. Distinguish between the process of sterilization and other processes that render objects clean
4. Explain the Spaulding system of classification for selecting a reprocessing system
5. Describe the steps of reprocessing from the point of use to sterilization
6. Describe the principles and processes of decontamination

7. Describe the different methods of sterilization used for instruments
8. Explain the rationale for proper wrapping of instruments and loading of the steam sterilizer
9. Explain the principles of gas sterilization
10. Describe special processing required for instruments exposed to CJD
11. Distinguish between disinfection and sterilization
12. Recognize the hazards associated with the use of chemical disinfectants
13. Describe terminal decontamination of the operating room environment and equipment

TERMINOLOGY

Association for the Advancement of Medical Instrumentation (AAMI): The AAMI is an authoritative source of standards for sterilization and disinfection.

Antisepsis: A process that greatly reduces the number of microorganisms on skin or other tissue.

Bactericidal: Able to kill bacteria.

Bacteriostatic: Chemical agent capable of inhibiting the growth of bacteria.

Biofilms: Dense colonies of bacteria that adhere tightly to surfaces. Biofilms, which are resistant to chemical disinfectants and scrubbing, are a matrix of extracellular polymers produced by microorganisms. These substances bind the microorganisms tightly to a living or nonliving surface, making them highly resistant to antimicrobial action.

Biological indicator: A quality control mechanism used in the process of sterilization. It consists of a closed system containing harmless, spore-forming bacteria that can be rapidly cultured after the sterilization process.

Case cart system: A method of receiving clean and sterile equipment and preparing it for transportation to a central decontamination area. All equipment is contained within a covered movable storage cart.

Cavitation: A process in which air bubbles are imploded (burst inward), releasing particles of soil or tissue debris.

Central Processing (CP) department: The area of the hospital where medical devices and equipment are processed; also called Central Surgical Supply or the Surgical Processing department.

Central Processing technicians: Skilled professionals who specialize in processing and maintenance of medical devices used in the health care facility.

Chemical indicator: A method of testing a sterilization parameter. Chemical strips sensitive to physical conditions, such as temperature, are placed with the item being sterilized and change color when the parameter is reached; sometimes called a chemical monitor.

Chemical sterilization: A process that uses chemical agents to achieve sterilization.

-cidal: A suffix indicating death. For example, *bactericidal* means "able to kill bacteria."

Cleaning: A process that removes organic or inorganic soil or debris using detergent and washing.

Cobalt-60 radiation: A method of institutional bulk sterilization used by manufacturers to sterilize prepackaged equipment using ionizing radiation.

TERMINOLOGY (cont.)

Contaminated: Rendered nonsterile and unacceptable for use in critical areas of the body.

Decontamination: A process in which recently used and soiled medical devices, including instruments, are rendered safe for personnel to handle.

Detergent: A chemical that breaks down organic debris by emulsification (separation into small particles) to aid in cleaning.

Disinfection: Destruction of microorganisms by heat or chemical means. Spores usually are not destroyed by disinfection.

Enzymatic cleaner: A specific chemical used in detergents and cleaners to penetrate and break down biological debris, such as blood and tissue.

Ethylene oxide (EO): A highly flammable gas that is capable of sterilizing an object.

Event-related sterility: A wrapped sterile item may become contaminated by environmental conditions or events, such as a puncture in the wrapper. Event-related sterility refers to sterility based on the absence of such events. The shelf life of a sterilized pack is event related, not time related.

Evidence-based practices: Methods and procedures proven to be valid by rigorous testing and professional research.

Exposure time: This is the amount of time goods are held at a specific time, temperature, and pressure during a sterilization process. Exposure time varies with the size of the load, type of materials being sterilized, and type of sterilizer. Exposure time is sometimes called the hold time.

Fungicidal: Able to kill fungi.

Gas plasma sterilization: A process that uses the form of matter known as plasma (e.g., hydrogen peroxide plasma) to sterilize an item. Also referred to as plasma sterilization.

Germicidal: Able to kill germs (bacteria).

Gravity displacement sterilizer: A type of sterilizer that removes air by gravity.

High level disinfection (HLD): A process that reduces the bioburden to an absolute minimum.

High-vacuum sterilizer: A type of steam sterilizer that removes air in the chamber by vacuum and refills it with pressurized steam. Also known as a prevacuum sterilizer.

Inanimate: Nonliving.

Implant: Defined by the U.S. Food and Drug Administration (FDA) as "a device that is placed into a surgically or naturally formed cavity of the human body if it is intended to remain there for a period of 30 days or more."

Immediate-use sterilization: Items to be sterilized shortly before surgery must be processed so they are ready as close to the time of surgery as possible. This is referred to as immediate-use sterilization, previously called *flash sterilization*.

International Association of Healthcare Central Service Material Management (IAHCSMM): International organization that represents Central Service Technicians by providing opportunities for continuing education, professional development, and communication among its members. IAHCSMM offers certification programs for Certified Registered Central Service Technician (CRCST), Certified Instrument Specialist (CIS), and Certified in Healthcare Leadership (CHL).

Material Safety Data Sheet (MSDS): A government-mandated requirement for all chemicals used in the workplace. The MSDS describes the formulation, safe use, precautions, and emergency response. The MSDS must be available for each chemical an employee is required to handle in his or her work.

Medical device: Any equipment, instrument, implant, material, or apparatus used for the diagnosis, treatment, or monitoring of patients.

Noncritical items: Items that are not required to be sterile because they do not penetrate intact tissues. Patient care items such as a blood pressure cuff and a stethoscope are noncritical.

Nonwoven: A fabric or material that is bonded together as opposed to a process of interweaving individual threads.

Peracetic acid: A chemical used in the sterilization of critical items.

Personal protective equipment (PPE): Approved attire worn during the reprocessing of medical devices and the cleaning of patient areas. PPE protects the wearer from contamination by microorganisms.

Prion: Proteinaceous infectious particle, a unique pathogenic substance that contains no nucleic acid. The prion is transmitted by direct contact or ingestion and is resistant to all forms of disinfection and sterilization normally used in the health care setting.

Process challenge monitoring: A sealed, harmless bacteriological sample included in a load of goods to be sterilized. The sample is recovered following the sterilization process and cultured to test for viability. This process is also called biological monitoring.

Reprocessing: Activities or tasks that prepare used medical devices for use on another patient; these activities include cleaning, disinfection, decontamination, and sterilization.

Reusable: A designation used by manufacturers to indicate that a medical device can be reprocessed for use on more than one patient.

Sanitation: A method that reduces the number of bacteria in the environment to a safe level.

Sharps: Any objects used in health care that are capable of penetrating the skin, causing injury.

Shelf life: The length of time a wrapped item remains sterile after it has been subjected to a sterilization process.

Single-use items: Instruments and devices intended for use on one patient only; sometimes called disposable items.

Spaulding system: A system used to determine the level of microbial destruction required for medical devices and supplies based on the risk of infection associated with the area of the body where the device is used. Categories include critical, semicritical, and noncritical.

Sporicidal: Able to kill spores.

Sterilization: A process by which all microorganisms, including spores, are destroyed.

Terminal decontamination: Thorough cleaning and disinfection of supplies or an environment such as the operating room suite after patient use. Specific protocols and procedures are used during terminal decontamination.

Ultrasonic cleaner: Equipment that cleans instruments using ultrasonic waves.

Viricidal: Able to kill viruses.

Washer-sterilizer/disinfector: Equipment that washes and decontaminates instruments after an operative procedure.

Woven wrappers: Also called linen or cloth wrappers, these are fabric cloths used to wrap clean, disinfected supplies in preparation for a sterilization process.

INTRODUCTION

In the community, people avoid infection through hygiene practices, public health measures such as vaccination, and healthy lifestyle behaviors. In the perioperative setting, patients are vulnerable to infection by instruments, equipment, surgical drapes, and medical supplies used during a surgical procedure. The environment, including operating room furniture (e.g., instrument tables, operating table), floors, and even the air, is also a potential source of infection. This chapter provides the knowledge and methods required to prevent disease transmission by instruments, medical devices, supplies, and the surgical environment. The concepts and practices presented in this chapter bring together the science of microbiology and the recommended processes and practices for reducing the risk of infection through decontamination, disinfection, and sterilization. The health facility is a congested setting in which pathogens have ample opportunity to thrive. The purpose of decontamination, disinfection, and sterilization is to control the spread of disease by eliminating or reducing the number of microbes and preventing their proliferation on the equipment used in patient care. All procedures for decontamination of equipment and the surgical environment are performed to prevent disease transmission, and apply to patients and staff.

STANDARDS AND REGULATIONS

Standards for sterilization and disinfection of instruments, devices, and equipment in the perioperative environment are based on evidence established only after research has been conducted to prove the validity of a practice. The following organizations are responsible for performing the research or validating standards based on the evidence. The organizations are listed in alphabetical order:

- *Association for the Advancement of Medical Instrumentation (AAMI):* The AAMI provides recommended practices and technical information for the U.S. medical professions. Standards are developed with the support of the U.S. Food and Drug Administration (FDA). http://www.aami.org.
- *Association of periOperative Registered Nurses (AORN):* AORN is the professional association for perioperative nurses that publishes standards and guidelines of practice for all areas of perioperative care. http://www.aorn.org.
- *Association of Surgical Technologists:* The AST is the professional organization of surgical technologists that publishes guidelines for many practices in the perioperative setting. http://www.ast.org.
- *Centers for Disease Control and Prevention (CDC):* The federal agency that provides research and protocols in all areas of public health. http://www.cdc.gov.
- *Centers for Disease Control and Prevention and Prevention-Healthcare Infection Control Practices Advisory Committee (CDC-HICPAC):* Joint federal agencies that provide research and protocols in all areas of public health and infection control, including those in the professional environment. http://www.cdc.gov/hipac.
- *ECRI Institute:* Research and consulting organization that applies scientific research to determine which medical procedures, devices, drugs, and processes are best for patient care. http://www.ecri.org.
- *The Joint Commission (TJC):* The accreditation agency for all health care organizations in the United States. It oversees compliance with environmental and patient safety regulations and enforces compliance with standards. http://www.jointcommission.org.
- *U.S. Food and Drug Administration (FDA):* The federal agency responsible for the regulation of medical devices, drugs, food, and cosmetics. http://www.fda.gov/default.htm.

Standards are established to maintain evidence-based practice. Evidence-based practice means that practices and results are based on sound research and professionally conducted studies. Standards also provide us with precise definitions so that professionals can communicate clearly using a common set of terms.

Standards and regulations are implemented through the policies of the health care provider. Management teams in infection control in the Central Processing (CP) and surgical departments develop ways to implement the standards and monitor the outcomes. The actual tasks are performed by perioperative and CP staff. These tasks are set out in the health care facility's procedures manual.

Surgical technologists have a very large role in implementing standards related to infection control. It is important for students and certified technologists to keep up with changing standards and help others become aware of any changes that are implemented.

PRINCIPLES OF DECONTAMINATION, STERILIZATION, AND DISINFECTION

BASIC TERMS

Before studying the material in this chapter, the reader should become familiar with basic terminology related to the processes discussed. Ongoing research and new technology often produce new terms. It is important to learn updated terms because they accurately describe current technology that has been validated by standards agencies. The following are basic definitions used throughout the chapter.

- An *antiseptic* is a chemical used to remove microorganisms *on skin* or other tissue. This process is referred to as **antisepsis**. Surgical handrubs and soaps contain an antiseptic. The patient's skin is cleaned with an antiseptic just before surgery to reduce the number of microorganisms. Some chemicals have dual-purpose qualities (i.e., they may be used on tissue and objects). However, if a chemical is labeled a *disinfectant,* it is intended for **inanimate** (nonliving) surfaces only.
- **Bacteriostatic** refers to an agent that inhibits bacterial colonization (growth) but does not destroy bacteria. On the other hand, a *bactericidal* is an agent that kills bacterial.
- As discussed in Chapter 10, *bioburden* is the number of live bacterial colonies on a surface before it is sterilized. For example, endoscopes used in gastrointestinal procedures contain a high level of bioburden and require meticulous

cleaning and high level disinfection after use. **Biofilms** are dense colonies of microbes that are attached to surfaces. These films are extremely resistant to physical cleaning and chemical removal. They can also cause a surgical site infection.

- **Contaminated** refers to any surface or tissue that has come in contact with a *potential* or actual source of microorganisms. A sterile item is considered contaminated even if the surface it touches is clean but not sterile.
- **Cleaning** is the process of removing surface soil, blood, body fluids, and other kinds of organic debris, usually with detergents and mechanical action (scrubbing or washing).
- **Decontamination** is a process in which instruments and supplies are first cleaned and then processed through chemical or mechanical means so that they are safe for handling. The decontamination process must kill all pathogens.
- **Disinfection** is a process that removes most but not all microbes on inanimate (nonliving) surfaces. Most disinfectants are not safe for use on tissues. Some disinfectants are formulated for use on surgical equipment, whereas others are used for environmental cleaning.
- **Reprocessing** refers to all the steps necessary to render soiled **medical devices**, including surgical instruments, safe for use on the next patient.
- **Sterilization** is a process that results in the complete destruction of all forms of life on an object. An object is either sterile or not sterile. There are no "levels" of sterility.

APPLICATION OF TERMS

The terms just listed are used every day in the health care environment, especially in the operating room. Before and after a surgical case, the floors, walls, and tables are *cleaned* using a **detergent**. The floor is wet-vacuumed to loosen all soil and debris and remove it completely. Perioperative staff put on *clean* scrub attire, which is freshly laundered at the start of each working day. Clean scrub attire is put on at the start of every workday and changed whenever it becomes soiled or wet. Instruments are cleaned thoroughly before disinfection.

Instruments are *disinfected* after use so they can be safely handled by staff members. This reduces the bioburden, so that instrument trays and other equipment can be *sterilized* for a surgical case.

Before surgery begins, the surgical technologist dons *sterile* gloves and gown. The surgical technologist then proceeds to arrange the sterile instruments and supplies on the instrument tables. Sterile supplies and instruments are prevented from touching *contaminated* surfaces or objects. Touching a contaminated object will contaminate the sterile object, which then must not be used in surgery unless it is resterilized.

At the close of the case, the used instruments are removed from the perioperative environment for extensive cleaning and decontamination. After this process, the instruments can be safely handled.

SPAULDING CLASSIFICATION SYSTEM

The **Spaulding system** provides health care professionals a way to determine if a patient care device requires sterilization, disinfection, or cleaning (washing). The system separates patient care items by the risk of that item causing an infection in the patient. The Spaulding category associates high risk with *critical devices.* Intermediate risk is assigned to *semicritical devices,* and low risk devices are *noncritical.*

- Each classification requires specific methods for sterilization or disinfection, according to the level of microbial destruction required. *Critical items* are those that come in contact with *sterile body tissues* and internal organ systems, including the vascular system. Examples are surgical instruments, vascular cannulas, and hypodermic needles. All medical devices in this category must be sterile.
- *Semicritical* devices are those used on the *mucous membrane or nonintact skin* such as a bronchoscope, thermometer, or otoscope. Any device in this category requires high level disinfection.
- **Noncritical items** are those that are used *only on intact skin.* Examples are blood pressure cuffs and examination tables. This category of items requires intermediate disinfection. Items that have not been exposed to body fluids or patient skin may be treated by low level disinfection methods.

Table 11-1 shows the three levels of the Spaulding classification with examples of items in that category.

THE PRINCIPLES OF REPROCESSING

All instruments and equipment used on one patient must be cleaned, disinfected, sterilized, and protected from contamination for the next patient. The following form the basis of safe reprocessing:

1. Soiled instruments and other surgical equipment are reprocessed in a designated area of the health care facility. This area is separated from the surgical suites and the patient care areas to prevent cross-contamination. The reprocessing area is separated into sections, one for soiled instruments and the other for handling and assembly of clean instruments.
2. Staff members are fully trained in the standards and approved methods of reprocessing.
3. Staff members understand the rationale (the "why") used in reprocessing.
4. The health care facility provides written policies and procedures based on the accepted standards of professional and accrediting organizations.
5. Evidence-based methods for quality control are used to validate and monitor the efficacy of the reprocessing methods.

THE REPROCESSING CYCLE

All equipment used in providing patient care is potentially contaminated with pathogenic microorganisms and must be

Table **11-1**	Spaulding Classification System for Medical Devices			
Device Classification	**Examples of Devices**	**Level of Disinfection**	**Requirements For Disinfection**	**Examples**
Critical: These devices come in contact with sterile tissues or are used to convey blood or blood products	• Surgical instruments used within the abdominal, thoracic, cranial, pelvic cavities • Intravenous cannulas • Implants	Sterility	Method must completely destroy microbes including bacterial spores	Sterilization processes such as high pressure steam, ethylene oxide, ozone, gas plasma, peracetic acid
Semicritical: Devices come in contact with mucous membrane or nonintact skin only	• Laryngoscope • Bronchoscope • Vaginal retractor • Tongue blade	High level disinfection	Method must destroy all microbes except bacterial spores	Liquid chemical disinfectants such as glutaraldehyde, peracetic acid, sodium hypochlorite
Noncritical: Devices contact skin and may be exposed to body fluids	• Pneumatic tourniquet • Pulse oximeter • External Doppler • Operating table accessories	Intermediate level disinfection	Disinfection method must kills mycobacteria, viruses, fungi, and vegetative bacteria, but not necessarily spores	Liquid chemical disinfectant, phenolics, sodium hypochlorite

reprocessed for safe use on the next patient. Reprocessing is a step-by-step procedure that follows an exact protocol, starting from the point of use and ending with the assembly and sterilization of equipment used for surgery (Figure 11-1). During the cycle, the equipment is:

1. Maintained in a clean and orderly way at the point of use; transferred to the processing area in a way that protects it so as to prevent contamination of the environment or personnel
2. Decontaminated for safe handling
3. Prepared for sterilization or disinfection
4. Subjected to a sterilization or disinfection process, with simultaneous monitoring and validation of the process
5. Stored in a way that maintains its sterility

These steps are consistent whether an item is to be disinfected or sterilized. Sterilized items must be wrapped or protected from contact with nonsterile surfaces during the preparation phase because the packs must be handled and stored after the process is complete.

CENTRAL PROCESSING DEPARTMENT

In most large health care facilities, high volume processing takes place in the health facility's **Central Processing (CP) department**. The personnel responsible for this are the **Central Processing technicians**. This is a skilled, certified profession that requires expertise in the science and practice of materials management, decontamination, and sterilization. In smaller facilities, surgical technologists may fill the role and perform tasks required for processing surgical equipment.

Nearly all instruments and equipment used in surgery are transferred to Central Processing for reprocessing. A high level of coordination is required between perioperative personnel and the CP staff to ensure a smooth turnover of supplies. Central Processing must make sure that equipment is safe and ready for scheduled surgery and that thousands of

instruments are organized and processed according to strict standards. Perioperative staff members are under pressure to deliver equipment fully intact with no missing parts, ready for immediate use in the surgical field. This collaboration works when staff members from the departments understand and respect each other's roles. A bond of trust exists as well. The CP staff must handle extremely sharp and potentially dangerous equipment that arrives directly from the operating room. The surgical technologist has a responsibility to prepare equipment for processing in a way that protects CP personnel from injury. CP staff members must appreciate the need for instrument trays to be complete and ready for use in time for a scheduled procedure.

Personnel in both departments also must understand the critical nature of their work—disease prevention and safety for patients and staff.

QUALITY CONTROL MONITORING

Procedures and methods for reprocessing medical devices must be monitored to ensure patient safety. Monitoring means *checking, recording, and reporting*. Quality control includes monitoring the *technologies* (such as the steam sterilizer, or instrument washer) used in reprocessing, as well as the *human* factor (is the person following the correct procedure, do they understand the process, are they protecting themselves from injury during the process?). Both the human and technical aspects are equally important.

Technology-Based Parameters

- The parameters of the sterilization or disinfection method, such as a maximum temperature, pressure, or chemical concentration, are verified by printed data generated by the system itself or by external testing methods.
- All batches of goods processed together in a single load are identified by batch number and date; these data are

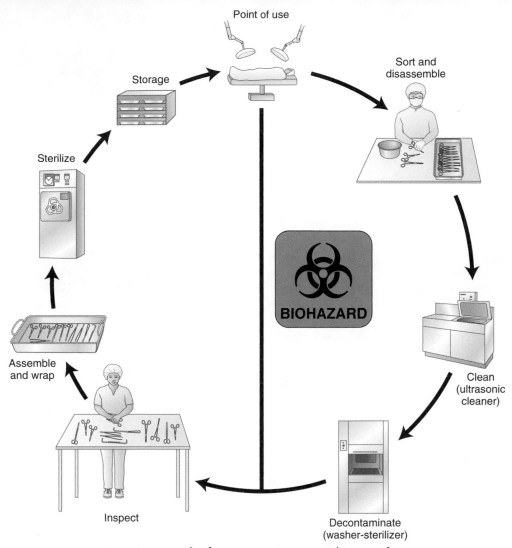

Figure 11-1 Cycle of reprocessing, starting at the point of use.

maintained to allow tracking of items in case of an adverse event related to system or equipment failure.

- Sterilization and disinfection systems undergo regular maintenance and inspection by biomedical engineering professionals.

Human (Personnel) Resources

- Central Processing and perioperative personnel are involved in coordinated roles and responsibilities that directly affect their safety.
- Personnel are provided with the tools and methods needed to meet the objectives of their work. They understand how to operate disinfection and sterilization equipment that is within their area of responsibility.
- Personnel document the procedures and results of specific reprocessing activities.
- Accurate records of responsibilities and tasks are maintained for the purpose of tracking adverse outcomes related to sterilization and disinfection.
- Staff members are offered and encouraged to participate in ongoing training as new technologies and **evidence-based practices** are introduced.

REPROCESSING DISPOSABLE DEVICES

Single-use, or disposable, medical devices and products have come into extremely widespread use in the past two decades. The debate over environmental damage, use of shrinking natural resources, and waste is a separate issue and should be an ongoing discussion. The trend favoring disposables is unlikely to change as long as patients and medical professionals create a demand for such products even though they are not environmentally-friendly.

The increased acceptance of single-use products has created a need for regulations and recommendations covering reprocessing of these items. **Single-use items** are those meant to be used on one patient only. These are manufactured under FDA approval for their intended use on one patient. However, many items opened for surgery are never used and eventually discarded as waste. To cut costs and retrieve the high cost of these items, some institutions reprocess the items. Commercial reprocessing services are available for instruments and equipment *approved for reprocessing* by the manufacturer. However, unless the manufacturer states specifically that the item can be reprocessed by the health care facility, the safety of a single-use device may be compromised. The health care facility is liable for any patient injury that occurs as a result of malfunction of a reprocessed single-use item that is not approved for multiple use.

DECONTAMINATION

CLEANING AT THE POINT OF USE

The preparation of equipment and instruments for patient use begins at the point of use in surgery. In the perioperative environment, this means during surgery and immediately afterward. During surgery, instruments and equipment exposed to blood and body tissue are periodically wiped free of blood and debris to prevent caking and drying. Dried blood and tissue debris make instruments difficult to operate and create a film on the instruments that is difficult to remove later. Also, dried blood and tissue must not be reintroduced into the surgical wound. A sponge moistened with water can be used for this purpose, or instruments may be placed in a basin of water. Suction tips should be periodically flushed with water. Saline is never used for cleaning or soaking instrument because it causes pitting, rusting, and corrosion.

Equipment that is not immersible should also be wiped down periodically during surgery. This includes digital or electronic cameras, light cables, pneumatic drills, and other power equipment. Wiping instruments during surgery reduces biofilm and prevents buildup of organic debris.

At the close of surgery, sharp instruments are separated out to prevent injury. Other instruments usually are placed in a separate basin with the heaviest ones on the bottom and lighter ones on top. The water used to soak the instruments is suctioned off before the equipment is transported out of the surgical suite; this prevents spills and contamination of the transport cart. The equipment is placed on a covered or closed transportation cart for transfer to the decontamination area.

TRANSPORT OF SOILED INSTRUMENTS TO DECONTAMINATION AREA

Most surgical departments use a **case cart system** to collect and transport instruments and equipment for a surgical procedure (Figure 11-2). Sterile instruments and supplies are loaded onto the cart before surgery and transported to the surgical suite. Immediately after surgery, instrument trays, basins, and any other soiled equipment are placed on the cart, which has closed shelving units. The covered cart then is transferred to the decontamination area for processing. If the health care facility has a cart decontamination system, basins and trays can be placed directly on the shelves at the point of use before transport to the decontamination area. If no such system is available, all soiled items must be contained in leak-proof bags to prevent gross contamination of the cart. Instruments and equipment are transported directly to the decontamination area by the scrubbed technologist or nurse.

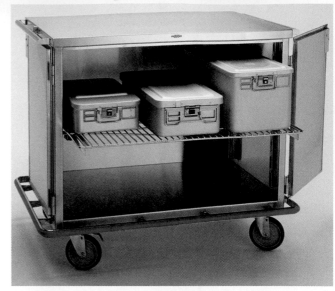

Figure 11-2 Case cart used to transport sterile packs to the surgical suite and return them to the decontamination area after surgery. A closed cart system is recommended. *(Courtesy Pedigo Products, Vancouver, Wash.)*

DECONTAMINATION ATTIRE

All staff members who work in the decontamination area must wear **personal protective equipment (PPE)** in compliance with government regulations (Figure 11-3). This is necessary in order to protect staff from potential infection from body fluids present on the equipment. PPE includes:

- Protective eyewear (i.e., goggles with side shields)
- Face shield
- Gloves approved for contact with chemical disinfectants (surgical or patient care gloves are not permitted)
- Full protective body suit or gown with waterproof apron and sleeves
- Waterproof shoes and covers

SORTING INSTRUMENTS

The first phase of reprocessing is sorting. This is done to prevent damage to delicate items and prevent injury during reprocessing. It is also important to gather the small parts of instruments (pins, gaskets, screws) and keep them together to prevent their loss during reprocessing.

Items are removed from the transport cart and grouped together by category:

- Nonimmersible equipment or instruments
- Instruments with sharp edges or points
- Small gaskets, screws, pins, and other small parts
- Heavy instruments
- Delicate instruments
- Heat- and pressure-sensitive instruments
- Instrument containers
- Basins and cups
- Tubing, suction tips, or other instruments with a lumen
- Instruments or equipment requiring repair or replacement

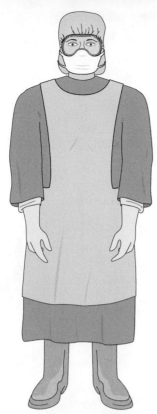

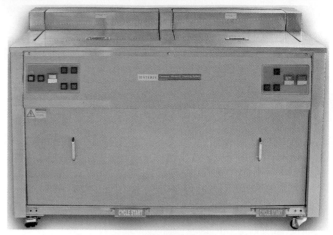

Figure 11-4 Ultrasonic cleaners remove tissue and other debris from instruments through a process called *cavitation*. (Courtesy STERIS Corporation, 2008. All rights reserved.)

Equipment and specialty instruments that are not immersible, such as those with lenses or electronic parts, are cleaned according to the manufacturer's specifications. After cleaning, instruments must be completely rinsed to remove all traces of detergent and debris. Some instruments require rinsing in distilled water. In this case the manufacturer's guidelines should be followed.

ULTRASONIC CLEANING

The **ultrasonic cleaner** removes debris from instruments by a process called **cavitation.** High-frequency sound waves are generated through a water bath. Cavitation causes tiny air spaces trapped within debris to implode (explode inwardly), and this releases the debris from the surface of the instrument. The ultrasonic cleaner has one or more recessed cavities that are filled with **enzymatic cleaner** intended for use in the system (Figure 11-4). Instruments may be exposed to ultrasonic cleaning before entering the automated washer-sterilizer-disinfectant process or as a stand-alone process. Many washer-sterilizer systems have an ultrasonic phase as part of the cycle. If this part of the process is a stand-alone procedure, only instruments that are free of gross debris are processed in the ultrasonic cleaner. Many instruments are damaged by ultrasound energy. Manufacturers of medical devices are careful to state whether the item can be cleaned by ultrasound. Ultrasound alone does *not* decontaminate or sterilize instruments.

SPECIAL HANDLING OF OPHTHALMIC INSTRUMENTS

Ophthalmic instruments require special handling in order to prevent toxic anterior segment syndrome (TASS). TASS can result in damage to the intraocular tissue and loss of vision. This condition occurs postoperatively after cataract surgery when various substances, including those not removed during reprocessing, enter the eye's anterior chamber

Instruments and equipment must be cleaned before they are disinfected or sterilized. Dried blood, body fluids, and tissue debris trap microorganisms and become contaminants. This debris can also cause instrument damage and malfunction. Cleaning is performed by hand, ultrasonic cleaner, and automated washer.

CLEANING INSTRUMENTS BY HAND

After the instruments have been sorted, selected instruments are soaked and hand cleaned using *cold* water and enzymatic detergent. Cold water is superior to hot water as a solvent for blood and other body fluids. Also, some enzymatic detergents are deactivated at temperatures over 140° F (90° C). The instruments are submerged during cleaning to prevent the release of contaminated airborne droplets (aerosol effect).

Areas that are difficult to clean must be scrubbed with a small brush. Particular attention is paid to hemostats and other clamps, orthopedic rasps, and other instruments that contain bits of trapped soft tissue or bone. Items with a lumen (e.g., hollow tube) are cleaned with a soft, narrow brush. The correct size brush must be used to be effective. Brushes that are bent or have sections of missing bristles are not efficient in removing tissue and biofilm. Suction tips are cleared with a *stylet*, a fine wire that can be passed through the instrument to push out debris. Instruments with channels and valves may require disassembly for complete cleaning.

- During surgery, instruments should be wiped clean with a lint-free sponge and water
- At the end of the procedure, the instruments must be immediately submersed in sterile water.
- Single-use cannulas (fine suction tubing) should be used if possible. If these are not available, the lumens of the cannulas must be flushed with sterile water immediately after the procedure.
- All phacoemulsification tips, tubing, handpiece, and other components must be flushed before they are disconnected at the close of surgery according to the manufacturer's instructions.
- Only single-use brushes and syringes are used to clean ophthalmic instruments. These should be discarded after use.
- Items that have been manually or ultrasonically cleaned should be wiped with alcohol before sterilization and according to manufacturer's instructions.
- All instruments should be inspected thoroughly for residue before sterilization.

For detailed guidelines on reprocessing ophthalmic equipment to prevent TASS, refer to Association for the Advancement of Medical Instrumentation standard, AAMI ST79 and the American Society of Cataract and Refractive Surgery (ASCRS).

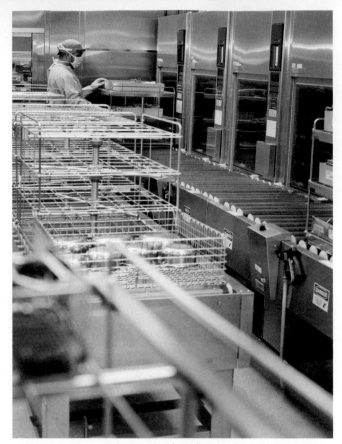

Figure 11-5 Processing area and washer-sterilizer or decontaminator used to process soiled instruments and equipment so that personnel can handle them for assembly, wrapping, and storage. (*Courtesy STERIS Corporation 2008. All rights reserved.*)

during or after surgery. These substances include residue from detergents and lubricants used on the instruments during the washing and decontamination process. Other agents that may cause TASS are topical antiseptic and lubricating agents and powder from surgical gloves. Mitomycin C and improperly reconstituted intraocular preparations are also implicated in TASS.

In order to prevent TASS, special reprocessing methods must be used (Box 11-1).

WASHER-STERILIZER/DISINFECTOR

The **washer-sterilizer/disinfector** is used to process instruments that can tolerate water turbulence and high pressure steam. Instruments are opened and hinges extended to their widest adjustment. The instruments are then placed on metal trays and loaded into the washer chamber (Figure 11-5).

Steel basins, bowls, and containers are also processed in an automatic washer. These are not placed in with instruments but handled separately to prevent damage to instruments and ensure complete contact with water and steam.

Washer-sterilizer/disinfectors are available in several different designs. They include a cleaning phase by immersion in a water bath with air injection or direct water spray wash. Newer systems include an ultrasonic phase. In the final stage, the instruments are sterilized by steam under pressure. At the conclusion of this process, the instruments can be handled by personnel. The correct detergent to use with any washer-sterilizer disinfectant is the one recommended by the manufacturer. This ensures that the detergent is compatible with the system and complies with safety standards.

LUBRICATION

Instruments are lubricated to ensure smooth mechanical action. This process is used on stainless steel instruments and other selected equipment according to the manufacturer's recommendations. Only lubricants approved for use on medical devices are used. *Oils are not used* for lubrication, because the sterilization process may not penetrate oil. Steel instruments may be dipped in a combined lubricating and protective instrument milk as the final stage in cleaning and decontamination. Instrument milk can be added to the rinse cycle of some sterilizer-disinfectors.

LOANER INSTRUMENTS

Specialty instruments and surgical implant sets used on loan from sources outside the health care facility may arrive through health care industry representatives or other sources. Sometimes instruments are wrapped and have undergone a sterilization process. *The sterility of these items must not be assumed.* This is because there is no way to track the conditions under which the instruments were stored or transported. Therefore all loaner instruments should be processed first by decontamination and then by a sterilization method approved for those particular instruments by the manufacturer. In most cases, the health care facility will have a contractual agreement

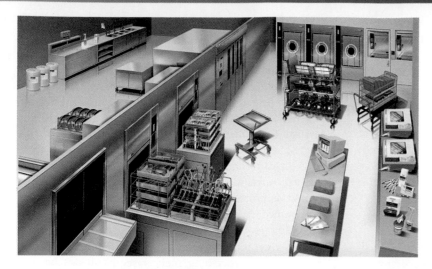

Figure 11-6 **Clean processing area.** This area is used for sorting, inspecting, tracking, and wrapping instruments. *(Courtesy STERIS Corporation 2008. All rights reserved.)*

with the industry representative covering how the instruments are transported and their care while on loan, including decontamination and sterilization before and after use.

SORTING AND HANDLING FOLLOWING DECONTAMINATION

Following the terminal decontamination just described, instruments are safe for handling. They are taken to the clean assembly area for sorting, inspection, and assembly (Figure 11-6). The clean processing area is separated from the decontamination area to prevent cross-contamination. The area includes a workroom with ample table space for sorting instruments and assembling instrument sets. Attire in the clean assembly area includes a clean scrub suit with long sleeves and a surgical cap.

Large-volume sterilizers are located adjacent to the clean work area for easy transfer of instruments once they have been arranged in sets and wrapped for a specific sterilization process.

NOTE: Instruments and equipment designated for semicritical and noncritical use (e.g., endoscopes and endoscopic instruments) may be processed and stored in another location near the point of use. These instruments often are processed by perioperative staff members within that department. (Chapter 24 presents a complete discussion of the processing of fiberoptic endoscopes.)

INSTRUMENT INSPECTION

Before instruments are assembled and wrapped for sterilization, they are inspected for soil, stains, corrosion, proper function, and structural soundness. Instruments that are not properly cleaned before the sterilization process harbor tissue fragments in the hinge or other areas. Microbes can survive in tissue fragments and cause infection in the patient. The shanks of instruments such as hemostats, needle holders, and scissors should be straight. The instrument should be opened and shut several times. If the hinge is stiff during opening and closing, it can be treated with an *approved* instrument lubricant. Mineral oil and silicone must not be used on surgical instruments because they can interfere with the sterilization process. While examining the instrument, look for the conditions of the ratchets and hinges. With time, hemostats and needle holders may spring open unexpectedly. To determine whether an instrument is "sprung" (i.e., will not stay closed), perform this test: Close the jaws and lock the ratchets in place. Then rap the edge of the finger rings gently on a firm surface. An instrument that is sprung will pop open when bumped.

Cutting instruments such as scissors, curettes, osteotomes, rongeurs, and shears should be examined for pitting along the cutting edge. Sharp instruments should be inspected to ensure that the blade surfaces meet smoothly and properly. Forceps must be tested for spring. When the tips are compressed and then released, they should immediately return to the open position. The tips of forceps should close freely and align precisely.

Microsurgical instruments are very expensive to purchase, repair, and replace. These instruments should never be mixed with heavier ones. The tips of microsurgical instruments should be inspected under magnification to ensure that the sharp points are smooth, sharp, and in proper alignment. Any instrument found to be malfunctioning should not be packaged and sterilized; rather, it should be sent for repair. A more detailed discussion of instrument inspection can be found in Chapter 12.

ASSEMBLING INSTRUMENT SETS

After inspection, the instruments are ready for assembly and wrapping. Lists of all instruments and equipment usually are maintained in a computer database or hard copy file. Materials management systems allow CP personnel to track both individual instruments and instrument sets. Standardized trays are assembled so that staff members know what is included in an instrument tray at the point of use. Lists are printed out so that they can be checked at the time of tray assembly.

Guidelines for Instrument Set Assembly

Instruments are assembled in a way that protects them and allows the sterilization method to reach all surfaces:

1. Hinged instruments are opened (unlocked) and strung together with an instrument stringer or in racks designed to hold the instruments in an open position during the sterilization process (Figure 11-7).

2. When assembling instrument sets, make sure any sharp or pointed items are turned downward to prevent injury and sterile wrapper puncture.

3. Sharp and pointed instrument tips may be covered with plastic tip protectors to protect them from injury.

4. Instruments that have movable parts intended for disassembly must be disassembled before sterilization. Any instrument that was not disassembled before disinfection may not be clean and should be returned for disinfection.

5. Instrument trays have a perforated bottom that allows steam to circulate up through the tray and adequately cover all surfaces of the instruments. Make sure no instrument tips are caught in the perforations, where they could be damaged. A cloth towel may be placed on the bottom of the tray to prevent damage to the instrument tips during the sterilization process.

6. Heavy instruments are placed on the bottom of the tray, and the others are packed or nested so that they cannot shift and damage each other during processing.

7. For items with a lumen, a small amount of sterile, deionized (distilled) water should be flushed through the item immediately before sterilization. This water vaporizes during sterilization and forces air out of the lumen. Any air that is left in the lumen may prevent sterilization of its inner surface. Remove stylets from suction tips for assembly so that the sterilant can freely circulate inside the lumen.

8. Instrument trays should not contain separate items wrapped in peel pouch packages. Air can become trapped inside the pouches and prevent steam from reaching all surfaces of the items inside.

9. Rubber bands must not be used to group instruments, as these cannot be sterilized effectively.

10. Do not use nonwoven disposable wrapping material to separate instruments inside the tray or for lining the tray bottom. The material may prevent penetration of the sterilant to the instruments. Power-driven surgical instruments (e.g., drills and saws) should be disassembled before steam sterilization. Hoses can be coiled loosely during packaging, and all delicate switches and parts should be protected during preparation. Before sterilization, power-driven instruments should be lubricated according to the manufacturer's specifications. Power-driven instruments should be tested before wrapping. Finally, before processing, make sure that all switches and control devices are in the safety position.

11. Container devices that allow systematic organization and separation of specialty instruments such as ophthalmic and microsurgery sets must be safe for surgical use. Make sure that the specifications of the device meet AAMI and FDA standards.

WRAPPING INSTRUMENTS FOR STERILIZATION

All items to be sterilized by pressurized steam, ethylene oxide, ozone, or gas plasma methods must be wrapped according to approved methods. The purpose of wrapping an item before sterilization is to protect it from contamination after the sterilization process. Two broad categories of wrappers are woven and nonwoven paper or polymer material. Combination polypropylene-paper pouches are also used to wrap small items.

Qualities of a Wrapping System

A quality wrapping system accomplishes the following:

- Allows the sterilant to penetrate the wrapper and reach all parts of the device
- Allows complete dissipation of the sterilant when the process is finished
- Contains no toxic ingredients or nonfast dyes
- Does not create lint
- Resists destruction by the sterilizing process (e.g., melting, delamination, blistering, and alteration of the chemical structure of an item)
- Permits complete enclosure of the package contents
- Produces a package strong enough to withstand storage and handling
- Is convenient to work with (i.e., pliable and easy to handle)
- Facilitates a method of opening and distributing the device that prevents contamination at the point of use
- Is cost-effective
- Matches the method of sterilization to be used

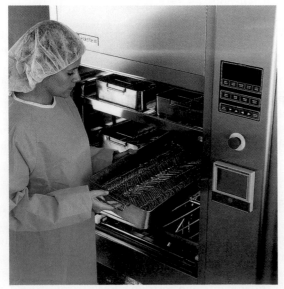

Figure 11-7　Instrument tray ready for wrapping. Instruments must be secured to prevent damage but are opened to allow the sterilant to flow to all surfaces. *(Courtesy STERIS Corporation 2008. All rights reserved.)*

Woven Wrappers

Reusable cloth wrappers are woven from high quality cotton or a combination of cotton and polyester. **Woven wrappers**

are sufficiently dense to protect goods from contamination, yet porous enough to allow penetration of steam or gas. The thread count (number of threads per square inch) must be at least 140 for an effective wrapper. Two double-thickness muslin wrappers or the equivalent (one double-thickness wrapper of 280-count muslin) are used to wrap items. Before use, all cloth wrappers must be laundered and the lint must be removed. The rationale for fresh laundering is to ensure a minimum level of moisture in the cloth, which prevents superheating during sterilization. Wrappers are inspected on a light table for any pinholes or tears in the cloth, which must be repaired before use for sterilization processes.

Single-Use Nonwoven Materials

Disposable **nonwoven** wrappers are intended for one-time use only. These materials are manufactured from spun, heat-bonded fibers such as polypropylene. Nonwoven fabrics must be used in accordance with their thickness. Lightweight fabrics require the same treatment as muslin (i.e., four thicknesses for complete protection). Heavier fabrics may be used according to the manufacturer's specifications. These are valuable for wrapping heavy instruments and flat-surfaced items such as basins and trays or heavy linen packs.

Paper derived from cellulose is *not* used for wrapping items for sterilization because paper recoils when the package is opened, making it difficult to distribute the goods inside aseptically. Also, paper is incompatible with many sterilization processes.

Wrapping Methods Using Flat Sheets

When goods are wrapped in cloth or synthetic material, the most common method is the envelope technique (Figure 11-8) and square wrap. Items may be single wrapped or double wrapped, according to the specifications of the *wrapper* and in accordance with standard protocols for wrapping.

Peel Pouch

Combination synthetic and paper wrappers, commonly called *sterilization pouches* or *peel pouches,* are available in various compositions and styles (Figure 11-9). Pouches are made of a number of different synthetic materials (e.g., Tyvek), that meet the standards for the sterilization process. The item

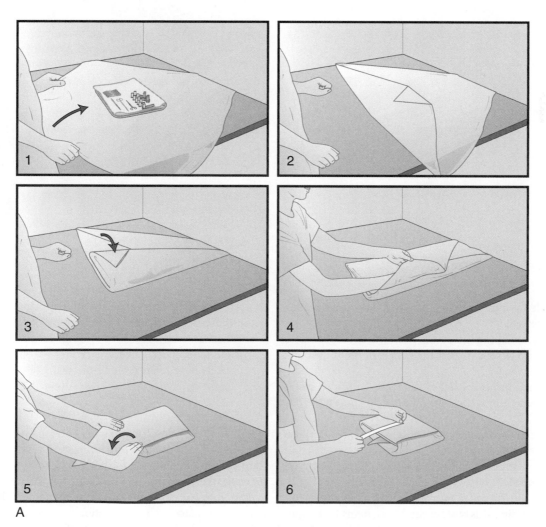

A

Figure 11-8 A, Envelope-style wrapping.

Continued

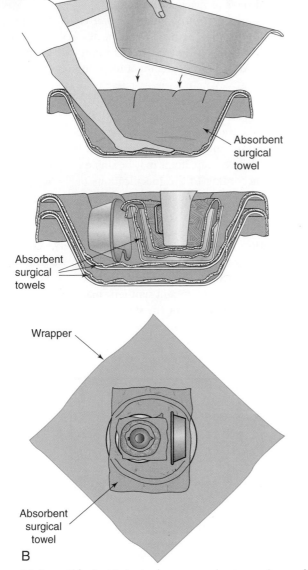

Absorbent surgical towel

Absorbent surgical towels

Wrapper

Absorbent surgical towel

B

Figure 11-8, cont'd   **B,** Method of wrapping basins and cups for steam sterilization. Note the absorbent towel placed between objects to distribute steam evenly through the pack.

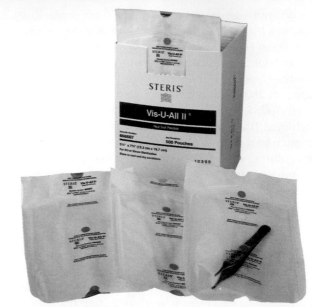

Figure 11-9   Peel pouch wrapping system used for lightweight items. *(Courtesy STERIS Corporation, 2008. All rights reserved.)*

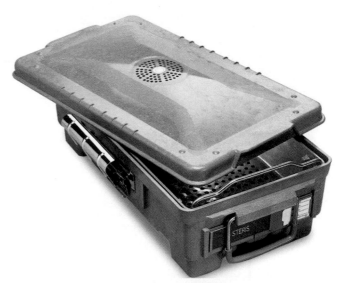

Figure 11-10   Closed sterilization container.

is placed inside the pouch, which is closed with a self-sealing strip or heat-sealed.

Peel pouch wrapping must be performed according to accepted standards to ensure that the item is sterile at the point of delivery:

- Items wrapped in peel pouches must not be placed inside an instrument tray. The sterilant might not penetrate the pouch.
- Double pouches are unnecessary and may prevent sterilization of the item.
- The item in the pouch should clear the seal by at least 1 inch (2.5 cm).
- Peel pouches are intended only for lightweight instruments and devices. Using this system for heavy items (e.g., bone rongeurs, rasps, and multiple instruments) usually leads to tearing and loss of integrity of the pouch.

- Air should be evacuated from the pouch before it is sealed. Otherwise, the package may rupture during sterilization.
- When a mechanical heat-sealing device is used, the seal should be checked very carefully to ensure that no air pockets have formed along the seal.

Sterilization Containers

Manufactured closed containers (also called cases) also are used to hold equipment for sterilization (Figure 11-10). These are convenient and safe for both gas and conventional steam sterilization. Sterilization containers incorporate disposable filters into the construction of the container, and these must remain in place after sterilization to maintain the sterility of the enclosed items. A tamper-proof seal is used to verify that the cover of the container was not removed before use. When sterilization containers are used, the manufacturer's recommendations must be followed. Some containers are suitable only for a single method, whereas others are suitable for a number of different sterilization methods.

EQUIPMENT TRACKING

Regardless of the type of packaging or wrapping system used, each package must be properly labeled. The date of processing, name of the item, a lot control number, batch number, employee initials, and the department to recevie the package must be included on the label. The lot control number is used to identify items that have been included in a sterilization load that may have yielded a positive biological or mechanical control test. Any information written by hand on the outside of a wrapped package usually is placed on the sealing tape, the main purpose of which is to verify the parameters of the sterilization process (discussed in following sections).

A variety of computer-based technologies allow for accurate management and tracking of surgical supplies and equipment. Bar code scanning allows the CP department to track specific instrument sets and identify their location at any given time (Figure 11-11). These programs identify instrument sets that have been used a certain number of times and automatically advise CP personnel to take a routine action, such as holding an instrument set for sharpening of scissors or replacing certain reusable items.

To improve the management of single-use items, special cabinets and carts have been designed to allow personnel to obtain items through a computerized system. Items are stored in the cabinet and retrieved by pushing the button associated with that item. A computer printout in a central inventory office tells the supply or stock personnel to replace that item. These systems may be connected to the hospital billing system. In this way, equipment charges are automatically assigned to individual patients.

STERILIZATION

Instruments and equipment used in critical areas of the body must be sterile before use. This means the instruments must be completely free of all forms of microorganisms. Common methods of sterilization in the patient health care setting include:

- High-temperature steam
- Ethylene oxide (EO) gas
- Gas plasma sterilization
- Peracetic acid processing
- Ozone
- Dry heat
- Ionizing radiation (used in commercial manufacturing of sterile goods). This method is used outside the health care facility and commonly used for bulk sterilization of equipment and supplies.

SELECTING A METHOD

In the past, surgical technologists and nurses have been confronted with decisions about which sterilization method to use for items such as wooden tongue depressors, petroleum-based gauze, liquid in glass bottles, dry powders, and even surgical gloves. These products are now safely sterilized by the manufacturer using technology such as cobalt-60 ionizing radiation.

The selection criteria for the modern perioperative environment have changed with advances in technology and economics and with the increased focus on patient and personnel safety. Whereas in the past "instrument nurses" were relied on to choose the correct sterilization method for a given item, now the responsibility has been given over to the manufacturer. The enormous variety of instruments and equipment used in surgery does not fit easily into a generalized protocol for selecting a sterilization method. This complexity of methods also means that the manufacturer's recommendations must be followed exactly. These methods can also change quickly when new models are marketed. For example, some endoscopic instruments must be hand-cleaned and gas-sterilized, whereas others, even those with digital imaging capability, can be safely sterilized by high pressure steam. The current line of robotic instruments (discussed in Chapter 24) is disassembled, cleaned, decontaminated, and sterilized in an exact manner. These instruments can be steam-sterilized, but only according to the manufacturer's detailed instructions.

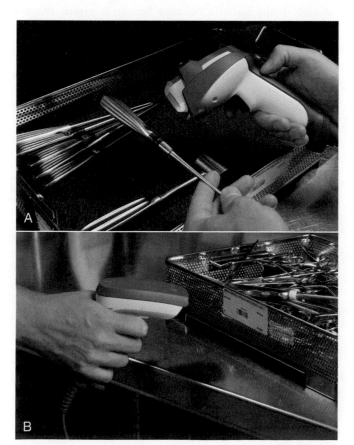

Figure 11-11   **A,** Scanning system for tracking instruments. **B,** Tracking codes are recorded in a central database, which can be used to verify the location and status of equipment. *(Courtsey STERIS Corporation, 2008. All rights reserved.)*

Charts and reference guides are available for most equipment, and these should be readily available in the processing area for staff members to consult.

Safety, Efficiency, and Economic Considerations

Because steam sterilization is the most efficient method of sterilization, this is the first choice whenever possible. However, many delicate items, or those with a complex structure that does not allow steam to reach all surfaces of the item, may require alternative methods.

- All devices used in the health care setting, including surgery, are sold or leased by manufacturers with instructions and recommendations for their care, including methods of reprocessing. These devices include a wide range of digital, electronic, electric, pneumatic, and lensed instruments and equipment.
- Patient safety cannot be ensured unless devices are handled according to the manufacturer's recommendations. Manufacturers are liable for any injury caused by their products as long as the products are used according to exact specifications. This includes the method of reprocessing. Consequently, reprocessing methods are specified exactly.
- Specific categories of devices, such as stainless steel (or other alloy) instruments, are processed according to standards established by professional organizations, such as the AAMI.
- The structure of a device and its composition help determine the method of reprocessing. The complexity and variety of manufactured materials are greater than in the past. Parameters for reprocessing are established according to the *exact type of material* used in the manufacture of the device, including plastics and elastomers such as silicone, polypropylene copolymer, and ethylene-propylene rubber. Compatible reprocessing methods for these materials are widely referenced and easily available.
- Speed of processing for use is an important consideration in the selection of a method. A need for rapid turnover disqualifies many items for gas sterilization. Manufacturers are well aware of this constraint, and newer models of digital and electronic equipment that can be sterilized more quickly are being developed for rapid turnover.

As the student or newly hired technologist becomes familiar with his or her hospital's routines, these decisions will become second nature.

PARAMETERS FOR STERILIZATION

A method of sterilization is effective only when certain conditions are met. Microbial destruction depends on the individual phases of the process itself and on the bioburden, virulence, and resistance of the microorganisms.

- *Time:* Items must be exposed to the process long enough to destroy microorganisms.
- *Saturation and surface exposure:* All parts of the item must be exposed to the sterilization process.
- *Temperature:* Some processes depend on the temperature to which the items are exposed.

- *Quality of the sterilant, air, and water:* The agent must be pure, as must the air and water used in conjunction with it. Chemical or elemental residue in water can reduce the efficacy of the process.
- *Presence of moisture:* Humidity is necessary in most sterilization processes.
- *Method of packing (where applicable) and loading the sterilizer:* This is related to saturation and exposure. Instruments and supplies that have multiple parts or complex design may require disassembly before processing and wrapping. Items must be loaded in a manner that allows the sterilant to penetrate all surfaces. The choice of packaging materials must be suitable for the process.

QUALITY ASSURANCE IN STERILIZATION PRACTICES

A number of different methods are used to determine whether the *parameters* for any method of sterilization have been met. Parameters must be regularly tested for all sterilization methods; the fact that items have been subjected to a sterilization process does not ensure that there was no mechanical or human error that may have prevented actual sterilization. This type of monitoring is called a *challenge* or *challenge test.* By monitoring the parameters, we know that the conditions for sterilization have been reached. The final challenge is to culture harmless bacteria that have been processed with the load. If the bacteria colonize (grow), it means that the process failed.

Objective testing or monitoring is needed to verify both the process and the outcome. Some tests involve the use of chemically impregnated materials (tape or paper indicator) that are placed on the outside and inside of a wrapped sterile pack. When opening the pack on the field during surgery, the scrubbed technologist retrieves this indicator and interprets it. Other indicators involve more complex tests and methods that are explained in the following section.

NOTE: *Standards for monitoring steam sterilization are classified according to type. These are shown in Box 11-2.*

Modern sterilizers have microprocessors that provide a feedback of the parameters of each phase of the sterilization cycle. These quality assurance methods provide valuable information and the means to detect a malfunction. Everyone involved in steam sterilization, including surgical technologists, must understand the information output from the sterilizer. In the event a malfunction is detected, the load is *rejected* (not released for use), and the cause must be immediately investigated to ensure patient safety.

Chemical Indicators

A **chemical indicator** (monitor) is a chemically treated strip that changes color when exposed to a specific temperature, pressure, and humidity (Figure 11-12). The pellet form of this indicator is contained in a glass vial. Chemical monitors are available for both steam and EO sterilization. The chemical responds to high temperature, pressure, and humidity but

Box 11-2 Monitoring Indicators for Steam Sterilization

Steam uses a system of six classes of indicators for quality assurance. Although the different classes are numbered, there is no associated ranking of the indicators. Each type produces different information about the performance of the sterilizer, and each type has a specific use.

- Class 1 (single parameter): These are process indicators. This can be tape or a label indicating only that an individual item or unit was directly exposed to the sterilization process. An example is tape that changes color when exposed to the critical temperature required in steam sterilization.
- Class 2 (specialty indicators): These are used for specific tests that measure parameters. Examples include the Bowie-Dick and daily air removal tests for the presence of pure air (no steam) in the sterilization chamber.
- Class 3 (single parameter): This class includes indicators that respond to only one critical parameter with an exact value. An example is a heat-sensitive pellet (encased in a glass tube) that melts only at a certain temperature that is consistent with the sterilization method. The pellet is placed in specific areas of the sterilization chamber.
- Class 4 (multiparameter): These are represented by multivariable indicators that react to two or more parameters. An example is internal chemical indicators printed on a paper strip.
- Class 5 (integrating parameters): This class includes indicators that react to all critical values over a specified range in the sterilization process. These are the most exacting and accurate of all indicators.
- Class 6 (emulating indicators): Class 6 indicators are used for internal pack control of each cycle run, not for the overall performance of the sterilizer for all cycles.

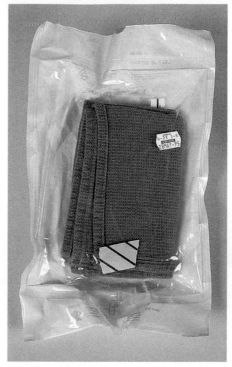

Figure 11-12 Chemical monitor. The striped monitor changes color when exposed to specific parameters used in the sterilization process. (From Elkin MK, Perry AG, Potter PA: Nursing interventions and clinical skills, ed 3, St Louis, 2004, Mosby.)

- Hydrogen peroxide gas plasma: *Bacillus subtilis*
- Peracetic acid: According to the manufacturer's specifications
- High-speed steam sterilizer: *Geobacillus stearothermophilus* enzyme (fluorescence testing)
- Ozone sterilization: *Geobacillus stearothermophilus*

The test bacteria are encased in a self-contained unit that usually is placed in the most challenging area of the load—that is, near the outlet drain of the chamber (steam sterilizer). For EO monitoring, the biological test pack is positioned in the center of the load. After the sterilization process, the bacterial spores are cultured. The growth of bacteria in the test culture indicates that the sterilization process probably was ineffective. If no bacteria grow, all items in the load are presumed to be sterile.

Biological controls should be administered at least once weekly in all sterilizers and daily if possible. Biological monitors are always used when an artificial **implant** or prosthesis is sterilized. If any **biological indicator** shows a positive result, all items included in that load are withdrawn from use. The infection control department will be notified and the event documented. If the items have already been used in patient treatment, additional safety precautions are immediately implemented, including notification of the surgeon or other primary health care provider who used the items during patient care.

Figure 11-13 shows examples of biological monitors.

Rapid biological monitoring uses an enzyme that binds to spores. After the sterilization process, the level of enzyme is

does not register **exposure time**, which is critical to the sterilization process. A chemical monitor should be placed inside and outside all packs to be sterilized. After the cycle, the indicator must be retrieved and interpreted.

Biological Indicators

Biological monitoring is a highly reliable method of determining whether the conditions inside the sterilizer met the parameters (pressure and heat) for sterilization. The sterility of an item cannot be *guaranteed*, because errors can prevent some items in a load from being exposed to the process. The load might be too compact, or air pockets that prevent steam from reaching all surfaces of the contents may be present in the sterilization chamber. However, a bacterial sample can be exposed to the sterilization process and tested for viability. This is called **process challenge monitoring** or biological monitoring. The bacteria used during biological monitoring can differ according to the sterilization process. The harmless bacteria are contained in a vial that is recovered after the cycle and observed for bacterial colony growth. The following bacteria are used according to the sterilization process:

- Steam sterilization: *Geobacillus stearothermophilus*
- Dry heat and EO sterilization: *Bacillus subtilis*

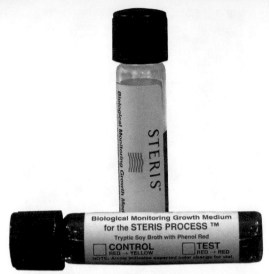

Figure 11-13 Biological indicators (BIs) contain harmless, spore-forming bacteria that can be quickly cultured after the sterilization process to monitor the load. *(Courtsey STERIS Corporation, 2008. All rights reserved.)*

measured. This corresponds with destruction of the bacterial spores. The monitoring system is used for both high pressure steam and EO sterilization. Results can be obtained in 1 to 4 hours, depending on the sterilization process.

Air Detection Testing

To test and monitor the efficiency of the high-vacuum steam sterilizer, a test called the daily air removal test (DART) is performed. Bowie-Dick tests also are commercially available for this purpose. High-vacuum sterilizers are monitored to detect air in the chamber during the exposure phase. In these tests, a special package of properly wrapped towels is taped with heat-sensitive chemical monitor tape and stacked to a height of 10 or 11 inches (25 to 27.5 cm). The package is then placed by itself in the sterilization chamber and run for the appropriate time. An unsatisfactory DART indicates a failure in the vacuum pump system or a defect in the gasket of the sterilizer door. Unsatisfactory results must be reported to the biomedical engineering staff so that they can inspect the sterilizer, especially the vacuum system and door seals.

STEAM STERILIZATION

Steam sterilization is the most widely used, effective, and efficient method of sterilization in the health care setting. Normal atmospheric steam is not hot enough to completely destroy microbes and spores. However, steam under pressure reaches the extremely high temperatures necessary for sterilization. Steam under pressure coagulates the nucleic acids and protein that make up the cell's genetic and enzymatic material. Pressurized steam also destroys the cell's resilient outer wall and bacterial spores.

Steam sterilization is achieved according to the temperature, pressure, and exposure time. These depend on the type of steam sterilizer, the size of the load, the temperature, whether items are wrapped, and the type of materials or supplies being processed. The entire process of heating, pressurizing, and timing the load is called a cycle. Modern steam sterilizers have preprogrammed cycles for these parameters. A steam sterilizer has a central chamber where goods are placed and a mechanism for creating extremely high pressure. Steam enters the chamber, air is removed, and the internal pressure increases. This process heats the steam to the very high temperatures required for sterilization. The full cycle may differ slightly among models and manufacturers.

However, there are three distinct phases in all types of steam sterilizers:

1. *Conditioning (sometimes called preconditioning):* Air is removed from the chamber and replaced with steam.
2. *Exposure or holding time:* Goods in the chamber are exposed to superheated steam at a precise temperature and duration. This duration depends on the size of the load, complexity of materials being sterilized, and whether or not the items were wrapped before sterilization.
3. *Exhaust and drying:* Pressure in the chamber is reduced and the load is exposed to cool air.

Two types of steam sterilizers are used in the clinical setting, gravity displacement and dynamic (also called pre-vacuum or **high-vacuum sterilizers**).

The main difference in these types is the actual process of removing air and replacing it with steam. The gravity displacement system injects steam into the chamber and displaces the air, which escapes by gravity (downward) through a drain. Dynamic air removal sterilizers use a high-vacuum system to quickly and forcefully evacuate air from the chamber and replace it with bursts or pulses of steam.

Gravity Displacement Sterilizer

The **gravity displacement sterilizer** (also called a *downward displacement sterilizer*) operates on the principle that air is heavier than steam (Figure 11-14). All the air must be removed from the inner chamber, because all surfaces of the items must be exposed to the pressurized steam to ensure sterilization. Any air in the inner chamber blocks the passage of pressurized steam to the goods and prevents sterilization. The sterilizer is constructed in such a way that air is displaced downward by gravity (hence the name *gravity displacement sterilizer*) and is replaced by steam.

Dynamic Air Removal (Prevacuum) Sterilizer

The dynamic air removal (prevacuum) sterilizer pulls air from the chamber with vacuum force and replaces it with steam. As air is pumped into the chamber, steam enters in pulsed phases. Air is completely removed with positive- and negative-pressure pulses. As the pressure increases, so does the temperature of the steam inside the sterilizer. Superheated steam is possible only with extremely high pressure. The chamber pressure and temperature are held according to the specified program, then the steam is removed through a filter, and the chamber pressure is reduced to normal (atmospheric) temperature. A cool cycle reduces the temperature to a level at which personnel may safely handle the sterilized goods.

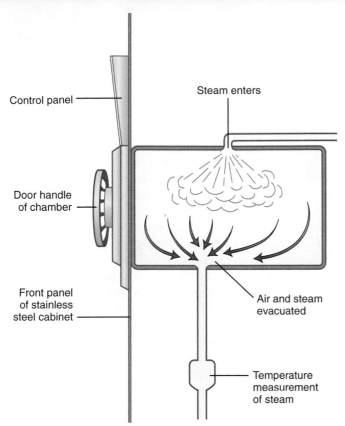

Figure 11-14 **Prevacuum steam sterilizer.** *(Redrawn from Phillips N: Berry and Kohn's operating room technique, ed 10, St Louis, 2004, Mosby.)*

Selection of Items for Steam Sterilization

Stainless steel instruments, other items made of stainless steel, and woven materials are routinely sterilized with steam. However, many items used in surgery cannot tolerate high pressure, high temperature, and exposure to steam. The appropriate processing method should always be verified directly with the manufacturer's manuals or company representative. Many power-driven instruments and those that contain an optical system or microprocessor cannot be steam-sterilized. Some synthetic materials, such as Silastic, Teflon, polyethylene, polypropylene, and other complex polymers, may also be altered during steam sterilization.

Moisture Concentration (Steam Quality)

Effective steam sterilization requires a specific concentration of moisture. If too little moisture is present, items become superheated and eventually can be burned. Too much moisture leaves items wet after removal from the chamber; this can result in contamination of the item. The amount of moisture in the steam is referred to as the *steam quality*. Water is converted to steam at 212° F (100° C). At this temperature, steam is ineffective for sterilization. Steam that contains more than 97% water is necessary for sterilization to be achieved.

Water Quality

Although the water used during steam sterilization is filtered, contaminants are still present. These usually consist of mineral particles that are too small to be trapped by filters. These minerals are deposited on the surfaces of sterilized items and on the internal surfaces of the sterilizers. The presence of orange, white, brown, or black spots on sterilized items may indicate the presence of excess minerals in the water supply. As these minerals become deposited in the box locks of surgical instruments, they can impair the function of these instruments.

Loading and Operation of a Large-Capacity Steam Sterilizer

Large steam sterilizers are used for bulk processing of hospital equipment, including surgical instruments, basins, linen, drapes, and towels. They usually are located in the Central Processing department. Loading techniques for any sterilizer influence the outcome. Large sterilizers used for bulk linens, basins, and complex instruments multiply the problems of air pockets, overheating, and proper steam drainage. Careful loading of items in the steam sterilizer is critical, because if the load is too dense or improperly positioned, air may become trapped in pockets. Items in these air pockets will not be sterilized.

- Instrument pans with mesh or wire bottoms are placed flat on the sterilizer shelf.
- Linen packs, because of their density, require special attention. Linen packs are best sterilized by placing the packs on their sides.
- Packs and instrument trays should be placed so that they do not touch, or touch only loosely, and small items should be placed crosswise over each other.
- Heavy packs should be placed at the periphery of the load, where steam enters the chamber.
- Basins, jars, cups, or other containers should be placed on their sides with the lids slightly ajar so that the air can flow out of them and steam can enter.
- Any item with a smooth surface on which water can collect and drip during the cooling phase of the sterilization cycle should be placed at the bottom of the load. Figure 11-15 shows the proper methods of loading a gravity displacement sterilizer.

Modern steam sterilizers are preprogrammed for specific cycles that can be selected by the operator. Information about each load is stored in memory, and hard copies are maintained for quality assurance. The total time necessary to expose goods to pressurized steam and sterilize them depends on the density of the goods and the temperature in the sterilizer. Tables 11-2 and 11-3 show cycle times for the gravity displacement and dynamic (high-vacuum) sterilizers. These exposure times and temperatures do not reflect the entire time needed to include all phases of the sterilization process. These minimum standards apply only to the amount of time necessary for the pressurized steam to contact all surfaces of the load. Total time includes the preconditioning phase, holding or exposure phase (sometimes called the *kill time*), a factor of safety time, and an exhaust phase. Some sterilizers also include a drying phase. Because these times may vary from load to load, depending on the items to be sterilized, the operator should always check the

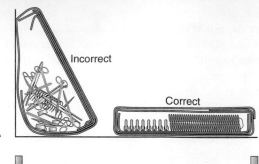

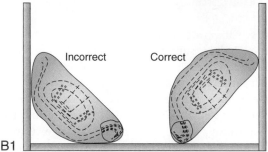

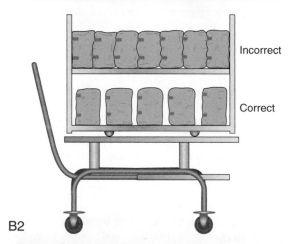

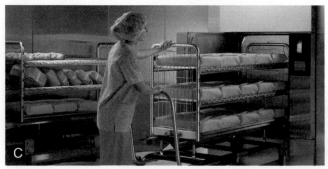

Figure 11-15 **A,** Proper method of placing instrument trays in a steam sterilizer. **B,** Proper method of loading basins and packs for steam sterilization. **C,** Loading trays into a steam sterilizer. *(Redrawn from STERIS Corp., Mentor, Ohio.)*

specifications of the item's manufacturer, not the sterilizer's manufacturer, for recommended sterilization times and temperatures. Many items, especially dense instruments and power-driven orthopedic tools, require longer periods of sterilization and cooling.

To assist in the removal of moisture and to prevent wet packs, the sterilizer operator may use a dry cycle as part of the steam sterilization process. Regardless of whether a dry cycle is used, items that have been steam sterilized should be allowed to remain in the sterilizer chamber for 15 to 30 minutes after the cycle to prevent the formation of condensate. Do not crack the door of the sterilizer during drying phase, as this can result in inefficient cooling and drying of the load.

FLASH (IMMEDIATE-USE) STERILIZER

A high-speed prevacuum sterilizer is used in the operating room and in other areas of the hospital to sterilize items for immediate use. Steam sterilization using an abbreviated cycle at a high temperature is necessary for rapid sterilization. However, advanced technology leading to new materials and complex equipment has led to equally complex guidelines for ensuring patient safety. In the past, the term *flash sterilization* was used to describe the process of a shortened sterilization cycle for uncovered items. Now, however, there are situations in which items are covered in a variety of ways, even for immediate use following sterilization.

A standards committee composed of members of accreditation bodies, research professionals, and key health professionals agreed in 2010 that the term *flash sterilization* does not reflect the complexity of sterilization for immediate use. The term has been replaced with **immediate-use sterilization**. Standards for immediate-use sterilization have been adapted by the Association of Surgical Technologists as well as other professional organizations.

The statement on adaptation to the new terminology can be found on the AAMI website, http://www.aami.org/publications/standards/ST79_Immediate_Use_Statement.pdf. This website also provides references for the standards and practices currently approved by accrediting and professional agencies.

Sterilizers employed for immediate use are usually located just outside the operating suite, in the substerile or core area. This type of sterilizer is used *only when no alternative is available.* Items are sterilized just before use. Ideally, items to be sterilized for immediate use should be in a covered metal tray. However, some immediate-use sterilizers can be used with a drying cycle that is suitable for items wrapped in a single layer of woven material. Unwrapped items coming from the immediate-use sterilizer will be wet, as there is no drying cycle for unwrapped goods.

Recommended Practices for Immediate-Use Sterilization (AAMI)

1. Implants must never be sterilized immediately before use except in a documented emergency situation when no other option is available. If an implant must be sterilized in an emergency, a rapid readout biological indicator must be used.
2. The manufacturer's specifications for exposure time and temperature must be followed.
3. If a covered sterilization container is used to sterilize instruments immediately before use, parameter values

Table 11-2 Cycle Times for Gravity Displacement Steam Sterilization

Item	Exposure Time at 250° F (121° C)	Minimum Drying Time	Exposure Time at 270° F (132° C)	Minimum Drying Time	Exposure Time at 275° F (135° C)*	Minimum Drying Time*
Wrapped instruments	30 min	15 to 30 min	15 min	15 to 30 min	10 min	30 min
Textile packs	30 min	25 min	25 min	15 min	10 min	30 min
Wrapped utensils	30 min	30 min	15 min	15 to 30 min	10 min	10 min

From Rutala W, Weber D, and the Healthcare Infection Control Practices Advisory Committee (HICPAC), Atlanta, 2008, Centers for Disease Control and Prevention.
*From AORN, *Perioperative standards and recommended practices, 2011 edition.* Denver, 2011, AORN.

Table 11-3 Cycle Times for Dynamic Air Removal (Prevacuum) Steam Sterilization

Items	Exposure Time at 250° F (121° C)	Minimum Drying Time	Exposure Time at 270° F (132°C)	Minimum Drying Time	Exposure Time at 275° F (135° C)*	Minimum Drying Time*
Wrapped instruments	NA		4 min	15 to 30 min	3 min	16 min
Textile packs	NA		4 min	5 to 20 min	3 min	3 min
Wrapped utensils	NA		4 min	20 min	3 min	16 min

Note: Exposure and drying times for enclosed rigid sterilization containers are specified by the manufacturer and vary according to design. Always check manufacturer's specifications for sterilization.
From Rutala W, Weber D, and the Healthcare Infection Control Practices Advisory Committee (HICPAC), Atlanta, 2008, Centers for Disease Control and Prevention.
*From AORN, *Perioperative standards and recommended practices, 2011 edition.* Denver, 2011, AORN.

specified by the manufacturers of the container *and* the instrument must be followed.

4. Power-driven equipment and cords are never sterilized without first verifying the manufacturer's recommendations.
5. Immediate-use sterilizers must be located in an area where unwrapped sterile items can be transported directly from the sterilizer to the sterile field.
6. Items for flash sterilization are never wrapped unless this is permitted by the manufacturer's specifications.
7. Sterilization monitors must be used with every load.
8. Immediate-use sterilization is never performed for postprocedure decontamination of instruments used on patients who may have Creutzfeldt-Jakob disease (CJD) or similar disorders.
9. Items that are sold from the manufacturer as sterile devices intended for single use only must never be sterilized for immediate use.
10. Sterilization containers with tamper-proof seals may be used for immediate-use sterilization. Always follow the manufacturer's instructions for use.

Table 11-4 shows the parameters for immediate-use (flash) sterilization.

Removing Items from the Flash Sterilizer

To remove items from in the sterilizer chamber, the circulator dons sterile gloves and grasps the edges of the tray using sterile transfer handles. The tray is offered to the scrub, who removes the sterile items from the tray with care to prevent contamination of her or his gown or gloves. The tray should not be transferred to the sterile field, and the scrub should not leave the sterile field or the room to retrieve the item from the sterilizer, as this is poor aseptic technique.

Table 11-4 Flash Steam Sterilizer (for Immediate Use) Parameters

Type of Sterilizer	Load	Temperature	Exposure Time
Gravity displacement	Metal instruments (nonporous, without lumens) only	270° to 275° F (132° to 135° C)	3 min
	Porous items with lumens; complex power instruments (always consults manufacturer)	270° to 275° F (132° to 135° C)	10 min
Dynamic (prevacuum)	Metal instruments (non porous without lumens)	270° to 275° F (132° to 135° C)	4 min
Pressure pulse/ steam flush	Nonporous / mixed porous and nonporous	270° to 275° F (132° to 135° C)	4 min

Note: Exposure and for enclosed rigid sterilization containers are specified by the manufacturer and vary according to design. Always check manufacturer's specifications for sterilization using these systems.
From Rutala W, Weber D, and the Healthcare Infection Control Practices Advisory Committee (HICPAC), Atlanta, 2008, Centers for Disease Control and Prevention.

ETHYLENE OXIDE STERILIZATION

Ethylene oxide (EO) is used to sterilize objects that cannot tolerate the heat, moisture, and pressure of steam sterilization. It can be used for delicate instruments, including microsurgical instruments and those with optical systems. It is highly penetrating, which makes it ideal for complex instruments with delicate inner components.

EO is a highly flammable liquid that when blended with inert gas, produces effective sterilization by destroying the deoxyribonucleic acid (DNA) and protein structure of micro-organisms. EO is used in a 100% pure form, blended with carbon dioxide gas, or mixed with hydrochlorofluorocarbons.

EO kills microorganisms and their spores by interfering with the metabolic and reproductive processes of the cell. The process is intensified with both heat and moisture. The EO sterilizer operates at a *low temperature*. The temperature of the gas directly affects the penetration of items in the chamber. Operating temperatures range from 85° to 100° F (29° to 388° C) for a "cold" cycle and 130° to 145° F (54° to 63° C) for a "warm" cycle.

Humidity is required to make spores less resistant to the EO gas. The preferred moisture content for EO sterilization is 25% to 80%. The length of exposure depends on the type and density of material to be sterilized, temperature, humidity, and concentration of the gas.

Precautions and Hazards

A number of environmental and safety hazards are associated with EO. Exposure to the gas can cause burns to skin and mucous membranes. Prolonged occupational exposure to EO gas is known to cause respiratory damage. EO is a stable com-pound with a long half-life. Its advantage as a penetrating sterilant also poses hazards. It is difficult to remove, and the level of EO residue is not the same in different materials. In addition, it reacts with many different substances, causing them to disintegrate or creating other toxic compounds, such as ethylene glycol and ethylene chlorohydrins. These chemi-cals also are difficult to remove from the environment.

To prevent injury from EO exposure, the Occupational Safety and Health Administration (OSHA) requires air sam-pling in areas likely to contain high concentrations of EO. The level of EO must not exceed 0.5 ppm in any area. Personal dosimeter badges measure EO exposure. Air samples should be taken regularly in the sterilization area. Other safety pre-cautions include the installation of an exhaust system that vents the gas to the outside of the building through an exhaust vent located above the chamber door. Six to 10 exchanges of fresh air per hour are delivered to the sterilization area.

Observing the following precautions reduces occupational and patient risk:

- After the sterilization process is finished, keep the sterilizer door opened slightly for about 15 minutes.
- Make sure goods transported from the sterilizer to the aerator (discussed later) remain on a transport cart.
- Always wear protective gloves when handling unaerated items.
- Never retrieve an instrument from the aerator before com-pletion of the approved aeration period. Do not ask anyone else to do this, even if a surgeon requests it.
- Always pull the transport cart rather than pushing it. Pushing the cart places personnel in back of the air flowing from the unaerated items.
- Follow the manufacturer's exact specifications for aeration.

Preparation of Items for Gas Sterilization

All items to be gas-sterilized must be clean and dry. Any water left on equipment bonds with EO gas and produces a toxic residue, which can cause burns or a toxic reaction in those who come in contact with it. Any organic material or soil exposed to EO also may produce toxic residues. Therefore, all items processed for EO gas must be completely clean. Items are loaded in the sterilizer loosely so that the gas is free to circulate over every surface.

Every attempt should be made to load items that have similar aeration requirements. Some items must not be gas-sterilized. These include acrylics and some pharmaceu-tical items.

Because EO does not penetrate glass, solutions in a glass vial or bottle cannot be sterilized by this method. Any instru-ments with fittings or parts should be disassembled before EO sterilization to facilitate exposure to the gas.

Wrapping techniques for EO sterilization are the same as for high pressure steam sterilization. However, some materials are not suitable for EO processing. These include wrappers made of natural fiber combined with nylon and rayon, poly-ester, and polyvinyl chloride. Double-wrapped peel pouches are not suitable for some EO sterilizers. The manufacturer's recommendations should always be followed.

Loading and Sterilization

The EO sterilizer is loaded in such a way that gas can penetrate all surfaces of the packages. Packages must not touch the bottom or top of the chamber and must be placed loosely on their sides. The EO sterilizer is preprogrammed for exposure time, temperature, and aeration parameters. The sterilizer is operated from the control panel by trained CP technologists.

Aeration

Unlike steam sterilization, items sterilized with EO require aeration to dissipate any residual gas remaining on the items. The manufacturer's recommendations for aeration are critical to the safety of both the patient and the hospital personnel handling equipment that has been gas-sterilized. Aeration takes place in a special aeration chamber or by room air, pro-vided that safety precautions are followed. In many newer models, aeration takes place within the sterilizer chamber through the addition of an aerator that evacuates the gas from the chamber and flushes the chamber with room air. The aeration time for an object depends on its porosity and size (Table 11-5). Aeration can require up to 12 hours for some items.

GAS PLASMA

Gas plasma sterilization is used on items that are heat and moisture sensitive. The time required for gas plasma steriliza-tion is much shorter than that required for EO sterilization. Gas plasma is made up of ionized gases. During the steriliza-tion process, hydrogen peroxide is exposed to a vacuum. This creates a vapor, which is forced into the central chamber where goods have been loaded. Radiofrequency energy is transmitted through the vapor, which excites the hydrogen

Table **11-5**	Minimum Aeration Times after Ethylene Oxide Sterilization at Different Temperatures		
Materials	**Ambient Room Air** 65°-72° F (18°-22° C)	**Mechanical Aerator** 122° F (50° C)	140° F (60° C)
Metal and glass	May be used immediately		
Unwrapped	2 hr	2 hr	2 hr
Wrapped			
Rubber for external use—not sealed in plastic	24 hr	8 hr	5 hr
Polyethylene and polypropylene for external use—not sealed in plastic	48 hr	12 hr	8 hr
Plastics except polyvinyl chloride items—not sealed in plastic	96 hr (4 days)	12 hr	8 hr
Polyvinyl chloride	168 hr (7 days)	12 hr	8 hr
Plastic and rubber items—those sealed in plastic and/ or those that will come in contact with body tissues	168 hr (7 days)	12 hr	8 hr
Internal pacemaker	504 hr (21 days)	32 hr	24 hr

From Phillips N: *Berry and Kohn's operating room technique,* ed 10, St Louis, 2004, Mosby.

peroxide molecules. This action destroys microorganisms by interfering with the cell membrane, genetic material, and cell enzymes.

The gas plasma sterilization cycle has four phases:

1. *Vacuum phase:* Air is evacuated from the chamber to reduce the pressure.
2. *Injection phase:* Liquid hydrogen peroxide is injected into the central chamber, where it is vaporized.
3. *Diffusion phase:* Hydrogen peroxide vapor disperses throughout the load.
4. *Plasma phase:* Radiofrequency energy breaks apart the hydrogen peroxide vapor, creating a plasma cloud containing free radicals and ultraviolet light. The compounds recombine into oxygen and water and are dissipated from the chamber. This completes the cycle.

The exposure time depends on the type and size of the load but ranges from 30 to 60 minutes. No toxic chemicals are created by this process, and aeration time is not necessary. After the sterilization cycle, hydrogen peroxide gas is converted to its molecular components, water, and oxygen.

Cloth and cellulose products cannot be processed by gas plasma sterilization. Only specific nonwoven wrapping materials can be used (e.g., Tyvek or Mylar wrappers). Materials compatible with gas plasma sterilization are listed in Box 11-3.

Preparation of materials for gas plasma sterilization is the same as for EO sterilization. Items are decontaminated as usual, dried, assembled, and wrapped according to the manufacturer's specifications. Quality control indicators to verify sterilization parameters are used just as with other sterilization procedures (see later discussion).

LIQUID PERACETIC ACID

Peracetic acid solution is a liquid chemical made up of 35% peracetic acid, hydrogen peroxide, acetic acid, sufuric acid, and water. This system is an alternative to cold sterilization processing, commonly performed with a glutaraldehyde solution. During the sterilization process, peracetic acid inactivates many cell systems through a chemical process called *oxidation.* As the peracetic acid decomposes after the sterilization process, it converts to acetic acid (vinegar) and oxygen. Peracetic acid does not leave a chemical residue, but it must be rinsed thoroughly from instruments.

Box **11-3**	**Materials Compatible with Gas Plasma Sterilization**

Metals
- Stainless steel 300 series
- Aluminum 6000 series
- Titanium

Nonmetals
- Glass
- Silica
- Ceramic

Plastics and Elastomers
- Acrylonitrile-butadiene-styrene (ABS)
- Chlorinated polyvinyl chloride (CPVC)
- Ethylene propylene diene monomer rubber (EPDM)
- Polycarbonate (PC)
- Polyetherketone (PEEK)
- Polyetherimide (Ultem)
- Polyethersulfone (PES)
- Polyethylene
- Polymethyl methacrylate (PMMA)
- Polymethylpentene (PMP)
- Polyphenylene oxide (Noryl, PPO)
- Polypropylene (LDPP, HDPP)
- Polypropylene copolymer (PPCO)
- Polysulfone (PSF)
- Polyvinyl chloride (PVC)
- Polyvinylidene fluoride (PVDF)
- Teflon (PTFE, PFA, FEP)
- Tefzel (ETFE)
- Most silicones and fluorinated silicones

From Johnson & Johnson: *Material compatibility for STERRAD system.*

Peracetic acid is used in a closed commercial processing system manufactured by the STERIS Corporation (Mentor, Ohio).

OZONE

Ozone sterilization utilizes a molecular form of oxygen (three oxygen atoms) at low heat for sterilization of moisture- and heat-sensitive instruments and equipment through a process of oxidation. The process has four separate phases that are repeated in the sterilization process. Following the cycle, ozone is converted back to oxygen and water. This method is environmentally friendly and safer than EO but as yet has not been approved for many materials and instruments. The process can be used for rigid diagnostic instruments, stainless steel, and synthetic substances such as polyvinyl chloride (PVC), silicone, and polytetrafluoroethylene (PTFE [Teflon]). It is not approved for implants. Sterilization time exceeds 4 hours. This method is used only on equipment whose manufacturer has approved it for ozone sterilization, usually in closed containers or nonwoven pouches approved for exposure to ozone.

COBALT-60 RADIATION

Most equipment available prepackaged from a manufacturer has been sterilized by ionizing radiation (cobalt-60 radiation), which destroys all microorganisms through destruction of the DNA. Items such as **sharps**, sutures, sponges, and disposable drapes are just a few of the many types of presterilized products available.

Also included are anhydrous materials such as powders and petroleum goods. These products traditionally have been sterilized by dry heat in the hospital setting. However, the current trend is away from dry heat sterilization because of its inconvenience and because these substances now are available as **single-use items**, packaged in one-dose containers to prevent cross-contamination. Items intended for single use, whether supplies for use in the surgical field or other substances meant to be used only once, must never be resterilized by conventional methods (steam sterilization, EO, or **chemical sterilization**) without the manufacturer's express recommendation to do so. The item might change in composition or deteriorate and could become a hazard to the patient or personnel.

INSTRUMENTS EXPOSED TO CREUTZFELDT-JAKOB DISEASE PRIONS

CJD and variant CJD are fatal diseases caused by prions. A **prion** is a protein particle that is not a cell and is not related to bacteria or viruses. These prions are highly infective in central nervous system tissue, and they are of special concern in the processing of instruments and equipment. Prions are not destroyed by normal means of mechanical or chemical sterilization. Specific procedures are necessary to control and destroy the prion on medical devices in the clinical setting (Table 11-6 presents general guidelines).

Perioperative staff members can update their knowledge of the recommended procedures by consulting the CDC website (http://www.cdc.gov) and the AORN website (http://www.aorn.org).

STORAGE OF WRAPPED STERILE GOODS

After an item has been decontaminated, sorted, wrapped, and sterilized, consideration must be given to how the item can be kept sterile. Time-related sterility measures (based on the length of time since sterilization) are not considered valid. **Event-related sterility** or terminal sterilization is the accepted standard.

Event-related sterility or terminal sterilization is based on the principle that sterilized items are assumed sterile between uses unless environmental conditions or events interfere with the integrity of the package.

Guidelines for Storage

Items should be stored according to the following guidelines:

- Sterile items should be stored in areas that are separate from those used to store clean nonsterile items.
- Sterile items must never be stored near sinks or other areas where they can be exposed to water.
- Sterile items should be stored in critical areas or in the sterile core when possible. They should be placed in a draft-free area away from vents and windows. The area must be dust- and lint- free.
- Closed cabinets are preferred to open storage areas.
- If items are stored in open bins, the bins or drawers should be shallow to prevent excess handling of the items.
- Mesh or basket containers are preferable to those with a solid surface where dust and bacteria can collect.
- Packages should be placed loosely on shelves to prevent crushing, tearing, or damage to items and wrappers.
- Heavy items must never be stacked on top of lighter ones. Stacking heavy instrument trays poses a risk that wrappers will be torn as the top tray is removed.
- Seldom-used items can be wrapped in protective dust covers.
- Wrappers should be inspected for damage and expiration before they are opened for use.
- Items commercially prepared and sterilized by manufacturers may be considered sterile indefinitely as long as the wrapper is intact. An expiration date printed on the package shows the maximum time the manufacturer can guarantee product stability and sterility.

DISINFECTION

TERMS RELATED TO DISINFECTION

Disinfection is the destruction of some but not all types of microorganisms. Common terms used to describe chemicals and the process of disinfection help distinguish chemicals and also clarify their action.

Table 11-6   Care of Items Exposed to Creutzfeldt-Jakob Disease (CJD) Prions

Tissue Infectivity	Item/Device (Spaulding Classification System)	Cleanable	Heat/Moisture Stable	Disposition
High infectivity	Critical/semicritical instruments and devices	If easily cleaned	If yes	1. Thoroughly clean with antiseptic detergent 2. Process at 272°F (134°C) immersed in water in prevacuum sterilizer for 18 min (extended cycle) *or* 3. Process instruments immersed in water at 250°F (121°C) in gravity sterilizer for 20 min; 60 min if not immersed in water *or* 4. Immerse in 1 N NaOH (1 normal sodium hydroxide) for 60 min at room temperature. After 60 min, remove items from NaOH, rinse, and steam-sterilize at 250°F (121°C) in gravity sterilizer for 30 min. 5. After processing as selected from 1-4, prepare instruments in the usual fashion and sterilize for future use.
			If no	Discard

	Critical/semicritical instruments and devices	If difficult to clean	If yes	1. Discard *or*
				2. Decontaminate initially by:
				  a. Steam sterilization at 272°F (134°C) in prevacuum sterilizer for 18 min *or*
				  b. Steam sterilization at 250°F (121°C) in gravity sterilizer for 60 min *or*
				  c. Immersing in 1 NaOH for 60 min at room temperature. After 60 min, remove items from NaOH, rinse, and steam-sterilize at 250°F (121°C) in gravity sterilizer for 30 min.
				3. After initial decontamination as above, thoroughly clean, wrap, and sterilize by conventional methods for future use.

			If no	Discard
	Critical/semicritical instruments and devices Noncritical instruments and devices	If impossible to clean	NA	Discard
	Noncritical instruments and devices	If cleanable	NA	1. Clean according to routine procedures. 2. Disinfect with 1:10 dilution of sodium hypochlorite or 1 N NaOH, depending on which solution would be least damaging to the items. 3. Continue processing according to routine procedures.
		Noncleanable	NA	Discard
	Environmental surfaces	NA	NA	1. Cover surface with disposable, impermeable material. 2. Incinerate material after use. 3. Disinfect surface with 1:10 dilution of sodium hypochlorite (bleach). 4. Wipe entire surface using routine facility decontamination procedures for surface decontamination.
Medium/low/no infectivity	Critical/semicritical/noncritical instruments and devices	Cleanable	NA	1. Clean, disinfect, or sterilize according to routine procedures.
		Noncleanable	NA	Discard
	Environmental surfaces	NA	NA	1. Cover surface with disposable, impermeable material. 2. Dispose of material according to facility policy. 3. Disinfect surface with OSHA-recommended agent for decontamination of blood-contaminated surfaces (e.g., 1:10 or 1:100 dilution of sodium hypochlorite).

Data from Favaro MS, Bond WW: Chemical disinfection of medical and surgical materials. In Block SS, editor: *Disinfection, sterilization, and preservation*, ed 5, Philadelphia, 2001, Lippincott Williams & Wilkins; New clues on how to inactivate prions, *OR Manager* 20:23, 2004; Rutala WA, Weber DJ: Creutzfeldt-Jakob disease: recommendations for disinfection and sterilization, *Clinical Infectious Diseases* 32:1348, 2001; World Health Organization, Department of Communicable Disease Surveillance and Response: WHO infection control guidelines for transmissible spongiform encephalopathies. Report of a WHO consultation. Geneva, Switzerland, 23-26 March 1999. Accessed April 18, 2012, at http://www.who.int/csr/resources/publications/bse/whocdscsraph2003.pdf.

NA, Not applicable; *OSHA*, Occupational Safety and Health Administration.

The suffix -cidal means to kill. A **bactericidal** chemical is one that kills bacteria, and a **viricidal** chemical kills viruses. A **sporicidal** chemical destroys bacterial spores, and a **fungicidal** agent is one that kills fungi. The term *germicide* ("germ killing," or **germicidal**) is commonly used by the general public but not in medicine. *Germ* is the lay term for infectious microorganism.

USE OF CHEMICAL DISINFECTANTS

Disinfectants commonly used in patient care are categorized by chemical type (Table 11-7). The selection of a disinfectant is based on the result required. Some disinfectants are effective at destroying a limited number of microorganisms; others are very effective at killing all organisms, including bacterial spores. Some are extremely corrosive, whereas others are relatively harmless to common materials found in the hospital.

Factors that affect a disinfectant's activity (or "-cidal" ability) include the following:

1. *Concentration of the solution:* Every chemical disinfectant is used at a prescribed dilution. Chemicals may require premixing with water. This must be done with a measuring device.
2. *The bioburden on the object:* As the bioburden increases, the effectiveness of the disinfectant may decrease.
3. *Water hardness and pH:* The mineral content and pH of the water used for dilution may alter the action of the chemical.
4. *Presence or absence of organic matter on the item:* Nearly all disinfectants are weakened in the presence of organic material such as blood, sputum, or tissue residue. Therefore, items to be disinfected must undergo cleaning (removal of organic debris and soil) and thorough drying before the disinfection process.

Precautions and Hazards

Many disinfectants are unsafe for use on human tissue, including skin. This means that employees must be extremely cautious when handling them. Warnings and instructions for use must be strictly followed. Do not be misled by the mild odor of some disinfectants. Many chemicals do not emit noxious fumes but they are still toxic.

Every health care facility is required by law to provide employees with information about hazards in their work environment. This includes specific training and information about the chemicals they handle. Every chemical used in the workplace has a corresponding **Material Safety Data Sheet (MSDS)**, as mandated by OSHA. The MSDS describes the chemical, potential hazards, and what to do if the chemical comes in contact with the skin or is splashed into the eyes. The MSDS for each chemical is easily accessed and should be read by all who work in the perioperative environment. (A more complete discussion of chemical safety is presented in Chapter 8.)

Safety Guidelines for Disinfectants

- All disinfectants should be stored in well-ventilated rooms, and their containers should be kept covered.

- All personnel handling disinfectants must wear personal protective equipment.
- The dilution ratio of a liquid chemical should never be changed except by hospital protocol.
- A measuring device designated for mixing liquid disinfectants with water should always be used. Personnel should not rely on haphazard techniques or guesswork when preparing solutions.
- Two disinfectants should never be mixed; this could create toxic fumes or unstable and dangerous compounds.
- Liquid chemicals should be disposed of as directed by hospital policy and the chemical's label instructions. Some chemicals are unsafe for disposal through standard sewage systems.
- An unlabeled bottle or container should never be used and should be discarded. Personnel should always be aware of what chemical is being used and its specific purpose.

CHEMICAL DISINFECTANTS FOR MEDICAL DEVICES

The chemicals most commonly used in high level disinfection are glutaraldehyde and orthophthalaldehyde (commercially prepared as Cidex and Cidex OPA).

Glutaraldehyde

Glutaraldehyde is a high level disinfectant that is sporicidal, bactericidal, and viricidal. It is tuberculocidal in 20 minutes. This disinfectant is weakened considerably by unintentional dilution, which occurs if instruments are wet when placed in the immersion tank. Glutaraldehyde is also weakened by the presence of organic matter (tissue debris or body fluids). When glutaraldehyde solutions are mixed and kept for repetitive use, the solution must be completely renewed after 14 days because it is ineffective after that time. In addition, during its time in use, the solution must be evaluated often with test strips to ensure that the proper concentration is maintained (2% glutaraldehyde).

Occupational hazards of glutaraldehyde most commonly arise when the solution is kept in open immersion baths in a poorly ventilated work area. The safe levels of formaldehyde or glutaraldehyde in the air are under 0.2 ppm. Any amount over that causes irritation of the eyes and nasal passages. Glutaraldehyde is toxic to tissue; items that have been disinfected or sterilized in glutaraldehyde must be completely rinsed with sterile distilled water before they are used on a patient.

Orthophthalaldehyde

Orthophthalaldehyde 0.55% (Cidex OPA) is a non–glutaraldehyde-based, high level disinfectant that can be used for immersible medical devices. Instruments and equipment are thoroughly cleaned, dried, and placed in the solution for 12 minutes. The items must be thoroughly rinsed with water three times. Items not properly rinsed will stain the skin of the handler or the patient. Orthophthaldehyde has a **shelf life** of 14 days; daily testing is required to ensure that the concentration of the disinfectant is at the required level.

Table **11-7**	**Properties of Disinfectants**						
Chemical	Level of Disinfection	Kills Spores	Kills HIV	Kills *M. tuberculosis*	Kills HBV	Uses	Risk
Isopropyl alcohol (70% to 90%)	Intermediate (some semicritical and noncritical items)	No	Yes	Yes	Yes	Limited; no longer used as a general disinfectant.	Flammable; can damage lensed instruments.
Phenolic detergent compounds	Low	No	Yes	Yes	No	Environmental cleaning only.	Highly toxic.
Glutaraldehyde (2%)	High (critical items)	Yes	Yes	Yes	Yes	Endoscopes, respiratory equipment, anesthesia equipment, immersible items. Long shelf life. Disinfectant active for long periods when used properly.	Vapor causes eye, skin, and nasal irritation. Improperly rinsed endoscopes can cause tissue damage.
Stabilized hydrogen peroxide (6%)	High (critical items)	Yes	Yes	Yes	Yes	Must contact all surfaces when used as a sterilant.	Can cause tissue irritation.
Formalin (37% formaldehyde)	High	Yes	Yes	Yes	Yes	Currently used for specimen preservation.	Highly noxious fumes; carcinogenic.
Iodophor (free iodine in a detergent-disinfectant solution)	Intermediate to low, depending on concentration	No	Yes	Yes	Yes	As a disinfectant, limited to use in cleaning hydrotherapy tanks and thermometers, environmental cleaning.	May cause reaction in sensitive individuals.
Quaternary ammonium detergent	Low (noncritical items)	No	Yes	No	No	Limited effectiveness; used for low level environmental disinfection.	May cause reaction in sensitive individuals.
Sodium hypochlorite (5%, 500 ppm)	Low (noncritical items)	No	Yes	No	Yes	1:100 ppm for spot disinfection and blood spills; environmental cleaning.	Fumes can irritate skin and mucous membranes.

HBV, Hepatitis B virus; *HIV,* human immunodeficiency virus.

HIGH LEVEL DISINFECTION

High level disinfection (HLD) is a process in which most but not all microorganisms are killed with a liquid disinfectant. HLD does not usually destroy bacterial spores; therefore it is used only for instruments that will be used in semicritical areas of the body (e.g., nonintact skin and mucous membranes). Instruments and other items that are semicritical include:

- Anesthesia equipment
- Gastrointestinal endoscopes
- Bronchoscopes
- Respiratory therapy equipment

HLD is used for flexible and rigid endoscopes that are used in noncritical areas of the body. Processing takes place in a special area of the operating room adjacent to or near the point of use, such as the endoscopy department or cystoscopy suite.

The process uses a commercial reprocessing unit, or the instrument is simply soaked in a large basin or tray. Before any instrument is disinfected, it must be thoroughly cleaned to remove all traces of blood, tissue, and body fluids. Cleaning proceeds in a systematic fashion so that no areas are overlooked.

A complete discussion of the techniques used in the reprocessing of endoscopes can be found in Chapter 24. Important guidelines are listed in Box 11-4.

LOW LEVEL DISINFECTION: NONCRITICAL AREAS

Low level disinfection is performed on equipment that comes in contact with skin but not mucous membranes or any other tissue. The process of low level disinfection kills most, but not all, bacteria and viruses. This category of disinfection is

Box 11-4　Important Guidelines for Processing Endoscopes

Manual Cleaning

- Always wear personal protective equipment when reprocessing instruments in a chemical solution.
- Always leak-test any flexible endoscope before cleaning.
- Submerge the instrument in detergent solution and clean all surfaces with a clean cloth.
- Use a suction pump and syringe to flush detergent through the instrument channels and ports.
- A soft brush can be used to clean channels.
- After cleaning the instrument completely, rinse it in deionized water to remove all traces of detergent.
- Inspect the instrument for any soil or debris missed during cleaning. If any debris remains, repeat the cleaning process, including all channels, valves, and stopcocks.
- Remove all water from the instrument channels and exterior. Low level compressed air may be used to dry channels, valves, and stopcocks.

High Level Disinfection

- Processing should be done just before use.
- If an automatic reprocessor is used, following the manufacturer's guidelines exactly.
- Make sure the instrument is completely dry before submerging it in disinfectant.
- For manual processing of items in a tray or basin, make sure all channels are filled with solution.
- Cover the tray and start timing.
- Do not add any instruments or change the dilution after processing has begun.
- When timing is complete, remove the item and rinse thoroughly according to operating room policy at least three times to remove all traces of disinfectant.

performed on patient care items, transport devices, and furniture, such as:

- Operating room table and accessories
- Furniture in the surgical suite
- Floors and walls
- Intravenous (IV) stands
- Stretchers
- Blood pressure cuffs
- Stethoscopes

Low level disinfection is performed as part of routine decontamination of the operating room and in all patient care settings.

ENVIRONMENTAL DISINFECTANTS

Environmental disinfectants are used for routine low level disinfection and terminal decontamination. These disinfectants contain enzymes and other chemicals that destroy or inhibit microbes by changing cell proteins (denaturation) or by drying (desiccation) them.

PHENOLICS

Phenol (carbolic acid) is formulated as a detergent for hospital cleaning. It is not sporicidal, but it is tuberculocidal, fungicidal, viricidal, and bactericidal. Because scant information is available on the specific effects of phenol on microorganisms, its use is restricted to disinfection of *noncritical items*. It is extremely important to follow the manufacturer's instructions for dilution and mixing, because phenolic mixtures can be very toxic. Phenol has a very noxious odor and causes skin lesions and respiratory irritation in some individuals.

QUATERNARY AMMONIUM COMPOUNDS

Quaternary ammonium compounds, or *quats*, are fungicidal and bactericidal but not effective at killing spores. This group of disinfectants is less effective in hard water, which can limit their use in some regions. Benzalkonium chloride and dimethyl benzyl ammonium chloride are common quaternary ammonium compounds widely used as disinfectants.

HYPOCHLORITE

Hypochlorite is sporicidal and tuberculocidal and effective against the human immunodeficiency virus (HIV). The CDC recommends this product for use in spot cleaning of blood spills, because it is very fast acting. However, it is deactivated in the presence of organic material; therefore, the area must be cleaned before hypochlorite is applied. The chemicals in the hypochlorite family are not used on instruments, because they are corrosive. However, they are widely used for environmental cleaning, because they are effective and inexpensive. Sodium hypochlorite, for example, is common household bleach. Hypochlorite must be diluted properly to prevent respiratory irritation and skin burns.

ALCOHOL

Alcohol is a commonly used disinfectant that is composed of two components: ethyl alcohol and isopropyl alcohol. Both are water-soluble (mix easily in water). Alcohol is not sporicidal, but it is bactericidal, tuberculocidal, and viricidal. It is effective against cytomegalovirus and HIV. Alcohol's optimum disinfection ability occurs at a 60% to 70% dilution. Alcohol must never be used on surgical instruments, because it is not sporicidal and is very corrosive to stainless steel.

Alcohol greatly reduces the number of bacteria on skin when used as a surgical handrub. However, it also removes fatty acids from the skin and has a drying effect when used routinely.

Because it is highly flammable and volatile, alcohol must never be used around electrosurgery instruments or lasers. It must be stored in a cool, well-ventilated area. Skin preparation solutions that contain alcohol must be allowed to dry completely before draping.

ENVIRONMENTAL CLEANING

The perioperative environment is cleaned with disinfectants to reduce the bioburden to a safe minimum. Cleaning should be the responsibility of everyone in the department. In certain settings, the responsibility belongs to specific personnel assigned by the nurse manager or by the job description given to them by the hospital. The duties and tasks associated with sanitation and decontamination must never be taken lightly.

Disinfection or **sanitation** is the process by which surfaces, materials, and equipment are cleaned with specific substances (disinfectants) that render them safe for their intended use. Any item that is soiled with organic matter such as blood, tissue, or any body fluid is considered contaminated. The process that renders the surface or item safe is decontamination. The disinfection or sanitation process may achieve the same result as decontamination. One must assume that all items are contaminated and clean all items properly. *Cleaning* refers to the process by which any type of soil, including organic material, is removed. This is accomplished with detergent, water, and mechanical action. Cleaning precedes all disinfection processes. The purpose of sanitation and disinfection is to prevent cross-contamination between patients and personnel.

ROUTINE DECONTAMINATION OF THE SURGICAL SUITE

Before the Workday

The recommended practice before the first case of the day is damp dusting of surgical lights, furniture, and fixed equipment in the operating suite. A clean, lint-free cloth and a hospital-grade chemical disinfectant are used.

During Surgery

The principles of Standard Precautions apply to all surgical procedures, and all cases are considered contaminated and treated accordingly. During surgery, the circulator and his or her assistants are responsible for ensuring that the environment in the surgical suite is kept as disease-free as possible. They do this by confining and containing all potential contaminants. The following activities, which are part of the Standard Precautions, must be performed to prevent cross-contamination with blood-borne pathogens.

- Any blood spills or contamination by other organic material should be removed promptly with a hospital-grade disinfectant. Household bleach should not be used for this purpose because of its potential to damage certain equipment and instruments.
- All articles used and discarded in the course of surgery must be placed in leak-proof containers. This prevents spilling of contaminated liquid onto other surfaces.
- Any contaminated or suspect item must be handled in a manner that protects personnel from contamination. Non-scrubbed personnel must wear PPE. This includes cap, gloves, a cover gown, a face shield or mask, and protective eyewear. An instrument can be used to transfer contaminated articles to a waste or other receptacle (this is called the *no-touch method*).
- Tissue specimens, blood, and all other body fluids must be placed in a leak-proof container for transport out of the department. The outside of any specimen container that is passed off the surgical field to the circulator must be cleaned with a hospital-grade disinfectant.
- Because paper products are difficult or impossible to decontaminate, every effort should be made to keep patients' charts, laboratory slips, radiograph reports and radiographs, and any paper documentation free of contamination.
- Contaminated sponges must be collected in a kick bucket in which a plastic bag or liner has been previously placed. Sponges must not be lined up on the floor for counting. Sponges should be counted and immediately placed in plastic bags representing increment numbers such as 5 or 10 sponges.
- Instruments that fall off the surgical field must be retrieved by the circulator (with gloves protecting the hands) and placed in a basin containing a noncorrosive disinfectant. In this way, organic debris on the instrument is prevented from drying and becoming airborne.
- During surgery, the scrubbed surgical technologist should periodically wipe blood and tissue from instruments. Those that are difficult to clean (e.g., orthopedic rasps, drill bits, and suction tips) should be kept moist at all times to prevent blood, tissue, and body fluids from drying on the surface.
- Small-bore cannulas and suction tip lumens should be flushed frequently to prevent interior buildup of debris. If a suction tip becomes completely occluded, a metal stylet should be used to remove the debris before flushing. When blood and tissue are allowed to dry on an instrument, they stick to the surface and may pass intact through subsequent phases of processing, including vigorous mechanical washing.
- Any organic debris or residue that remains is a potential source of pathogenic microorganisms, even if the item has been through the sterilization or disinfection process. A basin of sterile water should be available during surgery to aid in keeping instruments clean. Instruments should never be soaked in saline, because it causes the metal to corrode.

Terminal Decontamination

The process of **terminal decontamination** follows every surgical case. This is the thorough cleaning and disinfection of all equipment and soiled surfaces in the operating room. It follows the removal of instruments and contaminated disposable items used during surgery.

The goal of terminal decontamination is to prevent disease transmission. A systematic routine is followed to ensure that no step in decontamination is missed. Rapid turnover of patients is important in a busy operating room. However, environmental safety takes priority over scheduling. After a surgical procedure, duties are shared between the scrub person, who handles equipment and instruments directly related to the performance of the surgery, and the personnel responsible for case cleanup. These can be housekeeping personnel, scrub persons, circulators, or surgical aides. Regardless of the type of personnel participating in the cleanup, all should be attired in PPE.

During decontamination, an approved disinfectant is used to clean surfaces and fixtures. High level disinfectants are not used in terminal disinfection.

The steps in the procedure are described below:

1. After surgery, the scrub prepares equipment and instruments for transport out of the surgical suite. Any instrument exposed to the sterile field must be processed whether it appears soiled or not. All instruments are placed in leakproof containers and placed into a closed cart for transport to the decontamination area.

2. All disposable sharp instruments (e.g., knife blades, sutures, trocars) are placed in a designated sharps container in a manner that prevents injury to the personnel who next handle the container. If other personnel are responsible for cleaning up the back table, the scrub person should verbally communicate the presence of sharps on the table and visually identify them to the other personnel.

3. All disposable anesthesia equipment is removed in closed bags.

4. Suctioned blood and body fluids may be treated with a hypochlorite solidifier and then placed in leak-proof biohazard bags or containers.

5. Soiled linens and/or single-use drapes are gathered from the outer edges inward to contain contaminants. Linen is placed in waterproof biohazard bags in such a way as to prevent the soiled areas from touching bare skin. Open bags should not be compacted, because this releases contaminated particles into the air.

6. All disposable items contaminated with blood must be placed in waterproof bags or containers and clearly labeled as biohazardous waste. If any items are likely to leak blood or body fluids, they must be removed from the operating room in a closed container system.

7. All soiled equipment that is routinely kept in the operating suite is removed to the decontamination area or safe disposal area.

After instruments, supplies and contaminated equipment have been removed from the surgical suite, the walls, floors, furniture, and fixtures are cleaned.

- Floors are cleaned with disinfectant and may be wet-vacuumed. A 3- to 4-foot area (about 1 to 1.2 m) around the sterile field is considered efficient for routine decontamination between cases.
- The pads of the operating table are removed to expose the undersurface of the table. All surfaces of the table and pads are cleaned, with particular attention to hinges, pivotal points, and castors.
- The operating table is moved aside for cleaning underneath and to check for any items that may have dropped to the floor during surgery.

- All soiled operating room equipment is cleaned with disinfectant.
- Walls, doors, surgical lights, and ceilings are spot-cleaned if they are soiled with blood, tissue, or body fluids. Additional attention is given to supply cabinet doors, especially the latches and handles.
- All contaminated items used during the cleaning process are removed from the room.

After decontamination, all furniture is repositioned, and clean linen is placed on the operating table. Clean covers are also placed over table accessories. Clean liner bags are placed in kick buckets and linen frames.

HISTORICAL HIGHLIGHTS

- "Dry heat" sterilizers used to be found in most operating rooms before the 1960s. These were essentially large ovens used to sterilize powders (e.g., glove powder), wood, glass (including glass syringes), and other items that could withstand high heat without melting or oxidizing. Dry heat sterilization is now used in chemical and biological laboratories rather than the patient care setting.
- Before the 1980s, instruments were routinely hand-washed, then processed in a single-unit washer-sterilizer. This resulted in instruments with baked-on blood and tissue that then had to be removed by handcleaning and resterilization. The washer-decontaminator used now replaces this older system with a more efficient and much safer method of decontaminating surgical instruments and supplies.

KEY CONCEPTS

- The practice of aseptic technique is based on the separation between sterile and nonsterile surfaces. The purpose of practicing aseptic technique is preventing infection.
- Correct use of terms related to sterility and disinfection demonstrates understanding of the concepts and their importance in preventing infection.
- The Spaulding system separates medical devices and instruments according to the location of their use in the body and thus the level of asepsis required—sterilization, disinfection, or cleaning.
- Systematic methods are used in the sterilization and disinfection of surgical devices and instruments so that no step is missed in the process. All surgical technologists are required to know what method to use, and how to perform that method.
- Decontamination of instruments and devices is critical to prevent the transmission of infection from one individual to another.
- Surgical instruments and devices are made of many different types of materials whose physical properties require specific methods of cleaning, disinfection, and sterilization. One of the primary goals in reprocessing is to use the most effective means while also considering safety and economics.

- Correct wrapping of surgical equipment and loading in the steam sterilizer are essential to achieve and maintain sterility of an item. If this phase of the process is incorrect, the whole process will be invalid.
- Biological monitoring during sterilization is performed by exposing the load to harmless bacterial spores, which are then recovered and cultured.
- Steam under pressure is the most common and economical method of sterilizing surgical equipment.
- The flash sterilizer is used to rapidly sterilize clean decontaminated equipment for immediate use. This method is used only when no other method is available. Implants are not flashed sterilized except in an emergency and must be monitored with a biological control system.
- Other methods of sterilization include ethylene oxide gas, gas plasma, liquid peracetic acid, and ionizing radiation (commercial use only).
- All equipment used on a patient must be cleaned and decontaminated before sterilization.
- Disinfection is performed on equipment used in semicritical areas of the body. High level disinfectants are capable of destroying bacteria and their spores.
- Low level disinfection is used for environmental cleaning.
- Terminal decontamination of the operating room is performed after each case according to established methods and protocols.

REVIEW QUESTIONS

1. What is *bioburden*?
2. What three conditions are necessary for any sterilization or disinfection process to be effective?
3. Why are instruments processed in the washer-decontaminator sterilizer?
4. What is the purpose of wrapping instruments for steam sterilization?
5. What disinfectant is approved for cleaning blood spills in the surgical suite?
6. Why doesn't a control monitor determine that sterilized goods are sterile?
7. What is DART?
8. Describe each of the three levels of the Spaulding classification system.
9. What is immediate-use processing?
10. What is terminal disinfection?
11. Why are sterile packages given a lot number?

CASE STUDIES

Case 1

While scrubbed, you open a basin set and find a small amount of water pooled in the bottom of the basin. What are the possible causes of this? What will you do?

Case 2

During the setup for a case, you notice that one of the indicator strips in a pan of instruments on your back table has not changed color. What should you do?

Case 3

You are employed in a small community hospital. In your first week, you are scrubbed on a laparotomy case. The circulator opens a single-use electrosurgery pencil that has been resterilized with EO in the hospital's Central Processing department. What will you do?

Case 4

You are the afternoon shift relief scrub on a plastic surgery case. About an hour into the case on which you have relieved, you happen to notice the chemical sterilization monitor at the bottom of the instrument tray, which is on the sterile back table. The monitor has not changed color. The surgeon is using instruments from this tray. What do you do?

Case 5

You are about to scrub on an orthopedic case in which a stainless steel implant will be inserted into the patient's hip. The surgeon wants to see the implant before surgery. He opens the package and examines it with bare hands. He then instructs you to flash-sterilize the implant. What will you do? Who is responsible? What are the risks associated with flash sterilization of implants?

Case 6

You have been assigned to work in the endoscopy room for the day. You will use gastrointestinal endoscopes. When you arrive in the laboratory, you notice that the endoscope to be used first is soaking in disinfectant solution that has expired (has been held beyond the date approved for disinfection). The physician tells you that he will use the endoscope anyway. What is your response?

Case 7

While opening sterile goods for a case, you find a basin set that has been wrapped in one double-thickness wrapper. You are able to open the basin set using sterile technique. Is it sterile?

BIBLIOGRAPHY

American Society of Cataract and Refractive Surgery and the American Society of Ophthalmic Registered Nurses: Recommended practices for cleaning and sterilizing intraocular surgical instruments, Accessed July 24, 2011, at http://www.ncbi.hlm.nih.gov/pubmed/17883207#.

AORN, *Standards, recommended practices, and guidelines,* 2011.

Association for the Advancement of Medical Instrumentation: *Comprehensive guide to steam sterilization and sterility assurance in health care facilities.* ANSI/AAMI ST79: 2006.

Association of periOperative Registered Nurses: Recommended practices for environmental cleaning in the surgical practice setting. In *Standards, recommended practices and guidelines, 2007 edition,* Denver, 2007, AORN.

Association of periOperative Registered Nurses: Recommended practices for sterilization in the perioperative practice setting. In *Standards, recommended practices and guidelines, 2007 edition,* Denver, 2007, AORN.

Association of periOperative Registered Nurses: Sterilization in the perioperative practice setting. In *Standards, recommended practices and guidelines, 2007 edition*, Denver, 2007, AORN.

Association of Surgical Technologists: Aseptic technique, in *Standards of practice*. Accessed March 19, 2009, at http://www.ast.org/educators/standards_table_of_contents.aspx.

Carlo A: The new era of flash sterilization, *AORN Journal* 86:1, 2007.

International Association of Healthcare Central Processing Materiel Management: *Enhancing cooperation between the central service and operating room departments*. Accessed May 20, 2008, at http://www.iahcsmm.org.

Medical Device and Diagnostic Industry: *Global sterilization: making the standards standard*. Accessed November 13, 2007, at http://www.devicelink.com/mddi/archive/05/03/008.html.

Spry C: Care and handling of basic surgical instruments, *AORN Journal* 86(Suppl 1):77, 2007.

U.S. Department of Labor: *Hazard communication: foundation of workplace chemical safety programs*. Accessed November 13, 2007, at http://www.osha.org.

Surgical Instruments

12

CHAPTER OUTLINE

Introduction	Common Types of	Use of Instruments by	Inspecting Surgical
Instrument Names	Instruments by	Tissue Type	Instruments
Instrument Manufacturing	Function		

LEARNING OBJECTIVES

After studying this chapter the reader will be able to:

1. Understand how instrument names are used in the operating room
2. Review information on instrument manufacturing
3. Identify the different types of finishes on surgical instruments
4. Differentiate types of instruments by their design
5. Differentiate types of instruments by their function
6. Classify instruments by tissue type
7. Describe how to inspect instruments for defects

TERMINOLOGY

Alloy: A combination of several different kinds of metals. Alloys are used in the manufacture of stainless steel.

Box lock: The hinge point of many surgical instruments.

Chisel: An orthopedic instrument used to slice bone; one side is straight and the other is beveled.

Curettage: The removal of tissue by scraping with a surgical curette.

Dilator: Graduated, smooth instrument that is used to increase the diameter of an anatomical opening in tissue.

Double-action rongeur: A bone-cutting instrument with two hinges in the middle. This increases leverage and strength of the instrument.

Elevator: A straight instrument with curved sharp or dull tip used to separate tissue layers such as periosteum from bone.

Gouge: A V-shaped bone chisel.

Hemostat: A surgical clamp most often used to occlude a blood vessel.

Rongeur: A hinged instrument with sharp, cup-shaped tips that is used to extract pieces of bone or other connective tissue.

Serosa: The delicate outer layer of tissue of most organs.

Shank: The area of a surgical instrument between the box lock and the finger ring.

Single-action rongeur: A heavy cutting instrument that has one hinge.

Tenaculum: A grasping instrument with sharp pointed tips, generally used to manipulate or grasp tissue such as the thyroid or cervix.

INTRODUCTION

Expertise in surgical instrumentation is among the most important roles of the surgical technologist. Familiarity with instruments and their names (sometimes different from one region to another, and even among health facilities) is *also one of the most difficult* learning curves for students in surgery.

The purpose of this chapter is not to provide a catalog for memorization of instruments Instead, the chapter provides the basis for understanding how instruments are made and the relationship between design and function of the instrument. The most useful way to learn the *names* and use of instruments is to study them in association with the surgeries they are used in rather than in isolation, such as in a catalog. This is because a relatively small number of instruments are used compared to the thousands contained in different catalogs. In this text, surgical instruments are illustrated within their specialty chapter to reinforce the association and aid in memorization. Some common nicknames are given but because of the regional variation in nicknames, technologists are usually required to learn these on the job.

NOTE: Microsurgical and endoscopic instruments are discussed in Chapter 24. Ophthalmic instruments are illustrated in Chapter 27.

Classification of instruments in groups according to function and association with tissue types encourages critical thinking during surgery. Finally, students need to know how to evaluate surgical instruments for soundness. This is an important role that has implications for patient safety and a technically smooth surgical procedure.

INSTRUMENT NAMES

Learning instruments by name is one of the challenging tasks of all surgical students. However, the task is not as complicated as it first seems in the early weeks of working in the operating room. The following steps provide general guidelines for learning instrument names:

1. Each health care facility has a limited number of instruments, which are assembled in sets according to surgical specialty and case.
2. Within each prepared set, only a fraction of the instruments included will be used. The others are there to complete the set and because some surgeons might need them.
3. Surgeons have favorite instruments, according to individual skills and techniques used.
4. The most important instruments to focus learning at the beginning are instruments used *commonly* and those that are the *favorites* of specific surgeons you are likely to scrub with.
5. Many instruments have multiple catalog names that are also the name of the person who invented them. For example, in gynecology surgery you will find many instruments named "Sims" and "Heaney," including curettes, retractors, needle holders, and clamps. Both Sims and Heaney invented many of the prototype gynecological and obstetrical instruments used today. When the name of an instrument consists of two or more hyphenated parts, such as Beckman-Adson retractor, usually only the first name is used (e.g., Beckman).
6. Many surgeons do not know the exact names of instruments, or they have come to call the instrument a made-up name. This can complicate learning instruments, but usually there are only a few examples of invented names in each health care facility.
7. Surgeons often call for an instrument by type rather than name. For example, a surgeon may ask for "a self-retaining." This refers to a self-retaining retractor. There will be a limited number of self-retaining retractors available on an instrument set, and perhaps only one. In this case, the technologist must pass the most appropriate retractor according to the size of the surgical incision, type of tissue,

and depth of the tissue to be retracted, all of which come with experience.

INSTRUMENT MANUFACTURING

The manufacturing process, the origin of the materials, and the quality control on the finished product determine the quality and safety of surgical instruments. High quality surgical instruments are constructed using specific types of metals. Stainless steel contains iron, carbon, chromium, nickel, manganese, and other metal combinations. Such a combination is called an **alloy**. In general, higher quality instruments contain a greater percentage of chromium. This results in greater *passivation*, which is decreased reactivity and increased resistance to corrosion. Poor quality steel does not have this quality and tends to develop hairline fractures that are sometimes not visible without magnification. These fractures become deeper with repeated use, finally causing the instrument to break. Soldering defects can cause breakage or microscopic burrs and sharp points that puncture and cut tissue. This is especially critical for eye surgery and microsurgery. Microscopic ridges and troughs in the surface of the steel can slice through delicate tissue and collect tissue debris. Biofilm in these small defects may not be removed in the disinfection and sterilization process, increasing the risk for patient infection. Metal flaking is another problem encountered with cheap, poorly made instruments.

INSTRUMENT GRADES

Within the stainless steel and surgical instrument industry, grades are assigned according to the quality of the steel. In the current global market, surgical instruments can be assembled in one country with steel obtained from another. Quality may not be consistent, and poorly made instruments that have not been properly calibrated for precision or metal defects are widely available. Surgical instruments are used in a variety of settings besides surgery. These settings include biological science laboratories, classrooms, and goods manufacturing. The highest quality instruments, suitable for human surgery, are *surgical grade*. Those of lower quality are usually referred to as *economy* or *floor grade*. The quality of the steel used in the manufacturing of an instrument is as important as the assembly and inspection process.

INSTRUMENT FINISHES

High quality stainless steel resists corrosion and is the most commonly used metal for instruments. However, even high quality instruments can become damaged when subjected to harsh chemicals, frequent ultrasonic cleaning, and repeated sterilization. Different types of finishes on instruments protect them from environmental damage. The most common finishes are easy to recognize:

1. *Highly polished* or *mirror finish* instruments resist staining. However, they are highly reflective and produce glare under strong lighting.
2. *Satin finish* reduces glare but is also prone to staining.

3. *Black chromium finish* is used on laser surgery instruments. The black finish absorbs all light and prevents reflection of laser energy into adjacent tissues.

4. *Titanium anodizing* is a method that imparts color and hardness to the surface of titanium. Anodizing is performed by passing an electric current through the surface metal, resulting in oxidation. Different colors are achieved by adjusting the oxide level of the coating. This process is commonly used in the manufacture of orthopedic implants such as plates and screws. Color coding allows easy matching of implant components and specialized tools. Titanium is extremely hard and resistant to corrosion and pitting, a quality that is essential in orthopedics.

5. *Anodizing* is used in the manufacturing of lightweight aluminum instrument sterilization trays. Without the anodizing process, aluminum trays would easily scratch. The process allows the manufacturing of large instrument trays without the added weight of stainless steel.

6. *Gold dip* or *black finish* on the handles (finger rings) and shanks of scissors or needle holders means that the working tip or edge of the instrument has tungsten carbide inserts that are highly resistant to scratching, pitting, and dulling. Tungsten carbide scissors hold their cutting edge much longer than conventional scissors. The tungsten carbide inserts in needle holders prevent the needle from slipping or rotating.

INSTRUMENT DESIGN

Surgical instruments are designed for specific functions and use with specific tissue types. An understanding of design features can help in passing the right instrument at the right time, even if the surgeon does not specify the exact name of the instrument needed. This is one of the most important skills in surgical technology and one that can also be the most difficult to learn.

If we examine some common design/function relationships in instruments, it clarifies understanding of instrument technology as a whole. Much of this information has to do with surgical technique. Remember that in good surgical technique, tissues are usually handled with instruments, not with the hands. The exception is when the surgeon needs to palpate or feel the tissue for assessment purposes. The instrument is a tactile interface between the tissue and the surgeon's hand.

- *Finger rings for precision:* Instruments used for general dissection (delicate cutting), clamping, or holding soft tissue have a finger ring design that allows dexterity and precision. This is true whether the instrument is short or long.
- *Overall length:* Short instruments are used on surface tissues—those that are not deep inside the body. For example, ophthalmic surgery requires the hand to be very close to the anatomy for the greatest control. Because the surgeon performs the procedure using an operating microscope, handles like those on most instruments would be awkward and get in the way of the focal point. Therefore, ophthalmic instruments are designed to be cradled in the palm. On the other hand, long instruments are needed for use deep in body cavities or in very deep-bodied patients.

- *Weight and thickness:* The heavier an instrument is, the *less* precise the instrument will be at the working end (tips). Lightweight instruments are used for the most delicate tissue so that the surgeon has immediate *tactile feedback*. Even long instruments used in minimally invasive surgery must have delicate tips. The **shank** (long portion) of the instrument must also be somewhat delicate in order to provide the tactile feedback needed for precision surgery. Surgical scissors with moderately heavy blades are generally used on fibrous tissue (e.g., dissecting the uterine ligaments), whereas those with short delicate blades (even if the shanks are very long) are intended for dissection of delicate tissues.
- *Points or teeth:* Toothed or sharp-pointed instruments are used to grip fibrous tissue that would otherwise slip through the instrument's jaws. Tissue forceps or "pickups" with one or more teeth are used only on connective tissues such as ligament, fascia, or skin, but never on delicate tissue (e.g., a blood vessel or a duct such as the fallopian tube). Vascular forceps contain one or two *smooth ridges* along the tips. These can grasp delicate tissue without tearing it. Retractors with sharp teeth are placed only in tissue that is avascular, such as adipose and fascia.
- *Shape:* The overall shape of the instrument is a clue to its specific use. Long shanks are necessary for instruments used deep in the body. The "bayonet"-shaped instruments are almost always used in nasal or neurosurgery. Shorter instruments are used on superficial tissues. Few instruments are perfectly straight, because the contours and bends of anatomy require instruments that can reach around and under structures.

COMMON TYPES OF INSTRUMENTS BY FUNCTION

CLAMP

The term *clamp* can refer to any instrument that closes over tissue to hold or occlude it. Most ring finger instruments are joined at the center by a **box lock**. This is a single-pin design that provides balance and reduces weight. A locking ratchet mechanism secures the clamp and remains locked when closed tightly (Figure 12-1). Microsurgical and ophthalmic instruments use a spring lock mechanism that is much more delicate than a ratchet system. A **hemostat** is a particular kind of clamp used to stop blood flow through a vessel. A hemostat can be long or short, straight or curved. Other types of holding clamps are used to handle and manipulate tissue in the surgical wound. Examples of common hemostats are the mosquito, Kelly, Crile, Mayo, right angle or Mixter, and Schnidt clamps (Figure 12-2). The Kelly and Crile clamps are nearly identical; the Schnidt (also called a tonsil clamp) has a slight curve at the tip, and the right angle clamp has a distinctly short right angle at the end of a medium or long shank.

Partial Occlusion Clamp

A partial occlusion or atraumatic clamp has locking ratchets, but the tips and shanks do not close tightly over the tissue.

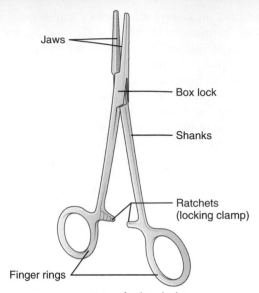

Figure 12-1   Parts of a box lock instrument.

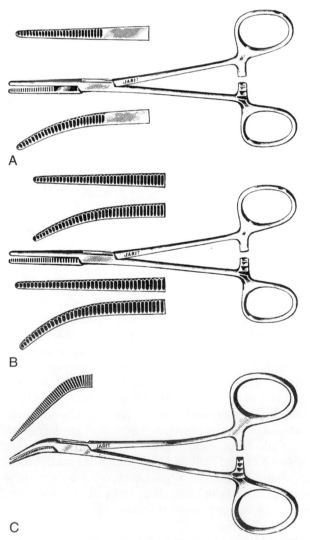

Figure 12-2   **Hemostats. A,** Kelly hemostats. **B,** Crile hemostats. **C,** Mosquito hemostats. *(Courtesy Jarit Surgical Instruments, Hawthorne, NY.)*

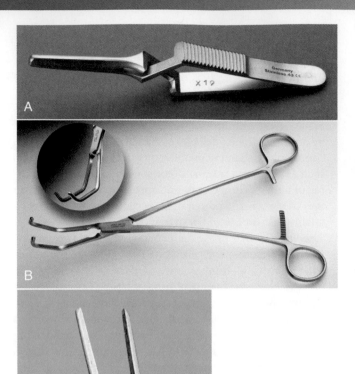

Figure 12-3   **Vascular clamps. A,** Bulldog clamp (actual size, 2 inches [5 cm]). **B,** Satinsky vena cava clamp. **C,** Fogarty clamp. *(**A** courtesy Jarit Surgical Instruments, Hawthorne, NY; **B** from Nemitz R: Surgical instrumentation: an interactive approach, St Louis, 2010, Saunders. Photo by Frank Pronesti; **C** from Tighe S: Surgical instrumentation, ed 7, St Louis, 2007, Mosby.)*

During vascular surgery, blood flow must be temporarily stopped without damaging the vessel. *Vascular clamps* rather than hemostats are used in this case. These partially occluding clamps have enough pressure to slow or stop blood flow, but do not bruise or crush the vessel. These are recognizable by their relatively light weight, delicate structure, and single or double ridges that run longitudinally for the length of the tips. Examples of vascular clamps include bulldog, Satinsky, Fogarty, Craoord, and Cooley clamps (Figure 12-3).

Other tissues also require partial occlusion. The Duval lung clamp is used to gently grasp segments of the lung. The Babcock clamp is an atraumatic noncrushing clamp used to manipulate the bowel or fallopian tubes. The Bainbridge and Doyen intestinal clamps are used during intestinal resection to cross-clamp bowel segments (Figure 12-4).

Biting Clamps

A biting clamp has teeth or sharp serrations in the jaws that penetrate the tissue to hold it securely. Because this type of

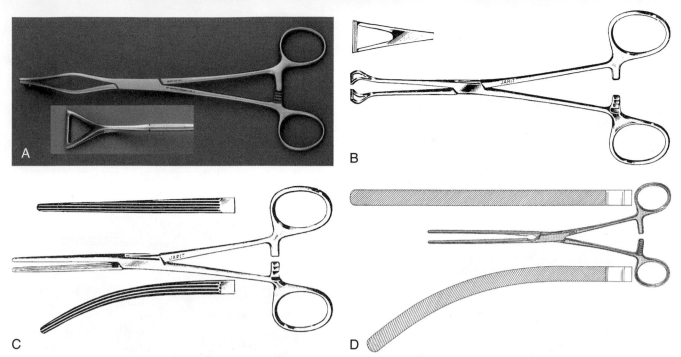

Figure 12-4 **Atraumatic clamps. A,** Duval clamp (lung surgery). **B,** Babcock clamp (fallopian tubes, intestines). **C,** Bainbridge clamp (intestine). **D,** Doyen clamp (intestine). *(Courtesy Jarit Surgical Instruments, Hawthorne, NY.)*

clamp can damage the tissue, it is mainly used on tissue that will be removed as part of the surgical procedure or on tissue that is extremely tough and resilient, such as fascia or ligament. The *Kocher* is a very common biting clamp used in a variety of general, gynecologic, and orthopedic procedures. The *Heaney* clamp is used specifically in gynecological surgery to grasp the uterine ligaments. Examples of biting clamps used in various specialties are shown in Figure 12-5.

A **tenaculum** has one or more needle-sharp teeth in jaws that can be delicate or heavy. This instrument penetrates the tissue on both sides of the jaws, in a pincer hold. Examples are the cervical tenaculum used in vaginal procedures and the Lahey tenaculum used on the thyroid. The *towel clamp* is another type of tenaculum used to secure towels in the draping process.

THUMB FORCEPS

The thumb forceps is a nonlocking instrument used for grasping tissue and suture needles during suturing and for general tissue manipulation. Thumb forceps often are called "pickups." Toothed forceps have one or more teeth in the jaws and are described by the number and type of teeth that mesh with slots on the opposite tine. For example, 1 × 2 forceps have one tooth and two slots; 2 × 3 forceps have two teeth and three slots. Examples of toothed forceps include Adson forceps with teeth, Bonney tissue forceps, and Cushing forceps. Toothed forceps are used on skin, fascia, and other connective tissues.

Smooth forceps (no teeth) are used on delicate tissue such as serosa, bowel, blood vessels, or ducts. Examples include smooth Adson forceps and smooth Cushing forceps. Vascular

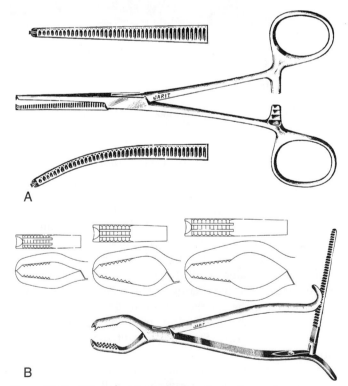

Figure 12-5 **Biting clamps. A,** Kocher clamps (general and gynecological surgery). **B,** Lane bone clamp (orthopedics). *(Courtesy Jarit Surgical Instruments, Hawthorne, NY.)*

forceps are recognized by their single or double rows of fine rounded serrations on each tine of the forceps.

Bayonet forceps are angled and typically are used in neurosurgical and nasal procedures. Figures 12-6 and 12-7 show common tissue forceps.

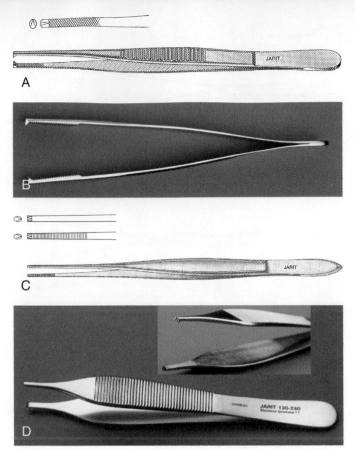

Figure 12-6 Tissue forceps. A and **B,** Single-toothed forceps. **C,** Cushing forceps. **D,** Adson tissue forceps. *(Courtesy Jarit Surgical Instruments, Hawthorne, NY.)*

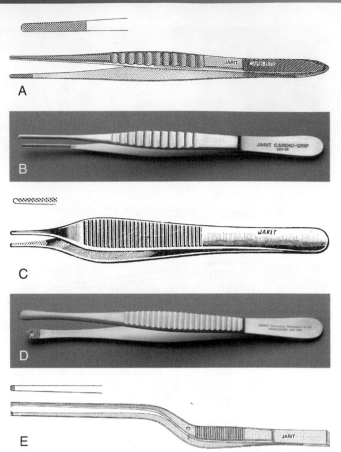

Figure 12-7 Smooth or nontoothed forceps. A, General surgery forceps. **B,** DeBakey vascular forceps. **C,** Adson forceps. **D,** Russian forceps. **E,** Bayonet forceps. *(Courtesy Jarit Surgical Instruments, Hawthorne, NY.)*

CUTTING INSTRUMENTS

Surgical Blade

The common surgical blade or scalpel (commonly called "the knife") is used whenever razor sharp cutting is required for tissue dissection. A scalpel blade is detachable from the knife handle, although single-use scalpels are available and these do not detach. Surgical blade handles are numbered according to their size and shape (Figure 12-8), known as the Bard-Parker system (for the company that first manufactured them). Each specific number handle is designed for only certain blades. This numbering system is consistent across all manufacturers. The number of the blade corresponds to a specific size and shape. The most common surgical blades are shown in Figure 12-9. Scalpel blades fit specific handles as shown in Table 12-1.

Another system of blades and handles, separate from the one just described, is the Beaver system. Beaver blades and handles are smaller and more delicate than those used in general surgery (Figure 12-10). These blades are designed for use in plastic, ophthalmic, and ear surgery and in general microsurgery.

Scissors

Scissors are among the most frequently used and important instruments in surgery. Careful handling and processing of scissors are necessary to maintain blade alignment and

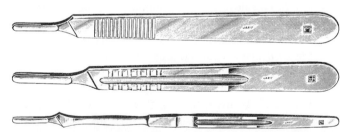

Figure 12-8 Scalpel handles. Handles *(top to bottom)*: 3, 4, and 7. *(Courtesy Jarit Surgical Instruments, Hawthorne, NY.)*

sharpness. High quality surgical scissors are distinguished by the sharpness of the cutting edges, balance, metal composition, and design of the point. Scissors with extremely sharp points are intended to sever very small points of tissue during dissection. The blades of the high quality scissor are coated with tungsten or other hardened alloy to maintain sharpness. Surgical scissors are available in a wide variety of sizes and types (Figure 12-11).

- Small, sharp-tipped scissors, such as iris scissors, are used for extremely fine dissection in plastic surgery.
- Castroviejo scissors are commonly used in microsurgery.
- Round-tipped, light dissecting scissors, such as Metzenbaum scissors, are used extensively on delicate tissue in general surgery. These are the most commonly used scissors in general surgery.

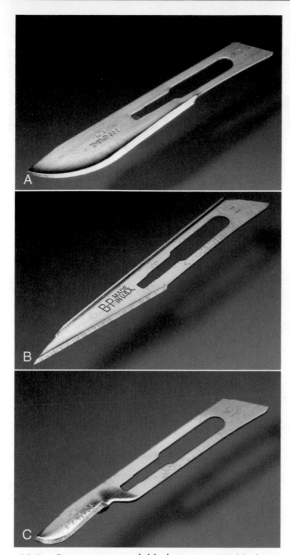

Figure 12-9 **Common surgical blades.** A, #10 blade, B, #11 blade, C, #15 blade. *(From Nemitz R: Surgical instrumentation: An interactive approach, St Louis, 2010, Saunders Elsevier.)*

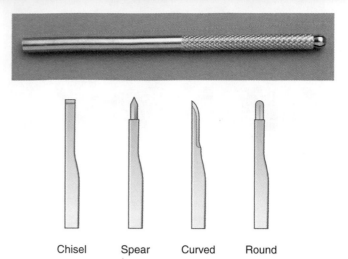

| Chisel | Spear | Curved | Round |

Figure 12-10 **Beaver blades.** *(Courtesy Jarit Surgical Instruments, Hawthorne, NY.)*

Table **12-1**	**Commonly Used Surgical Blades and Handles**	
Handle Size	**Fits Blade**	**Features**
3, 3L (long), 7, 9	10	Curved edge, curved tip
	11	Straight edge, pointed tip
	12	Hook edge, pointed tip
	15	Narrow, curved edge, curved tip
4, 4L	20	Same as 10; larger one often used for skin incision
	23	Slightly curved edge, sharp tip

Note: Handles 4 and 4L are used with blade nos. 21 through 28.

- Fibrous connective tissue requires heavier scissors, such as the curved Mayo scissors.
- Straight Mayo scissors are used for cutting suture. Note that tissue scissors must never be used to cut suture because it dulls them quickly.
- Wire-cutting scissors are used for stainless steel and other metal suture materials.

Rongeur

A **rongeur** is used to cut and extract tissue and is distinguished by having a *spring-loaded* hinge. The tips are cupped or beveled and the edges are sharp. A rongeur may have a single hinge (**single-action rongeur**) or two hinges (**double-action rongeur**). A double-action rongeur creates twice the leverage of a single-action rongeur. A heavier rongeur used in orthopedic and neurosurgical procedures is called a *Stille rongeur*. A long-handled delicate rongeur, such as the Kerrison rongeur, often is used in spinal surgery. Long, fine-tipped rongeurs, such as the pituitary rongeur, are used to remove tissue in areas that are difficult to reach, such as the vertebral column and nasal sinus.

Fine-tipped rongeurs such as the Kerrison are categorized by the angle of their tips and described as either *up-biting* or *down-biting*. The angle of the rongeur tips allows the surgeon to cut and remove tissue in areas that are difficult to reach, such as around the spinous processes.

Shears

Shears are large cutting instruments used to sever bone tissue. Their most common use is during thoracic surgery when one or more ribs must be cut for access to the chest cavity. Some shears are designed so that the cutting edge is left or right of the hinge. These are called side-cutting shears. Rongeurs and bone shears are shown in Figure 12-12.

Curette

The curette is a small cup with a sharpened, serrated, or smooth rim at the end of the handle. The curette is used in many specialties for scooping out tissue, including bone and soft tissue.

Very fine curettes are used in ear, paranasal, and spinal surgery. Larger heavier curettes are used in orthopedic procedures. Soft tissue curettes are used in gynecological surgery for endometrial **curettage**.

When asked for a curette during surgery, the technologist will usually be told which type is needed. In some cases,

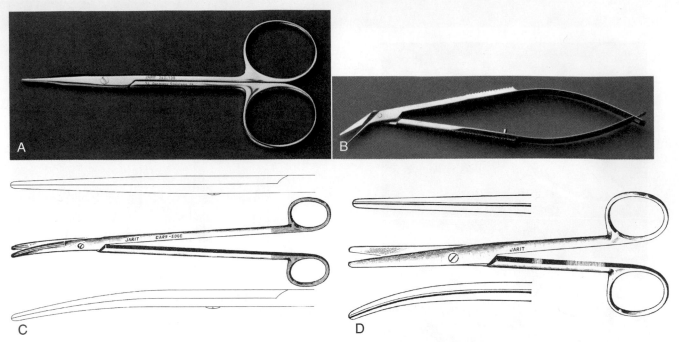

Figure 12-11 **Scissors. A,** Stevens tenotomy scissors (plastic surgery). **B,** Castroviejo scissors (eye and plastic surgery). **C,** Metzenbaum scissors. **D,** Mayo scissors (straight and curved shown). *(Courtesy Jarit Surgical Instruments, Hawthorne, NY.)*

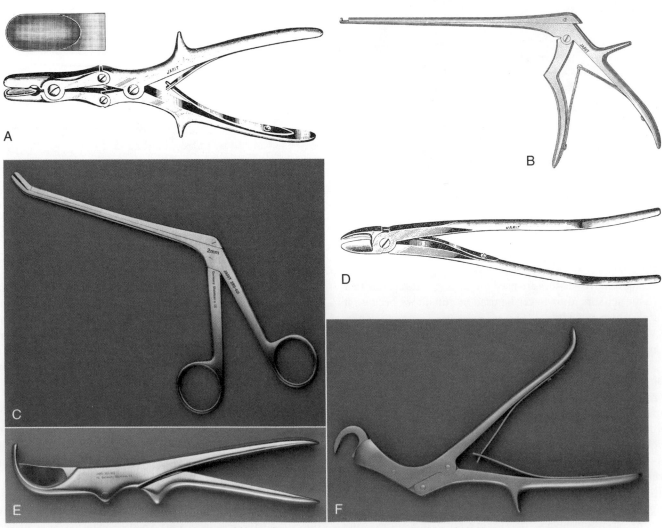

Figure 12-12 **Rongeurs and bone shears. A,** Stille-Luer rongeurs (orthopedics). **B,** Kerrison rongeurs (neurosurgery; ear, nose, and throat [ENT] surgery). **C,** Pituitary rongeurs (neurosurgery, ENT surgery). **D,** Bethune rib shears. **E,** Gluck rib shears. **F,** Stille-Giertz rib shears. *(Courtesy Jarit Surgical Instruments, Hawthorne, NY.)*

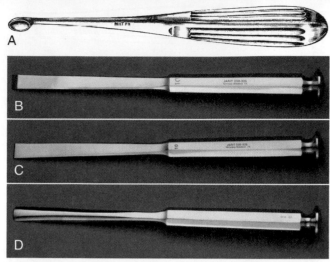

Figure 12-13 Curette, chisel, osteotome, and gouge. A, Curette. B, Chisel. C, Osteotome. D, Gouge. (A courtesy Integra Miltex, York, Pa; B to D courtesy Jarit Surgical Instruments, Hawthorne, NY.)

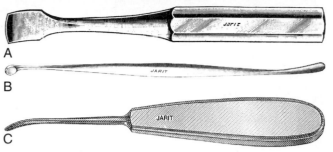

Figure 12-14 Elevators. A, Key periosteal elevator. B, Penfield elevator (neurosurgery, ENT, plastic surgery). C, Joker elevator (multiple specialties). (Courtesy Jarit Surgical Instruments, Hawthorne, NY.)

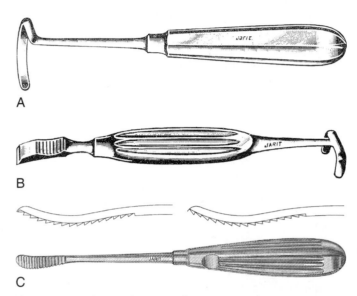

Figure 12-15 Rasps. A, Doyen rib stripper (used to remove periosteum). B, Matson elevator and stripper. C, Aufricht nasal rasp (ear, nose, and throat surgery). (Courtesy Jarit Surgical Instruments, Hawthorne, NY.)

however, it will be apparent that only a sharp curette is required—for example, in orthopedic work, sharp curettes are required to scoop out portions of diseased or obstructing bone.

Osteotome, Chisel, and Gouge

A **chisel** is an orthopedic cutting instrument that is used with a mallet (like chisels used in sculpting or carpentry). Chisels are available in many widths and sizes that fit a particular specialty. For example, a chisel used in paranasal surgery is much more delicate than one designed for the tibia. Chisels and osteotomes are often confused with one another. Remember that the osteotome is beveled on both sides, whereas a chisel blade is sloped on one side only. A large osteotome often is used to remove bone from the iliac crest for use as a graft elsewhere in the body. The chisel produces a straight-sided cut. Both instruments' tips must be protected from damage. When the blade becomes pitted or chipped, it loses its precision and becomes a hazard. Both types of instruments are quite heavy and should be kept in a metal rack where their blades cannot touch each other.

A **gouge** is a V-shaped bone chisel. Its cut looks like a small trough. Figure 12-13 shows the curette, chisel, osteotome, and gouge.

Elevator

An **elevator** is used to separate or "lift" tissue (Figure 12-14). The most common use is in separating the periosteum from bone and in vascular surgery. The heavy, round cutting elevator, such as the *Lambotte* elevator, slices tissue as it elevates. The small, square-tipped *Key* elevator also has a sharp edge but is much more delicate. Very finely balanced elevators, such as the *Penfield* and *Freer* elevators, are used in soft tissue surgery such as neural and vascular procedures. In vascular surgery, the elevators are used to separate atherosclerotic plaque from the inside of a blood vessel. These delicate elevators are well balanced convey excellent tactile information from the working end to the surgeon's hand. The *joker* is a

very commonly used elevator. Its short handle and strong tip make it ideal for separating connective tissue layers without causing bleeding.

Rasp

A rasp is used to remodel bone (Figure 12-15). Many sizes, shapes, and surfaces are available. Fine rasps are used in ear, nose, and throat surgery for the delicate bones and surfaces of the nasal sinuses and ear. Heavy rasps are used to ream the medullary canal of long bones in preparation for an implant or to prepare the surface of the humerus before sutures are attached. A rib stripper is a type of rasp used to scrape tough connective tissue from the surface of a rib before it is cut with rib shears. Examples of rib strippers include *Matson*, *Alexander*, and *Doyen* rib rasps.

Saw

Saws are used in procedures that require bone cutting. Although almost all saws and other bone-cutting instruments are powered pneumatically, one unpowered type is still commonly used during amputation. This is the Gigli saw, which is a flexible wire with cutting barbs along its length. The Gigli is used by mounting its ends on hook handles and drawing it through the bone. Refer to Chapter 31 for a further discussion and illustrations.

RETRACTION INSTRUMENTS

Retractors are used to hold back tissue layers. The body contains many complex tissue layers with individual structures penetrating at different angles. Even a shallow incision requires retraction of the upper tissue layers in order to expose deeper structures. Most retractors have a right angle or curved design. One end lies more or less flat and parallel to the body surface (the handle) while the other end curves down and inward to hold back the tissue within the surgical wound. The working end can be deep or shallow, depending on the depth of the surgical incision. The tips are sharp or rounded, depending on the type of tissue being retracted. The overall size of the instrument can be very large or minute, self-retaining with a spring or ratchet mechanism, or handheld.

Handheld versus Self-Retaining Retractors

Handheld retractors range in size from the very fragile skin hook used in plastic surgery to the large, 4-inch (10-cm) wide Deaver retractor used in abdominal procedures. Other common retractors are the Army-Navy retractor (also called a U.S. retractor), vein retractor, Goelet retractor, and Richardson, ribbon, and Harrington ("sweetheart") retractors. The rake retractor generally is used only for connective tissue. Sharp rakes or hooks are designed to grasp the undersurface of superficial tissues. The small Senn retractor is used in plastic or superficial surgery. This is a very commonly used instrument that is double-ended (either end can be used). One end is an atraumatic right angle and the other has sharp rake teeth. This retractor is also called a "cat's paw" because of its small sharp teeth and overall size.

Dull hooks and rakes are used in areas close to nerves or near blood vessels. Common handheld retractors are shown in Figure 12-16.

Self-retaining retractors hold tissue against the walls of the surgical wound by *mechanical action* (Figure 12-17). They can have many attachments suited to the needs of the surgery. The O'Sullivan-O'Connor, Bookwalter, and Balfour retractors are examples. Blades of various sizes and shapes can be attached to the frame to accommodate the specific needs of the procedure. Other examples include the Finochietto self-retaining retractor, which is used in cardiothoracic surgery, and the smaller Gelpi and Weitlaner retractors, which are used for superficial incisions, such as in the groin during hernia procedures. Very delicate self-retaining retractors are spring-loaded similar to the action of a common safety pin. An example is the McPherson self-retaining lid speculum that is used to retract the eyelids.

By definition, the self-retaining retractor works by a ratchet or other locking mechanism to hold the retractor blades in place in the surgical wound. This means the retractor is first positioned against the tissue to be retracted, and then opened manually. From that point, it is not held in place by anyone on the sterile team. The potential for bruising, nerve, and vessel

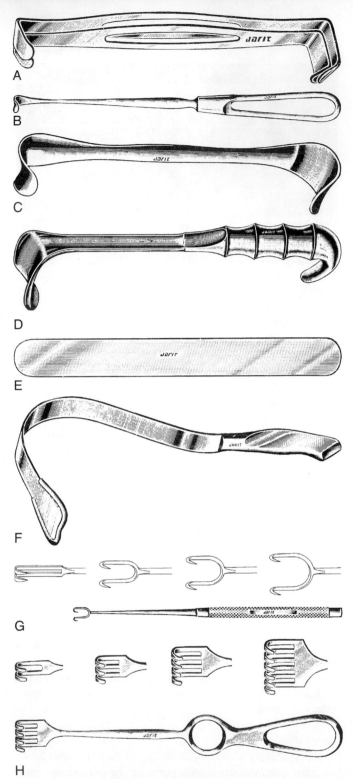

Figure 12-16 **Handheld retractors. A,** Army-Navy retractor (also called U.S. retractor). **B,** Vein retractor. **C,** Goelet retractor. **D,** Richardson retractor. **E,** Ribbon, or malleable, retractor. **F,** Harrington retractor (also called a *sweetheart retractor*). **G,** Skin hook. **H,** Rake. (Courtesy Jarit Surgical Instruments, Hawthorne, NY.)

damage, and even serious injury, exists for any mechanical device used on living tissue. For this reason the retractor is placed carefully and usually cushioned using laparotomy (lap) sponges so that the bare blades do not press against the tissue. However, a sharp-tipped or superficial self-retaining retractor

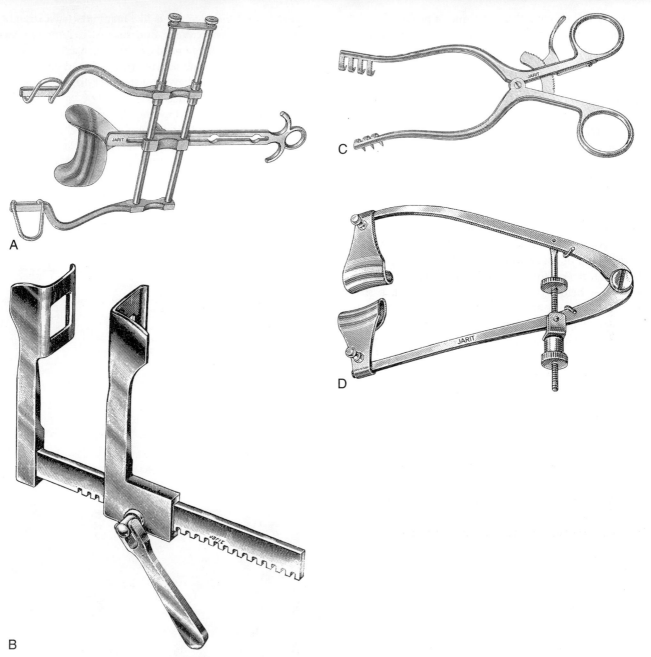

Figure 12-17 **Self-retaining retractors. A,** Balfour retractor (abdominal surgery). **B,** Finochietto retractor (thoracic surgery). **C,** Weitlaner retractor (superficial surgery [e.g., inguinal area or limb]). **D,** McPherson eye speculum. *(Courtesy Jarit Surgical Instruments, Hawthorne, NY.)*

such as a *Gelpi* or *sharp Weitlaner* is used without the aid of sponges, because sponges would defeat the retractors' purpose of penetrating and gripping the tissue as it is retracted.

Selection of Retractors

The selection of a retractor is based on the length and depth of the incision. At the beginning of a procedure, superficial retractors are used, and as the incision is carried deeper, a longer blade or deeper retractor is required to create exposure. The *width* of the retractor blade is determined by the size of the incision and the tissue to be retracted. The retractor blade can be curved, right-angled, or malleable (bendable to any angle).

DILATORS AND PROBING INSTRUMENTS

The **dilator** is a cylindrical instrument used to increase the inside diameter of a tubular structure. Very delicate dilators are used in tear duct surgery, whereas the larger cervical dilators are used to dilate the cervix so that instruments can be passed into the uterus. Urethral dilators are used to open a stricture of the urethra. Dilators are used in *sets* containing individual instruments that are graduated in their diameter from small to large. A probe is used to explore an anatomical structure for patency (open) passage through tissue or structures (such as the tear duct, or a fistula), or in dentistry to determine the nature of bone and enamel by touching it gently with a sharp instrument. The technique of probing tissue has been largely replaced by imaging technology which provides a more accurate assessment of tissue. Refer to Chapter 27 for images of tear duct probes.

MEASURING INSTRUMENTS

Tissue and hollow structures are measured for many purposes. For example, the uterine sound is inserted into the cervix to measure the depth of the uterus from the cervix to the fundus. This is done to prevent uterine perforation during curettage. Orthopedic calipers are used to prepare the bone for a joint implant. A depth gauge is used in orthopedic surgery to determine the length of screws to be implanted into bone.

A *sizer* is a trial, reusable replica of an implantable prosthesis. Rather than opening and contaminating many expensive implants, the sizer allows the surgeon to test a replica first. For example, before a cardiac valve is inserted, a sizer is used to determine the correct size. A surgeon may use a basic sterile ruler to measure tissue or specimens removed from the patient. Assorted measuring instruments are shown in Figure 12-18.

SUTURING INSTRUMENTS

A needle holder is used to grasp a curved needle during suturing (Figure 12-19). The length, weight, and type of tip must be matched to the suture and tissue. Using a heavy needle holder, such as a Heaney or Mayo-Hegar needle holder, to

suture a small blood vessel is like manipulating a straight pin with a pipe wrench. Very fine sutures require fine needle holders. A sharp-tipped needle holder, such as the Sarot needle holder, is used for fine sutures (i.e., 4-0 and smaller). High quality needle holders have tungsten carbon inserts in the jaws for added durability and grip.

If the needle holder is too heavy, the surgeon will lose the "feel" of the needle. On the other hand, a lightweight or fine-tipped needle holder (e.g., the Webster needle holder) does not have enough surface area at the tip to grasp a heavy needle. A needle holder that is too delicate for the needle will cause the needle to twist during use. Most needle holders are ratchet- or spring-locked. Always test the ratchets before the needle holder is used. If they do not mesh correctly, the

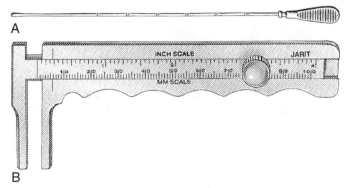

Figure 12-18 **Measuring instruments. A,** Uterine sound. **B,** Caliper (orthopedics). *(Courtesy Jarit Surgical Instruments, Hawthorne, NY.)*

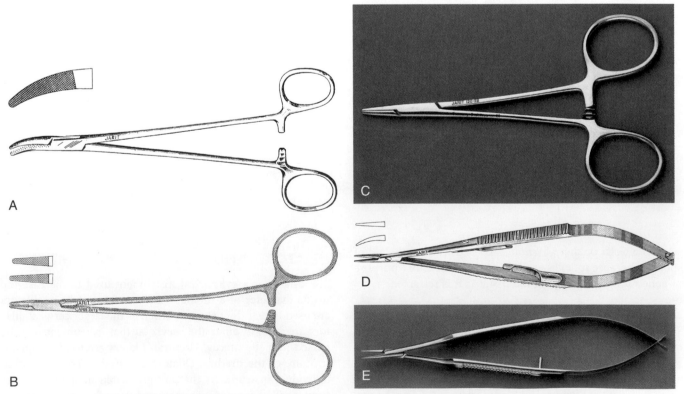

Figure 12-19 **Commonly used needle holders. A,** Heaney (broad tip) needle holder. **B,** Sarot (fine tip) needle holder. **C,** Webster needle holder (plastic surgery). **D,** Castroviejo needle holder with spring lock. **E,** Castroviejo needle holder without lock. *(Courtesy Jarit Surgical Instruments, Hawthorne, NY.)*

needle holder may spring open unexpectedly, resulting in tissue damage or needle loss. The smallest needle holders, such as the Castroviejo used in eye surgery and microsurgery, have a spring catch and may be locking or nonlocking. Only gentle pressure is needed to open and close a spring catch.

SURGICAL STAPLING AND LIGATING DEVICES

Stapling

Surgical stapling instruments (Figure 12-20) are used to perform multiple suture and resection maneuvers. Staplers are available as single-use medical devices or as stainless steel instruments. Both types use manufactured cartridges or staples made of steel, nylon, or absorbable polymer for use in open or endoscopic surgery. The cutting assembly includes an anvil, which clamps the tissue against the staple cartridge. The cartridge contains staples that fire individually or together in single, double, triple, or quadruple lines. Surgical staples have many advantages:

- Tissue handling is greatly minimized, reducing trauma from manipulation and exposure.
- The suture lines are strong and dependable.
- The staples are nonreactive in tissue.
- The staples are noncrushing, preventing tissue necrosis from compromised blood and nutrient supply to the tissue edges.

The surgical technologist must become familiar with the proper handling of staplers and the loading of staple cartridges. Much aggravation can be prevented during surgery if the instruments are studied carefully before they are needed. There are wide variations in assembly and component parts and the surgical technologist is urged to become familiar with those used in his or her facility. Reusable staplers must be completely disassembled for cleaning, terminal disinfection, and sterilization and all parts accounted for during the process.

Several manufacturers make surgical stapling instruments. Each type of stapler is intended for a specific surgical technique and use. When passing a surgical stapling device, make sure any safety catch is activated to prevent accidental firing of staples. Any loose staples must be removed from the surgical site to prevent their loss in the wound. Remember that staples are sharp and must be handled with care. The most common types of surgical staplers are:

1. *Skin stapler:* Places a single line of staples across the incision border and is used for closing a skin incision.
2. *Gastrointestinal anastomosis (GIA) stapler:* Used for linear resection, transection (division or cutting), and anastomosis.
3. *Ligating-dividing stapler (LDS):* Places a double row containing two staples in each row and severs the tissue between rows when fired.
4. *Circular or end-to-end anastomosis (EEA) stapler:* Used for end-to-end intestinal resection (cutting and rejoining). It joins two arms of intestine with a double row of staples.
5. *Thoracoabdominal (TA) stapler:* Has a right-angled firing section that fits around deep structures for resection and

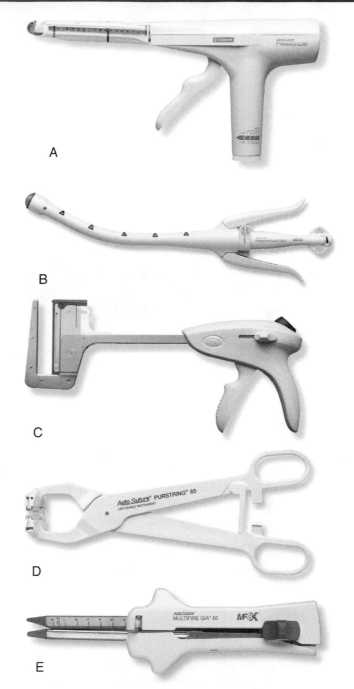

Figure 12-20 Surgical stapling instruments. **A,** Ligating-dividing (LDS). **B,** Circular or end-to-end anastomosis (EEA) stapler. **C,** Thoracoabdominal (TA) stapler. **D,** Purse-string stapler. **E,** Gastrointestinal anastomosis (GIA) stapler. *(Copyright ©2012 Covidien. All rights reserved. Used with the permission of Covidien.)*

anastomosis. It is commonly used in lung or abdominal surgery.
6. *Purse-string stapler:* Performs the same function as a purse-string suture and places circumferential nylon sutures and staples.

Hemostatic Clips

Hemostatic or vessel clips are small, V-shaped staples that close down and occlude a vessel or duct. Small, medium, and

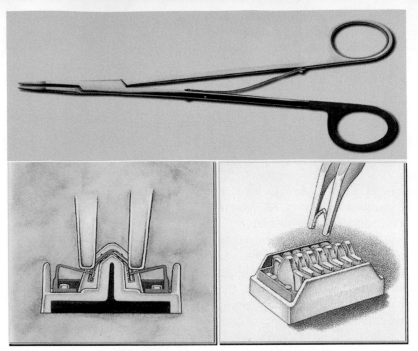

Figure 12-21   **Loading the WECK® Horizon™.** *(Courtesy of Teleflex, Research Triangle Park, NC).*

large clips are available in cartridges that are color-coded by size. Disposable and reusable systems are available. Clips may be made of stainless steel, titanium, tantalum or absorbable polymer. The size of the applier must be matched to the size of the clip. To load the vessel clip, grasp the proper-sized clip applier at the hinge. Press the open jaws of the applier straight down over the clip; this locks the clip into the jaws (Figure 12-21). Pass the clip applier with the tip down, taking care not to squeeze the handles, which would release the clip prematurely. Clips are also available in biosynthetic materials.

SUCTION INSTRUMENTS

Suction (aspiration) is needed during a surgical procedure to clear blood, fluids, and small bits of tissue debris from the surgical site and provide an unobstructed view of the anatomy. Suction is provided using sterile plastic tubing, which attaches to a suction tip (instrument) at one end and a closed suction canister (nonsterile) at the other.

The instrument itself varies in length and diameter from very small (for eye surgery and microsurgery) to larger tips for general surgery and orthopedics. Tips are straight or angled and may have a removable tip or shield or guard that reduces the suction pressure. For example, the Poole suction tip is designed for abdominal surgery and has a removable perforated guard that protects bowel and intestinal organs from injury by spreading the suction pressure over many small holes in the guard. The Yankauer or tonsil suction tip is designed to suction in the chest cavity and throat. The more delicate Frazier tip is designed to suction in superficial areas in the face, neck, and ear and in neurological and some peripheral vascular procedures.

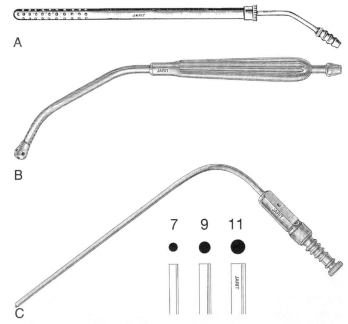

Figure 12-22   **Commonly used suction tips.** A, Poole. B, Yankauer. C, Frazier. *(Courtesy Jarit Surgical Instruments, Hawthorne, NY.)*

Depending on the diameter of the lumen of the suction tip, the scrub may need to clear the suction tip frequently to remove clotted blood or debris, such as bone chips and dust. These are produced when orthopedic saws and drills are used. This is done by dipping the suction tip in sterile water or by inserting a stylet (flexible wire) into the lumen. Three commonly used suction tips are shown in Figure 12-22.

USE OF INSTRUMENTS BY TISSUE TYPE

The selection of a particular surgical instrument is based on the tissue type, the depth of the surgical wound, the technical requirements of the instrument, and the surgeon's preference or experience. Tissues vary in texture, strength, elasticity, water, fat content, and permeability. If all body tissues were the same, far fewer instruments would be required. Table 12-2 shows a basic guideline for different types of tissues and the common types of instrument used on these tissues. Naturally there will be exceptions, and the list is not exhaustive. The names of the instruments are cross-referenced in illustrations.

SKIN

Skin is elastic, relatively fibrous, and strong. In most surgical procedures, skin is incised rather than cut with scissors. This is because the elastic quality of skin makes it difficult to cut an exact straight line with scissors. The scalpel (commonly called the "knife") is more precise, and extremely sharp to prevent the skin from dragging through the instrument as it cuts. As a general rule, only toothed, hooked, or serrated instruments are used to grasp the skin. This is because skin is relatively tough compared with other tissue types, and smooth instruments such as smooth tissue forceps do not have enough "bite" to hold skin.

VISCERAL SEROSA

The viscera, or organs of the body, are each covered by a fine membrane called the **serosa**. This membrane is easily punctured, and the underlying tissue layers can bleed profusely. Therefore, atraumatic instruments are needed when handling this tissue. These include nonpenetrating forceps (smooth forceps), wide retractors that do not cut into the tissue, and suction tips that have a guard to decrease the suction pressure

Table 12-2 | Tissue Types and Appropriate Instruments

Type Tissue	Type Instrument			
Connective	Thumb Forceps	Scissors	Tissue Clamp	Retraction
Skin • Elastic • Resilient	Toothed, delicate, such as Adson Short to medium length, single-toothed	Use scalpel for incision Use fine-tipped short scissors, such as Westcott or tenotomy scissors for trimming and fine dissection	Not used on skin	Skin only, small rakes, sharp or rounded tips, such as Senn or double hook Plastic surgery skin hooks Self-retaining small spring, such as Green Skin plus fat layer—use rake retractors, Army-Navy
Adipose (loose connective tissue) • Lobular • Sparse blood vessels • Oily • Tends to break apart when clamped	Toothed if used on body wall fat, medium length	Metzenbaum curved ESU (electrosurgical unit)	For controlling bleeders use mosquito, Kelly, Crile, or Mayo clamps	Handheld rake size depends on depth of incision Shallow—Weitlaner self-retaining or small rake Israel rake for deep adipose layers Large abdominal retractor for very deep layers: use Deaver or Richardson
Ligament • Strong • Fibrous • Elastic	Toothed Broad-tipped or heavy for large ligaments	*Mayo* scissor for broad ligaments May require incising with knife	Use strong ligament clamps, such as Heaney, for uterine ligaments Joint surgery, use Kocher clamp for grasping Hemostasis, use Mayo clamp	Fibrous sheath: use nonslip self-retaining retractor Single ligament: use loop
Tendon • Tough • Stringy • Extremely strong • Avascular	Toothed forceps Heavy for large tendons, lighter for finer ones	Metzenbaum scissors for larger tendon Tenotomy scissors for delicate tendon	Use tendon clamp where available Avoid crimping tendon with hemostatic clamps	Tendon retractor when available Can use rubber loop to retract

Continued

Table **12-2** | **Tissue Types and Appropriate Instruments—cont'd**

Type Tissue	Type Instrument			
Connective	**Thumb Forceps**	**Scissors**	**Tissue Clamp**	**Retraction**
Abdominal viscera • Delicate • Each encapsulated by thin, strong serous tissue	Use long, smooth tissue forceps or vascular forceps for suturing Babcock clamps for intestine, reproductive organs Allis clamps may be used on stomach borders	Always use fine Metzenbaum scissors for dissection, medium or long sometimes used for incising serosa Spleen, liver, pancreas, uses ESU for dissecting	Nonocclusive clamps including Bainbridge, Babcock, Doyen, and Duval are used on abdominal organs	Use broad, smooth, handheld retractors with adequate sponge packs to prevent injury to organ. Use Deaver, Richardson, Harrington, retractors.
Bone • Strong • Resilient • Springy or spongy • Covered with tough periosteal layer	Forceps not commonly used on bone Use broad-toothed forceps when needed	Bone rongeurs and single- and double-action cutters with various tips Saw, Gigli manual or power saws Drills Shaver Reamer Osteotome Chisel Elevator Knives, such as meniscus knife	Bone clamps, Lewin Bone hook	Handheld retractors for specific parts of the anatomy • Bennet—hip • Blount—knee • Meyerding—shoulder • Smilie—knee
Muscle • Fibrous • Vascular • Strong	Toothed forceps used for general manipulation	Heavy or lightweight dissection scissors (Mayo or Metzenbaum)	Striated muscle not normally clamped except to grasp bleeders	Handheld retractor for isolated muscle groups

(level of "pull") on the tissue. Babcock clamps are favored by most surgeons for use on viscera.

LUNG, SPLEEN, LIVER, THYROID

These highly vascular tissues are very delicate, bleed profusely, tear easily, and have little or no elasticity. A strong membrane covers and protects these organs. However, these tissues must be handled by hand or with atraumatic (nonpiercing) instruments. The liver and spleen can "break" or develop fissures when traumatized. Only partially occluding clamps and smooth tissue forceps are used on these tissues. However, during dissection of adjacent tissues, very fine-toothed forceps and long curve-tipped clamps are used (e.g., *Schnidt* or *right angle* clamps). When the spleen, liver, and intestines are retracted, the retractor blade must be sufficiently wide to distribute the pressure. Edges must be protected with sponges to prevent the retractor edge from cutting into the tissue. A wide *Deaver, Richardson,* or *Harrington* retractor is often used for liver and spleen. Lung tissue is held with broad-tipped, partially occluding clamps such the *dual lung clamp*.

PERITONEUM

The lining of the body cavities is smooth, elastic, and strong. Normal peritoneal tissue is dissected with the *Metzenbaum*

scissors (the most commonly used scissors in general surgery) and may be grasped with *toothed* forceps or *Allis* clamps. The right angle of an abdominal retractor is placed over the edge of the peritoneum or with folded damp sponges to provide cushioning.

ADIPOSE TISSUE

Loose connective tissue, such as the subcutaneous tissue of the abdomen, has a high fat content. It does not compress well and tends to fragment into small pieces when clamped. Adipose tissue has few blood vessels compared with other types of tissue. This allows the use of penetrating retractors, such as a sharp rake or Weitlaner (self-retaining). The Allis clamp, which has a T tip with fine serrations at the tip, often is used to clamp or grasp adipose tissue. The high fat content of this tissue can cause instruments to become slippery and difficult to handle. In this case they can be frequently wiped down with a damp sponge during surgery. Toothed forceps are used for suturing adipose tissue.

MUSCLE

Striated muscle tissue is moved aside or the muscle bundles are manually separated rather than cut whenever possible during surgery. This is because muscles are normally slow to regain function when severed, and nearly all surgical incisions are oriented on the long axis of the muscle. Large muscles are elastic and fibrous, allowing for the use of toothed forceps and clamps. On rare occasions when muscle tissue must be severed, it is often grasped with Allis clamps and severed with heavy Mayo scissors or an electrosurgical unit.

BONE

Bone tissue is resilient and somewhat springy. Large bones are manipulated using traction or leverage rather than direct pulling. Bone retractors, such as the Bennett and Scoville retractors, have a toothed tip or a reverse curve that can be inserted under another bone for leverage. Other types of bone clamps, such as the Lewin clamp, wrap around the bone for manual traction.

CARTILAGE, TENDON, AND FASCIA

Cartilage, tendon, and fascia are extremely strong and resilient. The cartilaginous joint surfaces (those with a capsule) are naturally lubricated with synovial fluid, which has an oily consistency. These tissues can be quite slippery, requiring toothed clamps or those with ridges to maintain the hold. Tendons are also covered by a sheath that is strong and smooth. These connective tissues are handled using Kocher clamps, which have a single or double tooth at the tip increasing the instrument's gripping ability. More specialized tendon clamps, such as the Martin clamp, have double rows of heavy teeth and are frequently used in knee surgery for grasping the medial and lateral tendons. Fascia is grasped with Kocher clamps. Strong dissecting scissors such curved Mayo scissors are used on fascia and large tendons.

INSPECTING SURGICAL INSTRUMENTS

The surgical technologist takes a proactive role in checking instruments for safety and correct operation. This can be done while instruments are being prepared for a procedure, or after the procedure when instruments are sorted and prepared for terminal disinfection. Stainless steel instruments can be damaged mechanically or structurally, or there can be defects on the surface that lead to weakness or cross-infection. Damaged instruments must be withdrawn from service because they can lead to patient injury, lost operating time, and increased expense.

The following discussion, along with Figures 12-23 through 12-26, illustrate instruments and areas of instrument damage and how to look for dangerous defects.

SCISSORS

1. Look for pitting, chipping, and fractures along the blade edges. Vertical cracks in the blade tine are serious and may mean that the instrument cannot be repaired.
2. Check that the scissor tips meet precisely and are not bent or chipped. Sharp dissection scissors can develop burrs on the tips, usually from misuse or rough handling with

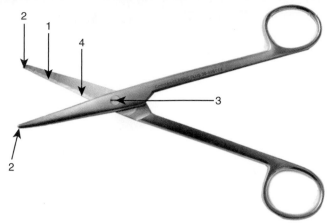

Figure 12-23 **Tissue scissors.** *1,* Chips, cracks, and pitting in the finish impair the performance of the instrument and can eventually result in breakage. Cracked blades can result in serious injury to tissue. *2,* Bent tips cause a distinct rub of metal on metal when the scissors are opened and closed. *3,* A loose hinge screw or one that is worn creates a sloppy feel during operation. Check also for cracks in the screw. *4,* Check for dull blades by cutting through a latex glove, using only the tips of the blades. Sharps blades will cut easily whereas dull blades may require tension on the material being cut. *(Courtesy Bramstedt Surgical Inc., Lino Lakes, Minn.)*

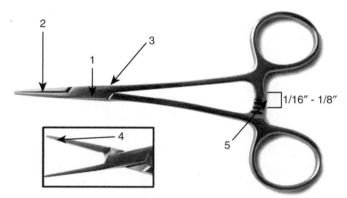

Figure 12-24 **Clamp.** *1,* Cracks in the box lock impair the function of the clamp and are a result of normal wear of the instrument, but can also be caused by using a clamp on tissue that is too thick or fibrous for the clamp. *2,* Jaw alignment can be checked by opening and closing the instrument and visually inspecting the points of contact. Misalignment can also cause the jaws to snag on each other. *3,* A loose box lock is a common result of stress and wear. To check for a loose box lock grasp the ring handles using both hands and gently push one handle up and down. A slight amount of play is normal, but a sloppy feel is an indication of a loose box lock. *4,* Check the ratchet fit for secure closure. There should be $\frac{1}{16}$ to $\frac{1}{8}$ inch of space between the ratchets, which should stay tightly locked when closed in the first ratchet position. *(Courtesy Bramstedt Surgical Inc., Lino Lakes, Minn.)*

heavier instruments. When the scissors are opened and closed, there should be no grinding of tips or shanks, which would indicate rough edges or bent tines.
3. The center screw of the scissors can become worn with time. When the scissors are opened and closed, they should feel snug but not tight at the center screw.
4. Test the blades for sharpness by cutting through a surgical glove. There should be no resistance, and the blade should cut a straight line. Remove dull scissors from active use as soon as a defect is noticed.

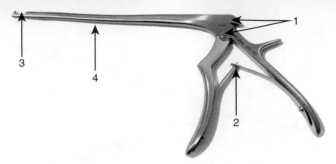

Figure 12-25   Rongeur. *1,* The rongeur is a complex instrument with multiple pins and screws that if damaged or loose can be lost in the surgical wound during use. The screw connecting the handle to the body must be secure in order to use the instrument effectively. Test this screw by gently pushing the handles back and forth. Vibration in the front handle indicates a loose screw at the hinge shown. The top shaft is secured with a drive pin. A loose or faulty pin prevents the rongeur from opening and closing. *2,* The rongeur is closed over tissue by the action of an internal spring, which also allows the instrument to snap back into open position when the handles are released. A broken or worn-out spring prevents the blades from returning to the open position whereas a normal spring feels somewhat tight when compressed and releases quickly when the handle is opened. *3,* The cutting blades can be tested for sharpness by cutting through thin card paper such as a business card. The blades should easily cut a section from the card. *4,* A sticky top shaft may indicate a worn spring or, more likely, tissue debris that has not been removed during previous reprocessing. Debris collects between the top shaft and guide during use and may become baked into the mechanism during sterilization. The resulting debris and biofilm can contaminate the surgical wound and also cause instrument failure. *(Courtesy Bramstedt Surgical Inc., Lino Lakes, Minn.)*

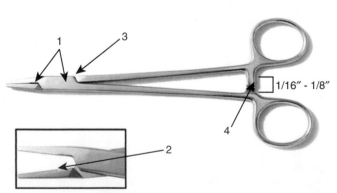

Figure 12-26   Needle holder. *1,* A crack in the box lock or jaw can lead to breakage. Needle holders with carbide inserts are designed so that the insert will fail before the box lock. However, a crack may occur in either location, an indication for immediate repair. *2,* Examine the inserts before use to check for defects. A smooth insert indicates one that is worn and needs to be replaced. A normal insert has a coarse appearance and secure grip on the suture needle. Another reliable test for worn inserts is to hold the closed tips to the light and check for light passing between the inserts. There should be no gap between the inserts. *3,* A loose box lock occurs with normal use. See instructions for testing the box lock in Figure 12-24. *4,* A faulty ratchet will may cause the needle holder to snap open unexpectedly during use, releasing the needle. The closed instrument should have $\frac{1}{16}$ to $\frac{1}{8}$ inch of space between the ratchets in order to maintain the correct pressure. The needle holder should remain secure in the first ratchet position. *(Courtesy Bramstedt Surgical Inc., Lino Lakes, Minn.)*

CLAMP

1. Examine the box lock closely for cracks, pitting, and even tissue debris. Small cracks in the surface can lead to breakage with repeated use.
2. The jaws of the clamp should be aligned, with serrations meshed properly. Close the instrument and examine it in this position to check for irregularities on the surface or teeth that do not mesh.
3. Check for loose box lock. Open the instrument and examine for "play" in the box lock. A very small amount is normal, but if the box is loose, it needs repair.
4. Fractured or broken teeth and serrations are dangerous on tissue because they can sever and tear delicate tissue.
5. Check that ratchets are aligned and that they do not spring open unexpectedly. The instrument should close easily and the ratchets click into place with moderate pressure. Loose or worn ratchets close *too* easily and do not hold the instrument closed. There should be $\frac{1}{16}$ to $\frac{1}{8}$ inch of space between the ratchets.

RONGEUR

1. Look for loose or missing screws and pins. Rongeurs are complex instruments with multiple pins, springs, and screws. Test the screw connecting the handle to the body by gently pushing the handles back and forth. The front handle should not rattle. The top shaft is secured to the body by a pin, which must be intact.
2. The spring in the center of the handle allows the handle to snap back to neutral position after closing. A worn spring causes the handles to lose tension.
3. The rongeur's cutting edge at the tip must be sharpened periodically. Make sure there are no pits or cracks and that the tips do not stick or grind when opened and closed. Tissue not removed during reprocessing can easily build up in the tip, causing an infection hazard as well as damage to the instrument. The tip should be visually inspected and should be able to cut through a thin strip of paper, approximately the same thickness as a business card.
4. The tip of the rongeur opens and closes by a sliding pin mechanism in the shaft. The central screw connects the handle to the body. All of these mechanisms must slide smoothly, with no "stickiness."

NEEDLE HOLDER

1. Needle holders and dissection scissors are the most frequently used instruments. They must be checked frequently for mechanical breakdown and signs of wear that can lead to breakage. Look for cracks in the box lock and in the jaws of the instruments. Even small hairline fractures are enough to take an instrument out of service for repair.
2. The tungsten carbide inserts can wear down and require replacement. The insert should feel uniformly coarse all along their length. Test the inserts to see if they mesh together when the instrument is locked by holding the

closed instrument up to the light and looking for gaps along the length of the inserts.

3. Like other instruments with a box lock, the needle holder can lose accuracy when the box lock is worn or loose. When the instrument is opened and closed, it should feel smooth and responsive, but not tight or sticky.
4. Check the ratchets for alignment and fit.

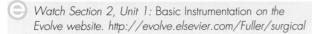 *Watch Section 2, Unit 1: Basic Instrumentation on the Evolve website. http://evolve.elsevier.com/Fuller/surgical*

KEY CONCEPTS

- Knowing the names of surgical instruments and how they are used is a fundamental skill in surgical technology. Instruments are generally named according to type and shape, and often include the name of the of the instrument's designer.
- Modern surgical instruments are manufactured in a global market where materials may be derived from one country, while assembly and distribution take place elsewhere. Quality control varies and there is a wide variety of workmanship among instrument manufacturers worldwide.
- Metal finishes have significance in the quality of an instrument and in its function. Surgical technologists must be knowledgeable about the relationship between a particular metal finish and function of the instrument.
- One of the most important ways in which a surgical instrument is classified is by type, which also identifies its function, or use in surgery. The ability to identify types of instruments is the first step in more complex differentiation.
- Structural, functional, and surface defects in a surgical instrument are associated with significant patient injury. The surgical technologist is responsible for identifying defects, including incomplete cleaning, cracks, chips, broken parts, and insulation failure before an instrument is used in surgery.

REVIEW QUESTIONS

1. What is the relationship between the characteristics of a particular type of tissue and the instruments that are used on that tissue?
2. On what types of tissue would you *not* use an instrument with teeth (one that punctures)?
3. What is the advantage of having a right-angled instrument?
4. What is the most efficient way to learn the names of surgical instruments?
5. Describe a tenaculum.
6. List the correct scalpel blade numbers and their handles.
7. How would you protect the cutting edges of instruments from damage during surgery?
8. What is the function of a self-retaining retractor?
9. Describe your personal plan for learning the names and uses of instruments.

CASE STUDIES

Case 1

As a student, you are scrubbed on a large case. Your preceptor has shown you which instruments will be needed during the case. As the preceptor names the instruments, you remember only a few of the names. To make matters more difficult, the preceptor does not tell you the technical name of the instruments but refers to them by the nicknames used at this hospital. What strategies might you use to pass the correct instrument even though you do not know the name?

Case 2

You are scrubbed on a large case. Loud music is playing, and it is difficult to hear the surgeon's requests for instruments. You know the instruments but have not had much experience with them. You make many mistakes, and the surgeon becomes irritated. What will you do?

Case 3

You have finished a case and are now preparing supplies to be taken to the decontamination area for processing. You have placed all instruments in appropriate containers for reprocessing and discarded disposable and sharp items in the correct disposal containers. You are about to take your case cart to the decontamination area when the circulator asks whether you have a particular part for an instrument. You realize that you have discarded it in the sharps box, thinking it was disposable. What is the proper action?

Case 4

You have opened a case and are now scrubbed, preparing instruments for the start of surgery. Among the sterile goods is a complex instrument that you have not seen before. The instrument has been disassembled for sterilization, and you must now put it together. Little time is left, and you have 12 separate parts to assemble. What is the correct action? Consider the importance of not wasting operating time, the need for your attention at the sterile field, and prioritization of your time.

Case 5

The surgeon asks for a particular instrument during a stressful procedure. You pass the instrument she requested. She states, "Don't give me what I ask for, give me what I need here." What does this mean?

BIBLIOGRAPHY

Nilsen E: Managing equipment and instruments in the operating room, *AORN Journal* 81:349, 2005.

Spry C: Care and handling of basic surgical instruments, *AORN Journal* 86:S77, 2007.

13

Perioperative Pharmacology

CHAPTER OUTLINE

Introduction
SECTION I: PRINCIPLES OF PHARMACOLOGY
Sources of Drugs
Drug Information Resources
Regulation of Drugs, Substances, and Devices
Drug Nomenclature
Pharmaceutical Formulation
Drug Labeling
SECTION II: THE MEDICATION PROCESS
Preventing Drug Errors

Prescriptions and Drug Orders
Selection of Drugs
Dispensing Drugs to the Sterile Field
Medical Measurement Systems
Delivery Devices
Managing Drugs on the Sterile Field
Drug Administration
Assessment
Documentation

SECTION III: DRUG ACTION
Pharmacokinetics
Pharmacodynamics
SECTION IV: SELECTED DRUG CATEGORIES
Antiinfective Agents
Antineoplastic Agents
Autonomic Drugs
Blood and Blood Derivatives
Blood Coagulation
Cardiac Drugs
Central Nervous System Agents

Sedatives and Hypnotics
Local Anesthetics Diagnostics
Fluid Balance and Electrolytes
Gastrointestinal Drugs
Hormones and Synthetic Substitutes
Emergency Drugs
Drug Calculations

LEARNING OBJECTIVES

After studying this chapter the reader will be able to:
1. List the sources of drugs
2. Explain the different drug resources available
3. Discuss the importance of drug regulation
4. Understand how drugs are named and formulated
5. Correctly identify and interpret the components of a drug label
6. Discuss ways to prevent drug errors
7. List and use the seven rights of the medication process
8. Recognize the elements of a prescription and the types of drug orders

9. Apply the correct protocol for receiving drugs on the sterile field
10. Accurately convert values within and between measurement systems
11. List and describe the different delivery devices
12. Describe the role of the surgical technologist in handling drugs
13. List drug administration routes
14. Describe the principles of pharmacokinetics
15. Describe the principles of pharmacodynamics
16. Explain the different drug categories and give examples of drugs in each category

TERMINOLOGY

Adverse reaction: An unexpected harmful reaction to a drug.
Agonist: A drug that produces a response in the body by binding to a receptor.
Allergy: Hypersensitivity to a substance, a response produced by the immune system.
Antagonist: A drug or chemical that blocks a receptor mediated response.
Antibiotics: Drugs that inhibit the growth of or kill bacteria.
Bioavailability: The extent and rate at which a drug or its metabolites (products of breakdown) enter the systemic circulation and reach the site of action.
Chemical name: The name of a drug that reflects its molecular structure.

Concentration: A measure of the quantity of a substance per unit of volume or weight.
Contraindications: Contraindications to a protocol, drug, or procedure are circumstances that make its use medically inadvisable because it increases the risk of injury or harm.
Contrast media: Radiopaque solutions (i.e., not penetrated by x-rays) that are introduced into body cavities and vessels to outline their inside surfaces.
Controlled substances: Drugs that have the potential for abuse. Controlled substances are rated according to their risk potential; these ratings are called *schedules*.
Diluent: The liquid component of a drug that must be reconstituted from a powder to a solution for purposes of administration.

TERMINOLOGY (cont.)

Dosage: The regulated administration of prescribed amounts of a drug. Dosage is expressed as a quantity of drug per unit of time.

Dose: The quantity of a drug to be taken at one time or the stated amount of drug per unit of distribution (e.g., 0.5 mg per milliliter of solution).

Drug: A chemical substance that when taken into the body, changes one or more of the body's functions.

Drug administration: The giving of a drug to a person by any route.

Generation: In pharmacology, refers to a drug group that was developed from a previous prototype (e.g., first-generation cephalosporin).

Generic name: The formulary name of a drug that is assigned by the U.S. Adopted Names Council.

Half-life: The time required for one half of a drug to be cleared from the body.

Hypersensitivity: Allergic immune response to a substance causing a range of symptoms from mild inflammation to anaphylactic shock and death.

Intraosseous: Refers to administration of a drug directly into the bone marrow.

Intrathecal: Refers to administration of a drug into the spinal canal.

Parenteral: Refers to administration of a drug by injection.

Peak effect: The period of maximum effect of a drug.

Pharmacodynamics: The biochemical and physiological effects of drugs and their mechanisms of action in the body.

Pharmacokinetics: The movement of a drug through the tissues and cells of the body, including the processes of absorption, distribution, and localization in tissues; biotransformation; and excretion by mechanical and chemical means.

Pharmacology: The study of drugs and their action in the body.

Prescription: An order for a drug written by a qualified medical staff member.

Proprietary name: The patented name given to a drug by its manufacturer.

Side effects: Anticipated effects of a drug other than those intended. Side effects may be uncomfortable for the patient or may have a positive outcome.

Therapeutic window: Range of drug doses that can treat disease effectively while staying within the safety range.

Topical: Refers to application of a drug to the skin or mucous membranes.

Trade name: The name given to a drug by the company that produces and sells it.

Transdermal: Refers to administration of a drug by absorption through the skin, such as with ointments or patches impregnated with the drug.

U.S. Pharmacopeia (USP): An organization that establishes standards for drugs approved by the U.S. Food and Drug Administration (FDA) for their labeled use. All approved drugs have been tested for consumer safety, and written information is available about their pharmacological action, use, risks, and dosage.

INTRODUCTION

The study of drugs is called **pharmacology**. The term **drug** is defined in U.S. law as a substance intended for use in the diagnosis, cure, relief, treatment, or prevention of disease or intended to affect the structure or function of the body.[1] This qualification is associated with regulations that protect the public from harm resulting from medical or pharmacological intervention.

This chapter focuses on the *medication process* and the role of the surgical technologist in drug handling. The medication process begins with an order or prescription for the drug and includes selection of the correct drug, measurement and mixing, distribution or dispensing, administration and finally, assessment of the patient and documentation.

This chapter emphasizes drugs used on the surgical field. Other drugs are referenced to give the student a broad understanding of pharmacology. Anesthetic and adjunct drugs are also discussed in preparation for the study of anesthesia in the next chapter.

Pharmacological terms used in the chapter have been standardized to match the FDA terminology so that students can research topics easily and accurately. The classification system and proper drug categories follow the American Hospital Formulary Service (AHFS), which is the current system used in the United States. Students are urged to become familiar with and this use professional system rather than lay pharmaceutical terminology.

Some drug categories are discussed in association with their surgical specialty as follows:

- Ophthalmic drugs: Chapter 27
- Drugs used in ear surgery: Chapter 28
- Tissue adhesives: Chapter 22

SECTION I: PRINCIPLES OF PHARMACOLOGY

SOURCES OF DRUGS

Drugs used in modern medicine are derived from a number of natural and synthetic (human-made) sources:

- Synthetic chemicals
- Animal and human proteins
- Minerals
- Elemental metals
- Plants

Most drugs are derived from synthetic molecules. These may mimic, or act like, substances found in nature, but have been modified to alter particular physiological effects or to make them safer to use. Many of the plant-based drugs provide

---

[1]Federal Food, Drug, and Cosmetic Act. Sec.201. [21 U.S.C. 321] Chapter II—Definitions 1. Available at http://www.fda.gov/RegulatoryInformation/Legislation/FederalFoodDrugandCosmeticActFDCAct/FDCActChaptersIandIIShortTitleandDefinitions/ucm086297.htm

drug manufacturers with the formulas for their synthetic counterparts.

Throughout history, healers of all cultures have used biological (natural) substances in the treatment of medical and psychological illness. Traditional healing with plants has guided the development of modern pharmaceuticals. Today, herbal medicines have returned to modern therapy as a component of healing. Other biological substances include proteins and hormones derived from animal or human sources. These are used in many different medicinal and immunological agents and also for tissue grafting.

Purified metals, salts, and other elements are also used alone or as components of drugs. For example, barium is used for diagnostic procedures, and electrolytes, which are necessary for life, are administered to balance cell function, which depends on electrochemical reactions.

The pharmaceutical industry also uses biotechnology to manufacture certain drugs, including those derived from human-made molecules and natural sources such as animal or plant substances. Biotechnology is not the source of the drug; it is the *process* used in manufacturing. Biotechnology in drug manufacturing uses genetically modified microorganisms for the production of chemicals that are purified to form a product.

DRUG INFORMATION RESOURCES

REFERENCES

Drug information, including a drug's biochemical action, the correct dosage, and other technical data, is widely available in books and online. Reference books are used by clinicians to find out technical information about a drug—its action, dose, and form, how the drug is metabolized, its interaction with other drugs, and other details important for the prescriber and other health care providers.

- *The Physicians' Desk Reference (PDR)* is used by many primary health care providers—especially prescribers and pharmacists. It contains detailed information about prescription and over-the-counter (OTC) drugs needed for safe administration. The PDR is updated yearly, and the entries are made by subscription. This means that only those companies that wish to be listed publish information about their products.
- *The United States Pharmacopoeia–National Formulary (USP-NF)* is the complete reference of all drugs, dietary supplements, and devices marketed for medical use in the United States. This reference is published by the official standards agency for the manufacture of drugs, medical devices, dietary supplements, and other substances sold for use on or in the body. The reference is composed of many different standards sections, which describe packaging, storage, and labeling requirements for drugs.
- *The American Hospital Formulary Service* publishes a number of products related to safe use of drugs. These include drug handbooks and references related to prescribing, consumer drug resources, indexing and categories of drugs, drug licensing, and poisoning.

Box **13-1** Drug Information Resources Online

FDA Orange Book:
    http://www.accessdata.fda.gov/scripts/cder/ob/
      default.cfm
    or search "FDA Orange Book"
DEA List of Controlled Substances:
    http://www.justice.gov/dea/index.htm
Institute for Safe Medication Practices:
    http://www.ismp.org
National Coordinating Council for Medication Error Reporting and Prevention:
    http://www.nccmerp.org
TJC National Safety Goals:
    http://www.jointcommission.org/standards_information/
      npsgs.aspx

- Reputable *online drug resources* are often a good way to research drugs at all levels. A starter list of organizations and their websites useful for health care workers is given in Box 13-1.

TEXTBOOKS

Pharmacology textbooks are written according to the intended audience. Texts may focus on specific areas of health care, such as allied health (including the surgical technologist), cancer medicine, and pain management. There are many reference texts on pharmacology subspecialties such as pharmacokinetics and pharmacodynamics.

PUBLIC HEALTH EDUCATION

The public also needs information about drugs and other substances. Many books have been published to guide consumers, and popular websites are also used by the lay public to learn more about the drugs they are prescribed. However, these websites are not regulated. The best information is probably available from pharmacists, who are trained to assist the public and can answer questions accurately.

REGULATION OF DRUGS, SUBSTANCES, AND DEVICES

LAW AND INSTITUTIONAL POLICY

The laws pertaining to prescriptions, dispensing, and administration of drugs are defined by each state's *practice acts*. The Joint Commission requires health care organizations to develop policies that are in compliance with state laws regulating who may handle drugs and how. This means that health care institutions or organizations may not establish independent policies or guidelines that violate state practice acts regarding drugs. It is important for the surgical technologist to know both the health care institution's policy and the state's laws regarding prescriptions, dispensing, and administration of drugs. To find out your state's laws regarding drug dispensing and administration, search "practice act," plus the state, plus the profession. For example, to research the practice acts for surgical technologists in Utah, type "practice acts Utah surgical technologist." When researching practice acts, be sure to look for the current version of the law.

The following roles and who may perform them are regulated by law:

- Procurement and secure storage
- Prescription, ordering, and transcription of drug orders
- Preparation and dispensing of drugs
- Administration of drugs

FDA REGULATION

The FDA maintains strict regulatory control on devices and substances used on or in the body. This includes the following:

- Prescription drugs
- Nonprescription—OTC—drugs
- Food supplements
- Cosmetics
- Medical devices, including implants and equipment used in the delivery of drugs
- Wound closure materials, such as suture and tissue sealants
- Biologicals (materials for immunization against disease)
- Devices that deliver potentially harmful levels of radiation

In the United States, drugs are approved for medical use only after rigid testing and application to the FDA. The FDA authorizes the sale and distribution of drugs and is responsible for ensuring that approved drugs meet consumer safety requirements. It approves drug literature and labeling so that health care providers and the public are informed of the nature and use of a drug and any risks associated with it.

To protect the public from harm, prescription and OTC medicines must meet standards for quality, purity, identity, and strength. These standards are set by the **U.S. Pharmacopeia (USP)**. All substances that meet these standards have the initials *USP* after their generic (nonproprietary) name. Approved substances are published in the *U.S. Pharmacopeia–National Formulary* (USP-NF). The World Health Organization (WHO) publishes an international formulary, the *International Pharmacopoeia*.

PRESCRIPTION AND OVER-THE-COUNTER DRUGS

A **prescription** is authorization to obtain a licensed drug. Only certain state-licensed professionals (e.g., a doctor, dentist, osteopath, advanced practice nurse, or physician's assistant) are allowed to provide a prescription. Prescription drugs are differentiated from OTC drugs, which are available to the public without authorization. OTC drugs are considered by the FDA to be effective and safe to use without medical supervision.

CONTROLLED SUBSTANCES

Controlled substances are drugs that carry a high risk of abuse or addiction and are specifically designated and regu-

---

Box 13-2 Federal Drug Schedules of Controlled Substances

- Schedule I:
  The drug has a high potential for abuse
  There is no accepted safety for use of the drug under medical supervision
- Schedule II:
  The drug has a high potential for abuse
  It has an accepted medical use with restrictions in the United States
  Abuse may lead to severe psychological or physical dependence
- Schedule III
  The drug has less abuse potential than Schedules I and II
  It has an accepted medical use in the United States
  Abuse of the drug can lead to low or moderate physical dependence or high psychological dependence
- Schedule IV
  The drug or other substance has a low potential for abuse relative to the drugs or other substances in Schedule III
  The drug has a currently accepted medical use in treatment in the United States
  Abuse of the drug may lead to limited physical or psychological dependence relative to the drugs in Schedule III
- Schedule V
  The drug has low abuse potential compared with Schedule IV
  It has an accepted medical use
  Abuse can lead to limited physical or psychological dependence as compared to substances in Schedule IV

From the Controlled Substances Act 1/07/2011. Accessed September 1, 2011, at http://uscode.house.gov/download/pls/21C13.txt.

---

lated by state and federal law. The designation (called a **schedule**) is based on the risk of abuse or dependency. Controlled drugs include both prescription and illegal substances. The regulating body for controlled substances is the federal Drug Enforcement Administration (DEA) (http://www.justice.gov/dea/index.htm). The regulations for controlled prescription drugs apply to all stages of the prescription and dispensing process. Controlled drug schedules are shown in Box 13-2. Schedule I drugs carry the highest risk of abuse.

A full list of controlled substances can be viewed at http://www.justice.gov/dea/pubs/scheduling.html.

PREGNANCY CATEGORIES

Drugs are classified by pregnancy category (A, B, C, D, and X) to inform health care workers and patients of the potential risk to the fetus if a pregnant woman takes the drug. The categories are described as follows:

- A: No demonstrated risk to the fetus
- B: Animal studies have not demonstrated risk and there are no adequate and well-controlled studies in pregnant

women, or studies in animals show risk to the fetus; but well-designed studies in people do not

- C: Inadequate studies have been done in animals and people; some studies show risk to the fetus in animals
- D: There is risk to the human fetus, but the benefits may outweigh risks in certain situations
- X: Drugs have been proven to pose a risk that outweighs the benefit of the drug

Most drugs are listed as category D, because it is not known whether they pose a risk and testing would be unethical under any circumstances.

HERBAL REMEDIES AND FOOD SUPPLEMENTS

The FDA does not regulate herbal substances as drugs and classifies them as food rather than medicine. Companies both within and outside the United States may market substances to the American public without the stringent testing and quality control required for prescriptions and OTC drugs. Some herbal drugs can produce physiological changes in the body and may interfere with the action of regulated medicines. However, lack of scientific data on the exact content and effects of marketed substances prevents effective regulation.

The FDA regulates dietary substances such as vitamins and minerals less stringently than it does prescription and OTC drugs. Some supplements such as folic acid and vitamin A are known to be beneficial in the treatment or prevention of specific diseases. However, the manufacturer of dietary supplements does not have to *prove* efficacy of a supplement in order to market it. Manufacturers do have to prove that the products meet safe manufacturing standards. All food supplements produced in the United States are monitored for safety, and a substance can be withdrawn if it is found to be unsafe.

DRUG NOMENCLATURE

Drug *nomenclature* is a system of identifying drugs by name. Three methods are used in the international nomenclature system—generic name, trade name, and chemical formula.

GENERIC NAME

The **generic name** of a drug is assigned by the United States Adopted Names council (USAN) at the time the drug is patented. The USAN ensures that generic drug names do not sound or look alike in order to prevent drug errors. Generic drugs are substantially cheaper (sometimes up to 10 times less expensive) for the consumer. By law, drugs with the same generic name must have the same chemical composition as the identical drug with a trade name, regardless of how many companies produce it. Generic drugs are tested and regulated by the same standards as identical brand-name drugs. By law, they are the same as branded drugs in dosage form, strength, safety, performance, and intended use. In general, generic drugs are much more widely available than

Table **13-1**	**Drug Nomenclature**	
Trade Name	**Generic Name**	**Chemical Name**
Zoloft	sertraline HCl	(1S,4S)-4-(3,4-dichlorophenyl)-N-methyl-1,2,3,4-tetrahydronaphthalen-1-amine
Cipro Ciproxin	ciprofloxacin	1-cyclopropyl-6-fluoro-7-piperazin-1-yl-quinoline-3-carboxylic acid
Lasix	furosemide	4-chloro-2-(furan-2-ylmethylamino)-5-sulfamoylbenzoic acid

branded equivalents. The WHO, FDA, and patient advocacy groups have campaigned rigorously for many years to promote the use of generic drugs and educate consumers about their safety, effectiveness, and affordability.

TRADE (PROPRIETARY) NAME

When a drug is developed, the company that produces the drug obtains a patent for it and gives it a **trade name** (known also as the brand name or **proprietary name**) under which the drug is marketed. Trade names apply to both prescription and OTC drugs. Drug patents and their names are currently granted for 20 years. After that time, the exclusive rights to the drug formula and name expire, allowing other companies to produce the same drug with their own trade names or as a generic drug.

CHEMICAL FORMULA

The **chemical name** of a drug is derived from its molecular formula following international convention. Some examples of drug nomenclature are shown in Table 13-1. The chemical formula is listed in the package insert and usually referred to for scientific purposes only rather than during the medication process. The chemical is the *active ingredient*. This is the specific chemical or compound that provides the drug's therapeutic or other medical properties. This includes diagnosis, cure, treatment, or prevention of disease. Drugs also contain *inactive ingredients* that have no therapeutic effect. These are added to the drug formula for preservation, for color, or to bind the other ingredients.

PHARMACEUTICAL FORMULATION

Drugs and other medical substances are manufactured in a formulation that is compatible with how the drug is administered and how it reaches the target tissue. The formulation is also called the *dosage form* or therapeutic presentation (e.g., tablet, liquid, or cream). For example, drugs that are intended to reach the central nervous system (CNS) quickly might be in the form of a liquid intravenous injection, or a tablet placed under the tongue where it is rapidly absorbed into the bloodstream through the mucous membrane. Tablets meant for oral administration must be resistant to breakdown until they reach the gastrointestinal system, where they will be absorbed through the stomach lining. Skin patches or films impregnated with medication keep the drug in contact with skin, which slowly absorbs the drug at the start of the metabolic pathway.

The FDA lists more than 100 different pharmaceutical forms (formats). These can be seen on the main FDA website under the link "Dosage and Form." Only a small number of these forms are encountered in the health care facility. Lists of common forms are shown in Table 13-2.

DRUG LABELING

All pharmaceutical products, including implants, are *labeled* with specific information mandated by the FDA. Labeling means not only the physical label and package insert, but also the information itself. For example, we say that a drug is labeled for topical use only or is labeled for use in patients with hypertension. Drugs must be labeled for specific use to prevent injury or misuse when prescribed for reasons other than those for which the drug was approved. Drug labeling is complex

Table **13-2**	Pharmaceutical Dosage Forms
Form	**Description**
Aerosol	A product that is packaged under pressure and contains therapeutically active ingredients that are released on activation of an appropriate valve system; it is intended for topical application to the skin as well as local application into the nose (nasal aerosols), mouth (lingual aerosols), or lungs (inhalation aerosols).
Capsule	A solid oral dosage form consisting of a shell and filling.
Cement	A substance that produces a solid union between two surfaces.
Concentrate	A liquid preparation of increased strength and reduced volume that is usually diluted before administration.
Cream	An emulsion, semisolid dosage form used for external application to the skin or mucous membranes.
Emulsion	A dosage form consisting of at least two immiscible liquids, one of which is dispersed as droplets within the other liquid.
Film	A thin layer or coating.
Gel	A semisolid dosage form that contains a gelling agent to provide stiffness to a solution or colloidal solution or dispersion.
Graft	A slip of skin or other tissue for implantation.
Implant	A material containing drug intended to be inserted securely or deeply in tissue for growth, slow release, or formation of an organic union.
Inhalant	A class of inhalations consisting of a drug or combination of drugs that are carried into the respiratory tract where they exert their effect.
Injection	A sterile preparation intended for parenteral use. Five classes of injections are defined by the USP.
Irrigant	A sterile solution intended to bathe or flush open wounds or body cavities; used topically, never parenterally.
Packing	A material usually covered by or impregnated with a drug that is inserted into a body cavity.
Patch	A drug delivery system that often contains an adhesive backing that is applied to an external site on the body.
Pellet	A small sterile solid mass consisting of a highly purified drug intended for implantation in the body.
Pill	A small round solid dosage form containing a medicinal agent intended for oral administration.
Plaster	Substance intended for external application of consistency to adhere to the skin and attach to a dressing, intended to afford protection and support.
Powder for solution	A mixture of dry drugs or chemicals that on addition of a suitable vehicle yields a solution.
Solution	A clear homogeneous liquid that contains one or more chemical substances dissolved in a solvent.
Solution for slush	A solution for the preparation of an iced saline slush, which is administered by irrigation and used to induce regional hypothermia (in conditions such as certain open heart and kidney procedures) by its direct application.
Sponge	A porous interlacing, absorbent material that contains a drug.
Spray	A liquid minutely divided as by a jet of air or stream. Suspension: A liquid dosage form that contains solid particles dispersed in a liquid medium.
Suspension	A liquid dosage form that contains solid particles dispersed in a liquid medium.
Swab	A small piece of flat absorbent material that contains a drug.
Tablet	A solid dosage form containing medicinal substances.
Tincture	An alcoholic or hydroalcoholic solution.

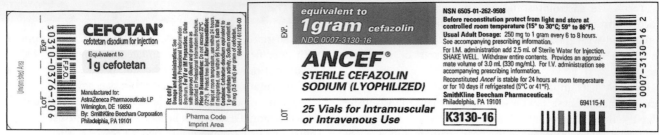

Figure 13-1   Drug labels. Note dose, strength, bar code, and use. *(From Kee J, Hayes E, McCuiston L: Pharmacology, ed 5, Philadelphia, 2006, WB Saunders.)*

because it contains information about all aspects of the drug—its composition, action, adverse reactions, warnings, dosage forms, and other information needed for all phases of the medication process. Highlights of the prescription drug labeling process include the following:

1. *Name of the drug including proprietary and generic name:* The drug formula is also included in the package insert.
2. *Dosage form:* For example, solution, capsule, dry powder for reconstitution.
3. *Amount contained in the package:* For example, 1 gram, or 2 mg per mL.
4. *Indications:* The labeled purpose of the drug.
5. **Dosage** *and route of administration:* The amount to use and route of administration (e.g., intravenous, intramuscular injection).
6. **Contraindications:** Information included in the package insert. This may be a special warning such as "Do not use in patients with a history of hepatic disease."
7. *Lot number:* When each drug batch is mixed in the drug laboratory, it is assigned a lot number in case a batch must be recalled from use.
8. *Expiration date:* The date beyond which the drug must not be used.

All information contained on the label or drug insert is important to the medication process, including the indication, which has recently been added to the "drug rights." Health care providers who administer drugs are required to know why the drug is being used and when it should *not* be used to avoid injury to the patient.

Other important information includes the expiration date. Drugs must not be used beyond the specified expiration date. Over time, many drugs lose their efficacy or may become toxic. The expiration date indicates when the drug must be withdrawn from the market and destroyed. Administration of drugs that have passed their expiration date is a drug error.

Every drug has a labeled *route of administration* (e.g., intravenous, topical, oral). It is critical that drugs intended for one route are not administered by another. For example, heparin, which is a high risk drug, is manufactured for intravenous use and also as a topical irrigation fluid. The formulation and strengths are different for each route. The surgical technologist is directly responsible for knowing the difference between these two drugs and passing the correct one when it is required on the sterile field. Drugs labeled for topical use must never be administered by any other route. Figure 13-1 illustrates two different drug labels.

SECTION II: THE MEDICATION PROCESS

The medication process is a prescribed way of handling drugs in the health care environment. The following individual practices make up the whole process:

- Prescription or drug order by a licensed health care provider
- Correct interpretation of the drug prescription or order
- Selection of the drug
- Drug preparation, mixing, measuring (can also take place on the sterile field)
- Drug dispensing
- Correct administration of the drug
- Patient assessment
- Documentation

PREVENTING DRUG ERRORS

A drug error is a mistake made at *any stage* in the medication process. A study carried out in 2008 revealed that preventable adverse drug events are responsible for the deaths of 7,000 patients each year. The medication process involves many different steps and involves multiple health care workers. Medication errors are often attributed to fatigue, stress, and distraction in the workplace—all prevalent in the perioperative environment. Some of the more common errors made in the perioperative area are negligence in labeling drugs or inability to read the label, incorrect knowledge about the drug, misidentification, and passing the wrong drug to the surgeon. Some of these errors have resulted in death or severe injury to patients. The problem of medication errors is so serious that recent changes have been made in standards and guidelines to try to reduce the number and severity of drug errors in all areas of care. Increased pressure for surgical technologists to become involved in the medication process now places them in a position of individual responsibility and accountability for patient outcomes, including drug errors that occur during surgery.

The Institute for Safe Medication Practices (ISMP), in coordination with TJC's National Patient Safety Goals, has published a list of 10 elements that have the most influence on drug errors. These are:

1. Patient information—including age, weight, height, allergies, lab results that can affect routes of administration and dosage.

2. Drug information—lack of knowledge about the drug, its action, its intended use, appropriate dosage individualized according to the patient, drug interactions. Drug information available to all surgery team members must be up to date.

NOTE: *Surgical technologists have a responsibility to become familiar with drug alert information provided by the ISMP. These can be obtained through the ISMP website and email alerts.*

3. Communication of drug information—a common cause of drug errors. Communication "barriers" must be eliminated for communication to flow.
4. Drug packaging, labeling, and nomenclature—including look-alike, sound-alike drugs, confusing labels (including those made by the scrub during surgery), nondistinct packaging
5. Medication storage, stock, standardization, and distribution—nonstandardized methods used within the care facility or department can result in errors.
6. Environmental factors—including poor lighting (e.g., when operating room lights are dimmed during endoscopic surgery), loud conversation, music, and other distracting environmental conditions that prevent concentration.
7. Drug device acquisition, use, and monitoring—includes any devices used for drug delivery. These must be proven safe and monitored in the clinical area to prevent device errors.
8. Staff competency and education—all staff must focus on new medications being used at their health care facility, high-alert medications, and protocols, policies, and procedures related to medication use.
9. Patient education on medications—remains the responsibility of the licensed primary health care provider.
10. Quality processes and risk management—this focuses attention on improving practice as a means of attaining greater reduction in drug errors.

DRUG RIGHTS

One method that has proven successful in reducing drug errors is the drug "rights." This is a verification tool that is used to guide health care workers in the medication process. It is important to note that this method is only partially effective, because it does not account for errors outside of the administration process. The seven rights have evolved from an original five (detailed later). Recently added is "the right indication," because a number of serious incidents have involved health care personnel not knowing what a drug's actions were and why it was being given. "The right documentation" was also added recently to remind all health care workers that they must communicate detailed information about drugs they administer so that the next person in the care team has a complete picture of the patient's condition. Deaths in this area have occurred when improper or inadequate documentation was performed during surgery and the next health care worker

in the chain of care gave similar or the same drugs, resulting in overdose.

- *The right drug* is the one that has been ordered by the surgeon or other health care provider. This means that the correct drug must be selected from the operating room or pharmacy stock. Verbal orders are repeated back to the surgeon to verify accuracy. The scrubbed surgical technologist receives drugs from the circulator at the start of surgery or during the procedure. During this exchange the drug is verified again. After receiving the drug on the sterile field, the scrubbed surgical technologist labels the drug and then again selects the correct one when it is requested by the surgeon. Many drug errors made in surgery occur at this point and are related to lack of labeling or poor labeling.
- *The right patient* means that the surgical patient is identified on entering the surgical holding area and again when the individual is brought into the surgical suite. Before surgery begins, patient identification is again verified during the TIME OUT (see Chapter 21).
- *The right dose* means the correct **dose** (amount and strength of drug) is administered for that particular patient. Throughout the medication process, the dose is checked by each person handling the drug. Verifying the correct dose and strength before the drug is administered to the patient is one of the most important responsibilities of the surgical team. The surgical technologist must also keep track of the amount of drug given throughout the surgical procedure.
- *The right route* is the one intended for that drug and is labeled accordingly (e.g., "For topical use only" or "Not for use in the eyes"). A drug may not be administered by any route other than the one approved and labeled. Some drugs are formulated for different routes but have the same name. The route must be verified by the label.
- *The right time* refers to a schedule of administration according to the prescription or order.
- *The right indication* of a drug is the condition for which the drug is intended. This right has been added by patient safety advocate organizations in recent years because of numerous drug errors committed when the person administering the drug lacked the appropriate knowledge about indications, resulting in injury or death of the patient. The Joint Commission and other standards organizations recognize that patients are cared for by teams of individuals who are jointly responsible for patient safety. In the case of drug administration, drugs are contraindicated (must not be administered) under specific conditions.
- *The right documentation* means that drug administration must be documented in the patient chart. Drugs used by the anesthesia care provider are documented in the anesthesia record, whereas those used in or on the operative site are documented in the surgical report (see details of documentation, later). All documentation must identify the name of the drug, the strength, who administered the drug, the time, the route, and a report of patient assessment after administration.

LOOK-ALIKE, SOUND-ALIKE DRUGS

A significant number of adverse drug events have been caused by drugs whose names look and sound alike. The Institute for Safe Medication Practices has published a list of more than 100 of these drugs on their website at http://www.ismp.org/Tools/confuseddrugnames.pdf. It is best to visit the site frequently in order to remain up to date on surgical drugs recently released by the FDA. Each individual health care facility is also required to produce its own look-alike, sound-alike list of drugs used in that particular organization.

HIGH-ALERT DRUGS

High-alert drugs are those that have been implicated in an extraordinarily high number of errors—many of them with fatal consequences, as reported to the National Medication Errors Reporting Program. The drugs on this list are those that are frequently cited in drug errors and are also those that have the carry a great risk of adverse consequences when errors are made. Extra high-alert drugs in the perioperative area include the different formulations of heparin, thrombin, epinephrine, and local anesthetics. The surgical technologist must know the difference between these drugs and their maximum dose (calculated by the anesthesia care provider) and must be able to differentiate them clearly in the operative setting.

Box 13-3 lists high-alert drugs.

Box **13-3**   High-Alert Medications

Drug Classes/Categories
Adrenergic agonists, intravenous
   Epinephrine, phenylephrine, norepinephrine
Adrenergic antagonists, intravenous
   Propranolol, metoprolol, labetalol
Anesthetic agents, general, inhaled and intravenous
Antiarrhythmics, intravenous
   Lidocaine, amiodarone
Antithrombotics (anticoagulants)
   Warfarin, low-molecular-weight heparin, intravenous,
      unfractionated heparin, factor Xa inhibitors, direct
      thrombin inhibitors, thrombolytics, glycoprotein IIb/IIIa
      inhibitors
Cardioplegic solutions
Chemotherapeutic agents, parenteral and oral
Dextrose, hypertonic, 20% or greater
Dialysis solutions, peritoneal and hemodialysis
Epidural or intrathecal medications
Hypoglycemics, oral
Inotropic medications, intravenous
Liposomal forms of drugs
Moderate sedation agents, intravenous
Moderate sedation agents, pediatrics
Narcotics/opiates, intravenous, transdermal, and oral
Neuromuscular blocking agents
Radiocontrast agents, intravenous
Total parenteral nutrition solution

<small>From Institute for Safe Medication Practices, 2011. Report medication errors or near misses to the ISMP Medication Errors Reporting Program (MERP) at 1-800-FAIL-SAF(E) or online at HYPERLINK "http://www.ismp.org/" www.ismp.org.</small>

PRESCRIPTIONS AND DRUG ORDERS

A prescription is the authorization by a licensed health care provider for a licensed pharmacist to dispense a drug. The elements of a prescription are:

- Name of the patient
- Name of the drug
- Strength of the drug
- Dose (amount)
- Route
- Time or frequency of administration

The prescription must be dated, and the name of the person prescribing must be noted on the documentation.

In a clinical setting such as a health care facility, drugs are administered only after a drug *order* has been issued by the licensed health care provider. This can be the attending physician, surgeon, anesthesiologist, nurse practitioner, or physician assistant. Giving and receiving drug orders are roles in which a high number of errors are made. Mistaking one drug for another (as with look-alike, sound-alike drugs), ordering drugs that are contraindicated for the patient, interpreting extra zeros in the dose, and orders for drugs for which the patient has an allergy are all drug errors that commonly occur and lead to injury or death of the patient. According to the Agency for Healthcare Research and Quality (U.S. Department of Health and Human Services), poor communication and inadequate knowledge are the basis of many drug errors.

A drug order may be verbal, written, emailed, given over the phone, or faxed. Whatever the method used, the drug order must be communicated clearly and precisely. Hospital policy determines which health care professionals may receive a drug order, and which kind applies. For example, some health facilities may permit only a licensed nurse or physician to take phone orders.

The types of orders are:

- *Verbal order:* Directed to the person who will fill the order, who verifies the information by reciting it back to the prescriber. Verbal orders are made in person or on the phone.
- *Written order:* This can be in longhand, typed, or submitted electronically.
- *Standing order:* The order that remains in effect until the prescriber withdraws it. In the surgical context, standing orders are those included in the surgeon's preference cards, which are maintained electronically or written by hand for a particular surgical procedure. The elements of a drug order are the same as the prescription, except that the name of the patient may be omitted for standing orders where it is understood who is to receive the drug (e.g., the surgical patient).
- *Stat order:* The drug is to be administered "right away."
- *PRN order:* The drug is to be given *as needed.*

SELECTION OF DRUGS

Once a drug order has been issued, the medication is selected from the operating room stock or facility pharmacy. This may be in a separate room in the department, or a drug stock within the operating suite itself. Regardless of where the stock is kept, the correct ("right") drug must be selected. The amount, dose, strength, and expiration date of the drug are also checked at this time. The package and contents are checked for any signs of leakage, damage, or discoloration. After this initial check, the drug is taken to the room or area where it will be dispensed. Errors occur even when the drugs are stored in computer-controlled systems that are prestocked and accessed through a code or scanning system. The drug can be stocked in error, or the code mismatched to the drug; therefore, health care staff must never assume that the drug is correct as delivered by a computer storage system.

DISPENSING DRUGS TO THE STERILE FIELD

Before or during surgery, the circulating nurse dispenses medications needed on the sterile field to the scrubbed surgical technologist, who manages the drugs throughout the procedure. Drugs are received and contained on the sterile field in metal or plastic medicine cups and containers. Medicine containers are not used as measuring devices for drugs because the calibrations are not sufficiently accurate. Instead, the calibrated syringe is used.

PROTOCOL FOR DISPENSING AND RECEIVING DRUGS

1. Immediately before receiving a drug, the scrubbed surgical technologist selects an appropriate size and type of container for the drug.
2. The circulator holds the drug container so that the scrub can read it easily.
3. The nurse and scrub observe the commercial drug container and contents for integrity and safety such as discoloration, leaking, unusual sediment, or other impurities.
4. The scrubbed surgical technologist reads out loud the name, dose, amount, strength, route of administration, and expiration date.
5. The circulator verifies the information at the same time. Both verbal and visual verification are necessary.
6. The circulator dispenses the drug into a sterile container using sterile technique and a sterile transfer device.
7. The circulator again shows the drug container to the scrub, and both acknowledge the information.
8. The circulator or anesthesia care provider confirms the maximum dose limit of the drug.
9. All syringes or other devices used to contain drugs on the sterile field are immediately labeled by the scrub (see details later).
10. When the scrub passes the drug to the surgeon, the name and strength are again repeated out loud so that the surgeon knows exactly what is being dispensed.
    See Figure 13-2.

GLASS VIAL

Liquid drugs are dispensed to the sterile field by the circulator, who draws up the medication from its vial using a needle and

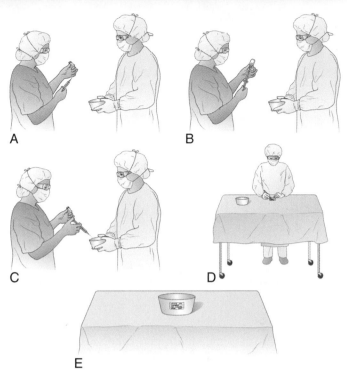

Figure 13-2 Protocol for receiving drugs on the sterile field; drug delivery to the field. **A,** The circulator shows the drug label to the scrub for verification. **B,** The circulator draws up the drug. **C,** The circulator distributes the drug into a sterile container. The circulator again shows the label to the scrub. **D** and **E,** The scrub immediately labels the drug.

syringe or needleless transfer device. The scrub can hold the container or place it near the edge of the back table while the drug is being dispensed. Regardless of which method is used, the protocol for dispensing the drug is followed precisely.

Never insert a needle into a vial held by another person. This increases the risk of needle injury to the person holding the vial. Always use a syringe or transfer device. Do not remove the vial cap and pour the drug out directly into the receiving basin, because sterility cannot be ensured.

GLASS AMPULE

The glass ampule is a small, hollow, one-piece container with a narrow neck. It is opened by breaking the tip at the neck. This type of container requires the use of an ampule breaker and transfer device, or the tip can be broken by placing a sponge over the top of the ampule and snapping it off away from the face. A syringe fitted with a transfer filter is used to withdraw the drug while excluding any small glass shards. The drug is injected into a small sterile container on the field as described earlier. The broken pieces and empty vial are discarded in the sharps box. The sponge is discarded because it contains glass chips. Glass ampules are used in the sterile and nonsterile settings. If the ampule has been processed by a sterilization method, the ampule can be distributed to the scrubbed technologist, who then opens it on the sterile field, taking care to contain glass shards and dispose of them properly. Only glass-filtering needles should be used to withdraw liquid from a glass ampule. Figure 13-3 shows a glass vial and a glass ampule.

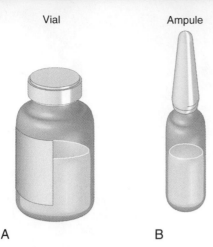

Vial   Ampule

A   B

Figure 13-3 **A**, Glass vial. **B**, Glass ampule. *(From Kee JL, Marchal SM: Clinical calculations: application to general and specialty areas, ed 5, Philadelphia, 2004, WB Saunders.)*

RECONSTITUTED DRUGS

Some drugs are dispensed in dry form and must be reconstituted to liquid form before administration. The liquid portion of the drug is called the **diluent**. Common drugs that must be reconstituted are bacitracin (an antibacterial used for irrigation) and topical thrombin (a coagulant).

Only *sterile injectable saline* is used to reconstitute a drug requiring saline as a diluent. The surgical technologist and circulator participate jointly in drug reconstitution so that both parts of the mixture can be identified correctly using the drug transfer protocol.

1. The circulator prepares the drug vial and sterile injectable saline vial for aseptic dispensing.
2. The injectable saline is injected into the vial containing the dry drug. The vial is gently agitated until no particles of dry agent are visible.
3. A sterile transfer device is attached to the vial.
4. The scrubbed surgical technologist receives the reconstituted drug in a container after the verification process.

IRRIGATION FLUIDS

Irrigation fluid is used during surgery to clear away blood and tissue debris in the surgical wound and to keep tissues moist. Topical *normal saline* is used for general irrigation in body cavities and large wounds. The most common general irrigation devices for this purpose are the Asepto syringe and bulb syringe (illustrated in Chapter 22).

Specialized procedures require specific irrigation fluids and mixtures such as heparin sodium in small quantities. Irrigation devices used to flush body cavities, such as the abdominal or thoracic cavity, hold relatively large amounts of solution. However, for small incisions, such as procedures on the blood vessels, a calibrated syringe or commercially prepared irrigation system is used. Smaller irrigation devices are required for microsurgery (e.g., eye, ear, and vascular or nerve tissue). In these procedures, the solution is used directly from its plastic container, which is fitted with a fine irrigating tip. A conventional syringe and specialized tip may also be used for fine irrigation.

Irrigation solutions are maintained at body temperature to prevent hypothermia. This is especially important for pediatric, older, and very thin patients. Sterile saline for irrigation can be kept at a controlled temperature in a solution warmer. Chilled solutions for cardiac and transplant surgery are maintained as sterile ice slush.

Sterile irrigation fluids are delivered to the sterile field directly into a basin or bowl on the field. When irrigation fluids are poured, the flow is never interrupted. *The entire contents of the container must be delivered at one time.* The rationale for this is that the lip of the container cannot be guaranteed to be sterile once the container has been recapped. Note that specific irrigation fluids, used for injection of blood vessels or ducts (e.g., saline solution for reconstitution with heparin or iodinated contrast media), require *injectable* saline. Saline for irrigation is never used for injection. High-alert irrigation fluids such as heparin and topical thrombin require particularly astute attention to handling and distribution.

MEDICAL MEASUREMENT SYSTEMS

The surgical technologist is required to measure drugs on the sterile field before handover to the surgeon for administration to the patient. This process often involves making calculations involving the strength of the drug, the amount needed, and the amount already administered. For example, the total amount of drug such as a local anesthetic given intermittently must be recalculated each time more is administered in order to prevent overdose. Drugs formulated as a combination of more than one substance (e.g., local anesthetic with epinephrine added) must be calculated separately even though they are given as one agent. Drug measurement requires familiarity with current measurement systems.

Two measurement systems were historically used in pharmacology, the metric system and the apothecary system. The now-obsolete "household system" is not used in medicine because it lacks precision and can cause drug errors. *This system must not be used for any form of medical measurement.* The apothecary system is also obsolete (see later discussion).

METRIC SYSTEM

The metric system of weights and measures is an international system. It is commonly used for all measurements in every country except the United States and is the accepted standard for scientific measurement. It was introduced in 1960 to standardize world trade and science. The system is based on units or powers of 10 (Table 13-3), which are applied to each type of quantity measured (volume, mass, and length). Box 13-4 shows mass and volume equivalents in the metric system.

Prefixes are used to express multiples of the metric system. Therefore, to arrive at an amount, the base unit is multiplied by the amount associated with its prefix. The prefixes are:

Kilo—1,000
Hecto—100
Deca—10
Deci—0.1 (one tenth)
Centi—0.01 (one hundredth)
Milli—0.001 (one thousandth)

Table 13-3 Metric Equivalents

%	Ratio	g/L	g/dL	mg/mL	mg/dL	mcg/mL
10	1:10	100	10	100	10,000	100,000
1	1:100	10	1	10	1,000	10,000
0.1	1:1,000	1	0.1	1	100	1,000
0.01	1:10,000	0.1	0.01	0.1	10	100
0.001	1:100,000	0.01	0.001	0.01	1	10
0.0001	1:1,000,000	0.001	0.0001	0.001	0.1	1

Box 13-4 Metric System: Mass and Volume

Units of Mass
1 kilogram (kg) = 1,000 grams (g)
1 gram (g) = 1,000 milligrams (mg)
1 milligram = 1,000 micrograms

Units of Volume
1 liter (L) = 1,000 milliliters (mL)
1 mL = 1,000 microliters

Examples:
1 *kilo*meter = 1,000 meters
1 *kilo*gram = 1,000 grams
1 *milli*gram = $\frac{1}{1,000}$ of a gram
1 *milli*liter = $\frac{1}{1,000}$ of a liter
5 *milli*liters = $\frac{5}{1,000}$ of a liter

APOTHECARY SYSTEM

The apothecary system is an antiquated system that is rarely encountered. It has been replaced in all countries by metric measurements and is mentioned here only for historical interest. The system employs Roman numerals to represent measurements and symbols to represent units of measure. The basic units of weight in the apothecary system are grains (not to be confused with *grams*) and ounces. Volume is expressed in drams and minims. Because of errors in measurement and lack of familiarity with the apothecary system, the metric system is now the common system of measurement.

INTERNATIONAL UNITS

International units are used in the measurement of selected drugs only. Any measure that is expressed as units describes the number of units per milliliter after addition of a diluent. For example, if a label states that a vial contains 400,000 international units of a drug, the concentrations of the drug can be altered by adding different amounts of diluent. Remember, however, that the same number of units is contained in the vial, regardless of how much diluent is added. Only the concentration changes.

ROMAN NUMERALS

Roman numerals were used in the past for writing prescriptions. This system has been phased out in medicine but is still used in some types of general numerical communication.

Table 13-4 Roman Numeral to Arabic Conversion

Roman Numeral	Arabic Number
I	1
V	5
X	10
L	50
C	100
D	500
M	1,000

Roman numerals are based on units of 10 and uses *letters* to represent numbers. The numeral is a symbol that represents a number in the Arabic system (0 to 9) as shown in Table 13-4.

When numerals are printed in succession, they are added:

$$III = 3$$

$$XXX = 30$$

When a smaller value is positioned in front of a larger one, the smaller one is subtracted from the larger one:

$$IX = 9$$

$$IV = 4$$

Other rules apply for subtracting numerals:
- Subtract only powers of 10 (e.g., XLV = 45).
- Subtract only a single numeral from another single numeral (e.g., 19 = XIX, not IXX).
- Do not subtract a numeral from one that is more than 10 times greater.

INTERNATIONAL TIME

International time is used in health care to prevent errors that occur when the same number is used for night and day. International time is based on a 24-hour clock. When international time is written, the colon (:) and common references to time of day (AM and PM) are unnecessary.

In this system, the 24 hours of the day begin with 0100, "zero one hundred hours," which corresponds to 1 AM, and end at 2400, "twenty-four hundred hours," or 12 midnight. To convert to international time, remove the colon from customary time and use the total number of hours and minutes elapsed from 1200 for daytime and 2400 for nighttime (Figure 13-4). Note that international time was historically called "military time." This term is no longer used.

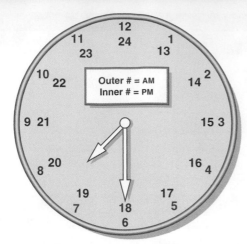

Figure 13-4 **Reading international time.** *(From Kee J, Hayes E, McCuiston L: Pharmacology, ed 5, Philadelphia, 2006, WB Saunders.)*

DELIVERY DEVICES

Drug delivery devices are used to *measure* and *administer* medications using aseptic technique. Drugs are manufactured in multiple- or single-dose containers with the content labeled in volume or weight. During surgery, the circulator dispenses the entire contents of the drug container or package to the scrubbed surgical technologist because incremental distribution does not ensure sterility of the product. This means that incremental doses must be measured by the surgical technologist on the sterile field. The amount is measured again before administration to the patient.

Although various pitchers, cups, and irrigation devices are calibrated in milliliters, these should not be used for measuring drugs because the calibrations are not precise enough and are not intended to be used except for gross determination of liquid amounts.

SYRINGE

The syringe is used to measure, dispense, and administer a drug. This is the most accurate method for measuring liquids. Two types of syringe tips are the locking (Luer-Lok) and catheter tips (also called plain tip or slip tip). The syringe tip accepts a variety of different medical devices including a hypodermic needle, intravenous tubing, stopcock, or extension device fitted with the same type of tip. The Luer-Lok system is locked in place by twisting it while the catheter tip connects by simply pushing it onto the needle or other device (Figure 13-5).

Syringes are available in many sizes and types. All syringes are calibrated in milliliters (mL) with increment hashes inscribed on the barrel. The most common syringe sizes are 1, 3, 5, and 10 mL. The largest syringe is 50 mL, used for flushing and irrigation, not usually for measuring drugs because the increments are too wide for safe calculation. The tuberculin syringe is the smallest metric syringe, which has a total volume of 0.5 or 1 mL and is used for doses less than 1 mL. The insulin syringe and needle is a one-piece unit, calibrated in both

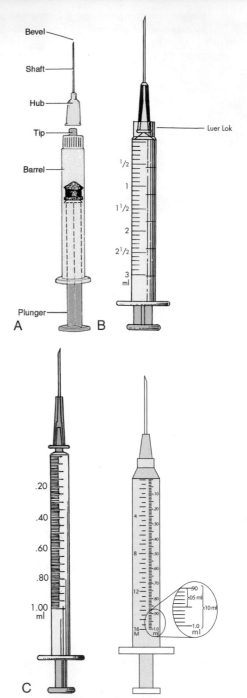

Figure 13-5 **A,** Catheter tip syringe. **B,** Luer-Lok syringe. **C,** *Left,* tuberculin syringe; *right,* normal syringe showing incremental subunits contained with the entire tuberculin syringe. *(A from Elkin M, Perry A, Potter P: Nursing interventions and clinical skills, ed 2, St Louis, 2000, Mosby; B from Potter PA, Perry AG: Fundamentals of nursing, ed 5, St Louis, 2001, Mosby; and C from Clayton B, Stock Y: Basic pharmacology for nurses, ed 12, St Louis, 2001, Mosby.)*

insulin units and milliliters. This syringe is intended for use with insulin only.

NEEDLES

Hypodermic needles are sized according to gauge (lumen size) and length. The larger the gauge, the smaller the needle size. For example, an 18-gauge needle has a larger lumen than a 22-gauge. Because of the risk of blood-borne diseases, the National Institute for Occupational Safety and Health (NIOSH) requires that syringes have some feature that allows the needle to be retracted or protected so that personnel are not punctured during or after use. It is acceptable to place the cap on the table and scoop it up with the point of the needle or use a needle-capping device. With this device, the cap is held in a rigid container and the needle and syringe combination is pushed down into the cap. *Needles must never be recapped using two hands* because of the increased risk of needlestick injury.

CONNECTION TUBING AND STOPCOCKS

Intravenous connection tubes and valves are often used in surgery as an attachment to a syringe for administration. The short, flexible tubing allows easier handling of the syringe and more precise direction in the flow of the medication. A two-way or three-way standard stopcock is used to turn the flow on and off. The important aspect of this device is to always use one device with the same drug during a procedure to prevent mixing of drugs not intended to be mixed. A stopcock also allows two syringes to be attached to one delivery tube for intentional alternate injection of the two drugs. Like all syringes, these must be clearly labeled, as directed later.

INFUSION PUMP

The infusion pump is an electronic device that delivers a programmed amount of drug in a specific time period. Pumps are external or may be implanted for long-term care in pain management. Epidural anesthesia may be delivered through an intrathecal infusion pump, and intravenous fluids are routinely administered this way. Infusion pumps are managed by the anesthesia care provider or licensed nurse.

CENTRAL VENOUS CATHETERS

Long term administration of drugs including chemotherapeutic agents, IV solutions, perenteral nutritional solutions, and blood is facilitated by placing a temporary or semi-permanent intravenous catheter into a major vein. This type of device spares the patient repeated venipuncture over long periods of treatment which can last for days, weeks, or months. A venous catheter may be left in place as long as it is carefully monitored for infection, fracture, and blockage. Refer to Chapter 32 for more details on central line equipment and procedures.

MANAGING DRUGS ON THE STERILE FIELD

Management of drugs and other pharmaceutical materials on the surgical field requires labeling, organization, and care of the materials, measuring, mixing, and dispensing to the surgeon. These roles should be carried out systematically to prevent drug error. Concentration on the task at hand is an important part of the role. The Joint Commission has issued specific directives for the management of drugs in the acute care setting, which includes surgery both on and off the sterile field.

LABELING

Removal of a drug from its commercial container and transfer to an unlabeled container makes the drug unidentifiable. To reduce drug error, every drug container or device must be labeled. Labels are made as soon as a drug is received. Commercially prepared labels are available for most drugs used on the sterile field, or these can be custom ordered by the health facility. All drugs and their delivery devices are labeled, even if there is only one. The label must state the following information:

1. Medication name
2. Strength
3. Quantity
4. Diluent and volume (if not apparent from the container)
5. Preparation date when not used within 24 hours
6. Expiration time (when expiration occurs within less than 24 hours of distribution)
7. Expiration date and time are not necessary for short procedures as defined by the health care facility

Standard of Practice for Labeling

- Labels must be printed with waterproof ink on an adhesive sticker.
- Write legibly and follow the Joint Commission ruling on "do not use" abbreviations (see Chapter 3).
- If any doubt exists about the identification of a drug, *the drug must be discarded* and a fresh drug distributed to the sterile field.
- The verification process is repeated with a change of scrubbed personnel, such as during shift changes. Any drugs not labeled are discarded.

ORGANIZATION OF DRUGS

Following distribution to the sterile field and labeling, the scrub places drugs in one designated area of the back table. Each drug should have a designated delivery device that is also labeled to avoid mixing drugs in a common delivery device. Take care not to mix syringe or irrigation tips. Even the residual amount of drug remaining in the device can have an effect. High-alert drugs such as intravenous heparin and epinephrine can be flagged using commercial markers. When there are two formulations of the same drug, try to avoid placing them next to each other where one might be accidentally mistaken for the other. The scrub must always check the label before passing any drug. In spite of efforts to alert perioperative personnel about this hazard, it continues to be a common source of drug errors that result in the patient being given the wrong drug, sometimes with fatal results. Extra precaution can prevent this.

MIXING AND PREPARATION OF DRUGS

Some drugs require mixing on the sterile field. In this case, the scrubbed surgical technologist receives the components separately, calculates the correct ratio of mixture needed, mixes the drugs accordingly, and puts them in the correct delivery device. Calculations must be performed accurately and checked before releasing the drug to the surgeon. If necessary, the scrub may ask another person on the team to validate the calculation, and this may be a requirement in some facilities.

Drugs and pharmaceuticals are prepared on the back table by the scrubbed surgical technologist. It is helpful to clear away a space on the back table to provide easy access to instruments needed for mixing drugs and loading syringes for dispensing. A variety of stainless steel bowls, basins, and cups are distributed at the start of a surgical case. These can be used to compartmentalize items on the field and for some liquids. Nonreactive plastic cups should be used for small amounts of medication received, especially local anesthetic, which may undergo a chemical reaction in contact with metal.

Drugs are measured by drawing up the components separately (not in the same syringe) and putting them in a *dry* basin or medicine cup of appropriate size. A new delivery device must be prepared for the combination drug, which now has different properties from its individual components. Drug components less than 1 mL must be measured using a tuberculin syringe to achieve accuracy.

Careful mixing of drugs prevents the introduction of air in the mixture. This is very important for precise measurement and also to prevent potentially fatal air embolism in vessels and ducts. Box 13-5 provides methods to prevent the introduction of air into a syringe or narrow delivery device.

Box **13-5**	Tips for Preventing the Introduction of Air into a Syringe or Other Delivery Device

- It is much easier to prevent air from entering a device than to remove it once it is there.
- Before drawing up the solution, make sure that the tip (catheter, needle, irrigation tip) of the syringe is attached tightly to the syringe. A loose tip can allow air to be aspirated into the device.
- Ensure that the tip attachment of the delivery device (catheter tip, needle, transfer device) is inserted into the liquid and remains in the liquid while withdrawing the drug. Remember to withdraw the needle slightly as the level decreases to prevent air from entering the syringe.
- When mixing dry and liquid drugs in a vial, do not shake the vial. This creates foam. Instead, hold the vial between your palms and gently roll it back and forth.
- When mixing a dry component with a water-based diluent, do not use force to inject the diluent into the dry component. Instead, inject the fluid slowly.
- To remove air from a delivery device before use, use gravity allow the air to float to the top of the fluid. Gently eject the air. If this does not work, gently tap or flick the tubing or syringe tip. It is very difficult to remove air from small-bore tubing or a syringe. It may be necessary to remove the needle or syringe tip in order to break the surface tension and release air.
- Be aware that when air is removed, a small amount of drug may be accidentally ejected. This might require recalculation of the total amount required.

DISPENSING A DRUG TO THE SURGEON

Drugs are passed to the surgeon when requested or when their need is anticipated by the scrub. When passing the drug, the concentration and amount must be verbally stated by the scrub and acknowledged by the surgeon. This is particularly important for high-alert drugs but should be carried out each time a drug is passed. This not only provides a safety check, but also informs the anesthesiologist and circulating nurse that a drug is being administered for assessment and documentation purposes. Note that the maximum safe dose of a drug is determined by the patient's individual condition, and also by weight. The surgical technologist is expected to validate the maximum dosage with the anesthesia care provider before surgery.

DRUG ADMINISTRATION

Drug administration is the introduction of a drug into the patient. There are many different methods and routes used for drug administration. The recommended route for a drug is based on its chemical composition, the target tissue, and the condition of the patient. The route of administration is indicated by the prescribing health practitioner. A drug intended for one route may not be given by another route. The drug may be available for administration in another form, but it must be approved and labeled for that use.

The usual clinical routes of administration are as follows:
1. **Parenteral**—by injection
   a. Intravenous—injection directly into a vein
   b. **Intraosseous** (IO)—injection into the bone marrow; used when an intravenous line cannot be initiated or maintained
   c. Intramuscular (IM)—injection into a muscle
   d. Subcutaneous—injection into the connective tissue directly beneath the skin
   e. Intradermal (ID)—injection between the dermis and epidermis
   f. Intraspinal—injection into the spinal canal (**intrathecal**) or epidural space (epidural injection)
   g. Intraperitoneal—injected into the peritoneal cavity
2. Oral (enteral)—by mouth (PO, *per os*)
   a. Ingestion—swallowing
   b. Buccal—tablet placed between the gum and mucous membrane of the cheek
   c. Sublingual—tablet placed under the tongue
3. **Topical**—on surface tissue
   a. Instillation—administration of drops into the eye or ear
   b. **Transdermal**—drug is absorbed through a skin patch
   c. Rectal—topical effect or systemic absorption through rectal mucosa
   d. Vaginal—topical effect or absorption through mucous membrane
   e. Nasal—on nasal mucosa
   f. Inhalant—drug is inhaled as an aerosol and absorbed through the bronchial tree and lungs

It is important to remember that drugs are administered through a specific route based on the nature of the chemical, on the physical characteristics of the drug, and on the rate of absorption required by the patient's condition. Every drug is labeled for a specific delivery method (e.g., injected, topical, by mouth.) Administration by any route other than that intended is a medication error and may lead to serious harm or even death.

ASSESSMENT

Following administration of a drug, the patient is assessed for physiological changes, including adverse reactions. In all clinical situations, assessment is made by the medical or nursing staff, who can quickly respond to the medical needs of the patient in the event of emergency.

ADVERSE REACTION TO A DRUG

Whenever a drug is administered, many physiological changes can take place in the body. Some of these are therapeutic (desirable) effects, whereas others may be undesirable or potentially harmful. Precautions against taking a drug under circumstances known to be harmful are stated as *contraindications*. An **adverse reaction** is an undesirable or intolerable reaction to a drug administered at the *normal dosage*. It is important to remember that the adverse reaction occurs when the drug is given at the normal dose. Adverse reactions are *unexpected*, although they may be predictable in certain individuals. When a drug is tested before its release, adverse reactions are documented, and this becomes part of the drug information available to clinicians and patients. Examples of mild adverse effects include nausea and dizziness. This type of effect is usually transient and ceases when the drug is stopped. More serious adverse reactions might include difficulty breathing or increased heart rate.

Medical and nursing personnel are trained to recognize the clinical signs and symptoms of an adverse drug event. Allied health personnel have two important roles in this process:

1. Keen observation of a patient's normal behavior and appearance
2. Immediately reporting to medical or nursing personnel any signs and symptoms that seem abnormal

When reporting a suspected drug reaction, follow these guidelines:

- What sign or signs do you observe that you believe are not normal for that patient?
- When did it start?
- What does the patient report (if applicable)?
- What comfort measures did you initiate (e.g., providing warmth, reassurance)?

DRUG ALLERGY

True **allergy** to a drug is mediated by the immune system and requires previous exposure to substances in the drug or a genetic predisposition to allergy. An immune response that causes irritation, respiratory failure, or death is called **hypersensitivity**. Hypersensitivity can be mild, producing only a

---

Box 13-6 | **Allergic Reactions**

- *Type I:* Characterized by tissue inflammation caused by the release of histamine in the body. This causes increased permeability of blood vessels and constriction of bronchioles, leading to difficulty breathing. The most extreme form of sensitivity is anaphylactic shock, which can lead to death.
- *Type II:* Called a *cytotoxic reaction*, the results of interaction between two antibodies and cell surface antigens. Results in the activation of powerful immune defense mechanisms, causing injury or death. Mismatched blood transfusion reactions and hemolytic disease in newborns are type II reactions.
- *Type III:* Caused by antigen-antibody complexes, which cause tissue damage when they trigger immune response. Allergy to antibiotics is an example of a type III response. Symptoms include itching, rash, severe tissue swelling, and fever. This type of reaction usually resolves in several days.
- *Type IV:* Cell-mediated reactions (not related to antibodies) that occur 24 to 72 hours after exposure to the agent. An example of this type of delayed hypersensitivity is a positive reaction to the tuberculin skin test in which a small amount of killed *Mycobacterium tuberculosis* is injected.

---

rash or wheezing, or it can be severe, resulting in respiratory failure and death caused by anaphylactic shock.

Allergic reactions are characterized as immediate or delayed. Delayed sensitivity can occur up to 12 hours after exposure to a drug and is mediated by T lymphocytes. Immediate reactions are mediated by antibodies. All allergic reactions are divided into the categories shown in Box 13-6.

DOCUMENTATION

Documentation is required following administration of any drug or pharmaceutical (including implants). Documentation may be included in the patient's electronic chart, written surgical report, or anesthesia record, depending on the situation. All elements of the drug administration must be included:

- The name of the drug
- Dose
- Amount
- The route (e.g., intravenous, intraperitoneal) and location
- Time of administration
- Name of person who administered the drug
- Patient assessment following administration

"DO NOT USE" ABBREVIATIONS

The Joint Commission has developed a list of abbreviations that can lead to drug errors. The "do not use" abbreviations are shown in Table 13-5. Health facilities are also advised to make additions to their own "do not use" list. This list applies to any documentation, including prescriptions, patient charts, and order transcriptions.

Table **13-5**	Joint Commission's "Do Not Use" Symbols in Documentation*	
Do Not Use	**Potential Problem**	**Use Instead**
U (unit)	Mistaken for "O" (zero), the number "4" (four) or "mL"	Write "unit"
IU (international unit)	Mistaken for IV (intravenous) or the number 10 (ten)	Write "international unit"
Q.D., QD, q.d., qd (daily) Q.E.D., QOD, q.o.d., qod (every other day)	Mistaken for each other	Write "daily" Write "every other day"
Trailing zero (X.0 mg)† Lack of leading zero (.X mg)	Decimal point is missed	Write X mg Write 0.X mg
MS MSO₄ and MgSO₄	Can mean morphine sulfate or magnesium sulfate Confused for one another	Write "morphine sulfate" Write "magnesium sulfate"

*Applies to all orders and all medication-related documentation that are handwritten (including free-text computer entry) or on preprinted forms.

†Exception: A "trailing zero" may be used only where required to demonstrate the level of precision of the value being reported, such as for laboratory results, imaging studies that report size of lesions, or catheter/tube sizes. It may not be used in medication orders or other medication-related documentation.

SECTION III: DRUG ACTION

When a drug enters the body by any route, *both the body and the drug undergo changes.* That is, the drug is broken down chemically (change in the drug), and the drug has a physiological effect on the patient (change in the body).

PHARMACOKINETICS

Pharmacokinetics is the study of movement of drugs through the body (what the body does to the drug). Once a drug is introduced, it moves through physiological paths. The individual's age, genetics, physical condition, and many other factors determine how quickly the drug moves through the body.

Pharmacokinetics is described by mathematical formulas that take into account the rate of absorption, the amount of drug in the body, and the **concentration** of the drug in the plasma.

For purposes of general study, the entire process of pharmacokinetics is divided into four processes:

- Absorption
- Distribution
- Biotransformation (metabolism)
- Excretion (elimination)

ABSORPTION

Absorption is the process by which a drug enters the body tissues following administration. The rate of absorption and the amount of drug that actually reaches the target tissue depend on many factors such as the chemical structure of the drug, the method of administration, and the condition of the patient. Absorption involves chemical and physical breakdown of the drug. For example, oral drugs must dissolve before passing through the wall of the small intestine and liver. The substance then enters the bloodstream, where it is carried to the target tissue. Drugs that are injected directly into a blood vessel do not require absorption and thus reach the target tissue almost immediately, whereas one injected into the muscle or connective tissue usually takes 15 to 30 minutes to take effect. Many drugs contain components or additives that enhance (increase the rate or amount) or delay absorption.

DISTRIBUTION

After the drug enters the bloodstream, it is carried (distributed) to body tissues, where it exerts its pharmacological effect. Not all of the drug administered reaches the target tissue. The amount of drug available and the rate of availability are called the **bioavailability**. For example, some drugs may become tightly bound to blood proteins and are released to the target tissue very slowly. Fat-soluble drugs move rapidly across the cell membranes and take effect quickly but also tend to accumulate in fatty tissue, which prolongs their effect. Water-soluble substances are much slower to act because they stay in the bloodstream longer than those that are fat-soluble. In all cases, only the free unbound drug is available to tissues for pharmacological effect.

BIOTRANSFORMATION (METABOLISM)

Biotransformation, or drug metabolism, is the chemical breakdown of a drug in the body. Most drugs are broken down into smaller, less complex chemical components by enzymes. This occurs mainly in the liver. Biotransformation prepares the drug for *excretion,* or elimination from the body. Because most biotransformation occurs in the liver, conditions that decrease liver function can alter drug metabolism, resulting in toxicity. Liver disease and advanced age are two causes of altered liver metabolism, which can affect drug metabolism.

In pharmacology and medicine, it is critical to know how long a drug is active. This is related to its rate of biotransformation, which is measured by the drug's half-life. The **half-life** is the time it takes for one half of the drug to be cleared from the body. Some drugs, such as antibiotics, have a short half-life and must be given repeatedly over a short period of time so that the therapeutic amount stays constant for the duration of treatment. Other drugs have a long half-life and can be given less frequently to maintain therapeutic levels.

The point in time when the drug first takes effect is called the *onset.* The point when the drug has the greatest effect is called the *peak.* From that point the effects diminish until the drug is cleared from tissues. The total time the drug is active is called the *duration of action*.

EXCRETION (ELIMINATION)

Drugs are mainly eliminated or cleared from the body through the kidneys. A small percentage is excreted through the biliary tract, breast milk, saliva, and intestine. Volatile drugs and anesthetics are excreted through the lungs during exhalation. Just as liver disease can alter drug metabolism, kidney disease can severely retard or block drug elimination and result in life-threatening toxicity.

Drugs are mainly eliminated as the products of metabolism. In this process, chemical reactions cause the drug to break down into smaller molecules or components. Metabolic components of the drug are called *metabolites*. In a healthy individual, the entire drug is excreted— in its intact form, or as metabolites— as smaller components resulting from breakdown of the drug.

PHARMACODYNAMICS

RECEPTORS, ANTAGONISTS, AND AGONISTS

Changes (both intended and unintended) in the body as a result of a drug are called **pharmacodynamics**. The changes occur with many drugs because of the drug's ability to "lock on" to certain target receptor sites on the cells. Normally, the receptor sites receive the body's own (endogenous) chemicals (e.g., hormones, neurotransmitters) that cause specific physiological changes in the body. However, when the drug occupies these sites, the endogenous chemicals are blocked. The drug may not have any function except blocking the site. An increased dose of the drug results in many more receptor sites being taken, and this severely affects the cell's ability to receive the endogenous chemical. A drug or substance that blocks endogenous substances is called an **antagonist**.

Some drugs, instead of blocking the effects of the body's chemicals, lock on to the receptor site and stimulate a particular response in the cell which has far reaching effects on physiology. These drugs are called **agonists**.

THERAPEUTIC WINDOW

Drug action is related not only to the amount of time it is in the body, but also to the amount of drug administered and its concentration (the amount of actual drug per unit dose). Although the drug may have a positive effect at a given level, increasing the amount of drug beyond the therapeutic (effective) level results in toxicity. The practical application of drug therapy is to give only the amount of drug that brings about the positive change desired without also causing toxicity in the body. The range of drug doses that can treat disease effectively while staying within the safety range is known as the **therapeutic window**. Drugs in which the difference between the therapeutic dose and toxicity or lethal effects is small are said to have a "narrow therapeutic window." The dose of a drug must therefore be carefully measured and administered properly to ensure that the safe, prescribed amount is administered. This is very important for the surgical technologist who handles dose-dependent drugs on the surgical field. Some drugs handled in surgery are extremely toxic and even lethal at high levels. This is why there is so much importance placed on identification of the drug strength and on the amount being delivered.

Drug *synergy* occurs when drugs given simultaneously cause an effect that is greater than any one of the drugs would have by itself. This allows certain synergistic drugs to be given in lower doses which is safer for the patient. However, drug synergy must also be considered when the greater effect has undesired results.

SECTION IV: SELECTED DRUG CATEGORIES

The scrubbed technologist is required to handle and deliver a number of different categories of drugs used on the sterile field. Naturally, these categories are only a fraction of all drugs. In practical terms, the surgical technologist should give priority to learning these particular drugs and agents. (Refer to Appendix B for a list of medications and other pharmaceuticals commonly used in surgery and their actions.)

In the United States drugs are classified through the AHFS. This is a tiered system based on therapeutic action of the drug and is used throughout the health care system. Drug categories and their subcategories are assigned a code number that can be researched easily by health care providers. Surgical technologists should become familiar with the system in order to use the correct professional terminology. The first-tier categories are shown in Box 13-7. The AHFS system is used to identify perioperative drugs in the following discussion.

ANTIINFECTIVE AGENTS

This category includes all drugs used in the treatment of infectious diseases caused by pathogenic organisms. Many drugs are differentiated in their second tier of identification by the type of organism they affect, such as antifungal, antiretroviral, or antibiotic. Categories are listed in Appendix B. The largest category of antiinfectives is the **antibiotics**, which are used to treat bacterial infections. There are many types of antibiotics that differ in their action against bacteria. The indication of one antibiotic over another is based on the type of infection, the drug resistance of the bacteria, and the condition of the patient. Many antibiotics developed decades ago are no longer effective because of drug resistance. As a result, newer drugs are in constant development. Antiinfectives are used in the perioperative setting in several ways:

- As a preoperative medication in selected cases. The patient may be started on intravenous antibiotics a few hours before surgery to prevent postoperative infection.
- As an irrigant in the surgical wound. Topical antibiotics such as bacitracin may be used to irrigate tissues of body cavities and spaces, especially when the risk of postoperative wound infection is high.
- Bacteriostatic agents (those that arrest the proliferation of bacteria) are impregnated into some types of dressings such as gauze strips and packing material, used in the nasal cavity following surgery.

Box 13-7　First-Tier Drug Categories

No.	Drug Category
4:00	Antihistamine Drugs
8:00	Antiinfective Agents
10:00	Antineoplastic Agents
12:00	Autonomic Drugs
16:00	Blood Derivatives
20:00	Blood Formation, Coagulation, and Thrombosis Agents
24:00	Cardiovascular Drugs
26:00	Cellular Therapy
28:00	Central Nervous System Agents
32:00	Contraceptives (foams, devices)
34:00	Dental Agents
36:00	Diagnostic Agents
38:00	Disinfectants (for agents used on objects other than skin)
40:00	Electrolytic, Caloric, and Water Balance
44:00	Enzymes
48:00	Respiratory Tract Agents
52:00	Eye, Ear, Nose, and Throat (EENT) Preparations
56:00	Gastrointestinal Drugs
60:00	Gold Compounds
64:00	Heavy Metal Antagonists
68:00	Hormones and Synthetic Substitutes
72:00	Local Anesthetics
76:00	Oxytocics
78:00	Radioactive Agents
80:00	Serums, Toxoids, and Vaccines
84:00	Skin and Mucous Membrane Agents
86:00	Smooth Muscle Relaxants
88:00	Vitamins
92:00	Miscellaneous Therapeutic Agents
94:00	Devices
96:00	Pharmaceutical Aids

From the American Hospital Forumlary Service, http://www.ahfsdruginformation.com. Retrieved December 2011. © American Society of Health-System Pharmacists, Inc. Reproduced with permission.

- Postoperatively, many patients are prescribed antibiotics to prevent infection.

Antiretroviral medications are in the antiinfective group of drugs. These are used in the treatment of human immunodeficiency virus/acquired immunodeficiency syndrome (HIV/AIDS) and are also prescribed as part of postexposure prophylaxis (PEP) immediately following exposure to body fluids such as a sharps injury in the medical workplace

MECHANISMS OF ACTION

The mechanisms of antibacterial action can include but are not limited to:

- Inhibition of synthesis of the cell wall
- Alteration in the permeability of the cell membrane
- Prevention of the synthesis of cellular proteins
- Inhibition of the cell's genetic material, deoxyribonucleic acid (DNA) and ribonucleic acid (RNA), which is needed for replication
- Interference with cell metabolism

PENICILLIN

Penicillin was developed during the early 1940s. It was the first true antibiotic, and many different categories of penicillin have emerged, all arising from the prototype. Penicillins are divided into two types: broad spectrum (effective on gram-positive and some gram-negative bacteria) and narrow spectrum (effective only on gram-positive bacteria). Other classes of penicillin are distinguished by their ability to target specific bacterial defense mechanisms or groups of bacteria.

Examples:
- Procaine penicillin
- Benzathine penicillin
- Penicillin V potassium
- Ampicillin
- Piperacillin

CEPHALOSPORINS

Cephalosporins were first developed in the 1960s. Each subsequent group has been broader in spectrum than the previous group. These groups are called generations of cephalosporins, because they emerged from the previous parent prototype. First-, second-, third-, and fourth-**generation** cephalosporins have been developed.

MACROLIDES

Macrolides are bacteriostatic at low levels and bactericidal in high doses. These are broad-spectrum drugs, but they are most active against gram-positive bacteria. They most commonly are used to treat respiratory tract infections and sexually transmitted diseases.

Examples:
- Azithromycin
- Clarithromycin
- Erythromycin

LINCOSAMIDES, VANCOMYCIN, AND KETOLIDES

Lincosamides, vancomycin, and ketolides have a similar action. They are bacteriostatic and bactericidal, and they inhibit protein synthesis in bacteria. Vancomycin was used extensively in the 1950s, but its use is now limited because it can cause auditory and cranial nerve damage.

Examples:
- Clindamycin
- Vancomycin
- Telithromycin

TETRACYCLINES

Tetracyclines are broad-spectrum antimicrobials that inhibit bacterial protein synthesis. They are supplied almost exclusively for oral administration against specific microbes such as rickettsiae and mycobacteria.

Examples:
- Doxycycline
- Minocycline
- Tigecycline

AMINOGLYCOSIDES

Aminoglycosides are effective against gram-negative bacteria, in which they inhibit protein synthesis. This group of antibiotics is used selectively and carefully because of adverse reactions.

Examples:
- Gentamicin
- Paromomycin
- Amikacin

QUINOLONES

These are broad-spectrum antibacterials that inhibit DNA synthesis. They are used in a variety of infections, including respiratory, arthritic, urinary tract, and gastrointestinal conditions.

Examples:
- Ciprofloxacin
- Levofloxacin

SULFONAMIDES

Sulfonamides were first introduced in the 1930s. They are bacteriostatic only. Because of their limited use and the emergence of increasingly drug-resistant bacterial strains, they have been replaced by drugs that are more effective. Sulfonamides are most commonly used to treat acute urinary tract infections.

Example:
- Sulfamethoxazole-trimethoprim

ANTIFUNGALS

Antifungal drugs are used for superficial and systemic fungal disease. Skin infections are treated mainly with OTC topical medications, although resistant strains may require oral administration. Systemic fungal infection is difficult to treat and can be fatal. Intravenous administration is required for many antifungal medications.

Examples:
- Amphotericin
- Miconazole
- Flucytosine

ANTINEOPLASTIC AGENTS

Cancer treatment may include the use of antineoplastic (anticancer) drugs that are occasionally used in the surgical setting. Intravesical treatment for urinary bladder cancer is a common procedure in which the antineoplastic drug is instilled directly into the bladder using a urinary catheter. This may follow tumor resection or as a stand-alone procedure. Intravesical instillation may also be performed in surgery or in the postanesthesia care unit (PACU).

Health care personnel can be injured through exposure to hazardous antineoplastic drugs. Risks include a higher incidence of leukemia and lymphoma, DNA damage, and miscarriage. Pregnant care workers are excluded from procedures in which there is a risk of contamination.

Safety precautions and standards for the handling and storage of antineoplastic drugs include the following:
- Storage of hazardous drugs
- Appropriate personal protective equipment
- Disposal of equipment contaminated by hazardous drugs
- Staff teaching on topics related to safe handling of hazardous drugs

Antineoplastic drugs are normally mixed by the facility's pharmacist and prepared ahead of the procedure.

AUTONOMIC DRUGS

Autonomic drugs affect neurotransmission in the autonomic nervous system. This category of drugs is used therapeutically in many different specialties to alter nerve transmission, especially in cardiac, respiratory, and ophthalmic medicine. A review of the autonomic nervous system explains the basics of how these drugs work.

AUTONOMIC NERVOUS SYSTEM

The central nervous system is composed of the brain and spinal cord. In order to exert action in the body systems, nerve impulses are sent from the CNS to the peripheral nervous system (PNS). The PNS is composed of major nerve pathways and their divisions, which extend into all tissues outside the brain and spinal cord. The PNS is divided into two separate systems, the somatic and autonomic nervous systems.

The *somatic nervous system* is under voluntary control. For example, nerve transmission to the striated muscles is somatic. However, the *autonomic nervous system* is involuntary. Stimuli to these nerves produce specific responses in body organs and tissues such as the heart, smooth muscle, and glands. Examples of autonomic responses are changes in heartbeat, the release of glandular secretions (e.g., insulin in the pancreas), and intestinal contractions (peristalsis).

Sympathetic and Parasympathetic Responses

The autonomic system can produce two different types of responses, sympathetic and *parasympathetic* (Figure 13-6). They are often referred to as fight-or-flight responses. However, a more accurate description would be related to stress and nonstress responses. During physiological and emotional stress, the sympathetic system takes priority, so digestion activity is delayed, but heart rate is increased to supply more oxygen to tissues. The parasympathetic system is most active when the body is at rest. For example, under the parasympathetic system the heart rate is slower and cardiac output is decreased, but digestion increases to allow

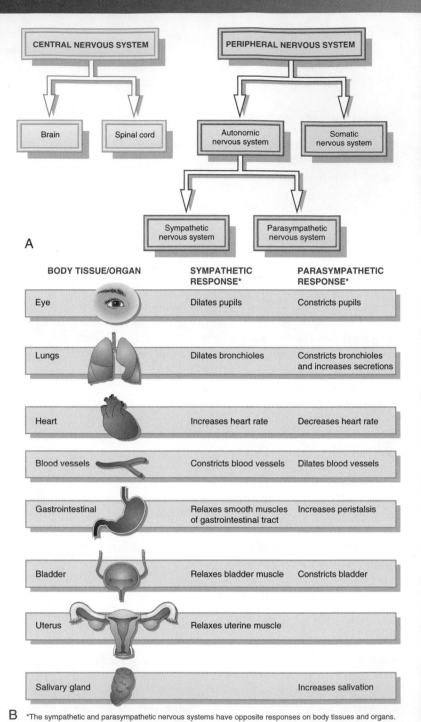

Figure 13-6 A, Divisions of the peripheral nervous system. **B,** Sympathetic and parasympathetic responses. *(From Kee J, Hayes E, McCuiston L: Pharmacology, ed 5, Philadelphia, 2006, WB Saunders.)*

greater storage of energy. The two parts of the autonomic system are constantly at work balancing body systems and physiology.

Separate neurotransmitters and receptors are responsible for the sympathetic and parasympathetic responses. *Noradrenalin* is the primary neurotransmitter for the sympathetic system. Certain receptors can also receive *adrenaline* and *dopamine. Acetylcholine* is the primary neurotransmitter of the parasympathetic system.

Receptors at the cellular level bind and interact with specific neurotransmitters. There are two main types of sympathetic (adrenergic) receptors: alpha (α) and beta (β). These are further classified into a number of different subtypes.

Receptors for the parasympathetic system are called *cholinergic* receptors.

Autonomic drugs are classified according to the type of receptor and neurotransmitter they interact with. To understand a specific drug, it is necessary to know where the receptor is located in the body (which tissue), its subtype, and whether it is an agonist (acting to increase the effect of the neurotransmitter) or an antagonist (blocking the effect of the neurotransmitter).

- *Adrenergic* agonists increase the effect of the sympathetic neurotransmitter (includes both alpha and beta agonists)
- *Adrenergic* antagonists block the effect of the sympathetic neurotransmitter (includes alpha and beta blockers)

- *Cholinergics* increase the effect of the parasympathetic neurotransmitter acetylcholine.
- *Anticholinergics* block the effects of acetylcholine.

ANTICHOLINERGICS

Anticholinergic drugs are frequently used during general anesthesia. In the past, potent anticholinergics such as scopolamine and atropine were given routinely to all surgical patients. Now, however, these agents are used more selectively and can be administered intravenously during surgery for rapid results. They are used to control airway secretions and to regulate the heart rate in selected patients. In ophthalmic surgery they are used to produce mydriasis (dilation of the pupil) and cycloplegia (paralysis of the ciliary muscles). Examples of anticholinergic agents include:

- Atropine sulfate
- Scopolamine
- Glycopyrrolate

The effects of anticholinergics include the following:

- Increase in the heart rate
- Relaxation of smooth muscles in selected ophthalmic procedures
- Reduction of gastrointestinal, bronchial, and nasopharyngeal secretions
- Emergency treatment of cardiac conduction block and sinus bradycardia
- Prevention of bronchospasm

ADRENERGICS

Adrenergic (also called sympathomimetic) drugs are used in many different specialties. In the respiratory system, the smooth muscles of the airways contain adrenoreceptors activated by adrenaline, which causes relaxation of the muscle fibers and dilation of the airways. Adrenergics are therefore used in the treatment of asthma and during respiratory emergencies such as anaphylactic shock. Some drugs are adrenergic to both the lungs and the heart, resulting in increase heart rate and expansion of the airways.

BLOOD AND BLOOD DERIVATIVES

Blood and blood derivatives (also called blood products) are used in the treatment of blood loss or for specific blood disorders that result in loss or destruction of a blood component. Whole blood replacement may be used if a significant amount of blood has been lost due to trauma or disease. It is normally used only when the patient's blood loss exceeds 30% of total blood volume (approximately 1,500 mL in an adult).

Whole blood and products are packed in collapsible bags that are labeled to include the type, amount, and number. When blood and blood products are used, an exact protocol must be followed. Cross-checking of products that are ABO-Rh specific is performed by two people (medical or nursing staff) before administration. Blood products must be stored at temperatures between 33.8° and 42.8° F (1° and 6° C). External temperature tape may be used to monitor the temperature of individual units. Units must be used within 30 minutes in a noncontrolled environment. Unused blood and blood products are returned to the blood bank.

EXAMPLES OF BLOOD AND DERIVATIVES

- *Whole blood* contains serum and blood cells plus anticoagulant and preservative. Whole blood is not commonly given because it can be broken down into components that can be administered separately. This prevents waste of blood products that are not needed.
- *Red blood cells*—a unit of red blood cells (RBCs) contains 150 to 210 mL of red cells, plus a small amount of plasma and preservative. Packed red blood cells (PRBCs) are administered to increase the oxygen-carrying capacity of the blood. A combination of PRBCs and plasma expanders is effective in increasing the total intravascular volume and oxygen-carrying capacity. All cell transfusions must be ABO-Rh compatible with the recipient. Packed cells are handled and monitored in the same way as whole blood.
- *Washed red blood cells* are normal RBCs that have been washed to remove the plasma and are administered to patients who demonstrate repeated hypersensitivity to blood or components.
- *Leukoreduced red blood cells* contain leukocytes in reduced volume within red blood cells. Leukoreduced RBCs are used in patients with a history of nonhemolytic febrile transfusion reactions.
- *Platelets* are essential for blood coagulation and contain coagulation factors, RBCs, and white blood cells. Platelets are administered to patients with bleeding disorders such as thrombocytopenia and platelet dysfunction.
- *Granulocytes (neutrophils)* are obtained from an ABO-Rh compatible donor and used in the treatment of severe neutropenia.
- *Fresh frozen plasma (FFP)* is extracted from whole blood and contains normal amounts of coagulation factors. This blood product is used for patients who have coagulation disorders and active bleeding and require invasive procedures.
- *Cryoprecipitate* is a concentration of several hemostatic proteins that have been prepared from whole blood. The hemostatic proteins contained in cryoprecipitate are factor VIII, von Willebrand factor, factor XIII, and fibrinogen. Cryoprecipitate is used for patients with significantly decreased fibrinogen who are actively bleeding or require invasive procedures. Cryoprecipitate is also used in the preparation of fibrin glue, orthopedic procedures, and ear, nose, and throat and neurosurgical procedures.
- *Factor concentrates* contain factor VIII, IS, and antithrombin III. This product is used in patients with hemophilia who require invasive procedures.

BLOOD COAGULATION

This category of drugs includes coagulants and anticoagulants used systemically and topically in medical treatment and surgery. These are high-alert drugs that must be very carefully handled on and off the sterile field to avoid drug error.

ANTICOAGULANTS

An anticoagulant is a drug that inhibits blood clot formation, but does not dissolve clots. There are several types of anticoagulant drugs.

Heparins

These are used for prevention of venous thromboembolism.
- *Unfractionated heparin* (UFH) has been largely replaced with safer low-molecular-weight heparin.
- *Low-molecular-weight heparin* (LMWH) is administered by injection to prevent venous thromboembolism after major orthopedic and gynecological surgery. It is also used in the prevention of coagulation during renal dialysis and cardiac surgery.

Warfarin (Coumadin)

Oral anticoagulant therapy using vitamin K antagonists (warfarin) is used in the treatment of venous thromboembolism, pulmonary embolism, and cardiac abnormalities that increase the risk of embolism in conditions such as valve disease. Patients on warfarin are usually required to stop therapy before surgery and then resume it on the first postoperative day.

Thrombolytic Agents

Thrombolytic drugs are used for the immediate breakdown of systemic blood clots, particularly in myocardial infarction, ischemic stroke, and pulmonary embolism. These drugs are usually administered in combination with heparin therapy. Common fibrinolytic drugs are:
- Recombinant tissue plasminogen activator, alteplase
- Urokinase

COAGULANTS

Topical coagulant is used on the surgical field to arrest bleeding when ligation, suturing, or electrosurgery is not possible. *Topical thrombin* in solution is used in combination with surface hemostatic materials such as gelatin sponge for application to capillary surfaces and vascular anastomosis sites to control bleeding. Thrombin is a high-alert drug.

NOTE: *Topical hemostatic agents such as gelatin foam and bone putty are classified as medical devices. Some formulations of gelatin sponge (such as Gelfoam Extra) do contain thrombin. The preparation and use of topical hemostatic agents is described fully in Chapter 22.*

CARDIAC DRUGS

Cardiac drugs are divided in categories according to their action (pharmacodynamics). Some are used for acute cardiac conditions, whereas others are part of a long-term treatment plan for patients with heart disease as indirectly affecting the cardiac system. Cardiac drugs used during surgery are given as needed to regulate heart muscle action, maintain arterial pressure, and prevent thromboembolus. Emergency cardiac drugs are also found on the emergency *crash cart*, which is a self-contained unit with drugs and equipment immediately available for physiological emergencies including cardiac or respiratory arrest. Common cardiac drug categories include:
- *Inotrope:* Increases (positive inotrope) or decrease (negative inotrope) heart contractility
- *Chronotropic:* Affects heart rate
- *Antiarrhythmic agents:* Used to treat abnormal cardiac rhythm
- *Antianginal drugs:* Used to treat *angina*, which is chest pain associated with decreased oxygen supply to the heart muscle. Blood flow to the heart is supplied by the coronary arteries. Antianginal agents increase oxygen supply by decreasing cardiac demand for oxygen or by vasodilation
- *Diuretic:* Increases urine output to balance sodium and intravascular volume
- *Antilipemic:* Cholesterol-lowering drug used in long-term treatment of hypercholesterolemia
- *Antihypertensive:* Lowers blood pressure

CENTRAL NERVOUS SYSTEM AGENTS

Knowledge of nerve transmission is basic to an understanding of how anesthetics and other CNS drugs work. The following basic description of how stimuli are transmitted provides useful background for the study of anesthetic drugs.

The transmission of nerve impulses (signals) is a complex biochemical process. In simple terms, impulses are chemical and electrical. Chemicals that carry impulses from nerve cell to nerve cell are called *neurotransmitters*. The biochemical work of the neurotransmitter is to transport the signal from one nerve cell to the next until the signal reaches the target tissue.

Each nerve cell (neuron) is separated from an adjacent nerve cell by a synapse (also called the *synaptic cleft*). The synapse is the small space in which the neurotransmitter passes from one nerve cell to another. For the neurotransmitter to transport a signal, it must be released from the presynaptic neuron (the neuron before the synapse) and received by the next neuron in line (the postsynaptic neuron). The neurotransmitter is contained in small vesicles (cell sacs). The receptor for a particular neurotransmitter is a specific molecule in the postsynaptic neuron (Figure 13-7).

NEUROTRANSMISSION

The body has many different types of neurotransmitters, each carrying a different type of impulse. About 30 known neurotransmitters occur in specific tissues of the body.

One type of neurotransmitter can be blocked without affecting the others. For example, the neurotransmitter for motor control can be inactivated by a neuromuscular blocking agent while the neurotransmitter for pain remains unaffected. This would result in the ability to feel pain but the inability to

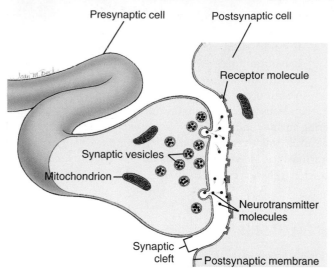

Figure 13-7 Neuron junction and neurotransmitter molecules. *(From Thibodeau GA, Patton KT: Anatomy and physiology, ed 6, St Louis 2007, Mosby.)*

move in response. Likewise, sedation or loss of consciousness can be achieved without reducing the sensation of pain.

One method of blocking neurotransmission is to administer a competitive antagonist drug that has an affinity for the postsynaptic receptor. These drugs limit the number of receptors available for the neurotransmitter molecule. When the drug attaches to the receptor site, the neurotransmitter cannot continue on its path, because no unbound receptors are available. The neurotransmitter remains in the space between the two neurons (the synapse) and eventually is reabsorbed by the presynaptic cell or broken down by enzymes. In this way, the path of transmission is broken. Antagonist CNS drugs increase the availability of postsynaptic receptors and the movement of neurotransmitters by increasing the release or uptake (or both) of a particular neurotransmitter.

ANESTHETICS

CNS anesthetics provide the physiological conditions necessary for surgery. This category of drugs causes the loss of primary CNS functions such as consciousness, sensation (including pain), some autonomic responses, and recall of events that occur while the drug is present in the body. The depth of the effect is dose dependent. However, selected adjunct agents are administered during general anesthesia to produce a more profound effect while protecting the patient from the risk of high-dose anesthetic.

Inhalation Anesthetics

Inhalation (volatile) anesthetics are formulated as liquids and administered as a vapor (gas). Only nitrous oxide is both formulated and delivered in gaseous form. All other agents must be vaporized in the anesthesia machine for administration by mask or through an artificial airway inserted into the patient's own upper airway. The agent enters the lungs, where it crosses the alveoli, enters the circulatory system, and is made available to the nervous system, producing deep sedation and unconsciousness.

Inhalation anesthetics are used to *maintain* a surgical level of anesthesia after a fast-acting intravenous anesthetic (discussed later) has been used to induce unconsciousness. Induction (the process of becoming unconscious) by gas anesthetic is slow and can result in delirium and other adverse reactions. However, this method is sometimes used in pediatric patients for whom an intravenous injection might be difficult.

In the past, anesthetic gases such as cyclopropane and vaporized ether were commonly used during surgery. These agents were highly flammable and explosive. Conductive shoes, nonstatic flooring, and high environmental humidity were necessary to prevent surgical fires, which were relatively common compared with today. These potent agents caused serious **side effects**, and the risk of anesthesia using them was significant. Flammable anesthetic agents are no longer permitted in surgery, and modern agents have created a much safer environment for both patients and personnel. However, extended exposure to small amounts of modern vaporized (gas) anesthetics is unsafe, so all anesthetic machines are manufactured with scavenging systems that collect and remove waste anesthetic gas from the operative environment.

NITROUS OXIDE Nitrous oxide is a colorless odorless gas in its natural state. It has low potency, but adjusting its concentration provides a range of anesthetic effects. It has strong analgesic properties and is quickly dissipated from the body, usually within minutes. Nitrous oxide is not flammable, but it supports combustion.

In some patients nitrous oxide can cause severe cardiovascular depression, leading to shock. It does not affect the respiratory system or the action of neuromuscular blocking agents. It can be used for induction, but is commonly mixed with other agents. The main advantages of nitrous oxide are minimal incidence of nausea and rapid absorption and clearance from the body. Disadvantages are low potency and lack of muscle relaxation.

ISOFLURANE Isoflurane is widely used for many different types of surgery. It causes rapid smooth induction and good muscle relaxation. It is nonflammable and has a strong odor. The systemic effects of isoflurane are superior to those of other inhalation agents. Cardiac and respiratory depression is minimal. Unlike many other agents, it does not cause bronchial spasm.

SEVOFLURANE Sevoflurane is very similar to isoflurane in action. It can be used safely for induction in both pediatric and adult patients. Patients emerge rapidly from sevoflurane, making it useful for outpatient surgery. It does cause increased postoperative nausea and vomiting compared with other agents.

DESFLURANE Desflurane provides rapid emergence, making it suitable for outpatient surgery when a short recovery time is important. It can be used as an induction agent in adults, but not in pediatric patients, because of the high incidence of bronchial spasm and laryngospasm associated with it. Desflurane must be heated during vaporization.

ENFLURANE Enflurane (Ethrane) is used for induction and maintenance. It can also be used in low doses for short surgical procedures that do not require unconsciousness. It produces rapid induction and emergence and also has excellent muscle-relaxing properties.

Dissociative Anesthesia

Ketamine is a rapidly acting sedative that produces isolation of the sensory parts of the brain, resulting in a trancelike state (dissociative anesthesia) and amnesia. Ketamine is valuable for sedation requiring profound short-term analgesia, such as during debridement of burns. However, it has distinctive adverse effects such as increased intracranial pressure, delirium, and hypertension. It is generally not used in adults because it may precipitate emergence delirium.

NEUROMUSCULAR BLOCKADE

Neuromuscular blocking agents are used to paralyze skeletal muscles, an essential component of general anesthesia. Even during profound general anesthesia, autonomic muscle responses can interfere with the manipulation of tissues such as during intubation and mechanical ventilation. Neuromuscular blocking is a complex, controlled process that is chemically reversed at the close of surgery or whenever necessary during an emergency. The drugs cause paralysis of the respiratory muscles, and mechanical ventilation is required during their use. The effect of neuromuscular blocking drugs is adjusted during surgery according to the level of relaxation needed.

Normal Nerve Transmission

Nerve transmission to striated muscles occurs at the neuromuscular junction where the motor neuron (nerve cell to the skeletal muscle) and muscle cell communicate. The nerve cell and muscle (motor end plate) do not touch. They are separated by a small gap called the synaptic cleft, as described earlier. Activation of the muscle cell occurs when the neurotransmitter *acetylcholine* (ACh) is released by the nerve cell where it crosses the cleft and binds to the ACh receptors at the motor end plate. This causes *depolarization* (electrochemical change necessary for cell activation) of the muscle cells and muscle contraction.

Neuromuscular Blocking Agents

Neuromuscular blocking drugs are used to interfere with normal muscle cell depolarization, which results in muscle relaxation. Two types of drugs are used to prevent muscle contractions. Both types attach to the acetylcholine binding sites and prevent ACh from attaching. An agonist (depolarizing) drug has some of the properties of ACh but does not permit the electrochemical changes (particularly the resting phase of the muscle fiber) necessary for muscle activation. A nondepolarizing agent (antagonist) also binds to the motor end plate but works by simply blocking ACh. Only one depolarizing agent is available—succinylcholine, which is used primarily for intubation because it is short-acting.

Examples of nondepolarizing blocking agents:
- Atracurium
- Cisatracurium
- Pancuronium
- Rocuronium
- Vecuronium

Neuromuscular blocking agents are reversed by administering an anticholinesterase. *Neostigmine* is the primary reversal drug and has replaced *edrophonium* which was used previously as a reversal agent in surgery. *Sugammadex* is used to selectively reverse rocuronium.

ANALGESICS

This group of drugs is used to control pain. Pain is a complex sensation that can be controlled through a number of different neurological pathways. It is important to note that in terms of nerve transmission and the use of analgesic drugs, there are significant differences among analgesia (lack of pain), sedation (sleep), and relaxation. For example, it is possible to produce a level of sedation (sleepiness or somnolence) while retaining the sensation of pain.

Opiates

Opiates are among the most common drugs used for moderate and severe pain control. All opiates (also known as *narcotics*) produce analgesia by altering the perception of pain. Because they reduce the work of the heart, morphine is often given in specific cardiac emergencies.

Opiates are derived directly from the natural psychoactive substance in the opium plant, whereas opioids are synthetic and semisynthetic drugs that resemble opiates in pharmacological action. The most common opiate used in health care is morphine. Other opiate drugs are often described by their relative strength as an analgesic when compared to natural morphine sulfate.

Examples of natural opiates are:
- Morphine
- Codeine

The semisynthetic opiates include:
- Hydromorphone
- Hydrocodone
- Oxycodone
- Oxymorphone
- Sunfentanil
- Alfentanil
- Remifentanil
- Pethidine (meperidine)
- Tramadol

Completely synthetic opiates include fentanyl, pethidine (also known as meperidine), and tramadol. All opiates are addictive and, in high doses cause depression of the CNS, hypotension, respiratory depression, profound sedation, and coma.

The *opiate antagonists* are used to treat opiate toxicity and overdose. These include naloxone, nalmefene, and naltrexone.

Nonopiate Analgesics

Nonopiate drugs are used for mild and moderate pain. These may be prescribed for mild postoperative pain following superficial procedures under local anesthesia. Ibuprofen and diclofenac are nonopiate antiinflammatory agents. Acetaminophen is used for mild pain and as an antipyretic.

SEDATIVES AND HYPNOTICS

Sedative or hypnotic drugs are used in a variety of medical and surgical situations to depress consciousness and induce drowsiness. Most do not have analgesic effects. Categories of sedative drugs include the sedative-hypnotics, barbiturates, and benzodiazepines. Sedatives are used to relax patients in the acute care setting and in behavioral emergencies. Oral sedative-hypnotic drugs are prescribed for short-term insomnia and to reduce anxiety in the preoperative period. They are also used during induction of general anesthesia to allow intubation (placement of an artificial airway) at the start of general anesthesia or in emergency situations requiring intubation.

Intravenous sedatives are used with or without analgesics for procedural sedation or *moderate sedation* (previously called conscious sedation) for short procedures when profound anesthesia is not required. Under mild and moderate sedation, a person can respond to verbal commands, and respiratory and cardiovascular functions remain intact. However, a deeply sedated patient cannot be easily roused, and ventilation may be decreased. Modern sedatives are rapidly cleared from the body, making them ideal for procedural sedation and anesthesia. Propofol is the most common intravenous sedative used for induction and maintenance of general anesthesia and also as a general sedative.

Examples:
- Propofol
- Etomidate
- Dexmedetomidine

BARBITURATES

This group of drugs was among the first to be used in clinical situations requiring profound depression of the CNS. Oral barbiturates are still used in the treatment of seizure disorders. Intravenous barbiturates are commonly used for induction of general anesthesia. They are rapidly effective, causing unconsciousness in 10 to 20 seconds. Recovery from thiopental, which is the most commonly used agent, is 20 to 30 minutes. Barbiturates cause dose-related respiratory depression and apnea (absence of breathing), which is transient during initial administration. Laryngospasm and bronchospasm can occur with thiopental.

Examples of intravenous barbiturates:
- Thiopental
- Methohexital

BENZODIAZEPINES

Benzodiazepines have many clinical uses because of their versatility. This category of drugs is anxiolytic (reduce anxiety) and also provides muscle relaxation. They cause desirable *anterograde amnesia* (loss of recall of events) for up to 6 hours from the onset of drug action and are commonly given intravenously during procedures requring sedation .

Examples of benzodiazepines:
- Midazolam
- Lorazepam
- Alprazolam
- Diazepam

The benzodiazepine antagonist *flumazenil* is used to reverse the effects of this category of drugs.

LOCAL ANESTHETICS

Local anesthetics are used in regional anesthesia to block sensation with or without sedative drugs that provide anxiolysis and relaxation. The process and specific role of the surgical technologist in assisting during regional anesthesia of local anesthetic agents are described fully in Chapter 14. These drugs are formulated for a variety of applications, including:

- *Infiltration injection:* The drug is injected directly into the operative site in small increments.
- *Regional nerve block:* A major nerve is anesthetized to affect a larger region.
- *Topical:* Anesthetic is applied to the skin or mucous membrane for short-term superficial procedures.
- *Spinal or epidural:* Anesthetic is injected into the spinal canal or epidural space for regional blockade of the lower body.

Handling local anesthetics on the surgical field requires extra attention because of their high-alert status. Many agents are formulated with the addition of epinephrine. As an adrenergic agonist, epinephrine causes vasoconstriction and increased heart rate. It is used in conjunction with local anesthetic to prevent the anesthetic from entering the vascular system, which would shorten the **peak effect** of the drug. *Epinephrine injection directly into blood vessels can be fatal, and both epinephrine and local anesthetic have definite dose limits.* Therefore, extra attention must be given to labeling and keeping track of the amount injected throughout the procedure.

When the scrubbed surgical technologist dispenses local anesthetic to the surgeon, he or she should share responsibility for ensuring that maximum dosage is not exceeded. The maximum dosage is therefore confirmed with the anesthesia care provider before the case, and incremental amounts injected are documented in real time by the circulator.

Local anesthetic agents are formulated as short- or long-acting, with or without added epinephrine or other vasoconstrictor. The safe maximum dosage for agents depends on the patient's specific condition and its exact use. Agents with added vasoconstrictors are not used for infiltration at end-arterial sites such as the digits, because this can result in ischemia and necrosis of the area. Common local anesthetic agents are listed in Appendix B.

Topical anesthetics are used on surface tissues such as mucous membranes, the surface of the eye, and the urogenital tract. These agents do require an order by a licensed primary care provider. This includes instillation of lidocaine gel to the urethra before catheterization. Topical cocaine is frequently used in nasal surgery to block pain receptors in the mucous membrane before injection with regional anesthetic. Cocaine is never injected—to do so can be fatal. It is a controlled substance, and protocols for handling it are guided by hospital policy and state law.

DIAGNOSTICS

CONTRAST MEDIA

Contrast media are diagnostic agents injected into tissue or hollow spaces of the body in conjunction with imaging studies. These substances enable clinicians to observe and document the interior margins or path of a hollow organ, vessels, or ducts. In many cases, a radiology technologist is responsible for handling and administering these substances in a diagnostic clinic or unit of the health facility. The surgical technologist may be asked to assist in these procedures. Contrast media are also used occasionally in surgical procedures to verify patency of a duct, organ, or vessel.

An *iodinated contrast medium* (ICM) is a clear, injectable liquid that is *radiopaque* (opaque on radiographs). An ICM is commonly used in radiography, computed tomography, and fluoroscopy. Agents differ in *osmolality* (the amount of solute, in this case iodine, by weight in solution). Contrast media with high levels of iodine are associated with increased adverse effects, whereas those with lower levels of iodine are safer. Allergic reaction can occur, and patients must be monitored during use. *(Note: There is no scientific basis for association of shellfish allergy with an adverse reaction to ICM.)* The modern ICMs are generally very safe as compared to prototypes used in the past. The patient may experience allergy or sensitivity to contrast media, but this is not related to shellfish.

As with all drugs used in surgery and interventional radiology, the surgical technologist must keep track of the total amount and concentration (dose) of contrast medium used. There are literally hundreds of types of contrast media available for use in medicine. The main categories for safety purposes are whether the substance is *high molecular weight* or *low molecular weight*. The lower molecular weight substances are much safer. Examples of iodinated contrast media are diatrizoate and metrizoate.

Gadolinium-based contrast media are used for magnetic resonance imaging and magnetic resonance angiography. These agents work by intensifying the magnetic field of protons, which in turn creates more contrast.

Perfluorocarbon microsphere contrast media are used in echocardiography and ultrasound. These consist of compressible shells filled with gas that resonate at the frequency of the ultrasound waves.

Barium sulfate is an opaque contrast medium used in radiological studies of the gastrointestinal (GI) tract (barium enema or barium swallow). These studies are performed in the GI clinic or interventional radiology department and are not part of a sterile procedure. However, the surgical technologist may occasionally work in these areas of the health care facility and should be familiar with the use of barium. Barium is supplied as a liquid for oral administration or rectal infusion. Following ingestion or infusion, barium radiographs reveal well-defined areas where the substance has filled the GI tract, including small surface irregularities, outpockets of tissue, strictures, and other anomalies. Barium is not absorbed through the tissues but is excreted through the normal GI tract in its intact form.

TISSUE DYES AND STAINS

Colored tissue dyes and tissue stains are used to differentiate microbes and tissue specimens for observation under the microscope. They are also used in medicine and surgery to distinguish borders and to determine patency (an open passageway) through tissue.

A dye is a colored substance that can be infused into a duct or natural passage such as the fallopian tube or into a tract such as that created by infection (called a *sinus tract*); the path is followed by simply observing the colored liquid as it passes through the tissue or opening. Another common use of tissue dye is in the manufacturing of skin marking pens used to delineate or identify the location of a skin incision and in plastic and reconstructive surgery to create landmarks that might be obscured once the incisions have been made.

Colored dyes are usually dispensed to the sterile field in glass vials. The most common types are:

- Gentian violet
- Methylene blue
- Indigo carmine

A *stain* is used as a diagnostic tool to differentiate normal cells from abnormal ones. Clinical laboratories use a variety of staining agents. In the surgical setting, several types of stains are used to enable surgeons to see areas of diseased tissue appropriate for destruction or excision. Stains typically are applied under direct visualization with a sterile sponge or cotton-tipped applicator. The stain generally is absorbed by the abnormal cells, giving these cells a different appearance from the healthy surrounding cells.

- Lugol solution is used to perform the Schiller test to identify cervical dysplasia.
- Monsel solution is used to identify abnormal tissue cells in gynecological and urogenital procedures.
- Acetic acid is used to enhance the detection of cervical neoplasia during colposcopy.

FLUID BALANCE AND ELECTROLYTES

INTRAVENOUS SOLUTIONS

Approximately two thirds of the body mass is made up of water. Water is gained normally through ingestion (eating and drinking) and lost through normal physiological processes, trauma, or disease (vomiting, diarrhea, burns, and hemorrhage). Surgery and anesthesia also result in shifts in fluid balance. Although surgery does not directly alter fluid balance, the anesthesia process can suppress some autonomic responses that do. Total body water is contained in three spaces: the intracellular spaces (inside the cells), interstitial space (between the cells), and intravascular space (within the blood vessels). Fluid shifts from one compartment (space) to another as the body maintains homeostasis. This is controlled by oncotic pressure (movement controlled by the presence of large molecules such as plasma proteins) and by the process of osmosis. The total volume of body fluid must remain stable in order to sustain life.

In surgery, fluid loss is monitored by measuring urine and blood loss. If fluids are needed, the choice is very specific according to the patient's physiological state at the time. Errors in fluid administration can result in fluid overload and heart failure. Administering the wrong dilution (osmolarity) of an electrolyte solution can cause serious injury or death related to the chemical reactions caused (or prevented) by the presence of the electrolytes.

Intravenous fluids are administered routinely in surgery and medicine. There are two general categories of intravenous fluids—crystalloids and colloids.

Crystalloids are solutions that contain a small amount of electrolyte solutes (dissolved substances). These solutions are mainly administered to correct physiological imbalance related to electrolytes and blood pH and to restore fluids lost through disease (dehydration).

Crystalloids are classified as:

- *Isotonic:* Solute concentration equal to the physiological environment
- *Hypertonic:* Solute concentration higher than that of the physiological environment
- *Hypotonic:* Solute concentration lower than that of the physiological environment

Commonly used crystalloids are 0.9% saline solution (also called normal saline) and dextrose solution. Another crystalloid used frequently is lactated Ringer's, the chemical composition of which is close to that of human plasma. Other crystalloids contain specific electrolytes such as potassium and calcium, which are prescribed according to the patient's electrolyte needs.

Alterations in blood pH can occur with trauma, shock, and disease. *Acidosis* is lower than normal blood pH. Respiratory acidosis occurs with hypercapnia (buildup of carbon dioxide), which can be caused by head injury, some anesthetics, and pulmonary diseases. Metabolic acidosis can be the result of kidney disease or low production of bicarbonate. *Alkalosis* is higher than normal blood pH. This can occur as respiratory alkalosis from elevated carbon dioxide concentration or as metabolic alkalosis caused by decreased hydrogen ion concentration. Crystalloids may be used in severe cases of pH imbalance.

Colloids are crystalloid-based water and electrolytes. However, they also have additional components that cause the fluid to move into and out of body spaces in a specific way. A colloid is a particle or substance that is dispersed throughout the fluid but not dissolved in it. In medicine, colloids are administered to prevent fluids from escaping the closed vascular system across the cell membrane. Patients who require intravascular fluid replacement may be administered a colloid; however, their use is somewhat controversial. This solution increases the intravascular (oncotic) pressure, but the colloid particles do not allow the fluid to escape into the other body compartments.

Common colloids are blood, plasma, and synthetic substances that have large *macromolecules* to prevent the escape of the fluid outside the vascular system. A colloid may be given, for example, as a lifesaving measure when blood is not immediately available. In this case normal saline cannot be used because it would quickly become dispersed among the other body compartments and would not exert oncotic pressure in the vascular system. During massive blood or plasma loss (as occurs during trauma or in burn patients), the oncotic pressure of the vascular system must be raised to enable the heart to move the blood through the body effectively. Colloids are vascular volume expanders. *Dextran* solutions have properties similar to those of human albumin. *Hetastarch* is a hypertonic synthetic starch. These colloidal fluids increase osmotic pressure, which controls the movement of water into and out of the intravascular space.

IRRIGATION FLUIDS

Irrigation fluids (described earlier) must be compatible with the physiological environment in which they are used. All irrigation solutions are saline-based, and they are labeled as *topical* or *intravenous*. *A topical solution must not be used in or around open blood vessels.* Only intravenous solutions are used to irrigate blood vessels or near open blood vessels. Differences in osmolarity among irrigation solutions can result in abnormal movement of fluid across the cell membrane. Ophthalmic and otology solutions are also specifically labeled in order to be compatible with these delicate tissues.

DIURETICS

Diuretics stimulate the production of urine by the kidneys. This creates a shift of body fluids. They are most commonly used in the treatment of hypertension and pulmonary edema. However, they are also used for emergency treatment of intraocular pressure and increased intracranial pressure (ICP). Diuretics reduce the total vascular volume by depressing reabsorption of sodium in the kidneys and increasing water excretion from the nephron. This results in increased *diuresis* (increased urinary excretion).

Specific classes of diuretics function differently. Many cause excess excretion of potassium, an electrolyte necessary for cardiac and cell function. Potassium-sparing diuretics are preferred for this reason. Loop diuretics are extremely potent and cause rapid diuresis and loss of electrolytes. The osmotic diuretics also are very potent and are used to reduce intraocular pressure and cerebral edema. This class of diuretics is given during neurosurgical procedures. Carbonic anhydrase inhibitors are used specifically for reducing intraocular pressure in patients with open angle glaucoma. They inhibit the enzyme carbonic anhydrase, which partly controls the acid-base balance in the blood. Thiazide diuretics are weaker and do not cause immediate diuresis. They are used in the treatment of hypertension because they cause arteriolar dilation and reduce cardiac output.

Examples of diuretics are:

- Hydrochlorothiazide
- Bumetanide
- Furosemide
- Mannitol
- Acetazolamide

GASTROINTESTINAL DRUGS

The stomach contains a number of different glands that secrete substances to maintain the integrity of the stomach lining and contribute to the digestion process. Mucoid cells produce protective mucus; the parietal cells secrete hydrochloric acid (HCl); and the chief cells produce pepsinogen, which is converted to pepsin on exposure to HCl for the breakdown of proteins. Activation of the glands is a complex process mediated by the autonomic nervous system.

Neutralization of stomach acid is an important goal before and during surgery in order to prevent lung damage in the event of regurgitation and aspiration during general anesthesia. Normally the pyloric sphincter and cardiac sphincters prevent regurgitation. However, the action is suppressed with unconsciousness. Regurgitation and aspiration are a particular concern in high risk cases such as emergency trauma, pregnancy, morbidly obese patients, and those with gastroesophageal reflux disease (GERD). To prevent potentially fatal aspiration, gastric drugs are administered selectively in the preoperative and intraoperative period. These drugs reduce the volume and acidity of gastric fluid.

HISTAMINE-2 RECEPTOR ANTAGONISTS AND PROTON PUMP INHIBITORS

Histamine-2 receptor (H_2 receptor) antagonists reduce gastric acidity by blocking the release of gastric acid in the parietal cells. The drugs do not change the acidity of contents already in the stomach. Examples of H_2 receptor antagonists are:

- Cimetidine
- Famotidine
- Ranitidine

Gastric proton pump inhibitors suppress action of the parietal cells that release hydrogen ions for the production of HCl. Examples are:

- Lansoprazole
- Omeprazole
- Rabeprazole
- Pantoprazole
- Esomeprazole

ANTACIDS

Antacids reduce gastric fluid acidity and volume. These are given on the day of surgery as preoperative medication. Calcium, aluminum, and magnesium salts that are available as OTC antacids are *not* used because they may cause an

increase in acid secretion and are also contraindicated in renal disease. Instead, prostaglandin drugs such as *misoprostol* are used to suppress acid secretion of the parietal cells. This drug may only be used in nonpregnant patients, because it is an abortive agent. *Sucralfate* is administered to increase the production of mucosal prostaglandin and form a barrier over the stomach lining. It does not influence the production of gastric fluid.

ANTIEMETIC AGENTS

Postoperative nausea and vomiting (PONV) is a significant problem in the immediate postoperative period. Antiemetic agents are used to prevent or reduce vomiting. These drugs are administered in the PACU. Medications used to control PONV include:

- Dolasetron
- Droperidol
- Granisetron
- Metoclopramide
- Ondansetron

HORMONES AND SYNTHETIC SUBSTITUTES

Hormones are naturally occurring substances produced by the endocrine system. Their function in the body is to regulate specific cellular and systemic functions. Natural and synthetic hormones are used in the treatment of specific deficiency diseases, to enhance certain processes such as the antiinflammatory response, to counteract neoplasms sensitive to hormonal control, and also in reproductive health. There are many hundreds of hormones used in long- and short-term therapy. Recognizing drug groups is important to an overall understanding of pharmacology.

Hormone substances are classified by their origin and action. The major groups are shown in Box 13-8.

CORTICOSTEROIDS

This group of drugs is used to reduce the body's immune response, especially in the treatment of autoimmune disease manifestations, asthma, and adrenal insufficiency. However,

Box **13-8** Classification of Hormones and Synthetic Substitutes
Adrenal corticosteroids
Contraceptives
Estrogens
Estrogen agonists-antagonists
Gonadotropins
Antidiabetic drugs (insulins, oral hypoglycemics)
Parathyroid substances
Pituitary agents
Progestins
Thyroid agents
Antithyroid agents

they are associated with many serious side effects such as adrenal cortex suppression, decreased immune response to infection, and muscle atrophy when used long term.

Examples of corticosteroids are:

- Dexamethasone
- Prednisone
- Betamethasone
- Methylprednisolone
- Triamcinolone

ANTIDIABETIC DRUGS

Diabetes mellitus is a metabolic disease in which beta cells that produce natural insulin are destroyed by an autoimmune disorder (type 1) or natural insulin is not regulated in the body and cells are resistant to insulin (type 2).

Diabetes treatment includes administration of insulin (for type 1 and often type 2) and drugs that increase cellular uptake of insulin as needed, usually in type 2. Exogenous insulin for injection is available in different strengths and differing duration of action.

There are eight types of oral hypoglycemic drugs used in the treatment of type 2 diabetes:

- Sulfonylureas—includes *glipizide* and others
- Alpha-glucosidase inhibitors—*acarbose* and *miglitol*
- Biguanides—includes *metformin* and others
- Glitazones—includes *pioglitazone* and *rosiglitazone*
- Meglitinides—nonsulfonylureas *repaglinide* and *nateglinide*
- Dipeptidyl-peptidase 4 inhibitors—includes *sitagliptin* and others
- Bile acid resin—includes *colesevelam*
- Dopamine agonist—includes *bromocriptine*

PROSTAGLANDINS

Prostaglandins are not endocrine hormones. That is, they do not originate in endocrine glands. Instead, they are chemicals synthesized within the cell, and their effect is within the same cell.

There are many types of prostaglandins that mediate various effects in the body, such as:

- Vasodilation
- Platelet and leukocyte aggregation
- Smooth muscle contraction
- Vascular permeability
- Softening and effacement of the cervix during labor

DRUGS USED IN OBSTETRICS

Drugs used in obstetrics are administered to induce or maintain the tone of the uterus.

- *Dinoprostone* pessary tablets are used to induce labor.
- *Oxytocin* is used for augmentation of labor.
- *Syntometrine* is a combination of oxytocin and ergometrine maleate used in third-stage labor and for incomplete abortion to induce uterine contractions.

- *Ergometrine* is used for treatment of postpartum hemorrhage.

GONADAL STEROIDS

The gonadal steroids include estrogen in the female and testosterone in the male. In the female, estrogen, progesterone, and synthetic substitutes are used in contraception. Testosterone is used in deficiencies in the male.

EMERGENCY DRUGS

A special group of drugs used in response to physiological emergencies include mainly those that affect the autonomic nervous system and others used in cardiac and respiratory arrest. These drugs, along with intubation and airway equipment, electrocardiograph, defibrillator, and other devices, are maintained on a department crash cart that is checked on each shift for completeness and maintained in all departments of the health care facility. A list of drugs found on the emergency crash cart is located in Appendix C.

DRUG CALCULATIONS

The surgical technologist is required to perform drug calculations when mixing drugs on the sterile field and for other circumstances when one unit of measurement must be converted to another.

 A review of arithmetic, including sample problems, is available on the Evolve website. http://evolve.elsevier.com/fuller/surgical

KEY CONCEPTS

- The manufacturing of drugs is a complicated process which is highly regulated and monitored. Drugs are derived from many different sources using increasingly complex technologies. The source or origin of a drug can relate to adverse reactions such as patient allergy and sensitivity.
- Drug regulations protect the public from harm by establishing quality standards in manufacturing, packaging, storage, transport, dispensing, prescribing, and administration. Every health care worker involved in these practices must be familiar with the rules and regulations associated with their specific role in the drug process.
- The identification (naming) of drugs follows rigorous international standards that contribute to public safety and establish a common language among health professionals worldwide.
- The drug process involves many people in multiple health care settings. Surgical technologists have a significant role in preventing errors in surgery. Knowing and practicing the protocols is part of a collaborative process with other members of the surgical team.
- Identification and interpretation of drug labels is one part of the drug process. Surgical technologists must be familiar with the drug label, its package insert, use, and precautions associated with any drugs they handle.

- Prescription drug errors are responsible for over 7,000 deaths per year in the United States. Methods to prevent drug errors have been established at every stage of the drug process.
- Drug errors most commonly relate to miscommunication and lack of knowledge on the part of health care workers who handle drugs. Errors are preventable by a conscious effort to learn and act on strategies that have been specifically developed to prevent death and disability from drug errors.
- Inaccuracy in basic drug computation is a significant cause of drug errors. Health care workers must be able to perform conversions among units of measure used in medicine, and demonstrate accuracy in drug computation.
- Drug prescriptions or orders are provided by health care providers licensed to do so. In order to deliver the correct drug, in the correct strength and dosage, and in the correct form to the right patient, the surgical technologist must be familiar with the process and terminology of drug orders.
- A specific protocol (method) is used to receive and deliver drugs to the sterile field. This protocol has been created to reduce the risk of drug errors and is followed strictly for every drug in every situation.
- Drug delivery devices such as syringes are calibrated in small increments to provide a high level of accuracy. Devices not specifically calibrated for exact dosages must not be used in the drug process.
- The role of the surgical technologist in the medication process must be precisely identified by the health care facility and be in accordance with state law, especially state practice acts. Surgical technologists in every state deliver medications to the surgeon after receiving them from the licensed circulating nurse.
- As a participant in the drug process, surgical technologists are mandated to demonstrate competence and knowledge in the specific tasks and roles they perform.
- The route of administration for any drug is critical knowledge for all health care workers involved in the drug process. An error in the route of administration can have fatal consequences.
- An understanding of pharmacokinetics and pharmcodynamics demonstrates advanced knowledge about how drugs work and their specific effects on the body. Even if this knowledge is not directly applied to a particular phase of the drug process, an understanding of the principles demonstrates the advanced professional capacity required to participate in the entire process.

REVIEW QUESTIONS

1. What particular drug policies are regulated by the Joint Commission?
2. What is a generic drug?
3. If the surgical technologist suspects that a patient is having an adverse reaction to a drug, what information is most important to give the surgeon or nursing personnel in the room?
4. What is an allergy?
5. Outline the headings of the medication process and describe them briefly.
6. How does the surgical technologist ensure that a drug is given by the right route?
7. What units are marked on an insulin syringe?
8. What is the rationale for pouring all of a liquid from its sterile container when it is distributed to the scrub?
9. What is the difference between a contrast medium and a dye?
10. As the scrub, how might you collaborate with the circulator to keep track of the amount of irrigation solution used during a surgical procedure?

CASE STUDIES

Case 1

Discuss how the concepts of team cooperation, shared communication, and adhering to required protocols for drug handling in the operating room could have changed the outcome of the following *real case scenarios*:

- A pediatric patient undergoing surgery was injected with pure epinephrine during the procedure because neither the medicine cup nor the syringe was labeled. The child died.
- A pediatric patient underwent surgery under local anesthetic with epinephrine added. The correct dose was calculated and administered in the operating room. At the close of surgery, the child was admitted to the postanesthesia care unit for observation. However, during her stay in the PACU, she required additional administration of epinephrine. The patient died in PACU as a result of epinephrine overdose. The surgical team had failed to properly document the administration of anesthetic with epinephrine during surgery.

Case 2

One of the most common sources of drug error is failure to properly label syringes and other drug delivery devices. The Joint Commission's "do not use" list of documentation errors was created to ensure that transcription of drug names and amounts are accurate. Analyze the case of a surgical technologist who labeled his medicine containers "heparin 100 u" and another "heparin 10 u." The actual label should have been 100 units per mL and 10 units per mL.

- What possible consequences might there be?
- Why does the Joint Commission require "units" to be spelled out rather than just using "u?"

REFERENCE

1. U.S. Food and Drug Administration: Sec. 201.[21 U.S.C. 321] Chapter II – Definitions 1. Available at http://www.fda.gov/RegulatoryInformation/Legislation/ FederalFoodDrugandCosmeticActFDCAct/ FDCActChaptersIandIIShortTitleandDefinitions/ucm086297.htm. Accessed April 7, 2012.

BIBLIOGRAPHY

American College of Radiology: *Manual on contrast media, version 6.* Accessed June 1, 2008, at http://www.acr.org.

Association of periOperative Registered Nurses (AORN): Guidance statements: safe medication practices in perioperative practice settings. In *Standards, recommended practices and guidelines*, Denver, 2011, AORN.

Hendrickson T: Verbal medication orders in the OR, *Journal of AORN* 86·4, 2007.

Kee J, Hayes E, McCuistion L: *Pharmacology: a nursing process approach*, ed 5, St Louis, 2006, Mosby.

Porth C: *Pathophysiology: concepts of altered health states*, ed 6, Philadelphia, 2007, Lippincott Williams & Wilkins.

Wanzer L: Perioperative initiatives for medication safety, *Journal of AORN* 82:4, 2005.

14 Anesthesia and Physiological Monitoring

CHAPTER OUTLINE

Introduction

Important Anesthesia Concepts

Anesthesia Personnel

Preoperative Evaluation of the Patient

Anesthesia Selection

Immediate Preoperative Preparation of the Patient

Physiological Monitoring During Surgery

Methods of Anesthesia

Airway Management

Phases of General Anesthesia

Dissociative Anesthesia

Conscious Sedation

Regional Anesthesia

Emergencies

Historical Highlights

LEARNING OBJECTIVES

After studying this chapter the reader will be able to:

1. Explain terms used to describe important anesthesia concepts
2. Identify anesthesia personnel
3. Describe the components of an anesthesia evaluation
4. Discuss the anesthesia selection process
5. Explain the preparation of the patient for anesthesia
6. Describe the components of physiological monitoring
7. Describe basic anesthesia equipment and its use
8. Describe the concepts of airway management

9. Define general anesthesia and describe induction, maintenance, and emergence
10. Discuss the difference between dissociative anesthesia and conscious sedation
11. Explain how regional anesthesia is used
12. Define common types of regional anesthesia
13. Define the role of the surgical technologist during the use of regional anesthesia
14. List common anesthesia emergencies

TERMINOLOGY

Airway: The anatomical passageway or artificial tube through which the patient breathes.

Amnesia: The loss of recall of events or sensations.

Analgesia: The absence of pain, produced by specific drugs.

Anesthesia: The absence of sensory awareness or medically induced unconsciousness.

Anesthesia care provider (ACP): A professional who is licensed to administer anesthetic agents and manage the patient throughout the period of anesthesia.

Anesthesia machine: A biotechnical device used to deliver anesthetic gases or volatile liquids and provide physiological monitoring.

Anesthesia technologist: An allied health professional trained to assist the anesthesia care provider.

Anesthesiologist: A physician specialist in the administration of anesthetics and pain management.

Anesthetic: A drug that reduces or blocks sensation or induces unconsciousness.

Anterograde amnesia: In anesthesia, the patient's inability to recall events that occur after the administration of specific drugs. After the drug is metabolized and cleared from the body, normal recall returns.

Anxiolytic: A drug that reduces anxiety.

Apnea: Absence of breathing.

Bier block: Regional anesthesia in which the anesthetic agent is injected into a vein.

Bispectral index system (BIS): A monitoring method used to determine the patient's level of consciousness and prevent intraoperative awareness.

Breathing bag: The reservoir breathing apparatus of the anesthesia machine. Gases are titrated and shunted into the breathing bag, which is connected to the patient's airway.

Central nervous system depression: This refers to a decrease in sensory awareness caused by drugs or a pathologic condition.

Coma: The deepest state of unconsciousness, in which most brain activity ceases.

Consciousness: Neurological state in which a patient is able to sense environmental stimuli such as sight, sound, touch, pressure, pain, heat, and cold.

Delirium: A state of confusion and disorientation. In the past delirium was defined as a distinct stage of induction and emergence from general anesthesia. However, this stage is rarely demonstrated in association with modern anesthetics.

Emergence: The stage in general anesthesia in which the anesthetic agent is withdrawn and the patient regains consciousness.

Endotracheal tube: An artificial airway (tube) that is inserted into the patient's trachea to maintain patency.

TERMINOLOGY (cont.)

Esmarch bandage: A rolled bandage made of rubber or latex that is used to exsanguinate blood from a limb.

Extubation: Withdrawal of an artificial airway.

Gas scavenging: The capture and safe removal of extraneous anesthetic gases from the anesthesia machine.

General anesthesia: Anesthesia associated with a state of unconsciousness. General anesthesia is not a fixed state of unconsciousness, but rather ranges along a continuum from semiresponsiveness to profound unresponsiveness.

Homeostasis: A state of balance in physiological functions.

Hypothermia: A subnormal body temperature.

Induction: Initiation of general anesthesia with a drug that causes unconsciousness.

Intraoperative awareness (IOA): A rare condition in which a patient undergoing general anesthesia is able to feel pain and other noxious stimuli but unable to respond.

Intravascular volume: Fluid volume within the blood vessels.

Intubation: The process of inserting an invasive artificial airway.

Laryngeal mask airway (LMA): An airway consisting of a tube and small mask that is fitted internally over the patient's larynx.

Laryngoscope: A lighted instrument used to assist endotracheal intubation.

Malignant hyperthermia: A rare state of hypermetabolism that occurs in association with inhalation anesthetics and neuromuscular blocking agents. In extreme cases, the condition causes hyperpyrexia, seizures, and cardiac arrhythmia.

Monitored anesthesia care (MAC): Monitoring of vital functions during regional anesthesia to ensure the patient's safety and comfort.

Nasopharyngeal airway: Artificial airway between the nostril and the nasopharynx; used in semiconscious patients or when an oral airway is contraindicated.

Neuromuscular blocking agent: A drug that blocks nerve conduction in striated muscle tissue.

Oropharyngeal airway (OPA): Artificial airway that is inserted over the tongue into the larynx; used in patients in whom endotracheal intubation is difficult or contraindicated.

Perfusion: Circulation of blood to specific tissue, organ, system, or the whole body. Perfusion is necessary to maintain life in the cells.

Physiological monitoring: Assessment of the patient's vital metabolic functions.

Pneumatic tourniquet: An air-filled tourniquet used to prevent blood flow to an extremity during surgery.

Postanesthesia recovery unit (PACU): The critical care area in which patients recover from the sedation of general anesthesia.

Preoperative medication: One or more drugs administered before surgery to prevent complications related to the surgical procedure or anesthesia.

Protective reflexes: Nervous system responses to harmful environmental stimuli, such as pain, obstruction of the airway, and extreme temperature. Coughing, blinking, shivering, and withdrawal (from pain) are protective reflexes.

Pulmonary embolism (PE): An obstruction in a pulmonary vessel caused by a blood clot, air bubble, or foreign body. Causes sudden pain and possible pulmonary arrest.

Pulse oximeter: A monitoring device that measures the patient's hemoglobin oxygen saturation by means of spectrometry.

Regional block: Anesthesia in a specific area of the body, achieved by injection of an anesthetic around a major nerve or group of nerves.

Sedation: An arousable state in which an individual is unaware of sensory stimuli. Depression of the central nervous system.

Sedative: A drug that induces a range of unconscious states. The effects are dose dependent. At low doses, sedatives cause some drowsiness. Increasing the dose causes central nervous system depression, ending in loss of consciousness.

Sensation: The ability to feel stimuli in the environment (e.g., pain, heat, touch, visual stimuli, sound).

Topical anesthesia: Anesthesia of superficial nerves of the skin or mucous membranes.

Unconsciousness: Neurological state in which the person is unable to respond to external stimuli. Unconsciousness can be induced with drugs or may be caused by trauma or disease.

Ventilation: The physical act of taking air into the lungs by inflation and releasing carbon dioxide from the lungs by deflation.

Vital signs: Minimum assessment of heart rate, temperature, and respiratory rate. In actual practice, a qualitative assessment of these indicators is necessary to provide a more meaningful picture of the patient's cardiac, ventilatory, and perfusion status.

INTRODUCTION

Anesthesia means "without sensation." The goal of *surgical anesthesia* is to allow the patient to tolerate surgery and maintain the body in a balanced physiological state, called **homeostasis**. These processes cannot be isolated from the principles of surgical technique because one cannot exist without the other. Anesthesia personnel are responsible for physiological management of the patient before, during, and after surgery. They provide the techniques and means to achieve anesthesia and work closely with the other members of the surgical team to maintain safety in techniques such as positioning and handling the patient. The anesthesia care provider (ACP) uses highly technical physiological monitoring devices to provide continuous feedback on vital physiological mechanisms that are affected by drugs used in the anesthesia process, the surgery, and the patient's condition coming into surgery. Continuous monitoring provides information on physiological changes that require immediate attention, including emergency situations.

This chapter is an introduction to the process of anesthesia and physiological monitoring. The primary purpose is to familiarize the surgical technologist with basic concepts and terms associated with anesthesia and basic monitoring and to describe basic procedures and techniques in which the surgical technologist may be required to assist. The pharmacology of anesthetic and adjunct drugs is fully discussed in Chapter 13.

IMPORTANT ANESTHESIA CONCEPTS

Anesthesia is achieved by altering the patient's level of consciousness, by interrupting nerve pathways that transmit sensation, or a combination of the two.

1. **Sensation** is the awareness of stimuli. The nervous system is capable of many sensations, including hearing, sight, smell, taste, touch, temperature (heat and cold), pressure, and pain.
2. **Analgesia** is loss of pain sensation. Specialized nerves transmit signals from the source of pain to the brain. Analgesic drugs interrupt these pain nerve pathways.
3. **Consciousness** is a state of awareness in which a person is able to *sense the environment and respond to it*. In a fully conscious person, all autonomic and sensory functions are intact and the patient is "awake."
4. **Sedation** is a *state of consciousness* described along a continuum. At one end, a person is fully aware of the surroundings and able to respond to stimuli. At the other end is unconsciousness, in which the patient is not aware of the environment and cannot respond to external stimuli including those that are noxious (e.g., pain, cold, heat).
5. **Central nervous system depression** refers to diminished mental, sensory, and physical capacity. It is another way of expressing sedation.
6. **Unconsciousness** is severe depression of the central nervous system (CNS) resulting in the *inability to respond to external stimuli*. Deep unconsciousness, such as that achieved during general anesthesia, results in the absence of **protective mechanisms**, such as swallowing, coughing, blinking, and shivering. General (surgical) anesthesia produces reversible unconsciousness.
7. **Coma** is the deepest state of unconsciousness, in which most brain activity ceases.
8. **Amnesia** is the loss of recall (memory) of events. Drugs that produce amnesia are used during the process of anesthesia.

ANESTHESIA PERSONNEL

ANESTHESIA CARE PROVIDER

The **anesthesia care provider (ACP)** administers anesthetic agents, performs physiological monitoring, and responds to anesthetic and surgical emergencies. An **anesthesiologist** is a medical doctor with specialist training in anesthesia (MDA). The certified registered nurse anesthetist (CRNA) is licensed to deliver anesthesia after achieving a master of science degree in nursing and obtaining certification in anesthesia. Specialty areas in the field of anesthesia care include chronic pain management and clinical anesthesia specialties, such as obstetrical, cardiac, pediatric, and ambulatory anesthesia.

Role of the Anesthesia Care Provider

The primary role of the ACP is to provide an adequate level of anesthesia while assessing and managing the patient's physiological responses to the surgery and anesthesia. The primary role of the ACP includes the following:

- Protects and manage the patient's vital functions during surgery.
- Manages the patient's level of consciousness and ability to sense pain and other external stimuli.
- Provides an adequate level of muscle relaxation during general anesthesia.
- Provides sedation as needed during regional anesthesia.
- Communicates with the surgeon about the patient's responses to intraoperative stimuli. This includes information on homodynamic changes, fluid and electrolyte balance, level of muscle relaxation, and level of consciousness.
- Reports and responds to any physiolgoical or anesthetic emergency.
- Provides psychological support to the patient throughout the perioperative experience.

The ACP monitors the patient from the time he or she enters the surgical suite until discharge from the hospital. Intraoperative care begins when the patient arrives in surgery and continues through the duration of the procedure and into the next phase, postoperative care. This begins when the patient is transported to the postanesthesia care unit and continues until discharge. The ACP is available to respond to medical problems related to the anesthesia, including management of postoperative pain.

ANESTHESIA ASSISTANT

The anesthesia assistant (AA) assists the anesthesia care provider in tasks that are delegated according to the AA's practice skills and knowledge. The AA, who has a master's degree, performs a variety of functions on the anesthesia care team. These include obtaining the patient history and performing the presurgical examination of the patient. During surgery, the AA performs invasive and noninvasive procedures such as drawing blood samples, administering induction and adjunct agents, and applying invasive and noninvasive physiological monitoring devices. The AA may also apply and interpret electroencephalographic spectral analysis, evoked potential, and echocardiography. The AA also performs and monitors regional anesthesia such as spinal, epidural, intravenous (IV), regional, and other techniques under the direction of the supervising anesthesiologist and according to state law.

ANESTHESIA TECHNOLOGIST

The **anesthesia technologist** is a health professional trained to assist the ACP in the delivery of anesthesia during surgery. This includes maintaining anesthesia and physiological monitoring equipment, preparing drugs and supplies, and providing assistance during anesthesia delivery. The anesthesia technologist is knowledgeable about **anesthetic** agents and adjunct drugs, advanced pharmacology, all airway and related anesthesia equipment, emergency response techniques, clinical monitoring, and anesthesia procedures. He or she assists the ACP directly during surgery and is responsible for the preparation and maintenance of anesthesia supplies and devices. Certification is granted after graduation from an approved 4-year college or university program and successful certification examination.

PREOPERATIVE EVALUATION OF THE PATIENT

Before surgery, the ACP or other qualified personnel (e.g., nurse practitioner, physician assistant, anesthesia assistant) performs a complete assessment of the patient, including history and physical examination. This usually takes place 1 to 3 days before the date of surgery. In an emergency, the assessment is performed just before the procedure and may be done in the patient holding area. Emergency cases can increase anesthetic risks related to a lack of information available preoperatively. At the very least, the patient's baseline **vital signs**, body mass index, and airway risk are assessed preoperatively. The purpose of the preoperative assessment is to determine the patient's specific medical needs and risk factors for anesthesia based on any history of anesthesia, and on his or her current physical and physiological status. The decision on the type of anesthesia to be used (general, sedation, regional) may also be discussed with the patient at this time. During the preoperative evaluation, patients have the opportunity to discuss specific concerns about their physical or psychological well-being as it relates to the anesthesia and postoperative care. Patient education during the assessment often resolves many fears and misconceptions about the effects of anesthesia and pain control. The preoperative assessment is modified according to the type of surgery and known risks such as difficult airway, sensitivity or allergy to particular drugs, and previous anesthetic complications.

COMORBIDITY AND ANESTHESIA CLASSIFICATION

A review of systems and screening for specific conditions reduces the risk of complications related to anesthesia and provides the basis of the **anesthesia classification**. This system, created by the American Society of Anesthesiologists, places patients in a specific category that corresponds to anesthetic risk (Box 14-1). The preoperative evaluation includes a current or past history of the most significant systemic disorders. These are shown in Table 14-1.

CURRENT MEDICATIONS AND ALLERGIES

The patient's current medications include prescription, over-the-counter medications, and herbal remedies. Drugs and agents the patient takes routinely may interfere with, block, or increase the effect of drugs used during surgery. The patient's normal medications may be altered (decreased or increased) before surgery. Known allergies are very important, and these are clearly documented according to facility protocol. The patient also is asked about illegal or recreational use of drugs and alcohol and about tobacco use.

Box 14-1 Classification of Patients by Risk of Anesthesia-Related Complications (American Society of Anesthesiologists [ASA])

ASA 1: The patient is normal and healthy.
ASA 2: The patient has mild systemic disease that does not limit the individual's activities (e.g., controlled hypertension or controlled diabetes without systemic sequelae).
ASA 3: The patient has moderate or severe systemic disease that does limit the individual's activities (e.g., stable angina or diabetes with systemic sequelae).
ASA 4: The patient has severe systemic disease that is a constant potential threat to life (e.g., severe congestive heart failure, end-stage renal failure).
ASA 5: The patient is morbid and is at substantial risk of death within 24 hours, with or without intervention.
E: Emergency status; any patient undergoing an emergency procedure is identified by adding "E" to the underlying ASA status (1-5). Therefore, a fundamentally healthy patient undergoing an emergency procedure would be classified as E-1.

Modified from Hata T et al: *Guidelines, education, and testing for procedural sedation and analgesia,* Iowa City, 1992-2003, University of Iowa.

PREVIOUS HISTORY OF ANESTHESIA

A history of previous general anesthesia or conscious sedation is important, especially if the patient experienced any adverse event during the procedure or postoperatively. A history of poor drug clearance, cardiovascular problems, difficult airway, or drug sensitivity is significant to the choice of drugs and anesthesia methods under consideration. Attempts should be made to determine the cause of the complications and plan the anesthesia accordingly. All findings are documented in the patient's chart so that other caregivers are aware of possible risks.

AIRWAY AND DENTAL STATUS

Any abnormality of the **airway** or potential obstruction can create an anesthesia emergency. General anesthesia requires complete assessment of the airway to evaluate conditions that might lead to an airway obstruction or make intubation difficult and may represent the most important aspect of the preoperative assessment. This is particularly true for obese patients, who often have difficult airways because of neck circumference and distortion of the laryngeal structures related to excess fat and muscle in the neck. Range of motion of the head and neck are also negatively affected by obesity. This may prevent the hyperextension of the neck that is necessary for intubation. Loose teeth or crowns may break loose and become an airway obstruction. Jewelry implanted in the tongue, lips, cheeks, or teeth also create a risk. Such jewelry can easily become a tracheal or bronchial obstruction, especially during placement of an artificial airway, which requires manipulation of structures in the mouth, pharynx, and larynx. Even during local or conductive anesthesia, a patient may need emergency

Table **14-1**	Comorbid Conditions Important to Risk Assessment in Anesthesia
Category	**Conditions**
Cardiovascular disease	Hypertension Ischemic heart disease Heart failure Murmurs and valve deformities Hypertrophic cardiomyopathy Prosthetic heart valve Rhythm disturbances
Pulmonary disorder	Asthma Chronic obstructive pulmonary disease Restrictive pulmonary disorder Dyspnea Pulmonary hypertension Smokers (and secondhand smokers)
Endocrine disorder	Diabetes mellitus Thyroid or parathyroid disease Hypothalamic pituitary adrenal disorder
Renal disease	Acute renal failure
Hepatic disease	Hepatitis Obstructive jaundice Cirrhosis Remote history hepatitis
Hematological disorder	Anemia Sickle cell disease Coagulopathies Von Willebrand disease Thrombocytopenia Thrombocytosis Polycythemia Risk of thromboembolism
Neurological disease	Cerebrovascular disease Asymptomatic bruit Seizure disorder Multiple sclerosis Aneurysms Parkinson disease Muscular dystrophies Neuromuscular junction disorder
Musculoskeletal or connective tissue disorder	Rheumatoid arthritis Ankylosing spondylitis Systemic lupus erythematosus Systemic sclerosis
Cancer or tumor	Carcinoid tumor Mediastinal mass

resuscitation, requiring placement of an artificial airway. The patient with a difficult airway presents a challenge during intubation and may require additional personnel or specific type of airway during general anesthesia (discussed later). The airway assessment includes the following:

- Neck circumference and length
- Range of motion of the head and neck
- Size or presence of the uvula
- Tongue size
- Position of the thyroid
- Ability to advance the mandible
- Condition of the teeth

MUSCULOSKELETAL ASSESSMENT

Impaired mobility, skeletal injuries, and other structural problems can result in restricted range of motion during surgical positioning. The ACP therefore documents any joint replacements, previous skeletal injury, disease, and areas of nerve damage. This information is available in the patient's chart, and the ACP may provide specific information to other perioperative team members before or during patient positioning.

MENTAL AND NEUROLOGICAL STATUS

An evaluation of the patient's mental and neurological status, including cognition, speech, gait, and motor and sensory functions, is important for the diagnosis and also for establishing a baseline before surgery. Baseline evaluation allows comparison of neurological deficit before surgery in order to establish or defend against claims or injury or adverse events during the procedure.

Many patients fear anesthesia and pain more than the surgery itself. Common concerns are that they will have inadequate medication for pain or that they will become addicted to pain medication. Misinformation from various media sources and lack of knowledge about the pharmacology of analgesics often contribute to these fears. The ACP or perioperative registered nurse can answer the patient's questions about the action and duration of postoperative medication, which frequently allays the patient's fears.

SOCIAL ASSESSMENT

The patient's emotional and social well-being is important to recovery. The ACP inquires about the patient's family and whether the patient will have a caregiver or helper after surgery. This affects not only the physical care of the patient, but also the psychological support available in the postoperative period. Patients who are fearful or anxious about their surgery and the possible consequences for work, family, and social environment may have a higher threshold for sedation and anxiolytic (anxiety-reducing) medications.

PREOPERATIVE INVESTIGATIONS

Diagnostic testing to determine the patient's risk level has been routine for many decades. In current practice, fewer investigations are performed than previously. This has been influenced by managed care and the streamlining of hospital stay and preoperative routines. Institutions vary in their requirements for preoperative assessment, and the rationale for ordering investigations generally is based on the patient's ASA (Anesthesia Society of America) classification, which considers the findings of the history and physical examination. In these cases, the tests are intended to confirm or elaborate on a finding or diagnosis rather than to discover an abnormality. The ASA has determined that there are no routine laboratory or diagnostic screening tests that are necessary for perioperative anesthetic care. However, specific tests may be performed to establish a baseline for known risk factors such as cardiac, respiratory, and renal disease. Basic tests include electrocardiography (ECG), complete blood count, kidney function tests, and specific electrolyte and blood pH tests.

ANESTHESIA SELECTION

Following the patient evaluation, an appropriate type and method of anesthesia are selected. This is a cooperative and informed decision made by the ACP, the surgeon, and the patient. The decision is based on the following:

- The patient's assigned ASA classification
- The patient's current physical status
- The presence or history of metabolic disease
- The patient's psychological status
- The type of surgery, including positioning requirements
- The length of the procedure
- Any history of adverse reactions to anesthetics and drug allergies

The patient's safety and well-being are always the primary considerations in the selection of the method of anesthesia. The medical and surgical goals are to provide the appropriate level of anesthesia without compromising the patient's safety. This means that not only the patient's physical condition and past history are considered, but also the requirements of the surgical procedure. The surgeon may participate in the decision based on his or her knowledge of the time required for surgery and the extent of the procedure.

Patients participate in their own anesthesia care by expressing preferences. However, these must be informed choices based on safety and environmental considerations. The ACP helps the patient choose among the "best choices." This is especially important for patients who have moderate or high risk factors to consider. Patients differ in their desire to be awake during the procedure, fully sedated, or only partly conscious. An informed consent to anesthesia including risks and alternatives is necessary for surgery to take place.

The choice between general anesthesia and regional (local) anesthesia often depends on the anatomical extent of the surgery and the anticipated anesthesia time required. Very long procedures and those involving the abdominal and thoracic cavities are not suitable for regional anesthesia. Superficial procedures and those of the limbs may be performed using regional anesthetics.

IMMEDIATE PREOPERATIVE PREPARATION OF THE PATIENT

ADMISSION DOCUMENTATION AND PREOPERATIVE CHECKLIST

Every precaution is taken to ensure the patient's safety in the perioperative period. When the patient arrives in surgery, the surgical checklist is used to ensure that all preoperative

procedures have been completed. This includes any special procedures such as evacuation of the bowel (bowel prep) before surgery. Patients are also advised to remove makeup, including nail polish, before surgery. The admission procedure is also important to the patient's emotional well-being. Reassurance and physical comfort are critical in this first encounter.

In the ambulatory setting, patient teaching is done before the day of surgery, and the patient is made aware of special precautions and procedures. Inpatients are prepared in the ward. Hospitals and other surgical facilities have individual check-in protocols. However, specific details are always verified:

1. *Patient identity* is meticulously checked. The health care provider asks the patient his or her name and verifies this with the patient's unique identifiers, the surgery schedule, and the medical records at hand.
2. *Correct procedure, side, and site* are validated with the patient, the medical record, the surgical schedule, and the consent form. Preoperative procedures include the surgeon's skin markings on the operative side showing the location of the incision. These are matched with all other information available.
3. *Surgical and anesthesia consent forms* must be signed according to facility protocol. (Details on legal aspects of the consent are described in Chapter 3.)
4. *Resuscitation orders* and any other legal documents are checked.
5. *Patient allergies* must be noted on all medical records, and the patient is asked about allergies again in the holding area.
6. *Preoperative medications* are documented in the patient's medical and preoperative records. Any medication ordered but not yet given may be administered in the holding area as directed by the surgeon or ACP.
7. *Prostheses,* including dentures and hearing aids, must be removed before surgery whenever possible. In the event a prosthesis is removed in the holding area, extreme care is taken to protect it from loss or misidentification.
8. *Jewelry,* including body-piercing jewelry, is removed before anesthesia or any procedure in which electrosurgery is used. Any jewelry removed in the holding area is placed in a container, labeled, and placed in a secure location until it can be safely returned to the patient. A wedding ring may be taped in place.
9. *Medical records* accompanying the patient are noted. Diagnostic results accompanying the patient, such as radiographs or other imaging studies, are clearly labeled.

PREOPERATIVE MEDICATION

Preoperative medication is administered as required, at home, on the inpatient ward, or in the perioperative holding area. Historically, preoperative drugs were given routinely while the patient was awaiting surgery on the hospital ward. In the past, patients were heavily sedated, and most arrived in the operating room disoriented and even unresponsive because of the sedative drugs. Heavy preoperative sedation can prolong anesthesia recovery, cause delirium, cardiovascular,

Table **14-2**	Summary of Fasting Recommendations for Healthy Patients*
Ingested Material	**Minimum Fasting**
Clear liquids	2 hr
Breast milk	4 hr
Infant formula	6 hr
Nonhuman milk	6 hr
Light meal	6 hr

*American Society of Anesthesiologists, 2011.

and respiratory risks, and produced many unpleasant side effects. Heavy sedation in the preoperative period is no longer used. Instead, specific drugs are used to lower metabolic and physiological risks and are prescribed according to the individual patient's needs and condition as they relate to anesthesia and the surgical procedure. Other drugs used routinely in the past have been removed from the ASA recommendations. These include antiemetics to reduce the risk of postoperative vomiting and anticholinergics to reduce the risk of pulmonary aspiration.

The current practice in anesthesiology is *selective* preoperative medication for patients with specific risks or conditions that can be mitigated by drugs, rather than a single drug routine for all patients. Adjunct drugs are given in all phases of the surgery to maintain physiological balance in cardiac, respiratory, and hemodynamic function as well as other metabolic states that require immediate pharmacological intervention. These functions are continually assessed through physiological monitoring.

PREOPERATIVE FASTING

Preoperative fasting is required to minimize aspiration (inhalation) of gastric contents during general anesthesia. In the past, all liquids and food were withheld after midnight the day of surgery. However, this rigid parameter is no longer standard practice. Strict fasting in pediatric and geriatric patients may lead to dehydration, headache, and irritability, especially when surgery is delayed. A safer and more realistic fasting period is now determined by the type of surgery and the patient's age and condition. A summary of the current (2011) fasting recommendations by the American Society of Anesthesiologists is shown in Table 14-2.

PHYSIOLOGICAL MONITORING DURING SURGERY

In a state of well-being, the body responds readily to stimuli to maintain life. Many complex biochemical, physical, and metabolic processes control the balance between stimuli and responses. Examples are *shivering* (uncontrollable muscle tremor) when the body's temperature drops and *vasoconstriction* (constriction of blood vessels) when blood pressure falls. This maintenance of physiological balance is called *homeostasis*.

Table **14-3**	Physiological Monitoring Devices and Use
Type of Monitoring	**Parameters Measured**
Pulse oximetry	• Blood oxygen saturation • Heart rate
Automatic blood pressure cuff	• Blood pressure
Electrocardiography	• Heart rhythm • Heart rate • Myocardial ischemia
Capnography	• Adequacy of ventilation • Airway pressure
Oxygen analyzer	• Delivered oxygen concentration
Ventilator pressure monitor	• Ventilator disconnection during general anesthesia and assisted ventilation • Monitor airway pressure
Temperature monitoring probe (Foley type)	• Core body temperature
Urine output using Foley catheter	• Gross indication of renal perfusion and intravascular volume
Central venous catheter	• Measures central venous pressure • Rapid administration of fluids and blood • Drug administration
Arterial catheter	• Measurement of arterial blood pressure • Obtain samples of arterial blood for analysis
Precordial Doppler	• Detects air embolism
Transesophageal echocardiography	• Evaluates myocardium • Assess valve function • Assess intravascular volume • Detection of air embolism
Esophageal Doppler	• Assessment of descending aortic flow • Assessment of cardiac preload
Transpulmonary indicator dilution	• Cardiac output • Cardiac preload
Esophageal and precordial stethoscope	• Auscultation of breathing and heart sounds

During surgery, the ACP and registered nurse assess and control the body's normal responses to noxious (harmful or painful) stimuli. Physiological monitoring provides the basis on which personnel assess homeostasis and respond to the patient's needs. Basic and special monitoring devices and their use are shown in Table 14-3.

Physiological monitoring is assessment of the patient's vital metabolic functions. All anesthetics (regional, general, or sedative) require physiological monitoring. However, the complexity and type of monitoring depend on the type of anesthesia, the patient's physical condition, the known risks, and the anticipated complications.

Monitoring is necessary because anesthetic drugs, position changes, and the trauma of surgery itself alter in some cases prevent normal body functions. **Protective reflexes** (e.g., respiration, gagging, swallowing, withdrawal from pain) are suppressed during general anesthesia. Rapid physiological changes can occur during positioning (e.g., tilting the patient's body, placing the legs in stirrups). Many types of anesthetic agents cause changes in the blood pressure and heart rate. Sedating and analgesic drugs can depress respiratory function.

MONITORING PROCESS

The standards for monitoring patients are set by the ASA. The level of monitoring—whether invasive methods are needed or not—depends on the patient's ASA numerical classification. The routine parameters that must be monitored include the following:

- *Oxygenation:* The oxygen-carrying capacity of the blood (also called oxygen saturation).
- *Ventilation:* The exchange of gases in the respiratory system. Two types of ventilation occur—alveolar and pulmonary. *Alveolar* refers to exchange of oxygen for carbon dioxide at the cellular level, whereas *pulmonary* refers to the exchange of environmental gas (air) for exhaled gas containing carbon dioxide.
- *Cardiac function:* Electrical activity of the heart, continuously monitored using a standard digital cardiac monitor or more invasive device according to the patient's physiological needs.
- *Perfusion:* Blood supply to the capillaries in the peripheral circulation where oxygen exchange takes place.
- *Body temperature:* The patient's core temperature; must be assessed and maintained within a range compatible with normal homeostasis.
- *Neuromuscular response:* Measured during surgery to determine the level of neuromuscular blockade resulting from specific drugs given to induce paralysis (neuromuscular blocking agents).
- *Fluid and electrolyte balance:* Electrolyte and fluid balance, including total intravascular fluid volume; continually monitored, especially during lengthy cases or in very ill patients.

Ventilation, Oxygenation, and Perfusion

Pulmonary **ventilation** is the total mechanism for drawing air into the lungs (muscular activity, negative pressure in the thoracic cavity, lung capacity). Adequate ventilation results in oxygen reaching the alveoli of the lungs where gas exchange takes place. Insufficient or poor ventilation results in low oxygen in the blood (hypoxia). **Perfusion** is the movement of oxygenated blood to the peripheral capillaries where oxygen is exchanged for carbon dioxide at the cellular level. Methods of monitoring ventilation and perfusion include:

- *Capnography:* The partial pressure of expired carbon dioxide, which is produced by the cells and expired during ventilation, is measured and the value displayed as a waveform on a monitor. The SARA (Smart Alarm Respiratory Analysis) is a branded capnography system used in some facilities.

- *Arterial blood gas (ABG):* Blood gases are measured using a sample of arterial blood. The parameters are partial pressure of carbon dioxide and oxygen and blood pH, which are indicators of blood gases.
- *Pulse oximetry:* The **pulse oximeter** is a digital sensor that detects oxygen saturation in the hemoglobin by spectrometry. The device is placed on a highly vascular area of the body (digit or earlobe) and provides continuous readings. A healthy individual should show a reading of 95% or higher saturation.

Fluid and Electrolyte Balance

The ACP maintains **intravascular volume** and pressure using adjunct drugs, IV solutions, and blood products as indicated. Fluids are replaced using an IV infusion pump, which delivers the amount of fluids at a programmed rate. The selection of fluids depends on specific physiological parameters measured by rapid blood tests and physiological monitoring of circulatory and respiratory function. Electrolyte balance is measured by a blood test, and fluid volume is indicated by arterial blood pressure and blood loss. Blood loss is calculated during surgery by measuring the amount of total fluids (blood and irrigation fluid) suctioned from the wound and subtracting the total amount of irrigation fluids used. Blood loss is also estimated by weighing surgical sponges.

Circulatory Function and Perfusion

Circulatory assessment includes monitoring of heart function and peripheral circulation. Two types of methods are used to monitor circulation: direct (invasive) methods and indirect (noninvasive) methods. Direct monitoring requires the insertion of a measuring device (e.g., internal pulmonary artery catheter) inside the patient's body. Noninvasive techniques are growing in popularity. Invasive intravascular devices such as Swan Ganz and other arterial catheters are now used infrequently, because newer technology has been developed that is much safer and more accurate.

- *Electrocardiography:* ECG measures the electrical activity of the heart, which is projected into a waveform. ECG leads are placed on the thorax in a pattern that accurately detects and transmits the electrical impulses of the heart to the monitor (Figure 14-1).
- *Arterial blood pressure monitoring:* Blood pressure is measured manually with a sphygmomanometer and blood pressure cuff or automatically using a digital blood pressure monitoring system. Noninvasive hemodynamic monitoring is used in selected patients.
- *Transesophageal monitoring:* A transesophageal stethoscope may be used to monitor the heart's rhythm, intensity, pitch, and frequency during general anesthesia. Respiratory sounds and rate also are monitored through the stethoscope, which is attached to a small earpiece worn by the ACP.
- *Intravascular monitoring:* Hemodynamic monitoring is used to measure central venous pressure, mean artery pressure, stroke volume, and cardiac output. Noninvasive electronic systems are now used that replace the older style pulmonary artery catheters (PACs) used in the past (see next item).

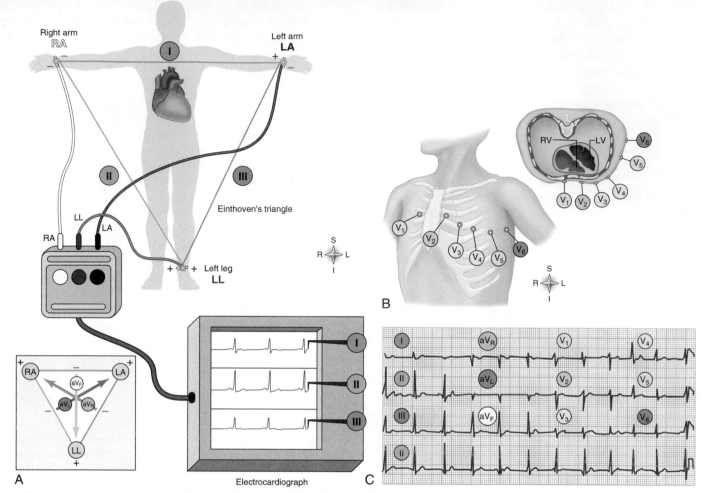

Figure 14-1 Electrocardiogram leads and output. Electrocardiography maps the electrical activity of heart through electrodes placed on the skin A. Electrodes are strategically placed to record, amplify, and display voltage (potentials). Here, the limb leads form a triangle which reflects the basic pattern of electrical potential generated by the heart's pacemaker cells. B. The chest leads produce a three dimensional picture of electrical activity represented by the ECG pattern. C. Each pair of leads is represented as specific patterns on a graph. Heart rate, rhythm, strength of conduction, location of impulses and other information from the readout is interpreted to assist in diagnosis. *(From Thibodeau GA, Patton KT: Anatomy and physiology, ed 3, St Louis, 2007, Mosby.)*

- *Pulmonary artery catheter:* The PAC is used for critical care monitoring in selected patients. The PAC is sometimes referred to as a Swan Ganz catheter, but this is only one of many different types of PACs. The PAC is no longer commonly used because safer and more advanced technology is available. The catheter provides direct assessment of pulmonary artery pressure and indirect left ventricular filling pressures. The PAC is inserted into the pulmonary artery via the subclavian, internal jugular, or femoral vein. Multiple ports (openings) are used for withdrawing blood or injecting drugs. Internally, the catheter measures pressure through a transducer and temperature via a thermistor. The PAC is used to assess the following:
  - Central venous pressure (CVP) (1 to 6 mm Hg)
  - Mean pulmonary artery pressure (PAP) (systolic 15 to 30 mm HG, diastolic 6 to 12 mm Hg)
  - Pulmonary capillary wedge pressure (PCWP) (6 to 12 mm Hg), which estimates the left arterial heart pressure and left ventricular end-diastolic pressure

- Cardiac output (CO) (3.5 to 7.5 L/min)
- Mixed venous partial pressure of oxygen (Svo$_2$) (70% to 75%) taken from the end of the PAC and used to calculate the efficiency of oxygen as it passes from the blood into the tissues

Renal Function

Kidney function can be grossly measured by observing renal output during surgery. More specific tests such as blood urea nitrogen (BUN) are used to measure substances in the blood that are not effectively filtered by the kidneys. Selected surgical patients are catheterized before surgery so that fluid balance (input and output) can be measured during lengthy procedures.

Body Temperature

The normal body temperature is 97° F to 99.5° F (36° to 37.5° C). The body can tolerate environmental temperatures outside this range, but only with protection. The core temperature must be maintained within a range compatible with life.

During general anesthesia, the body temperature is measured with various types of internal and external devices. During cardiac surgery, probes can be inserted into the myocardium to monitor the temperature of the heart. A temperature sensor may also be contained with the pulmonary artery catheter used for direct measurement of arterial pressure.

MAINTAINING NORMOTHERMIA The patient's normal temperature (normothermia) is maintained using medical devices that provide convectional heat. The most common method is with a forced air blanket. This is a baffled air mattress that rests lightly on the patient's body. Warmed air is pumped into sections of the blanket via a flexible hose. The warm air blanket must be monitored to prevent burns. These risks are greatest when the patient is unconscious or semiconscious and unable to respond to pain. The temperature setting and the air hose-to-blanket connection should be checked before the unit is activated and thereafter at regular intervals throughout the surgical procedure.

The device should be activated only after the correct temperature has been verified with the ACP. If the connection is loose and the air hose becomes detached during surgery, the patient's skin may be exposed to a column of heated air. This might go unnoticed under the surgical drapes. Pediatric and geriatric patients and patients who are thin or debilitated are at particular risk for burns. Meticulous attention to any device that creates heat is the collaborative responsibility of everyone on the operating team.

Other methods are also used to prevent heat loss from the patient's body during surgery. Irrigation solutions are warmed to a safe temperature before use in the body cavities. In preoperative and postoperative periods, the patient is kept warm using conventional linen blankets.

DELIBERATE HYPOTHERMIA Deliberate **hypothermia** (lowering of the patient's core body temperature) is used during **malignant hyperthermia**. This is a physiological reaction to specific anesthetics and neuromuscular blocking agents in which the body temperature is critically elevated (discussed later in the chapter). Hypothermia may also be initiated when normal blood flow presents a severe, uncontrollable risk. In cardiac surgery, surgical repair of large vessels, organ transplantation, and neurosurgery, *controlled hypothermia* produces a margin of safety while particular surgical procedures are performed.

METHODS OF ACHIEVING HYPOTHERMIA Hypothermia is obtained by a number of methods. Blood may be diverted to a cooling system, as during cardiopulmonary bypass. Other methods include IV administration of a cold solution and irrigation of body cavities with a cold fluid. During cardiac surgery, saline ice slush is packed around the heart to produce localized cooling. Target temperatures are no lower than 78.8° F (26° C).

Complications of induced hypothermia include cardiac arrhythmia, which occurs when normal conduction is interrupted. This can lead to heart block and cardiac arrest. Other organs of the body also may suffer damage as a result of inadequate blood supply.

Rewarming is achieved with a heating blanket, heating mattress, warm IV fluids, and warm cotton blankets. Shivering, which increases the body's requirements for oxygen, is controlled with muscle relaxants, selected analgesics, and further rewarming. The patient is rewarmed slowly to reduce the risk of circulatory collapse or sudden dilation or constriction of blood vessels.

Neuromuscular Response

During general anesthesia, neuromuscular blocking agents are administered to relax skeletal muscles. Without adequate muscle relaxation or paralysis, retraction of the body wall and other tissues is difficult, and this prevents adequate exposure of the operative site. Controlled (mechanical or manual) ventilation is required whenever a neuromuscular blocking agent is used, because the respiratory muscles are paralyzed.

A peripheral nerve stimulator is used to monitor the level of neuromuscular blocking. The stimulator delivers a series of painless electrical impulses. Muscle twitching in response to the stimuli produces a means of evaluating the degree of neuromuscular blockade.

Level of Consciousness

The patient's level of consciousness is monitored to prevent **intraoperative awareness (IOA)**. This is a rare phenomenon in which the patient retains some degree of consciousness (including sensory awareness) but lacks motor ability. The **bispectral index system (BIS)** is used to prevent patient recall of pain perceived during surgery. BIS electrodes are attached to the head to measure the level of hypnosis during anesthesia. Although intraoperative awareness is rare, the psychological consequences are serious and include posttraumatic symptoms.

METHODS OF ANESTHESIA

GENERAL ANESTHESIA

General anesthesia is *reversible loss of consciousness*, which is accompanied by the *absence* of:

- Pain
- Sensory perception
- Cognition (awareness, ability to interpret the environment)
- Memory of experiences during the period of unconsciousness
- Some autonomic reflexes

During general anesthesia, different types of drugs are used to achieve the effects needed for surgery. For example, the anesthetic may cause loss of consciousness but not muscle relaxation. In this case, a paralytic agent is administered during surgery. Other drugs are given to produce smooth emergence from the anesthesia. This combination of drugs and anesthetic agents is sometimes referred to as *balanced anesthesia*.

An *inhalation anesthetic* is used for prolonged surgery. IV agents are used to induce unconsciousness or to maintain

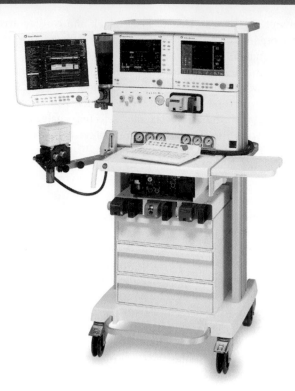

Figure 14-2 Anesthesia machine. (Courtesy Datex-Ohmeda, Madison, Wis.)

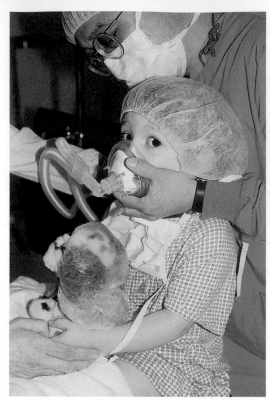

Figure 14-3   Pediatric patient with an anesthesia mask. (From Leibert PS: Color atlas of pediatric surgery, ed 2, Philadelphia, 1996, WB Saunders.)

deep sedation during short procedures. During inhalation anesthesia, an IV barbiturate drug is used for **induction** (causing unconsciousness), and the inhalation anesthetic is used to maintain unconsciousness.

Anesthesia Machine

General anesthesia requires the use of an anesthesia machine (Figure 14-2).

The **anesthesia machine** is a complex biotechnical device used in patient monitoring, respiratory function, and administration of inhalation anesthetics. An inhalation anesthetic is administered in the form of a volatile liquid that is changed into a gas in the vaporizer. The basic mechanism is a return flow system that includes the patient's inspiratory and expiratory functions. Important components are the vaporizer, ventilator, breathing apparatus, and **gas scavenging** system.

The anesthesia machine allows the patient to be mechanically ventilated or hand-ventilated with the **breathing bag**, which is part of the ventilator and valve system. Gases enter the bag and then are delivered to the patient through a tube, which is connected to an invasive airway or face mask. Exhaled carbon dioxide is captured from the system, measured, and absorbed by a soda lime reservoir.

The anesthesia face mask is used to deliver positive-pressure ventilation with anesthetic gas and oxygen. An anesthesia face mask generally is not used in place of an invasive airway device except for administration of oxygen or brief sedation or to induce anesthesia in pediatric patients (Figure 14-3).

Cleaning, disinfection, and basic troubleshooting of the anesthesia machine are the responsibilities of the anesthesia technologist. Maintenance and testing of the machine are performed by the bioengineering department. All equipment that comes in contact with the patient must be decontaminated to prevent cross-contamination. Standard Precautions are followed whenever equipment is handled and used. The hoses, soda canister, masks, and airways are sources of high bacterial contamination. The intricate valve mechanisms may also harbor large colonies of pathogenic bacteria. The use of disposable patient air hoses, masks, and airways is preferred whenever possible. Nondisposable items are decontaminated and sterilized before use.

SCAVENGING SYSTEM Escape of anesthetic gas into the surgical suite is an environmental hazard for health care workers. Scavenging systems capture escaped gases and vent them through a vacuum line. The National Institute for Occupational Safety and Health (NIOSH) and the Occupational Safety and Health Administration (OSHA) regulate the allowable percentage of environmental anesthetic agent in the air. Scavenging equipment can reduce health care worker exposure up to 95%.

More information on the hazards of environmental exposure to anesthetic gas is available at http://www.cdc.gov/niosh/docs/2007-151.

MEDICAL GASES Medical grade gases include oxygen, nitrogen, air, and nitrous oxide. These are obtained through an inline hose from wall outlets or from metal tanks (cylinders). Hoses for gas delivery to the anesthesia machine originate through inline sources. Portable oxygen cylinders are available for use during transportation of the patient recovering from anesthesia. (Chapter 8 presents a complete discussion on the safety and handling of gas cylinders.)

AIRWAY MANAGEMENT

Managing the patient's airway is a primary concern during general anesthesia or an emergency in which the patient is unable to maintain ventilation. During an emergency, such as cardiac or respiratory arrest, securing the patient's airway is the first priority. During surgery, the unconscious patient requires an invasive artificial airway to provide a sealed connection between the source of air, oxygen and anesthetic gases, and the patient's lungs. It also supports the patient's natural airway structures. The process of placing the invasive airway is called **intubation**. Less invasive airways are used to maintain the position of the tongue and support the soft tissues of the pharynx and larynx.

TYPES OF AIRWAYS

Endotracheal Tube

The **endotracheal tube** (ET tube) is an invasive airway that extends from the mouth to the trachea. It is inserted orally or, less commonly, through the nose. The tube has a balloon or cuff at the tip that acts as a barrier between the upper and lower airways and prevents aspiration of fluid into the respiratory tract (Figure 14-4). The ET tube is inserted with the aid of a rigid or flexible **laryngoscope**, a lighted instrument that is inserted into the trachea during intubation (Figure 14-5).

Laryngeal Mask

The **laryngeal mask airway (LMA)** is inserted without the aid of a laryngoscope and fits snugly over the larynx. The LMA is used in patients with a difficult airway condition. However, it does not protect against aspiration (Figure 14-6).

Oropharyngeal Airway

The **oropharyngeal airway (OPA)** is inserted over the tongue to prevent the tongue or epiglottis from falling back against the pharynx (Figure 14-7, *A*). The OPA is commonly used when the patient is semiconscious, such as during the recovery period in general anesthesia or during an airway emergency. The OPA is used in patients who have respiratory function but need upper airway support (Figure 14-7, *B*).

Nasopharyngeal Airway

The **nasopharyngeal airway** provides a passage between the nostril and the nasopharynx. This type of airway is used in a semiconscious patient when an OPA causes gagging or when a mouth injury (e.g., fracture) is present (Figure 14-7, *C*).

Oxygen Delivery

Patients who do not need assisted ventilation receive oxygen by a nonocclusive mask or nasal cannula (Figure 14-8). These systems deliver a small amount of oxygen combined with room air. Face masks cover both the nose and mouth and can

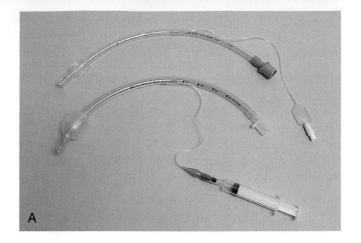

A

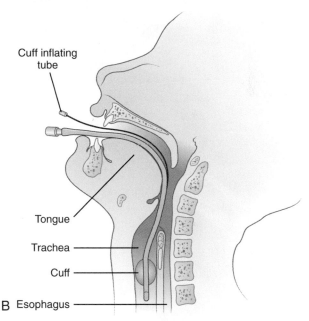

Cuff inflating tube

Tongue

Trachea

Cuff

B Esophagus

Figure 14-4 **A,** Endotracheal tubes. **B,** Endotracheal tube in position. (*A from Elkin MK, Perry PA:* Nursing interventions and clinical skills, *ed 3, St Louis, 2004, Mosby;* **B** *redrawn from Rothrock JC:* Alexander's care of the patient in surgery, *ed 12, St Louis, 2003, Mosby.*)

be adjusted to regulate the ratio of oxygen to air. This is passive delivery of oxygen, because the patient retains respiratory function.

INTUBATION

Intubation is a routine procedure during general anesthesia and is also performed as an emergency procedure to establish and maintain the airway. The patient usually is unconscious (e.g., during general anesthesia). However, conscious intubation also is performed when the patient is awake but requires airway support. Intubation with an ET tube requires a rigid or flexible laryngoscope to guide the ET tube into the trachea (Figure 14-9). A flexible metal stylet may be inserted into the tube to make it more rigid and facilitate placement. This procedure is also performed using a nasal laryngoscope.

During general anesthesia, the patient is intubated immediately after induction. Intubation is a critical process, because the patient's respiratory status may be unstable. During general anesthesia, the circulating nurse or anesthesia assistant stands at the patient's head and assists as needed during intubation.

The scrubbed surgical technologist should always be ready to assist in case of cardiac arrest, aspiration, or other anesthetic emergency during intubation. The exact role of the surgical technologist during any emergency depends on the nature of the event. This is a critical period during surgery, and the scrub shares responsibility for the patient's safety. Attention should be focused on the patient and ACP until an airway is secured and the patient is stabilized.

DIFFICULT AIRWAY

A difficult airway is one in which the usual methods of providing ventilation—placement of an artificial airway and mask ventilation—are extremely difficult. In the worst case, the outcome is failure to ventilate, even after many attempts.

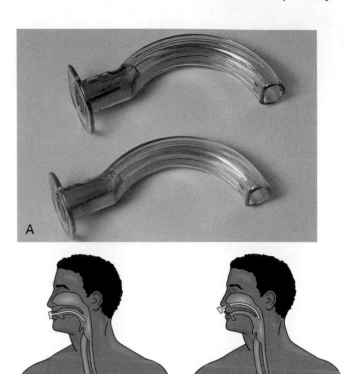

Figure 14-7 **A,** Oropharyngeal airway used in conscious patients who require support of the pharynx. **B,** Position of the oropharyngeal airway. **C,** Nasopharyngeal airway. *(A from Elkin MK, Perry PA: Nursing interventions and clinical skills, ed 4, St Louis, 2007, Mosby; B and C modified from Sorrentino SA: Mosby's textbook for nursing assistants, ed 5, St Louis, 2000, Mosby.)*

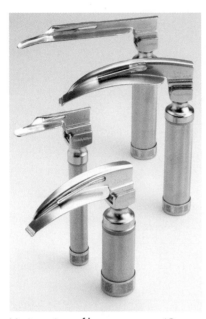

Figure 14-5 **Various sizes of laryngoscopes.** *(Courtesy Welch Allyn, Skaneateles Falls, NY.)*

Figure 14-6 **A,** Laryngeal mask. **B,** Laryngeal mask in place. Note the position over the larynx. *(A courtesy LMA North America; B redrawn from Phillips N: Berry and Kohn's operating room technique, ed 10, St Louis, 2004, Mosby.)*

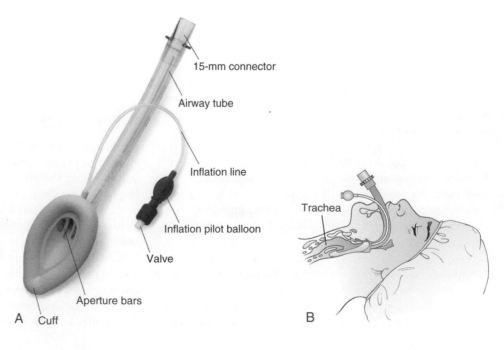

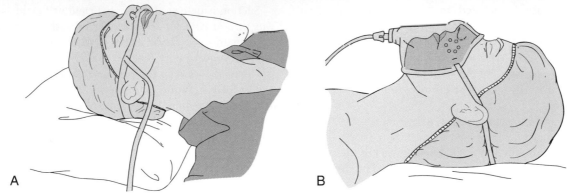

Figure 14-8 **Oxygen delivery. A,** Nasal cannula. **B,** Oxygen face mask for passive delivery of oxygen. *(Modified from Sorrentino SA: Mosby's textbook for nursing assistants, ed 5, St Louis, 2000, Mosby.)*

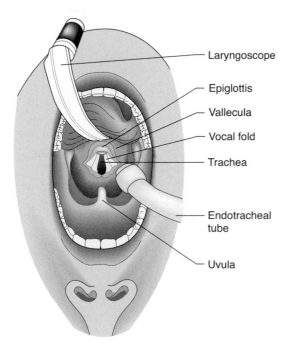

- Laryngoscope
- Epiglottis
- Vallecula
- Vocal fold
- Trachea
- Endotracheal tube
- Uvula

Figure 14-9 Endotracheal intubation is performed immediately after induction of general anesthesia. The airway is inserted with the aid of a laryngoscope. *(From Garden O, Bradbury A, Forsythe J, Parks R: Principles and practice of surgery, ed 5, Edinburgh, 2007, Churchill Livingstone.)*

has developed a grading system for airway difficulty and provides algorithms (stepwise decision tree for medical intervention) for establishing an airway in emergency situations. In the case of unexpected difficult airway, there may not be time to secure expert assistance. Having the emergency crash and airway carts available at all times decreases the risk of adverse events.

A difficult airway is usually related to the patient's specific neck anatomy. The patient with heavy muscle and fatty tissue in the throat and neck regions are prone to a difficult airway because of the pressure from these tissues collapsing on the airway during anesthesia induction or deep sedation. These conditions are most common in obese patients and in those who are of short, heavy stature. Other predisposing factors are neck and throat pathology including facial fractures. Patients who lack most of their teeth may also be difficult to intubate because without the support of teeth, the cheeks tend to collapse inward.

The most critical time for the patient with a difficult airway is during intubation and extubation. Patients known to have a difficult airway are positioned with the neck in hyperextension (sniffing position) with the head tilted back during intubation. Three anterior neck maneuvers for manipulating the larynx are recognized as beneficial for successful visualization of the throat structures and intubation in patients with difficult airway. *All three require training*, which anesthesia and nursing personnel undertake as part of perioperative study. Performed blindly without training, the maneuvers can result in poor patient outcomes. Poor technique that is ineffective can result in the loss of precious time, which quickly leads to hypoxia, hypercapnia, and brain damage. Other adverse outcomes include rupture of the tracheal structures.

The most effective of the three techniques is the bimanual or BURP technique. The least effective (except in some cases of emergency intubation) is direct **cricoid pressure** (CP or Sellick maneuver). This technique is intended to prevent regurgitation and improve visualization of the throat by depressing the esophagus. However, recent studies have shown that the Sellick maneuver, rather than actually compressing the esophagus, depresses the muscle lying directly

Adverse events related to a difficult airway are hypoxia leading to brain injury or death.

Patients undergoing elective surgery who are known to have or are at risk for a difficult airway are critically evaluated by the ACP before surgery to determine the extent of the risk and to prepare for interventions in the event of airway blockage. Preparations include having extra trained personnel available to assist and an emergency airway cart close to or in the operating room suite. Positioning devices that provide hyperextension of the neck are placed near the operating table before induction. The airway cart is managed by the ACP, anesthesia technologist, and circulator, who must be familiar with the types, names, and sizes of all equipment on the cart and also the emergency drugs that might be needed. The ASA behind it. Its use is debated in view of more modern techniques.[1,2]

1. Bimanual laryngoscopy or *optimal external laryngeal manipulation* (OELM) is pressure on the hyoid, thyroid, and cricoid cartilages by the ACP or laryngoscopist while simultaneously advancing the laryngoscope for placement of the airway.
2. *Backward upward right pressure* (BURP maneuver) on the thyroid cartilage for improved visualization.
3. *Backward pressure* (CP or Sellick maneuver) of the cricoid (intended to close the esophagus and prevent regurgitation and aspiration of stomach fluids).

PHASES OF GENERAL ANESTHESIA

The most prominent physiological effect of general anesthesia is reversible loss of consciousness, which is maintained while the anesthetic agent is administered. When the anesthetic is withdrawn, the patient quickly regains consciousness. The time- and event-related phases of general anesthesia are as follows:

1. *Induction:* General anesthesia begins with loss of consciousness. An induction agent (IV drug, inhalation gas, or combination of the two) is administered.
2. *Maintenance:* This phase involves continuation of the anesthetic agent; unconsciousness is maintained with the inhalation agent and adjunct agents.
3. *Emergence:* This phase is the cessation of the anesthetic. Reversal drugs may be administered, and the patient regains consciousness.
4. *Recovery:* Postanesthesia care is provided in this phase, which ends with clearance of anesthetic drugs from the body.

PREINDUCTION

The process of general anesthesia starts when all perioperative team members are present and preparations to start surgery have been completed. The patient is brought into the surgical suite, and noninvasive monitoring devices are put in place. If the patient does not have an IV line, the ACP inserts one when the patient arrives and ensures that the patient is comfortable and relaxed. The patient is positioned supine (lying face up), and the head is elevated slightly to facilitate respiration and immediate intubation after induction.

General anesthesia begins only after patient monitoring devices are in place and the operating team is present. The ACP assembles all needed drugs and equipment and reassures the patient while evaluating the individual's physiological status. Preoperative drugs that provide sedation and reduce anxiety may be given during this period.

Suction must be available to the ACP at all times. As long as the patient is in the operating suite, suction must remain operative. Inline suction is available from ceiling posts, cables, or wall outlets. When connecting suction cables, match the two ends of the connector, push, and turn the connector to secure it. This locking mechanism prevents the cables from separating.

Suction is delivered through a rigid or flexible suction tip. The *suction catheter* is a flexible tube that can be inserted through an airway (oral or nasal) to remove secretions below the pharyngeal cavity. The rigid suction tip has a blunt end and is used to sweep the oral and pharyngeal cavity.

Just before induction, the ACP may administer 100% oxygen to the patient through a face mask. The purpose of this is to ensure that tissues are fully oxygenated from the start of the procedure. If a temporary airway obstruction occurs, the reserve oxygen will already be in the system for rapid uptake into tissues.

INDUCTION

During induction, the patient passes through stages from consciousness to deep surgical anesthesia. Modern anesthetics and adjunct drugs allow the patient to pass through these stages very quickly, and they are seldom distinct. The stages are:

- *Stage 1:* Begins with the administration of induction drug and ends with loss of consciousness (usually within moments).
- *Stage 2:* Historically called the **delirium** stage, it is marked by unconsciousness and exaggerated reflexes. The airway remains intact and under the patient's control. Hearing is maintained. The pupils are dilated. This stage is almost never demonstrated with modern anesthetics.
- *Stage 3:* Surgical plane. The patient is relaxed, and protective reflexes (gagging, blinking, and swallowing) are lost. The patient is unable to maintain an open airway, and the respiratory response fails.
- *Stage 4:* Anesthesia overdose resulting in severe respiratory and circulatory collapse. This stage is never purposfully achieved because of its lethality.

The patient is induced with an inhalation anesthetic by mask or with an IV **sedative**, which causes unconsciousness within seconds. During induction, perioperative staff members must carry out their tasks as quietly as possible. Although induction takes place very quickly, the patient is able to hear well into the induction period. Conversation should stop, and care should be taken to minimize noise. The patient can easily misinterpret sounds and verbal exchanges during induction, because the ability to interpret the environment accurately recedes. Immediately after induction, the patient is intubated.

MAINTENANCE

Anesthesia maintenance begins when the patient's airway is secured and inhalation drugs can be administered. During maintenance, which represents the period of surgery itself, the ACP *titrates* (calculates and measures) the appropriate ratio of anesthetic agents and oxygen. These are delivered into the ventilatory system of the anesthesia machine and delivered to the patient via the airway. The levels of consciousness, analgesia, and sedation are continually monitored, along with physiological parameters. All drugs and procedures are documented in the anesthesia record throughout the procedure.

As the inhalation anesthetic is delivered through the airway (mask, laryngeal mask, or ET tube). The patient's ventilation is controlled by the ACP using a respirator. The ratio of oxygen to other anesthetic gases is adjusted and controlled through the anesthesia machine's ventilation system.

Neuromuscular Blockade ("Muscle Relaxation")

Adequate muscle relaxation is necessary during general anesthesia to allow manipulation of the body wall and other tissues in the operative site. Anesthetic agents vary in their effect on skeletal muscles. Most do not provide sufficient relaxation for surgery, and a separate drug must be administered. A muscle relaxant drug is called a **neuromuscular blocking agent**. This category of drugs causes paralysis by blocking neurotransmission to the muscle tissue. The level of paralysis is monitored continually throughout the procedure with a nerve stimulator. The level of relaxation is maintained at a minimum to prevent overdose. If increased relaxation is needed (e.g., during deep retraction), incremental doses can be administered.

EMERGENCE

Termination of anesthesia and the process of regaining consciousness is called **emergence**. The ACP controls emergence by withdrawing (stopping) the anesthetic agents and reversing the effects of adjunct drugs as necessary. When the patient regains consciousness, protective airway responses resume, and the ACP may remove the artificial airway. Removal of the airway is called **extubation**. A nasal or oral airway may be inserted at this time. Emergence can occur quickly and generally proceeds smoothly. Reversal drugs may be administered to hasten emergence. Occasionally the patient (especially a child) may enter a state of temporary delirium during emergence. The older person may experience persistent reversible delirium which might require several days to resolve. However, this is a postoperative complication, not a routine occurrence.

RECOVERY

When stable, the patient is transferred to a stretcher and transported to the **postanesthesia recovery unit (PACU)**. During transportation, oxygen may be administered from a portable tank. Patients who require continuous cardiac monitoring are transported with a portable monitoring unit. According to The Joint Commission policy, any patient requiring continuous cardiac monitoring must be accompanied to the PACU by a licensed perioperative nurse. On arrival in the PACU, the staff nurse receives the patient. Oxygen tubing is transferred from the portable unit to a wall outlet, and cardiac leads or other monitoring devices are connected to the PACU system. Suction is made immediately available for airway clearance. The nurse receives a report of the operative procedure, the patient's physiological status, and the anesthesia process from the ACP. The patient remains in the PACU until physiologically stable and conscious so that critical care personnel can respond to any emergency that may arise during recovery.

DISSOCIATIVE ANESTHESIA

Dissociative anesthesia is induced with the drug *ketamine*, which blocks sensory neurotransmission and associative pathways. The patient's eyes remain open and the person appears to be awake, but he or she is unaware of the environment. The drug also produces **anterograde** amnesia. Ketamine is administered intravenously or intramuscularly and is used for short procedures. It is used mainly in pediatric surgery in combination with other drugs to produce desired effects and reduce side effects such as excessive salivation and delirium during emergence. Muscle relaxants often are used in conjunction with ketamine to decrease muscle tone.

The advantages of ketamine are rapid induction and metabolism. The disadvantages are related mainly to cardiac stimulation and potential psychological effects, including delirium and hallucinations, which occur in adults more often than in children. Ketamine is contraindicated in surgery of the upper respiratory system because it does not suppress laryngeal and tracheal reflexes.

CONSCIOUS SEDATION

Conscious sedation is used for short diagnostic and minor surgical procedures that do not require deep anesthesia. In this process, a combination of sedatives, hypnotics, and analgesics is administered intravenously. The patient can respond to verbal commands and breathe independently but is sedated to tolerate the procedure. Patients undergoing conscious sedation are monitored continuously throughout the procedure.

Minimal sedation is a state in which the patient can respond to verbal commands. Cognitive function and muscular coordination may be impaired. The patient's ventilatory and cardiovascular systems remain unaffected.

In *moderate sedation*, the patient's consciousness is depressed. However, the person can respond to verbal commands when stimulated. Airway support is not needed, and the patient can breathe independently. The cardiovascular system usually is unaffected.

During *deep sedation*, the patient cannot be roused easily but responds to pain stimulation. Ventilatory function is intact but may be depressed. Cardiovascular functions remain intact.

Table 14-4 shows the levels of sedation.

REGIONAL ANESTHESIA

Regional anesthesia provides reversible loss of sensation in a specific area of the body without affecting consciousness. Regional anesthesia is also called *conductive* or *local anesthesia*. The term *regional* is preferred because it describes the process accurately. This type of anesthesia can be used in a small superficial area of skin and subcutaneous tissue or in an entire region of the body, such as during spinal anesthesia. Patient monitoring is always provided during regional anesthesia. The level and scope of monitoring depend on the

Table 14-4 Characteristics of Levels of Sedation

Sedation Level	Level of Consciousness	Airway	Verbal Response	Response to Touch
No sedation	Aware of environment and self	Normal or adequate	Normal or adequate	Normal or adequate
Light sedation	Sedated but aware of environment and self	Normal or adequate	Adequate or limited Abnormal	Normal or adequate
Moderate sedation	Sleepy but easily aroused; slight awareness of environment	May require airway support	Limited or none	Adequate or limited Abnormal
Deep sedation	Unaware of environment or self	May be mildly abnormal or absent	None	Only partially responsive to pain
Surgical general anesthesia	Unconscious; does not respond to pain	Limited or absent	None	No response to touch or pain

patient's condition and whether sedation is used during the procedure.

The most common uses of regional anesthesia are:

- Limb surgery in which complete nerve block is possible
- Procedures in which consciousness is desirable or required (e.g., obstetrical procedures)
- Minor superficial procedures
- Patients for whom general anesthesia poses a significant physiological risk

Regional anesthesia can be provided to a single nerve, to a group of nerves, or to an area of the spinal cord. When sensory nerve transmission is interrupted, tissues that transmit signals along that nerve are unable to receive pain signals. There are several types of regional anesthesia:

- *Topical anesthesia:* An anesthetic is applied directly to the eye, skin, or mucous membranes. This is done before injection of a regional anesthetic into sensitive areas of the body. Topical anesthesia may also be used before insertion of a tube or catheter.
- *Local infiltration:* A small amount of drug is introduced by multiple injections into the skin and subcutaneous and deeper tissue.
- *Nerve block:* A single nerve or nerve plexus (group) is anesthetized, blocking sensory stimuli to the tissue enervated by that nerve or group.
- *Spinal, caudal, and epidural anesthesia:* These are specific techniques for blocking transmission to the middle and lower body.

DRUG DOSAGE

The effective dosage of anesthetic is calculated according to the individual patient's ability to absorb and metabolize the drug. The "normal" or safe dosage depends on many factors. Therapeutic ranges for all local anesthetics are considered with knowledge of the patient's physical condition, especially the presence of cardiac disease, concurrent use of other drugs, and the patient's age, weight, and vascular status.

The rate of metabolism and response to the drug determine whether toxic levels are being reached. External monitoring is an objective method of detecting signs of toxicity. This is especially important in patients who require large amounts of anesthetic.

MONITORING

Monitored anesthesia care (MAC) is continuous patient monitoring provided during regional anesthesia. In addition to non invasive physiological monitoring, the ACP administers sedative and **anxiolytic** (antianxiety) drugs as needed and manages any anesthetic or physiological emergencies. Monitored care is particularly important for patients receiving regional anesthesia who have underlying systemic disease or respiratory or cardiovascular risks. Basic monitoring includes the parameters listed previously and may include others, depending on the type of drugs administered.

TYPES OF REGIONAL ANESTHESIA

Topical Anesthesia

Topical anesthesia is used on mucous membranes and on superficial eye tissues during ophthalmic surgery. Topical anesthetics are used before insertion of endotracheal and LMA devices and also before laryngoscopy and bronchoscopy to prevent reflexive gagging. During regional cystoscopic procedures, transurethral instruments may be coated with a topical anesthetic gel to ease insertion. Topical agents are readily absorbed through the mucous membranes. Although the amount of agent applied is limited, the patient is monitored for toxic reactions.

Local Infiltration

Local infiltration is injection of an anesthetic into superficial tissues to produce a small area of anesthesia. The combination of an anesthetic and epinephrine sometimes is used to constrict blood vessels at the infiltration site and prevent dissipation of the anesthetic through the vascular system. Epinephrine also facilitates entry of the anesthetic into the nerve cell. Examples of procedures performed with local infiltration are excision of a skin lesion and insertion of a chest tube.

ROLE OF THE SURGICAL TECHNOLOGIST Local infiltration takes place after the patient has been prepped and draped as part of the surgical procedure. The scrubbed technologist assists the surgeon during infiltration as follows:

- Make sure supplies (including the anesthetic) are available before the procedure.

- Receive the anesthetic drug from the circulator and verify the amount and strength using proper technique (described fully in Chapter 13).
- Label the drug and syringe on the instrument table and protect it from contamination.
- Provide the following:
    At least two 25-, 26-, or 30-gauge needles
    Two 10- or 25-mL syringes
    Gauze sponges
- Fill one syringe to capacity and have another ready to use as necessary. Do not fill syringes partway. This may cause confusion about the amount of anesthetic used during the procedure.
- Separate all syringes and needles used for infiltration from others on the instrument table. Do not use the equipment for any purpose except infiltration of the local anesthetic.
- Note the total amount of anesthetic used and report this to the surgeon or circulating nurse as required.

Nerve Block

A peripheral nerve block provides anesthesia to a specific area of the body supplied by a major nerve or nerve plexus (group). The anesthetic agent is injected into the adjacent tissue, not into the nerve itself. The difference between a peripheral nerve block and local infiltration is that the objective of the nerve block is to anesthetize a single nerve, which results in blockade of its branches. Local infiltration is used to anesthetize a group of fine, usually superficial nerves in a small area.

The surgical technologist assists in the procedure using the same techniques as described for infiltration.

PROCEDURE The peripheral block is performed after a surgical skin prep of the injection area. The nerve block may be performed as part of the surgical procedure or separately before the surgical skin prep and draping. The procedure for injection is similar to infiltration anesthesia. The scrub assists when the nerve block is carried out as part of the surgery.

Intravenous (Bier) Block

Intravenous regional anesthesia is often referred to as a **Bier block** (Figure 14-10). In this procedure, blood is temporarily displaced from a limb and replaced by a local anesthetic drug. To displace the venous blood, an air-filled **pneumatic tourniquet** is placed around the proximal end of the limb. The ACP then displaces blood in the limb using a latex bandage (**Esmarch bandage**). The bandage is wrapped around the entire length of the extremity, starting at the distal end and extending to the proximal end. The tourniquet is then inflated, and the Esmarch bandage is removed. Anesthetic is injected into the major vein through a previously placed IV catheter. Double tourniquets also may be used, one proximal and one distal. The tourniquet "time" starts at the beginning of inflation and continues until the tourniquet is released. The safe tourniquet time and pressure depend on the patient's age, general condition, and size and surgical site.

ROLE OF THE SURGICAL TECHNOLOGIST The circulating surgical technologist assists in a Bier block by having the necessary

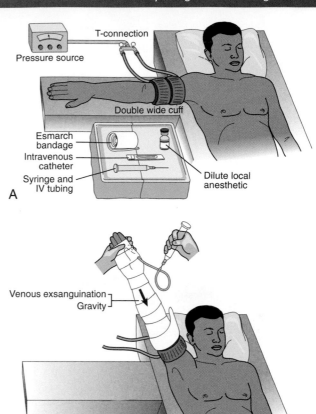

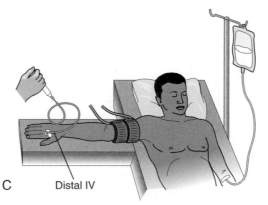

Figure 14-10 Intravenous (Bier) block. **A,** Equipment needed and position of double tourniquet. **B,** Venous exsanguination using Esmarch bandage and inflation of the tourniquet. **C,** Injection of the anesthetic into the vein. The upper tourniquet is then deflated. *(From Phillips N: Berry and Kohn's operating room technique, ed 10, St Louis, 2004, Mosby.)*

supplies and equipment prepared, and in the skin prep. The Bier block is an IV procedure and is performed using aseptic technique including skin prep and draping as described in Chapter 20. The hand may be excluded from the prep with an occlusive drape. The scrubbed technologist assists in draping the patient's arm and preparing the sterile equipment. The anesthesia care provider usually directs and performs the procedure. The surgeon or surgical technologist assists as required. The surgical technologist may be required to regown and reglove after the Bier block is performed and before the surgery begins.

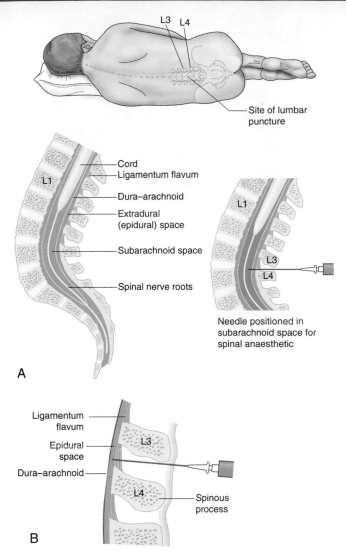

Figure 14-11 **A,** Area of injection for spinal anesthesia. The injection is made between L3 and L4 into the subarachnoid space. **B,** Epidural anesthesia. The injection is made into the epidural space. *(From Garden O, Bradbury A, Forsythe J, Parks R: Principles and practice of surgery, ed 5, Edinburgh, 2007, Churchill Livingstone.)*

Spinal Anesthesia

Spinal anesthesia is injection of anesthetic into the intrathecal (subarachnoid) space (Figure 14-11). To help facilitate correct placement of the anesthetic in the spinal canal, dextrose sometimes is added to the agent. This makes the drug heavier than the cerebrospinal fluid. In accordance with the patient's position, the drug settles in the dependent areas (those affected by gravity) and is absorbed at a specific site along the spinal cord.

Conduction along the nerve roots that emerge from that location is blocked, and anesthesia is achieved. The anesthetic can be directed up, down, or laterally by tilting the operating table. Spinal anesthesia can be used for many procedures but is most often used for gynecological, obstetrical, orthopedic, and genitourinary surgery.

PATIENT PREPARATION To facilitate exact placement of the spinal needle for injection, the patient must be positioned in a way that opens the intervertebral space. Two positions are

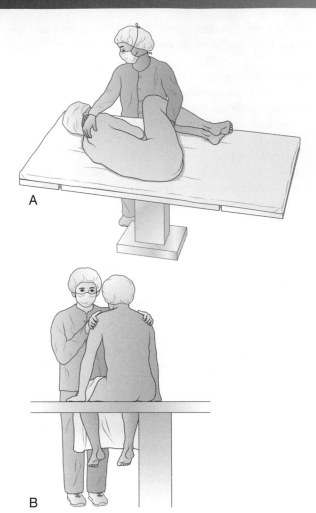

Figure 14-12 Position of the patient for spinal anesthesia. **A,** The patient is side lying with the lumbar area exposed. (The patient is shown without a blanket for clarification.) **B,** Sitting position. The circulator stabilizes the patient at the shoulders.

used to achieve this, lateral (side-lying) or sitting. A lateral position used with the patient's knees drawn up to facilitate exposure of the intervertebral spaces. The circulator stabilizes the patient's shoulders with one hand while providing support to the midleg with the other, as shown in Figure 14-12, *A*. The patient also may sit on the edge of the operating table and bend forward to create a rounded back. In this case, the circulator should support the patient as shown in Figure 14-12, *B*. The patient is covered with a blanket or sheet so that only the injection area is exposed. This provides warmth and protects the patient's modesty.

PROCEDURE When the patient has been positioned correctly, the ACP prepares the injection site with antiseptic and applies a small sterile drape. The spinal injection site is infiltrated with a small amount of anesthetic. A spinal needle is then inserted into intervertebral and subarachnoid space, and the anesthetic injected. The patient is placed in the supine position with a slight downward tilt (Trendelenburg position) to maintain a safe level of anesthesia. The patient given spinal anesthesia receives continuous physiological monitoring throughout the procedure and is given adjunct drugs to provide mild sedation and relaxation.

ROLE OF THE SURGICAL TECHNOLOGIST The surgical circulating surgical technologist assists in the procedure by preparing the spinal tray and correct size of spinal needles, prep solution, and drape as needed. The circulator helps the patient maintain his or her position during the procedure and verifies the type and strength of anesthetic used.

RISKS OF SPINAL ANESTHESIA Risks associated with spinal anesthesia include the following:

- *Hypotension:* A severe decrease in blood pressure may occur, resulting in pooling of blood in the lower extremities.
- *Postspinal headache:* This condition is related to decreased cerebrospinal pressure resulting from a leak at the injection site in the dura mater.
- *Total spinal anesthesia:* This occurs when the hyperbaric spinal anesthetic blocks the nerves controlling the diaphragm and accessory breathing muscles.

Epidural and Caudal Block

Epidural anesthesia is produced when the anesthetic agent is injected into the epidural space that surrounds the dural sac. The space contains connective tissue, an extensive vascular system, and the spinal nerve roots. Caudal and epidural anesthesia target the epidural space. However, in epidural anesthesia, the approach is through the lumbar interspace, whereas in caudal anesthesia, the caudal canal is used. A caudal epidural blockade produces analgesia of the perineum and groin and is therefore commonly administered during labor.

After injection, the anesthetic agent is very slowly absorbed into the cerebrospinal fluid through the dura mater. It spreads both caudally (toward the feet) and cephalad (toward the head). For a single-injection epidural, the patient's position and the molecular weight of the anesthetic have no effect on its distribution. However, with a continuous epidural, the position of the patient may affect the spread of the local anesthetic. Epidural anesthesia is often used in obstetrical, gynecological, urological, and rectal surgery. It also is used for postoperative pain control.

PROCEDURE The patient's skin is prepped as for spinal anesthesia. A thoracic, lumbar, or caudal puncture site is used, depending on the target site of anesthesia. The epidural needle is advanced through the skin until it enters the epidural space, and the anesthetic is injected (see Figure 14-12). Continuous or intermittent epidural anesthesia is provided through a small catheter placed in the epidural space for the duration of the surgery. This technique also is used for postoperative pain relief and for chronic pain management in selected patients.

In contrast to spinal anesthesia, epidural anesthesia requires a much larger amount of anesthetic agent. Accidental puncture of the dura mater can cause total spinal anesthesia. Also, because the epidural space has an extensive network of veins, overdose by accidental venous injection is a risk. If this occurs, the patient is immediately intubated and ventilated. Although the risk of hypotension exists with epidural anesthesia, the onset is slower than with spinal anesthesia and therefore easier to control and correct.

The role of the circulating surgical technologist is the same as for spinal anesthesia. All regional anesthetics are absorbed into the body and metabolized. This means that although regional anesthetics are relatively safe, exceeding the maximum dose may cause toxic reactions. If absorption is more rapid than metabolism, the risk of toxic reaction increases.

EMERGENCIES

The role of the surgical technologist at all times during an emergency is to protect the surgical field and provide assistance as directed. The surgical technologist may also be required to assist in cardiopulmonary resuscitation (CPR). However, CPR is meant to be a stopgap measure until biomedical intervention and medical care begin. Because these interventions are already in place in surgery, the patient is in the best location possible for a positive outcome.

REGIONAL DRUG TOXICITY AND ALLERGIC RESPONSE

Toxic reactions to local anesthetics arise most often during **regional block** and epidural anesthesia. This is because of the large amount of drug administered and the proximity to the vascular system. Toxic reactions related to regional anesthetics occur in two forms, central nervous system toxicity and cardiovascular toxicity.

Central Nervous System

CNS toxicity occurs in three phases. The *excitation phase* produces light headedness, restlessness, confusion, perioral tingling (tingling around the mouth), a metallic taste, tinnitus (ringing in the ears), and a sense of impending doom. The patient may become talkative. This phase is followed by the *convulsive phase*. Seizures can occur in this phase. The *depressive phase* is characterized by drowsiness, respiratory depression, and **apnea**.

Cardiovascular System

The first phase of cardiovascular toxicity is the *excitation phase*. The patient develops tachycardia, hypertension, and convulsions. This is followed by the *depressive phase*, which is characterized by decreased blood pressure, bradycardia, and possibly cardiac arrest.

Allergic Reaction

A true allergic reaction, which differs from reactions caused by toxicity, ranges from local skin irritation and itching to severe anaphylaxis, which produces life-threatening changes in the cardiovascular and respiratory systems. Maintaining verbal contact with the patient helps in the identification of symptoms. (Chapter 13 presents a complete discussion of drug hypersensitivity.)

Resuscitative equipment must be immediately available whenever a local anesthetic is administered. During any emergency, surgical technologists respond according to their training and scope of practice. Cardiopulmonary resuscitation is the minimum requirement for emergency response. Beyond this, the resuscitation team is responsible for administration of resuscitative drugs, airway maintenance, and advanced life support procedures.

CARDIOPULMONARY ARREST

All health care workers must maintain current certification in CPR and be able to respond in case of a cardiac or respiratory arrest. Personnel may not be employed in a health care facility without this certification. The goal of CPR is to support and restore oxygenation, ventilation, and circulation. Restoration of intact neurological function accompanies this process. Return of spontaneous circulation is accomplished with basic life support (BLS) or advanced cardiac life support (ACLS) measures. These follow distinct algorithms that depend on the nature of the emergency. Airway, breathing, and circulation are the most basic priorities, followed by administration of cardiac drugs and defibrillation as required. In the clinical setting, the defibrillator is immediately available on all crash carts. Automated external defibrillators are located throughout the healthcare facility for emergency treatment of specific conditions.

The signs and symptoms of cardiac arrest vary according to whether the patient is fully conscious at the time or sedated. A conscious patient may feel nausea, shortness of breath, chest pain or pressure, or pain radiating from the jaw, neck, or shoulder. Cardiac dysrhythmias are a warning of impending problems. Minor conduction changes are managed by the anesthesia care provider and all dysrhythmias are monitored carefully before, during, and after surgery. Sudden collapse and unresponsiveness may be the first signs of arrest. Resuscitative efforts must begin quickly to prevent neurological damage from lack of oxygen to the brain. Brain damage may occur as quickly as 3 minutes after circulatory collapse. Physiological monitoring during anesthesia permits immediate recognition of cardiac or respiratory failure. In these cases, medical assistance is immediately available.

Certification in CPR is the required method of ensuring complete knowledge and understanding of the procedure. All health care professionals and students are provided the opportunity for certification before beginning clinical work.

> *To obtain information about ACLS courses and certification, students should contact the American Heart Association or consult the organization's website at http:// www.americanheart.org/cpr.*

AIRWAY EMERGENCY

An airway emergency is one in which the unconscious patient cannot be intubated. In this case an artificial airway cannot be established as described earlier because of a difficult airway. The window of treatment to prevent hypoxia and subsequent brain damage is several minutes. The exact time depends on whether the patient was given extra oxygen before the event, such as during induction to general anesthesia.

Emergency response may include repeated attempts by more than one individual to intubate the patient either by endotracheal tube or LMA. An emergency airway cart containing all necessary equipment is maintained by the anesthesia department. If repeated attempts fail tracheotomy can be performed to establish the airway transcutaneously. In this case, the surgical technologist should be prepared to assist.

Emergency tracheotomy is an incision over the anterior wall of the trachea through the skin and strap muscles, and insertion of a tube to provide immediate access to air or anesthesia circuit. Refer to Chapter 28 for a description of a tracheotomy. An alternative treatment is the cricothyrotomy, in which an opening is made through the cricothyroid structures and a tracheotomy tube inserted. The procedure may have fewer complications than the tracheotomy and be faster to perform than the standard tracheotomy. In this procedure a 10-gauge needle is inserted across the cricothyroid membrane. The needle is used to ventilate the patient through the anesthesia circuit by *jet or high-velocity* ventilation (often referred to as transtracheal jet ventilation).

LARYNGOSPASM

Spasm of the larynx is usually is associated with airway secretions or stimulation of the laryngeal nerve during intubation or extubation. The condition may lead to complete airway obstruction. It is treated with mechanical ventilation or, in severe cases, administration of succinylcholine to paralyze the muscles. Laryngospasm constitutes an emergency when an airway cannot be immediately established by positive-pressure ventilation. Patients with a difficult airway, such as those who are obese, have the highest risk for laryngospasm.

ANAPHYLAXIS

Anaphylaxis is a true allergic reaction to a substance or drug that can lead to shock (see next section). In surgery, this is most commonly associated with regional anesthesia. Signs and symptoms include rash, abnormal lung sounds detected during auscultation, wheezing, and difficulty breathing. In the event of anaphylaxis, the ACP, nurse, or surgeon immediately administers multiple doses of epinephrine. Other respiratory drugs and antihistamines are administered as needed. Airway assistance may be required. The on-call resuscitation team is alerted if no physician is in the room, and an airway and oxygen administration are quickly established. The preoperative examination and preanesthesia evaluation often can predict allergic response to substances or drug groups, and preventive measures are very valuable.

SHOCK

During severe shock, the supply of oxygen and nutrients to all body tissues is inadequate. This is caused by a cascade of physiological events that begins with a variety of conditions in which the body's compensatory mechanisms focus on shunting blood (and oxygen) to the most vital organs. In hypovolemic shock (caused by decreased vascular volume), the heart rate increases initially, and there is widespread vasoconstriction. Capillary flow diminishes or is shut down. The body tries to conserve fluid by reducing renal blood flow and increasing water retention in the kidneys. Urinary output is diminished or ceases. Eventually multiple organ failure occurs as a result of oxygen and nutrient starvation at the cellular level.

Types of Shock

- *Circulatory shock* is a state of inadequate blood volume for supplying the whole body. This type of shock can be caused by hemorrhage, burns (in which a dramatic shift of body fluids occurs), or severe diuresis (excretion of fluids through the renal system).
- *Cardiogenic shock* is caused by heart failure, which disables the vascular system because blood cannot be pumped adequately throughout the body.
- *Anaphylactic shock* is caused by true allergy, resulting in vasodilation and pooling of blood, which slows or halts normal circulation.
- *Neurogenic shock* is caused by failure of the autonomic nervous system to maintain vascular tone. This type of shock can be caused by specific drugs, brain injury, anesthesia, or spinal cord injury.
- *Septic shock* is caused by severe infection, which results in hypovolemia. Bacterial infection most often is the cause of septic shock, which can be rapidly fatal. Disseminated intravascular coagulation (DIC) is a complication of septic shock in which microcoagulation occurs in the cells. This depletes the body's platelets and other clotting factors, leading to continuous hemorrhage and death.

Treatment for shock is targeted at restoring circulatory function, electrolyte balance, and oxygenation of tissues. The immediate emergency response is related to the cause. However, in all cases, *Anaphylaxis* circulatory balance is a priority. This may necessitate administration of fluid or blood components and drug therapy to improve the systemic blood pressure. The exact cause of the crisis is determined early in treatment so that appropriate emergency measures can be initiated.

MALIGNANT HYPERTHERMIA

Malignant hyperthermia (MH) is a rare physiological response to all volatile anesthetic agents and succinylcholine. MH causes a severe immediate or delayed hypermetabolism. The patient exhibits an extremely high core temperature, tachycardia, tachypnea, and increased muscle rigidity. Metabolic crises accompany the physical signs and include an increase in intracellular calcium ions, respiratory acidosis, metabolic acidosis, and hemodynamic instability, which may lead to cardiac arrest and death.

MH is related to a familial genetic trait. Patients with family members known to have experienced MH usually report this to the ACP during the preoperative evaluation. However, no method has been devised of predicting MH when the patient has no family or personal history of the condition.

A malignant hypothermia cart is maintained in the surgical department so that all emergency equipment and drugs can be brought in immediately, because time is extremely important. The cart contains cooling equipment, including Foley catheters, plastic bags, tubing, peritoneal lavage equipment, and nasogastric tubes. Emergency drugs for MH treatment include dantrolene (Dantrium) and agents to treat specific metabolic disorders.

If MH symptoms occur during surgery, the ACP alerts the team immediately. Treatment requires immediate cessation of anesthesia and drug therapy to treat the adverse metabolic symptoms. The scrub remains sterile to help protect the surgical incision. When immediate body cooling is required, the surgeon and ACP may initiate cold irrigation in open body cavities, ice packs, and a cold IV solution. The scrub receives sterile equipment, ice, and fluids to assist in lowering the body temperature. Therapy is continued until the patient is stabilized. The surgical wound is closed quickly when surgery must be halted. The patient is transported to the intensive care unit for further treatment and observation.

HEMORRHAGE

In the event of severe hemorrhage during surgery, blood volume is restored by giving blood substitutes, blood components, or autologous blood (the patient's own blood previously banked or harvested at the surgical site). Allogeneic (donor) blood transfusions may also be provided.

Packed red cells are mostly commonly used for transfusion, because the patient's immediate need is oxygen-carrying capacity. All blood products must be matched with the patient's blood type. A precise protocol has evolved to prevent the administration of blood of the wrong type. Whether the patient's own blood or banked blood is used, meticulous attention is given to patient identification, blood group, registration number, and date of expiration. Blood usually is brought from the blood bank shortly before surgery; in an emergency, it is brought immediately. Blood must be stored in a location known to all personnel and protected from direct heat. Unused blood must be returned to the blood bank as soon as possible.

Intraoperative cell salvage (autotransfusion) is the immediate harvesting of blood on the surgical field and reinfusion into the patient. This may be planned in advance of a high risk surgery or implemented in an emergency. Special equipment is required for this procedure. The prototype autotransfusion system is the Cell Saver. However, other systems have now been developed. Scrubs must be familiar with the cell salvage device used in their facility, because special training is required.

HEMOLYTIC REACTION

Hemolysis is the rupture of red blood cells. It is associated with ABO factor incompatibility during blood transfusion. Before any transfusion, the ABO and Rh systems are tested and crossmatched against the donor blood. However, mistakes in recording and reading blood registrations do occur, with serious consequences. Patients under anesthesia do not show the signs and symptoms seen in a fully conscious patient. ABO mismatch during transfusion outside of surgery produces the following symptoms:

- Back pain
- Chills
- Hypotension
- Dyspnea

These can lead to complete vascular collapse or renal failure. In surgery, the only symptoms likely to appear are oliguria (cessation of renal output) and generalized bleeding. Treatment requires stopping the transfusion and immediate hydration with IV fluids and forced diuresis.

DEEP VEIN THROMBOSIS

An embolus is any moving particle within the vascular system. Risk factors for emboli include trauma, orthopedic fracture, burns, surgical procedures involving flexion and rotation of the hip, and use of a pneumatic tourniquet. Venous stasis, or "pooling," occurs when the patient is immobile for long periods, which can lead to clotting. A thrombus may form in proximal deep veins and subsequently break loose, preventing circulation to a vital organ such as the lung (**pulmonary embolism [PE]**). Symptoms may become apparent at any point in the perioperative period. Prevention of deep vein thrombosis (DVT) includes preoperative application of anti-embolic stockings, use of a sequential compression device, and prophylactic medication when appropriate. Other preventive measures include slow, deliberate movement of limbs during positioning and following DVT and PE protocols according to hospital policy. Treatment for DVT includes drug therapy to prevent further embolization and treatment for the specific emergency condition, such as shock and respiratory arrest.

HISTORICAL HIGHLIGHTS

Neuroleptanalgesia and neuroleptanesthesia are two methods of pain control introduced in the late 1940s. This technique involved a combination of drugs (anxiolytics and powerful analgesics) that suppressed the autonomic nervous system and produced immobility. The method was retired from human medicine many years ago as much safer and more predictable drugs were developed for conscious sedation.

KEY CONCEPTS

- The principles and concepts of anesthesia are defined using specific terms that have detailed meanings. Many of these terms are unique to the process of anesthesia and must be used appropriately to avoid miscommunication.
- Terms used to describe the process and medical aspects of anesthesia differ from the lay terms, which are often vague and inaccurate. Accuracy in communication among health care workers is a fundamental necessity in safe patient care.

- Anesthesia is a subspecialty of medicine. Within the practice there are a number of different professional roles performed by physicians and nonphysician specialists. An understanding of these various roles and the credentialing necessary to perform them is important to team communication and appreciation of the professionals involved.
- The anesthesia evaluation is a critical assessment of the patient's physiological fitness for surgery. Information gathered during the assessment is of interest to all members of the surgical team, who must be informed about the patient's condition.
- The type of anesthesia selected for a particular patient is determined by many different criteria. An understanding of how these criteria are weighed is important to an overall understanding of the process of anesthesia.
- Preparation of the patient for anesthesia has changed dramatically in recent years. This is especially relevant to the use of preoperative medications and requirements for specific investigations and tests in the preoperative period. The surgical technologist should be aware of new trends and how these might affect patient care.
- Anesthesia equipment and devices used in physiological monitoring are increasingly complex. However, the most basic devices are those used to establish and maintain the airway. All team members must be familiar with basic airway technology in order to assist in the event of emergency.
- Airway management is the first of three (airway, breathing, circulation) critical interventions in a physiological emergency and in routine care of the patient. Surgical technologists should develop a basic understanding related to the problems of airway management, and how these are resolved.
- General anesthesia that produces unconsciousness is achieved and maintained using a variety of procedures and drugs. It is necessary to study the basics of anesthesia because the process relates directly to patient care and the surgical procedure itself.
- Manipulation of the patient's level of consciousness, sensory awareness, and physiological processes is possible using a variety of drugs and methods of anesthesia. All members of the surgical team need to be aware of the differences in these methods.
- The surgical technologist is directly involved in certain types of regional anesthesia. He or she must understand how the drugs are used, when they are used, and how they are delivered. Knowledge of all phases of the drug process and how it relates to the administration of regional anesthetic is necessary for safe practice.
- Anesthesia emergencies are those that occur as a direct result of the drugs used, or to a physiological emergency that occurs while the patient is under anesthetic. Some emergencies require action by the entire surgical team. Individual roles depend on the type of emergency.
- The surgical technologist has distinct roles during some types of emergencies with which he or she should be completely familiar. This includes knowledge of what to do,

when to do it, and what equipment is needed to provide emergency assistance.

REVIEW QUESTIONS

1. Under what medical circumstances might regional anesthesia be used?
2. What educational and certification processes differentiate an anesthesiologist from an anesthetist?
3. What is the purpose of the ASA risk assessment classification?
4. Why is a musculoskeletal assessment necessary for the preoperative patient?
5. What are some considerations in selecting an appropriate method of anesthesia?
6. Define *homeostasis*.
7. What is physiological monitoring?
8. Name and define the five parameters of physiological monitoring discussed in this chapter.
9. What is the normal core temperature range for an adult?
10. What are protective reflexes? Describe four or more protective reflexes.
11. Describe commonly used methods of regional anesthesia.
12. Into what specific tissue is a spinal anesthetic administered? An epidural anesthetic?
13. Describe deep vein thrombosis and pulmonary embolism. How are these conditions prevented?

CASE STUDIES

Case 1

A patient arrives in the operating room for surgery to be performed under general anesthesia. You have been assigned to assist the perioperative registered nurse circulator during the case. The anesthesiologist assists in settling the patient and preoperative medications are administered. The team is ready to start and the patient is induced. Immediately after intubation, the anesthesiologist hands you the patient's dentures, which she has just removed, and asks you to take care of them. What should you do with these? Should the dentures have been removed before the patient arrived in surgery?

Case 2

You are assigned to assist in circulator duties on a procedure requiring spinal anesthesia in your teaching hospital. Your immediate task is to help position the patient for the spinal and help the patient maintain the position while the spinal is administered. The patient states to you that she is afraid, but you reassure her that there will be little discomfort. The anesthesia care provider and anesthesia resident state that the patient should be placed in a side-lying position. The anesthesia procedure begins:

1. The anesthesia care provider tells the resident that he or she should go ahead and perform the procedure. The resident

steps forward and applies a cold prep solution to the injection site. The patient flinches and moves out of position. What do you do?
2. The local anesthetic has been injected into the spinal injection site and the resident searches for the correct insertion site for the spinal needle by palpating the intervertebral spaces. The patient asks you quietly if the needle is in yet. What do you reply?
3. Now the resident has made four attempts to enter the subarachnoid space. Fresh spinal needles have been brought into the room for more attempts. The patient is now very uncomfortable and feeling the pain of the repeated insertions of the spinal needle by the resident. Two more attempts are made without success. What should you say to your patient, who is visibly upset and trying to remain still?
4. What, if any, is your dialogue with the resident during these attempts?
5. Finally, after many attempts, the anesthesia care provider takes over and is able to insert the spinal needle at first try. Everyone is relieved. Think carefully about what you would say to the patient at this point.

Case 3

You are assigned to scrub on a case requiring local infiltration anesthetic with moderate sedation for removal of a skin lesion on the leg. The patient is positioned on the operating table and the anesthetist applies monitoring devices and administers light sedation. The surgeon arrives and states that he will inject the local anesthetic and then go out to scrub. You have prepared the local anesthetic and the surgeon puts on gloves and infiltrates the surgical site. He then leaves the room. You have completed your setup and are ready for the case. The circulator has left the room to check on the surgical schedule. The anesthetist states that he needs to step into the hallway to speak to a colleague, and asks you to keep an eye on the patient. Within moments, the patient appears restless. You note that the patient's heart rate has increased dramatically, as tracked by the cardiac monitor. The patient mumbles something and without contaminating your gown and gloves you come closer to try and understand what he is saying. You are alarmed to see that the patient is quite pale.

1. What should you do?
2. This scenario might be the beginning of an emergency. Was there any violation of patient care responsibilities? Think carefully about this.
3. After the situation is resolved you mention to the circulator that it might be necessary to fill out an incident report. He replies "Oh, that's not necessary, nothing bad happened." What is your response to this?

REFERENCES

1. Mace SE: Challenges and advances in intubation: airway evaluation and controversies with intubation, *Emerg Med Clin North Am* 26(4):977.
2. Miller R, Eriksson L, Fleisher L, et al: *Miller's anesthesia*, ed 7, Philadelphia, 2009, Churchill Livingstone.

BIBLIOGRAPHY

American Society of Anesthesiologists Committee on Standards and Practice Parameters: *Pulmonary aspiration: application to healthy patients undergoing elective procedures, Anesthesiology* 114:495, 2011.

Association of periOperative Registered Nurses (AORN): *Standards, recommended practices and guidelines, 2011 edition*, Denver, 2011, AORN.

Hemmings H, Hopkins P: *Foundations of anesthesia*, ed 2, St Louis, 2006, Elsevier/Saunders.

Kee J, Hayes E, McCuistion L: *Pharmacology: a nursing process approach*, ed 5, St Louis, 2006, Elsevier/Saunders.

Miller R, Eriksson L, Fleisher L, et al: *Miller's anesthesia*, ed 7, Philadelphia, 2009, Churchill Livingstone.

Nagelhout J, Zaglaniczny K: *Nurse anesthesia*, ed 3, St Louis, 2005, Elsevier/Saunders.

Phillips N: *Berry and Kohn's operating room technique*, ed 11, St Louis, 2007, Mosby.

Porth C: *Pathophysiology: concepts of altered health states*, ed 6, Philadelphia, 2002, Lippincott Williams & Wilkins.

The Joint Commission: *Preventing and managing the impact of anesthesia awareness*. Accessed August 27, 2011, at http://www.jointcommission.org/sentinel_event_alert_issue_32_preventing_and_managing_the_impact_of_anesthesia_awareness.

Thibodeau G, Patton K: *Anatomy and physiology*, ed 6, St Louis, 2007, Elsevier/Saunders.

Postanesthesia Recovery

CHAPTER OUTLINE

LEARNING OBJECTIVES

After studying this chapter the reader will be able to:

1. Describe the layout of the PACU
2. Discuss the elements of a handover from the circulating nurse to the PACU nurse
3. List the elements of patient assessment
4. Describe the Glasgow Coma Scale
5. Discuss selected types of postoperative complications
6. Define the purpose of discharge planning
7. Discuss the rationale for patient education
8. Discuss unanticipated PACU outcomes

TERMINOLOGY

Activities of daily living (ADLs): Basic activities and tasks necessary for day-to-day self care, such as dressing, bathing, toileting, and meal preparation.

Arterial blood gases (ABGs): A blood test that measures the level of oxygen and carbon dioxide and the pH of the blood.

Aspiration: Inhalation of fluid or solid matter.

Auscultation: Listening to the lungs, heart, or abdomen through the stethoscope.

Bronchospasm: Partial or complete closure of the bronchial tubes.

Discharge against medical advice (AMA): Self-discharge by a patient who has not necessarily met discharge criteria.

Discharge criteria: Objective criteria used to determine whether a patient is safe for discharge from the health care facility.

Glasgow Coma Scale (GCS): A standardized method of measuring a patient's response to external stimuli.

Handover (hand-off): A verbal and written report from one nurse to another to provide updated patient information.

Hypothermia: Body temperature that is below normal.

Hypoxia: Lack of oxygen in the tissue.

Laryngospasm: Muscular spasm of the larynx, resulting in obstruction.

Malignant hyperthermia (MH): A potentially fatal syndrome of hypermetabolism that results in an extremely high body temperature, cardiac dysrhythmia, and respiratory distress.

Perfusion: Flow of blood to tissue.

Prognosis: A prediction of the patient's medical outcome (e.g., poor prognosis, good prognosis).

INTRODUCTION

After surgery, patients are transported to the postanesthesia care unit (PACU) for recovery. Postoperative patients are at risk for immediate postoperative complications that may require an emergency medical response. The PACU is staffed by critical care nurses who are trained in postoperative recovery and emergency medicine. The unit is equipped with all necessary physiological monitoring equipment, drugs, and emergency supplies. The PACU is close to the surgical suites for rapid transfer of patients after surgery. In some facilities, the PACU also functions as an ambulatory patient recovery area.

PACU FACILITY

The floor plan of the PACU usually is one large room with separate patient stations along two or more perimeter walls. Patient beds (stretchers) are positioned in the individual care areas (or *cubicles*) on the perimeter wall in view of a central nursing station.

This arrangement allows the staff to attend to patients quickly and efficiently. Stretchers can be easily moved within the unit and around the cubicles. Because there are no walls between patients, diagnostic equipment such as portable radiograph machines, 12-lead electrocardiograph equipment, and emergency crash carts can be brought to the bedside quickly and with minimal maneuvering. The central nursing station is equipped with patient telemetry monitors, phones, and computers. Each patient cubicle has outlets for suction, oxygen, power, and high level lighting. Individual patient monitoring is transmitted through the department telemetry system so that staff members at the central nursing station can view each patient screen individually. Medication and supplies are dispensed from designated areas attached to the main patient area. Emergency airway equipment, including a tracheostomy tray, is kept in an easily accessible area and on crash carts.

The PACU is fully equipped with patient care supplies which would normally be found on any nursing unit. These include dressings, catheters, airways, and medication administration devices.

In addition to individual patient cubicles, an isolation area provides barrier protection for selected patients, such as those with an active infection. The PACU may also have a designated area for pediatric patients.

If ambulatory patients recover in the same department as inpatients, a designated area is provided with changing rooms, a lounge, and an ambulatory discharge area. Side rooms provide space for dictation, patient and family conferences, and staff lockers.

PACU PROCEDURES

ADMISSION

Patients are admitted to the PACU immediately after surgery. When the patient arrives at the unit, an assigned PACU nurse receives the individual and assists the circulating nurse and anesthesia care provider (ACP) in setting up the patient in a cubicle. Electrocardiogram (ECG) leads, the pulse oximeter sensor, oxygen, and suction are immediately engaged. The patient's level of pain and consciousness, airway, circulatory status, oxygen perfusion, and temperature are then assessed.

HANDOVER (HAND-OFF)

Once all monitoring devices are in place and the patient is stable, the circulating nurse performs a **handover** (also called a **hand-off**) to the PACU nurse. The circulator or ACP communicates all information needed to update the PACU nurse on the patient's physiological status before and during surgery. The ACP provides specific orders for continuation of care and a smooth recovery. The circulator and ACP remain with the patient until the handover is complete. The following verbal and written information is provided in the handover:

1. A brief patient history. This follows standard nursing and medical protocol and includes the patient's age, allergies, current medications, and existing pathology. This is the patient's preoperative status.

   Rationale: This information is relevant to proper assessment of current signs and symptoms and for continuity of nursing care.

2. The exact surgery that was performed, including the side and site (e.g., right colectomy with colostomy).

   Rationale: This is reported so that the PACU staff knows exactly where the surgical wounds are and the extent of the surgery for continuous postoperative care, monitoring, and assessment.

3. The total length of time anesthesia was delivered and the drugs given during that time. The amounts and routes are also reported.

   Rationale: Drugs given during the preoperative and intraoperative phase have a direct pharmacological effect on those administered postoperatively. The cumulative effect and drug interactions must be considered when additional medications are administered. The PACU nurse must know what drugs were given to anticipate physiological changes caused by the drugs.

4. Estimated blood loss and the amount and type of intravenous (IV) fluids or blood administered. If blood products were administered, the type and amount are reported.

   Rationale: The estimated blood loss is needed to determine the need for further action, such as transfusion. Total fluids given during surgery are balanced against output. This information contributes to the patient's overall medical "picture" so that evaluation is accurate. Blood loss or fluid imbalance explains specific physiological signs that trigger a nursing or medical response in the postoperative period.

5. Condition of the wound, drains, and other devices. If the surgical wound contains drains or a drainage device such as suction or closed water-seal drainage, this is reported in detail. The amount, color, and consistency of the drainage fluid are noted.

   Rationale: Wound assessment and care are of primary importance during the postoperative period. A baseline assessment provides information against which subsequent evaluations are compared. Changes in wound drainage may indicate bleeding, which requires an immediate medical response.

6. ASA score. Each patient is assigned a score according to the system established by the American Society of Anesthesiologists (ASA). This score reflects the patient's overall health status (see Chapter 14).

   Rationale: The ASA score is reported on postoperative records and is used in patient care planning.

7. Any surgical or medical complications that occurred during surgery.

   Rationale: This alerts the PACU staff to the patient's current condition and further complications. The information also is needed in case follow-up measures are required, such as radiographic films or blood tests.

8. Information about family members (e.g., contact numbers or location) who may be waiting in the family room.

   Rationale: The PACU staff maintains contact with the family during the postoperative period to update them on the patient's progress, condition, and discharge plans.

PATIENT ASSESSMENT AND CARE

After accepting the handover, the PACU nurse performs a patient assessment. This can be either a focused assessment or a head to toe assessment. The focused assessment, as the name implies, focuses on specific criteria, such as respiration, circulation, pain, and level of consciousness. The *head to toe assessment* covers all or most body systems. Standard procedures are used to assess specific functions. General assessment procedures are carried out to obtain baseline information. This may lead to more complex methods of testing, such as blood tests, a 12-lead ECG, or radiographs. All findings are documented in the PACU record (Figure 15-1).

Respiratory System

- The airway is assessed by **auscultation** (listening with a stethoscope) and by observation for signs of airway obstruction.
- The respiratory rate and rhythm (patterns) are measured by observation of the thorax and accessory muscles during breathing.

Circulation

- **Perfusion** (flow of blood to tissue) is measured by pulse oximeter.
- The color of the patient's skin and mucous membranes is observed for signs of **hypoxia** (inadequate oxygen to tissues).
- The heart is monitored for rate and rhythm using ECG leads and a cardiac monitor, which produces a digital waveform.
- Heart sounds are assessed with the stethoscope and may be amplified by the cardiac monitor.
- The arterial pressure is measured directly with an arterial line or indirectly by taking the patient's blood pressure with a digital sphygmomanometer.
- **Arterial blood gases (ABGs)** (the ratio of oxygen to carbon dioxide and the blood pH) may be measured by taking a blood sample from an artery. In the modern PACU, the sample can be analyzed immediately.
- The central venous pressure may be measured with an inline catheter or subjectively by observing the jugular veins.
- The presence or absence of a peripheral pulse is determined by palpation or by Doppler.

Core Temperature

- The patient's temperature is assessed continuously or intermittently using a digital thermometer or temperature probe.
- Hypothermia is a serious postoperative complication. The patient is continually observed for signs such as shivering.

Abdomen

- The abdomen is assessed for distention (which may indicate the presence of fluid, including blood or air). This is done by observation, palpation, and radiographs.

- Bowel sounds are assessed by auscultation. A persistent lack of bowel sounds may indicate surgical paralytic ileus—cessation of peristalsis in the bowel leading to obstruction. Persistent paralytic ileus is a serious postoperative complication.

Fluid and Electrolyte Balance

- Fluid shifts from the vascular space to the intracellular space can occur after surgery, and the patient must be evaluated carefully for this.
- Assessment for dehydration includes physical signs and symptoms. Replacement fluids are administered intravenously as needed.
- Electrolyte imbalance is assessed through blood tests and specific physiological signs of imbalance, such as alteration in consciousness or cardiac dysrhythmia.

Neurological Function
LEVEL OF CONSCIOUSNESS

- The patient's level of consciousness is assessed using the **Glasgow Coma Scale (GCS).** In this system, points are assigned to the response to specific stimuli (shown here). The GCS score is calculated as the total of all parameters. A score of 15 indicates the best **prognosis** (medical outcome), whereas a minimum score of 3 indicates a poor prognosis. The following parameters are evaluated:

Eye Opening
  (4) Spontaneously
  (3) To voice
  (2) To pain
  (1) No response

Best Verbal Response
  (5) Oriented and converses
  (4) Disoriented and converses
  (3) Inappropriate words
  (2) Incomprehensible sounds
  (1) No response

Best Motor Response
  (6) Obeys simple command
  (5) Localizes to pain
  (4) Flexion—withdrawal or abnormal
  (3) Abnormal flexion
  (2) Extension
  (1) No response

Pain

- Pain is assessed using the following tools:
  Alertness: Asleep to hyperalert
  Level of calmness: Calm to panicky
  Movement: No movement to vigorous movement
  Facial expression: Face relaxed to contortion or grimacing
  Blood pressure: Baseline or below to 15% or more elevation
  Heart rate: At or below baseline to 15% or more elevation
  Vocalization: No vocalization to crying out

FORREST GENERAL HOSPITAL
POST ANESTHESIA CARE UNIT RECORD

POST ANESTHESIA RECOVERY SCORE		MINUTES in	30	60	90	out
Activity						
Able to move 4 extremities voluntarily or on command	= 2					
Able to move 2 extremities voluntarily or on command	= 1					
Able to move 0 extremities voluntarily or on command	= 0					
Respiration						
Able to deep breathe and cough freely	= 2					
Dyspnea or limited breathing	= 1					
Apneic	= 0					
Circulation						
BP ± 20 of Preanesthetic level	= 2					
BP ± 20-50 of Preanesthetic level	= 1					
BP ± 50 of Preanesthetic level	= 0					
Consciousness						
Fully Awake	= 2					
Arousable on calling	= 1					
Not Responding	= 0					
O_2 Saturation						
Able to maintain O_2 Sat > 92% on room air	= 2					
Needs O_2 to maintain O_2 Sat > 90%	= 1					
O_2 Sat < 90% even with O_2	= 0					
TOTAL						

Pre-op B.P. ________
Allergy

Airway: On Adm.
Jawthrust ________
Chin Hold ________
Endotracheal ________
Oral Airway ________
Mask Oxygen ________
Nasal Oxygen ________
Trach ________
T-Tube ________
Nasal Airway ________
Ventilator Settings ________

Addressograph

Time In ________ Time Out ________
Accompanied by ________
Type of anesthesia ________
Surgical Procedure:

PULSE - RESPIRATION - BLOOD PRESSURE

	15	30	45	15	30	45	15	30	45	15	30	45
240												
220												
200												
180												
160												
140												
120												
100												
80												
60												
40												
20												
O_2 Sat.												
PAP												

CODES: ⊥ A-line, T B.P. | V Manual or Λ NBP | Pulse •, Resp. ○ | Siderails: Yes / No | Restraints: Yes / No

IV Type ________
Total IV in OR ________ cc
Blood in OR ________ units
Urinary Output in OR ________ cc
Est. Blood Loss ________ cc

Foley Cath. ________
Suprapubic ________
Ureteral ________
Levine ________

DRAINS

MEDICATIONS AND TREATMENTS

	AMT.	ROUTE	TIME
Demerol			
Morphine			
Phenergan			
Droperidol			
Zofran			
Toradol			

________ RN Signature

________ RN Signature

FORREST GENERAL HOSPITAL

DATE	TIME	DESCRIPTIVE NOTES (SIGN EACH ENTRY)

Report to Family: Time:	GU IRRIGANT	FOLEY OUTPUT
	TOTAL INFUSED:	TOTAL OUTPUT:

Figure 15-1 PACU record. *(Courtesy Forrest General Hospital, Hattiesburg, Miss.)*

PACU DISCHARGE SUMMARY

VITAL SIGNS ON DISCHARGE	PACU OUTCOME	COMFORT LEVEL
R/P: P. R: T:	UNEVENTFUL ☐	PAIN FREE ☐ PAIN CONTROLLED ☐ SLEEPING BUT C/O PAIN WHEN
OXIMETER: PAR SCORE:	COMPLICATIONS ☐	AWAKEN ☐

REPORT TO: TIME:	SKIN CONDITION WARM COOL DRY MOIST	COLOR PINK PALE JAUNDICED DUSKY

DRESSINGS / SURGICAL SITE / PUNCTURE SITE

X-RAYS TAKEN IN PACU	LABS DRAWN IN PACU	O₂ ORDERED YES NO _____ L/MIN PER _____ O₂ TRANSPORT YES NO

TOTAL IV IN PACU	TOTAL OUTPUT IN PACU		
	URINARY	LEVINE	DRAINS
TOTAL BLOOD IN PACU			
TOTAL PO INTAKE IN PACU	IV SITE:		

_____ cc LTC

ORDERS FAXED TO PHARMACY YES NO	EQUIPMENT ORDERED	TRANSPORT BY: AMBASSADOR RN LPN TECHNICIAN

DIAGNOSIS (Circle number of any diagnosis made)	GOAL	Goal Achieved	
		YES	NO
1 Alteration in neurological status			
2 Alteration in comfort level			
3 Alteration in emotional status			
4 Alteration in circulation			
5 Alteration in fluid volume			
6 Alteration in mobility			
7 Alteration in respiratory function			
8 Alteration in skin integrity			
9 Alteration in temperature			
10 Alteration in elimination			
11 Alteration in gastrointestinal function			
12 Alteration in injury			
13 Alteration in bleeding			
14 Other			

RHYTHM STRIPS

Figure 15-1, cont'd.

- The assessment of pain in a preverbal child is described in Table 15-1.

Muscular Response

- Patient able to move on command
- Muscular strength (also related to neurological function)

Renal Function

- Urinary output is measured in milliliters per hour (includes intraoperative measurements). Urinary retention may be caused by neurological deficit and requires more complex assessment and treatment.
- Appearance of urine
- Selected blood tests

Wound Assessment

- Drainage amount, color, and consistency
- Incision assessment
- Swelling noted, measured for baseline reference

Catheters and Tubing

- Drainage amount, color
- Drains and catheters intact, open
- Intravenous lines intact

PSYCHOSOCIAL CARE

The PACU staff provides continual emotional support to the patient. Patients often need reassurance and orientation to

Table **15-1**	**Comfort Scale for Infants**
Sign	**Assessment Score***
Alertness	1. Sleeping deeply
	2. Sleeping lightly
	3. Drowsy
	4. Fully alert
	5. Hypervigilant
Calmness	1. Calm
	2. Slightly anxious
	3. Anxious
	4. Appears panicky
	5. Panicky
Crying	1. Quiet breathing, no crying
	2. Sobbing or gasping
	3. Moaning
	4. Crying
	5. Screaming
Physical movement	1. No movement
	2. Occasional slight movement
	3. Frequent slight movement
	4. Vigorous movement
	5. Vigorous movement, including head and torso
Muscle tone	1. Muscles totally relaxed
	2. Reduced muscle tone
	3. Normal muscle tone
	4. Increased muscle tone with flexion of fingers, toes
	5. Extreme muscle rigidity with flexion of fingers, toes
Facial tension	1. Facial muscles relaxed
	2. Facial muscle tone normal
	3. Tension in some facial muscles
	4. Tension throughout facial muscles
	5. Grimacing or contortion of facial muscles
Blood pressure baseline	1. Below baseline
	2. Consistently at baseline
	3. Infrequent elevations 15% or more above baseline
	4. Frequent elevation 15% or more above baseline
	5. Sustained elevation 15% or more
Heart rate baseline	1. Below baseline
	2. Consistently at baseline
	3. Infrequent elevations of 15% or more above baseline
	4. Frequent elevation 15% or more above baseline
	5. Sustained elevation 15% or more

From the National Institutes of Health Warren Grant Magnuson Clinical Center, 2003.
*Scores are assessed as a total from 9 to 45.

their environment while emerging from general anesthesia or heavy sedation. Patients may be fearful of their diagnosis or the results of the surgery. Although not fully conscious, they may return emotionally to the preoperative state of anxiety. Patients need to know that although they may not be fully functioning, they are being cared for, and they need to know who is caring for them. In some cases, the surgeon may see the patient briefly and explain the results of the surgery.

Family awaiting the results of the surgery and the patient's emergence from anesthesia also need contact with the PACU staff. The nurse may visit the family (which includes friends) in the waiting area to let them know the patient's progress and estimated time of discharge from the unit.

POSTOPERATIVE COMPLICATIONS

Postanesthesia complications occur because patients are physiologically unstable during the immediate postoperative period and may react to the procedure or drugs administered intraoperatively. They are vulnerable to pain, hemorrhage, reaction to the anesthetic agents, and rapid changes in homeostasis. The PACU staff is specially trained in critical care monitoring and response. Note that the physiological complications discussed in Chapter 14 can occur during the postoperative period.

PAIN

Although pain is expected in the postsurgical phase, not all patients respond to pain in the same way. A patient's response to pain is affected by previous experience, level of anxiety, the drugs used during surgery, and environmental factors. Patients also respond to pain according to what is acceptable in their culture. For example, in some cultures, crying out is acceptable, whereas in others it is not. Pain management requires assessment and planning to ensure a smooth recovery. Analgesics are administered according to the patient's level of consciousness, cardiopulmonary status, and age.

RESPIRATORY

Respiratory problems are the most frequent life-threatening postoperative complication. Inadequate ventilation can be related to the effects of anesthetic drugs, pain, muscle relaxants, or fluid-electrolyte imbalance. Inadequate intake of air and oxygen results in the accumulation of carbon dioxide in the blood. Normally, a high carbon dioxide level triggers the autonomic nervous system to stimulate breathing. However, drugs administered during the intraoperative period suppress this reflex. Pain at the operative site is another cause of **hypoventilation,** resulting in low oxygen saturation. For example, patients with abdominal or thoracic incisions do not breathe deeply because of the pain at the operative site.

Airway Obstruction

Airway obstruction most often is caused by anatomical structures or by aspiration of fluids. The tongue or soft palate can obstruct the airway in a state of deep relaxation related to anesthetic agents and adjunct drugs.

Contraction of the laryngeal muscles (**laryngospasm**) can occur whenever the larynx is irritated or stimulated by secretions, intubation, extubation, or suctioning. **Bronchospasm** is partial or complete closure of the bronchial tubes. It can be triggered by airway suctioning, aspiration of fluid, or allergy. Both laryngospasm and bronchospasm can be caused by particular anesthetic agents.

Aspiration or inhalation of secretions or stomach contents is associated with a weak gag reflex related to the use of narcotics, sedatives, and anesthetic agents. Aspiration of gastric contents after vomiting can result in an obstructed airway and chemical pneumonia.

Atelectasis

Atelectasis is the collapse of the lung, which can occur suddenly (as in the case of trauma to the chest wall or pulmonary obstruction). Trapped mucus or fluid in the bronchial tree can result in pulmonary obstruction postoperatively. Smokers are particularly vulnerable to atelectasis in the postoperative period. The patient is encouraged to take deep breaths and to cough frequently in the immediate postoperative period to prevent obstruction.

Pulmonary Embolism

Pulmonary embolism is blockage of a pulmonary vessel by air, a blood clot, or other substance (e.g., fragments of atherosclerotic plaque). This results in *anoxia* (decreased oxygen to the lung tissue), which can cause death of lung tissue and right heart failure. The risk of pulmonary embolism is increased in patients with a history of deep vein thrombosis (DVT). Patients are assessed for signs of DVT and pulmonary embolism in the immediate postoperative period. The patient and family are also provided with information about the signs and symptoms of DVT and pulmonary embolism so that monitoring can continue at home after discharge.

CARDIOVASCULAR

Many anesthetic agents are cardiac irritants that can sensitize the heart muscle to disturbances in rhythm, rate, and cardiac output. Hypotension and hypertension can occur as a result of fluid or electrolyte imbalance.

Hemorrhage

Hemorrhage can occur during surgery or in the postoperative period. The patient is continually monitored for signs of hemorrhage, which include pallor, hypotension, an increased heart rate, *diaphoresis* (sweating), cool skin, restlessness, and pain. Hemorrhage may be caused by the loss of a ligature placed during surgery, inadequate hemostasis, leakage from a vascular anastomosis, or a clotting disorder. If hemorrhage is suspected, emergency assessment measures are initiated, and the patient may be returned to surgery. Chapter 14 presents a complete discussion of shock and hemorrhage.

METABOLIC COMPLICATIONS

Hypothermia

Hypothermia is a persistently low core body temperature (less than 98.6° F [37.5° C]). Older, pediatric, and frail patients are most vulnerable. Hypothermia can result in a longer postoperative recovery period, surgical wound infection, cardiac

ischemia, and reduced ability to metabolize drugs. Most patients undergoing general anesthesia experience some level of hypothermia. However, persistent or extreme hypothermia can occur as a result of the following:

- Exposure of the body cavities to the cold ambient temperature of the operating room
- Administration of cold IV fluids
- Patient exposure before draping
- Vasodilation related to medications administered during surgery
- Decreased metabolism
- Cold irrigation solutions

Risks related to hypothermia are due mainly to physiological stress. These include:

- Shivering, which increases oxygen demand and consumption by 400% to 500%
- Excessive demand on body energy
- Decreased immune response, leading to postoperative infection
- Increased risk of adverse cardiac events, especially in patients with coronary artery disease
- Depression of the coagulation pathway
- Decreased tissue healing

Treatment for hypothermia includes use of a forced air heating mattress or placement of warm water pads under the patient. Further loss of body heat is prevented by warming IV solutions. Patients who are hypothermic during the intraoperative period may be difficult to warm postoperatively. Preoperative and intraoperative care are essential to prevent complications related to this condition.

Malignant Hyperthermia

Malignant hyperthermia (MH) is a rare condition that results in an extremely high core body temperature, cardiac dysrhythmia, tachypnea (increased respiratory rate), hypoxia, and hypercarbia. The condition is potentially fatal and occurs most commonly at the time of administration of the anesthetic. However, symptoms may appear in the postoperative period. MH can be triggered by inhalation anesthetics and succinylcholine, an anesthetic adjunct used for muscle relaxation.

MH is an extreme emergency during and after surgery, and all perioperative staff members are trained to respond appropriately according to facility protocol. Dantrolene sodium is administered as soon as the diagnosis is made by the ACP. Additional management includes total body cooling with extracorporeal ice or a hypothermia blanket, iced IV saline, and iced irrigation fluid in an open body cavity (surgical wound site). Surgery is interrupted and the incision closed as quickly as possible. The patient is transferred immediately to the intensive care unit (ICU) for continuous care and monitoring.

NAUSEA AND VOMITING

Postoperative nausea and vomiting (PONV) are both a discomfort and a risk for the patient (see discussion of aspiration). PONV is controlled with medications in the preoperative period (as prevention) and in the postoperative period.

ALTERATIONS OF CONSCIOUSNESS

Anesthetic agents, adjunct medications, and environmental factors may cause patients to become disoriented, confused, or delirious during the immediate postoperative period. Preexisting psychiatric illness or drug abuse may contribute to these effects, which may also be due to organic causes such as electrolyte imbalance. Postoperative delirium is more common in pediatric patients and older patients. Risk factors include the following:

- Cognitive impairment
- Sleep deprivation
- Immobility
- Sensory impairment (e.g., vision, hearing)
- Advanced age
- Electrolyte imbalance
- Dehydration
- Substance abuse
- Depression

ELEMENTS OF DISCHARGE PLANNING

Before an ambulatory (day case) patient is discharged to home or to an extended care facility, the PACU staff, ACP, and surgeon must determine that the patient will be safe. The patient must be able to perform **activities of daily living (ADLs)** with some degree of independence or have help in dressing, eating, mobilizing, and toileting. Discharge planning is needed to prepare the patient and caregivers for possible problems.

Discharge planning and implementation follow established roles and tasks according to hospital policy:

1. *Discharge criteria:* These are standards that reflect the patient's physiological status and objectives for care once the patient leaves the facility.
2. *Transport or transfer plans:* Safe patient transportation is arranged, and an escort is identified.
3. *Home nursing care:* Home care objectives for the patient's recovery are established, and those who will be involved in the care are identified.
4. *Patient education:* Patients are informed and educated about their own care so that they can fully participate in their recovery. The family is instructed in specific care objectives and how to meet the patient's physical needs.
5. *Referral and follow-up:* The patient is informed of follow-up appointments. Referral numbers for emergencies or further advice are provided on a written document.
6. *Documentation:* Nursing care documentation is completed and signed off. Discharge checklists are prepared and completed.

DISCHARGE CRITERIA

Discharge criteria are physiological, psychological, and social conditions that serve as a measure of the patient's readiness for discharge. Patients are discharged from the PACU only when they meet discharge criteria. These are primarily

Box **15-1**	Modified Postanesthesia Discharge Scoring System	
Vital Signs		
Within 20% of the preoperative value		2
20%–40% of the preoperative value		1
40% of the preoperative value		0
Ambulation		
Steady gait/no dizziness		2
With assistance		1
No ambulation/dizziness		0
Nausea and Vomiting		
Minimal		2
Moderate		1
Severe		0
Surgical Bleeding		
Minimal		2
Moderate		1
Severe		0

From Miller R: *Miller's anesthesia,* ed 6, Philadelphia, 2005, Churchill Livingstone.

physiological objectives, which are necessary to ensure patient safety outside the critical care unit. The health care facility establishes the discharge criteria. A number of organizations have written suggested criteria; however, the *Aldrete scale* often is used to determine whether a patient is ready for discharge to the hospital ward or unit. This is a numerical scale used to evaluate activity, respiration, circulation, consciousness, and oxygen saturation. Box 15-1 shows an example of a scored discharge criteria system. Modified versions of the scale have been developed for special circumstances.

Criteria for discharge include physiological criteria and the patient's psychosocial status.

Physiological Criteria

1. Vital signs are stable and reflect the patient's baseline normal.
2. Nausea and vomiting are controlled.
3. Patient is mobile with assistance or by self (the patient must be able to walk without signs of dizziness or weakness).
4. Patient is able to void (this establishes that no evidence exists of urinary retention).
5. Skin color reflects patient's baseline normal.
6. Incision site is dry, and drainage is absent or within expected limits.
7. Patient is oriented to time, place, and person.
8. Pain is controlled (patients are discharged when the level of pain is acceptable to the patient).
9. Patient is able to drink fluids.
10. Discharge orders have been written and signed by the anesthesia care provider and surgeon.

Psychosocial Status

1. Patient has transportation home (not public transport).
2. Responsible escort is available.
3. Home care is available as needed.
4. Home environment is suitable for the recovering patient.

GENERAL PLANNING

Arrangements for discharge are sometimes complex. PACU nurses not only must care for the patient during the recovery period, they also must ensure that care is in place and that safe transport has been arranged.

Patients deserve a safe discharge and transfer from the providing facility. Discharge planning must be started at the time of admission to ensure a safe and event-free return home at the end of the recovery period. Home health service providers are notified, and a preoperative conference may be held with the family and discharge nurse.

When the patient is to be transferred to another care facility, a verbal and written hand-off is provided to a designated person at the receiving facility. The hand-off includes all information about the patient's physical and psychosocial status, the details of the surgery, and the care plan, including prescriptions, dressings, and drainage.

Transport

Patient transport to home or another care facility is arranged before surgery whenever possible. The patient is not discharged to public transportation, and a responsible escort must accompany the patient.

Home Nursing Care

In the past, patients anticipated a long recovery period, both in the hospital and at home. Because of advanced surgical technology and health care economics, patients are now discharged as soon as possible after surgery. Many procedures that used to require days of hospitalization are now performed as day surgery with discharge within 1 or 2 hours of recovery. Home care during the immediate postoperative period is now more focused and has specific outcome objectives.

Discharge planning includes specific written instructions for home care and goals for the patient. This new health care philosophy has shifted the responsibility of recovery from inpatient nursing to the patient and family. In the event the patient has no assistance available, community resources, including social services and professional home nursing services, must be brought in.

Patient Education

Patient teaching is the responsibility of trained nursing personnel. Current surgical practice with same-day discharge and fast tracking requires that patients understand all aspects of their recovery. In theory, this allows them to be active participants in their recovery. However, the postoperative patient may not be able to understand or remember new information. Therefore, patient teaching takes place before surgery and may include the family members who will assist in care.

The elements of patient teaching include both verbal and written instructions. In some facilities, video demonstration and education are available. Access to electronic information via the Internet has transformed the field of consumer medicine. However, not all patients have access to these types of resources or the ability to interpret them. Also, many more patients are too sick to achieve a level of self-education. For

these reasons, patients' family members (when applicable) are taken through the recovery process, step by step, with thorough explanations of what to expect and what to do. This is especially important for patients who will have drains, dressing changes, and surgical appliances to maintain.

Written information is intentionally simple and easy to understand. It is written in lay language, often with illustrations for clarification. It may include information about the surgery, what it entails, and exactly what anatomical changes were made (if any). All anticipated and unanticipated events are explained. Signs of infection or other complications are written out so that patients can refer to them. Knowing the expected effects of surgery helps give the patient confidence and eases anxiety when they occur.

Patients are educated fully about their prescriptions and how to take them. *Polypharmacy* is a clinical scenario in which patients are prescribed many different medications, sometimes by different primary health care providers who have no knowledge of other drugs the patient is taking. It is not unusual for a patient with a chronic disease to be taking 15 or 20 prescribed medications. Therefore, it is very important that education about drugs be covered fully.

The patient's ADLs are discussed in full. These activities of daily living often determine the patient's quality of life. Even if the recovery period is rapid, patients must be able to cope with activity restrictions, special toileting needs (or problems), and meal preparation.

Patients who require dressing changes or have appliances, drains, or catheters need particular assistance and teaching to prevent infection. Patients and family may be given supplies to take home with them at the time of discharge.

Patients and family receive referral numbers for emergency care or further information. Upcoming appointments for surgical follow-up are clearly written, along with any preparation for further testing or treatment.

UNANTICIPATED PACU OUTCOME

FAILURE TO MEET DISCHARGE CRITERIA

Some patients may not meet discharge criteria after ambulatory or inpatient recovery. Further observation and care may be required, especially if the patient entered the PACU in a deteriorated condition or an adverse event occurred during recovery. Examples of such individuals are patients who are hypothermic or posthemorrhagic, or those whose vital signs cannot be stabilized. Inpatients are transferred to the ICU for critical care observation and nursing. Ambulatory patients may be admitted to the ICU or surgical unit for overnight care (or longer if necessary).

DISCHARGE AGAINST MEDICAL ADVICE

Occasionally a patient may opt for self-discharge against the advice of medical and nursing personnel; this is known as **discharge against medical advice (AMA)**. Patients have a right to leave the health care facility as long as they do not pose a threat to themselves or others.

Unless evidence exists of potential harm, patients must be allowed to leave. However, if possible, the facility tries to obtain a signed waiver from the patient and explain the possible outcomes of both the surgery and the consequences of early discharge. The waiver states that the consequences of early discharge have been explained, that discharge was not advised, and that the patient takes responsibility for the consequences.

DEATH IN THE PACU

Death of a patient during surgery is unusual. In the event of impending death or a rapidly deteriorating patient, surgery may be terminated and the patient taken to the PACU. Death may be pronounced (formally) in the PACU after resuscitative means have been exhausted. The patient's family is notified, and PACU staff members arrange for an immediate conference with the family and surgeon. A designated staff member stays with the family to provide emotional support. Further care may be implemented through hospital chaplaincy and social services. Chapter 16 presents a complete discussion of death and dying.

KEY CONCEPTS

- The postanesthesia care unit is designed for immediate access to patients recovering from anesthesia. The open space design allows patient gurneys and large equipment to be positioned quickly and efficiently.
- Equipment and supplies used in the PACU are similar to other intensive care units. Inline oxygen, suction, and monitoring equipment are available in each patient bay for immediate use.
- As patients are admitted to the PACU, care of the patient is transferred from the anesthesia care provider to the PACU nurse. The protocol for handover includes details of the patient's condition, type of anesthesia, surgical procedure, medications and agents administered, drains and type of dressings placed, and any complications that occurred during surgery. The handover is a formal procedure that requires concise information and clear communication among professional staff.
- The Glasgow Coma Scale (GCS) is a basic assessment tool that can be used to determine level of consciousness.
- Postoperative complications can occur any time in the recovery period. Emergencies are handled according to hospital protocol using the normal emergency system. Acute hemorrhage may require the patient to be returned emergently to the operating room for wound exploration.
- Some health care facilities utilize the PACU for outpatient recovery and discharge. In this case, discharge planning must take place on the unit.
- Patient education is an important phase of discharge planning that requires thorough understanding of the patient's condition, healing process, and attention to the individual needs of patient.

- Unanticipated, usually uncommon patient outcomes include failure to meet criteria for discharge from the PACU, death of a patient, and discharge against medical advice.
- Early discharge is the patients' right, but they must sign a self-discharge release.

REVIEW QUESTIONS

1. Why is the PACU considered a critical care unit?
2. Why are the patient's vital signs taken immediately on arrival in the PACU?
3. What is the rationale for providing the PACU nurse with the names and amounts of all drugs administered to the patient in the preoperative and intraoperative periods?
4. Why is a patient assessment performed on arrival at the PACU, even though the patient has been under the immediate care of the surgeon and the ACP?
5. What is the Glasgow Coma Scale? What is its application in the postoperative recovery phase for a patient who has had general anesthesia?
6. Hypothermia is one of the most serious complications of surgery. What procedures are necessary during the *intraoperative period* to prevent hypothermia in the *postoperative period*?
7. Which are the specific duties of the *scrubbed* surgical technologist in preventing hypothermia?
8. What is the rationale for extensive patient teaching?

CASE STUDIES

Case 1

You are asked to transport a fully conscious and alert patient who has just undergone minor surgery under local anesthetic to the PACU. The handover will be provided by the circulating nurse, who will be delayed by a few minutes. When you arrive with your patient, you recognize that there is code (cardiac arrest) in the PACU and most of the staff is engaged in full resuscitation procedures. What should you do? What are the important considerations in this scenario? Think carefully about patient protection, priorities, and emotional impact on your patient.

Case 2

As a staff technologist in a busy ambulatory (outpatient) surgical facility, you are required to transport patients to the recovery area after surgery. Patients remain in this area for 1 to 2 hours until they are ready to be discharged home. One of your surgical patients has been waiting for a friend to pick her up from the facility. The friend is now 3 hours late. You are given the contact number for the friend. When you call, there is no answer. The patient states that she will just take a taxi home. What is your evaluation of the situation? What might be the next steps? Think carefully about discharge criteria, patient safety, and emotional support to your patient and facility policy. Who should be brought in to consult with you about this situation?

Case 3

Hospital policy states that patients who are transported with active cardiac monitoring in place must be accompanied to the PACU by a licensed perioperative nurse and anesthesia care provider. What do you think is the rationale for this? Among other things, think about patient safety and response in case of medical emergency en route.

BIBLIOGRAPHY

Association of periOperative Registered Nurses (AORN): Guidance statement: postoperative patient care in the ambulatory surgery setting. In *Standards, recommended practices and guidelines, 2011 edition*, Denver, 2011, AORN.

Barash P, Cullen B, Stoelting R: *Handbook of clinical anesthesia*, ed 5, Philadelphia, 2005, Lippincott Williams & Wilkins.

Good K, Verble G, Secrest J, Norwood B: Postoperative hypothermia: the chilling consequences, *AORN Journal* 83:5, 2006.

Kingon B, Newman K: Determining patient discharge criteria in an outpatient surgery setting, *AORN Journal* 83:4, 2006.

Miller R, Eriksson L, Fleisher L, Weiner-Kronish J, Young W: *Miller's anesthesia*, ed 7, 2009, Churchill Livingstone

Nagelhout J, Zaglaniczny K: *Nurse anesthesia*, ed 3, St Louis, 2005, Elsevier/Saunders.

Porth C: *Pathophysiology: concepts of altered health states*, ed 6, Philadelphia, 2002, Lippincott Williams & Wilkins.

Thibodeau G, Patton K: *Anatomy and physiology*, ed 6, St Louis, 2007, Elsevier/Saunders.

CHAPTER OUTLINE

LEARNING OBJECTIVES

After studying this chapter the reader will be able to:

1. Define the end of life period and brain death
2. Describe Kübler-Ross's stages of dying
3. Discuss ways to provide comfort and support to patients in the dying period
4. Understand the conflicts and stress families face during the dying period
5. Discuss significant ethical issues surrounding death and dying
6. Define cultural competence as it applies to the dying patient
7. Discuss the concept of determination of death and the physical changes in the body immediately after death
8. Give examples of a coroner's case
9. Discuss principles of organ recovery

TERMINOLOGY

Advance health care directive: A written document stating an individual's specific wishes regarding his or her health care to be enacted in the event the person is unable to make decisions.

Coroner's case: A patient death that requires investigation by the coroner, as well as an autopsy on the deceased.

Cultural competence: The ability to provide support and care to individuals of cultures and belief systems different from one's own.

Determination of death: A formal medical process to determine brain death.

DNAR: "Do not attempt resuscitation." Emphasizes the patient's desire to refuse intervention to resuscitate.

DNR: "Do not resuscitate." An official request to refrain from certain types of resuscitation, usually cardiopulmonary resuscitation.

End of life: A period within which death is expected, usually days to months.

Heart-beating cadaver: A cadaver maintained on cardiopulmonary support to provide tissue perfusion. This is done to maintain viability in organs for donation.

Kübler-Ross, Elisabeth: A Swiss psychiatrist who proposed a theory of developmental or psychological stages of the dying experience.

Living will: A legal document signed by the patient stating the conditions and limitations of medical assistance in the event of near death or a prognosis of death.

Non–heart-beating cadaver: A cadaver in which perfusion at and after death was not possible. Only certain tissues may be procured for donation.

Postmortem care: Physical care of the body to prepare it for viewing by the family and for mortuary procedures.

Required request law: A law requiring medical personnel to request organ recovery from a deceased's family.

Rigor mortis: The natural stiffening of the body that starts approximately 15 minutes after death and lasts about 24 hours.

INTRODUCTION

Death in the operating room is a relatively rare event. Training in death has only recently returned to the curriculum of health care workers. All allied health personnel benefit from a structured study on death, with the main focus on the psychosocial and procedural aspects.

This chapter is not intended to provide a course in death and dying. It is the basis for further study and exploration. This chapter discusses social, personal, ethical, legal, and medical perspectives on death. An understanding of the process of death and the events triggered by it can aid the surgical technologist in providing compassionate care to patients and their families. Knowledge and understanding also contribute to the health professional's beliefs and values.

The procedural aspects of death and the protocols that must be followed may seem "clinical" in nature; however, they are necessary to ensure dignity, order, and professionalism.

DEFINING THE END OF LIFE

Death and the end of life can be defined from many perspectives. The study and experience of different perspectives assists health professionals in their support of the dying patient and family.

From a medical point of view, the **end of life** is that period when death is expected. Most clinicians pronounce the patient's entry into a dying state when death is expected within days, weeks, or months. The dying period is marked by the inability to provide or the cessation of attempts to prolong life. However, this does not mean that comfort care is not provided in the dying period. It simply means that death cannot be avoided.

The diagnosis of *brain death* is used when the entire brain ceases to function without life support mechanisms in place. Some functions such as respiration and heartbeat can be maintained artificially even during brain death. However, in the United States, brain death means *real death*, and no other distinction is used for legal or medical purposes.

MODELS OF DEATH AND DYING

News that oneself or a loved one has begun the dying process triggers a cascade of emotional and psychological events. In the past few decades, a number of models have been presented that explain these events and processes. The best-known model was developed in the 1960s by Swiss psychiatrist **Elisabeth Kübler-Ross**, who described the stages of death. In her model, the stages of death are not discrete, nor are they predictable in all people of all cultures. The Kübler-Ross model proposed the following stages of grief and dying:

- **Denial:** The patient denies that he or she is dying. This is described by mental health professionals as a natural response to shocking events. Denial is a defense mechanism that forestalls the full impact of the fact of death until the mind is ready to accept it.
- **Anger:** Some patients express anger. Feelings of anger may be projected onto the family, oneself, health workers, or spiritual entity. Some patients feel great anger and remorse that they did not heed warnings to change lifestyle habits they knew were harmful. Others express anger at those who care for them or become very demanding in their care. Patients may express anger at themselves by refusing treatment or nutrition. These coping strategies may be an attempt to gain control over the environment.
- **Bargaining:** Kübler-Ross describes this stage as a way of postponing death. The patient may make an inner attempt to bargain with a spiritual entity, such as, "I just want to experience one pain-free day with my family" or "If I pray daily, maybe I will live."

- **Depression:** True clinical depression may occur during the dying process. In recent years there has been a trend away from accepting depression as a natural result of dying and to treat it clinically.
- **Acceptance:** In Kübler-Ross's theory, death is "accepted." The idea and interpretation of death are no longer a source of psychological conflict.

Critics of Kübler-Ross's model believe that the stage theory is too constricting and does not allow for individualism in the experience of death. However, the stages model provided a framework for psychologists and social workers to look at the process of dying in a way that had not been previously studied.

Many modern models have been developed since Kübler-Ross conducted her research. These appreciate individuals according to their situation, personality, culture, and life experiences. For example, William McDougall, a well-known social psychologist, emphasized the need to integrate the dying process into existing life experiences. Rather than focusing on particular tasks or psychological stages, he advocated maintaining a sense of self-awareness in relation to the environment. Social psychologist Charles Corr encouraged the dying to try different individual strategies and coping mechanisms based on their uniqueness as individuals and was a strong critic of the stage theory of death.

SUPPORT AND COMFORT FOR THE DYING AND BEREAVED PATIENT

Perioperative caregivers may have only brief encounters with the dying patient in the surgical environment, whereas contact between patients and palliative care specialists is frequent and the relationships can last weeks or months. Perioperative staff members should always be aware that no matter how brief their contact with the dying patient, all encounters provide an opportunity to support and care for the patient in the dying process.

Communication with the dying patient requires keen listening and observation skills. It is important to recognize and acknowledge the fact of death and what this means to the patient in that moment and time. As a surgical technologist, you should focus on what the patient is experiencing in the operating room or holding area. Observe facial expressions and gestures. Be alert to any changes in mood or signs of anxiety and fear related to death and isolation. Avoid communication that attempts to minimize, rationalize, or deny death. However, this does not imply blunt or insensitive communication. Focus on immediate physical and emotional comfort and acknowledgment, and above all, listen to the patient. Listening is sometimes the most effective source of comfort (but not always the easiest). A response may not be needed and should not be forced. Respect the patient's individuality and uniqueness in the present. Use the patient's verbal and physical cues as a guideline rather than making assumptions about what the patient feels or needs.

Never imply that a surgical procedure may "cure" the patient, but offer the possibility of a good outcome. Perhaps the patient is having surgery to reduce the size of a tumor or for treatment of intractable pain. These procedures offer hope for a longer survival period or one that is physically tolerable.

FAMILY

Families and friends react to dying and death in many different ways. Not only must they cope with the emotional and psychological impact of death, they also must make many significant decisions. They have a central role in the dying patient's emotional environment, and in sudden death they often need the assistance and guidance of health professionals.

The family's reactions of grief and sadness may be accompanied by bouts of anger and frustration with the health care system, each other, and even the dying family member. Death triggers large and sometimes unmanageable emotions, and these cannot always be contained in ways considered socially acceptable. This may be disconcerting to family members as they participate in the death and observe their own reactions as a family unit. The wise health professional recognizes when tensions are mounting and provides validation for these strong emotions. At the same time, the health professional can guide family members toward coping strategies to help defuse the tension and add order to the experience (e.g., support groups).

Families usually face many complex events associated with death and dying. The death may impose a financial burden. The dying patient may have children or other family members who rely on the individual for support, and these responsibilities must be shifted to other family members. Difficult decisions may need to be made about palliative care or "do not resuscitate" status. The administrative requirements, such as signing release forms or attending to the details of funeral arrangements, often seem too clinical or cold in the midst of grieving. Professionals who routinely care for the dying provide ongoing support in many areas. This includes not only management of the patient's medical needs, but also emotional support and even referral for counseling outside the medical and nursing environment.

SUDDEN UNEXPECTED DEATH

When death is sudden and unexpected, family and friends have many needs. In the clinical environment, these immediate needs are addressed by nurses, physicians, and spiritual counselors. Early reactions often focus on information about the cause and details of death. The need for cloistered privacy usually is very strong in the initial stages of shock and grief.

The surgical technologist should refrain from providing information to family or friends about the patient's medical condition. This is the responsibility of the physicians and nurses, and any discussions must be deferred to them. The surgical technologist may offer acknowledgment of the loss. He or she may also facilitate communication between the family and other professionals, such as showing the way to the consultation area and making sure the environment is appropriate.

ETHICAL CONSIDERATIONS IN DEATH AND DYING

The ethics of care and decision making in death and dying are highly personal, and there are many conflicting viewpoints. Beliefs and culture influence the decisions people make about how they want to die or how they would like others to go through the dying process. These beliefs are not universal. This means that whenever possible, an individual's personal wishes for his or her own death should be documented and validated by the individual and family.

SELF-DETERMINATION

Self-determination is the right of every individual to make decisions about how he or she lives and dies. Advance care planning provides an accepted method for individuals to define their needs and wishes about death and dying. Patients may refuse treatment at any point in the dying process. They may select which palliative measures are performed and which are withheld. Decisions can then be communicated and made official for health care providers. Ethical issues arise when the patient is not competent to communicate. Decisions about end of life care fall to the family when the patient is not able to communicate his or her wishes. In these cases, health care workers help provide information about choices, as well as ongoing support through the decision process. Ethical decisions that cannot be resolved by the family and health care professionals may be brought before the hospital ethics committee for review.

RIGHT TO DIE

An individual may believe that he or she has a "right to die" and may refuse treatment in order to fulfill this right. However, *not treating a dying patient* is a completely different process from *treating with intent to harm*. Assisted suicide is perceived by many as intent to harm and on that basis is rejected. *Assisted suicide* is intentional harm to a person, at their request, to promote or cause death. The arguments for and against assisted suicide continue in many states and countries. The Netherlands allows assisted suicide, as do Oregon, Washington, and Montana. The process involves stringent preconditions and extensive review by an ethics committee.

ADVANCE HEALTH CARE DIRECTIVES

The **advance health care directive** is a document in which an individual states his or her wishes with regard to health care. The document is used in the event that person is unable to communicate those wishes. This and other documents such as a *living will* that instruct others on how health care is to be delivered, as well as who should act on the patient's behalf and oversee that person's care, are generally referred to as a *power of attorney*. However, the names of the documents that reflect one's wishes regarding health matters differ according to state laws.

"Do not resuscitate" (**DNR**) and "do not attempt resuscitation" (**DNAR**) are two types of health directives that express the patient's decision to decline lifesaving efforts. In some cases the family makes this decision for the patient who is incompetent to do so at the time. The request not to resuscitate is made official when the patient signs a DNR order, which is charted in the patient's medical record. Explicit forms that define precisely the procedures that can and cannot be performed during resuscitation have been designed to alleviate ambiguity. However, ethical conflicts arise in spite of protocol. These usually occur when no DNR status has been stated and the decision is left for the family. The definition of *resuscitation* may also cause ambiguity. Active measures to prolong life are ethically different from those that do not halt the progression of death.

The individual's DNR status must be verified throughout the period of patient care. In most facilities, the DNR status must be renewed with each hospital admission. Health care providers may not realize that the patient has redefined his or her wishes at some point during illness. Admission to the surgical unit always includes verification of the DNR status.

CONFLICTS IN PALLIATIVE CARE

Palliative care is the medical and supportive care provided to the dying patient. Numerous types of surgical intervention may be included as a component of palliative care, such as debulking of a tumor or debridement of a pressure wound. Procedures for the implantation of biomedical devices, such as a gastric feeding tube or renal dialysis access, require anesthesia in the interventional radiology department or operating room. Medical interventions for the dying patient include extreme measures, such as respiratory support ("artificial respiration"), intravenous feeding, dialysis, drugs to maintain and regulate failed metabolic processes, and many others.

The ethics of palliative care involve reasoned arguments about the definition of particular interventions. Many patients have signed a **living will,** which specifies the exact nature of palliative care that they accept. In the absence of a living will, clinical decisions sometimes are made by consensus of the patient (when able), the family, and care providers. Most people intend to do the "right thing." They try to resolve the conflicts about quality of life. However, families may have trouble deciding when to prolong life by supportive measures and when to discontinue them based on the suffering they might cause. These decisions are extremely difficult and often fraught with emotion and conflict within the family.

An ethical discussion that often arises is whether withdrawal of care constitutes suffering. Intravenous maintenance (hydration) and feeding often are the most sensitive areas for families to resolve. In these cases the health professional makes every attempt to inform the family about the effects of withdrawing care without interfering with their right to decide.

Health care workers often face personal conflict about the decisions made by their patients or the families of patients. They may not agree with the decisions, but they are obliged to honor them. In extreme cases of ethical conflict, the health professional may ask to be excused from participation in the care of the patient. Although this resolves the conflict

temporarily, it does not offer long-term relief from an environment that frequently challenges beliefs and values. At some point in their careers, health care professionals usually need to define their own ethics and accept that others have differing perspectives.

CULTURAL RESPONSES TO DEATH AND DYING

SPIRITUAL AND RELIGIOUS CONCEPTS

Death, as perceived across cultures, often is defined through spiritual values and beliefs. Meaning in life and death often are linked to spiritual hope. The rituals and practices that people of different cultures observe are vital to the fulfillment of their duty to the dying person. In the United States, great efforts have been made to honor and respect the beliefs of others, but there is still a long way to go. Health care workers may question the validity of a belief or an expression of a patient's faith, often comparing it to their own. By definition, spiritual beliefs are valid for the believer and do not need approval or justification by others.

Support and care across cultures is called **cultural competence.** It is learned through experience and active learning. It begins with acceptance and respect. In many cultures, death is considered a natural phenomenon, a possible conclusion of serious illness and not a battle with the cause. Although grief and other deep emotions are present in all families at the time of death, these feelings often are mitigated by ritual and ceremony, which comfort as well as heal the living. In many cultures they also are believed to comfort the dead.

Handling of the body, especially its preparation for viewing by the family, may require special knowledge about the practices of certain cultures. As long as these practices do not conflict with health and safety standards, they should be carried out with dignity and respect. Notification of death to chosen religious clergy is generally left to the family.

DEATH IN THE CLINICAL SETTING

DETERMINATION OF DEATH

When death occurs in surgery, the surgeon and anesthesia care provider must verify that brain death has occurred; this is called **determination of death.** Death is determined by specific medical criteria, which have legal implications. To determine brain death, specific medical assessment may be carried out on the patient to determine absence of breathing and response to painful stimuli and the presence of cranial reflexes. More complex tests can be performed if necessary, such as electroencephalography or computed tomography (Box 16-1).

When death has been determined, the operating room supervisor communicates with other key individuals to prepare the morgue (or coroner in some cases) or the supervisor of the postanesthesia care unit (PACU). The deceased may be transported to the PACU for postmortem care. Arrangements are made for the family to meet with the surgeon or a designee in a quiet area near the surgical department or PACU.

The surgical wound is closed appropriately and dressed. Drapes are removed from the patient (if they were not removed during resuscitation), and instruments and supplies are prepared as they would be at the close of any case. The patient may then be transported to the PACU or another location in the surgical department for postmortem care.

Documentation for the surgical procedure is completed as usual, with accurate recording of the chain of events. Operative records for patient care, anesthesia, sponge counts, and all usual forms must be completed as for any case. Documentation related to the death of the patient is completed by the attending physician and anesthesiologist. Registration of the death is a separate legal document that is completed by the attending physician. Because death in the operating room is a sentinel event, the circulator must initial all forms as for any sentinel event. If death was pronounced in the operating room, members of the surgical team are named in the sentinel event documentation.

POSTMORTEM CARE

Postmortem care prepares the body for viewing by the family and assists in further handling procedures carried out by the morgue and mortuary. The exact protocol for postmortem care is carefully defined by every health care facility. All staff members who perform postmortem care must be completely familiar with the protocol, and there should be no ambiguity about the process. The protocol for coroner's cases is different, and this procedure also is clearly documented in each care health facility. General care of the body is based on the process of death.

NATURAL CHANGES IN THE BODY AFTER DEATH

Immediately after death, the body begins to cool. All sphincter muscles, including those controlling feces and urine, immediately lose tone. The eyes remain open, and the jaw drops down. Dependent areas of the body (those under pressure from body weight or gravity) begin to collect fluid, and the areas around the ears and cheeks may turn purple or red (a condition called *livor mortis*). The pooling of blood in these regions cannot be reversed in the embalming process. The sacrum and other pressure areas fill with fluid, possibly resulting in tissue rupture. **Rigor mortis,** the natural stiffening of the body, begins approximately 15 minutes after death and peaks at 8 to 10 hours. The exact time depends on the tissues and environmental temperature. At 18 hours the process regresses, and the body usually is relaxed after 24 hours. Rigor mortis begins at the head (eyelids) and progresses to the feet. When relaxation begins, it follows the reverse order of progression.

GENERAL POSTMORTEM PROCEDURES

All health care facilities have a postmortem kit, which contains the supplies needed to perform aftercare. During the aftercare procedure, the body is handled gently and with respect at all times. Postmortem care that conflicts with the patient's religious affiliation is not performed. In some facilities, with a death during surgery, the body must remain on the operating table, intact, until a decision is made about a coroner's investigation.

CORONER'S CASES

The circumstances of the patient's death determine whether the coroner must investigate the death; this process includes mandatory autopsy, and such a case is called a **coroner's case.** Most states have similar criteria for establishing coroner's cases, and the criteria may include the following circumstances of death:

- Death in the operating room or emergency department
- Unwitnessed death
- Death after admission from another facility
- Death in which criminal activity is suspected (the deceased may have been the perpetrator or the victim)
- Suicide
- Death of an incarcerated individual
- Death as a result of an infectious disease that might pose a public health risk

Other criteria may also apply, depending on state law. Coroner's cases require that the conditions of the body remain intact for examination and investigation. In the medical environment, all implanted or invasive devices are left in place. The patient's property may also be transferred to the coroner rather than returned to the family. Meticulous care and identification of specimens are always required, regardless of whether the specimens become part of the investigation. After a death in surgery, any specimens produced during surgery become the property of the coroner. They must be transferred directly from the operating room, as specified by hospital protocol, using universal precautions.

ORGAN RECOVERY

Organ recovery is the removal preservation and use of human organs and tissue from a recently deceased person for transplantation into a living individual. Once the decision has been made for organ recovery, exacting clinical protocols are followed to ensure the vitality of the organs.

Permission for Recovery

Before the issue arises, a person can make the decision to donate tissue or whole organs. In many states, this permission may be verified on an individual's driver's license or other identification card. Some states have a **required request law**, which requires medical professionals and other caregivers to ask the family for permission to recover organs from the deceased.

Protocols

The process of recovery is administered through tissue banks and organ recovery agencies, which locate donors, register recipients, and organize recovery. Many organizations are involved in the process which requires a high level of coordination and data exchange.

Donors are registered in different regions of the country, and the data are exchanged with recovery organizations (Box 16-2). The protocols for medical recovery, care of tissue, and identification of tissue are formulated by the American Association of Tissue Banks, a nonprofit scientific organization that accredits tissue banks and recovery organizations to ensure professional standards of practice.

Organs are collected and stored by regional organ banks and provided to facilities as needed. Services are available on call 24 hours a day. Data are constantly exchanged between tissue banks and the organ recovery registries to match donor organs with compatible recipients.

Organ recovery takes place as soon as possible after death because the vitality of some tissues is time dependent. Actual recovery takes place at the hospital or in a tissue bank organization. When recovery occurs at the host hospital, a transplant coordinator from the regional tissue bank arrives on site to ensure that medical, administrative, and supportive services are carried out according to set standards. The recovery team travels to the hospital as soon as possible after the death of a donor when time-sensitive tissue is to be procured.

Medical Criteria for Tissue Recovery

Different types of tissue require specific medical maintenance to remain viable after death. Donor cadavers generally are divided into two categories, heart-beating and non–heart-beating.

HEART-BEATING CADAVER A **heart-beating cadaver** is one in which tissue perfusion can be maintained during and immediately after death to preserve the life of the tissue. Cardiopulmonary support provides intact circulation to organs suitable for recovery. The availability of cardiopulmonary support depends on the exact location of death; it usually is restricted to the emergency department, operating room, or critical care unit, where equipment, supplies, and trained personnel are immediately available. The physiological parameters for recovery include renal output, vascular pressure, temperature, and perfusion.

NON–HEART-BEATING CADAVER Tissues from a non–heart-beating cadaver are restricted to those that do not need perfusion to sustain viability for later transplantation. These include the cornea, blood vessels, heart valves, bone, and skin.

ETHICAL DILEMMAS IN ORGAN RECOVERY Organ and tissue donation arise as an ethical issue when the patient has not left a clear directive before death. When no verifiable permission has been granted by the patient, the family may act as a surrogate for the patient.

Many cultures and faiths forbid organ removal after death, and these cases usually are straightforward for the family and patient. However, individuals often leave the question unresolved at the time of death. If no decision has been made by the patient, the attending physician must, *by law*, ask the patient and family to consider organ donation. In cases of sudden death without clear directives, conflicting views may be held by family members about organ donation. The ethical problem is whether the family can and should make such a decision for the deceased. Some families may feel very strongly opposed to organ donation, whereas others feel that it is a way of providing life.

HEALTH PROFESSIONALS CONFRONTING DEATH

The emotional and psychological events triggered by the sudden death of a patient vary in health care workers. The reactions and coping skills available to these professionals often are influenced by the following factors:
- Previous experience with death
- Support available in the environment
- The health care professional's beliefs and values
- Knowledge about the process of death
- The health care professional's emotional well-being

The types of emotions or even severe psychological events that health care workers experience may be similar to those of the dying patient. Shock and denial are common in sudden death, especially when the patient is young or the death was violent.

For many health care workers, care of the dying is extremely rewarding and leads to important knowledge about one's own values and beliefs. The ability to provide comfort to both the patient and the family often results in the discovery of a special ability to nurture. This quality is the reason many health care workers begin a career in patient care.

However, some health professionals may experience a crisis in connection with the death of a patient or in the care of the dying. Unresolved emotions related to previous loss or conflicts about beliefs and values may lead to depression or other severe psychological reactions. This is different from normal feelings of sadness, loss, and even frustration, which health professionals experience at various stages when caring for a dying patient. When these feelings arise, they can affect the quality of the health care worker's life and interfere with the individual's ability to cope with stress in the workplace.

A structured response may be required to help health care workers cope with death. This may involve planned "debriefing" periods, or spontaneous expressions of support and acknowledgment by individual team members. Organized support groups for team members can provide a forum for discussion and reflection. Health care workers often can benefit from coping skills that other professionals have found helpful:

- Often it is helpful for staff who were involved in the patient's care or death to discuss the details of the death, going over exactly what happened and why. This is not to "medicalize" the death, but rather to discern the limitations of medical care and the fact that medical professionals cannot control all situations. It helps people understand that human intervention has limits, especially in the face of inevitable death.
- Acknowledgment of one's feelings is helpful for many. Sometimes it is important to express the sadness, shock, and even anger that professionals feel after the death of a patient. It allows others to understand the feelings of their colleagues and to show acknowledgment and comfort. However, many people are not comfortable displaying their feelings or even discussing them, and this must be respected. No one should be coaxed into expressing that which is private and confidential.
- Distraction provides a healthy break from severe stress. The effects of a tragic death in the operating room can linger for weeks, and this can have a serious effect on team morale and individual coping ability. Sometimes it is good to "lighten the conversation" or plan activities that do not remind people of the death. This does not diminish the meaning or significance of the death; it simply provides time to step away from it.
- The health care worker must attend to self-care. At some point in their careers, all health care professionals must reflect on whether the stress of work is balanced by healthy coping mechanisms. This can be done through self-reflection or to a confidant (e.g., with a mentor or religious figure).

KEY CONCEPTS

- The terms *end of life* and *brain death* are precisely defined in medicine. Although it may seem that scientific definitions are uncompassionate, they are necessary in order to provide the basis of legal and ethical decisions surrounding the death of an individual.
- The Kübler-Ross stages of dying were among the first psychosocial descriptions of the experience of death. Since these were published in the 1960s, there has been more advanced work showing an appreciation of the individual nature of each person's response to the death experience. However, the Kübler-Ross model is frequently cited as a basic study.
- Surgical technologists may be required to communicate with the family of a patient who has died in care. Although this is a relatively rare occurrence, the surgical technologist should develop a method of communication that is supportive and comforting to the family.
- The families of dying patients face many challenges and difficulties in the end of life period. Effective and compassionate communication with the family and the patient is enhanced by understanding some of the more common problems families face. These not only include the psychological effects of grief, but can also be related to the patient's medical care or to the practical aspects of finances and estate issues.
- At some time in their career, nearly all health care workers are confronted with ethical issues involving death. Although they may not be required to make a decision themselves, they do witness others involved in choices and dilemmas. These are not easy topics and often touch on closely held values and traditions. However, awareness of events that might occur and reflection on the issues is worthwhile early in one's career.
- Death and dying are often accompanied by traditional practices, many of which are based in culture. Cultural competence in the subject of death area is extremely important to understanding how others interpret and respond to the experience. The process of learning about the traditions and rituals that are closely held by others helps to define the way we communicate and show empathy. Certain tradition may also directly affect the disposition of amputated limbs, or other tissues removed from the body.
- Specific circumstances under which a person dies determine whether a legal investigation, including an autopsy, is required. If the circumstances meet the legal criteria, the death is referred to as a *coroner's case*. Specific postmortem care and protection of evidence are also required in a coroner's case. The criteria and procedures for such a case vary from state to state. However the surgical technologist should be aware of the conditions that constitute a coroner's case in his or her state.
- Organ and tissue recovery may be performed after the death of a patient. The criteria for organ donation are previously established, and no organs are removed until the criteria have been met.

REVIEW QUESTIONS

1. Define the end of life from a medical perspective.
2. What are the five stages of death as defined by Kübler-Ross?
3. Name several administrative responsibilities of the family when death occurs in the clinical setting.
4. How can clinicians help families accomplish these administrative tasks while coping with the grief and shock of death?

5. What is self-determination? How does it apply to death and dying?

6. How can a patient express his or her "right to die?" How can this be carried out if the patient is unable to direct medical intervention?

7. Is there a difference between treating a dying patient for comfort measures and treating with intent to prolong life? Explain.

8. How can health professionals honor cultural practices and beliefs in caring for the dying and the dead?

9. What is a coroner's case?

10. What is rigor mortis?

11. What specimens may be collected from a non–heart-beating cadaver?

12. What kinds of self-care are appropriate for you in times of stress? Why is it important to know this?

CASE STUDY

Case 1

A patient who developed severe peritonitis following gastric surgery 1 week ago has been returned to the operating room for an exploratory laparotomy. Within the first 30 minutes of surgery the patient suddenly begins to hemorrhage from multiple sites within the abdomen, including blood vessels that were previously ligated. Although emergency attempts are made to halt the swift progression of this coagulopathy, the hemorrhaging worsens. When all attempts to reverse the condition have failed, the surgeon closes the abdominal wound and the patient is withdrawn from anesthesia. You now realize that the patient has died and will be quickly transported to the PACU.

1. Can you predict how this sudden death of a patient might affect your ability to carry on with necessary duties?

2. What are your initial responsibilities, assuming you will not be accompanying the anesthesia care provider to the PACU?

3. After you have been relieved for a break, you are just outside the surgical department when one of the patient's family members whom you met just before surgery approaches you. What will you say to her?

4. What particular documentation does the surgical technologist need to complete as a member of the sterile team in which a patient death occurred? Refer back to Chapter 3 for additional information on documentation.

5. Research the laws that establish a coroner's death in your state.

BIBLIOGRAPHY

American Academy of Hospice and Palliative Medicine: *General educational materials.* Accessed January 28, 2008, at http://www.aahpm.org/cgi-bin/wkcgi/browse?category=articlesion=CC.

Centers for Disease Control and Prevention, National Center for Health Statistics: *Physicians' handbook on medical certification of death, 2003 edition.* Accessed July 13, 2011, at http://unstats.un.org/unsd/vitalstatkb/Attachment277.aspx.

Eelco FMW, Panayiostis NV, et al: Evidence based guideline update: determining brain death in adults: report of the Quality Standards Subcommittee of the American Academy of Neurology. *Neurology* 2010;74:1911–1918, Accessed April 19, 2012, at www.learnicu.org/Docs/Guidelines/AANAdultBrainDeath.pdf

Kuebler K, Heidrich D, Esper P: *Palliative and end of life care*, ed 2, St Louis, 2007, WB Saunders/Elsevier.

Porth C: *Pathophysiology concepts of altered health states*, ed 6, Philadelphia, 2002, Lippincott Williams & Wilkins.

Thibodeau G, Patton K: *Anatomy and physiology*, ed 6, St Louis, 2007, Mosby/Saunders.

Physics and Information Technology

CHAPTER OUTLINE

LEARNING OBJECTIVES

After studying this chapter the reader will be able to:

1. Understand the relationship between technology and medicine
2. Describe the importance of atoms, molecules, elements, and matter
3. Describe the elements of motion
4. Discuss different types of energy
5. List the properties of waves
6. Discuss the principles of electricity and its application to surgery
7. Discuss alternating and direct current

8. Describe the principles of light
9. Discuss the methods of heat transfer and how they relate to patient safety
10. List and describe the properties of sound
11. Discuss how computers are used in the perioperative environment
12. Identify the physical components of a computer
13. Demonstrate computer motor skills
14. Discuss how computer networks and the Internet are used in a professional medical setting

TERMINOLOGY

Alternating current (AC): A type of electrical current in which electricity changes direction to complete its circuit.

Ampere: A unit measuring the amount of energy passing a given point in a stated period of time.

Amplitude: In electromagnetic wave energy, the height of a wave.

Atom: A discrete unit made of matter consisting of charged particles.

Boiling point: The temperature of a substance when its state changes from a liquid to a gas.

Central processing unit (CPU): The component of a computer that contains the circuitry, memory, and power controls.

Circuit: The path of free electrons as they move through conductive material. In a *closed circuit*, the electrons proceed unhindered and electrical energy is maintained; in an *open circuit*, the path of the electrons is interrupted, which stops the flow of current.

Coherent light waves: Light waves that are lined up so that the troughs and peaks are matched.

Conduction: The transfer of heat from one substance to another by the natural movement of molecules, which sets other molecules in motion.

Conductivity: The relative ability of a substance to transmit free electrons or electricity.

Convection: The displacement of cool air by warm air. Convection usually creates currents as the warm air rises and the cool air falls.

Database: In computer technology, a compilation of information, usually lists or numerical information, that can be manipulated or calculated.

Direct current (DC): A type of low-voltage electrical current in which electrons flow in one direction to complete a circuit. Battery power uses direct current.

Doppler effect: The effect perceived when the origin or receiver of sound waves moves. The perception is a change in the frequency of the waves and corresponding pitch.

Doppler ultrasound: A medical device that uses the Doppler effect and ultrasonic waves to measure and record blood flow as well as tissue density and shape.

Electromagnetic field: A three-dimensional pattern of force created by the attraction and repulsion of charged particles around a magnet.

Electromagnetic waves: The natural phenomenon of wave energy, such as electricity, light, and radio broadcasts. The type of energy is determined by the frequency of the waves.

Electron: A negatively charged particle that orbits the nucleus of an atom.

TERMINOLOGY (cont.)

Electrostatic discharge: The sudden release of electrical energy from surfaces where charged particles have accumulated because of friction.

Element: A pure substance composed of atoms, each with the same number of protons (e.g., iron, copper, uranium).

Focal point: The exact location where light rays converge after passing through a convex lens.

Frequency: In physics, the number of waves that pass a point in 1 second. The unit of measurement for frequency is the hertz (Hz).

Gravitational energy: The natural attractive force of masses in the universe.

Harmonics: The quality of sound related to the frequency of the sound waves.

Hot wire: In electrical circuits, the hot wire is the one that carries the electrical current.

Hyperlinks: In computer technology, electronic links between files and the electronic addresses for data associated with those links. Hyperlinks allow data to be obtained electronically and quickly from another computer through a computer network.

Insulator: A substance that does not conduct electrical current and is used to prevent electricity from seeking an alternate path.

Internal drives: Data storage devices that are an integral part of the computer.

Internet: A worldwide public network of computers that are connected by wires, fiberoptic cables, or satellite signals. Computers connected to this system can receive and transmit data to other computers in the system.

Intranet: A computer network within a facility or an organization that can be accessed only by those employed or affiliated with the organization.

Isotope: An atom of a specific element with the correct number of electrons and protons but a different number of neutrons.

Kinetic energy: The energy of motion; the kinetic energy of an object is mathematically related to its speed.

Magnetic field: A three-dimensional force pattern created by the positive and negative charges of a polar magnet.

Molecule: A specific substance made up of elements that are bonded together.

Momentum: The mathematical relationship between the weight and velocity of a mass.

Neutron: A subatomic particle located in the nucleus of the atom. It has no electrical charge.

Nucleus: The center of an atom.

Periodic table: A standardized chart of all known elements.

Photon: In physics, the name given to a light particle.

Plasma: A gaseous state in which the atom's nucleus becomes separated from the electrons.

Potential energy: Energy stored in the form of gravity, chemical bonds, nuclear particles, and mechanical springs.

Receptacle: An outlet in an electrical circuit that receives a plug containing live current, completing the circuit.

Reflection: The behavior of a wave when it reaches a nonabsorbent material. The wave reverses and is directed back toward the source.

Refraction: In optics, the behavior of light as it passes through a substance.

Resistance: In electricity, the measurement of a substance's ability to inhibit the flow of electricity.

Serial lenses: An optical system in which several lenses are lined up to produce a clear, well-defined image. Surgical endoscopes use serial lenses.

Solid: A state of matter in which the molecules are bonded very tightly. Characteristics of solids are hardness and the ability to break apart into other solid pieces.

States of matter: The physical forms of matter. The four states of matter are gas, liquid, solid, and plasma.

Static electricity: The buildup of charged particles on a surface.

Thermal conductivity: The ability of a substance to conduct heat. Different substances have different abilities to conduct or transmit heat.

Thermoregulation: A complex physiological process in which the body maintains a temperature that is optimal for survival.

Ultrasound: A technology that uses high-frequency wave energy to identify anatomical structures and anomalies. In ultrasound imaging, sound waves are transformed into visual images on a screen.

Voltage: The electrical force in a circuit, measured as the amount of force that passes a given point over a stated period. Voltage is measured in volts (V).

Wave: In physics, a naturally occurring phenomenon in which energy is transmitted in the form of peaks (high points) and troughs (low points).

Wavelength: The distance between peaks in a complete wave cycle.

World Wide Web: In computer technology, a network of links to data via an Internet system. The Web uses a special computer language protocol and is only one of many types of systems for transmitting data through a computer network.

INTRODUCTION

The field of medicine encompasses both human and technological principles. Rapid advances in technology in the past decade have been applied in all fields of medicine. Advances in surgery have been so rapid in the past 15 years that entire systems and methods of working have been changed, requiring continuous training and retraining. The human body has not changed, but the approach to medical and surgical problems often focuses on speed, efficiency, complete accuracy, and economics. Successes in technology have led to more and more complex machines and materials, as well as the use of computer technology to perform, analyze, record, and document medical procedures.

As a result of this shift, surgical technology has developed into a complex field of study and practice that follows two paths simultaneously: the human and the technological.

TECHNOLOGY AND MEDICINE

The nonhuman aspects of surgical technology draw most heavily from the field of mechanics. At a very basic level,

Table **17-1**	**Specialties in Mechanics and Physics**	
Area of Study	**Applied Theories**	**Surgical Applications**
Classic mechanics	Newton's laws of motion* Harmonic motion Gravity	• Any instrument or device that oscillates, rotates, flexes, pivots, bends, or flexes. • Work as it applies to potential energy in humans and devices. • The design of tools and instruments and its relationship to work (e.g., hinged instruments). • Any device or instrument that uses wave energy, such as light, heat, electricity, or sound.
Biomechanics	Various	• The principles of mechanics are used to explain and improve the function of the human body.
Thermodynamics	Laws of thermodynamics The nature of heat transfer States of matter	• Devices that create heat or cold (e.g., fluid warmer, patient thermal devices, sterilizers). • Compressed gas–powered equipment.
Particle, atomic physics	Nuclear physics Particle theory Wave motion	• Any device that uses electromagnetic radiation in the form of heat, light or electricity (e.g., ultrasound diagnostic devices, radiography, fluoroscopy).
Optical physics	Optics Light	• Any device with lenses (e.g., operating microscopes, endoscopes, lasers). • Equipment that uses or emits light (e.g., fiberoptic light sources). • Devices that produce an optical (not electronic) image.

*These theories are not always "intuitive" and often require mathematical expression for clarification.

mechanics is the study of motion and objects. Mechanics is involved in both the hand-held retractor and the computerized system that tells the surgeon how to remodel the patient's facial bones. Mechanics also is involved in heat, light, sound, electricity, and all the other forms of energy used in medical technology.

The origins of mechanics are found in the laws of physics. Physics is the complex study of matter, time, energy, force, and space. Physics describes the natural behavior of these concepts using complex mathematics. For example, without the mathematical formulas, we must simply accept that when an object is dropped from a height, it accelerates through space as it falls. The value of studying physics is that it helps us to better understand how the physical world behaves and why. In turn, the study of mechanics allows us to put that understanding to practical use.

Modern surgical technologists must ensure the safe use of electrical equipment, assemble and troubleshoot complex devices, and assist in their use on the surgical field. Many different applications of the principles of mechanics and physics are required. Likewise, their study is no longer simple or straightforward. Many different subspecialties have developed (Table 17-1).

SECTION I: PHYSICS

MATTER

ATOMIC STRUCTURE

The **atom** is the primary unit that makes up all physical matter. It behaves in very distinct and predictable ways. There are many types of *subatomic particles* (i.e., particles that are smaller than atoms). The ones discussed here are the proton

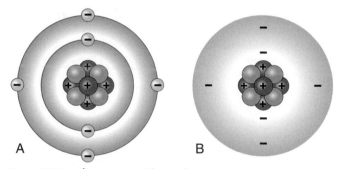

Figure 17-1   The atom. A, The nucleus contains positively charged protons and neutral neutrons. Negatively charged electrons surround the nucleus in energy "shells." **B,** Energy levels are not circular; rather, they resemble clouds. *(From Thibodeau G, Patton K: Anatomy and physiology, ed 6, St Louis, 2007, Mosby.)*

and the neutron, which are located in the center (**nucleus**) of the atom, and electrons, which occupy the atom's outer regions (Figure 17-1).

The average diameter of the nucleus atom is about 10^{-15} m. The relative distance between the nucleus and its electrons is extremely large, and the weight of the atom depends mainly on the number of particles in the nucleus. If we compare a golf ball to the nucleus of the atom, the distance from the nucleus to the electrons would be over 6.2 miles (10 km).

Nucleus

The nucleus of an atom contains two main particles, a neutron and a proton. A *proton* has a positive electrical charge and is the heaviest of the subatomic particles. A **neutron** has a neutral charge. The net charge of the nucleus is zero, because usually the number of protons and neutrons is the same. The nucleus is the center of the atom.

Electron

An **electron** is much smaller than a proton or neutron. Its weight is almost negligible compared with the nuclear particles. The number of electrons in the atom varies with the type of element. The electron has a negative charge and orbits the nucleus in discrete, three-dimensional energy levels. These energy levels are referred to as "clouds" because electrons move randomly within their discrete or separate energy level, not in a linear path, as was thought to be the case when atomic structure was first studied. Atoms that have more than two electrons have more energy levels. The more distant the energy level from the nucleus, the less energy is needed for an electron to separate from the nucleus. This is important to an understanding of electricity, which involves the movement of electrons from one atom to another.

ELEMENTS AND MOLECULES

An **element** is a pure substance in which each atom has the same number of protons (this number is referred to as the *atomic number*). Regardless of the number of electrons and neutrons an atom has, the atomic number of the element remains the same. For example, the element iron has 26 protons; therefore, the atomic number of iron is 26.

The *atomic weight* of an element is the sum of the weight of its protons and neutrons. An element can have a different number of neutrons. When this occurs, the substance is called an **isotope** of the element.

By international scientific convention, all known elements are classified and arranged on a standardized chart called the periodic table. The **periodic table** lists all known elements according to their mass and electronic behavior. The table, which was first developed in 1869 by Dmitri Mendeleev, has evolved as new elements have been discovered.

A **molecule** is two or more atoms held together by chemical bonds (Figure 17-2). Just as atoms of a particular element have the same number of protons and neutrons, molecules of a substance are identified by the different elements that compose them. For example, a molecule of water always contains one hydrogen atom and two oxygen atoms (H_2O). *Organic compounds* are those whose molecules contain the element carbon. Organic molecules are the basic structure of all living things.

STATES OF MATTER

We know from observing the physical world that substances take on different forms. These forms—liquid, solid, gas, and plasma—are referred to as the **states of matter**. Most substances can exist in a variety of states. For example, when water is heated to 212° F (100° C), it becomes steam, its gaseous state. The state of the water has changed from liquid to gas, but it retains its molecular structure.

A **solid** is a substance in which the molecules are tightly bound in rigid formation. A *liquid* is formed when heat (energy) is applied to a solid. Common experience teaches us that some substances melt more readily than others. This is because the bonds of some molecules are stronger in some substances than in others. The point at which a substance turns from solid to liquid is called the *melting point*.

A substance assumes a gaseous state when the energy applied to it is greater than the energy bonds that hold the molecules together. When heated, the molecules move away from each other in random directions. Different substances become gases at different temperatures. This is called the **boiling point** of the substance.

Plasma (in physics) is gas in which the atom's electrons are separated from its nucleus. For this to happen, the temperature of the molecules must be very high. Plasma is found in the arc of incandescent light produced by a welding torch; it also is present in the gaseous areas surrounding stars.

MOTION

ELEMENTS OF MOTION

Motion is the result of energy and work. We can describe motion in mathematical or conceptual terms. Some important qualities of motion are:

- *Speed:* Speed is a description of how fast an object travels from one point to another. In mathematical terms, the *rate* is the time it takes to cover a certain distance, or time over distance. For example, a car traveling 70 miles per hour is another way of stating the rate of 70 miles/1 hr. In surgical technology, the speed of some powered cutting instruments is measured in oscillations per second.
- *Distance:* Motion is the movement (displacement) of an object from one point to another or the return of the object to the point where it started. *Displacement*, therefore, describes how far the object went from its original position to its destination. *Distance*, a different concept, is the actual amount of space or ground the object covered during its period of motion.
- *Velocity:* Velocity is the speed of a moving object, measured as distance over time.

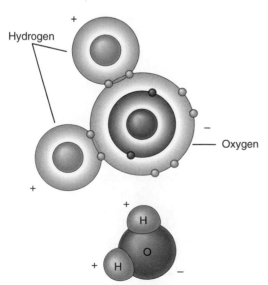

Figure 17-2 A molecule of water (H_2O) is composed of two elements: hydrogen (two atoms) and oxygen (one atom). *(From Thibodeau G, Patton K: Anatomy and physiology, ed 6, St Louis, 2007, Mosby.)*

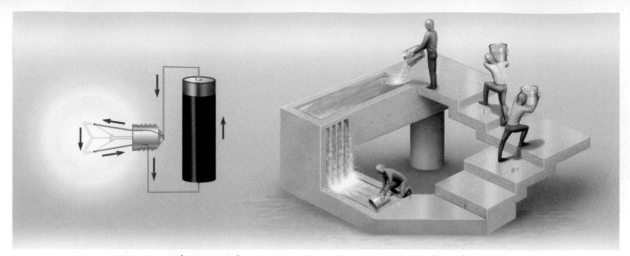

Figure 17-3 **Potential energy.** *Left,* A battery with stored energy. *Right,* The flow of water demonstrates the concept of potential energy. The potential energy is greatest at the top of the platform. *(From Giambattista A, Richardson BM, Richardson RC: College physics, ed 2, New York, 2007, McGraw-Hill. Reproduced with permission of the McGraw-Hill Companies.)*

- **Momentum:** A mathematical quantity that describes the amount and weight of matter (called the *mass*) and the velocity of the mass. In this relationship, the greater the mass and velocity, the greater the momentum: momentum = mass × velocity. In everyday terms, this means that the speed and mass of an object affect the amount of energy needed to change the momentum—that is, to stop it, change its direction, speed it up, or slow it down.
- *Force:* In mechanics, force is the pulling or pushing of one object on another.

CIRCULAR AND PROJECTILE MOTION

When an object travels in a circle, the length of its path around the circle is called a *circumference*. Satellites and planets have a particular kind of circular motion. Within our solar system, the sun is the center of the planets. A satellite accelerates toward the Earth because of the force of gravity (the force that pulls all objects with mass toward each other). However, because of the curvature of the planet, the satellite does not crash into the Earth (instead it falls around the planet in a circle).

When an object is thrown straight outward, it follows a curved path called *projectile motion*. This occurs because gravity pulls the object downward toward the ground.

ENERGY

All surgical devices and technologies depend on a form of *energy* for operation. The surgical technologist is required to have a fundamental understanding of these energy forms, especially as they relate to patient safety. The technologist must handle, assemble, and process the equipment in a way that protects it and prevents medical errors or malfunction. The first step in preventing accidents and errors with equipment is to understand the energy that powers the equipment or is emitted by it. Two types of energy are discussed, potential energy and electromagnetic energy. These classifications are used as an aid to comprehension. They are not rigid categorizations, but a general classification is helpful for learning about energy.

POTENTIAL ENERGY

Potential energy is also referred to as *stored energy.* Figure 17-3 illustrates the concept of potential energy.

GRAVITATIONAL ENERGY

Gravitational energy exists when a stationary mass or object is positioned such that gravity will cause it to move. A stationary rock on top of a cliff has potential gravitational energy because if it is pushed over the edge, it will fall. The **potential energy** of an object is measured by its mass (weight) and distance from the earth. This concept is vividly illustrated when we imagine a patient falling from the operating table. This can occur when the safety strap is not applied or the patient has not been positioned in a way that prevents sliding. In the case of the falling patient, the greater the weight (mass) of the patient, the greater the potential energy and the more forceful the impact from a fall.

MECHANICAL ENERGY

There are two types of mechanical energy—**kinetic** energy and potential energy. Objects in motion have kinetic energy that is translational (able to be transferred from one location to another). For example, an orthopedic drill uses circular motion to cut a hole in bone. The oscillating saw uses side to side motion in a straight line to cut or incise bone. Potential energy of an object is stored with the object in a static position. Potential energy can be seen in springs or elastic material. When these are compressed and then allowed to resume a neutral position, they exert force and produce energy. When energy is applied to a spring to compress it, the spring travels a distance, returns to its original position (neutral), and then moves in the opposite direction. This movement is called an *oscillation*. If the force is applied to the spring only once, the spring continues to oscillate at lower and lower levels and then comes to rest. However, if the force is applied at a continuous rate and strength, the spring keeps moving (oscillating) the same distance in a negative and positive direction.

CHEMICAL ENERGY

Molecules are bonded by several different kinds of forces. When these bonds are broken, energy is released. We can experience this when mixing components of methylmethacrylate bone cement. The chemical reaction of mixing the powder cement and liquid chemical together to form the end product creates heat. The same thing occurs when plaster cast material is mixed with water.

ELECTROMAGNETIC ENERGY

Many devices used in surgery derive their energy from electromagnetic radiation. Most of the wave energy studied in this chapter is electromagnetic energy. Electromagnetic waves exist in a very large range of frequencies. It is important to remember that *the frequency of the wave determines the type of energy and its capabilities.* (Chapter 18 presents additional information on specific energy sources used in surgery.) A brief explanation here will introduce this concept.

Electromagnetic energy exhibits wave behavior. The types of wave energy discussed in this chapter include:

- Electricity
- Light
- Heat
- Sound

WAVES

In simple terms, a **wave** can be described as a disturbance in a medium such as air, water, or a solid substance. Waves behave in predictable patterns, and their movements are measurable. Mechanical waves travel through a medium such as water or a solid. **Electromagnetic waves** move in the air or in a vacuum and are created by a vibrating electric charge. Another example is the frequency of waves transmitted by a radio station.

Properties of Waves

Waves can be drawn, or plotted, as shown in Figure 17-4. As you can see, a wave has crests and troughs. The *crest* is the highest point of disturbance, and the *trough* is the negative or lowest point of disturbance. The resting point is the area of no disturbance or movement and is represented by the straight line.

Waves move out from their source. An example is a stone thrown into a pool of water. The water is energized by the force of the stone disturbing it. This creates concentric waves. When the stone sinks, the energy source is no longer present, and the waves begin to diminish in size and finally stop.

Wavelength is a measurement of one complete wave cycle—that is, the length from one crest to the next.

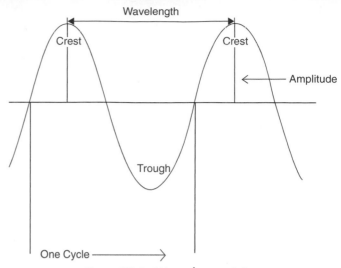

Figure 17-4   Wave characteristics.

Amplitude is the point of greatest disturbance, or the height of an individual wave. This is measured in meters from the top of the crest to the point of rest.

Frequency is the number of waves that pass a point in 1 second. The unit of measurement for electromagnetic frequency is the hertz (Hz). As the frequency of a wave increases, the units of measurement change to reflect these numbers. Kilohertz (kHz) is thousands of hertz, and megahertz (MHz) is millions of hertz. Radio waves are capable of producing the lowest frequency (but widest variation) while gamma rays have the highest frequency measured.

The speed of a wave is measured in meters per second. The speed of a wave depends on whether the wave energy is mechanical or electromagnetic.

NOTE: All electromagnetic waves travel at the same speed, regardless of the type of energy they produce.

Reflection

When a wave reaches a boundary, it may pass through the boundary or be reflected back (**reflection**), depending on the nature of the boundary and the type of wave energy. For example, light can pass through a glass lens because the optical density of glass is low. Gamma rays used in medical x-rays do not penetrate the lead aprons worn by the team. Sound waves are reflected as an echo when they reach a solid boundary.

Interference

Waves that have the same wavelength and are propagated at the same time can be lined up exactly. In this case, we say that the waves are coherent. An example of coherent waves is laser light. All the troughs and peaks match, and this creates a very intense white light. We know that laser light is very powerful—it is hot, bright, and penetrating. Technology that produces this coherent light has changed the way we perform surgery. When waves are superimposed, the amplitude of the resulting wave is greater than any one of the individual waves. However, if the waves are not lined up (the troughs and peaks are not in line), they will cancel each other out. Anyone who has seen waves on the shore has seen waves cancel each other when

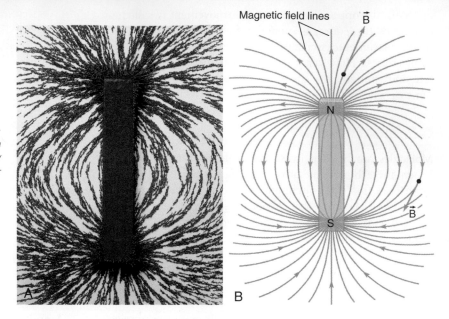

Figure 17-5 Force pattern of a bar magnet exhibited by iron filings. *(From Giambattista A, Richardson BM, Richardson RC: College physics, ed 2, New York, 2007, McGraw-Hill. Reproduced with permission of the McGraw-Hill Companies.)*

they come from different directions. This is mechanical interference, but the same thing occurs with other types of waves.

ELECTRICITY

APPLICATION IN SURGERY

Nearly all biomedical devices require electricity as their power source. Even optical instruments that use lenses, such as the endoscope and microscope, have imaging and power components that require electricity to move the equipment and provide light. Other complex devices, such as lasers, physiological monitoring equipment, diagnostic imaging equipment, and computer-assisted robotic systems, use complex circuits and high-voltage electricity.

Electricity is used directly to perform procedures in all forms of electrosurgery. Numerous risks and hazards are associated with electrosurgery. To ensure the safety of the patient and staff members, the surgical technologist and perioperative nurse are required to have more than a basic understanding of electricity. The following discussion of electricity forms the basis for a more advanced understanding of electrosurgery, which is discussed in later chapters.

NATURE OF ELECTRICITY

Recall that atoms contain positively charged protons, negatively charged electrons, and neutrons, which have no electric charge. The net charge on an atom is determined by the numbers of electrons and protons, which must be equal for the atom to be stable.

Electricity is created when electrons move from atom to atom. The movement of electrons and the energy this creates follow some basic laws, which are important to understand electricity:

1. Opposite charges attract each other, and like charges repel each other.

2. Energy is never lost or destroyed, but it can be transformed from one form to another.
3. Electricity flows out from a negative source seeking a positive conclusion.

MAGNETISM AND ELECTRICITY

Some naturally occurring metals, such as iron, attract and repel charged particles. The two poles of an iron bar or magnet exhibit opposite forces. This produces a **magnetic field**, a three-dimensional force pattern created by the positive and negative charges of a polar magnet (Figure 17-5).

It is important to remember that *magnetism* is not electricity; however, the two are closely related. When one pole of a magnet is passed over a rotating coil of conductive material, such as a copper wire, electric current is induced through the wire. An **electromagnetic field** is created around the rotating coil, and the energy that results can be captured and controlled to do work.

CONDUCTIVITY

Recall that the atom's electrons move randomly within discrete energy levels around the atom. In certain types of substances, especially metals, electrons are easily displaced from the outer energy levels. They become free electrons. When an atom loses one of its electrons, the atom is left with a positive charge. Another free electron in the vicinity is attracted to this positively charged atom and attaches to it. An atom that has lost or gained an electron is called an *ion*. You can imagine that the charged ion will pick up or lose electrons (depending on its overall charge) as it moves through a medium. In some elements, electrons move from atom to atom, balancing and unbalancing the charges. The ability of a material to release free electrons is called **conductivity**. Substances with low conductivity do not give up their electrons easily. Materials with high conductivity lose their outer electrons very easily.

Substances with low conductivity include rubber and glass, whereas metal is highly conductive. Temperature can alter the conductivity of a substance. For example, glass is non-conductive at low temperatures but conductive at very high temperatures.

It is important to remember that randomly moving free electrons are not the same as electricity. No work is being performed, and the net charge is usually neutral because the number of atoms losing electrons is equal to the number receiving them. Conductive material is simply the path through which the free electrons can be made to line up and move.

INSULATORS

A substance with low or no conductivity is called an **insulator**. Examples of materials used in modern electrical insulation are polyethylene, polyvinyl chloride (PVC), and Teflon. Insulators are used as protectors and to resist electric current. Surgical instruments used in minimally invasive surgery have insulated sheaths to protect the patient from being burned by stray electricity.

The concept of conductivity is directly related to operational safety in electrosurgery. For this reason, it is important to think of conductivity as it relates to a substance and its environment. Box 17-1 describes conductive and insulating materials.

STATIC ELECTRICITY

Under certain circumstances, such as friction and low humidity, charged particles tend to accumulate on surfaces. If two surfaces have the same net charge, they will repel each other. If the net charges are opposite, the surfaces will attract each other. This is called **static electricity**.

Electrostatic discharge occurs when the accumulation of charges on surfaces is so great that the air between the surfaces acts as a conductor. Air usually is not conductive; however, when the environment is very dry and sufficient friction exists between the materials, ions build up quickly and the air ignites. When a person's shoes accumulate static and the person then touches a conductive surface, such as a metal door

handle, the charges are suddenly transmitted. This can cause a perceptible electrical shock.

Electrostatic discharge is a significant problem in industry and biomedical technology. The sudden unexpected release of energy just described can be strong enough to ignite substances in the environment. In the past, when flammable anesthetic agents were commonly used, many precautions were taken to prevent static discharge. Although the phenomenon is less problematic now, with the regulated use of gases, static discharge is kept to a minimum with environmental controls such as low temperature and high humidity in the perioperative environment.

ELECTRIC GENERATORS

An *electric generator* converts mechanical energy into electricity. Generators provide the power to move electrical current through a conductive material. The generator does not produce the electrical current; it only provides the mechanical power to do the work. In simple terms, a generator is a coil of conductive material (usually metal wire) wound around a rotating shaft within a magnetic field. This creates electrical current.

ELECTRICAL CIRCUITS

Free electrons flow through conductive material in a continuous path, with each electron "pushing" the one ahead of it; this is called a **circuit**. As long as the path is not interrupted, the electrons will continue to flow, much as water flows through a tube. Electrical current always seeks the path of least resistance.

Direct Current

An electrical circuit that flows in one direction from one charged pole to the other is referred to as **direct current (DC)**. A battery is an example of a DC power source. The battery has a negative and a positive pole. When a wire is attached from one pole to the other, electrons flow through the wire from one pole to the other (Figure 17-6). The circuit is closed, because there is no break in the flow. Battery-powered instruments use low-voltage direct current.

Alternating Current

With **alternating current (AC)**, the direction of the flow changes back and forth within the circuit. The interval between directional changes is called a **cycle**. The rate at which the current changes directions is called the *frequency*. In the United States, the frequency of household power is 60 cycles per second.

AC is used for common municipal power and is the source of power for nearly every type of electrical device in medical technology. AC delivers high-voltage power. A clear understanding of alternating current paths, resistance, and conductivity is critical for all perioperative personnel. In this discussion, the basics of AC are explained. In Chapter 18, the use of electrosurgery and safety considerations are covered in detail.

Box **17-1** Conductors and Insulators	
Conductors	**Insulators**
Metal	Glass
Silver	Rubber
Copper	Fiberglass
Gold	Ceramic
Aluminum	Dry cotton
Iron	Wood
Steel	Plastic
Brass	Air
Other	Pure water
Water (with particles in solution)	
Concrete	

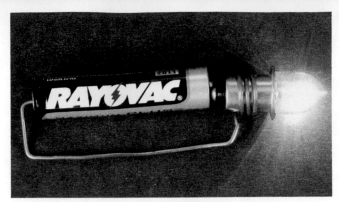
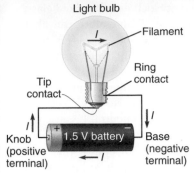
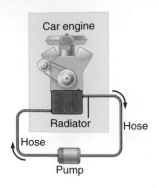

Figure 17-6   **Direct current (DC).** The battery has a negative pole and a positive pole. A wire attached to each end conducts electrons, which are condensed through a smaller wire filament, creating light. *(From Giambattista A, Richardson BM, Richardson RC: College physics, ed 2, New York, 2007, McGraw-Hill. Reproduced with permission of the McGraw-Hill Companies.)*

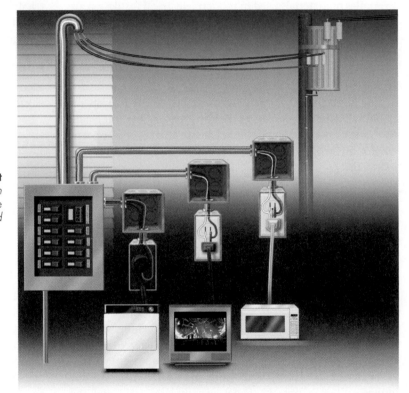

Figure 17-7   Household circuit using alternating current (AC) derived from a municipal electricity source. *(From Giambattista A, Richardson BM, Richardson RC: College physics, ed 2, New York, 2007, McGraw-Hill. Reproduced with permission of the McGraw-Hill Companies.)*

PATH OF ALTERNATING CURRENT Alternating current is brought into a facility such as a hospital or house from the municipal source through overhead or underground wires. The wires are collected and redirected at the facility's electrical grid. This is a complex system where all electrical connections coming into the facility meet, are metered, and then are directed to the appropriate sections of the facility. This is also where electricity leaves the facility and returns to the municipal source, completing the electrical circuit. Figure 17-7 shows alternating current from high-voltage lines and its path through a household electrical system.

Three wires make up the alternating current pathway through a building, terminating at the **receptacle**, or electrical outlet. Each of the three wires has a different function. The **hot wire** is the power source from the power grid to the receptacle. This wire usually is covered in black, nonconductive

material. The second wire, which usually is white, is called the neutral wire. It conducts electricity back to the grid and eventually out to the power pole or underground pathway. The third wire, which usually is green, is called the ground or ground wire. The *ground wire* protects the circuit from a "short" or fault in the system, such as when the active and neutral wires come into direct contact, resulting in sparks and heat. The ground wire receives the stray current and conducts it safely back to the facility's grid. A metal rod buried deep in the ground connects the grid to the ground, where electricity disperses and is rendered harmless.

Voltage

The force or power that pushes or drives electrons through the conductive material is called **voltage**. This is the potential energy expressed as units of charge. We measure the amount of charge that flows past a given point over a specific period. This unit of measurement is called an **ampere** or *amp*. Voltage can be increased or decreased with a device called a *transformer*.

Resistance

In electricity, **resistance** is any interruption of current through the conductive material. Resistance depends on properties such as the type and thickness of the material. Conductive materials are defined as having high or low resistance, depending on their ability to conduct electricity. Materials with low resistance have greater conductivity.

Resistance is used to transform one form of energy into another form. A common example is an incandescent light bulb. Current passes from a standard copper wire into the bulb's finer metal filament, which has a higher resistance than the wire conducting electricity to the bulb. Resistance at the filament causes it to become hot and glow. In this case, resistance is used purposefully to create a desired effect. The heating effect of the wire filament can be understood by comparing the electrons to water pressure. Water flowing through a hose remains at a constant pressure unless the diameter is decreased or increased. If you crimp the hose, reducing its diameter at that point, the pressure increases at the point of resistance. The point of resistance in an electrical circuit creates heat, which is analogous to the increased pressure in the hose.

Resistance is measured in units called *ohms*. We can measure the amount of resistance in conductive material with an ohm meter. Resistance is an important concept in surgery. In the perioperative environment, unintended resistance can result in injury to the patient. Electrical biomedical devices have a self-monitoring capability, which stops the current when resistance exceeds a specific level. However, this does not prevent patient injury in all cases.

NOTE: *When resistance occurs, an electrical current may seek an unintended alternative path, which can terminate at patient tissue, causing severe burns.*

LIGHT

PROPERTIES OF VISIBLE LIGHT

Light is a form of electromagnetic radiation, but it also has properties of a particle. The particle theory attributes the name **photon** to a light particle.

Visible light is actually white light and is made up of different wavelengths. When separated, these distinct wavelengths are perceived as different colors. White light, when transmitted through a prism, separates into distinct wavelengths, and its colors become visible. The same phenomenon takes place in a rainbow, in which the raindrops act as prisms.

SIGHT

We see an object because our eyes are able to interpret the image created when light encounters an object along our line of sight. The complexity of physiological interpretation is separate from the physical relationship between the object and light rays. We know intuitively that we can see objects directly only when they are "straight in front" of us. We can cause light rays to bend, such as in a fiberoptic cable, but under natural circumstances, the object must be within our line of sight to be seen.

REFRACTION

The ability to focus light through serial lenses, magnify the images, and transmit them to imaging systems is among the most important advances in modern surgical technology. Endoscopic minimally invasive surgery and microsurgery depend on these technologies, which include the manufacture of high-quality optical systems.

Light rays passing through a medium such as glass or plastic bend because the speed of the rays is decreased; this is called **refraction**. The more dense the material, the more slowly the light will pass through it. The term *refractive index* refers to the speed at which waves (light or sound) pass through a medium. Glass, sapphire, and other transparent media have high refractive indices.

REFLECTION

Light waves exhibit a property called *reflection*, which was described earlier as a wave property. This means that when light rays encounter some surfaces, they can reverse direction. Reflection occurs when light rays encounter a mirror or other surface that does not fully absorb the light. We know instinctively that sight requires light. The light rays are reflected at the same angle at which they contact the surface. Therefore, images seen in a mirror are those within the line of sight. The image in the mirror is a result of the light reversing direction—resulting in reflection of the image.

COHERENCE

Coherent light waves occur when propagated waves are lined up so that their peaks and troughs match. Under natural circumstances, light is emitted from its source in all directions. However, light rays can be focused through a lens or propagated through a medium such as a gas. When light is passed through a lasing gas, it becomes coherent and intensive enough to cut through many different types of material, including tissue. This is the basis of laser energy, which is discussed in detail in Chapter 18.

LENSES

Lenses are made of highly refractive material. They are manufactured in such a way that light rays passing through a lens are focused on one point or spread out over a large area. When the rays are focused in a single area, the area is called the **focal point**. The shape of a lens determines how the light rays bend as they pass through it. A simple *convex lens* is thinner at the edges than at the middle. A **concave** lens is thinner at the middle than around the edges and causes the light to diverge or spread.

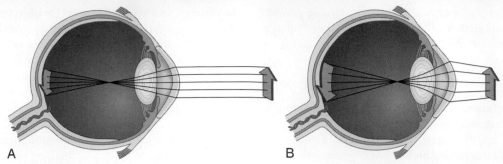

Figure 17-8 Focal points in the eye. Light converges inside the eye through the lens, which focuses the image on the retina. **A,** The focal distance is long resulting in a smaller image on the retina when compared with a shorter focal distance shown in **B. B,** A shortened focal length provides a larger image on the retina after the light rays converge and spread. *(From Thibodeau G, Patton K:* Anatomy and physiology, *ed 6, St Louis, 2007, Mosby.)*

Lenses used in surgery and microscopy refract light rays so that they converge (come together) in one area to produce a magnified image. The eye focuses an image on the retina as light passes through the lens (Figure 17-8). Endoscopes use **serial lenses** to achieve a high level of clarity and brightness. In this lens system, several lenses are lined up inside the endoscopic telescope.

HEAT

Heat is a form of energy that is quantitative (measurable) and transferable. In physics, temperature is a characteristic of matter and is related to the movement of atoms and molecules. Recall that energy is never lost but can be changed from one form to another. For example, electricity can be transformed into thermal (heat) energy and used in electrosurgery.

HEAT TRANSFER

Heat transfer is important in patient care and safety in the perioperative environment. The body maintains a constant temperature to sustain life through a process called **thermoregulation**. However, illness, medications, and trauma (including surgery) can alter the body's natural ability to maintain the correct temperature. During surgery, the patient's core temperature may be dangerously lowered by anesthetic agents, blood loss, and tissue trauma.

Heat is transferred in three ways:
- Conduction
- Convection
- Radiation

Conduction

Heat **conduction** is caused by the natural vibrations of the molecules that make up a substance. Warmer substances have more movement than cold ones. When a warm substance comes in contact with a cooler substance, the molecules collide, which increases movement in the cooler material, raising its temperature. Some substances conduct heat more efficiently than others; this quality is called **thermal conductivity**.

An example of thermal conduction occurs when a saline irrigation solution is placed in a fluid warmer. The fluid warmer, which is an electrical heating element, comes in contact with the basin holding the saline solution. Energy is transferred to the basin, which causes molecular movement in the saline solution. The thermal energy of the saline solution dissipates to the cooler room air, but as long as the fluid warmer is sufficiently heated to overcome this energy transfer, the saline will remain warm.

The patient can lose heat by conduction when exposed to cold air in the environment. Children and underweight patients are particularly at risk for hypothermia. This is prevented by using warm air blankets, which conduct heat at a controlled level.

Convection

Convection is heat transfer by the natural movement of heated air or water over a cooler surface. When air becomes warm, it rises, because the heated molecules become less dense and thus lighter. As the heated molecules rise, they carry energy.

An example of convection is seen when a radiator generates heat to the cool areas of a room. Warm air in the room is less dense and rises to the ceiling, where it displaces cooler air. A current occurs as the cooler room air sinks to the floor and the warm air rises. Figure 17-9 illustrates convection currents in the environment.

Radiation

Heat is given off from its source as electromagnetic energy; this is called *radiation*. This means that the energy behaves like all other waves. Some objects "glow" with heat, because these electromagnetic waves are in the visible spectrum. The eye perceives the energy as light, because the wavelength of the object is perceptible. Objects that are hot but do not glow also have radiant qualities, but their wavelength is outside the visible range.

SOUND

PROPERTIES OF SOUND

Sound is a type of energy generated by the movement of waves through a substance such as air or water. Because sound is wave energy, it has many of the properties of other waves: loudness, which is subjective interpretation of the intensity; frequency (the number of waves that pass a given

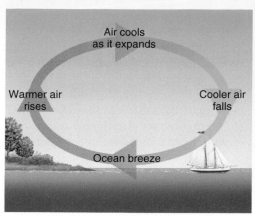 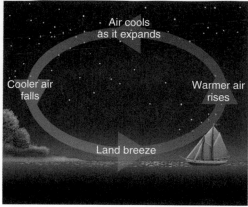

Figure 17-9 **Convection currents in the environment.** *(From Giambattista A, Richardson BM, Richardson RC: College physics, ed 2, New York, 2007, McGraw-Hill. Reproduced with permission of the McGraw-Hill Companies.)*

point in a given time); amplitude (the intensity of the sound as measured in decibels [dB]); and pitch (our perception of the different frequencies). Sound is characterized as a disturbance in a medium such as air or water. We perceive sound only when the vibrations are within the limits of the brain's ability to sense them.

REFLECTION

As wave energy, sound can be reflected, and this property is used in **ultrasound** technology, which is one of the most widely used diagnostic tools in medicine. In this process, sound waves with a frequency higher than those perceived by the human ear are transmitted through a medium, and the return signal is *transduced* (one energy form converted into another) into a visual image. The ultrasound wavelength is relatively short, which allows it to detect small targets. Advanced imaging techniques provide a concise picture of the ultrasound signal, which measures the density, size, and shape of the target anatomy. Echocardiography uses ultrasound technology to produce an image of the heart (Figure 17-10). Extremely high-energy sound waves are used in surgical technology to separate molecules and remodel tissue. This technique is discussed more fully in Chapter 18.

DOPPLER EFFECT

Mechanical or electromagnetic waves are perceived by the human senses (vision and hearing) or by equipment that can track and display the waveforms as data. When we hear an ambulance siren, the sound waves seem to change pitch as they approach us. The pitch seems to get higher as the ambulance approaches and lower as it moves away. This change in pitch is due to a phenomenon called the *Doppler effect.* The siren does not actually change pitch or frequency as it moves away. The waves become wider and wider (or more "stretched") as they move outward from the source. When the source of the waves is moving toward us, the waves are more compressed and therefore higher in frequency; that is, more waves can fit into a smaller interval. The ear perceives these wide (or tight) intervals as high and low pitch. This is the **Doppler effect**.

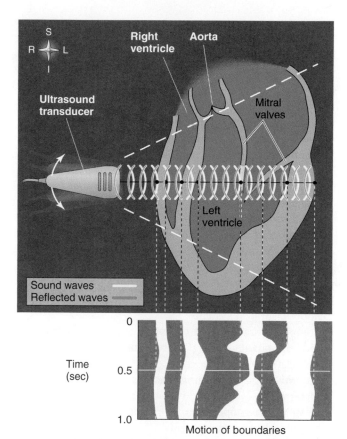

Figure 17-10 **Echocardiography uses ultrasound technology to produce an image of the heart.** *Sound waves are sent from a transducer to heart tissue, which reflects an accurate image. (From Thibodeau G, Patton K: Anatomy and physiology, ed 6, St Louis, 2007, Mosby.)*

Doppler ultrasound uses both the Doppler effect and ultrasound waves to detect narrowing or obstructions in blood vessels. The Doppler equipment emits a signal that is reflected by the moving blood cells. The reflected sound is measured and transduced to a visual image. More advanced systems transduce signals into color images, which provide detailed information about the velocity and direction of blood flow. Tissue Doppler imaging (TDI) uses the Doppler principle to detect movement in cardiac tissue (e.g., in valves) with ultrasonic imaging in cardiovascular assessment.

HARMONICS

Sound exhibits a property called **harmonics**, which is related to the frequency of the wavelength. Although wave harmonics can be measured in other forms of kinetic energy, harmonics produces a particular quality of sound, which we distinguish in the human voice or in musical instruments. For example, when force is applied to a string, the string oscillates back and forth (vibrates), creating wave energy. The oscillations of a string may be audible if their frequency is within hearing range. The quality of pitch is perceived as the oscillations move at greater or lesser frequency. The human voice is created by oscillations of the vocal cords, which are amplified by the larynx and other anatomical structures of the throat and mouth.

SECTION II: INFORMATION TECHNOLOGY

COMPUTERS IN THE PERIOPERATIVE ENVIRONMENT

Computer technology is incorporated into many different types of equipment and biomedical devices used in the perioperative environment. Some of these include:

- Secure computer systems for recording patient information (patient charts) and other medical records
- Preference cards for surgeons (indicates the surgeon's choice of equipment, supplies, positioning, and other important information)
- Diagnostic imaging equipment (e.g., radiography, magnetic resonance imaging [MRI], computed tomography [CT], fluoroscopy)
- Digital cameras and image output on monitors (screens) during surgical procedures
- Robotic surgical systems
- Computer tracking of hospital supplies, instruments, and equipment during reprocessing (e.g., disinfection, sterilization)
- Automatic patient billing systems for supplies used in surgery
- Computerized operation of sterilizers and instrument decontamination equipment

COMPUTER LEARNING TOOLS

As with any new skill, learning computer technology requires not only a basic understanding, but also time spent using the equipment and experiencing how it responds when commands are given (purposefully or accidentally). It is important and helpful to have someone who can coach the learner through the beginning phases of the learning process.

Many computer tasks are more easily understood by doing them rather than reading a description of them. Technology changes very rapidly, and information given in manuals and books can quickly become outdated. New technology commonly is developed and marketed within months.

HOW COMPUTERS WORK

The computer's main function is to store data and retrieve them using electrical signals. Most people have seen computers on which information is viewed on a screen and data are entered on a keyboard. The data are stored on *chips,* or small electrical circuits that are not readily visible. The microprocessor is another part of computer technology. Microprocessors provide computing power to everything from mobile phones to complex industrial and medical equipment.

COMPUTER TERMS AND LANGUAGE

Computer technology uses a particular terminology and language to describe the following:

- What the computer *does* (e.g., displaying an email)
- The *equipment* needed to perform the tasks (e.g., the keyboard or screen)
- The *process* used to make the equipment work (e.g., computer programs or the electrical signals that transmit information)

Computer terms mean very specific things. For example:

- Electronic information is called *data.*
- Pictures on a computer screen are called *images.*
- The process of entering information into the computer (by a human or another machine) is called *inputting.*
- Information received from the computer is called *output.* Output can be in any form—for example, a printed email or an actual radiograph that has been taken and processed by a computerized radiographic machine.

NOTE: *Data are input into the computer and can be seen as an image on the screen or printed as paper output.*

Try to learn basic computer terms as you learn how to use a computer. These will help you and others communicate clearly as you work.

HARDWARE (PHYSICAL COMPONENTS)

The physical parts of a computer are the central core unit and peripherals. The core unit contains the wiring and complex circuits that run the computer and store data. The peripherals are other types of equipment that *interface* with (work with) the computer and are part of its operation, such as the computer screen, keyboard, and mouse. The basic hardware components are described in Table 17-2.

COMPUTER SOFTWARE

The term *software* is used to describe programs that control the tasks a computer can perform. Software is stored in the electronic components of a computer. The computer needs instructions from the software to perform the tasks that individuals require it to do. Unlike a mechanical device, which performs physical work, the computer sorts and computes information electronically. These tasks are made possible through the computer software.

Table 17-2 | Basic Computer Hardware

Component	Description
Central processing unit (CPU)	The computer memory (internal) and electronic components that enable programming and output.
Memory	Also called **RAM** or random access memory, this connects with the main electrical circuits to perform all the tasks needed to operate the computer. Data placed in RAM must be saved on other hardware called the drive.
Motherboard	The primary circuits that run the computer.
Drive	Internal or external device that stores the computer's data. External data drives such as flash drives are portable and can be moved from one computer to another for reading. **Internal drives** are identified by a letter on some types of computers.
Monitor	The computer's screen where data are viewed by the user. The screen is also called the display or output display. Two types are commonly used—the liquid crystal display (LCD) and the cathode ray tube (CRT).
Modem/wireless card	An electronic device that makes the transmission to or from a computer via a communication line.
Keyboard	Alphanumeric device for inputting data to the computer.
Mouse	The user's steering component for inputting data on the monitor. It provides a visual cue on the monitor and signals the computer to perform a task associated with that cue.
Speakers	Like other types of speakers, these provide sound output from the computer.
Hard copy	Data computer output that has been reproduced in the form of a CD, DVD, or paper printout.
Printer/Scanner/Fax	Output and input devices that produce paper and electronic documentation.
USB Port	A type of serial port for connecting peripheral devices to a computer system.

To further define what software actually is, we need to know that the computer operates by reading a set of instructions that tell it what to do and how to do it. These instructions are contained in a code (called machine code), which is a series of billions of on-off switches. Combinations of on-off codes create endless possibilities for storing and manipulating information (data) based on the on-off switch codes.

Data in the memory of the computer are organized into blocks of eight switches. Each switch is called a bit, and each block is called a byte. Computer programs (software) are described as having a certain number of bytes that operate in an exact way, giving the computer instructions to perform different tasks associated with that program.

OPERATING SYSTEM

Computers are programmed to understand certain tasks through their operating system (OS). The OS is the electronic controller of all the data the computer needs to perform tasks. Several types of operating systems are commercially available. The most common are the Microsoft Windows, Macintosh, and Linux systems. In this discussion, the Microsoft system is used to describe basic functions and tasks.

COMPUTER PROGRAMS

Computer applications, or programs, perform specific tasks. An application is used to produce text documents, calculate mathematical equations, play music, or display photographs. Many kinds of programs are available for home computing and professional tasks. The most common types are:

- *Word processing:* This program performs the functions of a typewriter with many additional features. Documents can be created and formatted into simple or complex styles. The most common commercially used programs are Microsoft Word and Corel WordPerfect. An open-source version is called OpenOffice. Word processing usually is the first application a new user learns.
- **Database** or *spreadsheet:* This type of program allows the user to enter complex data involving items, lists, and numerical or arithmetic information. Calculations and formulas associated with the data are also computed. Examples of databases are statistical analysis and bookkeeping programs.
- *Graphic design:* This type of program provides the computing tools needed to "draw" and manipulate figures or to create complex images based on quantitative data. Examples are programs for designing engineering or architectural structures.
- *Interactive educational programs:* These programs are designed to help the user learn subjects such as mathematics, languages, and physical sciences. Educational programs are available for nearly any subject.

Although commercially sold programs are the most popular, many computer users are switching to *open-source software.* This type of software is noncommercial, and its intellectual property rights are in the public domain rather than belonging to a private corporation. These programs allow users to modify and openly share the processing information or language with others.

BASIC COMPUTER USE

COMPUTER MOTOR SKILLS

To work on a computer, an individual must learn a number of motor skills. These are not difficult, but they require instruction and practice. Typing skills are required to enter data into the computer quickly and with a minimum of errors. Another important skill is operation of the mouse.

Pointing and Selecting with the Mouse

The mouse is used to select and manipulate data on the computer screen. The interface between the mouse and the screen is either a graphic arrow or an "I," which shows where the mouse is pointed. This is called a *cursor* or *pointer*. A command or icon is activated by setting the cursor on the icon or text and pressing one of the mouse buttons (right or left). This is called *clicking* on an item. When a screen feature is clicked, the computer understands that it has been selected for some action. For example, if you want to start a computer program, you first must click on the icon representing that program. One click selects the item, and two clicks will open or retrieve the information associated with that item. The proper terms for the pressing the right and left buttons are *right click* and *left click*. A *double click* is two clicks of the same button.

Dragging

Dragging is a method of moving data icons and windows around on the monitor. To drag an item to a new location, place the cursor on the item. Left click and hold the button while moving the cursor, either by moving the mouse on the tabletop or with the mouse's trackball. When the item reaches the desired spot, release the button; this "drops" the item in the new location.

ELEMENTARY OPERATIONS

Start

To start a computer that is not already on, it is necessary to locate the power button on the **central processing unit (CPU)** or the keyboard. When the button is pressed, the computer begins to *boot up*, or start. The monitor lights up, and a logo appears on the screen. A password may be requested. If one is needed, a box appears on the screen asking for the password. The user must type the password in the box. Never share your password, and always *log off* after a computer session. This ensures that data are protected from manipulation by the next user (Box 17-2). When the computer accepts your password, another screen will appear.

Desktop

In graphics-based platforms, the desktop is the background for all computer program work (Figure 17-11). It displays the visual cues needed to start programs and perform tasks. It also is the visual "home base" of the computer; that is, it appears at the start and close of a computer session. The following sections discuss the items that appear on the desktop.

NOTE: The screen images and basic operations vary according to the year of publication for of the individual operating system and software.

Figure 17-11 Desktop.

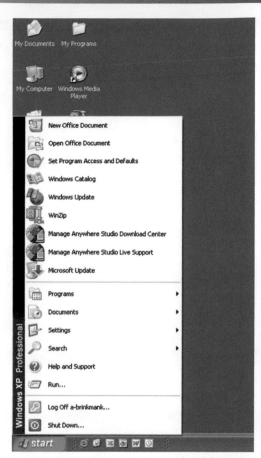

Figure 17-12 Start menu and task bar.

ICON An *icon* is a small picture or graphic cue associated with a program or data (see Figure 17-11). For example, particular information can be accessed through an icon that looks like a small file folder. Other examples of icons are those associated with documents, photographs, music, programs, Internet access, and power controls.

START MENU The Start menu is located at the bottom left corner of the desktop (Figure 17-12). This menu displays program icons and also a Help icon, where the user can access information on how to perform computer tasks. The Search icon is used to find data stored on the computer. This is also where you can log off to switch users and/or shut down.

TASK BAR The *task bar*, located at the bottom of the screen, displays applications and documents that are active, or *running*.

Files and Folders

A file is an electronic location where data are stored. Files are also graphic images that appear on the desktop or hard disk. To access all the files of the computer:

1. Right click on **START**.
2. Left click on **EXPLORE**.

This brings up a list of all the computer's files. Click on any file to select it. Double click to open the file and see the information. You can open a document inside the files by double

clicking on it. To close a file, click on the small box with the X in the upper right corner of the document.

Windows

A *window* is a rectangular frame that displays the boundaries of a document, graphic, or other image on the monitor. A window can be manipulated with the mouse. A window can be enlarged or reduced, or it can be moved around on the screen by dragging it with the mouse. To enlarge or reduce a window, look for three small boxes in the upper right corner. Left click on the middle box to reduce or enlarge the window. To change the size of a window, drag the edges of the window. You can also change the window by dragging the lower right corner.

To remove the window from the screen while keeping it active (in use), click on the far left box of the three boxes in the upper right corner. To restore the window to the screen, look for the tab associated with the window on the task bar and click on the tab.

The far right box will close the window and document completely. Do not close the window unless you have saved the document.

Toolbar

The *toolbar* is located at the top of a window (Figure 17-13). Many types of toolbars are available, each associated with specific programs. The toolbar displays icons and menus associated with tasks such as deleting text, saving documents to a file, or computing a formula. To change the toolbar or to see different toolbar options, look for the toolbar menus at the top of the screen:

1. Left click on **VIEW**.
2. Left click on **TOOLBARS**.
3. Select a toolbar and left click on it.

To remove a toolbar, left click on the active toolbar from the **VIEW** menu.

Menu

A *menu* is a list of optional commands the user can select while viewing or manipulating data. The menu appears as a list from which the user can select and execute a command. Menus appear as part of a computer program, on the Internet, or as a component of the standard desktop. To use a menu, left click on a word in the menu such as **WINDOW**, **FORMAT**, or **INSERT**. A list of options immediately appears on the screen. To use an option, left click on it. This executes a task or opens a box with further options to select.

Scrolling

Scrolling is the method used to "turn pages" on the computer screen. Windows-based programs have a rectangular border on the right and bottom of the window. Inside these borders are arrows. To move through pages of a document, place the cursor on one of the arrows and left click or hold the mouse button down. This causes the document to move page by page. To stop scrolling, release the mouse button. You may also scroll through pages by dragging the square located within the borders.

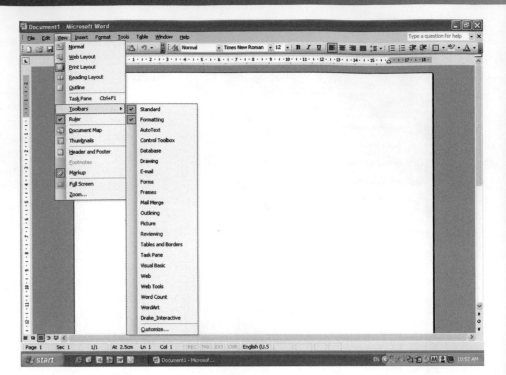

Figure 17-13   Toolbars.

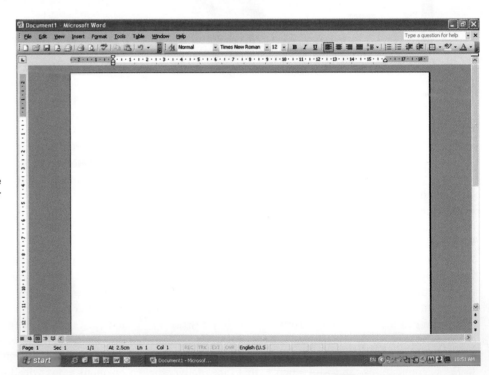

Figure 17-14 A window showing the boundaries of the document ready for typing and formatting.

WORD PROCESSING

Creating a Document

Word processing is a good way to learn how to use the computer. Many hundreds of options and formats are available on a word processing application. These can be learned over time with practice. The following are basic guidelines.

To start a new document in Microsoft Word, locate the **WORD** icon on the desktop or on the **START** menu. Click on this icon, and a new screen containing a blank "page" appears. The page is embedded inside a window (Figure 17-14). You can move the window around the screen by pointing and dragging it by the top of the frame.

Formatting Text

Text can be formatted and edited by using options on the **STANDARD** or **FORMATTING** toolbar (Figure 17-15).

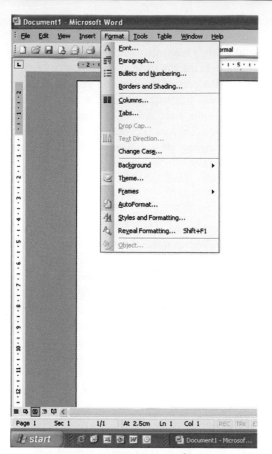

Figure 17-15 Formatting a document.

Font

To change a font (typeface):
1. Select **FORMAT/FONT**. A list of fonts and sizes appears.
2. Click on the font you prefer and then confirm the command by clicking OK.

The font selected now is applied to the document. Another way to select the font is to click on the font menu displayed in the toolbar. To adjust the size of the font from the toolbar, use the menu located next to the font style. Select and click on the size desired.

Changing Case

Letter case (capital or small letter) is established using the keyboard Shift key. To change a case once it is entered on the screen:
1. Select **FORMAT/CHANGE CASE**.
2. Select and click on the appropriate case in the box that appears.

Indents and Spacing

To adjust the space between lines in the text:
1. Select **FORMAT/PARAGRAPH** from the toolbar.
2. Select the desired spacing in **LINE SPACING**.
   To set the indent feature:
1. Select **FORMAT/PARAGRAPH**.
2. Choose the desired indentation feature from the menu displayed.

Page Numbers

To insert page numbers in the text:
1. Select **INSERT/PAGE NUMBERS** from the toolbar.

Selecting and Changing Text

To change the format or style of text that has already been entered in a document, you first must select the text with the mouse. This is done by positioning the cursor at the beginning of the word or sentence and then holding the left mouse button while moving the cursor over the text. Release the mouse button when all the desired text has been selected. Any format change will apply to the selected text. To *deselect* text, left click outside the selected area.

Editing Text

DELETE, MOVE, AND PASTE TEXT Sometimes text that has been entered must be deleted, or removed. To remove a word or small amount of text, place the cursor at the end of the area you want to delete and then backspace on the keyboard to remove. To remove large amounts of text, select the text with the mouse and press Delete or the backspace arrow on the keyboard. If you make a mistake in deleting text and you want to restore what was deleted, select **EDIT** and then **UNDO TYPING** from the toolbar.

To move text within a document:
1. Select the text.
2. Select **EDIT/CUT** from the toolbar.
3. Move the cursor to the desired location.
4. Left click.
5. Select **EDIT/PASTE**.

SPELL CHECK Spell check is a process in which the computer analyzes the spelling and grammar of the text and either suggests options for making corrections or makes them automatically. To use the spell check option:
1. Select **TOOLS/SPELLING** and **GRAMMAR** from the toolbar.

As the text is checked, a box with suggested corrections appears. To select one of the corrections, click on the option. The correction automatically replaces the error, and spell check continues until the entire text has been reviewed.

Graphics

Graphics are pictures used to enhance text documents. Pictures can be embedded into the text from many different sources. Bringing an image from one electronic source to another is called *importing*. Most word processing programs include a set of standard or "stock" images that can be imported into a document. These are called *clip art,* and they do not require copyright permission. Images also can be imported from other documents or files you have stored in the computer, or they can be obtained through the Internet. However, these imported images must not be used indiscriminately. Professional and medical images may require formal permission from the owner of the image. Graphic images can also be "drawn" using a graphics program.

To import an image to text:
1. Place the cursor where you want the image to appear in the text.

2. Select INSERT from the toolbar.
3. Select PICTURE.
4. Select the source of the image and follow the prompts in the dialogue box.

Saving Data

The computer does not automatically preserve or *save* data that the user enters. If the computer is turned off while a document is open, data may be lost. Different computer platforms use various methods and commands for saving data before closing a session or turning off the computer. Data can be saved on the computer's hard drive (memory) or on external drives and disks.

Data should be saved frequently during computer work. Power surges, other technical problems, and human error can result in permanent loss of data. The most secure way to save data involves two operations: saving to the computer memory and backing up data on another drive or output, such as a CD, external drive, or paper. To save a document to the hard drive while using Microsoft Office:

1. Select FILE/SAVE AS.
2. When the dialogue window appears, select the file or drive where you want the document saved and click on it. Confirm the command by selecting SAVE.
3. After selecting the location for saving the document, you may select FILE/SAVE.

Printing Documents

Documents can be printed from the computer screen using a color or black-and-white printer. The printer is connected to the computer by a cable and interfaces with it through its own software program. To print a document from the computer screen:

1. Select FILE on the toolbar.
2. Select PRINT. A dialogue box appears with options for style, paper size, and quality. Many other options become available by clicking on the PROPERTIES button. If no properties are selected, the computer reverts to its default settings.

COMPUTER NETWORKS

TYPES OF NETWORKS

The term *computer network* refers to two or more computers that are connected electronically. Networks allow the transfer of information from one computer to another.

The **Internet** is a vast computer network; the **World Wide Web** is part of the Internet. The Web is a method of exchanging files, documents, graphics, and other discrete packets of information through the Internet. The method used to exchange and transfer the data is complex and beyond the scope of this discussion. However, it is important to understand that the Web is only one of many types of information systems that use computer networking.

An **intranet** is a system of multiple computers within a facility or organization that allows communication only within that system. Medical facilities often have their own intranet, which transmits useful information such as medical references, articles, and announcements about upcoming events. More important, hospital intranets publish the facility's policies and safety protocols so that everyone on the staff can continually update information about safety issues and patient care. Email is also part of the intranet system in most organizations. To access the intranet, you must use a password. When you log onto your employer's intranet server, always remember to log off before you quit the session. This prevents others from accessing information that you have entered.

NAVIGATING THE INTERNET AND WORLD WIDE WEB

Internet Research

Research on the Web is done through a search engine. This is a computer program accessed through the World Wide Web. The search engine allows the user to type in a topic or phrase, which is sent out through the network. The program then returns information in data blocks called *links*, which are listed by their Internet title and address. The user can open these links and access the material within. An examples of a reliable search engine is Google. To search Google for information on a topic, proceed as follows:

1. Open the Internet browser installed on the computer by clicking on it.
2. Look for the address bar in the Internet toolbar.
3. Enter http://www.google.com in the address bar and click *OK* or *Go* to confirm. The Google website will open.
4. Enter the search topic in the search box (Figure 17-16). A list of **hyperlinks** will appear. Click on any of these to access the information.
5. Once you have accessed the pertinent information, you can add this reference site to your FAVORITES in your internet browser for future reference.

A vast amount of information is available on the Internet and World Wide Web. Traditional research sources (e.g., databases, periodicals, books, CD-ROMS, videos, DVDs) have largely moved to the internet. When these tools are used appropriately, research can be done quickly and efficiently. However, so much information is available that it sometimes is difficult to determine whether the source is reliable and the information is correct. Remember that anyone can post almost anything on the Internet, regardless of whether it is valid. It is up to the user to select information carefully and review the copyright restrictions. Always scan your choices before you start opening files on the Internet. If you are doing professional research, use professional sites. If you want to buy a product or research products for sale (e.g., surgical equipment), use the commercial sites.

For academic research, it is wise first to locate an academic institution or professional association most appropriate to the topic and then search for the desired topic. For example, if you want to research a disease, instead of simply typing the name of the disease in the search box, try locating a medical or academic link first. Use organizations such as the Centers for Disease Control and Prevention (CDC), the American Medical Association (AMA), or the Mayo Clinic. These organizations' websites have extensive search engines that will give you accurate and authoritative information. If you do not know any

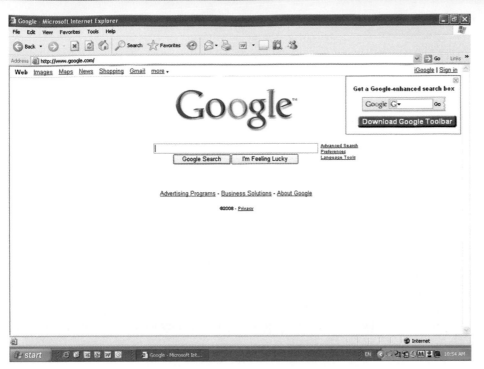

Figure 17-16 Google search engine and search box.

professional organizations, use the Internet search engine to find one. Key terms such as *surgical organizations, infectious diseases,* or *medical reference* will also give you authoritative links. Look at the Internet address of the link before you randomly click on any of the choices. Educational institutions have "edu" in the address. Professional organizations have "org" in the address. If the address ends in "com," the site is a commercial one, with a focus on products to sell.

When researching a topic, try to be as concise as possible. For example, searching the word *surgery* in place of a specific type of surgery would return many millions of documents, most of which would not be relevant. It is best to use combinations of words to research a topic. For example, use *orthopedic titanium knee* to obtain information about titanium implants used in orthopedic surgery of the knee. If you require additional help during your research, library resource centers can be a great asset.

Saving Internet Files

Information obtained through Internet searches can be saved on the computer in the same way that documents are saved. The best way to learn about saving and importing documents from the Internet is by studying and following the Internet tutorials, which are very easy to access on the toolbar. These tutorials and topical lists are designed to help both new learners and those who need more complex information. They are updated automatically by the Internet program itself and provide an excellent learning tool, especially when a more experienced person is available to answer questions that arise in the learning process.

EMAIL

Most people are familiar with email, even if they do not use it regularly. This process allows individuals or groups to contact each other through email programs on a network or the Internet and to send and receive messages, documents, and graphics electronically. When the user creates an email and sends it through the Internet, it is first received by an email server or agent, which processes and formats the data. The data are then sent electronically to the receiving agent, where the email is directed to the receiver's Internet address. To learn how to compose and send email, the new user should use the email tutorial on the computer and consult another person who can demonstrate the process.

Health care institutions often set up email systems for their employees as a means of communicating messages and sending documents. New employees are instructed in how to access their mail and send messages within the system.

KEY CONCEPTS

- The relationship between medicine and modern technology is one of increasing interdependence. As technology advances, medical procedures also become more technologically refined, with greater capacity to diagnose and treat disease and injury.
- Health care workers and providers are now challenged to balance the use of technology with the human side of medicine—empathy and care.
- The study of physics is fundamental to understanding the technological aspects of medicine. It is a prerequisite to safe handling and use of medical and surgical devices that are common in every operating room.
- The nature of matter, atoms, molecules, and elements may seem remote to the study of surgical technology but, knowledge about how particles and substances behave relates directly to energy sources and medical devices.
- There are many different sources of energy used to activate medical and surgical equipment. When we know what the

source of energy is, how it works, and why, we have the knowledge and confidence to use the energy safely.

- The way in which electromagnetic waves interact with substances such as tissue, air, and water is the basis of many surgical devices.

- Surgeons rely on electrosurgery for nearly every type of procedure. The technical aspects of this energy source have become very refined in the last few decades. With increasing complexity there is also a need for increased knowledge about the safe use of electrosurgery, because partial or incomplete understanding relates directly to greater patient risk.

- The principles of electrical current – how it behaves and how it can be stopped, started, and dispersed, are fundamental to the safe use of electrical equipment in the operating room.

- The use and manipulation of light in medicine and surgery allows us to magnify, see "around corners" using fiberoptics, focus tissue more clearly, cut and remodel tissue using lasers, and even determine the oxygen saturation of the blood through the use of pulse oxymetry.

- Many devices used in surgery generate heat that is used to perform tasks or simply maintain physiological processes. However, the body tolerates a fairly narrow range of temperatures.

- Sound can be a powerful tool for diagnosis and treatment. The properties of sound explain how this energy is used and how to manage it.

- Computer technology is now an integral part of many medical devices and is also a common method of documentation and communication in health care facilities. The surgical technologist is required to have fundamental computer skills needed to fulfill documentation requirements and, in many operating rooms, access to the surgeon's preference cards necessary to prepare for a case.

- The most basic physical components of the computer include the central processing unit, keyboard, mouse, and monitor. Entry level computing and digital communication require the use of these devices in order to access data stored in the computer.

- Health facilities use a computer network system or intranet to allow communication and access to important data by employees. The network, which requires a password to enter (log on), is a group of internally connected computers located throughout the health care facility. In many modern surgical departments computer stations are located inside or near each operating suite for convenient access. The Internet is an internationally connected network that is separate from an intranet. The Internet is accessible by the public whereas use of an intranet is restricted to facility employees.

REVIEW QUESTIONS

1. Surgical devices require energy sources to operate. What is the difference between mechanical energy and electromagnetic energy?

2. Define the properties of a wave.
3. Define *conductivity*.
4. What is insulation? How does it prevent the flow of electrons?
5. Why do electrons follow a conductive path?
6. What are the properties of visible light?
7. Describe three types of heat transfer. Give several examples of how heat transfer is directly related to patient safety.
8. Explain how ultrasound is used in diagnostic imaging.
9. How are data protected in institutional computers?

CASE STUDIES

Case 1

In your hospital, you are part of the orthopedic team, which includes the surgical technologists who specialize in this field and a team leader. Your team leader needs to notify you of upcoming courses to be held at the health care facility. What is the best way to communicate this to all members of the team?

Case 2

The Doppler ultrasound creates images based on signals through the unobstructed interface between the handheld transducer and the patient's skin. What might be the reasons for a distorted or incomplete image?

Case 3

You are setting up for a case in which electrosurgery will be used. Your colleague asks you to prepare a patient grounding pad for use with the electrosurgery unit. You know that only bipolar energy will be used during the case, but you do not want to look unprepared. Should you prepare the grounding pad or not?

Case 4

Discuss the importance of understanding of basic physics and computer technology in working as a surgical technologist.

BIBLIOGRAPHY

Halliday D, Resnick R, Walker J: *Fundamentals of physics*, ed 7, Danvers, Mass, 2005, Wiley.

Henderson T: *The physics classroom*. Accessed September 14, 2011, at http://www.physicsclassroom.com.

Microsoft Corporation: *Microsoft in education*. Accessed September 14, 2011, at http://www.microsoft.com/education/en-us/Pages/index.aspx.

Stutz M: *All about circuits. Basic concepts of electricity*. Accessed September 14, 2011, at http://www.allaboutcircuits.com.

Stutz M: *All about circuits, 1999-2000. Volume II: AC*. Accessed September 14, 2011 at http://www.allaboutcircuits.com.

Stutz M: *All about circuits, 1999-2000. Volume I: DC*. Accessed September 14, 2011, at www.allaboutcircuits.com.

Ulmar B: *The ValleyLab Institute of Clinical Education electrosurgery continuing education module*, 2011. Accessed September 14, 2011, at http://www.valleylab.com/education/poes/index.html.

Energy Sources in Surgery

LEARNING OBJECTIVES

After studying this chapter the reader will be able to:

1. Review the concepts of conduction, frequency, and impedance
2. Explain the relationship between electricity and some body functions
3. Describe the use and components of electrosurgery
4. Distinguish between monopolar and bipolar circuits used in electrosurgery
5. Discuss the safe use of the patient return electrode
6. List the primary hazards of electrosurgery and explain how to prevent accidents
7. Distinguish between capacitive coupling and indirect coupling
8. Describe the materials in a smoke plume and how to reduce exposure to the smoke plume
9. Describe how lasers are used in surgery
10. Recognize different types of laser media
11. Discuss safety precautions used during laser surgery

TERMINOLOGY

Ablation: The complete destruction of tissue.

Active electrode: In electrosurgery, the point of the electrosurgical instrument that delivers current to tissue.

Active electrode monitoring (AEM): An electrosurgical instrument system that monitors the impedance of the instruments and stops the flow of electricity when it reaches a critical level.

Alternating current (AC): Electrical current that changes directions and transmits high-voltage electricity.

Amplification: In wave science, the phenomenon of increasing wave height by lining up the peaks and troughs of individual waves.

Argon: An inert gas used in electrosurgery to direct and shroud the electrical current.

Bipolar circuit: An electrosurgical circuit in which current travels from the power unit through an instrument containing two opposite poles in contact with the tissue and then returns directly to the energy source.

Blended mode: In electrosurgery, a combination of intermediate frequency and intermediate wave intervals to produce a specific effect on tissue.

Capacitive coupling: A specific burn hazard of monopolar endoscopic surgery. It occurs when current passes unintentionally through instrument insulation and adjacent conductive material into tissue.

Carbon dioxide: An inert gas used as a lasing medium during laser surgery.

Cauterization: The use of a hot object to burn tissue to achieve coagulation.

Circuit: The flow of electricity through a conductive medium.

Coagulum: A sticky, semiliquid substance that forms when tissue is altered by electrical or ultrasonic energy.

Coherency: A quality of laser light in which all light waves are lined up with troughs and peaks matching.

Conductive: The quality of a material to give up electrons easily and thus transmit electrical current.

Continuous wave lasers: Lasers that emit the laser light continuously rather that in pulses.

Cryoablation: A method of tissue destruction in which a probe is inserted into a tumor or tissue mass. High-pressure argon gas is injected into the probe, causing the surrounding tissue to freeze and eventually slough.

Cryosurgery: The use of extremely low temperature to destroy diseased tissue.

Current: The flow of electricity.

Cavitron Ultrasonic Surgical Aspirator (CUSA): This instrument destroys tumors through the use of high-frequency sound waves (ultrasound).

Cutting mode: In electrosurgery, the use of high voltage and relatively low frequency to cut through tissue.

Desiccation: The removal of water from tissue, causing it to die.

Direct coupling: The transfer of electrical current from an active electrode to another conductive instrument by accident or as part of the electrosurgical process.

Direct current (DC): A type of low-voltage current generated by battery.

TERMINOLOGY (cont.)

Dispersive electrode: A component of the electrosurgical circuit that spreads current at the point where it exits the body and thus prevents injury.

Duty cycle: In electrosurgery, the duration of current flow sometimes is referred to as the duty cycle. The duty cycle can intermittently be applied to produce the desired effect on tissue.

Electrosurgery: The direct use of electricity to cut and coagulate tissue.

Electrosurgical unit (ESU): The power generator and control source in the electrosurgical system.

Electrosurgical vessel sealing: A type of bipolar electrosurgery in which tissue is welded together using low voltage, low temperature, and a high-frequency current.

Electrosurgical waveforms: The transduced or actual waves generated when frequency, voltage, and power are delivered in different combinations during electrosurgery.

Eschar: Charred and burned tissue created by a high-voltage current.

Excimer: A type of lasing energy that is created when electrons are removed from the lasing medium.

Excitation source: In laser technology, the energy that causes the atoms of a lasing medium (gas or solid) to vibrate.

Frequency: In electricity, the periodicity of electromagnetic waves.

Fulguration: A process of tissue surface destruction used in electrosurgery.

Grounding pad: An alternate name for the patient return electrode.

Holmium:YAG: A solid crystal lasing medium that penetrates a wide variety of substances, including renal and biliary stones and soft tissue.

Impedance: The constriction of electrical current by a nonconductive material or an area of high density. This results in the transformation of electricity into thermal energy.

Implanted electronic device (IED): An electronic device that monitors and corrects physiological conditions. Electrosurgery may interfere with the function of such devices, which include pacemakers, internal defibrillators, deep brain stimulators, ventricular assist devices, and others.

Inactive electrode: An alternate term for the patient return electrode.

Insulate: To cover or surround a conductive substance with nonconductive material.

Isolated circuit: An electrical circuit that has no ground reference or method of conducting current into the ground at the site of use. Current is directed from the energy source, through the patient, and back to the source.

Laser: Acronym for *light amplification by stimulated emission of radiation.*

Laser classifications: Industry and international system for grading laser energy according to its ability to cause injury.

Laser head: The component of the laser system that holds the lasing medium.

Laser medium: A solid or gas that is sensitive to atomic excitation by an energy source, which creates intense laser light and energy.

Lateral heat: The unintentional heating of tissue outside the direct area of electrosurgical application. Also called *thermal spread.*

Monochromatic: A characteristic of laser light in which the frequency of each wave is the same.

Monopolar circuit: In electrosurgery, a continuous path of electricity that flows from the electrosurgical unit to the active electrode, through the patient and the return electrode, and then back to the electrosurgical unit.

Neodymium:YAG: A solid lasing medium known for its attraction to protein and deep penetration into tissue.

Neutral electrode: An alternate term for the patient return electrode.

Nonconductive: The quality of a substance that resists the transfer of electrons and therefore electrical current.

Optical resonant cavity: The component of a laser system in which the lasing medium is contained and light is transformed.

Patient return electrode (PRE): A critical component of the monopolar electrosurgical circuit. The PRE is a conductive pad that captures electricity and shunts it safely out of the body and back to the electrosurgical unit.

Phacoemulsification: The destruction of cataracts using ultrasound technology.

Potassium-titanyl-phosphate (KTP): A low-power lasing medium that produces a very small diameter beam well suited to microsurgery.

Pulsed wave lasers: Lasers that apply the laser light intermittently to the target tissue.

Q-switched lasers: An alternate name for pulsed wave lasers.

Radiant exposure: In laser technology, the combination of the concentration of laser energy and the length of time tissue is exposed to it.

Radiofrequency: Electromagnetic energy in which the frequency is in the area of radio transmission. In electrosurgery, radiofrequency electromagnetic waves are used to produce the desired surgical effect.

Radiofrequency ablation (RFA): The use of radiofrequency waves to destroy a tissue mass or surface.

Resistance: The restriction of electron flow in a direct current circuit.

Return electrode monitoring (REM): A safety system used in electrosurgery in which the PRE transmits continuous feedback on the quality of impedance in the electrode and stops the current when it becomes dangerously high.

Selective absorption: The absorption of a lasing medium into tissue being lased, according to its color and density.

Smoke plume: Toxic smoke emitted by tissue during electrosurgery and laser surgery.

Spray coagulation: An alternate term for fulguration.

Tunable dye laser: A type of laser formed by the combination of argon gas and specific dyes that alter tissue absorption of the lasing beam.

Ultrasonic energy: High-frequency energy created by vibration or excitation of molecules. This type of energy destroys tissue by breaking molecular bonds.

INTRODUCTION

Many forms of energy are used during surgery to cut tissue, coagulate blood vessels, and destroy diseased tissue. The most common forms are electrical, **radiofrequency**, kinetic (movement), sound (ultrasonic waves), thermal (temperature), and laser energy. Although electricity may be used to power these advanced medical devices, the energy used to perform the surgical procedure is not always electrical. For example, an instrument that generates ultrasonic waves is used to coagulate tissue. The instrument is powered by electricity, but the effect on the tissue is caused by vibration and friction.

Figure 18-1 shows the electromagnetic spectrum, which is the source of most energy. The importance of this figure is that it demonstrates the relationship between the frequency of electromagnetic waves and the energies they produce. The type of energy produced is directly related to the frequency of the waves. Some types of energy (e.g., light and sound) can be perceived by the senses, whereas others are outside the range of human perception.

This chapter discusses common surgical devices that use electromagnetic energy and other types of energy. These devices are safe when used appropriately. However, they all carry the risk of serious injury. Surgical team members must understand the source of these risks to prevent serious accidents.

It is common practice for surgical personnel to identify a particular energy device by its proprietary name (company or trade name). However, these names do not identify the type of energy and, more important, the risks associated with that energy. A clear understanding of this concept is very important in the prevention of injury to patients and personnel. The surgical technologist is responsible for knowing exactly what type (classification) of energy is being used so as to provide appropriate safety measures on the sterile field and while circulating.

ELECTRICAL ENERGY

REVIEW OF ELECTRICITY

This discussion of electrical energy follows from the material found in Chapter 17, in which the nature of electricity and other physics concepts were discussed in detail. This chapter is dedicated to describing exactly how this and other energy sources are harnessed to perform surgery. It includes a brief review of the electricity concepts to enhance the reader's understanding of how electricity is used in surgery and its relationship to the human body. Note that many technical terms related to the *physics* of electricity can be found in Chapter 17.

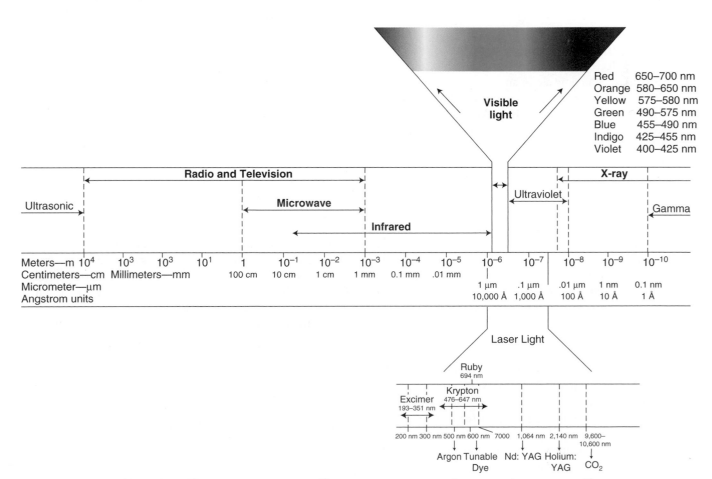

Figure 18-1 **Electromagnetic spectrum.** Electromagnetic waves are the source of most energy. The frequency of the wave determines the type of energy.

Conduction

Electricity is the flow of electrons through a **conductive** medium; this is called **current**. Atoms of a conductive medium give up electrons easily, allowing electrons to flow through the circuit. **Nonconductive** material does not accept or give up electrons easily and is not a good pathway for electricity. Electricity is similar to the flow of water through a tube. The flow can be regulated, stopped, and started.

CURRENT The two types of electrical current are direct current and alternating current.

- **Direct current (DC)** flows in one direction only. This is the type of current is found in low-voltage batteries such as AA batteries.
- **Alternating current (AC)** switches direction at a constant rate (in the United States, this rate is 60 cycles per second). This type of current is generated by municipal power plants and produces high-voltage power.

Frequency

Because electricity is electromagnetic wave energy, it has a **frequency**, which is the number of wave cycles that occur in 1 second. High-frequency energy in the electromagnetic spectrum includes ultrasonic and radiofrequency waves. Recall from Chapter 17 that the frequency of all wave energy determines its type (e.g., visible light, electrical, radiation, radiofrequency, ultrasonic).

Impedance

The path of electricity from its origin to the destination is the **circuit**. When electricity is introduced through a conductive circuit, it continues to flow along an unimpeded path. When the path is interrupted by a less conductive medium, the current seeks a path around the **impedance**. If no alternate path is available, the electrical energy is transformed into heat or light. This heat is used to perform electrosurgery.

Tissue impedance is the key to understanding electrosurgery.

Impedance to electricity is relative. A substance such as a copper wire can be very conductive, whereas glass and rubber are nonconductive. Nonconductive materials are used to **insulate** the conductive material carrying electricity to prevent injury and maintain the flow of electricity within its circuit. Thus, the insulator is a protective device or material. This is relevant to understanding how faults occur in electrosurgical devices and instruments that transmit electricity.

ELECTRICITY AND THE BODY

The human body uses electrical energy to perform many vital functions, such as conduction in the heart to pump blood and impulses from one nerve cell to another. These are internal changes created by the movement of ions (charged molecules and elements).

When electricity is applied to the body externally, the tissue reacts according to the **voltage** and frequency. High voltage is potentially more damaging than low voltage. The frequency of the current also influences tissue effects.

Table 18-1	Effects of Electricity on the Body		
Body Response	**Direct Current**	**Alternating Current (60 Hz)**	**Alternating Current (10 kHz)**
Slight perception	1 mA	0.4 mA	7 mA
Pain	5.2 mA	1.1 mA	55 mA
Severe pain and difficulty with respiration	90 mA	23 mA	94 mA
Fibrillation and possible cardiac arrest	500 mA	100 mA	—

Hz, Hertz; *kHz*, kilohertz; *mA*, milliampere.

Box 18-1	Key Concepts of Electrosurgery

Electrosurgery is the direct use of electrical energy to cut, coagulate, and weld tissue. The key concepts of electrosurgery are:

- Electrosurgery works by transmitting high-frequency electricity to tissue. The current is impeded at the point of contact with the tissue and this creates heat.
- High-frequency current does not interfere with the body's normal functions, whereas a low-frequency current can cause electrocution or cardiac arrest. Electrosurgery converts high-voltage, low-frequency electricity into very high-frequency energy, which does not cause electrocution.
- Voltage and frequency can be safely manipulated at the power source to produce different tissue effects.
- Cautery is the application of a hot object to living tissue. The electrosurgical unit (ESU) delivers electrical energy, which meets impedance (loss of conductivity) in the tissue. Heat is created in the tissue at the point of resistance.

Table 18-1 shows the effects of electricity at different voltages and frequencies.

The body is very sensitive to low-frequency electricity. *As the frequency increases, the body's response decreases.* Wave energy at frequencies above 100,000 cycles per second (*hertz,* abbreviated as *Hz*) does not interfere with the body's normal bioelectrical activity. Tissue can be burned at these frequencies, but the heart and other bioelectrical mechanisms are not affected. However, frequencies at or below 100 kHz *do* interfere with the body's bioelectrical activity and can result in electrocution and cardiac arrest.

Electrosurgical units operate at extremely high frequencies (300,000 to 1 million Hz). At this level, tissue is can be burned, coagulated, and cut without risk of electrocution or cardiac arrest. The key concepts of electrosurgery are shown in Box 18-1.

USES OF ELECTROSURGERY

Effects of Electrical Current on Tissue

The way tissue reacts to electrosurgery depends on a number of variables:

- *Tissue type:* The amount of water and collagen in the tissue and its density.
- *Exposure time:* The duration of contact with the electrical current.
- *Current density:* As current density increases, tissue response also increases. Current density increases when voltage is forced through a small area.
- *Frequency and voltage of the electrosurgical wave:* Specific combinations of frequency and voltage produce different effects in tissue.

Direct application of hot implements to tissue has been used throughout history to stop hemorrhage and sterilize wounds; this procedure is called **cauterization**. Cauterization differs from electrosurgery, which uses high-frequency energy to cut and coagulate tissue. The term *cautery* often is used incorrectly to describe any kind of electrosurgery. In fact, cautery refers only to the application of a superheated object (not electrical current) to tissue. The techniques associated with electrosurgery include:

- Incising tissue
- Coagulating blood vessels and stopping minor hemorrhage
- Destroying or removing diseased tissue
- Welding tissue together

COMPONENTS OF ELECTROSURGERY

Power Unit (Generator)

The ESU power source (also called a *generator*) is the control and power unit (Figure 18-2). The modern power source is digitally controlled and has both monopolar and bipolar capability (explained later). Power adjustments are programmable and controlled by push buttons on the screen panel. Digital waveforms showing the frequency, wavelength, amplitude, and other information are displayed on the screen. The ESU power source often is referred to as a *bovie*, which was the prototype ESU system introduced in the 1930s.

Active Electrode

The **active electrode** is the actual contact point at the tissue. It is contained at the tip of the ESU handpiece, or "pencil" (Figure 18-3). The handpiece is connected to the power source by a lightweight cable. Many types of active electrode tips and instruments are available because the devices are used in open surgery, minimally invasive surgery, and endoscopic procedures unit (Figure 18-4). The handpiece and cable are one closed unit.

Controls

Some types of ESU pencils have switches on the handpiece. However, the surgeon usually controls the ESU using a set of foot pedals, which is considered safer because it cannot be as easily activated in error.

Patient Return Electrode (Monopolar Circuit Only)

The **patient return electrode** (PRE) (or, simply, the return electrode) is a pad or thin plate that is placed close to the

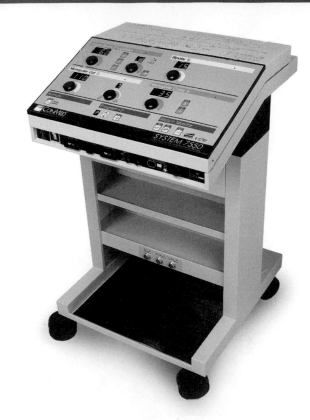

Figure 18-2 Electrosurgical power unit, also known as the *electrosurgical unit (ESU) generator.* *(Courtesy Conmed, Inc.)*

surgical wound site. It captures electrical current from the active electrode and transmits it back to the power unit (Figure 18-5). The return electrode is connected to the power source by a conductive cable fitted on the outside surface of the pad. This cable may attach to the return electrode using a secure fitting that cannot be accidently pulled out. The PRE shunts electrical current dispersed from the active electrode back to the ESU power unit (Figure 18-6). The return electrode is known by a number of different names, such as the **dispersive electrode**, **inactive electrode**, **neutral electrode**, or more commonly, the **grounding pad**.

When properly applied to the patient, the PRE prevents burns, because it spreads the current at the point where it exits the body. However, if it is not applied correctly or if it becomes dislodged during surgery, the patient can suffer serious injury. Box 18-2 lists safety guidelines for use of the return electrode.

MONOPOLAR AND BIPOLAR CIRCUITS

Two types of circuits are used in electrosurgery: the **monopolar circuit** and the **bipolar circuit**. Both circuits use alternating current and require the power unit described previously.

In monopolar mode, electricity flows from the ESU power unit through a power cable to the ESU pencil and active electrode (tip). The active electrode transmits energy in the form of heat and electrical impulses.

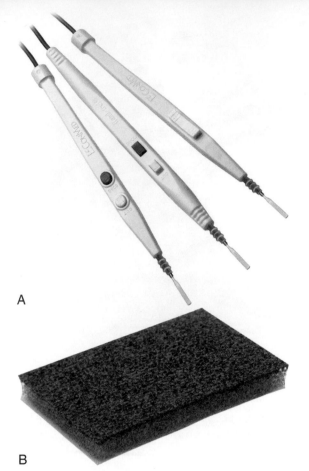

Figure 18-3 **A,** Monopolar active electrode pencil; also called the *bovie.* **B,** Cleaning pad for the electrosurgical unit (ESU) pencil. Accumulated tissue debris on the ESU pencil can serve as a source of burns and fire. The cleaning pad (also called a *scratch pad*) is used to wipe debris from the active electrode. *(Courtesy Conmed, Inc.)*

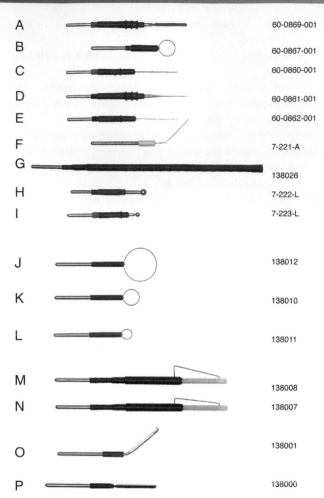

Figure 18-4 **Active electrode tips available for different types of monopolar electrosurgery.** *A,* Flat tip—general cutting and coagulation. *B,* Loop—biopsy and cutting. *C,* Fine needle—precise desiccation. *D,* Coarse needle. *E,* Blunt needle. *F,* Angled needle. *G,* Flat tip with extension—deep tissue general use. *H,* Ball tip, regular—fulguration. *I,* Ball tip, long—deep tissue fulguration. *J* to *L,* Cutting loops, long. *M* and *N,* Conization loop—endocervical cutting and coagulation. *O* and *P,* Straight and angled long flat tips. *(Courtesy Conmed, Inc.)*

When the activated tip touches the body tissue, electricity is impeded. This creates intense heat and produces the desired surgical effect, such as cutting or coagulation.

In **bipolar electrosurgery**, the surgeon uses a forceps or similar instrument that has two contact points. Current leaves the power unit and travels from one pole or contact point to the other in the instrument, passing only through the tissue held between the contact points. Next it returns to the ESU unit. No current passes through the patient's body; therefore, no PRE is needed to disperse the current. The voltage used in bipolar surgery is lower than that used for monopolar surgery, which makes the bipolar mode a safer technique with fewer risks for patient injury.

The bipolar unit is used mainly on low-impedance tissue because the low voltage is not strong enough to penetrate effectively through tissue such as bone or fat. An advantage of bipolar electrosurgery is that minimal heat is spread to surrounding tissues, which makes this technique safe for very delicate areas such as the brain and microvascular tissue. The bipolar unit delivers both cutting and coagulation modes and is especially useful for microsurgery, in which **lateral heat** spread would damage delicate nerves or blood vessels.

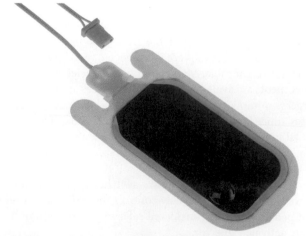

Figure 18-5 **Patient return electrode (PRE) used in monopolar electrosurgery.** The PRE is also known as a *patient grounding pad, dispersive electrode,* or *inactive electrode.* The purpose of the PRE is to provide a safe return path for electricity transmitted through the electrosurgical unit pencil and the patient's body. *(Courtesy Conmed, Inc.)*

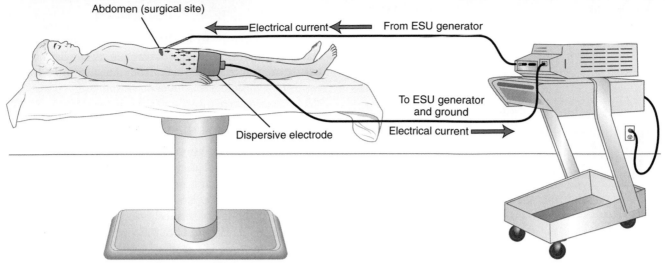

Figure 18-6 Monopolar electrosurgery circuit. With monopolar electrosurgical units, electrical current flows from the power source to the active electrode, through the patient's body, to the patient return electrode (PRE), which transmits it back to the power unit. This completes the circuit and prevents inadvertent patient burns.

Box 18-2 Safety Measures for Use of the Patient Return Electrode

- Always assess the patient's skin before and after applying the patient return electrode (PRE).
- The skin must be dry and free of hair. Moisture under the PRE can cause it to pull away from the skin. Shaving may be necessary for uniform contact with the skin.
- Use a PRE that has been stored in a sealed package only. The moisture content and quality of the conductive gel cannot be guaranteed with prolonged exposure to air.
- Inspect the PRE before applying it, and check the expiration date on the package. The electroconductive gel must be moist and should have been stored at the temperature specified by the manufacturer.
- Use the correct size PRE for the patient's surface area. Operating room protocol determines the appropriate pad size.
- Pediatric-size PREs are available. Never cut a PRE to fit the patient's size.
- The PRE must be placed close to the surgical site over a large muscle mass. Muscle has low impedance and is the best conductor. The PRE must not be placed over a prominent bony surface, scar, tattoo, hair, or fatty tissue; these increase impedance and can result in a burn.
- The PRE must be in complete contact with the skin, without tenting or buckling.
- Make sure the PRE cord has adequate slack to prevent pulling and displacement.
- Apply the PRE after final positioning to prevent dislodgment.
- Always check the PRE cable to make sure it is intact and undamaged. Check it from end to end, including the attachment clips and the plug or insertion point into the electrosurgical unit (ESU).
- Do not assume that single-use items are intact and free of damage. Inspect every device, every time.
- Do not use a PRE *if only bipolar electrosurgery* will be used.

ELECTROSURGICAL WORKING MODES

The specific effects of electrosurgery (e.g., cutting, coagulation) are related to whether the electrical current is delivered continuously or intermittently. These modes are displayed on the power unit as **electrosurgical waveforms** (Figure 18-7). The modes are preset and programmable with guidance from the manufacturer's technical advisor. The waveform itself is simply a visual representation of current transmission.

The duration of current flow sometimes is referred to as the **duty cycle**. When the duty cycle is pulsed or intermittently applied, waves are connected by a continuous line, which represents a period when the current stops. Continuous repetition of high-frequency waves at low voltage is characteristic of the cutting mode. The coagulation mode appears as intermittent waves at low frequency and high voltage.

The **blended mode** provides a combination of intermediate frequency and intermediate wave intervals. Radiofrequency electrosurgery and microprocessor technology combine to allow the surgeon many choices of waveform blending, with safety features that prevent voltage spikes and accidental tissue injury.

Cutting

The **cutting mode** is produced by high-voltage energy. In this mode, the electrode is held above the tissue and does not make contact. The air between the electrode and the tissue acts as a conductor (called a *spark gap*), allowing the high-voltage current to flow between the tissue and the electrode.

The cutting mode causes tissue **desiccation** (burning with the loss of water content). When a thin, narrow active electrode is used, the current is very concentrated. The tissue heats rapidly, causing the water in the cells to explode. This releases steam and dissipates the heat. As the superheated tissue releases its water content, it quickly dries.

Cutting electrodes are available in many designs and configurations. These include the standard blade electrode and

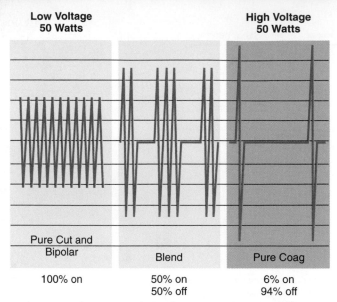

Low Voltage
50 Watts

High Voltage
50 Watts

Pure Cut and Bipolar

Blend

Pure Coag

100% on

50% on
50% off

6% on
94% off

Figure 18-7 **Electrosurgical waveforms.** The effects of electrosurgery on tissue are related to voltage and whether current is delivered continuously or intermittently. *(From Rothrock J: Alexander's care of the patient in surgery, ed 17, St Louis, 2007, Mosby.)*

others such as wire loops, spatulas, and needle tips. The spatula electrode is most commonly used.

Microbipolar cutting is among the newer modes available in bipolar electrosurgery. Fine-needle electrodes are used to sever tissue safely, using a blended frequency. Bipolar cutting probes are available in many designs, and bipolar scissors are also used to cut and coagulate tissue (see Figure 18-3).

Coagulation

The voltage is lower in the coagulation mode than in the cutting mode. The electrode is held in contact with the tissue or slightly above it. During contact, the active electrode is held in brief or pulsed contact with the blood vessel. Heating is slower, which results in tissue "welding" that seals blood vessels. Lengthy contact results in the formation of **eschar**, or blackened burned tissue. This can tear away from the surface and cause rebleeding. The buildup of eschar on the electrode increases impedance, which raises the temperature at the point of contact. Eschar also increases the risk of sparking at the point of tissue contact. Electrosurgical tips are coated with a protective substance such as Teflon or silicone to help prevent the formation of eschar.

The bipolar coagulation mode is safe for use on vessels when lateral spread is an important consideration, such as in microsurgery, vascular surgery, and neurosurgery. Bipolar forceps loops, probes, and hooks are used to cut and coagulate very delicate tissue.

Fulguration

Fulguration, or **spray coagulation**, is performed on tissue with pulsed or intermittent application of the active electrode. In this technique the current is pulsed through the active electrode, which is held just above the tissue. The high voltage creates an arc of current that spreads over a relatively large area compared to direct contact techniques. The effect is a combination of coagulation and superficial tissue cutting.

RADIOFREQUENCY ABLATION

Radiofrequency ablation (RFA) is the destruction of tissue using radiofrequency energy waves. This mode has numerous uses, including the destruction of tumors and endometrial tissue in gynecological surgery. During tumor ablation, an electrode is inserted directly into the diseased tissue. The high-frequency energy causes the molecules of the tissue to vibrate, which creates sufficient heat to destroy the tissue.

Bipolar RFA is used in conjunction with a conductive fluid medium to destroy diseased tissue. In this type of surgery, a hollow organ (e.g., the bladder or uterus) is filled with fluid, and the bipolar probe is used to destroy tissue in the fluid-filled cavity. The use of this technology as it applies to specific procedures is described more fully in Chapter 25 on gynecological surgery and in Chapter 26 on urological surgery. RFA is also used to treat heart disease in which cellular damage creates irregular conduction patterns.

ELECTROSURGICAL VESSEL SEALING

Electrosurgical vessel sealing uses high-frequency, bipolar electrosurgery, low voltage, and physical pressure to create a weld in tissue. A number of vessel sealing systems are available, such as LigaSure and Enseal. The elements of a vessel sealing system are:

- Transmission of radiofrequency waves to tissue through specialized grasping instruments
- Tissue impedance monitoring
- A microprocessor (programmable computer chip) that controls and programs the system
- An alarm system that automatically stops the current when the tissue seal is achieved

The vessel sealing system is used during resection procedures that traditionally require sequential clamping, suturing, and cutting. Whereas the traditional method of resection requires multiple instruments, the vessel sealing system accomplishes these tasks with only one instrument. This can reduce operating time and allow the surgeon to remain focused on the surgical site without the need for instrument exchange. The system is popular for selected patients in hysterectomy and some general surgery applications. A low temperature is used, which prevents charring and unintentional lateral heating. The instrument tip remains relatively cool, which prevents the tissue from tearing when the tips are released.

ARGON-ENHANCED ELECTROSURGERY

Argon gas is used in some electrosurgical procedures to focus the current during cutting and coagulation. Argon is inert and nonflammable but easily ionized. When a stream of argon gas is directed around the active electrode, it focuses the current and prevents sparking. Argon-enhanced electrosurgery also reduces the smoke plume and displaces oxygen along its path. This increases the safety and efficiency of the procedure. It is particularly useful during long fulguration procedures that require extended electrosurgery.

ELECTROSURGERY SAFETY

Electrosurgery historically has posed one of the greatest risks in the operating room. Recent advances in technology have lowered but not removed the risk of patient burns. Patient fires and burns related to electrosurgical devices still occur because safety protocols are not followed or personnel fail to recognize the danger signs. All perioperative personnel are responsible for preventing these accidents. Surgical technologists must be familiar with the safe use of specific devices and equipment in their facility.

Generator Safety

Modern generators now allow connections for both monopolar and bipolar functions. The system contains a self-check, which is activated before use. Power and blend settings can be preset and programmed into the unit. These features are convenient but may lead to safety risks when automatic settings are not appropriate for a specific tissue and impedance. During surgery, the perioperative team must suspect a problem if the surgeon repeatedly requests increases in power (voltage). This may indicate increased impedance, which can lead to fire or extensive burns.

Monopolar electrosurgery is performed through an **isolated circuit**. This means that the current travels only from the ESU generator, through the patient and the PRE, and back to the generator. There is no ground reference for discharge of electricity, as in older models of electrosurgery units.

Tissue impedance monitoring is available in many modern units. This safety feature provides automatic adjustments in voltage according to the impedance encountered in the tissue. Preprogramming of the automatic settings must ensure that the lowest power setting is used to achieve the desired surgical effect.

Generators must be used according to the manufacturer's specifications and within the guidelines of operating room policy. Written instructions and safety guidelines should be kept with the unit or close at hand to prevent misuse.

The surgeon is responsible for the direct use of active electrodes during surgery. However, if personnel have questions about power settings or other potentially harmful features, they must be able to participate in decision making from a firm knowledge base. This means that all staff members ultimately are responsible for the safe use of the ESU. Power settings must be used reasonably, and any alarms or other equipment warning systems require a response to prevent accident and injury. Alarm systems are designed to alert staff members to safety risks and should never be turned off or made barely audible. Loud music in the operating room has been identified as a barrier to hearing otherwise audible alarms. Box 18-3 presents safety guidelines for use of an ESU.

Active Electrode Safety

Active electrode safety includes precautions to prevent accidental burns at the surgical site and electrical faults that occur between the electrode tip, handpiece, and connecting cord.

Recall that the active electrode is the metal tip of the instrument that conducts energy directly into the target tissue. In

---

Box **18-3** **Safety Guidelines for Use of an Electrosurgical Unit**

1. Always inspect all power cords and cables before using the electrosurgical unit (ESU) generator.
2. Do not place items on top of the ESU generator. The unit's cooling system may not function properly, and this could result in overheating and malfunction.
3. Always allow the ESU to self-check, if this feature is available, before connecting cables.
4. Always ensure that the ESU generator is approved for the active electrodes and patient return electrodes in use. Do not attempt to use a return electrode monitoring system with a generator that does not recognize that feature.
5. Keep the generator away from other electronic and power sources because they may cause electrical interference.
6. Keep fluids and fluid sources away from the generator. Never place fluid or solution containers on top of the generator, even if the containers are sealed.
7. Each generator is designed to operate with different waveforms and power settings.
8. Become familiar with your facility's equipment and its capabilities.

---

monopolar electrosurgery, the tip transmits high-voltage power with powerful cutting and coagulation properties. The tip is capable of severing dense tissue, including bone. It also can cause inadvertent burns to the patient and scrubbed team members when used improperly.

Before surgery, the active electrode and cord must be examined for integrity. The scrub is responsible for ensuring that no defects are present in the insulation of the instrument and that the active electrode is seated tightly into the handpiece. Remember that disposable as well as reusable units can have defects. Do not connect the active electrode until the PRE is secure and connected to the ESU generator.

During surgery, the active electrode pencil must be kept in a nonconductive safety holster on the surgical field. The holster must be in plain sight of the team, and the ESU pencil must be replaced in it *after each use*. Never leave the pencil on top of the patient or drapes. Place the holster in a position that is convenient to the surgeon's reach so that the pencil can be easily stowed after each use. Do not attach the handpiece to the drapes by wrapping it around metal clamps or twisting the cord. Stray current can escape into the metal clamp. Twisting or tying the cord can break the conductive wires inside and put a strain on the insulation.

When eschar or **coagulum** (welded tissue) accumulates on the tip of the active electrode, the scrub should wipe it clean with a nonabrasive sponge. Abrasive materials or a scalpel blade should not be used to clean the electrode. Scraping the electrode causes abrasions and pitting, which make the tip more vulnerable to the buildup of tissue. Eschar creates increased impedance and heat, which causes sparking and lateral burns at the operative site. Combination suction-coagulation tips must also be kept free of debris. Always use water, not saline, to clear the inside of the suction tube, because water is nonconductive.

In some procedures, the surgeon may want to use a hemostat or other clamp to conduct current from the active electrode to tissue. This is called "buzzing the hemostat." This practice is not recommended by safety agencies but occurs nevertheless. The problems associated with this practice are accidental burns to the person holding the hemostat, lateral heat that extends beyond the area of the hemostat, and unintentional tissue burns (places where the clamp is in contact with tissue other than the intended site). The scrubbed surgical technologist may be asked to "buzz" a hemostat or other clamp during surgery. When carrying out this technique, make sure that only the tissue intended for coagulation is in contact with the ESU. Be aware that performing this skill does not release the surgical technologist from liability in the event of patient burn, even if the surgeon requests it. The variables that contribute to burns are the length of time the active electrode is in contact with the instrument (tissue), the power settings on the main unit, the type of tissue being coagulated (moisture content and density), the amount of tissue between the tines of the instrument, and the surface area of the active electrode.

ELECTRICAL HAZARDS IN MINIMALLY INVASIVE SURGERY

CAPACITIVE COUPLING

Capacitive coupling is a specific burn hazard of monopolar endoscopic surgery. It occurs when current passes inadvertently through instrument insulation and adjacent conductive material into tissue. Burns resulting from capacitive coupling are particularly dangerous in minimally invasive surgery, because the injury most often occurs outside the viewing area of the endoscope. The damage may go unnoticed until an infection develops at the burn site days later. Using only metal cannulas and active electrode monitoring (discussed later in the chapter) can prevent capacitive coupling.

DIRECTING COUPLING

Direct coupling is the flow of electricity from one conductive substance to another. This can occur when the insulation protecting the circuit has a defect or when an active electrode comes in contact with another conductive object. During minimally invasive surgery, direct coupling can occur when an active electrode touches the tip of another instrument in an instrument "collision." Direct coupling involving insulation failure can be more dangerous, because the resulting burn may not be detected immediately. In open surgery, direct coupling can occur whenever an active electrode insulator is inserted into a conductive metal sheath, such as a suction catheter. Direct coupling can be prevented by frequent inspection of insulation and proper care and handling of electrosurgical instruments. However, active electrode monitoring is the recommended method of preventing burns from insulation failure.

ACTIVE ELECTRODE MONITORING

Active electrode monitoring (AEM) is universally recommended by safety standard agencies to prevent accidental burns during electrosurgery. The system replaces nonmonitoring instruments with special AEM instruments designed to measure and react to impedance in the insulation. Recall that impedance along an electrical circuit results in heating. Defects in the insulation may cause current to escape through this pathway, but the flow is constricted or impeded, and this creates heat at the point of restriction. The AEM system measures impedance and immediately stops the flow of electricity when impedance reaches a critical level.

RETURN ELECTRODE MONITORING

Newer electrosurgical units use a safety feature that determines the impedance at the site of the PRE. The **return electrode monitoring (REM)** system, also known as the *return electrode contact quality monitoring system (RECQMS)*, automatically stops the flow of current when impedance reaches a preset level. An alarm system also alerts the user that impedance has exceeded a safe level. To function, the REM patient return electrode must be used with specific REM components.

PATIENTS WITH AN IMPLANTED ELECTRONIC DEVICE

A patient with an **implanted electronic device (IED)** requires special consideration when electrosurgery is planned. Implanted electronic devices include but are not limited to the following:

- Pacemaker
- Implanted cardiac defibrillator
- Deep brain stimulator
- Ventricular assist device (VAD)
- Spinal cord stimulator
- Programmable ventricular shunt
- Cochlear implant
- Auditory brainstem implant
- Bone conduction stimulator

These devices monitor and correct physiological dysfunctions and can be subject to interference from radiofrequency electromagnetic energy, including electrosurgical equipment. The monopolar ESU poses particular risks for patients with IEDs, which can malfunction during use of the ESU.

To prevent patient injury related to IED interference, staff members must know the specifications for the type of IED and its location before surgery. In some cases the IED manufacturer must be notified to provide expert information on the specific device and potential interference and sometimes the manufacturer's representative may be present to help reprogram and test the device in the perioperative period.

All patients with an IED are monitored per hospital protocols and standard procedures for ESU safety are followed.

SMOKE PLUME

During electrosurgery and laser surgery, tissue is destroyed or incised, and this process creates toxic smoke called **smoke plume**. Smoke plume contains about 95% water and 5% other products. The other products include chemicals, blood cells, and intact or fragmented bacteria and viruses. The potential hazards of these substances are infectious disease transmission, toxicity from chemicals, and allergy. The size of aerosol particles ranges from 0.1 to 0.8 μm. These droplets are capable of harboring much smaller viral and bacterial particles.

Smoke plume contains a number of toxic chemicals in concentrations that can potentially exceed those recommended by the Occupational Safety and Health Administration (OSHA). Among the chemicals found in smoke plume are toluene, acrolein, formaldehyde, and hydrogen cyanide. Both laser and electrosurgical plume contain living and dead cells. Disease transmission through smoke plume is a known risk to surgical personnel. Other transmissible biological particles, such as cancer cells, at laser and electrosurgical sites are an additional concern.

Risk Reduction

Smoke plume reduction or elimination is a mandatory process during electrosurgery and laser surgery. Normal room ventilation is not sufficient to capture chemical and biological particles from smoke plume. Two methods are used to prevent perioperative personnel from inhaling smoke, inline room suction systems and commercial smoke evacuation devices. Room suction is designed to carry liquids, not smoke. These systems pull at a much lower rate than commercial smoke evacuation systems and must have inline filters attached to be safe. Smoke evacuation systems are specifically designed to extract moist smoke plume from the surgical site.

Smoke Evacuation System

A smoke evacuation system contains a nozzle tip, suction tubing, filters, absorbers, and vacuum pump. Smoke plume is evacuated at a rate of about 100 to 150 feet (30 to 46 m) per minute at the site of generation. It then is carried through a high-efficiency particulate air (HEPA) filter and trapped in absorbers. The filters are considered biohazardous waste and must be disposed of according to hospital policy. When a smoke evacuator is used, the nozzle tip must be within 2 inches (5 cm) of the surgical site to be effective. Fresh filters and tubing must be used for each patient. Some ESU systems now have intrinsic smoke evacuation systems. Systems that attach directly to the ESU active electrode are now available.

KINETIC ENERGY

ULTRASONIC ENERGY

Ultrasonic energy is created when electricity is transformed into mechanical energy generated by high-frequency vibration and the forces of friction. The ultrasonic instrument simultaneously cuts and coagulates tissue by transmitting ultrasonic wave energy through specially designed forceps, scissors, or blades. The instrument vibrates at approximately 55,000 movements per second, and these vibrations cause protein molecules to rupture. One drawback of this type of energy is that it cannot cut tissue without coagulating it. When the instrument is applied, the tissue liquefies and forms coagulum, a sticky protein substance that congeals and welds the tissue in the same way that metal is melted to form solder.

Ultrasonic technology uses a very low temperature. Electrical current *does not* pass through the patient; therefore, no grounding pad (inactive electrode) is required for this type of energy. Examples of ultrasonic energy systems are the SonoSurg (Olympus America, Center Valley, Pa) and the Harmonic energy system (Ethicon, Somerville, NJ).

Although the ultrasonic scalpel does not transmit electrical current to the target tissue, the blades remain hot immediately after use. This is due to the vibration and friction produced by the instrument. The instrument must be held away from tissue during the cooling period to prevent accidental burns. The scrub should provide a moist towel on the surgical field where the instrument can be placed between applications.

Ultrasonic Ablation

Ultrasonic ablation is used as an alternative to electrosurgery. Tumor **ablation** is performed by inserting a series of needle probes directly into the tumor under direct fluoroscopic imaging. Other specialties that commonly use this technology are gynecology, endovascular surgery, neurological surgery, and ophthalmology. The **Cavitron Ultrasonic Surgical Aspirator (CUSA)** is commonly used for ultrasonic ablation and aspiration (suction) in tumor surgery. **Phacoemulsification** is a process employing a delicate ophthalmological instrument (phacoemulsifier) that uses ultrasonic energy for the destruction of cataracts.

COLD THERMAL ENERGY

CRYOSURGERY

Cryosurgery is the use of an extremely cold instrument or substance to destroy tissue. Cryosurgery has been used for many years to treat small skin lesions. Liquid nitrogen is applied to tissue, which freezes almost immediately and eventually sloughs.

Cryoablation is a newer technique in which a probe is inserted into a tumor or tissue mass. High-pressure argon gas is injected into the probe, causing the surrounding tissue to freeze. The tissue is destroyed and eventually absorbed by the body. This surgical technique is often performed in the outpatient setting under guided fluoroscopy.

LASER ENERGY

Laser is an acronym for *light amplification by stimulated emission of radiation*. Laser surgery uses an intensely hot, precisely focused beam of light to cut and coagulate tissue. Electricity does not pass through the patient during laser surgery.

Because lasers are high-energy, potentially damaging instruments in the operating room and health care facility, laser teams are established to oversee the training of staff and the appropriate implementation of rules and regulations regarding their use in the clinical setting. The Laser Safety Committee oversees the planning and implementation of the laser program, including its safety measures. The safety committee is also responsible for teaching and credentialing staff members who understand advanced courses in laser safety and technology. The Laser Safety Officer is responsible for fielding clinical questions and maintaining the highest level of safety standards in the health facility.

LASER STANDARDS AND REGULATIONS

The laser is a powerful instrument that has a variety of applications in manufacturing, engineering, biotechnology, and warfare. Laser technology has created a new field in medicine. However, lasers can also cause irreparable injury and destruction. Because of this, laser standards have been developed by governmental and private agencies. In health care, these standards are designed to protect both the patient and those who work with lasers. Some of the agencies involved in the regulation of laser safety are listed in Box 18-4.

HOW LASERS WORK

Laser Light

Recall that light has both particle and wave characteristics. Ordinary light is made up of many wavelengths and colors. When ordinary light is generated, the rays are transmitted from the source in infinite directions. However, laser light is unlike ordinary light. All the waves in the laser have exactly the same length and therefore are **monochromatic**. The waves are lined up so that their peaks and troughs are in exactly the same location, a quality called **coherency** (Figure 18-8).

The distinctive characteristics of laser energy are created when light is pumped into a sealed chamber and filled with a medium (i.e., a gas, solid, or liquid); this medium is called the **laser medium**. The chamber is called the **optical resonant cavity**. When photons of a specific energy enter the chamber, they stimulate the high-energy atoms in the chamber to vibrate or resonate in the same wave pattern. Mirrors in the laser system bounce the photons back and forth through the laser medium in the chamber. This increases the number of resonating parallel photons and is called **amplification** (Figure 18-9).

Lasers are grouped into two categories according to the duration of the output waves:

- **Continuous wave lasers** produce a steady stream of light.
- **Q-switched lasers** (also called **pulsed wave lasers**) emit light in bursts or pulses.

Laser Components

The main components of the laser delivery system are:

- The *optical resonator* (also called the **laser head**): Contains the lasing medium and mirrors needed to amplify the light waves.
- The **excitation source**: Supplies the energy needed to increase the resonance of the lasing medium.
- The *delivery system:* The instruments or devices that transmits the lasing energy to the operative site. The system depends on the type of laser and surgery. A laser *fiber* (filament) is commonly used.
- The *control panel* and *touch screen:* Contain the control system for the laser functions and operations.
- *Accessory equipment:* Includes the cooling system and vacuum pump, if required by the laser type.

The modern laser is controlled by microprocessing technology. The optical resonator and control system are contained in a single unit, and accessory equipment is attached

---

Box **18-4** | **Professional Resources in Laser Technology for Surgical Technologists**

- *American National Standards Institute (ANSI):* An organization of expert volunteers who develop the standards for laser use in specific professions.
- *Center for Devices and Radiological Health (CDRH):* A regulatory agency of the U.S. Food and Drug Administration and the Department of Health and Human Services. This agency standardizes the performance safety criteria for manufactured laser products.
- *Occupational Safety and Health Administration (OSHA):* A governmental regulatory body, OSHA follows accepted industry laser standards.
- *Association of periOperative Registered Nurses (AORN):* The professional organization of perioperative nurses, which publishes a review and expert guidelines for use of lasers by perioperative professionals.

Monochromatic:
All waves have exactly the same wavelength (one color)

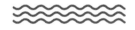

Parallel:
All waves move in columns

Ordinary light

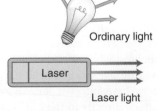

Laser light

Coherent:
All waves are exactly in step with each other (space and time)

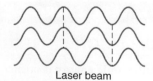

Laser beam

Figure 18-8 Comparison of normal and laser light. Ordinary light rays are transmitted in all directions. Laser waves are monochromatic, parallel, and coherent. They move in one direction and the waves are lined up, producing an extremely powerful source of energy.

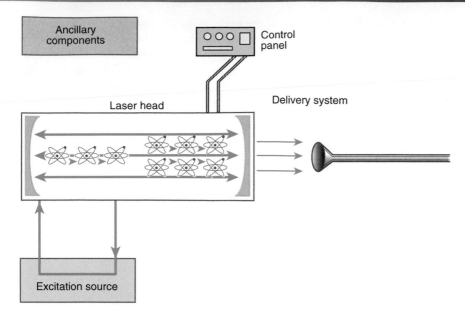

Figure 18-9 The characteristics of laser energy are created when light is pumped into a sealed chamber filled with a medium that excites the photons. *(From Rothrock J: Alexander's care of the patient in surgery, ed 17, St Louis, 2007, Mosby.)*

according to the requirements of the surgery. The actual laser housing is contained within the laser unit, along with the cooling system and vacuum pump. The controls of the modern laser include a touch panel or screen on which surgical options can be selected and adjustments made. A single foot pedal control is available to the operating surgeon. A registered nurse or surgical technologist is assigned to the console.

Effects of Lasers

When laser light is directed at a surface, any of the following can occur:

- Absorption
- Reflection
- Scattering
- Transmission

Lasers are distinguished by the functional or biophysical reaction of the target tissue. The tissue reaction depends on the following:

- The laser wavelength
- The power setting
- The absorption quality of the cells (e.g., color, density, moisture content)

The quality of the laser energy depends on its density, which is determined by the voltage, the diameter of the beam, and the exposure time on the tissue. The sum of these is called the **radiant exposure**.

When certain types of laser light contact tissue, the cells become extremely hot. Just as in electrosurgery, a high temperature causes cell destruction through vaporization. Laser light can also weld tissue.

Selective absorption is an important characteristic of laser energy. This means that some cells absorb the lasing medium, whereas others do not. This characteristic prevents the spread of heat (and damage) outside the target tissue.

The type of gas or other substance used to create specific laser energy determines its absorption by the tissue. The moisture content and density of a particular tissue are important factors in the choice of laser medium.

LASER MEDIA

Lasers are distinguished by the medium or the element activated to transmit photons. These include:

- Gases
- Solids
- Semiconductors (diode lasers)
- Excimers
- Solid-state media
- Liquid dyes

Argon (Gas)

Argon gas lasers produce a visible blue-green beam that is absorbed by red-brown pigmented tissue such as hemoglobin. The argon beam is not absorbed by clear or translucent tissue; therefore, the beam can pass through the cornea, vitreous, and lens of the eye without burning these tissues. The argon beam is used for coagulation and for sealing or welding tissue.

The argon laser is most often used in dermatological and ophthalmological procedures. In dermatology, it is used to remove pigmented lesions because it is not readily absorbed by light tissue. In ophthalmology, it is used in surgery for retinal tears, glaucoma, macular degeneration, retinopathy, and retinal vein occlusion. The argon beam is delivered through a laser fiber in combination with the surgical microscope, slit lamp, or handpiece attached to an articulated (jointed) arm.

Carbon Dioxide (Gas)

The **carbon dioxide** laser is invisible to the human eye. The beam has a high affinity for water and functions at a superficial depth. A helium-neon laser beam that produces a red light is added to the carbon dioxide laser beam to make it visible. The helium-neon beam is sometimes called the "pilot light" because of its guiding function. The carbon dioxide laser is extremely versatile and is used in many surgical specialties, including microsurgery. Krypton, another gas lasing medium, is used for the removal of superficial lesions in dermatology.

Holmium:YAG (Solid)

The holmium:yttrium-aluminum-garnet or **holmium:YAG** laser is a crystal containing holmium, thallium, and chromium. Its beam is outside the visible light range and able to penetrate all tissue types. This laser is used to cut, shave, contour, ablate, and coagulate tissue. It is extremely versatile and capable of ablating renal and biliary calculi as well as soft tissues. It has a low depth penetration to a maximum of 0.4 mm. The holmium:YAG laser is used in urological, orthopedic; ear, nose, and throat (ENT), gynecological, gastrointestinal, and general surgery. It also is suitable for use in minimally invasive surgery.

Neodymium:YAG (Solid)

The **neodymium:YAG** (Nd:YAG) laser is created from a solid-state crystal of neodymium, yttrium, aluminum, and garnet. As with the carbon dioxide laser, a helium-neon beam is used for visibility. The Nd:YAG laser beam has a high affinity for tissue protein but little for water. The beam is near the infrared region of the electromagnetic spectrum and has a penetration of 3 to 7 mm. Of all the laser types, the Nd:YAG has the greatest ability to coagulate blood vessels. Because of its deep penetration, it can coagulate vessels up to 4 mm in diameter. This laser can be used during endoscopic or flexible fiberoptic surgery. It is delivered through a laser fiber or probe in continuous or pulsed mode. The Erbium (Er:YAG) is similar to the Nd:YAG laser, except that it has a stronger affinity for water in tissue, which limits its use in surgery.

Ruby and Alexandrite (Solid)

Synthetic ruby crystals were the first substance to be used as a lasing medium. Initially used in industry and for military purposes, the ruby laser was also used to remove superficial skin defects and tattoos. The Q-switched ruby laser has been replaced with the Alexandrite, a solid lasing material which is more efficient for use in dermatology.

Potassium-Titanyl-Phosphate (Solid)

The **potassium-titanyl-phosphate (KTP)** laser is less powerful than the carbon dioxide or Nd:YAG laser, but it is capable of producing a minute beam that is well suited to microscopic surgery. The green laser light is readily absorbed by pigmented tissue and can be delivered by a number of different methods, including fiber, scanner, or microscope. The beam can also be transmitted through clear solutions. The KTP laser offers two wavelengths; this allows two separate sets of laser characteristics to be selected at any time. These provide hemostatic cutting and ablation as well as deep coagulation. The KTP laser is used in ENT, urological, gynecological, and general surgery and in dermatological procedures. KTP can also be combined with neodymium to double its frequency and increase versatility.

Excimer (Gas)

The **excimer** laser produces a cool beam by stripping electrons from the atoms of the medium in the chamber. This causes the energy bonds in the atom to break. The resulting shock waves stimulate short bursts of laser light. The light is delivered to the target tissue through fiberoptic bundles.

The beam of the excimer laser creates less heat than other laser types. This reduces damage to nearby tissues and also results in less carbonization of lased tissue. Specialized ultraviolet mirrors and optics are required to operate the laser safely. This laser is extremely precise and is commonly used in ophthalmological surgery and dermatology.

Tunable Dye (Solid)

The pulsed dye laser beam (**tunable dye laser**) is formed when fluorescent liquid or other dyes are exposed to argon laser light. The dye absorbs the light and produces a fluorescent broad-spectrum light. The spectrum of the light is then "tuned" to produce light of a particular wavelength (color). This provides versatility for a variety of tissue types and surgical specialties.

LASER SAFETY

Surgical lasers pose significant health and safety risks. These risks are manageable but require vigilance and attention to every detail of safety protocols. All perioperative personnel must know the protocols well and follow them carefully. The specific risks for patients and personnel are eye damage, tissue burns, fire, and smoke plume.

Laser classifications depend on the safety risks associated with their use:

- *Class 4:* Cause permanent eye damage if viewed directly or if viewed indirectly by reflection. These lasers can also ignite materials and cause skin burns. Most surgical lasers are class 4 lasers.
- *Class 3b:* Cause severe eye injury when viewed directly or by reflection. These lasers do not cause injury when the laser beam is diffused and do not normally present a fire hazard.
- *Class 3a:* Normally do not cause eye injury if viewed momentarily but present a hazard if viewed with collecting optics (e.g., fiberoptic cable, magnification loupe, or microscope).
- *Class 2:* Emit radiation in the visible range of the electromagnetic spectrum. These lasers do not normally cause harm when viewed briefly, although they can be hazardous when viewed for an extended period. Laser pointers and bar code scanners are class 2 lasers.
- *Class 1:* Are not hazardous for continuous viewing, are considered incapable of producing damaging radiation levels, and are exempt from control measures. Laser printers are in this category.

Note that class 3b and 4 lasers cause instantaneous retinal injury that may be irreparable. Class 4 lasers can penetrate the sclera and injure the retina. Turning the head away or turning away from the laser does not ensure protection because of the risk of scatter or reflection of the beam.

Recall the three specific characteristics of laser energy that distinguish it from ordinary white light: it is coherent (peaks and troughs match), monochromatic (all waves are of the same wavelength), and parallel (waves move in one direction only). These qualities make laser light extremely hazardous,

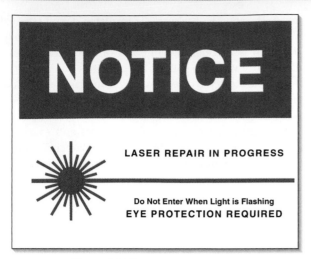

Figure 18-10   Laser warning sign.

because it can concentrate a tremendous amount of energy in one small area.

Precautions and Guidelines

- A laser safety officer is required to manage laser risks and define safety protocols.
- Lasers are key-locked when not in use.
- Lasers are a potent source of ignition in the operating room. All fire safety precautions must be in place before the start of surgery.
- Only personnel trained in and proven knowledgeable about laser use and precautions are allowed to participate in laser surgery. All reflective surfaces in the laser environment are covered, made nonreflective, or removed from the environment. Non-reflective, black matte finished instruments are to be used in laser surgery.
- Laser warning signs must be placed on all entrances to areas where laser surgery is being performed (Figure 18-10).
- All personnel entering a room in which lasers are in use must wear protective eyewear (see the next section).
- Only flame-retardant drapes are used during laser surgery.

The two most common injuries associated with unintentional laser exposure are eye injury and skin burn. Lasers in the ultraviolet and infrared areas of the spectrum are the most damaging. They can penetrate the sclera and enter the lens, cornea, and retina. Eye injury can be permanent, especially if the retina is involved. Injuries range from corneal burns to blindness, especially when the retina is involved.

Heat generated by the lasing light beam is the major cause of tissue damage. Intentional use of the laser results in incision or dissection, tissue vaporization, and welding. Unintentional exposure can have the same effects. These range from reddening of the skin to third-degree burns. The following criteria determine the degree of thermal damage:

- The sensitivity of the irradiated tissue
- The amount of tissue affected
- The wavelength of the laser beam
- The energy level of the laser beam
- The length of time the tissue was exposed

Eye Safety and Skin Protection

The eye is the tissue most vulnerable to accidental laser exposure and injury. To protect the eyes during laser use, personnel must shield them from the *specific wavelength* of light. Protective eyewear of the correct optical density is required for various types of lasers. Eyewear must wrap completely around the eyes, covering the sides, top, and bottom so that no diffuse laser energy can reach the eye. Regular prescription eyeglasses do not offer protection. Only eyewear that is specifically approved for laser use can be used during laser surgery. Protective eyewear is available commercially, and manufacturers offer different styles and lens colors for each type of laser.

The color of the laser lenses is not an indication of the level of protection. *The specific density of the lens, not the color, provides protection.* There is no color code associated with laser type.

The protective eyewear bears an inscription on the lens that details the optical density and the eyewear must be labeled for the specific laser type. In addition to protective eyewear for staff members, other precautions must be followed to prevent eye injury. These include but are not limited to the following:

- Lens filters are placed over any endoscope viewing port.
- The patient's eyes are covered with wet eye pads or eye cups that are laser-specific. Corneal eye shields are used for patients undergoing laser surgery of the eyelids.
- Appropriate laser backstops which stop the penetration of laser energy into normal tissue. A titanium quartz rob or guard is used as a backstop. Rhodium or stainless steel mirrors may also be used for backstopping.
- All patients undergoing surgery while awake wear protective eyewear.
- The windows to the operating room are covered with barrier material that stops the transmission of the laser beam being used in the room, and warning signs are posted outside to caution against unprotected entry during laser procedures (see Figure 18-10).
- Appropriate protective eyewear is available on the outside of each entryway leading to a room in which lasers are being used.
- The effective danger area where safety precautions must be observed, is a closed room where the laser surgery is being preformed called the Normal Hazard Zone (NHZ).

Skin injuries result from direct contact with the laser beam. Environmental precautions are necessary to prevent these injuries. In addition, anyone entering a room in which lasers are in use must remove any metallic jewelry, which can reflect the laser beam or absorb heat. The patient's tissues are protected from inadvertent laser injury. Wet towels are placed around the operative site to prevent burns in the area. When endoscopic lasers are in use the laser fiber must extend more than one inch beyond the tip of the endoscope to prevent back scatter of the beam and burning of the endoscope, and/or heating of the extension tube which can damage healthy tissues. Body cavities, such as the nasal cavity or rectal passage, may also be packed with moist sponges to prevent injury during laser use.

Airway Protection

In addition to routine precautions against fire, particular attention is given to anesthesia equipment, especially during laser surgery involving the head and neck. Endotracheal tubes and other anesthesia equipment can easily ignite in the presence of laser energy and oxygen-rich anesthetic agents. To minimize the risk of an endotracheal fire, a special metallic foil is wrapped around the endotracheal tube before laser surgery. Oxygen flow is reduced to a minimum and combustible gases are avoided.

Although an airway fire is a rare event, the possibility exists during laser surgery. When ignited, the endotracheal tube acts as a blowtorch, and flames may reach 5 to 10 inches (12.5 to 25 cm) within seconds. If a fire occurs, the tube may be removed or flushed with saline. The scrub and circulator should be prepared to offer emergency assistance to both the anesthesiologist and surgeons as needed.

KEY CONCEPTS

- The concepts of conduction, frequency, and impedance explain the fundamental properties of electricity. When we transfer this knowledge to electricity and the body, we can understand how heart contraction occurs, why electrolytes must be in physiological balance, how the kidney is able to filter waste products but retain fluid, and many other physiological processes.
- Electrosurgery is common in most surgical procedures. It is also one of the most frequent sources of patient injury. The surgical technologist must have a solid knowledge base in this area in order to protect patients against injury.
- The main components of electrosurgery are the power unit, the active electrode, which delivers the electrical energy to tissue, and the return electrode, which captures the current and conducts it safely back to the power unit.
- Monopolar and bipolar circuitry in electrosurgery give rise to two very different types of devices, each with its own properties and hazards. Monopolar electrosurgery produces an extremely powerful energy capable of incising all types of tissue including bone. The monopolar current passes through the patient's body before returning to the power unit to complete the circuit.
- Bipolar electrosurgery produces less powerful energy at a lower temperature. The energy passes from the control unit between the tips of the active electrode holding the tissue, and back to the power unit without passing through the patient's body.
- Specific terms are used to describe how electricity works, its behavior, and specific hazards. Examples are capacitative and indirect coupling, smoke plume, active electrode, and many others. Understanding the terms is the first stage of understanding how to handle electrosurgical devices.
- Many physiological processes occur normally as a result of electrochemical interactions at the cellular level. When electricity is applied to the body from an external source, such as during electrosurgery, the voltage and frequency of that source cause alterations in the tissue. Electricity is therefore an inherent hazard that must be controlled at all stages. The source of power, the insulated circuit (the path of the current), the active electrode, sources of stray electricity, areas of potential impedance, and all sources of interference with the path of the circuit.
- The smoke created by electrosurgical and laser energy contains chemical carcinogens, tissue fragments and potential bacterial contaminants that can be drawn into the lungs of the operating team. Smoke plume filters and evacuation systems are now required in all devices that create smoke. These are much more effective than normal suction devices, which should not be used for this purpose.
- Laser energy created when light is passed through particular kinds of media is among the most powerful types of energy used in surgery. Like electricity, it can be contained and directed for beneficial use, but when used incorrectly, can be a source of injury. Lasers are the most common cause of patient fires. There are many opportunities to learn how to reduce and mitigate risk by studying the types of laser media, how and when they are used, and what types of protective measures are required when lasers are in use.

REVIEW QUESTIONS

1. Discuss the difference between a bipolar circuit and a monopolar circuit.
2. Why do you place the patient return electrode over a large muscle mass?
3. What is active electrode monitoring (AEM)?
4. What kinds of electrosurgery require a patient return electrode?
5. Why doesn't the patient experience cardiac arrest when electrosurgical procedures are used?
6. What is the effect of impedance of electricity as it flows through a conductive medium?
7. What is cryoablation?
8. Why does eschar on the active electrode create a hazard?
9. What does the acronym *laser* stand for?
10. What precautions are needed during laser surgery of the throat?
11. A colleague asks you why the laser goggles are not color-coded. What would you say?

CASE STUDIES

Case 1

You are in a hurry to pass through a surgical suite where Nd:YAG laser surgery is in progress. You do not use protective eyewear, even though goggles are hanging on the door outside. You enter the room and turn your head away from the patient as you proceed to the other door. Just to be safe, you close your eyes for a few moments until you reach the door. Are you safe?

Case 2

You are asked to bring a 16-year-old from the holding area for surgery. When you arrive, you see that she has a metal ring through her lip. You explain to her that it is a hazard during electrosurgery. She tells you she cannot take it out because there is no way to remove it. How will you handle this situation?

Case 3

You are scrubbed during an emergency laparotomy in which monopolar electrosurgery is used extensively. Midway through the case, you notice that the power cord to the electrosurgical unit has been plugged into an extension cord to which the cardiac monitor is also connected. What should you do?

Case 4

You are at the scrub sink, preparing for an eye procedure in which laser surgery will be used. The surgeon's assistant is next to you at the sink. You notice that he is wearing a metal necklace. Can he tuck it into his scrub shirt?

Case 5

During surgery in which you are scrubbed, the surgeon asks you to hold a clamp that he has just placed over a vessel bundle. He proceeds to buzz the clamp. You suddenly feel a sharp burning pain on the hand holding the clamp. What caused this? What should you do?

BIBLIOGRAPHY

Ball K: *Lasers: the perioperative challenge*, ed 3, Denver, 2004, Association of periOperative Registered Nurses (AORN).

Fickling J, Loeffler C: *Electrosurgical considerations for the patient with an implanted electronic device.* Accessed September 20, 2011, at http://www.valleylab.com/education/hotline/pdfs/hotline_0706.pdf.

Fickling J, Loeffler C: *Using multiple accessories with one generator.* Accessed September 20, 2011, at http://www.valleylab.com/education/hotline/pdfs/hotline_0606.pdf.

Fickling J, Loeffler C: *Valleylab electrosurgical generators: general cautions and warnings for patient and operating room safety.* Accessed September 20, 2011, at http://www.valleylab.com/education/hotline/pdfs/hotline_0408.pdf.

Giesler C, Bowling M, Tobias D: *Abdominal hysterectomy with the harmonic wave coagulating shears.* Accessed September 20, 2011, at http://www.obgmanagement.com/MedEdLibr/PDFs/OBGSupp_HarmonicWave_0507.pdf.

Nagelhout J, Zaglaniczny K: *Nurse anesthesia*, ed 3, Philadelphia, 2005, Elsevier.

National Institutes of Health Clinical Center: *Overview for physicians: radiofrequency ablation.* Accessed September 20, 2011, at http://www.cc.nih.gov/drd/rfa.

Rothrock J: *Alexander's care of the patient in surgery*, ed 13, St Louis, 2007, Mosby.

Ulmer B: *The Valleylab Institute of Clinical Education electrosurgery continuing education module: electrosurgery continuing education module, July 2011.* Accessed September 11, 2011, at http://www.valleylab.com/education/poes/index.html.

LEARNING OBJECTIVES

After studying this chapter and laboratory practice, the reader will be able to:

1. Use the correct procedure to identify a patient
2. List and discuss the principles of safe patient transport and transfer
3. Demonstrate professional communication skills with families of patients being transported to surgery
4. Use safe body mechanics during patient transportation, transferring, and positioning
5. Discuss common methods of patient transport and lateral moving devices used in the perioperative environment
6. Demonstrate the different scenarios involving transferring and transporting ambulatory and wheelchair assisted patients

7. Describe guidelines for transporting special patient populations
8. Describe the responsibilities of the surgical technologist in patient positioning
9. Demonstrate the use of common operating table accessories
10. Describe how to prevent patient injury during positioning
11. Describe the principles of safe positioning
12. Demonstrate the different positions used in surgical procedures
13. Discuss the safety precautions for each position

TERMINOLOGY

Abduction: Movement of a joint or body part away from the body.

Compartment syndrome: Severe swelling and tissue injury caused by constriction of the blood and lymph. Compartment syndrome can progress to tissue necrosis.

Compression injury: Tissue injury caused by continuous pressure over an area.

Dependent areas of the body: Areas of the body subject to pressure from gravity and weight. For example, the sacrum is a dependent area when a person is in the supine position.

Embolism: A clot of blood, air, organic material, or a foreign body that moves freely in the vascular system. An embolus travels from larger to smaller vessels until it cannot pass through a vessel. At that level, it interrupts the flow of blood and may result in severe disease or death.

Fasciotomy: A surgical treatment for compartment syndrome in which the fascia is incised to release severe tissue swelling.

Footboard: Operating table attachment that braces the patient's weight when the table is tilted toward the feet.

Hyperextension: Extension of a joint beyond its normal anatomical range.

Hyperflexion: Flexion of a joint beyond its normal anatomical range.

Hypotension: Decreased blood pressure.

Ischemia: Loss of blood supply to a body part either by compression or as a result of a blockage in the blood vessels. Prolonged ischemia causes tissue death from lack of oxygen to the tissue.

Lateral transfer: Transferring the patient from one horizontal surface to another, such as from a bed to a stretcher.

Necrosis: Tissue death.

Neuropathy: Permanent or temporary nerve injury that results in numbness or loss of function of a part of the body.

Range of motion: The normal anatomical movement of an extremity.

Shear injury: Tissue injury or necrosis that results when two tissue planes are forcefully pulled in opposite directions. Shearing usually occurs when the body is pulled or slides by

TERMINOLOGY (cont.)

gravity across a high-friction surface, such as a bed sheet. Shearing can lead to a decubitus ulcer.

Thoracic outlet syndrome: A group of disorders attributed to compression of the subclavian vessels and nerves. Such compression can cause permanent injury to the arm and shoulder.

Thromboembolus (embolus): A blood clot that breaks loose and enters the systemic circulation, causing obstruction or occlusion of a blood vessel.

Traction injury: A nerve injury caused by stretching or compression of the nerve.

Transfer board: A thin Plexiglas, fiberglass, or roller board that is placed under the patient to move the person from the operating table to the stretcher or bed.

Trendelenburg position: The position in which a prone or supine patient is tilted with the head down.

INTRODUCTION

In the perioperative setting, patients must be transferred to and from a variety of conveyances, including gurneys, beds, wheelchairs, and the operating table. The transportation and positioning of patients are among the responsibilities that create the most risk for patients and health care providers alike. Patients may be unsteady, semiconscious, or unconscious and unable to use protective mechanisms that normally would prevent falls or other injuries. Diagnostic and operating room tables are narrow. Transfer vehicles, such as gurneys and wheelchairs, can slip unexpectedly. Perioperative work is physically demanding, and staff members may be tired or even themselves injured from the continual strain on the legs, back, and hips.

Moving and handling patients is one of the roles of the surgical technologist. In surgery the technologist is also required to assist in patient positioning under the supervision of the anesthesiologist and surgeon. While performing their duties, surgical technologists need to protect the patient from injury all times, while guarding their own health by using safe methods and protocols. This chapter provides an introduction to hands-on technique necessary to ensure the safety of patients and surgical team.

PATIENT IDENTIFICATION

The identity of the patient is verified before transporting and before any procedure. Patient identification is a critical issue in health care. The surgical technologist is responsible for patient identification according to facility policy and the mutual guidelines agreed on by all professional surgical organizations. No patient should be transported and no procedure should be initiated until the protocol for identification has been completed, even if the patient is known to the health care staff.

All patients are identified in at least three ways. The patient's wrist or ankle band is imprinted with the patient's name and other unique identifiers such as birth date and hospital number. If a scan or imprint card system is used, the patient's identification card is used to process all paperwork and matches the patient's identification bracelet. This card must be firmly attached to the chart during transport and must remain with the chart until the patient returns to his or her hospital unit. The patient's chart must accompany the patient whenever the individual is transported from the unit. Errors in patient identification usually occur when the necessary protocol has been bypassed.

To validate the patient's identity, follow these guidelines:

1. Examine the patient's identity band. Compare both the name and the number with those on the patient's chart.
2. Ask the patient to state his or her full name and date of birth. Do not call the patient by name before asking the patient to state his or her name.
3. Ask the patient to tell you what procedure he or she is undergoing and to point to the side on which the surgery will take place.
4. If the patient does not speak English, or seems to have difficulty understanding, you must seek assistance from an interpreter. This information can be determined ahead of time so that an appropriate interpreter is available.
5. Remember that patients may be anxious or worried before surgery and might answer closed-ended questions indiscriminately. It is necessary to question the patient without giving the answer.
6. Always check the chart, the identification band, and hospital ID number for each patient.

EXAMPLE 1

Wrong: "Are you Mr. X? I'm here to take you to surgery."

Correct: "Good morning, my name is _____. I'm here to take you to surgery. Can you state your full name and date of birth for me?"

EXAMPLE 2

Wrong: "So, Dr. X is planning to operate on your arm today."

Correct: "What surgery will you be having today?"

If the patient's name, hospital identification number, surgery, and surgical site do not match the chart or operative documents, you must report this to the unit charge nurse. Do not transport the patient if patient information does not match the chart. Call the operating room to let personnel know about the delay and the reason.

If the patient has no identification band, you must report this to the unit charge nurse or nurse manager. Under routine circumstances an identification band must be obtained before the patient leaves the unit.

PRINCIPLES OF SAFE PATIENT TRANSPORT AND TRANSFER

Specific risks are associated with patient transport and transfer. A weak, disoriented, or pediatric patient may attempt to climb out of the gurney or climb out of the crib and become entangled in side rails or climb over them and fall. Catheters, tubing, and other medical devices can cause tissue trauma or injury if pulled out of the body. The patient can sustain a shear injury (see the section on positioning injuries later in the chapter) if dragged across a high-friction surface such as bed linens or a draw sheet. Changes in posture can result in a sudden drop in blood pressure or elevated cerebral pressure. Even when transfers are done slowly and deliberately, accidents can occur.

Transport and transfer injuries occur more often in the following circumstances:

- There are not enough people to help with the move.
- Specialized moving and handling equipment is not available or is located too far away from the work area.
- Staff have not been trained adequately for safe moving and handling.
- Personnel assisting in the transfer or transport do not have a plan.
- Personnel feel rushed.
- The patient is disoriented.

The following principles apply to all types of patient transport and transfer:

- *Know the risks.* To keep the patient safe, you must understand exactly what the risks are and how to prevent injury.
- *Protect the patient's personal dignity at all times.* The patient has a right to be protected from exposure and embarrassment. Many patients fear that their personal rights, such as a right to modesty, are forfeited on admission to a health care facility. Try to avoid passing through crowded areas while transporting the patient. This is not always possible, but it is desirable. Use a patient elevator instead of visitor elevators during transportation.
- *Perform all patient movement deliberately and carefully.* You must have a plan before you begin. Prepare for the unexpected. Think ahead.
- *Coordinate with others when assisting in moving and handling.* When a patient is transferred, one person should be in charge of the move and guide the others.
- *Know your equipment.* Before moving any patient, know how to operate patient care equipment. Never use a mechanical lifting or transfer system without prior training and assistance.
- *Think about what you are doing while you are doing it.* As you move the patient, maintain your focus on the task at hand. Do not allow yourself to become distracted. Think ahead and be prepared for each step of the process.
- *Protect the patient from hypothermia.* The patient should be adequately covered with blankets. Corridors can be very cold and drafty. A patient who has become cold during transport is at higher risk for hypothermia during surgery.

- *Use approved protocol for patient identification at all times.* Check the name and number on the wrist or ankle band, identification card, permits, and chart.
- *Explain the process to the patient before and during the transfer.* This helps relieve the patient's anxiety and increases cooperation.

COMMUNICATION WITH FAMILIES

One or more family members may be present when the patient is transported to the operating room. Families are sensitive at this time and naturally concerned for their loved ones. They may accompany the patient on the way to the operating room up to the semirestricted area. At this point it is best to reassure the family that the patient will be well cared for and that a staff member, yourself, the nurse, or the surgeon will return to provide information on the progress of the surgery. Allow family members to express their concern and to speak privately with the patient before he or she enters the surgery doors.

SECTION I: TRANSFERRING AND TRANSPORTING THE PATIENT

SAFE MOVING AND HANDLING FOR HEALTH CARE PROVIDERS

All health care providers should normally receive facility training in safe patient moving and handling equipment used in their facility. Although all health care providers are at risk for skeletal injury, perioperative staff is required to move unconscious or semiconscious patients. A weak or sedated patient lacks muscle tone, which results in flaccid limbs and general unwieldiness. The adult human body is asymmetrical and heavy, and unlike a large inanimate object, the human body cannot always be held close to the health care provider's center of gravity while being moved.

Moving and handling always carries some level of risk to the patient. The patient can fall, equipment can become entangled during transfer, or a weak patient may pull the health care provider off balance. A sudden shift of weight may be required, and this can put unexpected strain on joints and tendons. Hospital rooms are often small and crowded, making movement awkward and sometimes difficult, especially when a gurney is introduced into a cramped cubicle.

Injuries are reduced when health care providers use proper body mechanics and patient transfer devices. Chapter 8 presents a complete discussion of body mechanics. The following guidelines can help prevent injuries during movement and handling patients:

- Prepare yourself and the patient before attempting a move. Assess the situation first. Have all equipment ready before you start.
- Ensure that you have sufficient help when moving a patient.
- Know your limits and try to remain within them while moving and handling patients.
- Use mechanical, hydrolic, or pneumatic moving and handling devices whenever possible.

- Maintain the spine in a neutral (natural) position whenever possible.
- Avoid twisting the spine, especially while lifting or bending.
- Position yourself as close to the patient as possible; this greatly reduces the spinal load.
- Keep your feet well apart to provide a wide base of support.
- When performing lateral transfers, such as moving the patient from one surface to another of equal height, *do not bend the knees.*
- For vertical moves (up or down), *do bend the knees.*
- Avoid positions that reduce your base of support.
- Never try to lift or maneuver the patient while reaching forward, away from your center of gravity. If necessary, place one knee on the bed to bring the patient closer to your center of gravity.
- Use abdominal, arm, and leg muscles when lifting the patient. The abdominal muscles can support the trunk much more efficiently than the lower back muscles.

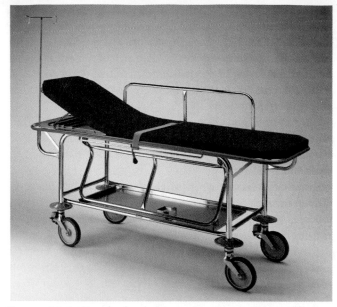

Figure 19-1 Standard gurney. *(Courtesy Pedigo Products, Vancouver, Wash.)*

TEAMWORK COUNTS

Teamwork is very important when positioning or transferring patients. The surgical technologist is often required to bring a patient from the hospital wards or other care areas into surgery. Teamwork begins from the moment the surgical technologist arrives on the patient care unit. He or she notifies the charge nurse that the patient is going to surgery. This sets others in action to help prepare the patient, talk to the family, and help secure the records. This is one of the occasions where the surgical technologist communicates directly with nursing and other colleagues outside the surgical department. Teamwork counts and is appreciated. Never take a patient off a ward without notifying the charge nurse or nurse manager. She or he is responsible for the whereabouts of all the patients and needs to know what is going on in the ward. Always keep in mind that good team relations increase safety in the workplace.

MOVING AND HANDLING DEVICES

Patients are transferred and moved in the clinical setting using a variety of different devices and conveyances. Many students will be familiar with these if they have worked previously in health care. It is best to learn how to use the device in training before being asked to actually transfer a patient.

Gurney (Stretcher)

The simplest gurney (Figure 19-1) has a removable mattress, an attachment for hanging intravenous (IV) solutions, side rails, a lower shelf for carrying oxygen tanks or other devices, and lockable wheels. The head can be raised, and there is a safety belt. The gurney is steered from the head end.

Wheelchair

The wheelchair is used to transport semimobile patients, usually in the ambulatory areas of the health care facility. The simple wheelchair must always be equipped with footboards

and a safety brake. More elaborate designs are able to tilt and raise the patient to a standing position and can accommodate medical devices such as an IV and oxygen tank.

Gait Device

A gait belt is a wide strap worn around the upper body and fitted with handles. It is sometimes used to guide and help stabilize ambulatory patients and prevent falls.

Lateral Transfer Devices

A **lateral transfer** is a move from a one surface such as a bed or gurney to another surface of equal height such as the operating table. Lateral transfers are most often carried out with a hydraulic, electric, or pneumatic transfer device. With the patient remaining in the supine position, the following transfer devices are commonly used in the surgical environment:

- An *air-assisted lateral transfer system* such as the HoverMatt device reduces friction during transfer. With the patient lying down, he or she is maneuvered onto the mat, which is then air-activated. Multiple air jets on the underside of the mat reduce the friction between the mat and the bed, allowing it to slide easily from one bed to another or from the bed to a gurney.
- A Plexiglas **transfer board** is placed under the patient and pulled from one surface to another (gurney to bed, or gurney to operating table). The board reduces friction and provides a stable surface for moving the patient. This device and air-assisted systems are the most commonly used lateral transfer devices in the modern operating room.
- A *roller board* is composed of multiple longitudinal rollers and covered with strong synthetic cloth The board is placed under the patient in the supine position and the board pulled from one horizontal surface to the other. The rollers provide the mechanism for movement.

- The *patient sling* is used to transfer the patient from a supine to sitting position to perform a lateral transfer or to rescue a heavy patient who has fallen to the floor. The cradle is made of heavy nylon material. It is placed underneath the patient and attached to a hydraulic frame, which is raised or lowered to suspend the patient during transfer.

The following websites provide useful information on patient moving and handling devices for students:

- United States Department of Labor: Ergonomics Equipment
  http://www.osha.gov/SLTC/etools/hospital/hazards/ergo/ergoequipment/ergoequip.html
- HoverTech
  http://www.hovermatt.com/reusable#reusable-video
- Entraco
  http://www.entracogroup.com/projects/ergo/flash/ergo_patient.swf

TRANSFERRING AMBULATORY AND WHEELCHAIR-ASSISTED PATIENTS

BED TO WHEELCHAIR

Transfer of a patient from a bed to a wheelchair is performed in distinct steps. During the transfer, reinforce your instructions and prepare the patient for each step. This increases the patient's confidence and reduces fear. Remember that weak or older patients often are often afraid of falling. Seek help from other staff when transferring a patient who is at high risk of falling (i.e., a patient who is obese, unstable, weak, or encumbered with medical devices).

Before beginning the transfer, familiarize yourself with the equipment. Make certain that the wheelchair's brakes and steering mechanism are functioning properly. Do not transport a patient in a wheelchair that has no foot supports or other safety attachments. The wheelchair must be able to accommodate the patient's size and weight.

Check the patient's identification as described previously. Free up any tubes or lines and make certain there is enough slack between the patient and the wheelchair to prevent entanglement or restriction during the transfer.

NOTE: Always remember to transfer and secure medical devices (tubing, oxygen tank, fluid collection bags) first, and then the patient.

LYING TO SITTING POSITION (PREPARATION FOR WHEELCHAIR)

Whenever you are responsible for transferring the patient, be aware of the location of the call bell in case you need assistance or emergency help.

To help a patient move from a lying position to a sitting position, follow these steps:

1. Bring the wheelchair to the side of the bed so that it is lined up with the bed. Lock the wheels. Make sure the bed's wheels also are locked. Place the bed in its lowest position.

2. If the patient is weak on one side, place the wheelchair on the opposite side of the bed. Raise the head of the bed slowly.
3. If the patient reports dizziness or any other changes, seek nursing help before proceeding. Dizziness may be caused by rapid **hypotension** that results in cardiac arrhythmia or a sudden loss of blood to the brain.
4. To assist the patient into a sitting position, support the patient under the shoulders and thighs if necessary.
5. Pull the patient's legs gently over the side of the bed to a sitting position. Allow the patient to remain in the sitting position for a few moments. Do not proceed if the patient shows or reports any physical or mental changes

SITTING TO STANDING POSITION

To help a patient move from a sitting position to a standing position, follow these steps:
1. Standing directly in front of the patient, place your hands around the patient's torso and under the arms to support the shoulder blades.
2. Slightly bend your forward leg while placing your opposite foot in a bracing position (Figure 19-2, *A*).
3. Slowly rock back and raise the patient to a standing position (Figure 19-2, *B*).

STANDING POSITION TO WHEELCHAIR

To help a patient move from a standing position to a sitting position in a wheelchair and then transport the patient, follow these steps:
1. Taking one small step at a time, rotate your entire body as the patient does the same until the patient's back is lined up with the wheelchair.
2. Slowly lower the patient into the wheelchair. Spread your feet so that they are approximately shoulder width apart. Use your abdominal muscles to support your back as you lower the patient. Do not allow the patient's weight to pull you downward.
3. Bend your knees, use the larger thigh muscles, and use your abdominal muscles to support your upper body. Lower the patient when your spine and body are in alignment with the patient and wheelchair (Figure 19-3).
4. Place the patient's feet on the footrests and cover the patient with a blanket or sheet. Secure the safety strap.
5. Make sure that you have the patient's chart and medical records.
6. Proceed to your destination. When entering an elevator or doorway, pull the wheelchair in backward into the elevator. Secure doorways in the open position before passing through them. Make sure you have the patient's chart before leaving the area.

WHEELCHAIR TO BED

To transfer a patient from a wheelchair to a bed or operating table, follow these steps:

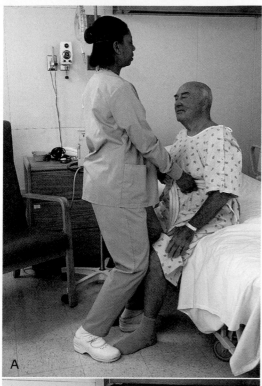

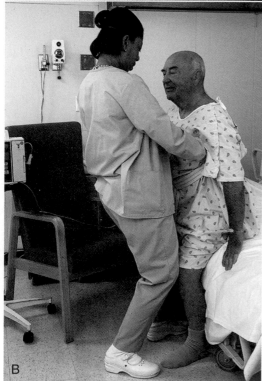

Figure 19-2 Lifting the patient from sitting to standing position. **A,** The surgical technologist positions herself to lift the patient. **B,** The surgical technologist lifts the patient safely. *(From Potter PA, Perry AG: Basic nursing: essentials for practice, ed 7, St Louis, 2009, Mosby.)*

1. Place the table or bed at its lowest height.
2. Reverse the steps used to transfer the patient to the wheelchair. Place the wheelchair in line with the bed and lock the wheels.
3. If the patient can put weight on the hands, ask the patient to push down. At the same time, assist the patient by

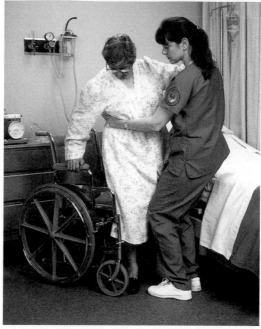

Figure 19-3 Lowering the patient into a wheelchair. *(From Harkreader H, Hogan MA: Fundamentals of nursing, ed 2, St Louis, 2004, WB Saunders.)*

placing your arms under the person's arms and securing your hands over the patient's shoulder blades.
4. Place your bracing foot back and rotated slightly outward.
5. As the patient stands up, rock back on your bracing foot and, step by step, rotate your body with the patient's until the person is positioned to sit on the edge of the bed.
6. Remember to keep your spine and the patient's back in alignment while turning. Ease the patient down to a sitting position on the bed.
7. One person should support the patient's back and head while another assists in bringing the legs to a horizontal position on the operating table or bed. A third assistant should stand at the opposite side of the operating table or bed to prevent the patient from falling.
8. Ease the patient to a lying position. Place a blanket or sheet over the patient and secure the side rails or safety strap.

ASSISTING A FALLING PATIENT

In the ambulatory care setting, patients walk or are transported by wheelchair from the holding area to the surgical area, and the surgical technologist may be responsible for assisting them. There is always a risk that the patient may fall during ambulation. The patient may suddenly experience a drop in blood pressure or become light-headed. Always anticipate the possibility of a fall, even when the patient is mobile and seems able to walk without assistance.

Patient falls can be dangerous for both the patient and the health care provider. The weight of the falling person can cause you to lose your own balance, which can result in a twisting injury or fracture. Patients who feel unsteady or insecure may take hold of the care provider and pull him or her off balance, causing injury to both.

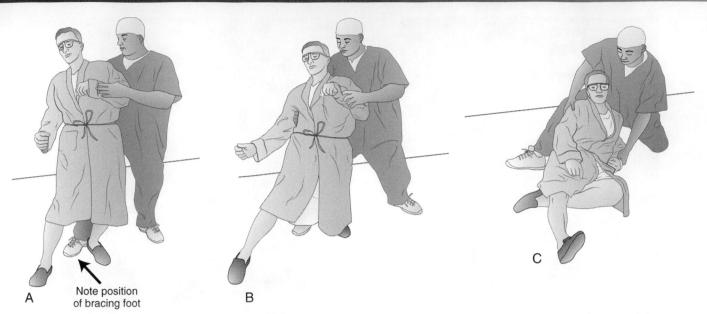

Figure 19-4 A to **C,** Preventing injury of a falling patient. *(Redrawn from Sorrentino SA: Mosby's textbook for nursing assistants, ed 7, St Louis, 2008, Mosby.)*

1. To assist the falling patient, *do not try to support the patient's weight.* Instead, ease the patient to the floor while protecting the person's head (Figure 19-4). Spread your feet to create a wide base of support. Bend your knees and use your thigh muscles for support.
2. Follow the patient's movements with your own body to prevent the patient from dropping.
3. Immediately call out for assistance while remaining with the patient.
4. Do not abandon the patient under any circumstances.

Guidelines for Assisting an Ambulatory Patient

1. Position yourself slightly behind the patient's shoulder while helping the person walk. This places you in a position to support the patient if the individual becomes weak or begins to fall. If the patient seems unsteady, use a wheelchair.
2. Allow the patient time to maneuver. Do not rush. Point out or otherwise orient the patient to where he or she is going, rather than simply guiding him or her to the location.

TRANSPORTING PATIENTS

USING A GURNEY

Use the following guidelines when transporting a patient by gurney:

1. Using a gurney requires some practice. In most systems, the wheels steer from the back, not the front, which means you must make sure the foot of the gurney leads in the direction of travel; otherwise the gurney will not go in the direction you are steering. Look toward the direction you want to travel, and this will help in steering.
2. IV bags and bottles must be suspended from an IV stand positioned at the patient's feet, not the head. Although most

IV solutions are contained in soft plastic bags, it is still important to adhere to this rule.
3. Patients who are on cardiac monitoring devices and are being moved from an intensive care unit (ICU) such as the postanesthesia care unit (PACU) must be accompanied by a registered nurse or anesthesia care provider. This meets normal standards for safety in an accredited health facility. Cardiac monitors are mounted at the foot of the patient gurney. Avoid placing a monitor between the patient's feet.
4. Oxygen and any other compressed gas cylinders are positioned underneath the gurney on a designated rack. No canisters are to be laid alongside the patient on the gurney mattress.
5. Try to anticipate obstructions, sudden hallway traffic, and corners. Use ceiling and mounted wall mirrors when approaching corners.
6. When rounding blind corners, be careful of oncoming traffic. Check first before proceeding. It is difficult to stop an occupied gurney, especially when the patient is heavy and medical devices are attached to the frame. If two people are available for transport, one person pushes from the head of the gurney and the other guides the gurney from the foot around difficult obstacles.
7. Be sure to remind the conscious patient to keep the hands and arms within the gurney rails. Anticipation prevents accidents. Gurney rails are not solid and do not protect the patient from injury. The patient can easily bruise or even fracture an elbow, fingers, or wrist on walls and doorways. Observe the patient during transport and remind him or her to keep the hands and arms well within the boundaries of the side rails.
8. Ramps, doors, and elevators must be negotiated carefully. Unless the patient is required to remain flat, raise the head of the gurney so that the patient can see where he or she is going.

9. Always warn the patient of bumps or other unfamiliar movements that will be encountered, such as entering or exiting an elevator.

Ramps

When rolling the gurney down a ramp, do not rely on your strength to hold the gurney against gravity. Ask for assistance. One person should stabilize the foot of the gurney while the second is at the head. Traveling up the ramp also requires two people—one to push, the other to pull.

Doors

When passing through manually operated doors, open the doors first and secure them open. *Do not use the foot of the gurney to open the doors. This is unacceptable patient care.*

Stand at the patient's head and push the gurney through the open doors or pull from the head of the gurney.

Elevators

1. Use the patient elevator. Do not transport the patient in an elevator full of visitors.
2. When the elevator doors open, lock the doors open.
3. Standing at the patient's head, pull the gurney headfirst into the elevator.
4. Do not unlock the doors until you are certain that the foot of the gurney has cleared the threshold.
5. Allow the doors to close.

EMERGENCY DURING TRANSPORT

Emergencies may occur during transport. The patient may suffer sudden hypotension, cardiac arrest, seizure, or another emergency during transport. The effects of moving the patient from bed to gurney can cause vascular or fluid shifts that may not manifest symptoms immediately.

If an emergency occurs during transport:

- Maintain verbal contact with the patient. If the person reports dizziness or light-headedness or if you suspect a problem, call for assistance from medical or nursing staff immediately.
- If you are in the corridor, request assistance from nursing or medical staff.
- If you are in an elevator, activate the emergency alarm system, which is clearly marked.

NOTE: Gurneys may be equipped with a back board used to place under the patient's thorax while performing CPR. Backboards are also located on crash carts.

LATERAL TRANSFERS

BED TO GURNEY

The patient with no physical restrictions can move from the bed to the gurney with limited assistance to ensure that any catheters or other medical devices in place are not dislodged and provide extra security. The patient with some mobility problems can be assisted with a draw sheet. The patient is transferred using the following procedure:

1. Before bringing the gurney into the patient's room, notify the unit clerk or nurse manager that you have arrived to transport the patient to surgery. Collect the patient's chart and any other documents required. Do this before entering the patient's room.
2. Knock on the patient's door or prepare the patient for your arrival before entering. Avoid simply entering the patient's room with the gurney and announcing that you are taking the individual to surgery.
3. After introducing yourself (family may be present), verify the patient's identity.
4. Arrange the furniture to make adequate space for the gurney. Patient rooms and cubicles often are very small. It is easier to make a path for the gurney before entering with it.
5. Lower the bed rails on the side where the gurney is located.
6. Align the gurney with the bed and lock the wheels on both the bed and the gurney. Under no circumstances should you move a patient to an unlocked gurney. Align the bed to the height of the gurney.
7. Identify and free up all tubing, drainage bags, or other devices that might restrain the patient or become dislodged during the transfer. Drainage collecting units (e.g., urinary or chest units) must remain lower than the patient's body at all times, and IV lines should be higher than the patient's body. Secure IV bags and other drainage units to the gurney.
8. Guide the patient slowly across the bed to the gurney. Prevent the bed sheets and other linens from entangling the patient. Maintain the top sheet to protect the patient from exposure. If the patient needs some help in moving across, a draw sheet or other lateral transfer device should be used (Figure 19-5).

MOVING A PATIENT USING A LATERAL TRANSFER DEVICE

A patient with limited mobility is transferred manually with a transfer board, draw sheet, slide sheet, air float, or other lateral transfer device to the gurney (Figure 19-6, *A* and *B*). This move may require four or more people. If the patient is unable to support his or her head, one person must guide the head and neck together, making sure that the cervical spine is in neutral position, with two people at each side of the patient and one at the feet.

1. Lower the bed rails on the gurney side.
2. Align the gurney with the bed and lock the wheels. Under no circumstances should a patient be moved to an unlocked gurney. Align the bed to the height of the gurney.
3. Make sure all tubing and medical devices have been freed.
4. Transfer medical equipment and devices first, and then transfer the patient.
5. If a draw sheet is used, roll the edges of the draw sheet toward the patient to provide a good grip and grasp the rolled edge firmly with both hands.
6. On the count of three, the patient is moved horizontally to the gurney in two stages. The first lift moves the patient to the edge of the bed. The person on the bed side may kneel on the bed and then proceed with a second lift to the

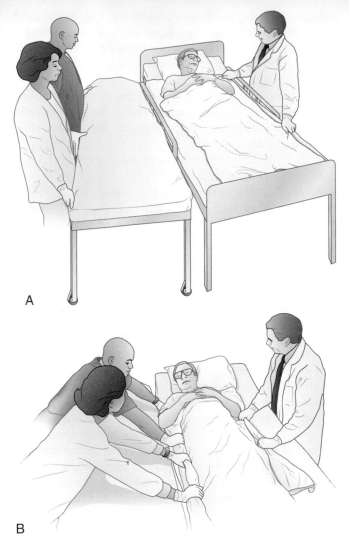

Figure 19-5 **A,** Aligning the bed with the gurney. **B,** Moving a conscious patient with a draw sheet. (**A** and **B** redrawn from Sorrentino SA: Mosby's textbook for nursing assistants, *ed 7, St Louis, 2008, Mosby.)*

gurney. If an air transport device is used, the move should be completed according to manufacturer's directions—usually in two moves.

7. Cover the patient and raise the side rails.

8. Place a pillow under the patient's head unless directed otherwise. Some patients must be transported flat.

9. Apply the safety strap midway between the knees and hips on top of the blanket or sheet. Allow two finger breadths between the strap and the patient. Do not place the safety strap over the patient's bare skin.

10. If the patient is cooperative, have him or her place the hands over the abdomen, with the elbows well inside the side rails. The patient's feet must not protrude over the edge of the gurney. Unlock the wheels and proceed to your destination.

11. Notify the charge nurse or other nursing staff that you are leaving the unit so this can be documented. (Never remove a patient from a ward without notifying a staff member.)

12. Proceed directly to your destination. If the patient is going to the operating room holding area, wait for the attending nurse to accept the patient before you leave. Do not leave the patient unattended at any time.

GURNEY TO OPERATING TABLE

The patient is transported to the operating room shortly before the start of the procedure. The circulator and anesthesia care provider should be present to receive the patient and assist in the transfer to the operating table. At least two and preferably three people should be present during the transfer of an alert patient. As the gurney is lined up next to the operating table, one person must stand on the opposite side to guide the patient and prevent a fall. The second person stands alongside the gurney to brace it against the operating table. A third person should stand at the head of the table. Make certain that the brakes on the gurney and the operating table are locked before beginning the transfer.

To transfer a conscious patient from a gurney to an operating table, follow these steps:

1. Align the head of the gurney with the head of the operating table. Lock the wheels of the gurney and the operating room table.

2. Free up IV lines and other tubing. Transfer medical equipment and devices first, and then transfer the patient.

3. Ask the patient to slide slowly onto the operating table, taking the top sheet along.

4. Open the back of the patient's gown to allow placement of cardiac leads or other monitoring devices.

5. Center the patient on the table and apply the safety strap immediately. Place the safety strap midway between the knees and hips on top of the blanket or sheet. Allow two finger breadths between the strap and the patient. Do not place the safety strap directly over the patient's bare skin. The patient should always remain secured on the operating table except during transfer.

TRANSFERRING THE PATIENT AFTER SURGERY

Following surgery, the patient is transferred from the operating table to a gurney for transport to the PACU or in some cases, to the ICU. An assisted transfer device is often used to move the postoperative patient. The anesthesia care provider directs the move.

If the patient has had a general anesthetic, he or she will remain in the operating room until extubation. After the anesthesia is withdrawn (halted), the patient is given oxygen and any reversal medications needed. Patient transfer to the gurney for transport to the PACU is not initiated until the patient is physiologically stable.

1. When it is safe to move the patient, the gurney is brought into the surgical suite. The circulator stands by to assist in the transfer. Before moving the patient to the gurney, all IV lines, drains, catheters, and any other devices attached to the patient are freed up, and the gurney is locked in place next to the operating table.

2. The patient safety strap is released. The IV, drainage bags, and any other devices are moved to the gurney. The patient transfer device is put in place and the patient is shifted to the gurney. The anesthesiologist and circulator then transport the patient immediately to the PACU.

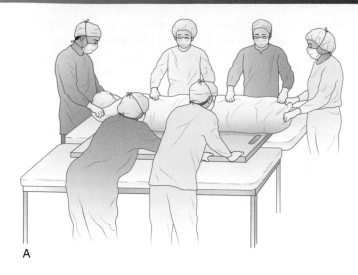

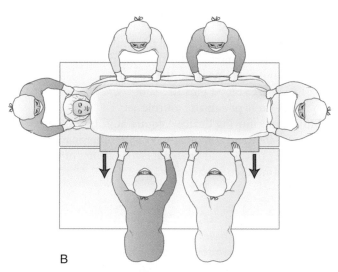

Figure 19-6 **A,** Log rolling the patient to slide the transfer board into position. **B,** Pulling the transfer board and patient in one or two coordinated moves.

3. If the patient is to be transferred immediately to the ICU, an ICU bed is used for transport. All cardiac and respiratory monitoring devices will be shifted from the anesthesia machine to a portable monitor next to the ICU bed. Normally a patient is not transferred until they are breathing without the need for a ventilator. However, if a ventilator is needed during transport, an additional person is needed to manage the equipment.

SPECIAL PATIENT POPULATIONS

PEDIATRIC PATIENTS

Children are transported to the operating room by gurney, crib, or bassinet. In some health care facilities, a small child's wagon is used to reduce the patient's fear of going to surgery. It is important to reduce anxiety in the preoperative period because in addition to the emotional effects of distress, a fearful, highly anxious child may experience difficulty during induction and emergence from anesthesia. For this reason,

health care facilities allow caregivers to accompany the child to the holding area, and in many hospitals a parent or other caregiver is permitted to stay in the operating suite during induction of anesthesia.

If the child is unaccompanied by a family member, the separation can be quite stressful. Most young children, especially toddlers and preschoolers, suffer extreme anxiety when separated from their caregivers.

- Talk with the child during transport and explain the environment in simple, nonthreatening terms. Remember that children understand the meanings of words in their most literal sense. The child's developmental age is critical to communication. Children from 5 to 9 years old are curious about their environment. Preteens want to take part in their care. Teenagers are likely to seem unconcerned but appreciate explanations of the environment.

- Do not treat the child like a small adult. Provide a calm, supportive presence, showing respect for the child at all times. Children are quick to understand when they are being falsely reassured. Instead of saying, "Oh, don't be afraid; this won't take long," evaluate the child's understanding of what is happening and try to clarify his or her perception in simple, concrete terms. Distraction may also be effective in allaying anxiety.

Cribs must always be equipped with a Plexiglas cover during transportation. Toddlers can climb and move with amazing speed and agility. Even a crib cover may not prevent a small toddler from attempting to climb between the top rail of the side bars and the crib cover. Crib bars can also be a source of danger, especially in health care institutions with older facilities. In recent years, regulations for cribs have become much more stringent. Problems with cribs arise from the width of the bars and from crib bumpers (pads). Deaths from bumpers have occurred in three ways:

- The child becomes wedged against the crib bumper and is strangled by the ties that attach it to the crib frame.

- The child becomes wedged between the crib bumper and the mattress and suffocates.

- The child climbs over the rail and falls to the floor or becomes entrapped by crib bars during the fall and fractures a limb.

The safest way to prevent these kinds of accidents is by never leaving the patient alone (abandonment). This cannot be stressed enough.

HEARING- OR SIGHT-IMPAIRED PATIENTS

Transporting the patient with a hearing or sight deficit may require more time and supportive personnel to help the patient understand the procedure. Patients with profound deafness should have an interpreter present to explain the process of transport to the operating room and the transfer to the operating table. Sight-impaired patients may be able to communicate verbally. However, if hearing is also impaired, an interpreter may be necessary. It is important for the patient to understand each part of any moving and handling procedure. This can be by visual or verbal cues, whichever is appropriate to the patient.

Guidelines for Caring for the Patient with a Hearing Deficit

- Allow patients to keep their hearing aids as long as possible.
- Use hand gestures to communicate.
- You may have to increase the volume of speech. Speak slowly.
- Articulate your words when speaking to the patient.
- Face the patient during communication.

Guidelines for Moving the Sight-Impaired Patient

- Allow the patient to keep glasses as long as possible.
- Provide verbal orientation before attempting any move.
- Explain the environment to the patient and remain in contact.
- Provide increased assistance during moves; the sight-impaired patient may also have problems with depth perception. Be aware of safety implications.

The lateral transfer may be frightening to patients with sensory deficit if performed too quickly or without warning. Make every attempt to communicate comfort to the patient before making any moves. During transport, and depending on the patient's needs and wishes, it is possible to maintain contact with the patient by touching his or her shoulder or hand periodically. Provide a full handover to the holding area staff on arrival in the operating room so that they understand the extent of the patient's deficit.

BARIATRIC PATIENTS

Obesity is defined by body mass index (BMI). Weight categories are shown in Box 19-1. The prevalence of obesity in the U.S. population and worldwide has caused a corresponding rise in surgery of obese persons. Many specialty health care institutions and surgical centers are trained and equipped to care for the needs of bariatric patients. Moving and handling the obese patient requires training, knowledge of the specific patient, and team planning. The objectives of these are not only to prevent patient and staff injury, but also to provide dignity and emotional support during patient care.

Care of the obese patient in surgery is complicated by comorbid conditions such as diabetes, heart disease, and airway obstruction and airway exchange problems. The lungs do not increase in size as the patient becomes heavier; therefore, the patient may have a "resting" hypoxia and hypercapnia. This is because pressure from the abdominal and chest wall restricts full lung expansion, resulting in poor ventilation. Obese patients also have a high incidence of pulmonary hypertension resulting in heart failure. Inability to move blood to all parts of the body results in poor peripheral circulation. Airway maintenance is a major challenge in the surgical setting because the obese patient has little neck flexibility and the usual landmarks for intubation are obscured by fatty tissue pushing inward on the neck structures. The obese patient is at high risk for deep vein thrombosis (DVT) because of circulatory stasis. All obese patients are fitted with a sequential compression device (SCD) to assist in venous return. Some of the primary challenges faced in the movement and handling of obese patients are practical. That is, patient conveyances, beds, elevators, and lifting equipment must all be capable of handling extreme weight and size.

Equipment needed for the obese patient includes:

- Bariatric patient gurney
- Bariatric operating table and accessories for surgical positioning
- Extra weight-bearing wheelchairs that are capable of tilting the patient to an upright standing position for transfer or ambulation
- Bariatric patient beds
- Slide sheets that reduce the friction between the patient and bed sheets, for adjusting the patient's position in bed, and for moving up the bed
- Extra-large blood pressure cuff
- Extra-large pneumatic tourniquet

Lifting and moving devices require staff training in order to be used safely and confidently. As with other manufactured devices, the protocol and procedures for safe use of the equipment vary among manufacturers.

PATIENTS IN POLICE CUSTODY

Health care facilities have a duty to cooperate with law enforcement agents and also provide appropriate care for patients in custody. Patients who are in police custody while in the health care facility are accompanied by one or two officers at all times. Unless the patient is a minor, the patient may be fitted with restraint devices (hand or leg cuffs). Law officers are responsible for protecting the patient from self-harm and harming others.

Communication between law officers and operating room personnel should follow the same protocol as for other staff on duty in the patient care area. Staff on the inpatient ward, emergency room, or other patient holding areas should be notified ahead of time that the patient will be transported to surgery. On arrival in the unit or room, introduce yourself to the custodial officers and patient and explain the procedure for transporting the patient (noting the need to check identity). The custodial police should cooperate with medical procedures, and health staff has a duty to comply with police procedures. If the patient is in physical restraints, you may expect the restraints to be maintained during transport to the operating room. Most police officers are cooperative. However, they are also required to perform their duties according to strict law enforcement protocol.

Box **19-1** Body Mass Index	
Weight Category	**BMI (kg/m²)**
Underweight	<18.5
Normal	18.5-24.9
Overweight	25-29.9
Mild obesity	27-30
Obese	>30

Data from Centers for Disease Control and Prevention.

Watch Section 3: Unit 2: Patient Transfer on the Evolve website. http://evolve.elsevier.com/fuller/surgical

SECTION II: POSITIONING THE SURGICAL PATIENT

The surgical patient is positioned on the operating table for a specific surgical procedure:

- To allow optimum access to the operative site
- To reduce adverse physiological effects and prevent injury during surgery
- To permit optimum access for anesthesia care (includes access to venous and arterial sites, airway, and monitoring sites)

The following elements are important in the safe positioning of patients:

- *Knowledge of anatomy, physiology, and the individual patient's specific medical condition.* Positioning is not a regimented routine. Each patient is unique and has specific considerations, such as age, joint mobility, and disease. Because of the high risk of serious and permanent injury, the surgical team must be guided and directed in the positioning process. The anesthesia care provider, surgeon, and circulator draw this direction from their knowledge of the patient's status.
- *Planning.* Planning promotes an organized and efficient effort by everyone involved. All necessary equipment must be assembled ahead of time. Pads, positioning devices, table accessories, and transfer devices must be on hand before positioning begins. Bariatric table extensions or special tables must be on hand before the patient arrives in the surgical suite. Adequate personnel must be available to complete the task safely.
- *Teamwork.* Teamwork is needed to create smooth, step-by-step coordination. Coordinated activities complement each other.

DUTIES OF THE SURGICAL TECHNOLOGIST

Surgical technologists have specific responsibilities during patient positioning:

- Understand common positions and the surgeries for which these positions are used
- Know ahead of time the position that will be used for each assigned surgical procedure
- Proactively prevent accident and injury during positioning
- Question any aspect of the patient's position that appears to have risk potential
- Remain alert and focused on patient safety
- Communicate clearly with other members of the team

GENERAL OPERATING TABLE

The general operating table is used for most surgical procedures (Figure 19-7, *A*). It can be configured into many positions and accommodates accessories for different types of surgery (Figure 19-7, *B* to *E*). The frame is stainless steel and attaches to a hydraulic lift. Weight restrictions for operating tables vary, and it is important to verify the table specifications *before* transfer and positioning. Some bariatric tables have an overall weight capacity of 1,200 pounds. The weight capacity of the table articulations must also be strong enough to safely accommodate the obese patient.

Table pads are covered with washable material. The pads are removable for cleaning. The top of the table can be rotated, flexed, tilted, or disassembled. Most table tops are radiolucent to allow intraoperative x-rays. A handheld remote control unit is used to operate the hydraulic components to change the angle and height. Normally, the anesthesia care provider manages the control unit. The headboard and footboard can be flexed or removed. The base is centered on the frame or may be offset to accommodate radiographic and C-arm fluoroscopy equipment. A perineal cutout allows unrestricted access when the patient is in the lithotomy position.

ATTACHMENTS AND ACCESSORIES: PADDING, WEDGES, ROLLS, AND LIFTS

Table accessories include different types of gel or foam pads, used to protect certain vulnerable areas of the body or to maintain the patient's position. Pads are usually made of gel, "bean bag" material, or dense foam to withstand day-to-day use in surgery. Pads of various shapes have different names with which the student will become quickly familiar. Cylindrical pads are used in the axillary region and also under the thorax. Head "doughnuts" are used to stabilize the patient's head for administration of anesthesia. Other pads are used to cradle the legs, feet, and arms. Wedges are used to tilt the patient from the side or for isolated areas of the body that require slight elevation.

The arm board is used to extend the arms away from the body at an angle less than 90 degrees (Figure 19-8, *A*). This provides access to IV and monitoring sites. The arm is secured by means of a padded strap, padded brace, or cradle. Professional safety organizations recommend that the arms should not be tucked at the patient's sides, because this can increase the risk of compartment syndrome. However, if this arm position must be used, take care that the arm is not constricted by a draw sheet or other device that holds the arm in place. It must be secure, but not tight (Figure 19-8, *B*).

Shoulder braces are *used only rarely and with extreme caution.* These are fixed to the head of the table to prevent the patient from sliding downward when he or she is in the extreme Trendelenburg position. Injury to the brachial plexus can be severe with improperly placed or poorly designed shoulder braces.

Abduction pads are used to separate the legs following hip fracture to maintain external rotation and minimize further trauma and pain.

Stirrups are used to elevate and abduct the legs for access to the perineal area in the lithotomy position. The type of stirrups used depends on the type of procedure and the patient's physiological tolerance for the position (see the section on the lithotomy position). Figure 19-9 shows two types of low lithotomy stirrups used for endoscopic, gynecological, genitourinary, and obstetrical procedures.

The headrest is attached to the operating table and stabilizes the head and neck during a craniotomy or when the

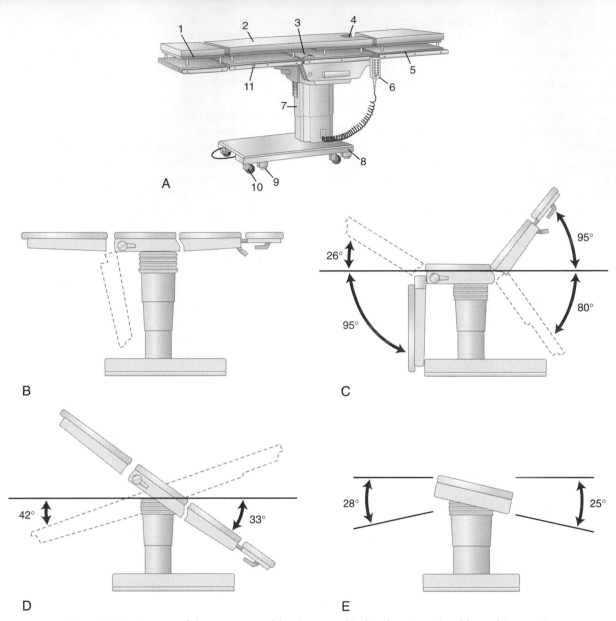

Figure 19-7 **A,** Parts of the operating table: *1,* removable head section; *2,* table pad (mattress); *3,* kidney lift; *4,* perineal cutout; *5,* radiolucent top and removable head section; *6,* hand control unit; *7,* hydraulic lift cylinder; *8,* table base; *9,* floor locks; *10,* locking swivel casters; *11,* side rail locking system. **B** to **E,** Positions of the operating table. *(Modified from Martin JT, Warner MA: Positioning in anesthesia and surgery, ed 3, Philadelphia, 1997, WB Saunders.)*

patient is in the Fowler (sitting) position. The horseshoe rest is a padded, U-shaped attachment that supports the forehead when the patient is in the prone position. Other attachments, such as the Gardner and Mayfield headrests, penetrate the skull with sterile pins and hold the head in precise position (see the section on the prone position).

The chest or back brace is an elevated pad or frame that lifts the thorax while flexing the spine to widen the intervertebral spaces. It is used when the patient is in the prone position to create access to the spine and back. Several types of patient braces have been designed to overcome the many risks of prone positioning. Most frames have two raised lateral pieces attached to a base that rests on the operating table. Other styles have lateral crosspieces that extend at right angles to the long axis of the body. The **footboard** attaches at a right

angle to the foot of the operating table. It prevents the patient from sliding downward when the table is tilted into a foot-down (reverse Trendelenburg) position.

Watch Section 3: Unit 1: The Operating Table on the Evolve website. http://evolve.elsevier.com/fuller/surgical

PREVENTING PATIENT INJURY DURING POSITIONING

PRINCIPLES OF SAFE POSITIONING

Positioning injuries usually are the result of pressure on neurovascular structures or moves made too quickly. These injuries are related to the failure of a mechanical accessory,

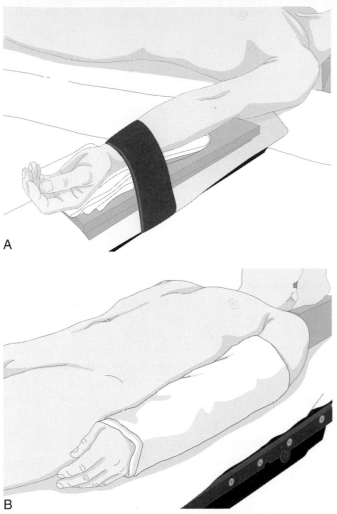

Figure 19-8 **Position of the patient's arm in supine position. A,** Position of the arm in supine position with abduction less than 90 degrees. Note that the arm is supinated and the elbow is adequately padded to prevent ulnar nerve damage. **B,** The arm at the patient's side loosely held within the draw sheet. *(From Miller R, Ericksson L, Fleisher L, et al: Miller's anesthesia, ed 7, Philadelphia, 2007, Churchill Livingstone.)*

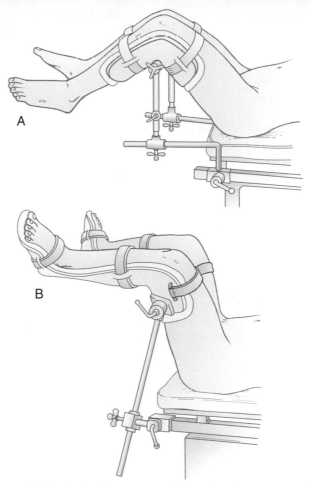

Figure 19-9 **A,** Crutch stirrups used in urology for access to the perineum. **B,** Multipurpose stirrups. *(Modified from Phillips N: Berry and Kohn's operating room technique, ed 11, St Louis, 2007, Mosby.)*

inattention to detail, haste in meeting the demands of a full (or unreasonable) schedule, and lack of adequate help. Injury awareness is the first step in prevention. Surgical technologists need specific knowledge about anatomy, range of motion, risks of pulmonary compromise, and effects of intravascular fluid shifts. Positioning is not a "cookbook" process. Although each position requires the body to assume a certain posture, the positioning team must have specific information about the patient's individual needs and medical conditions. The following guidelines apply to all positioning procedures:

- All equipment needed for positioning must be assembled and prepared for use before the patient is brought into the room.
- Adequate personnel must be available to assist before positioning begins. Do not risk the patient's safety because of a crowded surgical schedule.
- Before positioning begins, all team members should be familiar with the position and each person must understand his or her role in positioning.

- The patient should not be moved except on the instructions of the person directing the move. Everyone must be aware of the motion direction, movement process, and resting point of the body. Positioning is a collaborative task. Although everyone involved is responsible for the patient's safety, one person—usually the surgeon, anesthesia care provider, or surgical assistant—guides and directs the others. This ensures that movements are coordinated, which reduces injury to both the patient and team members. In general, the anesthesia care provider must give permission before any change is made in a patient's position because these can cause physiological alterations such as a drop in blood pressure.
- Always check equipment before using it. Tighten the locking devices of all weight-bearing accessories.
- Make sure the table is locked securely in position and do not assume that any accessory equipment is in working order.
- Move slowly when positioning the patient.
- Always move the body within its normal range of motion. This requires knowledge of joint types and anatomy.
- When positioning an unconscious, sedated, or weak patient, make certain that you have complete control of the part you are moving before you begin.

- Before moving the patient, make sure all tubing, leads, and other medical devices are untangled. Move devices first, then the patient.

CONDITIONS THAT INCREASE THE RISK OF INJURY

Physical examinations by the anesthesia care provider and physician can reveal preexisting conditions that predispose a patient for injury related to positioning. The anesthesiologist and surgeon, who have previously assessed the patient medically, usually guide the team during positioning based on their knowledge of the specific patient. Box 19-2 describes physical conditions that increase the risk of injury related to positioning.

Normal Range of Motion

The joints of the human body allow a specific type of movement, or **range of motion.** For example, the elbow joint is hinged; that is, it can move freely in only one direction. Its movement is described by the angle created by the upper and lower arm. The movement of this joint is called *extension* or *flexion.* As the elbow flexes, the angle becomes smaller. Extension results in a larger angle between the forearm and upper arm. Some joints, such as the ball-and-socket joint in the hip, allow rotation of a body part inward and outward. Such inward and outward rotation is called *internal* and *external rotation.*

During patient movement and handling, it is critical not to exceed the limits of a joint. Most joint movements are described in degrees of movement. For example, in the positioning of the patient's arm on an arm board, it is critical to restrict **abduction** to less than 90 degrees. This means that the angle

between the side of the patient's body and the arm is less than 90 degrees.

Nerve and Vascular Injury

Nerves are injured when they lose their blood supply, are stretched, or are compressed. Under general anesthesia, central nervous system depressants and muscle relaxants are administered, and muscles lose their normal tone. This allows the joints to assume exaggerated positions that the patient normally would not be able to tolerate. **Hyperextension** (greater than normal extension) and **hyperflexion** (greater than normal flexion) can result in a nerve injury called a **traction injury** (or stretching injury).

Continuous pressure on the nerve or its blood supply can cause **necrosis** (tissue death) within 2 hours. Nerve damage can result in loss of mobility or sensation.

Compression of vessels restricts the blood supply to the tissue, a condition called **ischemia.** Loss of oxygen to the tissue causes necrosis. Pressure injuries may not be readily apparent, because underlying tissues, such as muscle and fascia, are more susceptible to damage than skin (Box 19-3). Ischemia is time- and weight-related. To prevent ischemia and necrosis, all bony prominences and **dependent areas of the body** (areas of the body under gravitational force) must be adequately padded and the weight distributed over a large area.

LOCATIONS OF COMMON NERVE AND VESSEL INJURIES

Nerve and vessel injuries often occur at the following locations:

- The ulnar nerve where it passes through the condylar groove of the elbow. Here the nerve is covered only by skin

---

Box **19-2**	**Patient Conditions that Influence Positioning**

- Preexisting nerve compression syndrome
- Neuropathy (nerve disorder)
- Diabetes mellitus
- Osteoarthritis (progressive arthritic disease)
- Venous stasis (pooling of blood as a result of inactivity or cardiovascular disease)
- Preexisting decubitus ulcer (pressure sore)
- Previous traumatic injury
- Alcohol abuse
- Vitamin deficiencies
- Malnutrition
- Renal disease
- Hypothyroidism
- Previous joint fractures
- Rheumatoid arthritis
- Corticosteroid use
- Contractures (scar tissue that restricts joint movement)
- Poor skin turgor (lack of skin and tissue firmness)
- Peripheral edema (intracellular fluid swelling in the legs and arms)
- Reduced range of motion
- Weakness in the extremities

Modified from Martin JT, Warner MA: *Positioning in anesthesia and surgery,* ed 3, Philadelphia, 1997, WB Saunders.

Box **19-3**	**Classification of Pressure Damage and Stages of Pressure Ulcers**

The National Pressure Ulcer Advisory Panel has developed a ranking system for evaluating the extent of damage caused by pressure. Pressure damage is a risk for surgical patients and for bed-bound, debilitated, and older patients.

Stage I: Nonblanchable erythema of intact skin, the heralding lesion of skin ulceration. NOTE: Reactive hyperemia normally can be expected for one half to three fourths as long as the time that pressure occludes blood flow to the area.

Stage II: Partial-thickness skin loss involving the epidermis and/or dermis. A superficial ulcer evolves and develops clinically as an abrasion, a blister, or a shallow crater.

Stage III: Full-thickness skin loss, involving damage to or necrosis of subcutaneous tissue, that may extend down to but not through underlying fascia. The ulcer presents clinically as a deep crater with or without undermining of adjacent tissue.

Stage IV: Full-thickness skin loss with extensive destruction, tissue necrosis, or damage to muscle, bone, or supporting structures (e.g., the tendon of a joint capsule). NOTE: Undermining and sinus tracts also may be associated with stage IV pressure ulcers.

Modified from Martin JT, Warner MA: *Positioning in anesthesia and surgery,* ed 3, Philadelphia, 1997, WB Saunders.

and subcutaneous fat. There is risk of compression (pressure) injury when the elbow is tightly flexed or when the nerve is under direct pressure from the edge of the operating table.

- The ulnar nerve is exposed where it passes through the condylar groove and at the cubital tunnel. Injury in this area is the second most common cause of postoperative **neuropathy** (temporary or permanent nerve injury).
- The common peroneal and tibial nerves and vessels where they pass through the popliteal fossa at the back of the knee are common sites of injury.
- The brachial plexus is a complex anatomical area where the branches of nerve roots from C5 to T1 or T2 merge (Figure 19-10). It is vulnerable to injury because the nerves and blood vessels lie close to bony structures and are subject to direct compression. Injury in this area can be caused by shoulder braces and inappropriate placement of an axillary roll.
- The lumbosacral nerve roots at the base of the spine bear much of the weight of the torso and can be injured by continuous compression with inadequate padding.

PREVENTION OF COMPRESSION INJURY The following guidelines can help prevent **compression injury:**

- Padding can distribute weight over a larger surface area, or it can impinge on a vulnerable space. Make sure that in preventing one type of injury, you do not cause another. In general, bed pillows, sheets, blankets, and other linens should *not* be used for padding during surgery. Uneven folds in the outer covering may cause skin or compression injury, especially in older or debilitated patients. Axillary rolls must *never be placed in the axilla*, because this increases pressure on the axillary nerve and vessels. The axillary roll actually is positioned slightly inferior to the axilla when the patient is in the lateral position (Figure 19-11).
- Pressure on the "downside" shoulder of a patient in the lateral position is alleviated by shifting the upper arm and

shoulder slightly forward (also referred to as "pulling the shoulder through") and placing a foam or gel pad under the flank area. This prevents retroclavicular compression and nerve injury (Figure 19-12).

- Arm abduction must be limited to less than 90 degrees or less than the angle the patient can tolerate awake.
- Keep the cervical spine and head in neutral position at all times during positioning to prevent injury and protect the airway.

Shear Injury and Pressure Ulcers

Shear injury occurs when two parallel tissue planes are forced in opposite directions. The most common cause of shear injury is sliding the patient over a high-friction surface such as a bed sheet. Shearing is associated with extreme Trendelenburg and reverse Trendelenburg positions when the table is tilted head-down or feet-down and the patient slides slightly during the change of position. Shearing can result in tissue damage that may not be noticeable at the time of the injury but may easily progress to a pressure ulcer later.

Pressure ulcers are the result of continuous pressure over an area of the body. Tissue injury occurs because unrelieved compression impedes blood flow in the capillaries of the skin and deeper tissues, causing tissue necrosis and sloughing. Without skin protection, deep tissues can easily become infected. A pressure injury may begin to develop even after a short period of continuous compression and become deeper with subsequent pressure. Without capillary supply, the tissue can become infected and can become resistant to healing. In extreme cases, skin grafts are required to close the defect. Pressure ulcers are classified by stage, and they progress rapidly from mild to severe.

Continuous compression or extreme flexion can result in vessel compression and severe swelling within a muscle compartment. This is called **compartment syndrome.** In this situation, blood cannot return to the heart but pools in the extremity. As the surrounding tissues become more and more

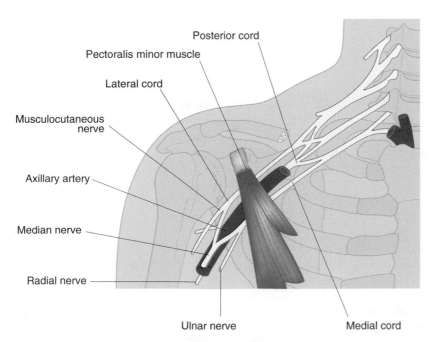

Figure 19-10 Brachial plexus. *(From Jacob S: Atlas of human anatomy, St Louis, 2002, Churchill Livingstone.)*

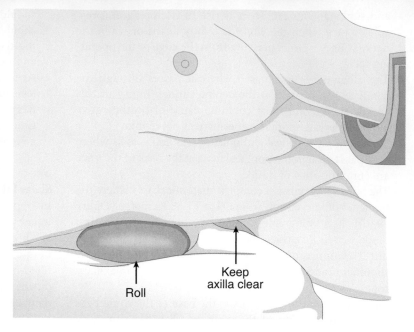

Figure 19-11 Preventing injury to the brachial plexus. The appropriate placement of a roll is inferior to the axilla, not at the axillary space. *(From Miller R, Eriksson L, Fleisher L, et al: Miller's anesthesia, ed 7, Philadelphia, 2009, Churchill Livingstone.)*

Roll

Keep axilla clear

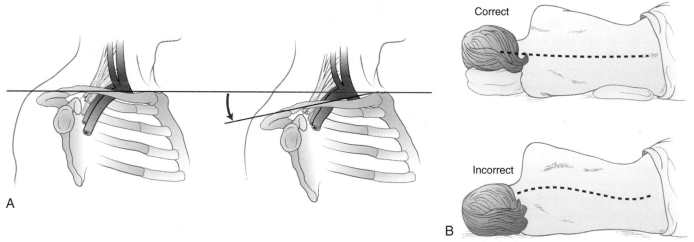

A

B

Correct

Incorrect

Figure 19-12 **A,** Potential injury to the retroclavicular space related to compression of the clavicle. **B,** Note the position of the padding to level the spine and prevent compression of the clavicle. *(**A** redrawn from Martin JT, Warner MA: Positioning in anesthesia and surgery, ed 3, Philadelphia, 1997, WB Saunders; **B** redrawn from Phillips N: Berry and Kohn's operating room technique, ed 11, St Louis, 2007, Mosby.)*

swollen, the risk arises of complete loss of blood supply to the whole limb and even distant organs. Treatment of compartment syndrome requires an emergency procedure called a fasciotomy to relieve the pressure on deep tissues. **Fasciotomy** involves making long incisions into the fascia and muscle to relieve pressure.

Skeletal Injury

Skeletal injury can occur during positioning when a joint is manipulated or forced beyond its normal range. Sudden dislocation can occur when the limb of a sedated or anesthetized patient is allowed to drop over the table edge. This can happen when positioning is hurried or too few personnel are available to maintain safety during positioning. Safe joint manipulation

requires a knowledge of the joint capacity, including its type and range of motion, and specific knowledge of the patient's condition. To avoid exceeding normal ranges of motion, one must know what those ranges are. Avoid skeletal injury by referring to the range-of-motion illustrations shown in Figure 19-13. Remember that the unconscious body can be manipulated into positions that would not be tolerable to a conscious patient and this must be avoided.

Embolism

A **thromboembolus** is a blood clot that circulates in the vascular system and lodges in a vessel, causing obstruction or occlusion. Circulating blood normally does not form clots. When blood is allowed to slow or pool, however, as can occur

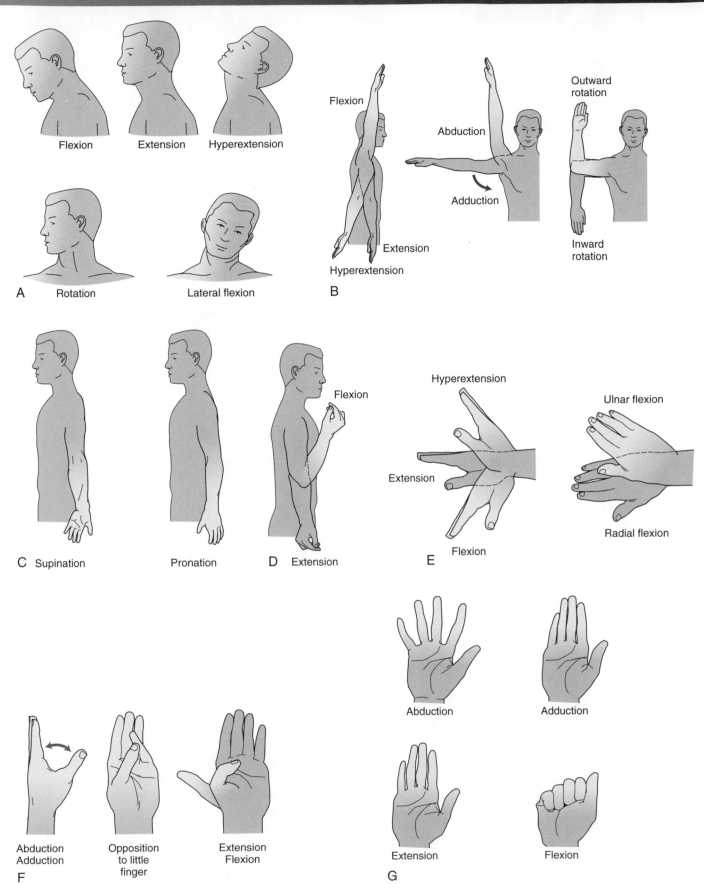

Figure 19-13   Normal range of motion. A, Neck. B, Shoulder. C, Elbow. D, Forearm. E, Wrist. F, Thumb. G, Fingers.

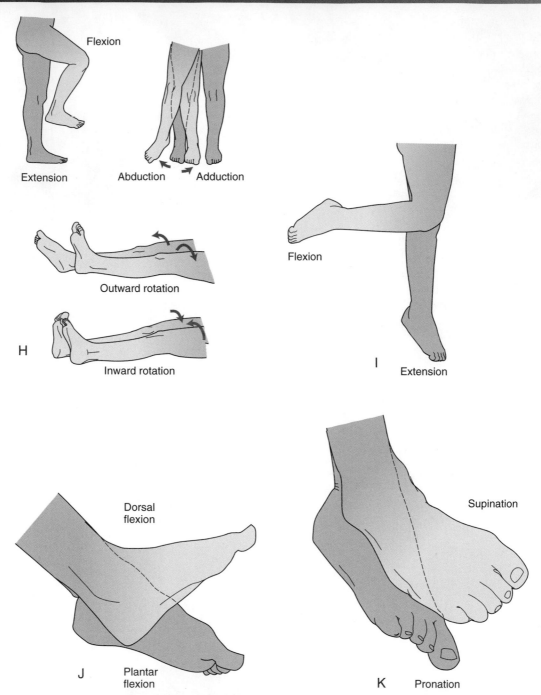

Figure 19-13, cont'd H, Hip. I, Knee. J, Ankle. K, Foot. *(From Sorrentino SA: Mosby's textbook for nursing assistants, ed 7, St Louis, 2008, Mosby.)*

during surgery, clots form in the lower extremities and migrate through the systemic circulation. A circulating thrombus (embolus) can lodge anywhere in the body. When it blocks blood supply to the lungs, brain, or heart, these vital tissues are deprived of oxygen and the tissue dies.

Embolism is a surgical risk, especially in the obese patient; in a patient with any circulatory disease that interferes with normal circulation; or in surgery in which large blood vessels are entered or exposed. Antiembolism stockings or a sequential compression device (SCD) is placed on patients' legs before long procedures or on patients predisposed to clot formation such as obese patients or those with vascular disease.

The SCD wraps around the leg, sequentially fills with air, and then deflates. During the inflation phase, the cuffs push venous blood toward the heart, and during deflation, the vessels refill. This reduces the risk of blood pooling (stasis) and thrombus formation.

Respiratory Compromise

Positioning can affect the patient's **ventilation** (ability to fill the lungs with air). Patients in the prone position and steep Trendelenburg position are particularly vulnerable to ventilation problems. Both gravity and the position of the chest wall can determine the amount of gas that enters the lungs.

Therefore, mechanical ventilation is used in these positions. Different types of open braces have been developed to raise the thorax from the operating table in prone position (see the section on the prone position). This increases ventilator capacity by relieving pressure on the chest wall.

Falls

Falls from the operating table are rare, but they do occur. Falls can result in major fractures and serious injury to the head and soft tissue. To prevent a patient fall, study and follow these guidelines:

- Never leave a patient unattended, not for any reason or any length of time.
- When transferring the patient between the gurney and the operating table, lock both the table and the gurney firmly in place. Never use a gurney that has a faulty locking system.
- Make sure that at least one person is standing at the receiving side of the operating table or gurney to prevent the patient from moving too far over the edge.
- Do not position or move the patient without adequate help. Administrative support may be necessary to establish strict safety standards.
- Do not rush while moving an unconscious patient. Likewise, allow a conscious patient to move slowly during any move from one surface to another.

- As soon as the patient has moved to the operating table, secure the safety strap midway between the knees and hips (as described earlier). Do not rely on the safety strap to hold the patient on the table. The strap is there as a precaution against movement, not to prevent a fall.
- Position a morbidly obese patient on a bariatric surgical table. Know the limits of the standard surgical table. A very heavy patient can tilt the tabletop to one side, which may cause the patient to roll off the side of the operating table.

POSITIONING THE PREGNANT PATIENT

When positioning the pregnant patient for transport on a gurney or on the operating table, a wedge pad is inserted under the right flank. This tilts the body to the left and prevents uterine compression on the vena cava and aorta, which can cause hypotension and compromise fetal circulation.

SURGICAL POSITIONS

SUPINE POSITION

The *supine position*, or dorsal recumbent position, is used for procedures of the abdomen, pelvis, thorax, and face and in orthopedic and vascular surgery (Figure 19-14). The patient is positioned with the head and spine in alignment. Arms

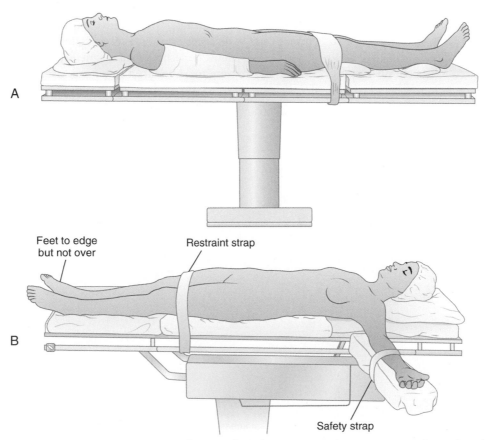

Figure 19-14 A, Supine position without arm board extension. **B,** Supine position with arm board extension. (**A** *redrawn from Phillips N: Berry and Kohn's operating room technique, ed 11, St Louis, 2007, Mosby;* **B** *from original artwork by Sandra McMahon.)*

should be placed on arm boards. The patient's feet must not extend over the edge of the table, and the legs must not be crossed one over the other.

The patient's weight is distributed over the occipital bone, back, sacrum, heels, and posterior legs. Patients with spinal or pelvic malformation or total joint prostheses may require padding to support irregular curvatures and prevent hyperextension. A foam or gel pad is used to support the head. The safety strap is placed midway between the knees and thighs.

Safety Precautions

1. Keep the cervical spine and head in neutral alignment.
2. Protect the ulnar nerve area.
3. Protect the brachial plexus. Arm boards must not be abducted more than 90 degrees.
4. Prevent decubitus ulcer formation at the lumbosacral area in older or debilitated patients.
5. Protect the popliteal fossa from impingement. Do not place pillows directly under the knee joint. Use gel pads placed proximal to the popliteal fossa under supervision of the anesthesiologist and surgeon.
6. Separate the patient's feet so that they do not touch each other. Padding under the heels or foam boots may be advised.
7. Do not use knee crutches (leg holders) that focus pressure in one area during surgery. Only approved leg holders intended for orthopedic surgery should be used. Some leg holders are only meant to be used during skin prep and draping, not for extended use. Maintain SCD or antiembolism stockings on the patient's legs to prevent an embolism.
9. Make sure the patient's legs are not crossed, because this puts pressure on the peroneal nerve and blood vessels of the posterior leg.

TRENDELENBURG POSITION

The **Trendelenburg position** is a variation of the supine position in which the operating table is tilted head down (Figure 19-15). This position permits greater access to the lower abdominal cavity and pelvic structures by allowing the abdominal organs to shift toward the head. The position is commonly used during lower gastrointestinal and pelvic surgery. It can cause hypertension, respiratory restriction, and increased intracranial pressure.

Safety Precautions

1. Distribute the weight of the elbow and upper arm evenly in the area of the ulnar nerve.
2. Protect the brachial plexus. Arm boards must not be abducted more than 90 degrees.
3. Prevent the Mayo stand tray from touching the patient's body. If the patient's position is altered in any way, always check the Mayo stand to make sure it is not touching the patient.
4. Anticipate the possible onset of hypertension during intraoperative positioning from level supine to Trendelenburg position. Surgery may be halted until the patient is stabilized.

REVERSE TRENDELENBURG POSITION

The **reverse Trendelenburg position,** or foot-down position (Figure 19-16), is used when the surgeon requires unobstructed access to the upper abdominal cavity and lower esophagus. When the operating table is tilted toward the patient's feet, gravity drops the viscera into the lower abdominal cavity, which allows a clear view of the diaphragm, cardiac sphincter, and esophagus.

During intraoperative positioning to the reverse Trendelenburg position, all instruments lying on the surgical field must be secured by a magnetic pad or pocket holders. Special care must be taken to ensure that endoscopes and all accessories are removed to prevent them from sliding to the floor. All tubing should be well secured at the beginning of surgery. The Mayo stand may be moved to accommodate the shift in the patient's position.

Safety Precautions

1. Follow all safety precautions applicable to the supine position.

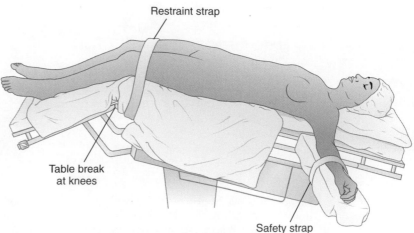

Figure 19-15 Trendelenburg position. *(From original artwork by Sandra McMahon.)*

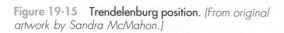

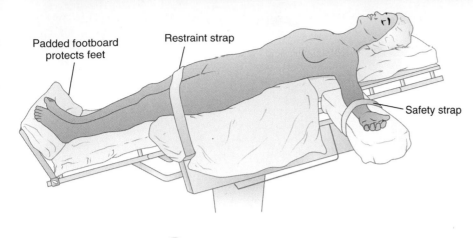

Padded footboard protects feet

Restraint strap

Safety strap

Figure 19-16 Reverse Trendelenburg position. *(From original artwork by Sandra McMahon.)*

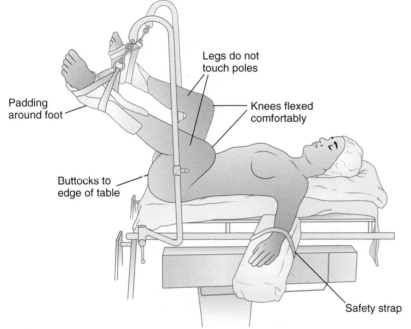

Legs do not touch poles

Padding around foot

Knees flexed comfortably

Buttocks to edge of table

Safety strap

Figure 19-17 Lithotomy position using sling stirrups. *(From original artwork by Sandra McMahon.)*

2. Prevent the patient's body from sliding toward the floor, which can cause a shear injury. Use a footboard if necessary, but use soft padding or protective foam boots to prevent nerve and vascular compression.
3. Make sure that the weight of each leg is distributed over a wide area at the popliteal fossa if the patient will be placed in the reverse Trendelenburg–lithotomy position. Do not rely on padding alone to protect the patient from compartment syndrome or nerve or vessel damage.

LITHOTOMY POSITION

The *lithotomy position* is a variation of the supine position. The patient's thighs are abducted and both the knees and hips are flexed. A low lithotomy position is achieved with the legs resting on low padded leg holders. The high lithotomy position is used for gynecological and radical perineal procedures (Figure 19-17). Incorrectly implemented, the lithotomy position can cause severe tissue injury, hypotension, and embolism; therefore, it is critical that protocol be followed. Attention to pressure points is very important. Patients with limited range of motion in the hip, spine, or knee joints are at

particular risk. Respect the patient's dignity by placing a cover sheet over the perineum during positioning.

Safety Precautions

1. Before anesthesia induction, the patient receiving a general or anesthetic or block is positioned with the sacrum at the lower table break. The offside stirrup or leg brace is secured to the table. The remaining stirrup is attached after the patient is transferred to the operating table.
2. When the patient is unconscious and sufficiently relaxed, the anesthesia care provider alerts the team when it is safe to elevate the legs. The lower portion of the table is flexed downward or the end section is removed.
3. The patient's arms should be secured on arm boards. However, if it is medically necessary to place the arms at the patient's sides, care must be taken to ensure that the patient's fingers do not become entrapped in the hinged table break as the lower section is flexed or raised.
4. When the legs are placed in stirrups, the knees must be flexed first, keeping them in midline position; then the thighs are abducted. Raising both legs at the same time

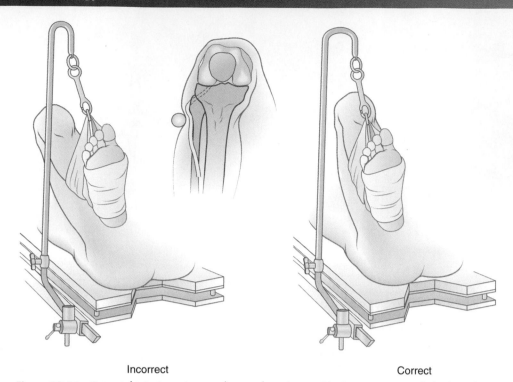

Incorrect   Correct

Figure 19-18 **Potential injuries using candy cane leg stirrups.** The leg must not touch the lateral part of the stirrup. Slings must be placed superior to the peroneal nerve. *(Redrawn from Martin JT, Warner MA: Positioning in anesthesia and surgery, ed 3, Philadelphia, 1997, WB Saunders.)*

keeps the body in alignment and prevents twisting of the lumbar spine.

5. If the angle of hip flexion is severe, the femoral vessels may be compressed, reducing blood supply to the lower legs.

6. Sudden shifts in blood pressure and spinal injury can occur as the legs are positioned in, or removed from, stirrups. To prevent this, the maneuver must be performed very slowly.

7. When attaching the stirrups and securing the patient's position, make sure the locking device is tight and that no portion of the patient's legs rests against the vertical extensions (Figure 19-18).

8. Protect the peroneal nerve (near the Achilles tendon) when sling stirrups are used. Do not place the stirrup sling directly over the Achilles tendon. Distribute the weight of the leg between both slings on the stirrup.

9. Two people are required to raise and lower the legs to prevent lumbar torsion. Release the feet from the stirrups or leg rests, slowly bring the knees together on the midline, and gradually extend the hips and knees.

10. Slow manipulation is necessary to allow blood to flow back into the limbs gradually. If the legs are lowered too quickly, a sudden shift of blood to the lower extremities and drop in blood pressure can occur.

11. Obese patients in the lithotomy position may experience a sudden hypovolemic episode on lowering the legs.

POSITIONING ON THE ORTHOPEDIC TABLE

The orthopedic or fracture table allows the patient to be positioned for hip and other orthopedic procedures of the lower extremities. The table allows circumferential access to the patient's leg (Figure 19-19). The patient rests with the injured leg restrained in a padded boot. The leg may be rotated, pulled into traction, or released as the surgery requires. The unaffected leg rests on an elevated leg holder with adequate padding to prevent pressure on the peroneal nerve or the foot may be placed in a foot holder (see Chapter 31, Orthopedic Surgery). The open structure of the table allows intraoperative fluoroscopy and radiography. Many different types of attachments are available, depending on the complexity and needs of the surgery. At least four people are required to position the patient on the orthopedic table. For surgical positions that allow access for other orthopedic procedures, refer to figures in Chapter 31, Orthopedic Surgery.

Safety Guidelines

1. When moving the patient from the gurney to the orthopedic table, maintain the spine and head in neutral position at all times.

2. The center post of the orthopedic table must be removed before the patient is moved. The post is repositioned and the patient's genitalia are protected with padding during positioning.

3. Pressure points on the sacrum, heels, and unaffected lower leg must be adequately padded, and weight must be distributed. The extended leg is held by a boot or a combination of boot and straps.

4. The perineal area and genital structures must not rest against the center post.

5. Traction on the affected leg is adjusted by the surgeon who directs the positioning team.

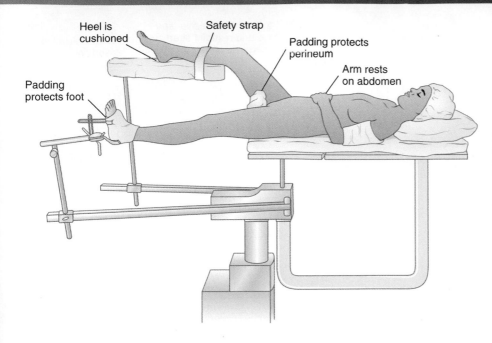

Heel is cushioned

Safety strap

Padding protects perineum

Arm rests on abdomen

Padding protects foot

Figure 19-19 Patient positioned on an orthopedic table. Here the patient is shown without arm boards. The unaffected leg may be cushioned on a raised leg holder or placed in a boot attachment. *(From original artwork by Sandra McMahon.)*

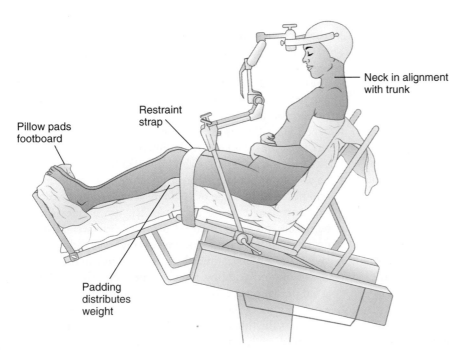

Neck in alignment with trunk

Restraint strap

Pillow pads footboard

Padding distributes weight

Figure 19-20 Sitting (Fowler's) position. *(From original artwork by Sandra McMahon.)*

6. Because of its design, this table is used for patients with fractures of the hip. Moving and transfer of the injured patient must be carried out slowly and carefully to prevent further injury.

SITTING (FOWLER'S) OR BEACH CHAIR POSITION

The sitting, beach chair, or *Fowler's position* is used for shoulder, facial, cranial, or reconstructive breast surgery (Figure 19-20). When this position is used, the general operating table is flexed to allow a beach chair position. The head may be secured by a craniotomy headrest or stabilized with a doughnut-shaped gel or foam pad.

LATERAL (SIMS) POSITION

The *lateral* or *Sims position* is used for surgical procedures that require access to the flank or lateral thorax (Figure 19-21). When the lateral position is described, the side named is the "down" side on the table. For example, in the left lateral position, the patient lies on his or her left side. The opposite side is the operative or "up" side.

When general anesthesia is used, the patient is anesthetized in the supine position and maneuvered into the lateral position after intubation. At least four people are needed for this maneuver.

1. The anesthesia care provider manages the head and cervical spine. If the patient does not have a risk of cervical injury,

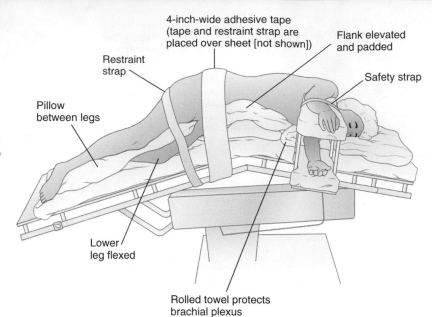

Restraint strap

4-inch-wide adhesive tape (tape and restraint strap are placed over sheet [not shown])

Flank elevated and padded

Safety strap

Pillow between legs

Lower leg flexed

Rolled towel protects brachial plexus

Figure 19-21 Lateral (Sims) position. *(From original artwork by Sandra McMahon.)*

the anesthesia care provider may rotate the head in advance of the body. The move is directed by the anesthesia care provider.

2. One person is responsible for the lower legs and feet, another for the pelvis, and one for the thorax, including the shoulders. All work in unison while maintaining the patient's spine in neutral position.

3. At the count of three, the assistants simultaneously pull the down-side hip and shoulder while pushing the up-side hip and shoulder. This effectively turns the patient while maintaining alignment.

4. Flex the lower leg and place padding between the legs. The upper leg remains extended.

5. Protect the brachial plexus with padding. The arms may be extended on double arm boards, or the down-side arm, which is the most vulnerable, may be placed in front of the body. An overhead arm sling also may be used.

6. Flank padding and a head stabilizer are also used.

Use of the flexed lateral position may require stabilization of the hips and/or shoulders with wide tape. The tape is placed on top of the top sheet, not on the patient's skin. It is secured to the table frame on both sides and passes over the pelvic rim or the shoulder. The tape is meant to stabilize, not to secure the patient's entire weight. Excess compression by the tape can cause tissue damage. The safety strap is placed midway between the thighs and knees. Flexing the middle table break increases the operative exposure. Some operating tables have a "kidney elevator," located under the table pad. This is used to lift the flank region but must be used with caution because it places excessive pressure on the deep blood vessels of the abdomen, resulting in vascular injury or hypotension.

Safety Precautions

1. During the move from supine to lateral position, the patient's shoulders and pelvis must be moved in the same plane without any torsion.

2. The anesthetized patient must be moved as one unit; that is, the head, neck, spine, pelvis, and legs all must be moved together to prevent twisting injury to joints.

3. The down side of the face should rest on an open horseshoe pad or pillow to protect the facial nerves, ear, and eye from compression.

4. When the patient is turned from supine to lateral, the head and neck must be kept in alignment at all times.

5. The patient's arms should be protected by extending them on double arm boards or positioning them with the up-side arm flexed at an angle of 90 degrees or less and the down-side arm lying close to the torso. The down-side arm can be flexed (no more than 90 degrees). The weight of the upper torso must be distributed evenly with padding.

6. When the patient is in a flexed lateral position, the angle of flexion and padding must be meticulously checked to avoid pressure on vessels and nerves in the flank.

7. Padding always should be placed between the legs so that it extends the full length of the leg. The up-side ankle must not rest directly on the down-side leg.

PRONE POSITION

A number of variations of the *prone position* are used to allow access to the spine, cranium, and perianal region. This position can compromise physiological and structural mechanisms in the body, and its use requires caution. The pressure exerted on the abdomen restricts normal ventilation, and the cervical spine may be forced into a position that would be intolerable to the patient if the person were conscious. There is risk to the nerves, eyes, genitalia, breasts, and spine. In the prone position, the patient's upper body rests on a raised padded frame or pads placed on each side of the patient's thorax.

When a patient is to be placed in the prone position, the person is anesthetized in the supine position on the gurney.

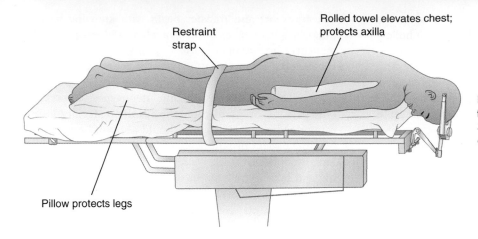

Restraint strap

Rolled towel elevates chest; protects axilla

Pillow protects legs

Figure 19-22 Positioning for a craniotomy in the prone position using a rigid head stabilizer. See text for detailed explanation. *(From original artwork by Sandra McMahon.)*

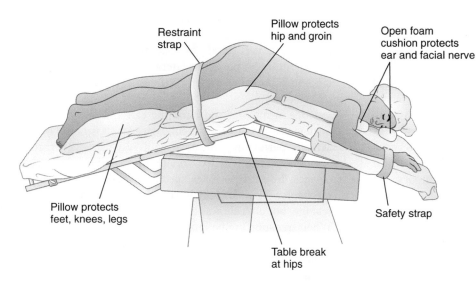

Restraint strap

Pillow protects hip and groin

Open foam cushion protects ear and facial nerve

Pillow protects feet, knees, legs

Safety strap

Table break at hips

Figure 19-23 Jackknife (Kraske) position. *(From original artwork by Sandra McMahon.)*

After intubation, the patient is repositioned on the operating table into the prone position. Four to six people are required to turn the patient. If the patient is turned on the operating table, two people lift and pull the patient close to them and then slowly rotate the body onto the arms of the other two helpers. The spine is maintained in alignment and the head is controlled by the anesthesia care provider. Check that the breasts are free of pressure from the chest brace. If the patient is a male, the genitalia must be assessed for pressure. To turn the patient into the prone position (pronation), follow these steps:

1. Align the gurney with the operating table.
2. If the patient is to be catheterized, perform catheterization before turning the patient.
3. When the anesthesia care provider is ready, he or she will temporarily disconnect the patient's ventilation circuit.
4. Two people positioned on the receiving side of the table reach across, while those on the other side slowly lift and rotate the patient's body onto the arms of the receiving personnel. The head is controlled by the anesthesia care provider and the feet by another helper.
5. The patient's shoulders are anatomically rotated and placed on arm boards.
6. Reconnect the airway and make adjustments in the position.
7. Place the arms on arm boards with the elbows flexed.

A laminectomy brace is used to elevate the trunk and allow expansion of the lungs during spinal or back surgery. The patient is turned from the gurney directly onto the padded lift or brace.

Surgery of the posterior spine or cranium often is performed with the patient in the prone position and the head supported by a headrest. The head is secured by sterile tongs that attach to the head brace (Figure 19-22).

JACKKNIFE (KRASKE) POSITION

The **jackknife (Kraske) position** is a modification of the prone position (Figure 19-23). The lower table break is flexed downward to achieve a simultaneous head-down and foot-down posture. This position may be used for anorectal surgery. The lower legs are elevated and rest on pads to distribute the weight.

Safety Precautions

1. The spine must be kept in a neutral position at all times during positioning.
2. There must be sufficient clearance to allow deep lung inflation. When a brace is used, the two sides of the brace should not impinge on the abdomen.

3. Corneal abrasion can result from compression on the globe of the eye. This can be prevented by using a hollow headrest.

4. A female patient's breasts must be protected. A patient with heavy breasts is likely to be unstable on the operating table because of the lack of firm support in the upper thorax.

5. Forcing the breasts laterally during positioning can cause bleeding and tearing of deep tissue at the breast margins.

6. Particular care must be given to positioning patients who have had a mastectomy or radiation treatment to the chest wall, because the skin and underlying tissues are tender and may be painful.

7. The male genitalia must be protected from compression. When a brace is used, the genitalia must be clear of any part of the frame. Pads placed across the thighs must not entrap the scrotum and penis.

8. If the patient has an intestinal stoma, this area must be completely free of contact with the brace or padding.

9. Pressure on the subclavian artery and brachial plexus when the head is turned to the side with the arms raised can lead to **thoracic outlet syndrome.** The result can be permanent injury, causing pain and loss of sensation along the ulnar nerve.

10. The risk of severe injury to the brachial plexus and cervical spine arises when the patient's arms are extended above the head. To prevent brachial plexus injury, the upper arms should be placed at an angle of 90 degrees or less to the trunk with the forearms parallel to the trunk.

11. When the patient's head is rotated to the side, the risk of a traction and compression injury to the brachial plexus is increased. Many patients cannot tolerate this degree of cervical rotation. Preoperative evaluation must include an assessment of this area to prevent temporary or permanent injury.

12. A wide area around the ulnar nerve must be amply padded.

HISTORICAL HIGHLIGHTS

The term *knee-chest position* has been used historically to describe an extreme variation of the prone position in which the patient kneeled on the examination table with legs flexed at the hips and the knees drawn up to the chest for access to the perineum. This extreme position is *not* used in surgery. Modern surgical beds provide safer positioning options for access to all areas of the body without endangering cardiac output. The knee-chest position is sometimes used in pediatric assessment and in obstetrics as a method of shifting the position of the fetus.

Watch Section 3: Unit 3: Patient Positioning on the Evolve website. http://evolve.elsevier.com/fuller/surgical

KEY CONCEPTS

- A systematic method of patient identification is used throughout the surgical process. The procedure for patient identification is intentionally precise to reduce the risk of error.

- Safe transport and transfer begin with knowing how to perform a maneuver, having a plan, and executing the maneuver by that plan.

- Professional communication with the patient and family is demonstrated by maintaining emotional and social boundaries and by showing respect and attentiveness. Expressing one's personal opinions about the health care facility, health care providers, or colleagues should also not be discussed with the patient or family.

- The risk of health worker injury can be mitigated by learning and taking the time to use safe body mechanics and patient lifting devices.

- Surgical patients are transported in the perioperative setting using a standard or specialty gurney or wheelchair. Lateral transfer devices are used to move a patient from one horizontal surface to another, such as the operating table to a gurney. A transfer device is used when the patient is unable to or it is unsafe to make the move without assistance. The most common lateral transfer devices are the air-assisted transfer system, Plexiglas transfer board, and roller board.

- Practice in moving and handling can and should be performed using nonpatients (colleagues or classmates) before actually performing the task with real patients. Practice should include a detailed orientation to moving and lifting devices, how to perform specific maneuvers, and body mechanics. This not only lowers the risk for the patient in real life, but also allows feedback from peers.

- When transporting patients, be aware of the special needs of particular patient populations such as children, the sight- or hearing-impaired, obese, and patients with severe physical impairment or injury. Consider the psychological needs and appropriate methods of communication in addition to particular safety measures to protect the patient from injury during transport.

- The surgical technologist may be required to assist in patient positioning. The specific role varies among health care facilities but is always performed under the direction of the anesthesia care provider or surgeon. The most important aspect of the role is attention to and prevention of injury.

- Practice sessions in the use of operating table accessories and patient positioning in a controlled environment are valuable learning tools. During practice, the principles of patient safety should be combined with a "dry run" using operating table accessories and equipment.

- Specific techniques and devices are used in positioning to prevent injury. The most common cause of injury during positioning is inadequate padding of superficial nerves and blood vessels, resulting in paralysis or ischemia, and losing control of a limb during positioning, which can result in dislocation or fracture. Injury prevention requires attention to the task at hand, knowledge of anatomy and range of motion, and specific knowledge of the patient's condition.

- Specific safety precautions are associated with standard surgical positions. Protection of superficial nerves and blood vessels, not exceeding range of motion in joints, and protecting the patient's airway are common to all positions;

the use of special positioning devices such as limb holders, a thoracic lift (brace), and stirrups compound the risks for injury. Positioning the patient safely requires expert knowledge and use of each type of device.

REVIEW QUESTIONS

1. What is a shear injury?
2. How can you best protect yourself from injury if a patient you are escorting begins to fall and leans into you?
3. Describe the proper method for identifying a patient.
4. What are the exact anatomical risks when moving a patient from a gurney into a prone position?
5. What are the anatomical risks in the lithotomy position?
6. Why is a sequential compression device used on patients during surgery?
7. Why are patients more prone to skeletal injury when under general anesthesia or unconscious sedation?
8. What is *thoracic outlet syndrome*?
9. What are the physiological risks of the Trendelenburg position?

CASE STUDIES

Case 1

You are asked to bring a patient from the medical unit to surgery. When you arrive on the unit, the patient is not in his room or in the hallway. What will you do?

Case 2

You are transporting a patient from the medical unit to the operating room. You discover that the patient elevator is out of order. What will you do?

Case 3

While turning the patient into the lateral position, you suddenly realize that the patient is falling off the table in your direction. What will you do? What precautions can be taken to prevent falls?

Case 4

You are assigned to act as circulator in a procedure in which the patient is placed in the lithotomy position. The patient emerges quickly from anesthesia and she begins to struggle. Her legs are still elevated in stirrups. What are the risks to the patient in this situation? What will you do?

Case 5

You are scrubbed on a laparotomy case. A number of medical students have been brought in to observe. One of the medical students is scrubbed and is holding a retractor. You notice the student has placed his elbow on the patient's shoulder, and he is resting his weight on the patient. The surgeon has said nothing. What will you do?

BIBLIOGRAPHY

Porth C: *Pathophysiology: concepts of altered health states*, ed 6, Philadelphia, 2009, Lippincott Williams & Williams.

Miller R, Ericksson L, Fleisher L, et al: *Miller's anesthesia*, ed 7, Philadelphia, 2007, Churchill Livingstone.

20

Surgical Skin Prep and Draping

LEARNING OBJECTIVES

After studying this chapter the reader will be able to:

1. Review the standards of practice for surgical prep and draping
2. Review the guidelines for patient hygiene before surgery
3. List the materials needed for urinary catheterization
4. Discuss the process and safety guidelines for urinary catheterization
5. Discuss the protocols for hair removal and skin marking in the surgical prep
6. List the FDA's approved antiseptics for the surgical prep
7. List the supplies needed for skin prep
8. Demonstrate the different procedures for skin prep
9. Discuss the elements of patient safety in regard to skin prep
10. Demonstrate skin prep on the standard prep sites
11. Discuss the rationale and techniques for surgical draping
12. Discuss how to maintain asepsis during draping
13. Demonstrate draping techniques of the surgical site
14. Discuss how to remove drapes at the end of a procedure

TERMINOLOGY

Antiseptic: Chemical agent approved for use on the skin that inhibits the growth and reproduction of microorganisms.

Debridement: The removal of devitalized tissue, debris, and foreign objects from a wound. Debridement is performed on trauma injuries, burns, and infected wounds either before surgery or as part of the surgical procedure.

Fenestrated drape: A sterile body sheet with a hole or "window" (*fenestration*) that exposes the incision site. The fenestrated drape is positioned after other drapes and towels have been placed in keeping with the procedure. Fenestrated drapes are differentiated by type (e.g., laparotomy, thyroid, kidney, eye, ear, and extremity drapes).

Impervious: Waterproof.

Incise drape: A plastic adhesive drape that is positioned over the incision site after the surgical skin prep. The incise drape creates a sterile surface over the skin.

Residual activity: The antimicrobial action of an antiseptic or a disinfectant that continues after the solution has dried.

Retention catheter: A type of urinary catheter that remains in place. Also called an *indwelling* or *Foley catheter*.

Solution: Any liquid antiseptic combined with water.

Single-stage prep: Also called a *paint prep*. The skin prep is performed using only antiseptic solution, which is painted on the skin at the operative site.

Straight catheter: A nonretention urinary catheter used to drain the bladder one time (sometimes called a or Robinson catheter).

Surgical site infection (SSI): Postoperative infection of the surgical wound, most commonly caused by the normal bacteria found on the patient's skin or shed from the skin or hair of members of the surgical team.

Tincture: Any liquid antiseptic combined with alcohol.

INTRODUCTION

The presurgical skin prep and draping procedure is one of the methods of preventing surgical site infection (SSI). Bacteria colonize all layers of the skin and its appendages (e.g., sweat and sebaceous glands and hair follicles). Before surgery the incision site and a wide area around it are cleansed with an **antiseptic** to reduce the number of transient and normal microorganisms to an absolute minimum. After skin prep, the patient is covered with sterile *drapes* that expose only the surgical site and create the center of the *sterile field*. The skin prep and draping procedures described in this chapter take place after the patient is positioned and immediately before surgery starts.

Skin prep and draping are discussed together in this chapter because the events are sequential. The guidelines presented here are presented in a timewise and stepwise way to help clarify who does what, and when.

Standards for practice in the surgical skin prep and draping come from the Surgical Care Improvement Project (SCIP) sponsored by the Centers for Medicaid Services and the Centers for Disease Control and Prevention (CDC).

PATIENT HYGIENE BEFORE SURGERY

At least 1 day before elective surgery, the patient is instructed to bathe twice with chlorhexidine gluconate (CHG) antiseptic soap (after validation that the patient has no history of allergy to CHG). This provides a thorough cleaning of the patient's skin and also reduces the number of resident and transient microbes. If surgery of the head or scalp is planned, the patient should also shampoo twice with CHG. Patients should be reminded to rinse the soap thoroughly. Patients should also be cautioned not to use any hair products after shampooing because they may interfere with the residual antiseptic action of the antiseptic.

Shortly before surgery, the patient is brought into the holding area and admitted to the department from the hospital ward or from outside the hospital for day surgery patients.

NOTE: The procedure for ensuring that all preoperative orders have been completed is explained in Chapter 21.

The patient is provided with clean hospital attire, which contributes to overall asepsis. When admission is completed, including the preoperative checklist, the patient is brought to the surgical suite and transferred to the operating table. Anesthesia preparations are begun, and if general anesthesia is planned, the patient is induced and intubated. At this stage the patient is ready for skin prep and draping, which take place immediately before the start of surgery. If the patient is having a regional or local anesthesia, this may be started, according to the surgeon's decision, before the skin prep and draping.

URINARY CATHETERIZATION

Urinary catheterization is a delegated invasive procedure that requires a specific order (physician orders are discussed in Chapter 13). The physician or other licensed professional can delegate catheterization electronically, verbally, or in writing. The order may be written on the surgeon's preference card and must include the type of catheter to be inserted and the date of the standing order.

Urinary catheterization is performed for certain types of procedures and circumstances:

- Continuous drainage prevents distention of the bladder during lengthy procedures.
- Surgery of the lower abdominal and pelvic cavity requires *decompression* (collapse) of the bladder to protect it from injury during procedures.
- Catheterization allows measurement of urine and thus assessment of renal output in patients at risk. The most common method of continuous drainage is a Foley urinary catheter (Figure 20-1, *A*). This is a **retention catheter**, which has a small inflatable balloon at the tip. After the catheter is inserted into the bladder, the balloon is inflated to keep the catheter in place. A **straight catheter** (without balloon for retention) is used when continuous urinary drainage is unnecessary (Figure 20-1, *B*). Catheterization often is performed immediately before the surgical skin prep. Other types of urinary catheters are indicated for

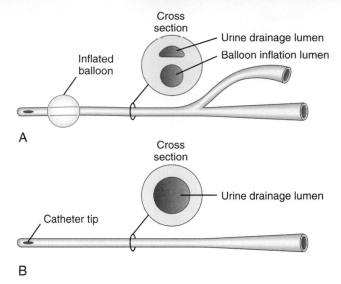

Figure 20-1   **A,** Foley catheter with balloon tip. **B,** Straight catheter.

specific conditions and circumstances and are discussed in Chapter 26, Genitourinary Surgery.

SUPPLIES

Prepackaged sterile catheter kits contain most of the supplies needed for catheterization. The correct catheter is selected based on the patient's age, size, and gender. A size 14 to 16 French (Fr) Foley catheter generally is appropriate for a female patient; males usually require a 16 or 18 Fr catheter. Pediatric patients require considerably smaller sizes, and this should be assessed by qualified personnel. The patient's allergy status must be verified before catheterization, because latex allergy is a risk of this procedure.

The standard catheter balloon inflates to 10 mL. When the catheter is in place, a Luer-Lok syringe is used to fill the balloon with 10 mL of sterile water. A valve prevents backflow and deflation of the balloon. The distal tip of the catheter is connected directly to the drainage tube, or a plastic connector is used. This tube is fitted to the drainage bag, which has graduated markers for measuring the amount of urine. After the catheter has been inserted and connected to the drainage device, the collection unit must remain below the level of the patient, because raising it would cause urine to drain back into the bladder. This can result in injury to the bladder or initiate an infection.

The supplies for catheterization must be gathered, checked, and opened before the patient is positioned. A small catheterization table is prepared and moved into place immediately before the procedure.

The following supplies are needed for catheterization:

- Containers for the antiseptic or saline
- Foley catheter
- Gauze prep sponges
- Antiseptic solution (water-based)
- Sterile lubricant
- Sterile gloves
- 10-mL syringe prefilled with water
- Perineal drape

- Forceps
- Cotton balls
- Drainage tubing and a urine collection unit

A prepackaged commercial kit used for catheterization contains most supplies needed for catheterization, except the catheter itself, which is selected according to appropriate size and type ordered.

PROCEDURE FOR CATHETERIZATION

Catheterization performed before surgery is performed only after the anesthesia care provider has indicated that it is safe. If the operative procedure requires the lithotomy position, the patient is positioned using the correct technique. A female patient is positioned with the knees slightly flexed and the hips externally rotated. A male patient is placed in the supine position for catheterization. Always keep the patient covered to protect their modesty.

The sterile technique required for catheterization entails keeping one hand sterile and the other nonsterile. The hand used to perform the skin prep and insert the catheter is referred to here as the *insertion hand*. The *assisting hand* is used to stabilize the genitalia and expose the urethral meatus. The assisting hand does not contact sterile supplies, including the catheter itself. The insertion hand remains sterile and is used to cleanse the area and guide the catheter into place.

If the insertion hand becomes contaminated, the procedure must be stopped and the contaminated glove changed. If the catheter becomes contaminated, a fresh sterile catheter must be obtained.

The following guidelines describe the step-by-step procedure for prep and insertion of a Foley catheter. Although catheterization is a sterile procedure, only the insertion hand remains sterile throughout. The catheterization kit is prepared by adding antiseptic solution, sterile lubricant, and the correct size of catheter.

Step-by-step illustrations for catheterization are presented in Figures 20-2 (female) and 20-3 (male), and listed here:

1. Position the patient. Don sterile gloves using the open gloving technique.
2. Before beginning the catheterization, check for body-piercing jewelry on the patient's genitalia. All jewelry must be removed before catheterization. Jewelry is secured in a closed labeled container and returned to the patient after surgery.
3. Place the prep sponges in the antiseptic.
4. The balloon may be tested before insertion. However, some manufacturers discourage this, because it can weaken the balloon and lead to rupture after insertion. Follow the facility's and manufacturer's recommendations. To test the balloon, inject 5 mL of sterile water from the prep syringe into the Luer-Lok tip of the catheter and observe for leakage. Withdraw the water back into the syringe and put it aside.
5. If the sterile lubricant is provided in a sealed pouch, open the pouch and place a small amount of lubricant in a sterile area of the prep tray or on the tip of the catheter. Position the catheter so that it can be easily grasped with one hand.

6. If the patient is already in the lithotomy position, an **impervious** (waterproof) drape is placed under the buttocks with the end or tails of the drape directed into a kick bucket.
7. If the patient is in the supine position, place a fenestrated barrier drape over the genitalia.
8. *Female prep:* With the *assisting hand*, spread the labia, using the thumb and forefinger to form a C. Then, use the *insertion* (sterile) *hand* to cleanse the genitalia. Grasp the prep sponge with the sterile forceps. Cleanse the meatus and internal labia by drawing the cotton prep sponge downward from the superior apex of the labia majora to the anus. Drop this sponge into the kick bucket. Do not allow the sponge to touch the area just prepped. Repeat this process several times.
9. *Male prep:* With the *assisting hand*, retract the foreskin and stabilize the penis just below the glans. Use the *insertion hand* to cleanse the penis. Grasp the prep sponge with the sterile forceps and, starting with the urethral meatus, draw it in a circular direction, widening the circle to include the outer portions of the glans. Do not draw the sponge back over the area just prepped. Discard the sponge and repeat this process several times.
10. Maintaining traction on the genitalia, grasp the insertion end of the catheter and lubricate the tip (if this was not done in step 5).
11. Guide the tip of the catheter into the urethra with slow, steady pressure. *Do not force the catheter into the urethra.* It should slide easily into place with little resistance. When the tip of the catheter reaches the bladder, urine will begin to flow through the tubing. (In male patients, replace the foreskin into its normal position.) Inflate the catheter balloon by attaching a 10 mL syringe into the luer lock connection of the catheter; inject 10 mL water and remove the syringe. The balloon will remain inflated. If blood returns through the urethra at any time during insertion, gently retract the catheter and request a medical assessment immediately.
12. Connect the distal end of the catheter to the sterile tubing and calibrated urine collection unit. Note that some collection devices may require an adapter.
13. Make sure no tension is placed on the catheter tubing once it is in place. This can traumatize the bladder neck and proximal urethra. Some institutions require that tape or a special strap be placed on the patient's thigh to secure the tubing.
14. Remove your gloves. Lower the drainage unit to allow gravity drainage. When urine stops flowing, secure the drainage unit to the operating table and measure the baseline amount. Document this amount according to policy.

PATIENT SAFETY

Catheterization is a routine procedure performed by (circulating) perioperative personnel. Recently the trend has been to reduce the number of catheterizations of hospitalized patients because of the risks involved. *Urinary catheterization is the most common cause of hospital-acquired infections in the United*

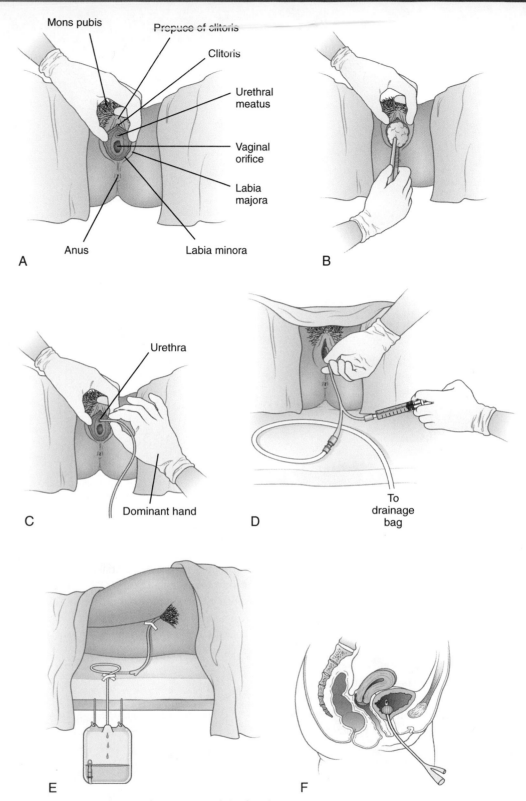

Figure 20-2 **Urinary catheterization of the female. A,** Exposure of the urethra using the assisting hand. **B,** Cleansing of the labia using the no-touch technique. **C,** Insertion of the catheter. **D,** Inflation of the balloon tip. **E,** Attachment of the drainage bag. **F,** Anatomical position of the catheter.

States. Two primary risks are associated with catheterization: infection and trauma to the genitourinary tract.

Urinary catheterization is a sterile procedure. The urinary bladder and proximal urethra are sterile, and contaminants introduced by catheterization increase the risk of urinary tract infection. Because of its proximity to the rectum (especially in female patients), the urinary meatus can be easily contaminated with *Escherichia coli*, which may be introduced into the urinary system during catheterization. Urinary tract infection can progress to systemic infection, with serious consequences. Strict aseptic technique is required to perform catheterization safely.

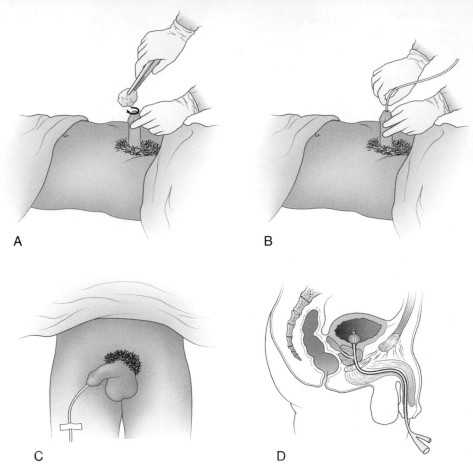

Figure 20-3   Urinary catheterization of the male. A, The assisting hand stabilizes the penis and draws back the foreskin. The insertion hand is used to cleanse the urethral meatus and glans. **B,** Insertion of the catheter. The assisting hand replaces the foreskin. **C,** The catheter is secured to the leg. **D,** Anatomical position of the catheter.

Repeated unsuccessful attempts at catheterization can cause mucosal abrasions that result in pain and increase the risk of infection. Damage to the urethra and sphincter muscle can result in prolonged urinary retention (inability to void).

SURGICAL SKIN PREP

Skin is the body's primary defense against infection. A surgical incision creates a portal of entry for microorganisms. Healthy skin contains colonies of microorganisms, which compete with and usually overcome foreign or transient bacteria. When normal or transient bacteria are introduced into the surgical wound, they can cause a **surgical site infection (SSI)**.

The surgical skin prep is performed immediately before surgery to reduce the bacteria on the skin and therefore reduce the risk of SSI. Skin cannot be sterilized, but the number of bacteria can be reduced significantly with antiseptic cleansing or a coating of antiseptic on the skin.

The surgical site and a wide area around the site are cleansed with antiseptic solution. If the prep area is soiled, it is scrubbed with antiseptic soap and then painted with antiseptic solution or tincture. In many facilities, only a *paint prep* is performed. Skin prep solutions selected for use in surgery are required by the U.S. Food and Drug Administration (FDA) to be

fast-acting, to provide persistent antimicrobial effect, and to be safe to use. The residual effect is important to maintain asepsis throughout the duration of the surgery.

An antiseptic prep solution is chosen according to the surgical site and any patient history of sensitivity or allergy to specific antiseptics.

NOTE: *There is no scientific evidence showing a relationship between allergy to fish (shellfish) and allergy to iodophor antiseptic.*

USE OF ANTISEPTICS ON MUCOUS MEMBRANES

At the time of this writing, only povidone-iodine (not tincture) and parachlorometaxylenol (PCMX) are *labeled for safe use* on mucous membranes. PCMX has minimal effectiveness in the presence of organic material, and the product is under review by the FDA.

HAIR REMOVAL

In modern surgery, hair is not removed from the surgical site unless the surgeon determines that it will interfere with the surgical procedure and then it can be clipped. In the past, the operative site was routinely shaved before surgery. Current research demonstrates that shaving the skin *increases* rather than decreases the risk of SSI. Shaving causes skin abrasions that may not be easily seen. These become a source of bacterial colonization by resident microbes, which are the most common source of SSI. Therefore, unless the patient's hair cannot be kept outside the wound, it is not removed. This recommendation includes craniotomy and facial procedures in which the hair can be braided and secured away from the incision site with elastic bands or water-based gel.

Hair clipping requires a verbal or written order by the surgeon. The following guidelines must be followed for this procedure:

- Hair should be removed as close to the time of surgery as possible.
- Hair is removed with single-use battery clippers or one with a head that can be resterilized. A chemical depilatory can be used only if the patient has had a skin test to ensure he or she is not sensitive to the product. This test must be performed at least 12 hours before the start of surgery.
- Hair is removed in an area away from the location where surgery is performed.
- Single-use clippers that come into contact with the patient are discarded in a biohazard container.
- Eyebrows are never shaved, because they may fail to regrow or may grow abnormally after removal. Eyelashes must also never be cut.

SURGICAL SKIN MARKING

The Joint Commission Guidelines for Universal Protocol for preventing wrong site, wrong procedure, and wrong person surgery require skin marking at the surgical site for procedures involving incisions, punctures, and insertions. This is to verify the side, levels (e.g., spinal location), and multiple sites such as fingers. The surgeon is required to mark the site before surgery so that the perioperative team can participate in the verification process from the time the patient arrives in the operating room until the start of surgery.

Surgeons use various types of pens for marking the site. The mark should be made with a surgical skin marker approved for this specific use. Gentian violet ink is the recommended product and the most effective because it is antiseptic, does not wash off, and is easily seen. The mark should *not be made with a ballpoint pen* or other inks that are not approved for presurgical use. Nonapproved inks can wash off during the skin prep, and some (e.g., felt marking pens used in labeling) are not FDA-approved as nontoxic on skin. If the skin marking has not been made with gentian violet or other long-lasting dye, care must be taken not to wash the mark off during the prep.

PREPPING AGENTS

Only antiseptic agents approved by the FDA for use on skin may be used for the prep. Approval of skin antiseptics for the surgical prep is based on research by the FDA and the

Association for Professionals in Infection Control and Epidemiology (APIC), which reviews the literature for all antiseptic testing trials and determines what is safe and effective in the perioperative environment. Some antiseptics cannot be used near the eyes or ears, and others must not be used on abraded skin or burns. Refer to Table 20-1 for a comparison of antiseptics.

Antiseptics used for the surgical prep are mainly evaluated according to the following criteria:

1. Effectiveness on microbes, especially gram-negative and gram-positive bacteria
2. Possible or actual toxicity
3. Ability to use in or around the eyes, ears, mucous membranes, and neural tissue
4. Flammability
5. Residual antimicrobial action after application and drying

Some of the challenges in preventing SSI are related to the preoperative prep of the surgical site. For example, alcohol is an excellent antiseptic, effective on both gram-positive and gram-negative bacteria. However, any product containing alcohol carries a high risk for surgical fire. There are no "perfect" antiseptics and no one solution for preventing SSI.

Alcohol

Alcohol solution contains isopropyl alcohol. It is used in the formulation of some preoperative prep mixtures but is rarely used alone except for small areas of the skin. At 70% concentration, isopropyl alcohol is 95% effective against both gram-negative and gram-positive bacteria, mycobacteria, fungi, and viruses. It is not completely effective against bacterial spores. Isopropyl alcohol is extremely flammable and volatile. It can be a source of fire in an oxygen-rich environment when lasers and electrosurgery are used. All traces of alcohol must be completely dry on the skin before drapes are applied. Alcohol mixed with any other liquid is referred to as a **tincture**.

Alcohol destroys microorganisms by *desiccation* (drying) of the cell proteins. For this reason, alcohol is never used on mucous membranes or the eyes or in any open wound. Alcohol preparations must not be used near the eye or ear because they can cause injury to the cornea or nerve damage.

Chlorhexidine Gluconate

Chlorhexidine gluconate (CHG) has not been approved as a first-choice skin prep by the Joint Commission or CDC. This antiseptic does provide some **residual activity**, which means that it continues to kill microorganisms for some time after application. It is not absorbed by the skin. A disadvantage of CHG is that it is not effective in the presence of soap and organic debris such as skin oils, blood, and body fluids. If it is used for preoperative bathing, the patient first must bathe normally, and chlorhexidine solution then is used as a final wash after all traces of soap have been removed from the skin and hair.

CHG has been linked to hearing loss when accidentally introduced into the middle ear. Therefore, it must never be used during prep of the ear or face. It is not recommended for use on large, open wounds, such as burns, *or in infants younger than 2 months.*

Table 20-1   Surgical Skin Prep Antiseptics

Chemical Name	Product	Action on Gram-Positive Bacteria	Action on Gram-Negative Bacteria	Residual Activity	Contraindicated (Do Not Use)
70% isopropyl alcohol HIGHLY FLAMMABLE	Alcohol	Excellent	Excellent	Little	Mucous membranes Eye Ear Wounds Infants
Chlorhexidine gluconate (CHG)	Hibiclens Exidine	Excellent	Good	Excellent	Eye Ear Mucous membranes Genitalia Brain or spinal tissues
70% alcohol/chlorhexidine gluconate HIGHLY FLAMMABLE	ChloraPrep	Excellent	Good		Infants younger than 2 mo. Open skin wounds Eyes, Ear Mouth Lumbar puncture Contact with meninges
Aqueous povidone-iodine	Betadine	Excellent	Good	Poor	Eye Infants younger than 2 mo May cause severe irritation
Iodine povacrylex (7% iodine)/ isopropyl alcohol HIGHLY FLAMMABLE	DuraPrep	Excellent	Good	Poor	Mucous membranes Eye Ear Wounds Infants
Parachlorometaxylenol (PCMX)	Surcide	Good	Fair	Moderate	Eye irritant

Iodophor

Iodine alone is irritating to tissue, but when combined with povidone (a synthetic dispersing agent), it becomes iodophor, a commonly used antiseptic. Iodophor is combined with detergent and used for the surgical hand scrub. Iodophor is commercially formulated with 70% alcohol as a tincture. It is effective against gram-positive bacteria but weaker against gram-negative organisms, mycobacteria, fungi, and viruses. It has some residual activity and retains its microbicidal action in the presence of organic substances.

Iodophor is absorbed through the skin and may cause toxicity. Although it normally is nonirritating to tissue, first-degree and second-degree chemical burns can result from improper prep technique or if the patient is sensitive to iodine. Iodophor cannot be used on infants younger than 2 months old because the skin of an infant of this age is highly absorbent, causing high blood levels of the chemical.

Triclosan

Triclosan 1% solution is an antiseptic commonly found in deodorants, antibacterial soaps, and other proprietary cosmetics. Its use in surgery is limited, because its full microbicidal effect occurs only with repeated application. It is safe to use as a prep solution in ophthalmic surgery and for use on the face.

Parachlorometaxylenol (Chloroxylenol)

Parachlorometaxylenol (PCMX) is labeled for use around the eye, mouth, or genital area, especially as an alternative to povidone-iodine. It is not used with alcohol, which interferes with the residual effects of PCMX. It has limited bactericidal, tuberculocidal, viricidal, and fungicidal properties.

Hexachlorophene

Hexachlorophene was popular as an infant bathing soap and antiacne wash in the 1960s. It quickly became a common surgical prep solution after coming on the market. However, in the 1970s, proven links were found between the active ingredient and central nervous system damage in infants. Hexachlorophene is readily absorbed through broken or damaged skin at all ages. Ingested, it can be fatal, and its use as a surgical skin prep solution has been officially retired. However, it is still found in some facilities and ordered by some surgeons. The FDA's most recent decision on hexachlorophene is that the antiseptic is not generally recognized as safe and effective for use as an antiseptic hand wash and should not be used to bathe patients with burns or extensive areas of susceptible, sensitive skin. This product is now available by prescription only and is not recommended by any safety agency for use as a preoperative skin prep.

PREP SUPPLIES

Supplies for the basic skin prep are available as prepackaged kits or may be assembled before the prep. If the surgeon's order is for a paint prep only, commercial sponge sticks with prep solution preloaded are used. The exact supplies required depend on the anatomical area of the prep. Specialty areas are described later in this chapter.

A **two-step prep** that includes skin scrub (wash) and antiseptic paint requires the following supplies, which are available as a commercially prepared kit or are assembled in the operating room before the prep:

- Sterile gloves
- Towels
- Gauze or foam prep sponges
- Sponge forceps
- Antiseptic prep solution
- Antiseptic scrub soap (as required)
- Sterile water or saline
- Several small basins
- Cotton-tipped applicators as needed

The skin prep is a sterile procedure. Sterile gloves are worn and supplies are sterile. Manufactured sterile prep trays are available that contain all or most of the supplies needed to perform the skin prep. Many different types of commercial prep systems are available, some with sponges on handles or other devices. The rationale and procedure for the prep remain the same, regardless of the system.

Before the prep is started, the prep kit is positioned on a small prep table near the patient, and the outer wrapper is opened using sterile technique. The sterile outside wrapper is folded down over the table, and a sterile field is created. Prep solutions such as antiseptic scrub soap and paint prep are poured into one of the small basins, and all other supplies are placed on the table.

When more than one procedure is planned during the same surgery, the circulator must prepare each site separately, using a different prep setup for each site. This can occur in cases of multiple trauma or in grafting procedures when the graft is taken from the patient's own tissues. Two people may prep simultaneously if enough staff members are available. More extensive sites such as multiple trauma or prep for cardiac surgery require a different setup. This is described later in the chapter.

X-ray detectable surgical sponges are never used to perform the patient prep. Surgical sponges are reserved for surgery and must never be used for the patient prep because they may be confused with the surgical sponges and count. Used prep sponges are discarded according to facility policy to keep them away from the surgical field and out of the incision. In some facilities, the kick bucket is used to collect prep sponges, which are then collected and bagged before surgery begins to keep them separate from surgical sponges.

PROCEDURE FOR THE SKIN PREP

There are two methods of prepping. In a two-stage prep, the skin is washed or scrubbed gently with antiseptic soap

---

Box 20-1   Checklist for Starting the Skin Prep

- **Prepare the patient.** Have you checked the patient's record for allergies? Has the patient been positioned properly? Has the surgical site been verified? Has all jewelry been removed? Has the anesthesia care provider given permission to start the prep? Are the surgeons present and available to start surgery?
- **Prepare the supplies.** Note which items are not included in the prep kit. Are sterile gloves available? Have the prep solutions been poured? Is the prep table positioned close to the patient? Is a receptacle at hand for soiled prep sponges? Do you have adequate light on the prep area?
- **Prepare yourself.** Do you have a plan? Do you know the exact boundaries of the prep area? Is your clothing contained so that it does not touch the prep area? (A loose warm-up jacket or baggy sleeves may drag across the prep area.)

---

solution followed by a coating of antiseptic. A single-stage prep uses antiseptic paint solution only. The type of prep used depends on the surgeon's preference, the condition of the skin, and the area of the body. For example, preparation of the foot and hand usually requires a two-stage prep to ensure that visible soil is removed.

Before starting the skin prep, the surgical technologist should perform a mental check of patient safety considerations. These are listed in Box 20-1.

Two-Stage Prep

1. The prep site must be assessed before the prep begins. Any lesion, rash, discoloration, or other skin condition must be medically documented in the patient's chart.
2. If the prep area is grossly contaminated with dirt, debris, industrial chemicals, or other foreign material, the site is cleansed as a separate procedure before the surgical skin prep. This procedure takes place before the patient comes to the operating room.
3. Prepare the prep supplies on a small table near the patient. If a scrub prep is planned, antiseptic scrub soap is added to sterile water in a small basin. The ratio of water to antiseptic soap is determined by facility policy and the manufacturer's recommendation. Do not alter the ratio. A small amount of paint prep solution is poured into a separate basin. This is painted on the skin following a scrub prep.
4. Before starting the prep, it is necessary to verify with the anesthesia care provider that it is safe to start.
5. Expose the prep area.
6. Don sterile gloves using the open gloving technique.
7. Position at least two sterile towels at the periphery of the prep site to absorb any prep solution that might pool between the patient and operating table. When placing the towels, make a wide cuff in the towel to protect your gloved hands from contamination.
8. Dip a prep sponge in the antiseptic solution and squeeze out any excess. Use one sponge at a time to perform the prep.

9. The prep is performed in a circular pattern starting at the incision site and moving outward. As the area of the prep is extended outward, do not bring the sponge back to an area already prepped. A new prep sponge is used to widen the circle as needed or to repeat the pattern. As each sponge reaches the periphery of the prep boundary, it is discarded.

10. Any area that is highly colonized with microorganisms (i.e., a contaminated area), such as a colostomy, skin ulcers, or foreign body, is prepped with fresh sponges *after* the surrounding area has been prepped. This limits the area of contamination.

11. After the scrub prep, use a towel to blot the soap from the skin.

12. Antiseptic paint prep solution is applied to the surgical site after the scrub prep. Dip fresh sponges into the paint solution and squeeze out the excess. Beginning with the incision site, apply paint prep in a circular motion from the center to the periphery. Apply the paint prep solution without allowing the sponge to return to an area previously prepped. When the periphery is reached, discard the sponge.

13. Allow the paint prep solution to air-dry. This enhances its bactericidal effect and is necessary whenever alcohol-based solutions are used to prevent possible ignition after drapes are applied.

14. Document the skin prep in the patient's chart, including the skin assessment, prep area, solutions, and name of the person who performed the prep.

Single-Stage Paint Prep

In a **single-stage prep**, the skin scrub is omitted and only antiseptic solution is applied. DuraPrep Surgical Solution is commonly used for patient prep. This solution contains iodine povacrylex and isopropyl alcohol. The solution is self-contained (preloaded) in an applicator sponge, which is applied to the surgical site using standard technique, moving from the center of the surgical site outward. The CDC recommends that pressure be used during the paint prep. This allows the solution to get into skin crevices, sebaceous glands, hair follicles, and pores more efficiently. It is a critical safety precaution to allow the solution to completely dry before applying drapes.

PATIENT SAFETY

As in all areas of surgical care, patient safety must be considered during the surgical prep and draping procedures. The use of chemical antiseptics and the flammability of alcohol on the surgical field are the primary concerns in the area of patient safety. Accredited health care institutions follow the recommendations of the Joint Commission, which defers to Association of periOperative Registered Nurses (AORN) guidelines.

Allergy

As part of the patient workup before surgery, a history of allergies to any medicines or solutions should have been documented by the admitting health care specialist. However, this is continually verified throughout the perioperative period. Surgical prep agents can cause skin irritation, rash, or other reactions. This does not mean that the patient is allergic to a solution; he or she may only be sensitive to it. However, an alternate prep solution must be used if the patient reports any adverse reactions in the past. Latex allergy should also have been noted well before the patient arrives for surgery and nonlatex equipment made available for use on that patient.

Chemical Burns

Serious chemical burns can occur when prep solutions are allowed to pool under the patient during surgery. Pressure and contact with the chemical over time can result in severe blistering and skin loss. To prevent burns, the prep area should be framed with sterile surgery towels that can absorb the excess solution at the periphery of the prep area. Towels must be tucked between the operating table and the patient to catch any runoff solution. Towels are removed after the prep. The circulator must check the entire site for pooling or dampness before drapes are applied. *All prep solution should be removed with water or saline at the close of surgery.*

Fire

Alcohol and alcohol-based prep solutions are volatile and flammable. When alcohol solution or volatile fumes come in contact with heat sources, they can easily cause a fire on or inside the patient. Approximately 100 surgical fires occur each year in the United States. These fires result in about 20 serious injuries and 2 deaths annually.[1]

In the presence of concentrated oxygen in an oxygen-enriched environment such as the operating room, the risk is even greater. Ignition can occur during electrosurgery or laser surgery. Closed cavities, such as the throat, are particularly at risk because they are small contained areas. Prevention of alcohol-related fires requires vigilance and proactive measures on the part of all members of the surgical team. To prevent a fire arising from a prep solution, make sure the prep area, towels, linens, and operating bed are dry before applying sterile drapes.

Thermal Burns

Prep solutions must never be prewarmed in a microwave or other method not specifically intended for patient solutions. Uncontrolled or unmonitored systems create a risk of thermal burns because the exact temperature is not known. When iodine is heated in a closed container, it combines with free oxygen, causing the iodine to be lost from the solution, which reduces its concentration.

STANDARD PREP SITES

Special procedures are needed for some surgical sites. Some of these procedures and precautions require supplies that are not included in a routine prep kit.

EYE

Surgical prep of the eye is performed after the patient has been anesthetized (if a general anesthesia is used). If a regional block is used, the prep may be continuous with the regional anesthetic procedure. Only prep solutions that are safe to use around mucous membranes, including the eye, can be used in the prep. Dilute (5% or less) povidone-iodine is the most common solution used in eye preps. The eye prep includes the eyelid, inner and outer canthus, brow, and face to the chin line, starting at the eyelid and working outward. When prepping the patient for an orbital injury, prep solution must not come in contact with the open orbital wounds. The surgeon usually performs the prep.

The eye prep usually includes irrigation of the eye with balanced saline solution for ophthalmic use. Other drugs may also be instilled according to the surgeon's orders.

NOTE: Among approved preoperative skin antiseptics, only two can be used around the eyes and ears. These are dilute povidone-iodine and parachlorometaxylenol (PCMX).

Supplies

- Adhesive barrier drape
- Lint-free cotton balls
- Small basins with warm saline solution and prep solution
- Towels
- Bulb syringe
- Eye sponges

NOTE: Eye prep solutions must be diluted according to the surgeon's orders.

TECHNIQUE

1. Explain the procedure to the conscious patient. Advise the patient not to touch the face during and after the prep.
2. Turn the patient's head slightly toward the operative side.
3. Start the prep at the eyelid. Prep in a circular pattern around the eye to within 1 inch (2.5 cm) of the hairline, including the nose, cheek, and jaw on the affected side. If the procedure includes both eyes, prep both sides of the face.
4. Prevent prep solutions from entering the patient's ear. Iodophor solutions can damage the inner ear. Although the tympanic membrane separates the external auditory canal from the middle ear, solutions may enter through a rupture or tear in the membrane. Place a cotton ball at the ear canal opening or an adhesive barrier drape along the side of the face to prevent solution from draining into the ear.
5. Discard each sponge after reaching the periphery of the prep area.
6. Repeat the prep at least three times, using fresh sponges each time.
7. Rinse the prepped area using warm saline and cotton balls. Discard each used cotton ball and obtain a fresh one. Rinse the area at least twice.
8. Use a bulb syringe and small basin to flush the conjunctiva. Using one finger, pull the conjunctival sac slightly downward while flushing with normal saline solution or a solution ordered by the surgeon.

Refer to Chapter 27, Ophthalmic Surgery, for further discussion on presurgical prep of the eye.

EAR

Supplies

- Occlusive towel drape
- Cotton balls
- Cotton-tipped applicators
- Prep solution labeled safe for use around the ear
- Prep towels

TECHNIQUE

1. Use a sterile plastic drape to exclude the eye on the affected side.
2. Exclude the hair using sterile plastic drapes or cloth towels secured with tape.
3. Place absorbent cotton in the external ear canal.
4. Cleanse the folds of the pinna (external ear) with cotton-tipped applicators.
5. Extend the prep area with sponges to the edge of the hairline, face, and jaw.
6. Remove the absorbent cotton from the external ear canal.

FACE

Surgery of the face may be performed as a reconstructive procedure, following trauma, or as an elective cosmetic procedure. Female patients are advised to remove all makeup before elective surgery. Any residual products should be removed because they can interfere with the antiseptic properties of the prep and may contaminate the surgical wound. Trauma procedures may require debridement and removal of embedded foreign material as part of the prep or just before it with the patient under sedation. In all cases, an antiseptic solution that is safe around the eyes is ordered by the surgeon. Only nonalcohol solutions are used.

The hair contains a high concentration of bacteria and is a contaminated area. Therefore, the hairline must be completely excluded from the prep and draping area. If the patient has long hair, it must be excluded using elastic bands (not metal hair pins) or nonalcohol water-soluble gel to hold it away from the face.

Supplies

- Nonalcohol prep solution (e.g., dilute povidone-iodine)
- Warm normal saline
- Cotton swabs
- Cotton-tipped applicators
- Towels
- Nonsterile comb and water-soluble hair gel

NOTE: Any prep sponge that touches the hairline must be discarded. Rinse the skin with cotton swabs dipped in warm normal saline solution.

TECHNIQUE

1. Use elastic bands as necessary to separate and contain hair strands away from the face and ears.
2. One or more occlusive towel drapes is placed at the hairline. The surgeon may require a cap or towel placed over the hair and secured with tape.
3. The prep includes the neck or chin upward to the hairline. The ears may be included in the face prep as ordered.
4. Place absorbent cotton at the external ear canal. Cleanse the folds of the pinna using cotton-tipped applicators. Do not allow prep solution to drain into the ear canal.
5. Prep the face from the incision area outward. Prep the incision site again with fresh sponges.

NECK

The neck and throat area is prepared for thyroid surgery, tracheotomy, carotid artery surgery, lymph node biopsy, or radical dissection of the mandible, shoulder plexus, and mediastinum. If radical dissection is anticipated or scheduled, the prep area extends from the chin to the nipple line or waist and around the side of the body to the operating table on each side (Figure 20-4).

TECHNIQUE

1. Place sterile towels at the periphery of the prep site.
2. An occlusive towel drape may be placed at the upper boundaries of the prep to exclude the face and airway.
3. Begin the prep at the incision site, applying prep solution in a circular motion to the periphery of the site.

BREAST

The boundary of the prep area for breast surgery depends on the extent of the surgery and the patient's position. The prep area for radical breast surgery extends from the chin to the umbilicus and includes the lateral thorax on each side.

When the surgery involves removal of a mass without the possibility of more extensive surgery, the breast is prepped from the clavicle to the midthorax and from the midline, including the sides of the thorax to the operating table on the affected side. The prep area is extended into the axilla for lesions in the upper lateral quadrant of the breast.

Surgery that includes both biopsy of a mass and the possibility of mastectomy requires a much wider prep area. A radical mastectomy requires a prep boundary that encompasses the neck, shoulder of the affected side, thorax to the operating table surface, and midpelvic region (Figure 20-5).

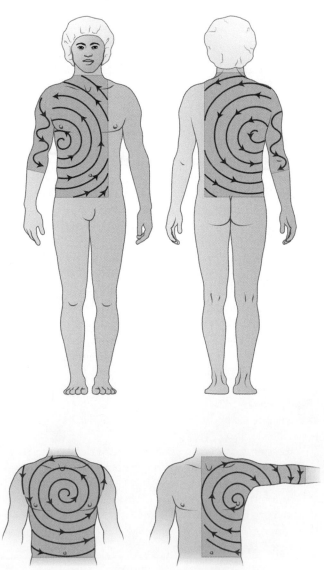

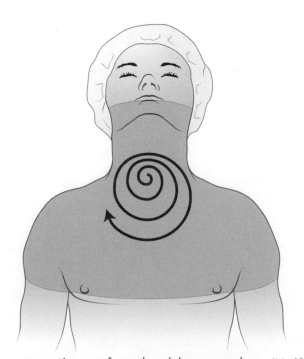

Figure 20-4 **Skin prep for neck and throat procedures.** (*Modified from Phillips N: Berry and Kohn's operating room technique, ed 10, St Louis, 2004, Mosby.*)

Figure 20-5 **Skin prep for the breast and thorax.** (*Modified from Phillips N: Berry and Kohn's operating room technique, ed 10, St Louis, 2004, Mosby.*)

In patients who have undergone an image-guided needle location procedure, great care is taken not to dislodge the needle, which is used to guide tissue excision during surgery.

Tissue that is suspected of being cancerous must be prepared gently. The area should be painted with as little friction and pressure as possible to prevent tumor cells from migrating into surrounding tissue. Skin prep for surgery of the thoracic cavity uses a bilateral extension of the boundaries for radical breast surgery.

TECHNIQUE

1. Square the prep boundary with sterile towels.
2. If the umbilicus is included in the prep, clean it with cotton-tipped applicators.
3. Prep the operative area, starting at the incision site.
4. If the shoulder is included in the prep, an assistant should abduct the arm so that solution can be applied circumferentially.

SHOULDER

The shoulder prep includes the neck, shoulder, upper arm, and scapula on the affected side (Figure 20-6). One assistant is required to elevate the patient's arm. The subscapular and midback areas also may be elevated on a pad.

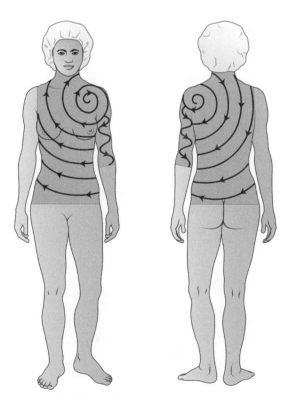

Figure 20-6 **Shoulder prep.** *(Modified from Phillips N: Berry and Kohn's operating room technique, ed 10, St Louis, 2004, Mosby.)*

TECHNIQUE

1. Remove the patient's gown to the umbilicus.
2. Place sterile prep towels at the periphery of the prep area.
3. Place an impervious sheet between the operating table and the subscapular area.
4. Have a gloved assistant elevate the arm.
5. The hand may be excluded from the prep. Some surgeons wrap the hand in an occlusive drape after the prep.
6. Do not pull the patient's shoulder laterally to expose the scapular area. This can cause injury. Seek guidance from the surgeon about the exact nature of the injury or repair to prevent damage.
7. Begin the prep at the incision site and extend it to the periphery.

ARM

Depending on the incision site, the arm is prepped in total or in one section. If a nerve block anesthesia will be performed, the entire arm usually is prepped. The hand is normally laden with transient and resident bacteria. It may be prepped but then excluded from the operative site by an occlusive drape. If the operative site is on the forearm, the prep extends several inches above the elbow.

In all cases, the arm or hand is prepped circumferentially. An assistant supports the arm and hand while another person performs the prep. If a pneumatic tourniquet is in use, it is important to prevent prep solutions from becoming trapped between the tourniquet and the patient's skin.

TECHNIQUE

1. Elevate the arm carefully, keeping it in anatomical alignment.
2. Place an impervious sheet under the arm, covering the operating table and the patient's torso.
3. Place sterile towels at the periphery of the prep site and under the shoulder. Towels are not required for hand prep.
4. Begin the prep at the incision site and move to the periphery.
5. When the prepped area is dry, remove the impervious sheet.
6. Continue to elevate the arm during draping.

HAND

Large colonies of resident and nonresident bacteria are present on the hand. The subungual area (under the nails) may contain debris and nonresident bacteria, requiring more thorough cleansing. The routine hand prep begins at the fingernails. A nail cleaner is used to cleanse the subungual area. After the hand is cleaned, prep solution is applied as usual, beginning at the incision site and moving outward and circumferentially. The upper boundary is a few inches above the elbow. If Bier block anesthesia is used, an upper arm prep is required to the level of the tourniquet.

Supplies

- Nail cleaner
- Scrub brush
- Impervious sheet
- Sterile gloves

TECHNIQUE

1. Elevate the hand carefully, keeping it in anatomical alignment.
2. Place an impervious sheet under the arm and hand.
3. Clean the subungual areas with a nail cleaner or soft brush.
4. Beginning at the incisional area, prep the hand in the usual manner, moving outward. Include the interdigital spaces, fingertips, and all four sides of each finger.
5. Extend the prep to the arm, covering all sides.
6. Blot excess antiseptic soap and paint with antiseptic solution.
7. Remove the impervious drape.
8. Support the hand until draping begins and the surgeon takes control of it.

ABDOMEN

The abdominal prep extends from the nipple line to midthigh and both sides of the body to the operating table (Figure 20-7). If a pelvic laparoscopy is planned, a vaginal prep may be included, and two separate preps are necessary.

TECHNIQUE

1. Square the abdomen with sterile towels. The upper towel is placed at the nipple line and the lower towel at the pubis.
2. Begin the prep at the umbilicus. Cleanse the umbilicus using cotton-tipped applicators dipped in prep solution to remove detritus (loose dead skin).
3. Prep the abdomen, starting at the incision site and moving to the periphery.
4. If soap solution is used, blot dry and apply prepping solution. Allow the prep solution to dry before applying drapes.

FLANK OR BACK

The flank and back areas are prepped in the same manner as the abdomen, starting at the incision site and moving outward. The sides of the body are prepped to the operating table. The back prep extends from the neck to the sacrum.

TECHNIQUE

1. Square the periphery of the prep site with sterile towels.
2. Begin at the incision area and apply prep solution in a circular pattern, continuing to the periphery. Complete this pattern at least twice, beginning again at the incision site and working outward to the surface of the operating table.

VAGINA

The vaginal prep is performed with the patient in the lithotomy position. After positioning, the lower table break is flexed downward. Before beginning the prep, place the kick bucket at the foot of the table to catch prep solution and used sponges.

An impervious drape is placed under the buttocks to prevent prep solution from seeping between the coccyx and the table. If a single impervious sheet is used, place the tail of the sheet in the kick bucket to drain excess prep solution. A perineal barrier drape with a self-adherent edge is placed across the perineum between the vagina and anus. This is done to prevent prep solution from seeping into the gluteal cleft. Place a prep towel above the pubis.

The vaginal prep is performed in two stages. The pelvis, labia, perineum, anus, and thighs are prepped first as one stage, and the vagina is prepped separately (Figure 20-8). Sponge forceps are used to prep the vaginal vault. The rationale for the two-step procedure is to ensure that bacteria from the external genitalia and perineum are not introduced into the vagina.

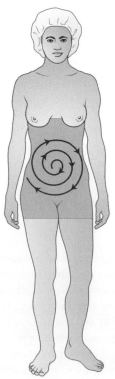

Figure 20-7 **Abdominal prep.** *(Redrawn from Phillips N: Berry and Kohn's operating room technique, ed 10, St Louis, 2004, Mosby.)*

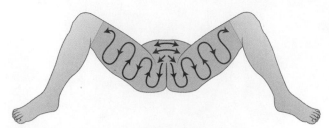

Figure 20-8 **Vaginal prep.** *(Redrawn from Phillips N: Berry and Kohn's operating room technique, ed 10, St Louis, 2004, Mosby.)*

NOTE: For combined abdominal-vaginal procedures, such as pelvic laparoscopy, the vaginal prep is done first, followed by the abdominal prep.

TECHNIQUE

1. Start the pelvic prep at the pubis, using back-and-forth strokes. This area is prepped to the level of the iliac crest.
2. Apply prep solution at the labia majora, using downward strokes only and including the perineum and anus. Discard the sponge after the anus is prepped. Do not return to the area previously prepped.
3. Using clean sponges, prep the inner aspects of the thighs. Start at the labia majora and move laterally, using back-and-forth strokes. Discard the sponge as it reaches the periphery.
4. Prep the vaginal vault last. Use sponges mounted on forceps and ample prep solution to reach the folds of the vaginal rugae. Discard the sponge and repeat.
5. Use a dry-mounted sponge to blot excess fluid from the vaginal vault and remaining prep area.

PENIS AND SCROTUM

Surgery of the male genitalia requires skin preparation of the penis, scrotum, upper legs, and inguinal areas. Minor procedures may require only prep of the penis and scrotum, excluding the peripheral areas. The patient is prepped in supine position.

Supplies

- Nonalcohol prep solution, sterile saline, or water
- Cotton balls
- Sponge forceps
- Sponges preimpregnated with prep solution or plain sponges.

TECHNIQUE

1. Place absorbent sterile towels on each side of the hips and under the scrotum. A barrier drape should be placed over the towel to prevent prep solution from seeping underneath the scrotum or legs.
2. If the patient has not been circumcised, the foreskin is retracted. The prep begins at the glans.
3. Using soft sponges or cotton balls and forceps, prep the external urethral meatus first and then extend the prep to the circumference of the penis to the base. This step is repeated with fresh cotton balls. Once the penis has been prepped, replace the foreskin to its normal position.
4. Prep the scrotum, ensuring that prep solution enters all folds and skin crevices.
5. The thighs and inguinal area are prepped beginning at each side of the groin, moving outward. The pelvis is prepped separately, beginning at the lower margin of the pubic bone and extending to the iliac crest bilaterally.

PERIANAL AREA

The perianal prep is performed with the patient in the prone position with a midpelvis break in the operating table. Because the anus is a contaminated area, the surrounding area is prepped first and the anus last. The anus is exposed by separating the buttocks with wide adhesive tape.

TECHNIQUE

1. Remove the patient's gown and the cover sheet to expose the lower trunk. Keep the patient's legs and upper body covered.
2. Begin the prep outside the anal mucosa and extend the prep area outward about 12 inches (30 cm) in all directions.
3. Prep the outer anus. In some institutions, the anal prep is omitted.

NOTE: For abdominoperineal resection, the patient is placed in the lithotomy position. The technique requires separate abdominal and perineal preps.

LEG AND FOOT

The leg prep is similar to that of the arm. The prep extends from the ankle to the groin (Figure 20-9). The limb must be elevated by an assistant or placed in a vertical leg holder attached to the operating table. Use a leg holder with extreme caution, because it can cause serious injuries. If the leg holder is not strong enough to support the leg of a heavy patient, it

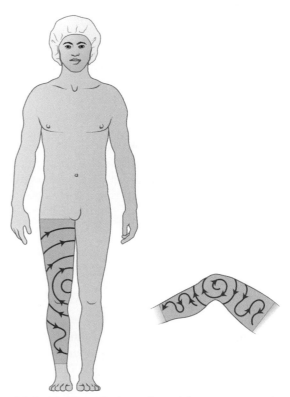

Figure 20-9 **Leg prep.** *(Redrawn from Phillips N: Berry and Kohn's operating room technique, ed 10, St Louis, 2004, Mosby.)*

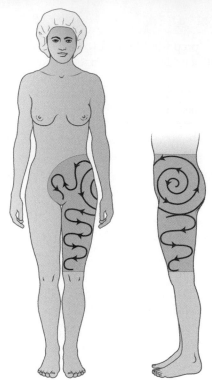

Figure 20-10   Hip prep. *(Redrawn from Phillips N: Berry and Kohn's operating room technique, ed 10, St Louis, 2004, Mosby.)*

can rotate or slip, causing injury. For knee surgery, the entire leg is prepped and the foot is wrapped in a separate drape. If a pneumatic tourniquet is in place, prevent prep solutions from seeping under the tourniquet cuff.

Hip surgery requires a circumferential prep from the midcalf to the iliac crest, excluding the groin (Figure 20-10).

TECHNIQUE

1. Place a towel between the groin and the fold of the upper leg.
2. Elevate the leg.
3. Place an impervious sheet over the operating table and the patient's nonoperative leg.
4. If the foot is to be included in the prep, scrub it as you would a hand. Remember that because the leg is elevated, the prep must begin at the highest level and move to the lowest level.
5. If the foot is excluded from the prep, perform wide skin prep around the operative site.

 Watch Section 3: Unit 4: Patient Prep on the Evolve website. http://evolve.elsevier.com/Fuller/surgical

TRAUMA AND DEBRIDEMENT

Trauma wounds are almost always contaminated because they are caused by external forces and often occur in environments that are mildly or grossly contaminated. These wounds are usually prepped by the surgeon. Penetrating traumatic wounds may contain small pieces of bone and foreign material that must be removed from the wound. A pressurized water system may be used to clean the wound with the patient under

sedation. This requires specialized drapes with drain pockets to collect and drain runoff solution. During the cleansing process, the surgeon removes all foreign material and trims away devitalized tissue (called **debridement**). Preliminary debridement is performed on a stable patient and takes place in the emergency department or in a separate treatment room to prevent gross contamination of the surgical environment. All tissue and foreign material are retained as specimens. After debridement, the wound can be prepped and draped. The prep area for traumatic wounds is larger than normal, and the draping procedure is usually led by the surgeon.

Debridement is used not only for wounds that are contaminated with foreign material, but also for infected wounds, including pressure sores and other chronic conditions resulting in dead tissue in and around the wound. If debridement is performed in the operating room, a minor plastic surgery set is needed. This includes several surgical blades of different sizes (15, 20, and possibly 11), plastic surgery scissors, and toothed pickups. An infected wound is usually cultured at the time of surgery (refer to Chapter 9 for details).

AUTOGRAFT

A tissue autograft is a graft that is removed from one site on the patient and grafted to another site. This requires two separate preps. Clear prep solutions are used on the donor site, especially for skin grafts. This is necessary to maintain a clear view of the vascular bed of the graft. It is important to maintain an aseptic barrier between the donor and recipient sites when grafting is performed in a contaminated or open wound.

CARDIOVASCULAR SURGERY

Cardiac and vascular surgery require a large area of exposure. In cardiac cases in which a saphenous graft is taken from the legs, a complete body prep is necessary, including the full circumference of the legs bilaterally. The feet may be excluded from the surgical site after full prep. The groin may also be excluded in the draping process. However, access to the deep femoral veins requires a full prep of the inguinal area.

In all cases requiring full body prep it is necessary to prepare the environment and solutions used on the patient to prevent hypothermia during the procedure. Prep solutions (saline and water), if used, are warmed in an approved device. Do not warm antiseptic solutions, because this can alter their effect. The operating room temperature must be monitored to ensure a normothermic environment. This is the joint responsibility of the circulator and anesthesiologist, who continually monitor the patient's core temperature.

DRAPING THE SURGICAL SITE

PRINCIPLES

Draping is performed immediately after the skin prep. The purpose of draping is to provide a wide sterile area around the surgical site. Drapes act as a barrier surface between nonsterile objects and the sterile field. They allow the sterile team to work in relative freedom without risk of contaminating the wound.

Once the patient is draped, the center of the sterile field is defined. Draped tables and equipment are moved into position close to the patient, and scrubbed team members work within the sterile area.

LEARNING TO DRAPE

Draping the surgical patient is one of the more difficult skills for surgical technologists to master. The principles of draping are not difficult to understand. However, the actual handling of drapes while maintaining aseptic technique sometimes is problematic. Drapes are folded in a specific way before sterilization so that they can be positioned over the operative site and unfolded in a way that prevents contamination. The orientation of the drape as it is first placed over the incision site is critical because once it is placed, it cannot be moved again without contaminating the site (which has just been prepped). To make the process more difficult, there are many variations on basic draping materials based on slightly different designs. However, all drapes and all draping procedures are based on the same principles. Understanding these principles can help clarify the practice.

DRAPING FABRICS AND MATERIALS

Drapes are large sheets of impervious material or bonded fabric, designed to fit the contours of the body and provide a large sterile surface that is both a barrier against the nonsurgical areas of the patient's body underneath and a large sterile surface on which to work (the top side of the drape). One area of the drape is cut out to accommodate the surgical wound or incision site. This is called the *fenestration* (window) of the drape. In order to accommodate different parts of the body, some drapes contain a U-shaped cutout instead of a window. The U portion is used to fit around the arm or leg. Other specialty drapes have windows that are more specific to specialty surgery, such as eye and ear drapes, which have much smaller fenestrations than an abdominal drape.

Drapes are available in all sizes and configurations. The draping routine for a surgical procedure is a *process*. Drapes are applied in layers, in a specific order around and over the surgical site using aseptic technique.

Drapes are made of woven material (cotton or cotton-synthetic blend) or nonwoven material (bonded synthetics). Sterile drapes must create a moisture barrier between the patient and the sterile field.

Nonwoven drapes are made from spun synthetic polymers as disposable, single-use items. They are impervious to moisture and breathable to prevent the patient from becoming hyperthermic. Many different types of nonwoven draping materials are available for specific uses and types of surgery.

Woven drapes are made of sewn cotton and synthetic cloth. This type of drape has become much less common than in the past because synthetic single-use materials have become more popular. Woven cloth drapes are reinforced around the fenestration and chemically treated for moisture resistance to prevent strike-through contamination. They are more pliable and easier to handle than synthetic drapes but require laundering, repair, and sterilization. This reprocessing may be more costly than single-use materials. However, the environmental impact may be less. Woven drapes must be carefully inspected for tears, holes, and fraying, which may become sources of contamination. Because the fabric is not waterproof, extra precautions, such as increased layers, are needed to prevent penetration with irrigation solutions, blood, and tissue debris during surgery.

Surgical *towels* are standard on all surgical setups. In addition to their use as towels, they are an integral part of most draping procedures. The surgical towel is soft, pliable, and very absorbent. Their primary use in draping is to "frame" the incision site and create the base layer for the larger drapes, which are placed over them. In the past, towel clamps were used to grasp the inside corners of the frame to keep the entire construction from sliding away from the operative site. These needlepoint clamps were also placed through the skin. This technique is no longer practiced.

TECHNIQUES USED IN DRAPING

1. Layering begins with a plain sheet, half-sheet, or body sheet. In upper body surgery, this is used to cover the patient's legs and lower torso. The plain sheet may also be called a half-sheet or cover sheet.
2. Surgical towels made of heavy absorbent cloth are used to make a frame around the incision site. Towels are folded along one edge before they are positioned on the patient. *Framing* the incision means providing a fenestration in the drapes for the incision. The fenestration can be square, oblong, or oval if a disposable **fenestrated drape** is used.
3. Plastic drapes and towels are used to cover the patient's skin and are used in many different applications. The towel drape, also called a *sticky drape,* is a sheet of smooth plastic or bonded draping material with one adhesive edge. The towel drape is commonly used to exclude an area from the prep. For example, during the skin prep for eye surgery, a towel drape can be applied to prevent prep solution from draining into the patient's ear on the affected side.
4. The plastic **incise drape** (Figure 20-11) is commonly placed over the entire surgical site on top of the towels and any bottom sheets and towels that form the fenestration. The sterile incise drape is coated with adhesive on one side and may be impregnated with iodophor. The drape is packaged with a paper backing on the adhesive side. The whole drape, including paper backing, is then folded lengthwise and contained in a plastic sleeve wrapping. During draping, the paper backing is peeled away while the drape is applied. This is done in a way that prevents the drape from tangling and sticking to itself. The surgical technologist and surgeon usually apply the drape together.
5. The last drape to be applied is the top drape, also called a *procedure* or *specialty drape.* Drapes are fan-folded to be compact and allow convenient unfolding over the patient. The folded drape must be positioned over the surgical site correctly before it is unfolded. It cannot be shifted once it is positioned; therefore, it must be correct the first time. The fenestration is centered over the incision site, and the

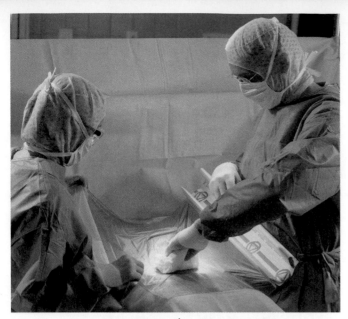

Figure 20-11   Incise drape. *(Courtesy 3M.)*

drape is unfolded over the patient's body. Many different specialty drapes are available (Figure 20-12). Printed directions are located on the edge of the fenestration for correct orientation.

ASEPTIC TECHNIQUE DURING DRAPING

The rules of asepsis are followed throughout all draping procedures. When draping, visualize the drape as having two surfaces or sides. One side is in direct contact with the patient and other nonsterile surfaces. The other side can contact only other sterile surfaces, such as the gloved hand or sterile instruments. This principle follows the rules of asepsis.

The following guidelines support the principles of asepsis and safety during draping:

- Handle drapes with as little movement as possible. This reduces the risk of contamination and prevents release of airborne particles that can become vehicles for bacteria.
- When placing a drape, do not touch the patient's body or any other nonsterile surface. Remain a safe distance from the patient to avoid contamination of your gown.
- After a drape has been placed, do not shift or move it. To protect the gloved hand during draping with flat sheets, grasp the edge of the sterile sheet and roll your hand inward. This forms a cuff. Position the drape and release the edge of the cuff, keeping your hands on the sterile side of the drape or towel.
- Use only nonpenetrating towel clamps for securing drapes. A hole in a drape creates a passageway for bacteria to contaminate the sterile field. When drapes are stapled to the patient's skin, the stapled area should be covered by an impervious (plastic) drape.
- To pass four towel drapes for framing the incision, fold down the top edge about 4 inches. Present the first three folded towels by grasping the top corners with both hands and the folded sides facing away from the surgeon. The

fourth towel is passed with the fold facing the surgeon. Adhesive towels are usually passed with the adhesive side facing away from the surgeon. After the surgeon has grasped the top edge, peel away the adhesive backing.
- After a drape has been placed, any portion that falls below the edge of the operating table is considered contaminated. If an area of the drape is suspected of being contaminated, the area may be covered with another impervious drape.
- After a drape has been placed, the edges are considered nonsterile.
- Do not reach over the prepped surgical site to place a towel or drape. Instead, move around the table to position yourself.
- Strike-through contamination occurs when a drape becomes soaked during surgery and solution penetrates to a nonsterile surface. Whenever possible, use only impervious drapes.
- Drapes fitted with a pocket reservoir and drainage system are used for cases in which extensive fluids or bleeding may cause strike-through contamination.
- Aluminum-coated drapes are used whenever laser surgery is planned. These deflect laser energy and prevent ignition in an oxygen-rich environment, especially in head and neck surgery.
- Plan ahead for draping. Verify the surgeon's procedure at the start of the case and stack drapes on the back table in reverse order of application. Have extra sterile towels and sheets available.

DRAPING TECHNIQUES OF THE SURGICAL SITE

ABDOMEN

The procedure for draping the abdomen can be used to drape many other surgical sites (Figure 20-13).

TECHNIQUE

1. Place a plain sheet over the patient's legs.
2. Place four towels (folded cloth, disposable nonwoven material) in a square to frame the operative site. These may be held in place with nonpenetrating towel clamps.
3. A plastic (adhesive) incise drape may be applied over the towels. Two people are required to perform this step. One person holds one end of the drape while the other pulls the paper backing away.
4. Smooth the plastic drape over the contours of the patient's skin.
5. Center a fenestrated body drape over the incision site and unfold it to provide a sterile field.

LITHOTOMY (PERINEAL) DRAPING

Lithotomy, or perineal, draping is used for gynecological surgery, transperineal surgery of the prostate, and combined abdominal-perineal resection of the colon (Figure 20-14). In most cases the anus is excluded from the surgical site with a

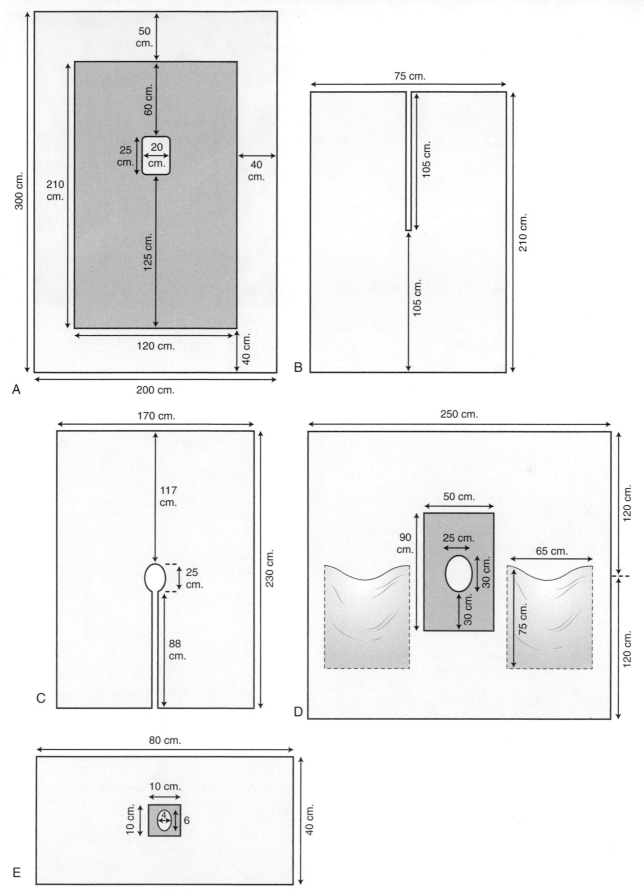

Figure 20-12 **Specialty or "top" drapes. A,** Laparotomy drape. **B,** Split sheet. **C,** Craniotomy drape. **D,** Lithotomy drape (leggings for draping stirrups included). **E,** Eye or ear drape.

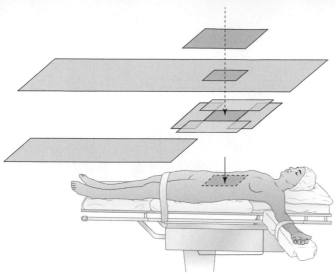

Figure 20-13 Basic draping layers shown in order of placement starting at the patient and moving upward on the figure. The first drape to be placed is the half-sheet (also called bottom sheet or plain sheet). Next, four surgical towels frame the incision site. The first towel to be placed is the one closest to the person placing it. The next layer is the procedure drape with fenestration (opening) placed directly over the exposed area created by the towels. Last to be placed is the transparent incise drape, which is self-adhereing on the skin side. This stabilizes the top drape. This drape may be omitted and skin staples used to hold the towels in place.

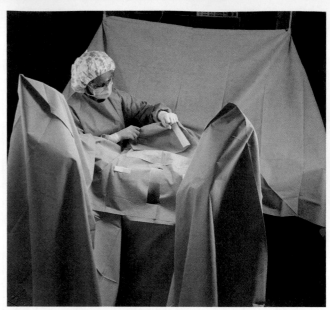

Figure 20-14   Lithotomy draping. *(Copyright Kimberly-Clark Worldwide, Inc. Used with permission.)*

barrier drape. An impervious drape is tucked under the patient's buttocks to begin draping. The bottom edge of this drape may be placed in the kick bucket to collect runoff fluids. Alternatively, a drainage bag drape may be used for this purpose.

TECHNIQUE

1. For gynecological surgery, a barrier is necessary between the anus and the vulva. Apply an adhesive towel across the perineum midway between the vulva and anus.
2. Use leggings to cover the patient's legs in stirrups (or the perineal drape may have inserts that extend over the stirrups and the patient's legs).
3. Center a fenestrated body sheet over the perineal area and extend it upward over the patient's abdomen and upper body. Secure the top to the anesthesia screen.

LEG

When draping the leg, the foot is excluded from the surgical site by wrapping it in a towel and then covering it with a tube drape (tube stockinet). The limb must be held up and away from the operating table while the stockinet is applied. With the limb suspended, a sterile impervious sheet is placed directly beneath the limb.

NOTE: *Chapter 17 contains a complete discussion of the pneumatic tourniquet, which is applied above (proximal to) the surgical wound site in limb surgery.*

TECHNIQUE

1. A towel is wrapped around the pneumatic tourniquet.
2. Place a rolled stockinet over the foot or hand and unroll it to cover the limb.
3. Secure a split drape around the proximal (upper) part of the limb.
4. Apply a fenestrated drape to complete the surgical field.

HAND OR ARM

Hand procedures are performed with the surgeon and assistant seated.

TECHNIQUE

1. After the skin prep, suspend the hand and forearm while the first drape is placed on the surgical arm board.
2. Use a towel to wrap the proximal arm and cover the pneumatic tourniquet.
3. A tube stockinet may be used to cover the arm.
4. Position a split sheet with the tails draped toward the patient's hand.
5. Place the arm through a fenestrated sheet and complete the sterile field (Figure 20-15).

SHOULDER

The shoulder is draped with the patient in beach chair (Fowler's) position. The arm is suspended away from the body with the hand and lower arm excluded from the surgical site. The arm is draped free so that it can be manipulated during surgery (Figure 20-16).

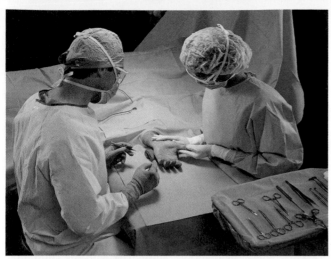

Figure 20-15 **Completed draping for the hand and upper arm.** The surgeon and assistant or surgical technologist are seated during hand surgery. *(Copyright Kimberly-Clark Worldwide, Inc. Used with permission.)*

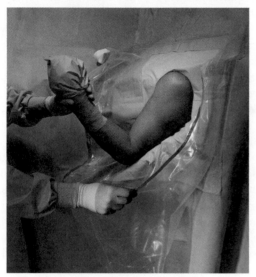

Figure 20-16 **Shoulder draping.** Note that the arm is draped free for manipulation during surgery. *(Copyright Kimberly-Clark Worldwide, Inc. Used with permission.)*

TECHNIQUE

1. Place an impervious drape between the upper torso and shoulder and the operating table.
2. Position a body or half-sheet over the torso.
3. The hand and lower arm may be occluded with towels and a stockinet applied over the arm. This may be secured with an impervious drape.
4. Use towels to frame the shoulder and cover them with an incise drape.
5. Apply a split drape.
6. Place the arm and shoulder through a fenestrated sheet.

Watch Section 3: Unit 5: Draping on the Evolve website. http://evolve.elsevier.com/Fuller/surgical

HEAD DRAPE

The **head drape** occasionally is used for nose and throat procedures to maintain a sterile barrier between the face and the

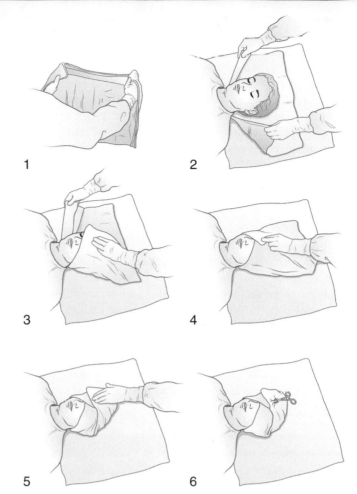

Figure 20-17 Application of a head drape, which is used to protect the eyes during nasal and oromaxillofacial surgery.

head. The head drape is created with two towels or plain draping sheets. The head is slightly elevated and both towels are placed under the patient's head, as shown in Figure 20-17. Each corner of the uppermost towel is brought to the center over the hairline and secured with a nonpenetrating towel clamp.

CRANIOTOMY

Draping for a cranial procedure is similar to that for other routines that require a large body sheet with a fenestration. Cranial access usually is obtained with the patient in the prone position using a Mayfield headrest or in beach chair (Fowler's) position. This allows the anesthesia care provider access to the patient's airway while providing access to the cranium.

TECHNIQUE

1. Position a body sheet at the neck and extend it to the legs.
2. Apply surgical draping towels to square the incision site. These may be secured to the scalp with skin staples.
3. An incise drape may be positioned on the scalp.
4. Center a large fenestrated procedure drape over the incision site and open it to cover the patient fully.

HOW TO DRAPE EQUIPMENT

Large equipment, such as the operating microscope, C-arm, and robotic equipment used within the sterile field, is draped before surgery. Most equipment drapes are designed to fit with cutouts and ample material to allow smooth draping. Adhesive strips and drape openings are imprinted with arrows and directions. The circulator assists during equipment draping by grasping the periphery of the drape and pulling it into place (the edge of a sterile drape is not considered sterile).

When the operating microscope is to be used right away during a case, it is draped before the patient prep. If it will not be used for an hour or more after the case begins, it can be draped during the procedure.

The single-use microscope drape is a continuous plastic sleeve that is fan-folded for easy application. The drape has "pockets" that cover the protruding parts of the scope. The scrub starts the draping. The circulator assists by pulling the drape down by holding the bottom portion, which will be outside the sterile field after the drape is in place. The ocular portions and optics of the microscope are not covered. The drape is secured over the lenses with sterile caps. After the drape is in place, it is loosely bound to the body of the microscope with adherent tapes that are an integral part of the drape itself.

REMOVING DRAPES

At the close of a procedure, all instruments and equipment are removed from the top drape, including the sterile sections of power cords, air hoses, and other devices that might become tangled in drapes as they are removed. One member of the sterile team holds any dressings in place while the drapes are slowly removed. When removing drapes, pull them away from the patient, starting at the patient's head, and proceeding to the feet.

Remove one layer at a time. Be sure not to dislodge any wound drains. Drapes should be contained with as little movement as possible, with the ends wrapped or rolled toward the inside, to confine blood and body fluids in the middle of the drape. The drapes are placed in a designated biohazard bag. No drapes are removed from the room until the final sponge, needle, and instrument count has been verified.

After removing the drapes, the circulator examines the prep area to assess the condition of the patient's skin and rule out a chemical burn.

KEY CONCEPTS

- The surgical prep and draping process follows specific standards, which have been set by the Centers for Disease Control and Prevention in coordination with other professional agencies. The primary focus of practice relates to shaving the skin before surgery and the use of specific antiseptics to perform the skin prep.
- It is not possible to sterilize the skin because it is living tissue. Skin and mucous membranes harbor resident bacteria beneficial to the immune system and nonresident

flora, which are potential causes of surgical site infection. Before surgery the incision site must be made as clean as possible to reduce the risk of postoperative infection.

- The materials needed for urinary catheterization must be assembled before the procedure and maintained on a small sterile field during the process. The exact type and size of catheter system is determined by the age and gender of the patient and surgeon's orders.
- Some surgical procedures require decompression of the bladder or intraoperative monitoring of urinary output. In these cases urinary catheterization is performed just before or during the surgical skin prep. Patient safety and risks associated with catheterization include injury to the urethra, damage to the sphincter muscle, and urinary tract infection. Prevention of these outcomes requires thorough knowledge of the anatomy, familiarity with the equipment used, and strict aseptic technique.
- Hair is not removed from the surgical site unless there is no possible way to exclude it from the surgical wound.
- It is required practice for the surgeon to mark the skin site of the incision before surgery. This documents the correct side, and location of the incision for comparison with the patient records and prevents wrong site surgery. These marks must be preserved during the skin prep.
- Drugs approved as antiseptics are labeled for use on skin. However, not all antiseptics can be used on all surface tissue or mucous membranes. Labeling includes warnings and contraindications that clearly indicate the safe and unsafe use of the antiseptic.
- Supplies for the skin prep include the prescribed antiseptic, sterile towels, and gloves and may include other items such as cotton balls, cotton-tipped applicators, or scrub sponges according to the type of prep.
- When the skin is prepped correctly, the area is antiseptically cleaned from the center of the incisional site to the periphery. Application of prep antiseptic in a spiral or circular pattern is used to prevent microbes from an unprepped area from contacting an area that has been prepped.
- Elements of the skin prep include obtaining and setting up sterile supplies, draping the prep site, and applying prep solution according to standards of practice. Specific details that may not be standard are prescribed by the surgeon.
- Skin burning and blistering occur when prep solution is not prevented from pooling between the patient's skin and operating table surface. This is prevented by placing sterile towels at the periphery of the prep area and making a conscious effort to prevent the solution from pooling on the skin.
- Surgical drapes are put in place after the prep antiseptic has dried thoroughly. The drape forms a sterile covering over the patient's body, leaving the incision site open through an opening in the drape. Drapes extend far beyond the incisional site so that sterile equipment, instruments, and the sterile team members have freedom of movement within the sterile field.
- Elements of the draping technique include preparation of the sterile drapes on the back table, delivering the drapes

to the surgeon in the correct order, assisting in correct placement of each drape, and maintaining sterility.

- Draping is a sterile process that is performed according to the rules of aseptic technique. It is important to remember the sterile boundaries that are consistent with any sterile surface. If a drape becomes contaminated within the sterile boundary during its placement, it must be discarded and a new sterile drape obtained. Likewise, if the sterile gloved hand comes in contact with a nonsterile surface, the glove must be changed.
- Drapes are removed at the close of surgery in a particular way to prevent contamination of the incision side and to contain blood and body fluids.

REVIEW QUESTIONS

1. Describe the risks of urinary catheterization.
2. Why is continuous urinary drainage required during surgery?
3. Explain how to maintain sterility while inserting the catheter.
4. Explain the rationale for the surgical skin prep.
5. During the skin prep for a contaminated region, the area of highest contamination is prepped last. Why is this?
6. What is the rationale for surgical draping?
7. What is the purpose of aluminum-coated drapes?
8. What parts of a drape are considered nonsterile after the drape is in place?
9. What techniques are used to prevent contamination of the gloved hand while draping the patient?

CASE STUDIES

Case 1

You are assisting in the circulator role and have been asked to perform the patient skin prep for a laparoscopy. When you expose the surgical site to begin the prep you see that a body piercing stud is imbedded in the patient's umbilicus. You do not see any wire or post attached to the stud. You have not encountered this type of body-piercing jewelry before and are unable to ascertain how to remove it safely. The patient has already been anesthetized. Using skills and knowledge learned in this and other chapters, what is your course of action? Consider carefully patient safety with regard to electrosurgery, aseptic technique, legal issues, and care of the patient's property.

Case 2

You have been asked to catheterize a male patient who is about to undergo suprapubic prostate surgery. After prepping the patient, you advance the urinary catheter a short distance into the urethra and encounter resistance. You apply slightly more pressure but the catheter will not advance. You decide to remove the catheter to be safe. As you withdraw the catheter you see fresh blood on the catheter tip. How would you evaluate this situation? What is your course of action? Was the procedure performed correctly?

REFERENCE

1. Association of periOperative Registered Nurses (AORN): Fire safety in perioperative settings, *AORN Journal* 86:2141, 2007.

BIBLIOGRAPHY

Association of periOperative Registered Nurses (AORN): Recommended practices for hand antisepsis/hand-scrubs. In *Standards, recommended practices and guidelines*, Denver, 2011, AORN.

Association of periOperative Registered Nurses (AORN): Recommended practices for preoperative patient skin antisepsis. In *2011 perioperative standards and recommended practices*, Denver, 2011, AORN.

Gould C, Umscheid C, Agarwal R, et al: HICPAC: *Guideline for the prevention of catheter associated urinary tract infections 2009.* Accessed August 26, 2011, at http://www.cdc.gov/hicpac/cauti/009_cauti2009_References.html.

Healthcare Infection Control Practices Advisory Committee: Recommendations from the CDC guideline for hand hygiene in healthcare settings. Accessed May 5, 2012, at http://solutions.3m.com/3MContentRetrievalAPI/BlobServlet?locale=en_US&lmd=1329821112000&assetId=1114284208573&assetType=MMM_Image&blobAttribute=ImageFile.

21

Case Planning and Intraoperative Routines

LEARNING OBJECTIVES

After studying this chapter the reader will be able to:
1. List and define common terms used in surgical technique
2. Discuss the elements of a case plan
3. Explain the four types of surgery and questions you should ask yourself for planning the procedure
4. Discuss preoperative case preparation
5. Describe the steps of sterile and nonsterile case setups
6. Describe the correct procedure for performing a count
7. Discuss the guidelines for preventing lost and retained items
8. Define the purpose and procedure for Universal Protocol

9. Demonstrate instrument handling and passing techniques, including neutral zone (no-hands) technique
10. Discuss specimen management during a surgical procedure, including the consequences of losing, mislabeling, or misidentifying a specimen
11. Identify different types of specimens
12. Identify methods of caring for specimens both on the sterile field and in preparation for transport
13. Explain the role of the surgical technologist at the end of surgery

TERMINOLOGY

Biopsy: Removal of a sample of tissue for pathological analysis.
Blunt dissection: The technique of separating tissue layers by teasing them apart with a rough sponge dissector, blunt instrument, or manually.
Case planning: The process of organizing and implementing the tasks and equipment required for a surgical procedure.
Count: A systematic method of accounting for all sponges, needles, instruments, and other items that can be retained in the patient.
Dissecting sponge: A small compact sponge used to dissect soft tissue planes; also referred to as a sponge dissector. The dissecting sponge is always mounted on a clamp for use in the surgical wound.
Event related: An activity or process linked with an event.
Frozen section: A procedure in which a tissue specimen is flash frozen and sectioned for examination under the microscope. The procedure is used to verify suspected malignancy during surgery.
Graft: An implant used to replace or augment existing tissue. A graft may be obtained from the patient, another person, an animal source, or synthetic or biosynthetic materials.
Implant: Any medical device placed in the body with intention to be permanent or semipermanent. Examples include

orthopedic hardware (e.g., plates, screws, rods), synthetic grafts, internal cardiac pacemakers, molded silicone used in plastic and reconstructive surgery, and intraocular implants used in cataract surgery.
Radiopaque: Any object that is not penetrable by x-rays.
Raytec: A surgical sponge folded to 4 inches by 4 inches. The Raytec derives its name from one of the companies that manufacture surgical sponges.
Sponge stick: A 4- × 4-inch sponge folded and mounted on a sponge forceps for use deep in the body.
Sterile setup: The process of organizing and arranging sterile supplies and equipment before surgery.
Surgeon's preference card: A database or card system listing the methods, materials, and techniques used by each surgeon for specific procedures.
TIMEOUT: A procedure for verifying the patient's identity, correct surgical procedure, site, and side. TIMEOUT takes place after the patient has been positioned, prepped, and draped but before the first incision. The procedure is promoted by the Association of Surgical Technologists (AST) and described in detail by the Association of periOperative Registered Nurses (AORN) and the World Health Organization (WHO).

INTRODUCTION

The purpose of this chapter is to orient the surgical technologist to the flow of a surgical procedure from the time of preparation to the close of surgery. This chapter also presents a portion of the fundamental skill set required for surgical technologists in surgery. Patient care and safety skills such as positioning, skin prep, and draping have been covered in previous chapters. The skills described here mainly relate to equipment, supplies, and activities carried on *outside* management of the surgical wound. Topics that relate to wound management in the intraoperative period are discussed in the following chapter. Many activities require coordination between the scrub person, the circulator, and other team members. Table 21-1 lists the activities of the scrubbed surgical technologist, circulator, and surgeon. Because of the many different contexts in which the surgical technologist works, it is meant to be a guideline only. Some of the tasks vary according to the setting and scope of the technologist's role, which may vary among regions and facilities.

SURGICAL TECHNIQUES

Throughout the history of surgery, certain terms have been developed to describe the techniques used to apply instruments to the body. They are used frequently in surgery and will appear in textbooks such as this one. Surgical technologists should learn these basic terms because they are the common language of surgery used in every operating room. These terms are particularly important as an introduction to surgical procedures, as described in the text.

- *Amputate:* This term usually refers to the removal of a limb or digit. When referring to other body parts, the term *remove* or *surgical removal* is used—for example, "The tumor spread to the spleen, which required surgical removal."
- *Anastomose (v.), anastomosis (n.):* This refers to the joining of two hollow anatomical structures (vessels, ducts, tubes, or hollow organs) using sutures or surgical staples. For example, "An anastomosis was created between the distal jejunum and colon." An anastomosis is performed to restore continuity, usually after a section has been surgically removed. When the term is used, it is preceded by the anatomical structures involved—for example, an arteriovenous anastomosis (between an artery and vein).
- *Approximate:* In surgical terms this means to "bring together" tissues by suturing or other means. For example, "The skin edges are approximated using fine nylon sutures." We *approximate* bone fragments in a fracture, tissues (especially the edges), and edges of hollow ducts and vessels.
- **Blunt dissection:** Separation of tissue without using sharp instruments. Blunt dissection is used to tease apart delicate tissue layers using a dissecting sponge, which has a relatively rough surface. The fingers are also used in blunt dissection during open procedures to manually separate tissue bands or fibers when sharp dissection is unnecessary and would cause excessive bleeding.
- *Debridement:* The use of sharp surgical instruments such as a scalpel and scissors to cut away dead tissue or remove nontissue debris embedded in a wound. Water under pressure is also used for this purpose. Traumatic wounds generally needed debriding in order to heal properly. Debridement is also performed on infected wounds or pressure sores to remove any tissue that is not viable (able to survive).
- *Dog ear:* In suture technique, a dog ear refers to an undesirable pucker in skin as a result of poor suture placement. A dog ear must be corrected because the puckered edges do not heal and can lead to infection.
- *Debulk:* In cancer surgery, to debulk means to remove a large portion, but not all, of a tumor. This is done to relieve pressure on nearby tissues and slow down metastasis. A tumor may also be surgically debulked before chemotherapy or radiotherapy to enable a reduction in these treatment modalities.
- *Dissect:* This term means to carefully separate anatomical structures by cutting with instruments, small firm sponges, or the fingers. For example, surgery on the large blood vessels requires meticulous separation of the vessels away from the surrounding connective tissue. This is called dissection. Sharp dissection is performed with scissors, whereas blunt dissection is performed with the fingers or dissecting sponges mounted on a clamp.
- *Elevate:* To raise or lift an anatomical structure, sometimes without removing it. Occasionally during surgery, it is necessary to lift a structure using a retractor or other instrument in order to pass sutures or instruments underneath, or for better visualization. Instruments called *elevators* are often used to peel away superficial tissue. For example, a periosteal elevator is used to lift away a portion of the periosteum that covers the long bones of the body. This is necessary before cutting or separating the bone. Elevators used in neurosurgery are used for fine separation, but not for cutting neural tissue. In facial reconstruction, fine-tipped elevators are used to separate delicate tissue layers such as the nasal submucosa from underlying cartilage.
- *Excise:* An excision is the removal of tissue, usually a tumor, or other small lesion using cutting instruments or electrosurgery. For example, "The tumor was excised using scissors and a #15 scalpel blade." This term generally applies to small or superficial lesions. For example, moles and small skin tumors are excised, but lobes of the lung are *removed.*
- *Expose (v.), exposure (n.):* This means to enable precise viewing of an anatomical area. For example, a retractor is used to move or hold tissue aside so that other structures underneath can be *exposed.* During surgery, the surgeon may say, "I need better exposure here." This usually means better retraction in order to see the tissues deep in the surgical wound.
- *Exteriorize:* To bring a tissue structure partially outside the body. For example, during bowel surgery, a section of intestine might be temporarily brought out of the surgical wound (exteriorized) for suturing or other surgical maneuvers. During cesarean section, the uterus may be exteriorized briefly to repair the muscle incision.
- *Ligate:* To constrict by tying. The most common use of this term is ligation of blood vessels. However, one may also ligate a duct or tissue bundle containing blood vessels.

Table **21-1**	**Tasks and Duties of the Scrubbed Technologist Circulator, and Surgeon**	
Scrubbed Technologist	**Circulator/Assistant Circulator**	**Surgeon**
Before Surgery		
Receives case cart for surgery or selects individual items needed from instrument and supply rooms.	Positions the operating table and prepares foam pads and accessories according to the surgery.	Greets patient in holding area.
Assembles all items needed for surgery according to surgeon's case information.	Assembles needed equipment.	Orients patient and family.
Orients furniture in the room in accordance with surgery.	Connects suction canisters to ceiling or wall mounts.	Answers patient's questions.
Opens sterile equipment and instruments using aseptic technique.	Tests suction and in-line gas.	Ensures that permits are signed and witnessed.
Protects the sterile equipment from contamination.	Keeps the operating room doors closed.	Identifies operative side and site.
Performs surgical hand scrub. After scrub, surgical technologist is a "sterile" team member.	Obtains x-rays or other diagnostic reports needed during surgery.	If patient is to be placed in prone position, assists in transfer after anesthesia induction. Patient undergoes induction in supine position and is then turned to prone.
	Opens sterile supplies.	
	*Selects medications and drugs for use during surgery.	
	*Reviews operative checklist.	
	Witnesses signing of operative or anesthesia permit.	Along with surgical assistants, performs surgical hand scrub or may scrub after positioning patient following induction.
	Checks all permits.	
	Notes operative side and surgeon's mark or signature on operative side.	
	*Assesses patient's psychosocial condition.	
	*Measures vital signs and performs assessment.	
	*Answers patient's questions about surgery and postoperative care.	
	Transfers patient to operating room.	
	Transfers patient to operating room bed using safe technique.	
	Applies safety strap over patient.	
	Provides warm blankets for patient.	
Before the Skin Incision Is Made		
Gowns and gloves self using aseptic technique.	Secures scrubbed surgical technologist's gown.	May perform skin preparation.
Drapes Mayo stand.	Secures surgeons' gowns.	
Places sterile instrument trays in position on back table.	Performs the instrument, sponge, and needle count with the scrubbed surgical technologist.	With assistants, enters operating suite from scrub area. Along with assistants, is gowned and gloved by surgical technologist.
Separates sharps (e.g., scalpel blades, needles) from other equipment to avoid injury during setup.	*Distributes medications to scrubbed surgical technologist.	
Sorts drapes and surgical gowns in order of use.	Prepares nonsterile equipment.	
According to the specific surgery, prepares instruments, sutures, devices, solutions, and medications.	*Assists anesthesiologist during anesthesia induction and intubation.	With assistants and surgical technologist, drapes patient.
Protects the surgical setup from contamination.	Assists in the correct positioning of the patient for surgery.	
Performs the initial instrument, sponge, and needle count.	*Carefully applies grounding pads to the patient for use of electrocautery.	
Receives medications from circulator using proper technique.	May perform skin preparation.	
When setup is complete, waits *within the sterile field*.	Completes connections to suction, power, electrosurgical unit, and other energy sources to be used.	
Hands each surgeon/assistant a sterile towel to dry hands.	Advocates for patient safety during the procedure.	
Gowns and gloves each sterile team member.		
Hands individual draping materials to surgeon and assistants. Participates in draping, maintaining sterility.		
Moves Mayo stand into position.		
Secures suction tubing and power and light cords to top drape.		
Hands or drops ends off operating table for attachment to power sources.		
Hands light handle covers to surgeon.		

Table 21-1 Tasks and Duties of the Scrubbed Technologist Circulator, and Surgeon—cont'd

Scrubbed Technologist	Circulator/Assistant Circulator	Surgeon
From Incision to End of Surgery		
Places two sponges on incision site.	*Records time of incision on patient record.	Marks incision area or begins skin incision.
Passes marking pen or scalpel to surgeon. Gives retractors to assistant after skin incision.	*Distributes sterile solutions and medications to scrubbed person.	Performs surgery according to plan and intraoperative events.
Participates in all instrument, sponge, and needle counts with circulator.	Provides additional equipment as needed by the surgical technologist and surgeons.	Directs the surgical team during emergency.
Passes sterile equipment to surgeons and assistants using correct orientation and technique.	Operates nonsterile equipment.	If count is incorrect and missing item is not found, takes responsibility for further action (e.g., x-ray, reopening of wound)
Listens for direction and anticipates each step of the surgery.	Adjusts lighting.	
Maintains a sterile field, notifying others when aseptic technique is broken.	Flash sterilizes instruments as needed.	
Deposits soiled sponges in designated receptacle.	Answers surgeon's pages and relays messages.	Removes gown and gloves, signs patient care documents, and gives any instructions to RN and ACP.
Maintains a safe surgical field by exercising all precautions when electrosurgical devices, lasers, and sharps are in use.	Anticipates flow of surgery and equipment needs of surgeon and surgical technologist.	
Requests additional equipment as needed.	*Monitors urinary output.	Assists in transferring patient to stretcher.
Secures intraoperative tissue and fluid specimens delivered by the surgeon.	Responds to medical emergencies.	
Obtains grafts and implants as required by the surgery.	Directs instrument, sponge, and needle counts at appropriate times.	
Prepares dressings and begins to separate soiled from clean instruments.	*Labels specimens obtained from the scrubbed person for the pathology department.	
Participates in final instrument, sponge, and needle count.	Wearing gloves, separates sponges and places them in counting area or isolates them in groups of 5 or 10.	
Notifies surgeon if count is incorrect.	Maintains safe environment. Keeps doors closed; maintains quiet.	
If count is incorrect, searches for missing item.	Replaces equipment that is unsafe or malfunctions.	
Applies sterile dressings as directed by surgeon.	Assesses the patient's physical status and assists ACP as needed.	
Maintains sterility until patient leaves the room.	Near completion of surgery, calls for next patient.	
Keeps basic instruments on Mayo stand in case of emergency. Prepares instruments on back table for decontamination.	Checks on equipment for next procedure.	
	Participates in count.	
	Notifies surgeon if count is incorrect.	
	At completion of surgery, assists in removing drapes and disconnecting hoses and tubing. Suction remains connected until patient leaves the room.	
	Applies tape to dressings and connects nonsterile ends of drainage devices.	
	Removes dispersive electrode pad and assesses site.	
	*Completes intraoperative record.	
	Transfers patient to stretcher.	
	Calls for orderlies to prepare for room turnover.	
	*Accompanies patient and ACP to postoperative recovery unit and gives report to PACU nurse.	

Continued

Table **21-1**	Tasks and Duties of the Scrubbed Technologist Circulator, and Surgeon—cont'd	
Scrubbed Technologist	**Circulator/Assistant Circulator**	**Surgeon**
After the Patient Leaves the Operating Room		
Separates single-use from reusable items. All soiled disposables are placed in biohazard bags. Linens are also placed in biohazard bags.	Checks on equipment for next case. May begin to open the next case after the operating suite is cleaned. Receives next patient in the holding area.	Notifies the family of the patient's condition. Dictates the operative report.
Aspirates all solutions in closed suction containers. Removes containers from room.		
Places sharps in secure closed sharps container.		
Places all contaminated materials in biohazard bags.		
Removes soiled gown and gloves and places them in biohazard waste bag.		
Removes mask by handling only strings. Removes face shield without touching bare skin.		
Puts on nonsterile gloves to transport covered equipment to decontamination area.		
Follows hospital policy for equipment decontamination. Is responsible for correct destination of instruments and supplies.		
Assists with proper cleaning of operating suite.		

ACP, Anesthesia care provider; *PACU,* postanesthesia care unit; *RN,* registered nurse.
*Licensed RN responsibility.

- *Resect:* A surgical procedure in which a large portion or segment of tissue is removed. The term is often associated with the accompanying reconstruction or repair of the remaining tissue. Bowel resection is removal of a section of bowel and joining the resulting segments by anastomosis. Resection of a tumor can mean simply removing the tumor and then using surgical means to repair the tissues involved in the dissection.

- *Undermine:* This refers to the separation of one flat tissue layer (such as the skin or fascia plane) from another. This is a somewhat blind procedure; the scissors are laid flat between the tissue planes and gently opened and closed, creating a space between the tissues. For example, the skin can be lifted from the fascia layer below by undermining it. Undermining is a technique used to extend the surface area of tissue. For example, in face lift procedures, the skin is undermined from the fascia in order to allow it to stretch and be reattached, thereby obliterating wrinkles.

- *Visualize, direct visualization:* In surgery and medicine means "see in detail." For example *the surgeon was able to visualize the tumor in the right fossa.* Direct visualization means without magnification—that is, with the naked eye.

SURGICAL CASE PLAN

The surgical technologist develops a *case plan* before surgery and implements it during the preoperative and intraoperative stages of the procedure. **Case planning** is preparation, both mental and physical, for the complex tasks involved in a surgical procedure. Just as the registered nurse is required to implement a *patient care plan* that includes a clinical pathway and nursing objectives, the surgical technologist must think strategically about the overall objectives of the surgery and the

technological requirements to meet the surgical objectives. At the same time, he or she must consider specific details about the patient in relation to the procedure. For example, a patient with a very high body mass index (BMI) may require mechanical moving and handling equipment, a high-capacity operating table, and extra-long instruments. Trauma patients may arrive with traction or other stabilizing equipment in place. Preparation for surgeries in which the expected blood loss is high might include orders for blood products or equipment for cell salvaging, in which the patient's own blood is recovered during the procedure and transfused back to the patient.

NOTE: *Case planning and case management are not the same. Case management, as defined in medicine and psychosocial work, refers to multidisciplinary collaborative teamwork involving medical management, rehabilitation, and other community services for patients coping with a complex medical illness, traumatic injury, mental health problems, or a combination of problems.*

The case plan is not mandatory; it is simply good practice. Using a case plan system, the surgical technologist can organize his or her activities into logical sequence. This contributes to a safer, smoother procedure. Students who master the case plan system demonstrate their organizational and strategic thinking skills, allowing them to advance more quickly in their careers.

ELEMENTS OF A CASE PLAN

Many of the elements of the case plan are included in the surgeon preference card (described later). However, the surgeon's preferences are usually generic and may not include provisions for patient populations who have special needs. Other elements are found in the patient chart, which may not be available until the patient has arrived in the holding area. However, the information must still be considered for proper case planning. Knowing the right questions to ask about a particular surgery is part of the learning process.

The basic elements of a case plan include the following:

- Name of the operative procedure
- Type of procedure
- Preoperative diagnosis as stated in the record
- Laboratory notified if frozen section or other consultation is necessary intraoperatively
- Patient BMI or weight category
- Patient age
- Mobility problems
- Sensory deficits
- Position and incision or entry site
- Skin prep and draping required
- Instruments needed, including "specials"
- Imaging required, including equipment
- Pneumatic, electric, electronic equipment required
- Implants planned, type, specifications if known
- Sutures, surgical staples required
- Drains needed
- Dressings
- Patient destination after surgery, such as postanesthesia care unit (PACU), intensive care unit (ICU), discharge to home

A case plan can be a simple checklist that reminds the technologist of what information is needed, or it may be a printed form that can be quickly filled in. An experienced technologist may know ahead of time exactly what instruments, equipment, and draping are needed for each surgery. However, the patient's condition and special needs are an unknown factor. In a busy operating room with little time for preparation between cases, case planning may be difficult, but without planning, some elements of the preparation may be overlooked, resulting in unnecessary delay or a disorganized case. Case planning combines knowledge about a surgical procedure (even if only basic) and understanding of the specific technical requirements of the procedure. As students become familiar with procedures, they start to think strategically about each case and link surgical goals with patient needs and technological needs.

TYPES OF SURGERY BY THEIR OBJECTIVE

There are a number of different ways to categorize surgical procedures for learning purposes. This and other textbooks usually focus on the anatomical specialty such as abdominal, genitourinary, or orthopedic surgery. This is a logical way to learn the regional anatomy, instruments, and techniques. Another method is to look at the surgical outcome or goals. The following categories are simply a tool for learning. There are obvious crossovers from one category to another (e.g., insertion of a pacemaker is a kind of implant; it does not replace an existing anatomical structure, but might replace a nonfunctioning implant battery). Understanding categories can aid case planning, because surgical procedures of a specific type require common skills and techniques. Suggested categories are:

1. Diagnostic
2. Reconstruction or implant
3. Repair
4. Removal

Diagnostic Procedure

The results of a diagnostic procedure provide information about the nature of a medical or surgical problem and the options available for treatment. Diagnostic procedures may be performed as a part of surgery or as a stand-alone procedure. Chapter 7 discusses many of the methods used in surgical diagnostic procedures and physiologic assessment. In many health care facilities, diagnostic procedures are performed in the *interventional radiology* department, which is equipped with advanced imaging equipment. The surgical technologist may be assigned to assist in invasive diagnostic procedures on a case by case basis in this setting. Surgical diagnostics usually involves techniques that produce images of the body so that the disease or problem can be assessed.

Invasive diagnostic procedures include biopsy, in which a portion of tissue is removed and prepared for microscopic examination, or injection of contrast medium, which produces images of tubes, ducts, or vessels. The common factor in diagnostic procedures is that the outcome is tangible and often visible. The process is almost always *multidisciplinary*—involving clinicians from other departments to assist in the process.

QUESTIONS FOR PLANNING

- What is the target structure or tissue? What technique will be used to perform the diagnosis (e.g., biopsy, dye study, magnetic resonance imaging, x-ray)?
- What special equipment is needed for the planned technique (e.g., endoscope and accessories, contrast medium)?
- Will there be tissue samples taken? Do they require any special handling?
- How will the information be documented (e.g., x-ray, pathologist's report, video record, fluoroscopic image)?
- Is the procedure scheduled to take place in a procedure room or in the operating room? Have other clinicians involved, such as x-ray and pathologist, been notified?
- Are previously performed imaging results available in the room or uploaded to the computer?
- What type of anesthesia will be required?

Reconstruction and Implant Surgery

In surgical reconstruction, tissue is remodeled or replaced for functional or aesthetic reasons. The procedure may be performed in a single operation or may be a multiple-stage procedure. This type of surgery often requires specialty instruments. For example, a maxillofacial reconstruction (reconstruction of a portion of the jaw and other facial structures) could require plastic surgery, oral, and fine orthopedic instruments. Breast reconstruction following mastectomy requires general surgery instruments with added special retractors.

Implant surgery often requires special techniques for determining the correct size of implant. In this case instruments called *trial sizers* are used. There are many different kinds of sizers, such as stainless steel or hard polymers for bone, or Silastic for plastic surgery or reconstruction of finger joints in the treatment of rheumatoid arthritis.

Reconstruction and implant surgery often require imaging techniques to determine the exact placement of the implant. Making sure that the operating suite is properly set up for fluoroscopy or x-ray is the responsibility of the surgical technologist and nurse circulator.

Surgery requiring a **graft** taken from the patient (autograft), from another biological source, or biosynthetic material requires knowledge about the type of graft and how it is handled on the sterile field. Autografts usually require multiple skin prep sites and may even involve two separate setups. Autografts are used in skin replacement surgery following injury, but also in orthopedic surgery and vascular replacement.

QUESTIONS FOR PLANNING

- What specialty instruments are needed for the surgery?
- What patient position will be used?
- Will grafts be taken? If so, what tissue will be selected? Are multiple prep setups necessary?
- What draping routine will be used for a multiple-site procedure?
- What is the autograft site (if appropriate), and how will it be prepped and draped?
- What is the age of the patient? Congenital defects often are corrected during infancy or childhood, and these procedures require pediatric-size instruments and other pediatric equipment such as positioning aids.
- Does the reconstruction require external support, such as special dressings, a rigid cast, or traction?
- If implants are to be used, what kind is needed? Are they available? Are trial sizers needed and available?

Repair

The goal of repair is to restore function to a structure, organ, or system. Repair can involve any type of tissue. The type of repair and the tissue involved determine which instruments or special equipment is needed. For example, repair of heart structures in the pediatric patient requires, at minimum, extensive cardiac equipment and pediatric chest instruments. Another example of soft tissue repair is hernia surgery, which may require synthetic mesh. Orthopedic repair usually involves implants of some type, even if just a simple plate or screw system. Imaging equipment will be used, and special dressings may be required for external stabilization after the repair.

QUESTIONS FOR PLANNING

- What will be repaired?
- What special instruments are needed?
- What materials will be used to make the repair (e.g., sutures, plates, synthetic mesh)?
- How will the repair be held in place (e.g., sutures, screws, fibrin glue)?
- Is the repair related to disease or injury? Does the patient have recent injuries and mobility limitations? If so, what specific techniques should be used in positioning?

- Will imaging (x-ray, fluoroscopy) be required?
- Is there a possibility of excess blood loss during the procedure? What preparation is necessary for this?

Removal

Removal may involve tissue, an organ, or a foreign body. Tissue removal surgeries (the *-ectomy* procedures) are performed to control or cure disease. Extensive cancer surgery practiced in the past often included radical removal of multiple structures. With modern diagnostic, chemotherapeutic, and radiological interventions, these surgeries, which included the radical Whipple, radical mastectomy, and pelvic exenteration, are seldom performed. However, removal of a single anatomical structure (e.g., gallbladder, appendix, or prostate gland) is common. Removal of a foreign body may include procedures following an industrial or workplace accident when items such as metal shards, wood, or glass are driven into the soft tissues. Forensic surgery involves removal of ballistic items such as bullets or shrapnel, or sharp weapons such as knife blades.

QUESTIONS FOR PLANNING

- What will be removed, and what tissue is involved?
- What surgical approach will be used (e.g., abdominal, thoracic)?
- Will a specimen be taken for frozen section analysis (immediate tissue analysis to determine malignancy)?
- Has the pathologist been scheduled to be available for surgery (if applicable)?
- Is the wound contaminated? (Procedures involving removal of foreign bodies are contaminated.)
- What special procedures need to be followed to submit forensic items removed from the patient?

PREOPERATIVE CASE PREPARATION

PREOPERATIVE SEQUENCE

Equipment and supplies for the surgical case are brought into the surgical suite.
1. The scrub and circulator open the case.
2. The patient arrives from the holding area and is transferred to the operating bed.
3. The anesthesia care provider and circulator prepare the patient for anesthesia.
4. The patient is positioned for surgery.
5. The scrub performs hand antisepsis or scrub.

ASSIGNMENTS

Surgical cases are assigned to individual staff members before the procedure, at the beginning of the day, or on a rolling basis. In most facilities assignments are posted on a schedule board (e.g., a white board), which lists cases and assigned personnel. This is usually located near the entrance to the restricted area. After receiving the schedule, the surgical technologist plans his or her time and tasks so that all instruments, supplies, and equipment are available and ready close to the time of surgery.

The schedule should be rechecked periodically in case there are cancellations or room changes.

SURGEON PREFERENCE CARD

The **surgeon preference card** is an electronic document or paper version of the specific supplies and other preferences required by each surgeon. Before computers became a common source of information sharing in the operating room, an index card file was kept in which records of specific surgeons and their routine cases were documented. Cards were usually kept in the clean workroom so all the staff had access to them. The system is still used, but most health care facilities have switched to an electronic system. However, the system is still referred to by its traditional name of *surgeon preference cards*. Each card or entry contains a list of the specific instruments, equipment, medications, suture, and other items that a particular surgeon uses on a specific surgery. The preference card also shows the surgeon's glove and gown size, draping routine, and other information that customizes case preparation according to that surgeon's usual practice.

The rationale of the preference card is to have everything ready *before* it is needed during surgery. This allows efficient use of time and prevents delays during the procedure. In general, surgeons are intolerant of delays caused by poor planning. Delay results in increased anesthesia time, which adds to patient risk, can upset the surgery schedule, and is also measured in financial cost. Many facilities have adopted elaborate computer programs used to create and archive surgeon preference cards that can be modified as needed and are also linked to patient billing and scheduling.

Surgeon preference cards in any form can also contain information that is misleading or even wrong. Their accuracy depends on efficient updating and making sure that it applies to all or most cases, not just some. Each individual using the system can contribute to keeping the information current. Good case planning is often directly related to the team effort in keeping preference cards updated and accurate.

ASSEMBLING SUPPLIES AND INSTRUMENTS

The method used to gather supplies for a case depends on the system established by the health care facility. The process is called "picking a case" or "pulling a case." The case cart method is most commonly used. In this system some or all of the sterile supplies are assembled in the central processing department and sent to surgery on a stainless steel *case cart* (introduced in Chapter 4). Prepared case carts are kept in the substerile area to protect them from contamination. Preassembly of case carts helps to decrease room turnaround time (the time between the end of one case and the start of another).

After the case cart is received in the operating room, the surgical technologist is responsible for checking it for completeness and adding equipment as required. For scheduled procedures, the surgical technologist works with the circulator to ensure that all supplies have been gathered, ready for opening no more than 1 hour before the start of surgery.

Selected case carts are kept ready for emergency cases, such as trauma, craniotomy, aneurysm, and cesarean section (C-section). These are high-priority emergencies in which every minute must be used efficiently to get the case underway. Basic items, such as instrument sets and linen packs, are preassembled on the emergency setup. Special items are quickly added shortly before surgery.

 Watch Section 2: Unit 3: Preparing the Operating Room for the Patient on the Evolve website. http://evolve.elsevier.com/ Fuller/surgical

OPENING A CASE

After sterile supplies have been gathered for a surgical case, the next step is *opening the case*. In this process the clean surgical suite is prepared—furniture and large equipment are put into place, and sterile instruments and equipment are opened up using aseptic technique to prevent contamination.

PREPARING NONSTERILE EQUIPMENT

The first step in preparing the surgical suite for a case is arrangement of bare furniture (instrument tables, Mayo stand, and other equipment). The surgical technologist and circulator arrange the furniture in the room in a logical manner to build the sterile field. Unless a dedicated room is already equipped with large nonsterile equipment such as the operating microscope or digital imaging cart, these are brought in during the nonsterile setup. As soon as the room is ready, the case cart and all supplies are brought into the room.

Essentials of the Nonsterile Room Setup

1. Place the operating table so that it can accommodate the anesthesia care provider, equipment that cannot be moved easily, and doors (Figure 21-1). The operating table may require rotation to accommodate large equipment such as an x-ray machine or C-arm fluoroscope. Make sure the operating table is positioned directly under the overhead surgical lights.
2. Arrange the room in a manner that prevents contamination of sterile surfaces by traffic from doorways and nonsterile equipment.
3. The electrosurgical power unit must be placed close enough to the operating table to accommodate the cables and patient connections so it can be moved into exact position after the start of surgery.
4. Suction canisters are positioned close to the operating table.
5. Kick bucket liners and trash receptacles should be in place. Usually this is done by the housekeeping team, but it should be checked by the surgical team ahead of time.
6. Place furniture so that draped (sterile) tables will be no closer than 18 inches (45 cm) from a nonsterile surface, equipment, or walls.
7. Place clean linen on the operating table and ensure that arm boards and other attachments are available in the room. Secure one end of the patient safety strap to the table.

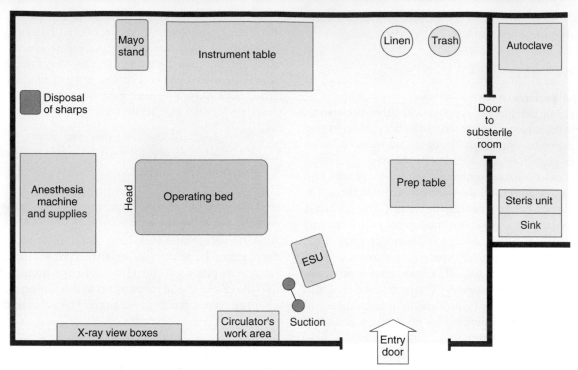

Figure 21-1   **Room setup for surgery.** (*Modified from Phillips N: Berry and Kohn's operating room technique, ed 10, St Louis, 2004, Mosby.*)

8. Have available specific positioning devices and aids, paying particular attention to patient age, size, and specific position to be used.

9. Connect suction tubing to canisters, making sure that the connections are tight. Pretest the suction lines for adequate and safe pressure.

10. Gather diagnostic studies (e.g., x-rays, magnetic resonance imaging scans) or other imaging data the surgeon will need during the case, or ensure that it has been uploaded to the computer.

11. If an anesthesia technician is unavailable, the circulator assembles monitoring equipment and other accessories, such as cardiac leads, airway equipment, compression devices, and warming or cooling blankets.

12. If pneumatic power equipment is to be used during surgery, the inline or tank gas sources must be tested and the gauges set according to the manufacturer's recommendations.

13. Other equipment such as portable imaging systems must be checked to ensure that all connections and leads are available.

14. Any other special equipment such as pneumatic tourniquet must be available in the room. Specialty carts must be available in the sterile core or corridor.

15. If lasers are to be used, make sure that warning signs are posted outside the room, and all equipment is available and ready.

OPENING STERILE SUPPLIES

Sterile supplies are opened within 1 hour of the time surgery begins. The surgical technologist participates in this activity until it is time to perform the surgical scrub or hand antisepsis (10 to 20 minutes before surgery, depending on the complexity of the case, or less in emergency cases). Sterile supplies are opened in logical sequence from large to small while avoiding a pyramid of supplies that can topple over and become contaminated. Refer to Chapter 10 to recall the boundaries of the sterile field and rules of asepsis. Keep in mind that anything that falls below table height is no longer sterile.

The basic pack containing towels, drapes, and gowns is centered on the back table and opened using aseptic technique. As the wrapper is unfolded, the inner sterile surface is exposed. This provides a sterile surface on which other items can be distributed. Remember that the edge of any sterile wrapper is not sterile. Small items are opened by removing the outer wrapper using aseptic technique. The item is then *gently but purposefully* ejected from the package onto the sterile table without allowing the item to touch the edge of the wrapper. Anticipate the need for smaller tables for supplementary sterile instrument trays or equipment and obtain sterile table covers as required for these.

RECOMMENDATIONS FOR OPENING A CASE

- Always maintain a safe distance from sterile surfaces to avoid contamination, but stand close enough to project the item you are opening accurately.
- While opening sterile goods, place clean single-use wrappers in clean trash receptacles. Do not use kick buckets or biohazard bags for clean waste.

- When opening packages sealed with tape, break the tape rather than tearing it. This prevents the outer wrapper from ripping and causing contamination. Always check the sterility monitor while opening a package.
- Packages wrapped in sealed pouches may contain an inner wrapper. Open the outer pouch and distribute the item with its inner wrapper intact.
- Avoid unwrapping a heavy item such as a large instrument tray while holding it in midair. Instead, place the item on a small table and open the wrapper, draping it over the edges of the table without touching the inside surface of the wrapper or sterile item, as shown in Chapter 10. Unless there is a shortage of tables, there is no benefit in trying to hold a heavy tray with one hand. Repetitive strain injury is a risk, as is simply dropping the entire tray of instruments or equipment.
- When opening instruments in closed sterilization trays, break the seal and lift the top straight up and away from the tray. Remember that the edges of the tray are not sterile. Do not open any sterile goods into this tray.
- Extra sutures, special equipment, and implants should be held unopened until the surgeon asks for them. This prevents waste.
- Sharps are opened onto a conspicuous location on the back table during the setup or held until the scrub can receive them (preferred method). This prevents the scrub from unexpectedly encountering or grabbing a sharp item. The circulator opens the outer package and the scrubbed technologist removes them and places them immediately in a sharps holder.
- Before performing hand asepsis for the case, the surgical technologist opens gown and gloves onto a small table away from where sterile items have been distributed (never on the back table) to prevent contaminating other supplies.

RECEIVING THE PATIENT

The patient is usually received in the operating room suite during the sterile setup (see description later). The circulator and assistant circulator are responsible for the patient, along with the anesthesia care provider. The patient is greeted and identified and then moved to the operating table and secured with a safety strap. The circulator is focused on patient safety at this time. Any items that still need to be opened or are found to be missing are the duty of the nonsterile circulator. However, timing is important. The scrubbed technologist performing the intraoperative sterile setup should avoid asking for items while the circulator is performing critical tasks such as documentation, ensuring patient normothermia, or attending to the psychological needs of the patient.

INTRAOPERATIVE STERILE SETUP

INTRAOPERATIVE SEQUENCE

1. Following hand antisepsis, the scrub gowns and gloves and immediately sets up sterile supplies.
2. The first sponge, sharps, and instrument count is performed.
3. General anesthesia is initiated (if applicable).
4. The circulator continues to distribute sterile supplies as needed.
5. The patient is positioned, prepped, and draped.
6. Sterile tables are moved into position.
7. Suction, the ESU, and sponges are secured on the surgical site.
8. A TIMEOUT is allowed for Universal Protocol.
9. Surgery is begun and the time noted.
10. The scrubbed technologist anticipates the need for instruments, equipment, and supplies for the surgeons.
11. Counts are performed per protocol.
12. Specimens may be collected at any time.
13. The wound is closed.
14. When the procedure is complete, anesthesia is withdrawn and the time noted.
15. Dressings are applied.
16. Drapes are removed and the dressings secured.
17. The patient is stabilized for transport.
18. The patient is transported to the PACU or other hospital area for recovery.

After the case has been opened, the surgical technologist or scrub performs the surgical scrub (or hand antisepsis). The scrub reenters the surgical suite without contaminating the hands or arms and proceeds to gown and glove.

Immediately after gowning and gloving, the scrubbed technologist must organize the sterile items on the back table, Mayo stand, and any other instrument tables. This is called the **sterile setup** or *setting up a case*. Students and even experienced surgical technologists in a new specialty can feel overwhelmed by the amount of equipment that must be organized and ready by the time the surgeons arrive to start the case. Using a methodical approach to all setups improves efficiency and greatly decreases stress and errors in the learning phase.

As you first approach the pile of sterile equipment, do not move anything until you have a plan. Do not begin moving things around aimlessly. This increases the chance of contamination and does not actually move the process forward. The following are general guidelines that can increase efficiency and decrease stress:

- *Increase the size of the sterile working area.* Before organizing and preparing supplies, increase the size of the sterile area. Drape the Mayo stand *first* (Figure 21-2). After draping the Mayo, place one or two towels over the tray on top of the Mayo cover. This provides some cushioning for the instruments and also helps decrease the possibility of penetrating the tray cover with a sharp instrument or needle.
- *If you need additional work space,* the circulator will provide smaller tables that can be draped. For example, power equipment or other specialty items can be placed on a separate table. If multiple tables are used, they should be placed close to the back table so that a continuous sterile field is created. This saves steps and excess motion.

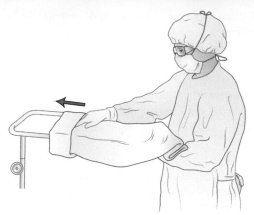

Figure 21-2 Draping the Mayo stand. *(Redrawn from Phillips N: Berry and Kohn's operating room technique, ed 10, St Louis, 2004, Mosby.)*

- *Check all sterilization indicators* placed in instrument and equipment packs at the time of their preparation for the sterilization process. (For a review of sterilization indicators, refer to Chapter 11.)
- *Avoid shifting the same items around from one place to another. Set a goal to handle an item only once or twice (one touch method).* Shifting items from one location to another without purpose is not productive. Start to build zones intended for specific types of equipment such as sutures, meds, sharps, and instrument stringers. Retrieve the item you need and place it in its final location once. Even if you have to push other things aside to make space for the item at hand, you will have started to establish zones.
- *Some facilities require a standardized setup.* This method is used to ensure that during a change of shift or breaks when more than one person uses the same setup, everyone is familiar with the arrangement of instruments and supplies.
- *Try to avoid doing several things at once.* Think and act strategically. Perform one task and then proceed to the next.
- *Start with items that are needed at the beginning of the procedure* and prepare them first. This serves two purposes—it helps in mental preparation for the case, and in the event there is not enough time to complete the setup before surgery starts, the supplies needed at the beginning of the case are ready. This is particularly useful in emergency cases when the patient may be brought very quickly with little time for the sterile setup.

The following list is the usual order of items needed on a routine case:

1. *Towels, gowns, gloves, drapes:* Pull the gowns out from the pile and stack them *in order of use* from the top down (e.g., towel, gown, towel, gown). Stack drapes with the first used on top and the last used on the bottom of the stack.
2. *Light handles, suction tubing, ESU pencil and holster:* You might place these in a dry instrument basin or on the Mayo stand. They will be placed on the field as soon as the patient is draped.

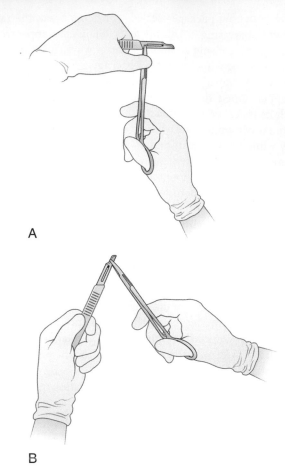

A

B

Figure 21-3 **A,** Mounting the knife blade on the handle. Brace the thumb against the clamp to stabilize it. **B,** Removing the knife blade. Always point the blade away from the body.

NOTE: If magnetic instrument pads are used in your facility, it is helpful to place this on the field immediately, especially if there is pressure to rush, which can result in instruments falling to the floor.

3. *Starting instruments:* These are scalpel (knife), scissors, clamps, shallow retractors, and suture ties. Locate knife handles, dissecting scissors, forceps, and superficial retractors. Mount knife blades (Figure 21-3). Place these, along with a few necessary instruments, on the Mayo stand. Prepare the ESU pencil and holster along with their holding clamp. These will go up as soon as the patient is draped. Place all other sharps together on a magnetic board or in a sharps holder (Figure 21-4).
4. *Sponges, sutures, sharps:* Put all sponges in one location on the back table, organized by type, so that you are ready to count when the circulator is free to do so. Do the same with suture packets and sharps. Sharps are placed on a magnetic board or sharps container ready for counting, and safely stored.
5. *You now have all the priority equipment you need to start a case.* All other equipment can be set up as "secondary preparation."

Watch Section 2: Unit 5: Preparation of the Sterile Field on the Evolve website. http://evolve.elsevier.com/Fuller/surgical

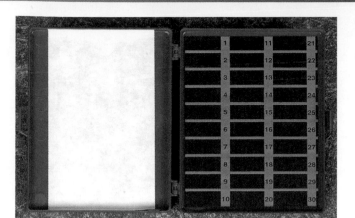

Figure 21-4 Magnetic sharps container with closing lid. *(Courtesy DeRoyal Industries, Powell, Tenn.)*

Watch Section 2: Unit 6: Monitoring the Sterile Field on the Evolve website. http://evolve.elsevier.com/Fuller/surgical

SUTURE PREPARATION

Suture material needed for a case is listed on the **surgeon's preference card**. If there is no preference card, it is possible to ask the surgeon at the start of the case. Although many different types of suture materials and needles may be opened during a case, not all of them need to be immediately available on the Mayo. Most sutures are kept on the back table and transferred to the Mayo as needed. After working in a particular specialty, you will become familiar with sutures used at a particular point in the procedure. It may be helpful to know that students, whether they are surgical technologists or interns starting surgical residency, are not expected to have complete competency in sutures. Some basic guidelines are essential to know when starting to work with sutures:

- *Suture ties* (strands) can be removed from their package, separated by size, and placed on the Mayo stand between the folds of a towel. Ties may also be maintained in the package, which is placed on the Mayo stand or in a small basin.
- *Suture reels* can remain on the Mayo stand, and individual ties can be removed as needed. Suture-needle combination packages can be placed in a small basin on the back table and brought to the Mayo as needed. Suture packets are designed to be opened quickly and easily. The needles are secured so that they can be grasped from the package using the needle holder. The suture attached to swaged needles should follow the needle smoothly as it is removed from the package. When arming the needle holder, try to position the needle correctly the first time. This saves having to handle the needle again before passing it to the surgeon. Empty suture wrappers should be placed in a paper suture bag taped to the back table cover, not dropped into the kick bucket, which is reserved for sponges.

NOTE: A complete discussion of sutures and suture use is located in Chapter 22.

INSTRUMENTS

Complex surgical cases require many instrument trays. This is why it is important to think about what instruments you need, locate them among all the supplies, and then put them in a specific place. If instrument trays must be stacked, place heavier ones on the bottom. The number of instruments available in the instrument sets usually far exceeds those needed on the case. The selection of instruments to have ready, or on the Mayo, is based on experience, help from mentors, and memory. During the first months of scrubbing, no one is expected to know exactly which instruments will be needed. Regardless of the method you use to learn, make sure you know each instrument's specific or general location on the back table to avoid delay during surgery. Your scrub mentors will help you locate what you need to prevent unnecessary delay during the case.

MAYO TRAY SETUP

The Mayo tray (called the *Mayo*) is the scrub's immediate personal work space for the rapid handing of instruments, suture, and other supplies to the surgeon during surgery. It is reserved for items needed immediately and frequently throughout the procedure. Part of the technologist's expertise is in knowing what is immediately needed in the surgery, but also the seamless exchange of items from the back table to the Mayo as the procedure progresses and the immediate needs change.

The Mayo setup is personal, and unless the health care facility requires a standard setup, technologists are free to develop a system and arrangement of items that works best for them. Regardless of the system used, the Mayo stand should be kept neat and orderly because a disorganized Mayo can lead to surgical errors such as lost needles, needlestick injury, and sluggish response to needs on the field. Figure 21-5 shows a classic general Mayo setup. However, students should try different setups to see what feels efficient and comfortable.

SOLUTIONS AND DRUGS

Medications and irrigation solutions usually are distributed after the case is underway or just before the case begins, *but only if there is a scrub person to receive them.* Solutions are distributed into basins or a temperature-controlled basin unit (Figure 21-6). One basin of sterile water is reserved for soaking instruments only. Instruments are never soaked in saline solution. The wound irrigation solution is kept separately. All irrigation fluid must be measured and recorded as it is used so that total blood loss can be calculated accurately.

The protocols for dispensing medications are discussed in detail in Chapter 13. A zone for labeled medications and labeling materials should be created on the back table so that they can be protected and well organized. During surgery, the scrubbed surgical technologist is responsible for all medications on the back table and for correct handover to the surgeon as needed.

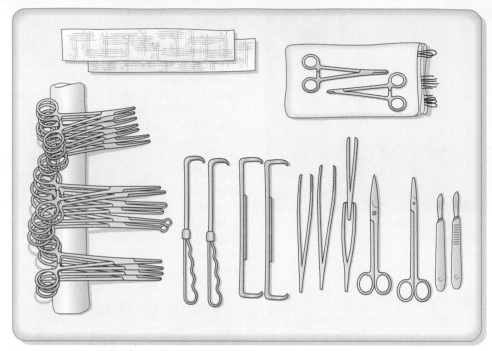

Figure 21-5   **Example of a Mayo tray setup.** *(Redrawn from Phillips N: Berry and Kohn's operating room technique, ed 10, St Louis, 2004, Mosby.)*

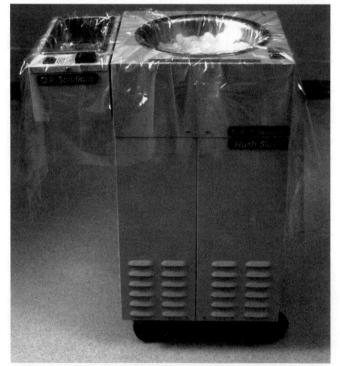

Figure 21-6   Slush basin draped with clear sterile plastic. *(Courtesy DeRoyal Industries, Powell, Tenn.)*

COMPLETING THE SETUP

Once the Mayo and back table have been set up for the start of the case, the remaining supplies can be arranged and prepared. The sponge, sharps, and instrument count is performed during the setup.

After the setup is complete, instruments and supplies should not be handled because this increases the risk of contamination. Questions often arise about how long the sterile setup remains sterile and whether it is permissible to leave the sterile setup in the event a case is delayed. Contamination of any sterile item is **event related**. The most recent guidelines on this topic, published in 2012, state that a sterile setup must be continuously monitored.[1] No research has demonstrated a specific period of time that a setup ceases to be sterile. Covering the sterile setup or taping operating room doors closed is unacceptable in all aseptic standards. In current guidelines, if a case is delayed such that trained personnel are not available to observe the setup, it must be *torn down* (disassembled) and the equipment reprocessed.

THE COUNT

Specific items opened for a surgical procedure are counted before, during, and after the surgery in a precise way to prevent their loss in the patient. The subject of *unintentionally retained foreign objects* during surgery was introduced in Chapter 3 as having safety, legal, and financial consequence.

Items to be counted are classified as follows:
1. Soft goods
2. Sharps
3. Instruments
4. Miscellaneous small items

Any item that can be retained in the surgical wound is included in the **count**. This includes sutures, surgical sponges, sharps, instruments, instrument parts, retraction devices (e.g., umbilical tapes, elastic vessel loops), instrument bolsters, suture reels, and any other small items used on the sterile field.

Retained surgical items continue to be among the most common sentinel events contributing to patient harm. A retained item can cause pain, infection, perforation of an organ, obstruction, and scarring. Repeat surgery for a retained item causes trauma, a longer recovery period, and additional expense. Severe infection or injury may result in death. Loss of an item is a sentinel event that may result in a negligence charge against any member of the surgical team.

Research shows that this event is often caused by not following established procedure. Excessive noise, lack of organization by the scrub person, and pressure to hurry through procedures were features of an operative environment incompatible with correct counts. The study also identified poor communication among surgical team members as a cause of poor counting and patient risk.[2]

RESPONSIBILITY FOR THE COUNT

Health care facilities create and enforce policies on the methodology or procedure for counts and appropriate documentation. The law does not state how counts are taken or who is to take them. The law *does* state that items not intended to remain in the patient must be removed. All team members are responsible for ensuring that no item is left in a patient. The scrubbed technologist or nurse and circulator normally perform the count together. In turn, they report the count to the surgeon, whether it is correct or incorrect. Action taken to resolve an incorrect count is then the entire team's responsibility. During surgery, the scrubbed technologist should know *at all times* how many sponges, instruments, and other items are inside the patient and the location of counted items on the back table and Mayo.

WHEN TO PERFORM THE COUNT

In general, counts are performed on all surgical or invasive procedures. Anyone on the surgical team may request a count at any time.

The health care facility determines policy for counting instruments, sharps, and miscellaneous items. All sponges (soft goods) are counted at the following times:

1. Before surgery begins to establish a baseline count and verify that the manufacturer's count is correct
2. Any time new soft goods are added to the sterile setup (the newly added sponges are counted upon distribution)
3. Before closure of any body cavity or cavity within a cavity, such as a hollow organ
4. At the start of wound closure
5. At skin closure or when counted items are no longer used on the sterile field
6. Whenever permanent relief staff enter the case (e.g., during a shift or other personnel change in either the scrub or circulator role)

Instruments, sharps, and miscellaneous items may also be counted at the same time, according to facility policy.

PROCEDURE FOR THE COUNT

Items are counted in a specific order:

1. Items on the immediate sterile field (i.e., those on or in the patient)
2. Items on the Mayo stand
3. Items on the back table
4. Items that have been discarded or dropped from the field

The count is performed in a systematic manner. Items should be counted according to their type. For example, count all laparotomy sponges, and then count all 4 × 4 (**Raytec**) sponges; continue to count all other types of sponges on the field according to their type.

Count suture needles, blades, and instruments (and their loose parts) as separate groups. The items being counted should be grouped together and accessible for the initial count.

The count is performed audibly, with the circulator and the scrub person participating equally. Both people participating in the count must *see the items* as they are counted. The circulator and scrub person are required to sign the count on the patient's operative record. This is a legal document that attests to the outcome of the count. Anyone who performs a count, including relief personnel, must sign off their count.

The standard procedure for the count is shown in Box 21-1.

COUNTING SYSTEMS

The most commonly retained item is the surgical sponge. Systems used to collect (confine), and count sponges are used to prevent errors. These include multipocket bags that can be suspended from an IV stand. Counts may be recorded during surgery using a white board. Electronic technology currently in use for the count includes bar coding and radiofrequency tagging, in which a chip is embedded in each sponge and can be tracked using a tracking device. This shows more promise than bar coding.[3] These devices are rapidly gaining the approval of professional organizations and may become mandatory in the future.

For information on approved electronic tracking devices, see http://clearcount.com.

Regardless of the system used, success requires the cooperation and communication of everyone on the surgical team.

EMERGENCY SETTINGS AND COUNTS

There may be extreme emergency cases in which the life of the patient is immediately endangered and a count is waived. The amount of time between the announcement of an incoming emergency and the arrival of the patient in the operating room may be less than 10 minutes. In these few minutes, the surgical team must prepare the operating room, open the case, perform hand antisepsis, and receive the patient. If an initial count is waived, documentation must reflect this and include the rationale. During the case, counts are taken as usual, as the situation permits. Imaging is performed at the conclusion of

| Box **21-1** | **Standard Procedure for the Surgical Count** |

What
- Soft goods (textiles) including radiopaque sponges of all types, surgical towels, and packing material (e.g., material used in the nasal cavity to absorb blood)
- Individual suture packages
- Sharps including intact knife blades, hypodermic needles, suture needles, trocars, and fragments, if broken
- Instruments
- Miscellaneous items such as electrosurgery tips, cranial (Raney type) clips and their cartridges, umbilical and vessel loops, electrosurgery cleaning pads, small bottles and their caps, medical device parts, and any other object that can be lost in the surgical wound

When
- Before the procedure (to establish a baseline)
- Whenever additional items are introduced to the sterile field intraoperatively
- At the start of wound closure
- Before closing any hollow organ
- Before closing a body cavity
- During closure of skin or other final tissue layer
- Whenever permanent relief personnel join the surgical team
- At the request of the surgeon or any other team member

How
- According to the healthcare institution's policy
- In a systematic, deliberate way, without distraction or interruption
- Without deviation from policy and protocol
- In an established sequence by the type of item being counted (e.g. instruments, sponges, sharps)
- By separating or pointing to each and every item and counting them individually
- Audibly and visually; both people performing the count do so aloud, as they see the items being counted

Who
- As designated by health care facility policy
- The circulator and scrubbed technologist or nurse
- Other members of the sterile team and circulator

the case to demonstrate that no item was seen. Each facility is responsible for publishing protocols and policies regarding waived counts.

DOCUMENTATION

All counts are documented in the patient record. Documentation includes names of the individuals who participated in the counts (including relief staff) and their signatures attesting to a correct or incorrect count. Count sheets on which real-time counts are documented may become part of the permanent record, according to facility policy.

A retained item is reported as a sentinel event (see Chapter 3), even if the item is eventually located and the count validated. This requires documentation on an incident report or by other facility protocol. If the item is found, it is documented as a *near miss*. The report must include steps taken to find the missing item.

LOST AND RETAINED ITEMS

Loss of sponges, needles, instruments, or other surgical equipment extends anesthesia time, increases patient risk, raises costs, and increases stress on the surgical team. If a surgical sponge or other item is left behind in the patient, it can often be spotted on x-ray. However, the extended anesthesia time required for x-ray to be called and an image made available can add substantial risk to the patient. The expense of extended time or medical consequences of a retained surgical item are not covered by insurance.

HOW ITEMS ARE LOST

The most recent studies on retained surgical items show that specific scenarios in surgery are more likely to lead to incorrect counts and discrepancies:
- The procedure lasts more than 8 hours.
- There is multiple staff turnover during a procedure.
- A sponge is used inappropriately (i.e., outside of the usual protocol). For example, a Raytec (4 × 4) sponge is not mounted on a clamp for use in a body cavity.
- There is failure to document items added to the field during surgery.
- The team has not kept track of sponges as they are used.
- The surgical field is cluttered or disorganized.
- The sponge count is performed improperly.

The scrub must be accountable for sponges *as they are used.* This requires keen attention to the operative site and concentration on what items are in use. Sponges (and instruments) can easily become "lost" in the body cavity of a deep-bodied or obese patient. Sponges often are found in the folds of drapes, under basins, among the skin prep sponges, or on the floor under the operating table. Small needles are lost when they snag on drapes or other linen and spring off the field. Small items, such as instrument parts, can easily drop into the wound.

HOW TO SEARCH FOR A LOST ITEM

If the count is incorrect, the surgeon is notified and the count is repeated. If the count is still incorrect, a search is initiated. Nonsterile team members search nonsterile areas while scrubbed team members search the wound and sterile field. Normally the surgical technologist is responsible for searching the back table, Mayo, and any other instrument tables. All trash and waste receptacles are emptied onto an impervious drape, and each piece is searched. As each bag is searched, the contents are rebagged systematically. Equipment on the back table must be shifted to allow a search under instrument trays and basins. The floor around the operating table is thoroughly examined, and team members are asked to step away from the field slightly because sponges often are found between the team member and the table or patient. A rolling magnet is used to search all floor spaces for metal items. Team members must show the soles of their shoes for inspection, another place where lost needles can be found. The smallest microsurgical needles cannot be seen on x-rays and may be very difficult to spot on or around the surgical field.

If a sponge or needle is not found, an x-ray usually is ordered. If the item is lost during closure, the procedure may be halted until the x-ray is read. However, not all retained items are easily seen on an x-ray. If a lost item is neither found in the room nor revealed on an x-ray, it may still be retained in the wound. In such a case, all layers of the surgical wound may be reopened and searched. If the surgeon is confident that the item has not been left in the wound, and the risk of extended anesthesia does not outweigh the risk of a retained object, the x-ray may be ordered in the PACU.

PREVENTING RETAINED ITEMS

The problem of retained items and the health consequences are of such significance that safety and professional organizations have instituted conferences, new research studies, and awareness campaigns to try and decrease the incidence. Among the most important messages to operating room teams are the following summary guidelines on preventing retained items, which are derived from both AST[4] and AORN[5] recommended practices:

- During the count, unnecessary activity and distraction should be curtailed to allow the scrub and RN circulator to focus on the task at hand.
- Standardized procedure should be used during all counts.
- Sharps must be contained within a specific area of the sterile field in a containment device.
- **Radiopaque** soft goods (e.g., sponges, towels, textiles) should be accounted for during all procedures in which soft goods are used.
- If the surgical sponge pack is banded, the band should be broken and discarded before the count.
- Items are counted as they are added to a case.
- Radiopaque sponges must not be used as wound dressings or in the patient prep.
- All counted items should stay in the operating room or procedure room until the close of surgery.
- The final count is not complete until all sponges used in the closing wound are accounted for.
- Sponges or other counted items dropped on the floor should be retrieved by the circulator and the item shown to the scrub.
- Sponges and other radiopaque items must not be cut for use in the wound.
- Small instrument components such as wing nuts, screws, and pins are counted separately.
- Broken instrument parts are isolated from the setup and accounted for.
- Trash and linen bags must remain in the operating room until the patient has left the room.

STARTING THE CASE

The start of surgery begins officially with the onset of anesthesia. The events that occur immediately before and after can take place in succession or simultaneously.

The patient usually is brought into the surgical suite during the latter part of the sterile setup. The anesthesia care provider and circulator then focus on preparing the patient for anesthesia. Anesthesia begins only after the surgeon has arrived and is ready to scrub. The surgeon and assistant perform hand antisepsis and enter the surgical suite to be gowned and gloved by the scrubbed technologist.

Patient positioning begins following intubation of the patient under general anesthesia and only when the patient is stable. These three events—intubation, arrival of the surgeons, and patient positioning—often occur in close succession.

The circulator performs the patient skin prep as soon as the patient position is secure and the anesthesia care provider has verified that the patient is stable. (If the surgeon performs the skin prep, he or she requires regloving.) Draping of the patient follows immediately afterward, performed by the sterile team. As soon as the drapes are secured, the Mayo and instrument tables are brought into position to complete the sterile field (Figure 21-7). Suction tubing, the ESU and holster, light cords, and tubing are secured to the top drape using one or more nonpenetrating clamps, allowing sufficient slack between the instruments and the edge of the sterile field. The technologist places one or two sponges on the field. At this point all activity stops so that TIMEOUT (Universal Protocol) can be completed.

TIMEOUT

Universal Protocol, also called **TIMEOUT**, is a method used to prevent serious error in patient identification, wrong site surgery, and wrong surgery. These "never" events occur frequently in the United States. Statistics from the Joint Commission indicate that wrong site surgery accounts for 13.1% of all sentinel events and represents the single largest group of

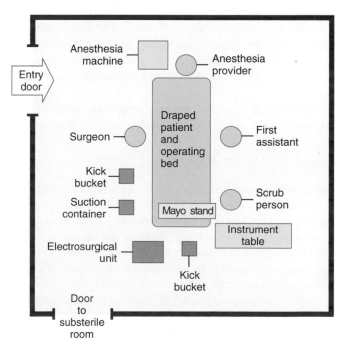

Figure 21-7 Completed surgical field. *(Redrawn from Phillips N: Berry and Kohn's operating room technique, ed 10, St Louis, 2004, Mosby.)*

sentinel events reported.[6] In human terms, this represents needless trauma and suffering for many patients. In 2004 the Joint Commission released a Universal Protocol for preventing wrong site surgery. The protocol establishes a TIMEOUT period for every surgical procedure to allow verification of information, which helps prevent wrong site surgery and other related events.

TIMEOUT is observed by surgeons, anesthesia care providers, nurses, and surgical technologists, all of whom are responsible for injury prevention and patient safety. TIMEOUT is a team event, with everyone participating. It takes place immediately before the start of surgery and includes but is not limited to the following information:

1. Verification of the patient's identity
2. Verification of the correct side and site as marked on the patient's skin
3. Agreement on the procedure to be done
4. Verification of the correct patient position
5. Verification of the availability of correct implants and any special equipment or requirements
6. Availability of laboratory or other test results in the room

TIMEOUT is preceded by the preoperative verification process and by marking of the operative site discussed in the previous chapter. Final verification of the site mark is done during TIMEOUT.

To view the entire protocol for presurgical verification and TIMEOUT, see the Joint Commission website at http://www3.aaos.org/member/safety/guidelines.cfm or search "Joint Commission Universal Protocol."

Documentation of the Universal Protocol is contained in a single document or in combination with the surgical safety checklist. A combined *Comprehensive Checklist* developed by AORN to represent both the WHO safety checklist and the Joint Commission universal protocol is shown in Figure 21-8. Note that the Joint Commission does not stipulate which team member initiates any section of the checklist except surgical site marking, nor does it stipulate where the activities occur.

Immediately after the surgical checklist including Universal Protocol has been verified, the skin incision is made.

MAINTAINING AN ORDERLY SETUP

Maintaining a clean and orderly setup is key to being organized and keeping pace with the surgery. Periodically remove paper wrappers and other items from the Mayo. Suture ends are cleared from the field and placed in the suture bag. Small bits of tissue should be removed from the drapes. If the drapes become soaked around the incision, a small impervious drape can be placed over the site.

Instruments should be kept off the patient when not in use. It is important to keep track of where specific instruments are on the field, Mayo, and back table. As instruments are passed back from the field, they should be wiped clean with a damp sponge to prevent blood and body fluids from drying on the surface. Suction tips are cleared by running small amounts of

water through them. An extra suction tip should be available for use while one is being cleared. A metal stylet is used to remove dried body fluids that cannot be removed with water. A sterile basin of water is placed near the back table for soaking soiled instruments during surgery.

Remove and replace sponges when they become soaked and can no longer be used, or if there are tissue fragments on the sponge that might be carried back into the wound. However, do this with as little movement as possible. When replacing a sponge, pick up the soiled sponge and lay the clean one on the field at the same time. Do not pull sponges out from under instruments or the surgeon's hand; this disrupts concentration and displaces instruments on the field. If instruments begin to pile up out of reach, wait for a pause in the surgery before asking the surgeon or assistant to place them within reach. Do not reach around behind the surgeon to retrieve the instruments.

NOTE: *Surgery requires extreme concentration. Sometimes the surgeon may ask for an instrument that is already at hand on the field. In this case, if it is within your reach, pick it up and place it in his or her hand. Do not simply state where it is unless it is out of your own reach.*

LIGHTING

Inadequate lighting increases the risk of surgery errors. The surgical technologist adjusts lights as needed. Overhead lights produce a small shadowless beam that spreads peripherally to focus on a large or small area as needed. If the surgeon is working high in the abdominal cavity or low in the pelvis, the light must be lowered vertically and directed horizontally to angle the beam correctly. Minimally invasive procedures that use concentrated fiberoptic light are performed with the operating room darkened. Some source of light must be available for surgical routines that require visual verification. Examples are reading medication labels and measuring drugs using a syringe. The surgical technologist should assert the need for a small light source to prevent these errors.

MANAGING SPONGES

Used laparotomy and 4×4 sponges are dropped into the kick bucket from the surgical field in a way that prevents splattering. The 4×4 sponge is never used "loose" on the field when a body cavity is open. These must be mounted on a sponge forcep. The mounted 4×4 is commonly called a **sponge stick** (or stick sponge). As soiled sponge sticks are retrieved from the surgical wound the scrubbed technologist removes the soiled 4×4 and drops it immediately into the kick bucket. The circulator retrieves all sponges with gloved hands or an instrument and isolates them in a pocketed sponge holder. Used dissection sponges are retained in their holders on the sterile field. Used, flat neurosurgical sponges are placed on a small container or towel on the back table or on a separate prep table near the back table.

Regardless of the type of sponge to be counted, the circulator places used sponges where the scrub can see them so that

COMPREHENSIVE SURGICAL CHECKLIST

Blue = World Health Organization (WHO)   Green = The Joint Commission - Universal Protocol (JC) 2010 National Patient Safety Goals   Orange = JC and WHO

PREPROCEDURE CHECK-IN	SIGN-IN	TIME-OUT	SIGN-OUT
In Holding Area	**Before Induction of Anesthesia**	**Before Skin Incision**	**Before the Patient Leaves the Operating Room**
Patient/patient representative actively confirms with Registered Nurse (RN):	RN and anesthesia care provider confirm:	Initiated by designated team member All other activities to be suspended (unless a life-threatening emergency)	RN confirms:
Identity □ Yes Procedure and procedure site □ Yes Consent(s) □ Yes Site marked □ Yes □ N/A by person performing the procedure	Confirmation of: identity, procedure, procedure site and consent(s) □ Yes Site marked □ Yes □ N/A by person performing the procedure	Introduction of team members □ Yes **All:** Confirmation of the following: identity, procedure, incision site, consent(s) □ Yes Site is marked and visible □ Yes □ N/A	Name of operative procedure Completion of sponge, sharp, and instrument counts □ Yes □ N/A Specimens identified and labeled □ Yes □ N/A Any equipment problems to be addressed? □ Yes □ N/A
RN confirms presence of:	Patient allergies □ Yes □ N/A	Relevant images properly labeled and displayed □ Yes □ N/A	
History and physical □ Yes	Difficult airway or aspiration risk? □ No □ Yes (preparation confirmed)	Any equipment concerns?	**To all team members:** What are the key concerns for recovery and management of this patient?
Preanesthesia assessment □ Yes	Risk of blood loss (> 500 ml) □ Yes □ N/A # of units available _____	**Anticipated Critical Events** **Surgeon:** States the following: □ critical or nonroutine steps □ case duration □ anticipated blood loss	
Diagnostic and radiologic test results □ Yes □ N/A	Anesthesia safety check completed □ Yes		
Blood products □ Yes □ N/A	**Briefing:**	**Anesthesia Provider:** □ Antibiotic prophylaxis within one hour before incision □ Yes □ N/A □ Additional concerns?	
Any special equipment, devices, implants □ Yes □ N/A	All members of the team have discussed care plan and addressed concerns □ Yes	**Scrub and circulating nurse:** □ Sterilization indicators have been confirmed □ Additional concerns?	
Include in Preprocedure check-in as per institutional custom: Beta blocker medication given (SCIP) □ Yes □ N/A Venous thromboembolism prophylaxis ordered (SCIP) □ Yes □ N/A Normothermia measures (SCIP) □ Yes □ N/A			April 2010

AORN

The JC does not stipulate which team member initiates any section of the checklist except for site marking.
The Joint commission also does not stipulate where these activities occur. See the Universal Protocol for details on the Joint Commission requirements.

Figure 21-8   Comprehensive Surgical Checklist. *(From AORN Correct Site Surgery Tool Kit.)*

both can participate in the counts. As additional sponges are needed during surgery, they are counted as soon as the scrub receives them. The circulator adds these to the count on the operative record. When blood loss must be estimated, the circulator may be required to weigh each sponge. The amount of irrigation fluid used is factored into this calculation.

NOTE: A full description of surgical sponges and their use is found in Chapter 22.

HANDLING AND PASSING INSTRUMENTS

Handling and passing instruments are important tasks of the scrubbed technologist. As with all manual skills, time is needed to develop speed and coordination. As you gain coordination, speed will follow naturally. Do not attempt to increase speed until coordination is secure. Rushing results in dropped instruments, mistakes on the field, hand collisions with other scrubbed team members, and injury. Try to find a rhythm and pace that feels safe and comfortable, even during the critical stages of the procedure. All instruments are passed in their closed (locked) position unless the surgeon requests otherwise. An instrument is oriented spatially so that the surgeon does not have to reposition it or look away from the operative site to receive it. From the surgeon's point of view, she or he is literally focused on a small area of complexity. Looking up and away from the surgical wound breaks this concentration. Even a few moments of distraction at the wrong time can create a problem.

The position of the instruments during passing is related to on which side of the table the surgeon stands, on the directional curve of the instrument itself, and on its immediate use in the wound. In general, when passing a curved or angled instrument, it is positioned so that the curved tip points at the incision. When the instrument is being passed, the surgeon usually opens his or her hand to receive it with the tip (working end) up. In this case, the technologist must still pass it so that the curve will point to the incision when the surgeon moves his or her hand back to the wound to use the instrument. Sometimes, the instrument is used in a "backhanded" way—that is, with the tip pointing in the opposite direction. In this case the surgeon will reposition the instrument after receiving it or state that he or she wants it passed backhanded. Retractors and other large or heavy instruments are passed in the position they will be placed in the wound. For example, a large self-retaining or handheld retractor is handed with the retractor blades pointed downward.

Try to avoid overmanaging the setup, including the instruments. Overmanaging is handling instruments and other sterile items when it is unnecessary. Try to avoid picking up an instrument with one hand and shifting it to the other hand to pass. Sometimes shifting the instrument is unavoidable but fewer motions result in increased efficiency.

Medium-weight to heavy instruments are passed firmly. When delicate instruments are passed, they are placed lightly in the surgeon's hand. When a specific instrument is required, the surgeon positions his or her hand as if using the instrument. Some surgeons use specific hand motions to indicate whether forceps, scissors, or suture is needed (Figures 21-9 through 21-14).

Long Instruments

When the surgical wound is deep, or the patient is large, long instruments are required. Some long instruments are passed

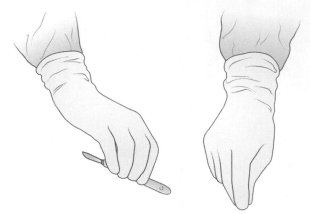

Figure 21-9   Passing the scalpel. The no-hands technique is used whenever possible.

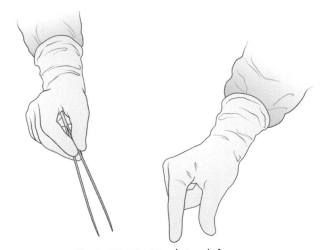

Figure 21-10   Hand signal: forceps.

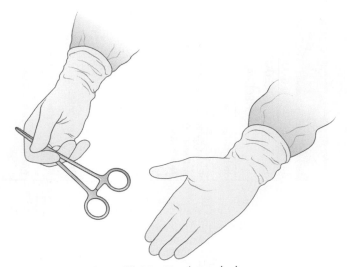

Figure 21-11   Hand signal: clamp.

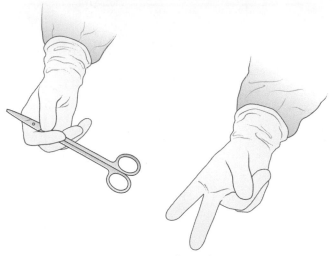

Figure 21-12 Hand signal: scissors.

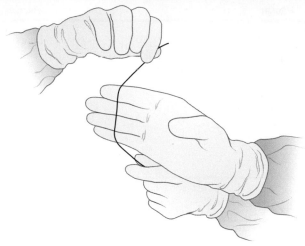

Figure 21-14 Hand signal: free tie suture.

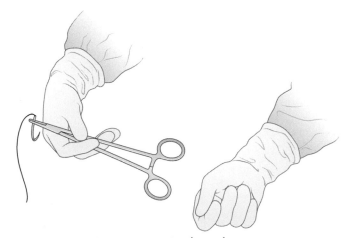

Figure 21-13 Hand signal: suture.

with the tips facing downward (e.g., ligation clips and mounted sponge clamps). If you see the surgeon repositioning an instrument each time you pass it, adjust your passing technique to match.

Microsurgical Instruments

When receiving microsurgical instruments, the surgeon does not remove his or her eyes from the microscope. The scrub must place the instrument in the surgeon's hand in exactly the correct position without touching the microscope.

Do not jar the microscope or the surgeon's hand when passing microsurgical instruments; the patient may be injured by an instrument in the surgeon's opposite hand or by sudden movement of the microscope. Jarring the microscope also moves the field of vision. Even a small unexpected movement of the lens can be disturbing for the surgeon and may require repositioning of the microscope.

Because instruments must be oriented according to use, the surgeon rotates the receiving hand into various positions. The technologist must adjust the instrument to complement the hand position. To determine the correct orientation, imagine yourself in the surgeon's place looking through the

microscope. For example, if the instrument tip is needed at the 12 o'clock position, the surgeon must reach around the front of the microscope ocular to receive it. If the instrument tip is needed at the 3 o'clock position, it is passed to the side of the focal point. The surgeon indicates the correct position of the instrument by the position of his or her hand.

Do not handle the tips when passing microsurgical instruments. Grasp the middle of the instrument (Figure 21-15, *A*). Bayonet forceps usually are oriented with the middle break of the instrument curved upward (Figure 21-15, *B*).

Neutral Zone

All sharp instruments or small sharps should be passed on the sterile field using the neutral zone (no-hands) technique. If hospital policy or an individual surgeon has not implemented this technique, the scrub must pass sharps in the traditional manner.

In the neutral zone technique, a designated area is established on the surgical field near the surgical wound. The site must be easily accessible to both the scrub and the surgeon. Whenever sharp instruments are exchanged, they are placed in this zone rather than directly into the hands of the team members. The neutral zone can be a magnetic pad with a recessed reservoir or a shallow basin used to receive the instruments. This eliminates hand-to-hand contact (Figure 21-16).

Establishing the practice of neutral zone instrument exchange requires collaboration among all team members. For the technique to be effective, everyone must agree that it is worthwhile, because use of the technique requires changing time-honored practices. The procedure for establishing and using a neutral zone is described in Box 21-2.

Scalpel

If operating room policy has not specified a neutral zone (no-hands) technique, the scrub passes the scalpel (commonly called the "knife") by grasping the handle in the middle with the cutting side of the blade down. Your hand should always be above the handle. The scalpel should not be released until the surgeon has complete control of the handle. The scalpel is

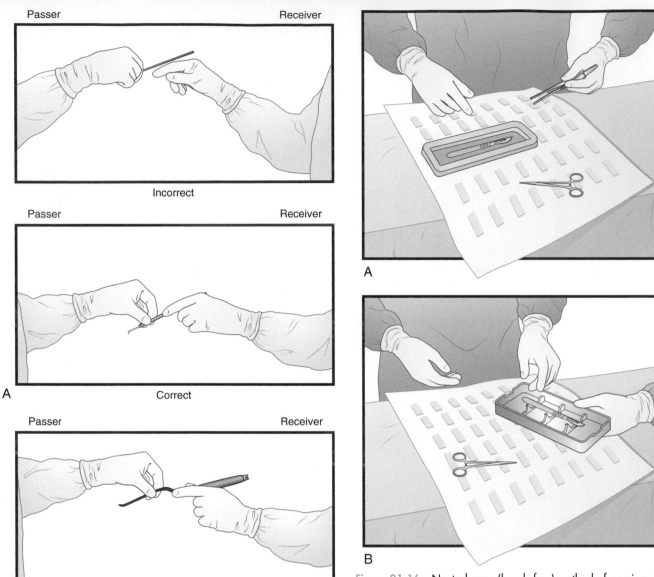

Passer   Receiver

Incorrect

Passer   Receiver

A   Correct

Passer   Receiver

B

Figure 21-15 **A,** Passing microinstruments. **B,** Bayonet forceps correct orientation.

A

B

Figure 21-16 Neutral zone (hands-free) method of passing sharps. A magnetic pad and square pan for scalpels are placed on the field.

returned by placing it on a folded towel or in a small basin. Never leave the knife on the surgical field. Some facilities have implemented a guideline for the surgeon to announce when the knife has been placed in the neutral zone by saying "Knife down," or in the case of a needle, "Needle down." This alerts the scrub person that the item must be removed from the field immediately.

If sharps are passed in the traditional manner, without regard to a neutral zone, extreme caution should be exercised. The surgical scalpel is a precision instrument, designed to cut smoothly and easily through tissue. A truly sharp scalpel should glide through tissue with minimal pressure.

The blade of the surgical scalpel loses its "buttery" feel after several passes through tissue, especially through skin and fibrous tissue, such as cartilage and periosteum. Surgeons who favor the scalpel over other cutting instruments may use many fresh blades during surgery. The surgical technologist should

know this in advance from working with a particular surgeon or from the surgeon's preference card.

Whenever you pass a scalpel with a new blade to the surgeon, you must announce, "new blade." This alerts the surgeon to exactly how much pressure is required to make a cut. There is almost no circumstance in which a dull blade is advantageous. Anticipate when a blade is getting dull and replace it. If you see the surgeon "sawing" through tissue with a scalpel blade, the blade probably is dull (or will be after being used in this manner).

In traditional surgical technique, one surgical blade is reserved for use on the skin and maintained separately during the procedure. The rationale is that the skin knife may have been contaminated by the patient's skin, which cannot be sterilized, whereas the deep tissues are sterile. There are no studies to confirm that the skin knife is contaminated, but the decision to use a separate skin knife rests with the surgeon.

- The location of the neutral zone is established by agreement between the surgeon and the scrub.
- Do not use a kidney basin or other small receptacle as a neutral zone. A small space with steep sides increases the risk of injury, because the hand must reach into the container for the instrument.
- Only sharps are to be placed in the neutral zone.
- The neutral zone should contain only one item at a time.
- Suture-needle combinations are exchanged one to one but never hand to hand. The prepared suture is placed in the neutral zone; the surgeon uses it and returns it to the zone.
- The scrub then replaces it with a fresh suture.
- Mounted suture needles and rakes should be turned downward but oriented correctly for use. The surgeon should not have to look away from the wound to pick up the instrument.
- When a sharp is placed in the zone, the person placing it calls it out, as in "Suture" or "Scalpel up" (i.e., up on the sterile field). A means of communication must be established by team members to prevent confusion.

Sharp Retractors

Skin hooks and rakes can easily puncture a glove or sleeve. When passing a sharp retractor, always keep the tips facing downward. Do not grasp the retractor near the sharp end. Remove the retractor from the field as soon as the surgeon removes it from the wound. Again, always make sure to pass sharp retractors with your hand above the instrument.

Suture Needles

Many needlestick injuries occur during suturing. To prevent injury, pass the needle holder to the surgeon on an exchange basis; that is, when the surgeon returns the needle holder and needle, pass another. Do not use more than two needle sutures on the field at one time unless two surgeons are suturing. If double-armed sutures are used (i.e., sutures with a needle at each end), clamp one needle in the needle holder and the other with a fine forceps to prevent snagging. (Refer to Chapter 22 for a complete discussion of suture handling techniques.)

MANAGEMENT OF SURGICAL SPECIMENS

Among the most important skills of the surgical technologist is proper handling of tissue, fluid, and other specimens removed from the patient during surgery. Nearly all types of tissue or items removed from a patient must be registered and submitted for analysis (a few exceptions exist, and these are discussed later). The surgical technologist participates in all intraoperative phases of the procedure. For ease of learning and appreciating the details of each phase of specimen handling, the process can be separated into the following stages:

1. Preparation
   - Pathology department is notified, if prescheduling is required
   - Appropriate containers are obtained before surgery
   - Method of transport to pathology is verified (chemical preservative, dry, other methods)
   - Requisition and laboratory forms are filled out
   - *No* prelabeling of specimen containers
2. Surgical removal of specimen and placement of markers (surgeon and surgical technologist role)
   - Some tissue specimens may be marked before surgery (e.g., core needle biopsy)
   - Specimen is marked during or after removal with sutures, clips, or tissue dye
   - Small specimens may be removed piecemeal
   - A portion of the suspect tissue is removed for analysis
   - The entire specimen (suspect tissue, organ, body part) is removed
3. Preservation and identification on the surgical field (surgical technologist's role)
   - Appropriate receptacle for the specimen(s) is made available
   - Correct specimen management protocol is followed (e.g., dry, saline float, saline Telfa)
   - Specimens are maintained separately and identified
   - Specimens are handed off the field to circulator using aseptic technique
4. Specimens not requiring frozen section are prepared for transport (circulator)
   - Specimen is placed in transport container and identified and labeled
   - Documentation is completed
   - Specimen is taken to designated area for transport

RESPONSIBILITY FOR SPECIMENS

Critical medical decisions are made based on specimen analysis. A decision to perform radical surgery or begin cancer therapy may depend on the pathology of a specimen. Damage, loss, and misidentification of specimens are a serious concern in patient safety. Mishaps related to specimen loss include incorrect identification, loss of a specimen in the laundry (a result of placing the specimen in a towel), specimens thrown away in the trash, and failure to correctly identify anatomical margins or the tissue of origin. The consequences of such negligence can be devastating. The result may be an incorrect diagnosis, repeated or needless surgery, delayed treatment for malignancy, or cancer treatment that was unnecessary. The patient's cultural practices involving body tissues must also be considered and assessed. Any deviation from normal pathology protocols may require the patient's signature and plans made to fulfill the patient and family needs on the matter.

In addition to ethical accountability for specimens, a legal responsibility exists. Losing, misidentifying, or damaging specimens can rapidly result in litigation. There are many guidelines and precautions related to the management of specimens. Most important are those for the facility, because these include the specific procedures and materials used in tissue preservation from the time it is removed until it reaches the pathology department for analysis. AST and AORN also publish guidelines for handling specimens (available online). It is important to remember that the exact preservatives and method of transporting specimens may change according to the surgical objective or method of analysis. The scrubbed surgical technologist is directly responsible for receiving and handling specimens on the surgical field. The surgeon communicates information about the exact site and tissue of origin, and the orientation of margins for malignancy (if applicable), to the scrubbed technologist and circulator. Other information needed for specimen labeling and registration, such as unique patient identifiers, is obtained from the patient chart.

PREPARATION FOR SPECIMEN REMOVAL

Preparation for specimen removal and analysis begins before surgery. Specific types of specimens require notification of the pathology department 24 hours before the procedure. The surgeon or ward administrator usually has the responsibility to contact the pathology department for advance notification.

Each type of specimen requires a specific method of transport and preservation from the time it leaves the body until it reaches the pathology department. Appropriate containers should be obtained before the start of surgery. The container must be large enough that all surfaces of the specimen are covered with preservative, if one is required. However, toxic preservative solutions must not be brought into the operating room. This includes formaldehyde (formalin), which is the most common preservative used. Formalin should only be handled in a well-ventilated environment and with protection to prevent exposure to skin, eyes, and the respiratory tract.

Accredited health facilities follow the guidelines of the College of American Pathologists (CAP), which advises on protocols related to specimen handling and preservation. The pathology department communicates with surgical staff about the appropriate preservative and procedure for specimen transport. These protocols should be available or surgery staff may contact the pathology department for verification.

DOCUMENTATION

Specimen handling and transport require documentation at all points in the specimen chain of custody. Before surgery begins, the appropriate laboratory requisition forms are obtained according to the type of specimen anticipated and which department will be responsible for analysis. Forms are specific to the type of analysis. For example, tissue analysis may require a different form than that used for bacterial culture. At least two *unique* patient identifiers (e.g., Social Security number or hospital number) must be verified for specimen documentation.

All specimens must be documented on the specimen container (discussed later), operative record, and pathology documents.

Postoperative documentation should include:
- Type of specimen
- Patient name, age, gender, health care organization, history, and preoperative diagnosis
- Analysis required
- Date and time of collection
- All information regarding the source of the tissue and its identification
- The surgeon's name and contact number
- The name of the person preparing and documenting the specimen for transport

NOTE: *The CAP cautions against prelabeling the containers. This prevents misidentification and mislabeling at the time the specimen is obtained.*

HANDLING SPECIMENS ON THE FIELD

The scrubbed surgical technologist may receive specimens on the field, or the surgeon may pass the specimen directly to the circulating nurse. When specimens are received on the sterile field, they must be immediately identified and protected from damage or loss.

The exact role of the surgical technologist during specimen removal depends on the type of tissue and the surgical procedure used for removal. Before studying these methods, certain general guidelines are important to learn:
1. The surgeon may place one or more sutures or clips in the specimen to indicate the anatomical margins of the tissue. Never remove any markers from a specimen. Handle specimens gently to prevent dislodging markers.
2. When multiple specimens are anticipated, the scrubbed surgical technologist must be prepared to identify each specimen separately.
3. Never remove a specimen from the sterile field without the surgeon's specific permission to do so.
4. *Do not use surgical sponges* or towels to wrap a specimen. This is a common cause of specimen loss because the tissue is hidden from view and can be disposed of accidentally. Place the specimen in a conspicuous protected area until it can be passed off the field to the circulator.
5. Maintain the specimen in a condition conducive to pathological examination per the facility's protocol. If you are unsure about the protocol, it is important to ask.
6. Never use water to preserve a specimen or keep it moist during surgery. Water can cause cell distortion. Use sterile saline instead.
7. Do not use bone clamps, hemostats, or other crushing instruments on tissue specimens, because this can damage the tissue and interfere with analysis. Use smooth tissue forceps, which are atraumatic.
8. After the surgeon approves it, the specimen should be handed off the field to the circulator as soon as possible after removal.
9. When a specimen is passed off the sterile field, there should be verbal verification of the origin, side (right or left), type of tissue, and any other special identifiers.

TYPES OF SPECIMENS

Tissue Biopsy

Tissue **biopsy** is the removal of tissue or cells for gross identification and microscopic analysis. Microscopic analysis results in a definitive diagnosis, such as malignancy, or is used to determine the nature of an abnormality. Biopsy is performed during endoscopic, image-guided surgery or as part of an open procedure.

Types of tissue biopsy:

- *Excisional biopsy* is removal of an entire mass or suspicious area of tissue. This refers to small lesions rather than removal of whole organs or limbs.
- *Incisional biopsy* is partial removal of a tissue mass.
- *Fine-needle aspiration (FNA)* uses a long, fine needle to aspirate (suction) small pieces of tissue from a mass.
- *Core needle biopsy* is similar to FNA, but a large-bore, hollow trocar or needle is used to collect tissue. The needle is inserted into an organ, such as the liver, and tissue is removed for analysis.

Small specimens removed for biopsy should be carefully maintained on the back table because they can easily become lost. Small samples of tissue also dehydrate rapidly. To prevent this, the surgical technologist should dip a Telfa strip in sterile saline and place it in a small specimen container. Tissue specimens are removed during endoscopic procedures using very small biopsy forceps. To collect the specimen, the surgeon removes the tissue with forceps and withdraws it from the endoscope. The surgical technologist must steady the end of the instrument and collect the tissue, which may be smaller than one millimeter across in size. This is best done using a needle or fine stylet. According to the surgeon's directions, the specimen may be transferred to a container partially filled with saline or Telfa saturated in saline. Core-needle and fine-needle biopsy tissue is extruded into the specimen container onto a saline Telfa, or floated in saline, according to the surgeon's request or directions from the pathology department.

Frozen Section

In surgical cases that require immediate analysis of tissue for malignancy, a **frozen section** is performed. This is done by flash-freezing the tissue and then making sectional slices that can be examined microscopically.

Frozen section analysis is scheduled ahead of the surgery to ensure that the pathologist is available. Once the pathologist has been scheduled, the circulator notifies him or her when the specimen is close to removal during surgery. The surgical technologist's role in frozen section depends on the complexity of the specimen. In order to verify the boundaries of a malignant lesion, the specimen may be taken in sections, which are marked according by orientation to the entire site. For example, a fine suture may be placed at the 3 o'clock position of the tissue sample. This creates a kind of mapping so that if additional tissue must be removed, the correct boundaries of the sample are known. This type of procedure is used in areas of the body where tissue removal causes loss of function or disfigurement. An alternative method is for the entire lesion to be removed at one time and the boundaries marked with sutures or surgical clips. If sutures are needed for marking, 3-0 or 4-0 nonabsorbable material on a small curved needle is commonly used.

Frozen section specimens are received on the surgical field in a small basin or bowl and kept moistened with a saline-soaked Telfa strip. Do not float the specimen in saline unless directed to do so by the surgeon. Always communicate clearly and precisely about the tissue origin and exact location, because this is critical information.

Frozen section specimens are usually passed off the sterile field immediately after they are surgically removed. Once the specimen has been transported to pathology, it usually takes 20 or 30 minutes for preparation and analysis. The pathologist may come into surgery to speak with the surgeon directly about the findings, or communicate through a speaker call to the operating room. The scrubbed technologist should be prepared for further dissection after the initial specimen has been analyzed. Following preparation and examination of frozen section specimens, permanent slides are made from the tissue.

Stones

Stones are removed from the urinary tract, salivary ducts, and gallbladder. The technologist receives these in a small dry basin. They should be kept dry and are transported in a dry container.

Bulk Tissue

Bulk tissue, organs, or partial organs are received in a container large enough to contain them on the field. This should be passed to the circulator as soon as possible after removal or kept moist with saline until transport.

Amputated Limb

The surgeon passes an amputated limb to the scrubbed technologist to pass off the field. In all cases the patient under local anesthesia must be protected from witnessing this. The limb can be wrapped in a paper drape and placed in a protected location on the back table until the circulator is prepared to receive it. It is then wrapped in plastic or according to hospital policy. Final disposition of the limb may be influenced by the patient's wishes and cultural practice. Initially the limb must be registered and sent for analysis, like other specimens. Special disposition is noted in the patient's record and documents accompanying the specimen.

Cells (Cytology)

Endoscopic procedures often include the collection of epithelial cells for cytological examination. This is usually performed to rule out carcinoma. Cells are removed using a soft biopsy brush, which is passed over the epithelium with the aid of the endoscope. The procedure is called a brush biopsy. As the surgeon withdraws the biopsy instrument, the scrubbed technologist assists by directing the brush end of the biopsy instrument into a small container of sterile saline. The tip is agitated slightly in the saline to release the tissue and cells, which might not be visible with the naked eye. Several containers should be prepared to receive the specimen. These must be clearly identified and labeled.

Cytology slides for microscope examination are prepared by the practitioner (usually in a clinic setting) and sprayed with a *fixative* before being sent to pathology. A fixative is a solution that stabilizes the cells for examination. An example of this type is a cervical smear that is fixed with fixative (98% alcohol). The patient's name is penciled on the slide before it is sent to pathology along with appropriate documentation.

Products of Conception

Embryonic and fetal tissue are registered and documented as *products of conception* and are treated with respect and dignity. States have individual reporting requirements for fetal death, and hospital policy is established around those requirements. The surgical technologist must become familiar with appropriate dispensation and specific documentation of fetal tissue for their facility and state.

Foreign Body

A *foreign body* is a nontissue item obtained from the patient's body. Some specimens, such as bullets and knife blades, are critical as forensic evidence and are used for legal purposes. Bullets and other metal objects removed from the body that can be scratched must not be handled with metal instruments, because these can damage the specimen and obscure analysis. A retained item from a previous surgery has obvious legal importance. Other items, such as implants and fragments of metal, glass, wood, or any other foreign material, may also be retained as specimens. All foreign bodies are submitted dry unless the surgeon requests another method.

Items that may be part of forensic evidence are handed over to the police for analysis. These must be registered according to hospital policy related to forensic evidence. No specimen can be released without specific documentation issued by the facility.

Clothes needed for forensic analysis are removed from the patient by cutting only along seams. Holes and tears should not be divided or cut because they may be significant for evidence.

Medical devices that were previously implanted are removed from the body because of failure, including breakage or fragmentation. All pieces of the device are kept dry and sent together in a dry container. The device is examined for identification and the manufacturer is notified. The device serial number or other identifiers should be included in specimen labeling and documentation along with the packaging, if it is available.

Cultures

Tissue or fluid suspected of being infected is cultured as described in Chapter 9. In this process, a small fluid sample is collected from the wound and transported by culture tube. Suspected infection is treated immediately until the confirmed diagnosis is returned.

The surgical technologist assists in collecting the culture sample. Sampling is performed with a special culture tube, containing one or two sterile swabs and culture medium. When the surgeon is ready to take the culture, the circulator removes the top of the culture transport tube, exposing the ends of the swabs. The technologist carefully removes them from the container and passes them to the surgeon, who swipes them across the tissue to be tested. The surgeon returns the swabs to the technologist who places them carefully back into the culture tube, which is still held by the circulator. Always use universal precautions when handling tissue and cultures. Two types of bacterial cultures are commonly taken during surgery, *aerobic* and *anaerobic* (discussed in Chapter 9). *Each requires a designated type of transfer tube.* Anaerobic sampling can be performed with a needle and syringe or using a Dacron swab as described earlier. Using the swab technique, more commonly performed in surgery, the transfer tube contains a small amount of preservative medium that is released into the swab when the tube is compressed.

Body Fluids

Sampling body fluids is usually performed in the clinical setting. However, occasionally the surgical technologist may be asked to assist in a procedure to obtain fluid samples, such as pericardial or synovial fluid sampling, which requires sterile technique. Fluid samples obtained by percutaneous methods (puncturing the skin) are removed using a needle and syringe. The fluid can be transported in the syringe, which is capped after the needle is removed. Never send a needle attached to a syringe, because the sample may be rejected by the pathology department as a safety hazard. Fluid samples may also be injected into a transport tube with stopper.

SPECIMENS REQUIRING SPECIAL PREPARATION

Some types of specimens require special protocol for collection and transport. Frozen section specimens were discussed previously. However, it is worth repeating that these tissues must be transported only on Telfa with saline. Other tissues that must not be preserved with formalin but are transported in a dry container (not floated) on Telfa with saline are:

- Cone biopsy of the cervix
- Lymph node for selected hematologic malignancy

These are transported immediately to the pathology department.

Advance notice is usually required by pathology for the following types of specimens:

- Muscle biopsy
- Kidney biopsy
- Frozen section

Muscle Biopsy

Muscle biopsy is a specific procedure for diagnosis of muscle or systemic disease. During muscle biopsy, a small section of muscle is removed from the *vastus lateralis* or other large muscle. However, the site depends on the pathology and whether there has been previous trauma to the area that might obscure analysis. The biopsy is performed routinely, like any small tissue excision. However, no electrosurgical instruments are used for cutting or coagulation.

Muscle tissue is ideally transported quickly to the pathology department on Telfa with saline—not floated in saline and never in formalin. The sample *must be kept cold* and the container (not the specimen) packed in ice. If the specimen cannot be transported within 30 minutes, it may require flash freezing. The method used for this will be directed by the pathology department according to their protocol.

Cord Blood, Umbilical Cord, Placenta

Blood remaining in the umbilical cord after birth is collected for simple laboratory analysis or for biobanking. Blood for laboratory analysis is collected in a small basin at the time the cord is severed during delivery. It is then transferred to the appropriate blood tubes according to laboratory requirements.

Cord blood banking is becoming increasingly popular and is performed to preserve hematopoietic stem cells, which may be beneficial in the treatment of blood-related diseases. The umbilical cord may also be preserved for use in the regeneration of organ tissues. Both blood and cord products are preserved in a tissue bank after they have been removed. Cord blood is removed following birth, before the placenta is removed. A blood collection kit containing collection bag, clamps, and tubing is used on the surgical field. After collection, the blood is sent to the pathology department according to facility protocol. The umbilical cord is removed and also transported according to facility policy. Placenta samples are collected and transported according to facility policy and disposition of the samples—whether for research or other use.

Radioactive Specimens

Patients who have undergone surgery to implant radioactive seeds or injection of radioactive material (e.g., sentinel lymph node biopsy) will have implants or tissue removed. Special precautions are required for handling and transport of radioactive tissue and implants. Each health care facility determines which departments may receive radioactive material and how it is to be transported there. Specimens are handled on and off the field using universal precautions. In general, solid radioactive materials are most commonly retrieved from prostate tissue. Radioactive implants have very low toxicity beyond the immediate area of the implant itself. However, precautions must be observed during transport and disposal. These procedures will be approved and published by the facility's radiation safety officer.

SPECIMEN TRANSPORT TO PATHOLOGY

All specimens, except those that are routinely discarded according to facility protocol, are sent to the pathology department for analysis. Depending on the type of tissue and the nature of the analysis, there are different methods for preserving tissue during transport.

Identification of Specimens

Specimen identification is a critical aspect of surgery. All tissues must be labeled before being transported from the operating room.

Each specimen must be identified with the following information:

1. Identification of the patient with two distinct identifiers (the patient's name and one other, such as the individual's hospital number)
2. Type of tissue
3. Origin (site) of the specimen (e.g., right breast, left leg, left tonsil)
4. Clinical diagnosis and other clinical information
5. Any special markings and their significance (e.g., suture at 1 o'clock)
6. Other registration information, date and time of removal, surgeon's name

Preservatives, Containers, and Labeling

Each type of specimen removed from the patient must be considered for the correct transport medium. Although most tissue is transported in formalin, using an incorrect transport medium can affect the ability to properly analyze the tissue and formulate a diagnosis. If there is any doubt about how to send a specimen, it is best to check with the surgeon or pathology department directly.

All specimen containers must be leak-proof and placed in an impervious bag for transport. Biohazard labeling is used on all specimens. When preparing specimens for transport, always place the label on the container itself, not on the lid, which might be separated from the container after arrival. Information on the label must be legible and written with water-resistant or waterproof ink. Before sending a specimen, check that the information on the label matches exactly with the requisition form and other documentation to be sent and that these match the patient's chart. Documents sent with the specimen must not be placed inside the bag in which the specimen has been placed in order to maintain universal precautions and prevent damage to the documents in case there is any seepage from a wet container. Always use designated transport containers, outer bags, and systems when sending specimens to the appropriate department.

WOUND CLOSURE

When the surgical procedure is complete, the wound is irrigated and closed. The surgical technologist begins preparing sutures for closure before they are needed. This occurs toward the end of surgery.

Before closure, all excess instruments are removed from the operative site. A clean surgical towel can be placed at the wound edge to prevent any tissue debris on the drapes from reentering the wound. Closure materials are placed on the Mayo stand, along with suture scissors and clean sponges. Drains and drain tubing are also prepared at this time. A complete discussion on the preparation and use of wound drains is located in Chapter 22. The wound then is closed according to the surgeon's protocol. Dressings are not brought to the Mayo stand until the superficial wound layers have been closed and the final sponge counts have been completed.

When closure is complete, the wound site is cleansed with moist sponges and the dressings are applied. These are held in place manually while drapes are removed. Dressings are secured and other wound materials are applied, depending on the procedure performed. All surgical instruments and supplies are sorted and assembled for transfer to the decontamination area.

NOTE: *The scrubbed surgical technologist is required to remain sterile with suction connected and working until the patient has left the operating room suite.*

END OF SURGERY

POSTOPERATIVE SEQUENCE

1. The patient is transferred out of the operating room in stable condition.
2. Surgical instruments and supplies are sorted and prepared for decontamination.
3. All disposable items are placed in designated containers.
4. Documentation is completed and signed off (circulator and scrubbed technologist).
5. Soiled instruments and reusable supplies are transported to the decontamination area.
6. Specimens are documented and transported to a designated area for pickup.
7. The surgical suite is cleaned and decontaminated for the next case.
8. Equipment and furniture are returned to their normal locations.

PATIENT TRANSFER

At the close of surgery, the patient is stabilized and prepared for transfer to the PACU or other unit in the health care facility. The anesthesia care provider is required to accompany the general anesthesia patient to the recovery area. The registered nurse circulator accompanies the patient and anesthesia care provider whenever physiological monitoring devices remain active or if oxygen is being administered during transport.

ROOM TURNOVER

The final process for room cleanup and turnover is the removal of soiled instruments and equipment, disposal of waste items in appropriate containers, and terminal disinfection of the room. This process is described in detail in Chapter 11.

HISTORICAL HIGHLIGHTS

- Before the manufacture of commercial surgical sponges, and even for some years after, a fabric loop was sewn into the corner of the laparotomy sponge. The scrub nurse or technologist attached a heavy metal ring (called a *lap ring*) to this loop as sponges were prepared. During surgery,

when a sponge was inserted into the wound, the ring and loop were left hanging outside the incision. The purpose of the ring was for x-ray detection in case a sponge was retained. After surgery the rings were removed (by the scrub) and sponges washed and resterilized to be used on the next procedure.

- Today we occasionally refer to laparotomy sponges as "lap tapes." The name comes from laparotomy sponges manufactured in the 1940s and 1950s, when sponges were not square, but long and rectangular—hence the name *tape*.
- Modern surgical gloves bear no resemblance to those used in the early half of the 1900s. At that time, only rubber was available for the manufacture of gloves. These were large, black, and very thick compared to today's surgical gloves. Before gloving, the surgeon's hands were doused with sterile talcum powder by the instrument nurse, spreading particles in the air where it settled on the instrument setup. The talcum power was purchased in bulk and was presterilized in small paper envelopes prepared by the instrument nurses as part of their duty.

KEY CONCEPTS

- A surgical case plan is a method for improving efficiency and accuracy in preparation for a surgical case. It is a way of thinking and doing that can enhance the surgical technologist's organizational skills and increase his or her ability to anticipate the technical requirements of the procedure.
- A surgical case plan contains distinct elements related to the technical and patient care requirements of the procedure. The elements may vary in complexity according to the type of procedure planned and the specific needs of the patient. The case plan elements can be formulated as distinct questions (e.g. do I need . . .?) or simply a list of points that must be considered to prepare for the procedure.
- The flow of a surgical procedure is dependent on a well-thought-out plan based on experience and logic. The case planning method greatly increases efficiency, which translates into safe patient care, cost-effectiveness, and appropriate use of materials.
- Surgery can be separated into preoperative, intraoperative, and postoperative phases. Planning ahead of time for each phase is one way to approach case planning. Some tasks and routines overlap through more than one phase (e.g., documentation), whereas others are closely associated with a specific phase, such as the universal protocol, which must immediately precede the first incision.
- The sterile setup can seem difficult at first, but can be made manageable by organizing each part of the setup into a sequence of tasks that can be used for most cases.
- The nonsterile case setup is the preparation of the operating room for a specific procedure. This includes positioning of furniture and nonsterile devices, correcting room temperature as needed, and testing and connection of energy and suction sources.
- The surgical count is performed at specific times using prescribed technique to decrease the risk of any surgical

device, instrument, or sponge being left behind in the wound. The count is both time and event related. For example, a count is always performed before surgery begins, before a hollow organ or body cavity is closed, and at the close of surgery before the skin incision is closed.

- Specific practices have been established to prevent retained surgical items. The surgical count is the primary practice. Other important standards identify the proper use, confinement, and detection of items that can be easily lost in the surgical wound.

- The surgical TIMEOUT (Universal Protocol) has been developed in response to the high rate of wrong site and wrong patient surgeries. The protocol is specific, precise, and mandatory in all accredited health care facilities.

- The neutral zone is a physical location on the sterile field designated and understood by the surgical team as a physical space (basin or magnetic board) where sharps are placed and retrieved. This prevents hand-to-hand contact with the surgical knife, suture needles, and other devices that can cause injury.

- The surgical specimen is tissue or objects removed from the patient's body as part of the surgical procedure. The surgical technologist is responsible for management and care of the specimen, which includes its preservation on the sterile field or back table, documentation of the type of tissue or object removed, where it was taken from in the body by tissue type and side, and preservation of orientation markers placed in the specimen by the surgeon. Specimen care also includes placing the specimen in the correct medium for transport to the pathologist, correct labeling, and additional documentation as required by the health care facility.

- The surgical technologist has specific duties at the close of surgery once the patient has been transported from the operating room. The primary duties include care of specimens, documentation, and preparing soiled instruments and other equipment for reprocessing. Cleanup and room turnover are performed using standard precautions for the confinement of body fluids and tissue.

REVIEW QUESTIONS

1. What do you think is the most difficult part of setting up a surgical case? What steps are you taking to overcoming this challenge?
2. What is the rationale for opening large, heavy items first when preparing for a surgical case?
3. During the surgical case setup, there often seems to be insufficient space to place items on the sterile table. What strategies can you use to solve this problem?
4. What is the rationale for handling sterile items as little as possible during the setup?
5. What is the rationale for surgical counts?
6. Who can perform a count?
7. When are counts performed?
8. Who is legally responsible for the surgical count?
9. What is the rationale for a hands-free technique when handling sharps?

10. What are the specific responsibilities of the scrubbed surgical technologist in handling tissue specimens?
11. Discuss the consequences of (a) losing a specimen; (b) misidentifying a specimen.

CASE STUDIES

Case 1

You have been assigned to scrub for an *exploratory laparotomy*. You have received the case cart from the central processing department and have the surgeon's preference card to pick the rest of the supplies noted on the card. You have about 30 minutes before the scheduled case and it normally takes you about 15 minutes to do the sterile set up for a laparotomy. After opening the case you proceed to the scrub area to perform the antiseptic hand rub. When you return to the suite, the anesthesiologist assistant is in the room preparing equipment and drugs. You proceed to gown and glove. *Consider the following events and describe your problem solving approach:*

1. After approximately 15 minutes you are finished with the set up and there the patient has not arrived and you are left alone in the room with the set up. The assistant arrives and states that the surgery is delayed. What will you do? Consider the options, the guidelines for leaving a sterile set up, and the uncertainty of the situation. The anesthesia assistant will not be able to help you make a decision.
2. You have decided to wait, still scrubbed, with the set up. The circulator arrives in another 15 minutes to tell you that case has been cancelled but another patient is coming in following a motor vehicle accident. The tentative procedure planned is *open reduction and internal fixation of a fractured tibia*. The case is scheduled to begin in 30 minutes. How can you use the sterile set up and still prepare for an orthopedic case? You have previously scrubbed only one minor orthopedic case. What is your *strategy* for case planning?

Case 2

You are assigned a large case to prepare for as a scrub and you will be assisted by a circulator and possibly a student circulator. Your case cart has arrived and you are almost sure that essential instrument trays, drapes, and basic equipment are all on the cart. However, there are special items – instruments, suture, equipment that you are not familiar with on the surgeon's preference card. By the time you are able to meet up with the circulator, she is occupied with checking the patient in, and other patient care duties. It is time for you to scrub and perform the set up. How should you communicate your needs and concern about the missing equipment?

Case 3

Universal Protocol (TIMEOUT) was developed because of the high rate of medical errors made in surgery including wrong site, wrong side, and even wrong patient. The protocols for sponge and needle counts (the *count*) and for the medication process were similarly created because of the number of deaths and injury related to these roles. Based on what you have learned and observed about human nature, job stress, and causes of surgical errors *what are the most important advantages to having such protocols?* Try to think about "near misses" you may have witnessed and what strategies you yourself use to prevent errors.

REFERENCES

1. Association of periOperative Registered Nurses (AORN): Recommended practices for maintaining a sterile field. In *AORN Perioperative Standards and Recommended Practices, 2011 edition*, Denver, 2011, AORN.

2. Rowland A, Steeves R: Incorrect surgical counts: a qualitative analysis, *AORN Journal* 92:410, 2010.

3. Norton E, Martin C, Micheli A: Patients count on it: an initiative to reduce incorrect counts and prevent retained surgical items, *AORN Journal* 95:109, 2012.

4. Association of Surgical Technologists: *Recommended standard of practice for counts (effective 2006)*. Accessed May 5, 2012, at http://www.ast.org/pdf/Standards_of_Practice/RSOP_Counts.pdf.

5. Association of periOperative Registered Nurses (AORN): Recommended practices for prevention of retained surgical items. In *AORN Perioperative Standards and Recommended Practices, 2011 edition*, Denver, 2011, AORN.

6. Joint Commission: *Facts about the universal protocol*. Accessed September 13, 2011, at http://www.jointcommission.org/facts_about_the_universal_protocol.

BIBLIOGRAPHY

American College of Surgeons: *ST-51 Statement on the prevention of retained foreign bodies after surgery*. Accessed September 13, 2011, at http://www.facs.org/fellows_info/statements/st-51.html.

Association of periOperative Registered Nurses (AORN): Guidance statements for sharps injury prevention in the perioperative setting. In *Standards, recommended practices and guidelines, 2011 edition*, Denver, 2011, AORN.

Association of periOperative Registered Nurses (AORN): Recommended practices for specimen care and handling. In *Standards, recommended practices and guidelines, 2011 edition*, Denver, 2011, AORN.

Association of periOperative Registered Nurses (AORN): Recommended practices for counts: sponges, sharps, and instruments. In *Standards, recommended practices and guidelines, 2007 edition*, Denver, 2007, AORN.

Barfield WD, Committee on Fetus and Newborn: Standard terminology for fetal, infant, and perinatal deaths. *Pediatrics* 128:177, 2011.

Dalstrom D, Venkatarayappa I, Manternach A, et al: Time-dependent contamination of opened sterile operating-room trays. *Journal of Bone and Joint Surgery (Am)* 90:1022, 2008.

Joint Commission: *Sentinel event statistics*, August 15, 2011. Accessed September 13, 2011, at http://www.jointcommission.org/sentinel_event_statistics_quarterly.

National Cancer Institute: *Laboratory of pathology online policy manual*. Accessed September 13, 2011, at http://home.ncifcrf.gov/ccr/lop/intranet/PolicyManual/SpecimenCollection/specimenhand.asp.

U.S. Department of Health and Human Services, Agency for Healthcare Research and Quality: *Initial clinical evaluation of a handheld device for detecting retained surgical gauze sponges using radiofrequency identification technology*. Accessed September 13, 2011, at http://psnet.ahrq.gov/resource.aspx?resourceID=4050.

Watson D: Improving specimen practices to reduce errors, *AORN Journal* 82:6, 2005.

Management of the Surgical Wound

22

LEARNING OBJECTIVES

After studying this chapter the reader will be able to:

1. Explain the role of the surgical technologist in wound management
2. Discuss Halstead's principles of surgery
3. Explain the importance of the following concepts and practices: preventing injuries, wound irrigation, retraction, thermal and high-frequency coagulation, the pneumatic tourniquet, and autotransfusion
4. Describe different methods of hemostasis
5. List and describe the different types of surgical sponges
6. Discuss the structure and properties of suture
7. Describe the sizing system used for sutures
8. List the types of absorbable and nonabsorbable sutures, and how these are used

9. Identify surgical needles by their shape and type of point
10. Describe the varieties of suture packing
11. Explain the varieties of suturing techniques, as well as specialty uses of sutures
12. Identify safety precautions to prevent needlestick injuries
13. List and describe different types of tissue and synthetic implants used in surgery
14. Describe common wound drains and how they are used
15. Discuss types of dressings and the indication of their use
16. Explain the process of healing
17. Discuss postoperative wound complications

TERMINOLOGY

Absorbable suture: Suture material that is broken down and metabolized by the body.

Adhesion: Scar formation of the abdominal viscera.

Anastomosis: The surgical creation of an opening between two blood vessels, hollow organs, or ducts.

Approximate: To bring tissues together by sutures or other means.

Autotransfusion: Also called *blood salvaging*. A method of retrieving blood lost at the operative site, reprocessing it, and infusing it back to the patient.

Capillary action: The ability of suture material to absorb fluid.

Contracture: Scar tissue that lacks flexibility, causing constriction and pain.

Debridement: Chemical or mechanical removal of necrotic or nonviable tissue and foreign bodies after infection or trauma.

Dehiscence: Separation of the edges of a surgical wound during healing.

Evisceration: The protrusion of abdominal viscera through a wound or surgical incision.

Fistula: A complication of wound infection in which one or more hollow, skin-lined tracts form at the wound site and continue to drain pus and fluid.

Hematoma: A blood-filled space in tissue, the result of a bleeding vessel.

Hemostatic agent: Substance applied to bleeding tissue in order to enhance clotting.

Inert: Causing little or no reaction in tissue or with other materials.

Interrupted sutures: A technique of bringing tissue together by placing individual sutures close together.

Ligate: To place a loop or tie around a blood vessel or duct.

Non absorbable suture: Suture material that resists breakdown in the body.

Primary intention: The wound-healing process after a clean surgical repair.

TERMINOLOGY (cont.)

Running suture: A method of suturing that uses one continuous suture strand for tissue approximation.

Serosanguineous fluid: Exudate or discharge containing serum and blood.

Swage: The area of an atraumatic suture where the suture strand is fused to the needle.

Tapered needle: A suture needle that has a round body that tapers to a sharp point.

Tensile strength: The amount of force or stress a suture can withstand before breaking.

Throw: A loop that forms a knot.

Tie on a passer: A strand of suture material attached to the tip of an instrument.

INTRODUCTION

The surgical incision, including all tissues from the most superficial to the deepest, is called the *surgical wound*. This is the focal area of a surgical procedure. Management of the surgical wound in the intraoperative period requires many skills related to operative (surgical) technique and technologies. Wound management is a team responsibility of the surgeon, surgeon's assistant, and scrubbed surgical technologist or nurse. Technical skills include handling tissues, retraction, hemostasis, and suturing. The surgeon must also choose appropriate instruments, wound products, implants, drainage devices, and dressings. The healing process cannot be separated from the events that occur during the procedure because wound management is directly related to healing.

This chapter covers important techniques and materials used in wound management with a focus on the role of the surgical technologist. The physiological process of wound healing and relationship between wound management and healing are also included to provide a holistic understanding of the surgical process.

THE ROLE OF THE SURGICAL TECHNOLOGIST IN WOUND MANAGEMENT

The surgical technologist participates directly in wound management. He or she must remain alert to the condition of the wound and the progress of the surgery in order to anticipate both routine and unexpected requirements on the field. The surgical technologist performs some of the surgical skills needed to manage the tissues. Retraction, irrigation, and many aspects of hemostasis are part of the technologist's skill set. Sudden hemorrhage in the wound requires quick action by the scrubbed technologist so that appropriate instruments and assistance are immediately available. Direct assistance in sponging and preparing suture and ligation materials are also the technologist's responsibility. Following is a summary of the primary features in wound management:

- Protecting the wound from contamination by any source—maintaining the sterile field
- Hemostasis—control of bleeding
- Exposure—providing an unobstructed view of the tissues and anatomy at hand

- Protecting the tissues from accidental injury by sharps or energy sources used on the field—keeping the area around the immediate wound site clear of instruments that are not in use. Removing sharps immediately after use.
- Contributing to tissue viability, including adequate hydration, gentle handling, and minimal trauma.
- Restoration of tissue planes, edges, and continuity using sutures or other mechanical means.
- Eliminating tissue *dead space* in the wound by providing adequate drainage in the postoperative period.

HALSTEAD'S PRINCIPLES OF SURGERY

Successful wound management is based on essential principles that were developed more than 100 years ago by the famous Johns Hopkins University surgeon William Halstead (also spelled Halsted). Halstead shocked his tutors by criticizing their lack (or absence) of aseptic technique and insisting that they handle tissues gently during surgery. (At the time Halstead was teaching, surgeons did not use gloves and operated in their street clothes.) Halstead also advocated for the use of very fine sutures placed close together with minimal tension on the tissue edges. The principles of surgical wound management that he developed are still considered to be the foundation of good surgical practice. As an essential member of the surgical team, the surgical technologist can benefit from studying these principles:

1. *Handle tissues gently:* Living tissues can be easily bruised, abraded, or crushed during surgery. This can be caused by the wrong instrument or by using an instrument incorrectly. Tissues must never be allowed to dry out during surgery. This can increase superficial abrasions and can result in tissue sloughing. Poor technique in retraction can also result in bruising, edema, or tearing the tissues. The wound edges are protected from injury during retraction by using sponges as a cushion between the instrument and the wound edge.

2. *Control bleeding as efficiently as possible:* Not only does hemorrhage in the surgical site result in loss of total blood volume, but small blood clots or hematomas can slow healing and promote postoperative infection. Meticulous hemostasis allows good visualization of the anatomy and a safer outcome.

3. *Preserve blood supply:* This refers to meticulous dissection, sacrificing as few blood vessels as possible. Without blood supply, tissues cannot heal.

4. *Observe strict aseptic technique:* This should not need emphasis in today's surgical environment. However, even in modern operating rooms, compromise in aseptic technique can be observed when staff are rushed, stressed, or tired.

5. *Minimize tissue tension:* In reference to suturing techniques, tissue tension is avoided. Tension on suture lines creates trauma, swelling, and compression on capillaries at the tissue edge. All of these prevent healing, cause pain, and may result in a surgical site infection.

6. *Eliminate dead space:* Dead space is a gap between tissue layers that normally lie in close contact. It promotes formation of hematoma and serum pockets, leading to infection or the necessity for a second surgery to drain the fluid. Dead space is minimized by careful suturing, hemostasis, and if necessary, insertion of a surgical drain to remove pockets of fluid in seeping wounds.

PREVENTING INJURY

Following Halstead's principles, gentle handling of tissues is one of the most important goals of wound management. Rough handling of deep tissues (e.g., bowel, blood vessels) and other delicate structures can cause extensive bruising, tissue swelling, and ischemia. This can result in an increased inflammatory response and delayed healing. Gentle handling of tissues and protection from drying, heat, and pressure leads to faster recovery. The surgical technologist can contribute to gentle handling of tissue by having the correct instruments in the correct size immediately available. Babcock forceps, smooth tissue pickups, and retractors with increased tactile response such as a Deaver over a Richardson for abdominal surgery must be available. Naturally in pediatric surgery, specific pediatric instruments must be used according to the scale and fragility of the organ systems and tissues.

The surgical technologist must continually retrieve instruments not in use from the surgical field. This is to protect the patient and team from injury and also to prevent instruments from falling to the floor. Surgeons generally do not place instruments back on the Mayo tray, out of courtesy to the scrub and to prevent "hand collisions." Instead, they usually lay them on the sterile field for retrieval by the scrub. Heavy instruments left on the surgical field can cause injury to the patient. Sharps not in use, including retractors with sharp teeth, must be retrieved immediately after use.

During surgery, tissue must be handled as little as possible. Physiological stress on the tissues causes an increased release of catecholamines (e.g., epinephrine). This produces local swelling and fluid accumulation. This serous fluid can become a reservoir for microorganisms in the postoperative period. Excessive or rough handling of bowel tissue can cause a sympathetic nerve response called *paralytic ileus,* in which peristalsis ceases. Paralytic ileus can be a serious postoperative complication when it leads to intestinal obstruction.

Scrubbed surgical team members must never lean on the patient. This sometimes occurs when a member of the team is required to provide retraction for a long period, resulting in fatigue. It is sometimes necessary to remind team members (especially staff new to surgery such as medical students and interns) not to lean on the patient.

WOUND IRRIGATION

Tissues must not be allowed to dehydrate during surgery. Dry tissues cannot withstand handling and may slough during the healing phase. Wound edges, bowel tissue, muscle, and subcutaneous tissue are particularly sensitive to dehydration and bruising. Intermittent irrigation is used to protect delicate tissues.

The technologist offers normal (0.9%) saline irrigation fluid when the surgeon asks for it and whenever tissues appear to be dehydrated. Signs of dehydration in internal tissues are surface dullness, loss of surface elasticity, and tissue fraying. Tissue is also irrigated to flush away very small bits of tissue that have sloughed during surgery. Antibiotic irrigation is used to prevent infection in selected cases.

A large wound is irrigated using an Asepto or a bulb syringe (Figure 22-1). Two syringes may be required; while one is in use, the other is being filled. Irrigation solution is removed from the wound using the inline suction with a suction tip, which is part of most instrument setups. When large amounts of saline are required, such as during orthopedic procedures or surgery of the major body cavities, a large suction tip such as the Yankauer (tonsil) suction or Poole suction tip is used. The Poole suction tip comes with a removable guard with multiple perforations that distribute the suction pressure and prevent damage to delicate tissue such as the spleen, lung, and intestine. When large amounts of irrigation fluid are used, the surgical technologist must keep track of the volume so that the estimated blood loss can be calculated.

Microsurgery, or any other small wound area such as eye and ear procedures, may not require suction, and only solutions labeled for these tissues are used. Irrigation during eye procedures is crucial to maintaining the cornea. Balanced salt solution is used for irrigation. It is supplied commercially in small plastic bottles to which the surgical technologist attaches

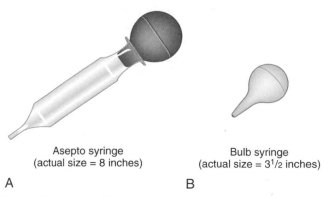

Asepto syringe
(actual size = 8 inches)

Bulb syringe
(actual size = 3½ inches)

A   B

Figure 22-1 Wound irrigation. A, Asepto syringe. B, Bulb syringe for smaller wounds.

an ophthalmic irrigation tip. This procedure is discussed more fully in Chapter 27.

Continuous irrigation is used in specific types of surgery of the joint capsule, genitourinary tract, and uterus. In these cases, the irrigation fluid is used as a medium through which surgery is performed. In bladder, uterine, and prostate surgery in which tumor tissue is removed piecemeal, continuous irrigation flushes the tissue specimens from the wound. In arthroscopic joint surgery, especially of the knee, continuous irrigation increases the joint space, providing better visualization through the arthroscope. (Refer to specific specialty chapters for a complete discussion.)

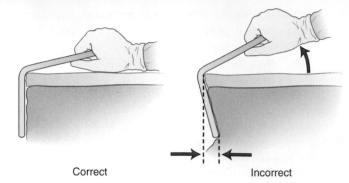

Correct   Incorrect

Figure 22-2   Correct technique for wound retraction.

RETRACTION

As tissue planes are dissected or opened, the surgical wound becomes increasingly deep. Retractors are placed at the wound edges to pull back the more superficial tissues and expose underlying anatomy. Categories of retractors are:

- Handheld
- Self-retaining (designed with a mechanism that holds them open)

Retractors are selected according to the depth of the retracting blade (the distance between the horizontal and vertical parts of the instrument), by their tips (blunt, curved, sharp, clawlike, gently tapered), and by overall size and weight. All of these variables are considered according to the type of tissue being retracted and the depth of the wound. Retractors are passed with the tip angled down, toward the wound. Self-retaining retractors with a ratchet mechanism are always passed in the fully closed position, ready for positioning in the wound.

As the superficial tissues are incised, the scrub anticipates the need for deeper retraction and selects the correct retractor as requested or required. Examples of large self-retaining retractors are the Balfour, the Omni used in abdominal procedures, and the Finochietto retractor designed for use in thoracic surgery. In back or hip surgery, the hinged Beckman retractor is often used.

The smaller self-retaining retractors (e.g., the Weitlaner retractor) are used in the groin and in other areas of the body that require superficial retraction. Small handheld retractors include the Senn, a very common double-ended retractor that has a small "rake" at one end and a superficial right angle at the other. This retractor is used in superficial wounds up to 1 inch in depth. Rake retractors come in many sizes, from very large (Israel retractor) to extremely small (simply referred to as a small rake). The tips of the rake retractor are dull or very sharp. The skin hook is a delicate handheld retractor that has a needle-sharp hook at the end. It is used only on skin for delicate retraction, usually in plastic surgery.

Localized retraction, as in moving a single blood vessel or nerve aside, is performed using premanufactured lengths of fabric or elastic. These are discussed in Chapter 32.

RETRACTION TECHNIQUES

The surgical technologist is often asked to retract during surgery. The blade of the retractor is used as a backstop to prevent tissue from obstructing the open incision. The usual method of retraction is for the surgeon to place the retractor and the surgical technologist to hold it in place without toeing the blade inward unless instructed by the surgeon (Figure 22-2). The blade should be maintained in position unless the surgeon asks for "toe in." The surgeon may take the retractor in hand for repositioning as needed. Retraction for a long period of time can cause stress on the operative hand and arm, which must be kept still the entire time (more so for delicate retraction). This can lead to distraction and slippage of the instrument. It may be necessary to switch hands when retracting for longer than a few minutes.

Retraction using skin hooks or small rakes requires concentration on the pressure at the tip in order to prevent accidental tearing of the tissue. Skin hooks should be held between the thumb and two or three fingers in the middle of the instrument for maximum control of the tip.

HEMOSTASIS

One of the most important technical objectives of surgery is to maintain hemostasis. *Hemostasis* means controlling bleeding by mechanical means such as sutures, sponges, surgical instruments, and electrosurgery, and by biochemical means using drugs or other pharmaceutical agents. (Do not confuse *hemostasis* with *homeostasis*, which is physiological equilibrium across all body systems, controlled by the central nervous system.) In physiological terms, *hemostasis* means conserving the body's total blood volume, which is necessary for life. Hemostasis is also a necessary component of good surgical technique. Pooling of blood and serum in the wound in the postsurgical period can increase the risk of infection. Fluid pockets also prevent healing, because they form a physical barrier between tissue edges that need to be in close approximation during healing. Uncontrolled oozing or insecure hemostasis can lead to a hematoma. This is a collection of blood that may need to be surgically removed, especially if the clot impinges on regional nerves and vessels.

METHODS OF HEMOSTASIS

Hemostasis is physiologically maintained by the process of coagulation, described later. During surgery, many techniques are used to control bleeding and prevent uncontrolled hemorrhage that would overwhelm the body's compensatory mechanisms. These techniques include:

- Clamping and ligating the bleeding vessel
- Sutures that bring tissue edges in close approximation and promote coagulation
- Use of electrosurgery to seal a vessel
- Use of **hemostatic agents**, which promote coagulation when directly applied to the bleeding tissue

Blood replacement (discussed later in the chapter) is a separate process. This may be performed using a blood product during transfusion or by autotransfusion when the patient's own blood is returned to the body during surgery.

THE PHYSIOLOGY OF COAGULATION

The natural (physiological) coagulation process takes place through a series, or *cascade*, of complex events, each triggered by the one preceding it. The *extrinsic* mechanism begins when a blood vessel is injured. The subsequent events are:

1. *Vasospasm:* The blood vessel retracts and constricts. This reduces blood flow through the vessel.
2. *A platelet plug forms:* Platelets aggregate in the area and form a plug. The presence of platelets initiates the release of coagulation factors in the plasma.
3. *Coagulation begins:* A meshwork of fibrin strands forms around the blood platelets, creating a clot. This process is initiated by coagulation *factors* (organic substances present in the blood) shown in Box 22-1. Coagulation is activated by two pathways, the *extrinsic pathway* and the *intrinsic pathway*. The intrinsic pathway is activated by factors present in the blood. The extrinsic pathway occurs in the tissues.

Coagulation involves many chemicals that interact in an elaborate feedback mechanism. If any of the factors are missing, through genetic anomaly or disease, hemostasis is altered. Severe hemorrhage may overwhelm the body's natural mechanisms for controlling bleeding, leading to shock and eventual death if the bleeding cannot be controlled.

Box **22-1**	**Coagulation Factors**
Factor	**Nomenclature**
I	Fibrinogen
II	Prothrombin
III	Thromboplastin, thrombokinase
IV*	—
V	Proaccelerin, labile factor
VI*	—
VII	Serum prothrombin conversion accelerator (SPCA)
VIII	Antihemophilic globulin (AGH)
IX	Plasma thromboplastin component
X	Christmas factor
XI	Stuart factor
XII	Hageman factor
XIII	Fibrin-stabilizing factor

*Factors IV and VI are now obsolete.

HEMOSTATIC AGENTS

Many different types of hemostatic agents have been developed in the past decade for use on bleeding surfaces during surgery. These include purified animal and human derivatives and also newer synthetic agents. Tissue sealants are a newer category of agents that are used as a coating over raw tissue surfaces to prevent capillary bleeding and in lung tissue to prevent air leakage. There are now several categories of topical agents available with which the surgical technologist should become familiar (refer to Table 22-1 for a complete listing of hemostatic agents and tissue sealants). These are:

- Active hemostats
- Flowables
- Fibrin sealants

Active Hemostats

An active hemostat stimulates the body's own coagulation process that converts fibrin to fibrinogen. These agents include topical (human) thrombin, bovine thrombin, and recombinant thrombin. *Topical thrombin USP* (U.S. Pharmacopoeia) is commercially prepared as a dry powder or solution derived from bovine or human sources (recombinant human thrombin). When applied to oozing tissue, it combines with the body's fibrinogen to promote coagulation.

Topical powder is applied directly to an oozing surface or mixed with injectable isotonic saline for use as a spray, by drop, or for soaking hemostatic sponges.

Topical thrombin is available as a sterile powder in vials containing 5,000 or 20,000 international units for reconstitution with sterile saline. Frozen thrombin *solution* is available in 800 and 1,200 international units per mL. When labeling these drugs on the sterile field, it is necessary to include the strength in international units per mL.

Note: Thrombin is never injected into blood vessels. It is a high-alert medication that must be carefully managed on the sterile field.

Mechanical Hemostatic Agents

Mechanical hemostatic agents enhance the normal coagulation (clotting) process by mechanical means, by providing a mesh, granular, or fluff matrix that promotes platelet aggregation on bleeding surfaces. These are formulated from gelatin, collagen, cellulose, and polysaccharides. They are manufactured without natural or synthetic drugs. However, some are prepared in combination with thrombin solution on the sterile field. The mechanical agent promotes hemostasis by forming a barrier on oozing surfaces. In contact with body fluid they instantly swell and form a physical matrix for coagulation.

ABSORBABLE GELATIN *Absorbable gelatin* is a dry sponge or film material derived from porcine tissue. When applied to tissue, it absorbs blood quickly and enhances clot formation. The clot is the result of mechanical rather than chemical action of the material. Absorbable gelatin is most commonly supplied under the proprietary names *Gelfoam, Gelfilm, and Surgifoam*. These are available in squares, which are cut to size as needed. The usual size used during surgery is $1/4$ to 1 inch square or rectangular pieces. Absorbable hemostatic

Table 22-1 Tissue Sealants and Hemostats

Names	Dosage Form	Use	Components	Qualities
Thrombin/Fibrinogen USP				
Topical Thrombin USP (Thrombin, Evithrom, Recothrom)	Solution or dry requiring saline diluent	Active hemostasis for topical use on bleeding tissues	Bovine or human origin thrombin	May cause severe coagulation disorder related to development of antibodies
Evicel	Solution	Active hemostasis	Fibrinogen concentrate and thrombin derived from pooled human plasma	Effective as spray or drip application
Gelatin Hemostats				
Gelfoam Surgifoam	Dry sponge sheets, powder	Mechanical hemostasis on tissue surface or vascular anastomosis	Gelatin sponge used with thrombin solution or saline	Can be soaked in thrombin; partially resorbable but usually removed to prevent granuloma
Collagen Hemostat				
Avitene EndoAvetine Instat MCH	Dry powder	Mechanical hemostasis	Collagen powder hemostat	Used in dry form
Oxidized Cellulose Hemostat				
Surgicel	Gauze fiber tuft or sponge	Mechanical hemostasis	Cellulose	Swells on contact with fluid Absorbs in 1 to 6 weeks
Fibrin Combination Sealants				
Tisseel	Gel	Capillary hemostasis Prevents air leaks; used to seal lung, liver; also in plastic surgery and skin grafting	Fibrinogen, CaCl, aprotinin, thrombin	Low bonding strength Requires 20 minutes preparation time
Floseal	Gel	Flowable topical hemostat	Bovine-derived gelatin matrix, human thrombin in calcium chloride solution	Resorbed in 6 to 8 weeks postop
Surgiflow	Gel	Flowable topical hemostat for use in surgery	Porcine-derived gelatin also available with thrombin	Effective with or without thrombin
CrossSeal	Gel	Flowable topical hemostasis	Crosslinked gelatin granules and thrombin	Crosslinked gelatin swells on application
Omnex	Liquid/gel	Vascular anastomosis site sealant	100% synthetic cyanoacrylates	Remains in place during healing
CoSeal	Liquid/gel	Used to mechanically seal vascular reconstruction site	100% synthetic; polyethylene glycol polymers	Remains in place during healing
Dermabond	Liquid	Used to close the skin (incisions and lacerations)	Synthetic cyanoacrylate	Fast setting with high strength; nonabsorbable
Other				
Platelet gel	Gel	Augments hemostasis provides additional platelets and growth factors	Autologous preparation from patient's plasma	Must be prepared for each individual patient
Ostene	Putty	Hemostatic agent used on bone surface	Combination of synthetics: ethylene oxide and propylene oxide	Safer than prototype bone wax made from beeswax combinations
BioGlue	Liquid	Tissue sealant used to seal leaks in vascular anastomosis	Bovine serum albumin plus glutaraldehyde	Creates flexible seal independent of suture anastomosis
Silver nitrate	Fluid or applicator	Creates thick eschar; stains tissue	Caustic chemical	Seldom used; used only for superficial bleeding

agents are not left in place over neural or bone tissue, because tissue injury can result.

The scrubbed surgical technologist prepares gelatin sponge on the surgical field. If thrombin is used as a soaking agent for gelatin, the circulator dispenses injectable saline diluent (liquid) and dry thrombin powder mix to the scrubbed technologist, using aseptic technique. The liquid drug is immediately labeled and used during the case to soak hemostatic gelatin.

Gelatin sponge is dispensed in 2- or 3-inch squares for cutting into smaller patches as requested by the surgeon. The pieces are placed in liquid topical thrombin or isotonic saline, or they may be used in dry form. After soaking, gelatin should swell and become soft. If this does not occur, the pieces can be removed from solution and compressed to remove the air. They then are returned to the solution and kept there until use. The technologist can dispense the sponge pieces to the surgeon in a small basin. All gelatin sponge squares are removed from the surgical wound after use. The technologist should collect these and remove them from the sterile field so they do not fall back into the wound.

OXIDIZED CELLULOSE *Oxidized cellulose USP* is available in mesh and powder form. It is always applied to tissue in dry form. On contact with blood, it rapidly forms a clot, which is absorbed by the body during the healing process. Oxidized cellulose is manufactured as *Surgicel*.

It must be kept dry until it is used on tissue. If allowed to become wet, it is difficult to handle and loses its shape. It is available in small strips or squares, which may need to be cut with suture scissors. The pieces can then be dispensed to the surgeon in a small basin or container. Any discarded material should be cleared from the surgical site so that it does not enter (or reenter) the wound accidentally.

COLLAGEN ABSORBABLE HEMOSTAT Collagen absorbable hemostat is manufactured from bovine collagen and supplied in dry form as powder, sheets, and sponges. *Avitene* is approved for use in all surgery and is also supplied in preloaded applicators for endoscopic use. In powder form, it is applied directly to capillary surfaces. The strips may be wrapped around the anastomosis connecting two vessels or hollow structures to form a hemostatic seal. This product is not approved for all surgical tissue. Preparation and use of collagen absorbable hemostat is the same as for oxidized cellulose. It must be kept dry before use.

BONE HEMOSTAT Hemostasis in bone is achieved by applying a waxy substance, commonly called *bone wax*, into the surface of a bleeding bone. This material, traditionally made from a combination of beeswax and other additives, has been replaced by more biocompatible agents. The current formulation of bone putty is derived from ethylene oxide and propylene oxide *(Ostene)*. Bone hemostatic materials must be warmed slightly before use. This is done by kneading small pieces between the gloved fingers. They are dispensed by mounting them on the edge of a small basin or container that can be placed on the sterile field.

Flowable Hemostats and Adhesives

Flowable hemostats are composed of porcine or bovine gelatin. They have a viscous quality (approximately the same as honey) and are used in areas that are difficult to access. Some products such as FloSeal (Baxter) and Surgiflow (Johnson & Johnson) also contain pooled human thrombin.

Fibrin Sealants

Fibrin sealants are applied to the surface of tissues to bind them together or to prevent air or blood leakage. A few sealants such as natural fibrin have been marketed for some time. Newer combination products and synthetic polymers are now formulated for use as sealants.

Common uses of sealants and adhesives are:
- In surgery of the respiratory system, they are used to close air leaks in on lung surfaces and to close bronchial tubes following anastomosis.
- Hemostatic sealant is used on liver and spleen surfaces that cannot be sutured easily.
- In vascular surgery, sealants or coagulants are used to bind together vessels in conjunction with sutures that connect blood vessels together (**anastomosis**).
- Other uses under experimentation are for use in the esophagus for bleeding esophageal varices, and in endoscopic surgery for hemostasis.
- Collagen-based adhesives are used for sealing anastomosies in vascular surgery and dura mater leaks.

Handling tissue sealants on the field is relatively straightforward. Components that must be mixed are dispensed in their own cartridges, and all are packaged as systems, including single-use applicators with easy use directions.

THERMAL AND HIGH-FREQUENCY COAGULATION

Coagulation is performed surgically using a number of technologies, including the electrosurgical unit (ESU), laser, high-frequency electricity, and ultrasound. These are discussed in detail in Chapter 18. Some state practice acts permit the certified surgical technologist to transmit electricity from the active electrosurgical electrode to live tissue in the surgical wound for coagulation. The technique for this procedure is also explained in Chapter 18, which provides a necessary explanation of the technology and patient safety considerations for the procedure.

PNEUMATIC TOURNIQUET

The pneumatic tourniquet (Figure 22-3) is used in limb surgery to create a bloodless surgical site. The tourniquet cuff is a nonlatex air bladder encased in a nylon cuff, much like a blood pressure cuff. Tourniquet cuffs are manufactured in a variety of sizes and widths. Before the tourniquet is placed on the limb, the area where the tourniquet is to be wrapped is padded with flat cotton bandaging material (Webril or Soft Roll) that conforms to the shape of the leg or arm as it is wrapped. The tourniquet is then applied over the cotton material (but not yet inflated).

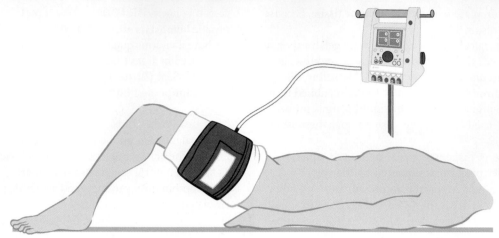

Figure 22-3 **Pneumatic tourniquet.** The tourniquet is applied to the limb, and the correct pressure is set on the digital control unit.

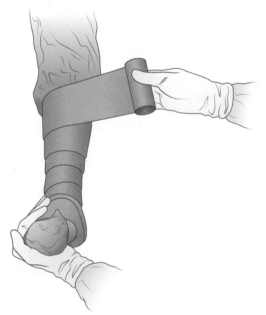

Figure 22-4 An Esmarch bandage is wrapped from distal to proximal to exsanguinate the limb before the pneumatic tourniquet is inflated.

To produce a bloodless surgical site, a flexible latex bandage (Esmarch bandage) is wrapped sequentially around the limb from distal to proximal up to the level of the tourniquet (Figure 22-4). This exsanguinates the limb, pushing the blood proximally away from the surgical site. The pneumatic tourniquet is inflated with the Esmarch bandage in place. This prevents blood from flowing back into the vessels. Once the tourniquet reaches the designated pressure, the Esmarch bandage is removed.

Misuse of a pneumatic tourniquet is associated with tissue necrosis and vascular and nerve damage. These tourniquets are applied and managed only by trained personnel, who observe the following safety precautions to prevent injury to the patient:

- When the pneumatic tourniquet is inflated, the period from cuff inflation to deflation is called *tourniquet time* and

is measured precisely. Both inflation and deflation times are documented in the patient's intraoperative chart.

- The tourniquet may remain inflated for up to 1 hour on an upper extremity and 1½ to 2 hours on a lower extremity. After that period, the patient is at risk for nerve and vascular damage and tissue necrosis related to ischemia.

- For an adult patient, the tourniquet pressure must not exceed 50 to 75 mm Hg above the patient's systolic blood pressure for an upper extremity or 100 to 150 mm Hg above the systolic pressure for a lower extremity. For a pediatric patient, the upper limit is 100 mm Hg above the patient's systolic pressure.

- Strict policies regarding the use of tourniquets are enforced in all facilities.

- Prep solutions and moisture must be prevented from seeping under the tourniquet cuff, because this can cause burns.

- The pressure gauge must be tested before the cuff is inflated.

- If surgery continues beyond the recommended inflation time, the tourniquet is deflated for 10 minutes and then reinflated. As soon as it is deflated, the field will fill with blood, and hemostasis must be maintained.

- The surgical technologist should always roll the Esmarch bandage after it is removed, because it may be needed again during the surgical procedure.

- The nurse circulator assesses the site for the tourniquet before it is applied. The site is assessed a second time and charted when the tourniquet is removed.

AUTOTRANSFUSION

Autotransfusion is the salvaging of blood at the operative or trauma site and reinfusion into the patient. Its primary use is during surgical cases in which large blood loss is anticipated, such as ruptured ectopic pregnancy and trauma cases. Autotransfusion equipment, such as the *Cell Saver* (Haemonetics, Braintree, Mass), is set up before or during surgery and sterile connections are passed to the scrubbed team. The concept of different autotransfusion devices is the same, with variations in technical aspects. Free blood is collected in the wound by

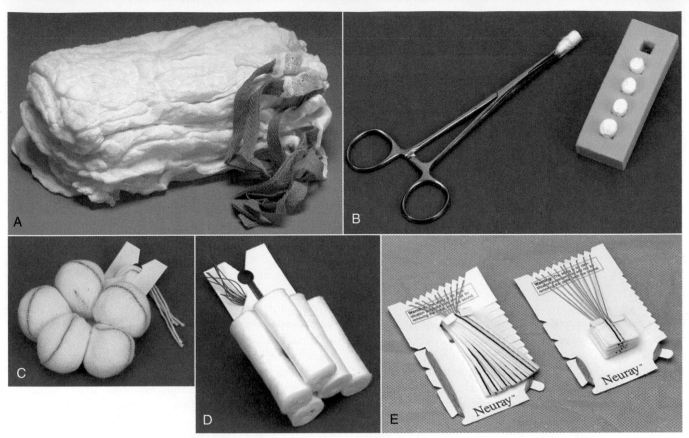

Figure 22-5 **Surgical sponges. A,** Laparotomy sponge. **B,** Small dissector. **C,** Tonsil sponge. **D,** Cotton roll. **E,** Neurosurgical patty. *(Courtesy DeRoyal Industries, Powell, Tenn.)*

suction and routed through blood tubing directly attached to the device, which rinses, anticoagulates, and filters the blood cells from unwanted components. Blood is then collected within the system and immediately available for reinfusion. Postoperative autotransfusion is performed with devices such as the cardioPAT and OrthoPAT (Haemonetics). The system collects blood in the postoperative wound through a closed system for reinfusion. Autotransfusion is acceptable to some patients who, for religious, cultural, or other reasons, decline transfusion of blood donated from another individual. Advantages of autotransfusion are decreased risk of communicable disease transmission by banked blood, increased hematocrit ratio in the blood, and immediate availability of blood during surgery. Autotransfusion systems include the power unit and cell washing system, blood tubing and bags, suction catheter, and filters. Equipment setup includes sterile and nonsterile components. Depending on the type and manufacturer, the setup is relatively straightforward. The surgical technologist may be trained on setup and use of a specific unit by the company representative or facility staff member who is familiar with the unit.

SURGICAL SPONGES

Surgical sponges are used for hemostasis and a variety of other purposes. They maintain a dry wound by soaking up blood and fluids. They are used to retract tissue in body cavities and as cushioning against instruments used to retract. Dissecting

sponges are used to separate tissue planes by flaying the tissue gently with the tip or edge of the sponge. Surgical sponges are available in a variety of sizes, shapes, and materials (Figure 22-5). Because of their compatibility with human tissue and their pliability when wet, sponges can become lodged in the surgical wound and become difficult to differentiate from tissue. As explained in the previous chapter, care of sponges on and off the sterile field is crucial to ensuring that no sponge is left behind in the wound.

4 × 4 (RAYTEC) SPONGE

The 4 × 4 sponge (also called a "four by four" or *Raytec*) is a large square of loosely woven gauze folded into a 4-inch-square pad. When used in a deep incision, the Raytec sponge is always mounted on a sponge forceps, commonly called a *sponge stick*. To mount a 4 × 4 sponge, fold it in equal thirds in one direction and in half in the other direction. Mount the sponge with the folded edge exposed at the tip of the sponge forceps.

NOTE: Only mounted 4 × 4 sponges are to be placed on the field when a body cavity is open.

LAPAROTOMY SPONGE

The laparotomy sponge, also called a *lap* or *tape,* is used in major surgery, including procedures in which the abdominal or thoracic cavity is opened, during major orthopedic surgery, and in procedures in which large blood vessels are encountered. Laparotomy sponges are used to absorb blood and fluids and for padding beneath the blades of large retractors. This helps prevent injury from direct contact with the retractor blade.

Lap sponges usually are moistened before use. A basin of warm saline is used for this purpose. The sponge is immersed in saline and then wrung dry.

SPONGE DISSECTOR

A sponge dissector (also called a *peanut*, a *pusher*, and various other names) is a small round or oval sponge covered with gauze. The sponge dissector is always mounted on a clamp and is used to separate or dissect tissue—, called *blunt dissection*.

ROUND SPONGE

A *tonsil sponge* is covered with gauze and has a string attached for retrieval. This sponge is commonly used in throat surgery and often is used to control bleeding in the tonsillar fossae after tonsillectomy. The string is draped outside the patient's mouth. Use of round sponges without strings is extremely dangerous in throat surgery. Such sponges can easily drop into the trachea and cause complete airway blockage. Asphyxia and death can occur very quickly, especially in pediatric patients. When the round sponge is returned after use, always make sure the string is attached.

SURGICAL COTTON BALLS

The surgical cotton ball is specially manufactured to resist shredding and is commonly used in neurosurgical procedures, especially around fragile brain and spinal cord tissues. Cotton balls may be dipped in normal saline or topical thrombin to aid hemostasis.

FLAT NEUROSURGICAL SPONGES

The flat sponge, also called a *cottonoid* or *patty*, is a compressed square of synthetic or cotton material with a string attached. Flat sponges are available in many different sizes for use during neurosurgical, ear, and vascular procedures. They usually are offered to the surgeon moistened with saline or topical thrombin rather than dry. The flat sponge is used to maintain hemostasis or as a filter over delicate tissue requiring suction. When flat sponges are exchanged on the field, make sure every sponge is returned intact with the string attached.

SUTURES

Suture materials are used to **approximate** tissues (i.e., bring tissue edges together by suture or other means) while healing takes place and to ligate (tie) blood vessels or tubal structures. In surgery, *suture* can refer to a length of suturing thread or a suture thread and needle combination. Packages of suture material are simply called "sutures." Suture material is made from synthesized chemicals, animal protein, metal, and natural fibers.

STUDYING AND LEARNING SUTURE USE

Learning the types and use of sutures is one of the most challenging skills for students in surgery. Familiarity with the many types of sutures and needles and the techniques for handling them is acquired over time with repetition and study. Suture manufacturers recognize that the scrub person and circulator need to identify a suture type quickly. Packages are color-coded by suture type, and needles often are pictured on the label for rapid selection and delivery to the sterile field.

Difficulties in learning sutures arise because of the many different types of sutures and needles, complicated by the fact that identical suture materials made by different companies have different trade names. Recall from Chapter 13 that the manufacturing company that creates a new drug formula receives a patent for that material. As with drugs, when the patent expires on suture material, (usually after 20 years), the material can be manufactured by any company with its own trade name. For example, Dexon suture (polyglycolic acid), which was patented in the early 1980s, is now off patent and is available by other names from many companies. The material is the same, but there are now multiple trade names. To complicate matters, suture-needle combinations are given a product number. These can be seen in any suture company's catalog. The same type of needle exists in other companies, but identified by their own catalog numbers. As an aid to comparing suture needle catalog numbers, companies now include a comparison chart that translates their catalog number to those of other manufacturers.

One of the ways to overcome some of these difficulties is to learn sutures and needles by their generic names, which never change (although new products are added). Mastery of technical aspects of sutures is an important skill for surgical technologists. Some of the difficulties are overcome by working with the same surgeons and becoming familiar with their preferences. It is generally not beneficial to memorize every company's trade name for a specific suture material. Health care facilities usually have a contract with one suture company to purchase their products in bulk. It is useful to become familiar with that company's suture products with focus on those that are used in your facility.

Overall, the learning process must include, in the beginning steps, types of suture materials and *why* that type and size is used in a specific tissue or circumstance. This is a professional approach that remains valid even if companies introduce new suture products.

REGULATION OF SUTURES

Like medications, suture materials used in the United States must be approved by the U.S. Food and Drug Administration (FDA) and the U.S. Pharmacopeia, discussed in Chapter 13. All substances, including suture products, that bear the USP label must meet minimum standards. The standards for suture materials include size conformity, tensile strength, and sterility. Additional standards cover packaging, dyes used in the suture, and the integrity of the needles. The European Pharmacopoeia (EP) sets standards for sutures used in European Union (EU) countries, including those sutures manufactured and distributed by U.S. companies.

PROPERTIES OF SUTURES

The properties and characteristics of sutures contribute to the surgeon's choice and application of a suture. The following terms relate to the properties of suture:

- *Physical characteristics*: The physical structure of the suture and its size.
- *Tensile strength:* The amount of tension a length of suture can withstand before breaking.
- *Fluid absorption:* The ability of a suture to take up fluid.
- *Knot strength:* The amount of force a knot can withstand before slipping or breaking. This is related to friction and plasticity.
- *Memory (recoil):* The ability of a suture to return or maintain its original shape. This is related to diameter, plasticity, and elasticity.
- *Plasticity:* The ability to withstand bending and crimping without breaking and to maintain the new shape after it is made. This applies to knot tying and the suture's tendency to untie, or to maintain the configuration of the knot.
- *Pliability:* A measure of the ease of handling, softness in the hand, and flat knotting.
- *Absorption quality:* The effect of the tissue on the suture, its resistance to breakdown (degradation of the material by the lysosomal action of enzymes), and absorption into the body.
- *Bioactivity*: The effect of the suture on the tissue.
- *Composition:* The chemical, molecular, or elemental makeup and origin of the substance used to manufacture the suture.

Physical Structure

Structurally, sutures are broadly divided into three categories:

- *Monofilament:* A single continuous fiber made of a polymer chemical (chains of the same molecule strung together) made by extrusion and stretching the material.
- *Multifilament:* Many filaments that together form one strand of suture. Multifilament suture in turn is divided into two types:
  - *Twisted:* Multiple fibers are twisted in the same direction.
  - *Braided:* Multiple fibers are intertwined.
- *Composite:* A core strand of one suture material is jacketed with another of a different type.

Figure 22-6 shows two basic suture structures.

Suture Size

The size of the suture is based on the diameter of a single strand. The USP numbering system indicates the suture's outside diameter and ensures that a stated size is the same regardless of the material. For example, size 2-0 silk suture has the same diameter as size 2-0 nylon suture. Although size contributes to strength, there are other factors involved. Selection of a particular size is based mainly on the type of tissue and the load or tension that will be placed on the sutures.

Suture ranges in size from 11-0 (thinnest) to 5 (thickest). The greater the diameter, the larger the designated size. For example, size 2 is thicker than size 0. Sutures smaller than 0 are designated by additional zeros. For example, size 2-0 is an average size for abdominal wall tissue. Size 11-0 is used in microsurgery. This suture is light enough to remain suspended in the air. Sutures of this size naturally are very delicate and expensive and must be handled with care.

Stainless steel suture historically has used the *Brown and Sharp (B & S) sizing system* rather than USP sizes. These numbers begin with size 38/40 gauge (the thinnest) up to 18 gauge (the thickest). Stainless steel now is sized according to USP standards. However, some surgeons may request the B & S number, which is printed on steel wire packages. Table 22-2 shows B & S sizes and their corresponding USP size.

Tensile Strength

The **tensile strength** of suture refers to the amount of force needed to break the suture. The linear strength of the suture can easily be tested by attempting to break a strand. However, its strength at the knot (the weakest point) and how resistant the suture is to breakage in the wound environment are more

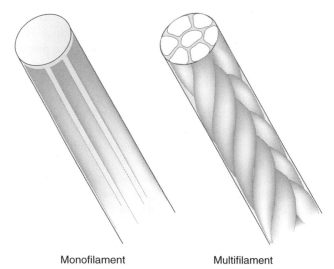

Monofilament   Multifilament

Figure 22-6 Extruded monofilament and braided multifilament sutures. *(Redrawn from Rothrock JC: Alexander's care of the patient in surgery, ed 12, St Louis, 2003, Mosby.)*

Table 22-2	Stainless Steel Suture Sizes										
B & S gauge (no.)	40	35	32	30	28	26	25	24	23	22	20
USP size	6-0	5-0	4-0	3-0	2-0	0	1	2	3	4	5

B & S, Brown and Sharp; USP, U.S. Pharmacopeia.

important. These characteristics are more difficult to predict and are influenced by many factors, such as:

- The *type of knot* used to tie the suture. Suture material becomes 10% to 40% weaker at the knot.
- The *biological environment* of the suture. Suture materials vary in strength when exposed to body fluids. Some resist breakdown, whereas others are quickly degraded and absorbed. The medical condition of the patient also influences suture strength. Most suture materials break down quickly in the presence of infection and in certain kinds of metabolic conditions.
- *Uniformity* (a quality control factor). Sutures must be uniform in diameter to maintain tensile strength.

Tensile strength is one of the most important qualities of a suture. Breakage during the process of suturing is frustrating and time consuming. *Breakage in the postoperative phase can lead to infection or injury* to the tissue.

Handling Qualities

The handling qualities of a suture determine its ease of use and may affect the technical quality of the wound closure. For these reasons, surgeons are careful to balance the handling qualities of a suture with its other characteristics.

Compliance or *pliability* is the ease of handling or softness in the hand. Pliability makes the suture material easier to manipulate. The knots lie flat and remain secure (called *tie-down*). Silk suture has traditionally been considered the gold standard of all suture materials for its pliability, tight knots, and ease of use. More inert suture materials have taken its place through the years, but silk's other qualities rank it high for handling and strength for size.

Memory describes the suture's tendency to retain its original shape or configuration after it is removed from the package. Most suture is packaged in coils or in "racetrack" formation (stainless steel is packaged straight to prevent kinking). High-memory suture is springy and tends to tangle during preparation and use. This also correlates with the ability of a suture to stay knotted. Material that is stiff or retains memory tends to loosen easily. This is both annoying and time-consuming for the surgeon. Extruded monofilament sutures have greater coil memory than braided or twisted fiber suture.

Plasticity refers to the material's ability to stretch and retain a new shape. Elasticity can be advantageous as long as the suture retains its strength when stretched. Increased plasticity contributes to secure knots when the suture material remains knotted and the strands resist sliding out of the knot.

Absorption

Suture materials are partly categorized according to their absorption characteristics and the origin of the material. Absorption is different from bioactivity, which describes how the body reacts to the suture. *Absorption* describes how the suture reacts in the presence of body tissue. Both **absorbable suture** and **non absorbable suture** are available in natural (biological) and synthetic (human-made) form.

The ideal suture would be one that retains its strength throughout the healing period and then dissolves (is absorbed) when healing is complete. However, the ideal suture does not exist.

Absorbable, protein-based suture is attacked by enzyme-releasing lysosomes that digest the suture. Absorbable synthetic sutures are degraded by *hydrolysis,* a chemical reaction that occurs in the presence of water. Non absorbable sutures become encapsulated in connective tissue, and some (e.g., nylon and silk) eventually are at least partly absorbed. All sutures, except stainless steel, can degrade if infection is present. Synethetic coating materials such as polytetrafluoroethylene (PTFE), and other complex synthetic polymers decrease suture drag and resist absorption.

Capillary Action

Sutures made of multifilament strands absorb moisture and hold body fluids (called *wicking* or **capillary action**). If bacteria are present, suture materials with high capillarity are able to retain and spread infection by means of the suture fibers. Suture with low capillarity is preferred in surgery when the risk of infection is high.

Some multifilament suture is coated with a chemical polymer to reduce tissue drag and wicking. In the past, absorbable suture was coated with a material such as beeswax, paraffin, or silicone. Modern sutures are coated with materials similar in composition to the suture itself, making them more biocompatible and lowering the risk of tissue reaction in the patient. Synethetic coating materials such as polytetrafluoroethylene (PTFE), and other complex synthetic polymers decrease suture drag and resist absorption.

Bioactivity

Bioactivity is the body's response to suture. The immune system reacts to suture as it would to any foreign material. The bioactivity depends on the chemical structure of the suture material and the condition of the patient. Sutures that cause little or no bioactivity are said to be highly **inert**, causing little or no inflammation. Stainless steel and titanium sutures are the most inert of all materials; natural fiber and protein-based sutures cause the most tissue reaction.

SUTURE TYPES

Suture is first classified by whether it is absorbable or nonabsorbable, and then by the size and chemical makeup of the suture material. In the past, classification included natural versus human-made or synthetic materials. Now, however, most sutures are human-made by complex bioengineering processes. The complex polymers—long-chain molecules that are molded or extruded into suture material—are the most popular. It is not necessary to memorize the chemical formulas for these compounds, but it is more useful to become familiar with the handling and absorption qualities of the more common types used in one's surgical facility. Note that suture products that have gone off patent are produced by different companies, using different trade names. The generic name, however, will provide a simple basis of comparison.

Absorbable Suture

SURGICAL GUT Surgical gut, also called *catgut,* is a protein collagen derived from the submucosal layer of beef or sheep intestine. It is the only naturally occurring absorbable suture available in the United States. It is used on tissues that heal rapidly. Surgical gut has been widely replaced by synthetic absorbable sutures, but may be occasionally used by oral surgeons.

Plain surgical gut is digested quickly and absorbed by tissues, but this rapid reaction can also cause inflammation. The suture retains tensile strength in the body for 7 to 10 days. It is used primarily in mucous membrane or in tissue where stones can form, such as the biliary or urinary systems. Plain gut is straw-colored in its natural bleached state. Chromic gut is treated with *chromic salt* to resist digestion and absorption. Chromic gut usually is absorbed in 7 to 21 days. Both types of gut are rapidly broken down in the presence of infection.

Gut requires special handling to preserve its strength and pliability. The sutures are packaged in an alcohol solution, which can be a source of fire on the surgical field. Packages must therefore be opened away from the surgical wound. Gut dries out quickly and can be dipped in saline just before use. This prevents the suture from breaking. However, gut should not be soaked, because it absorbs water readily and becomes swollen and weak. Dipping the strands in saline also softens them so that the coils can be removed. This is done by grasping the ends of the strand and pulling them gently. It is important to pull on the strands gently, especially when they are wet, because they can overstretch and become weak. Gut should be handled as little as possible, because contact with gloves causes the strands to fray.

ABSORBABLE POLYMERS Absorbable synthetic sutures are made of polymer or copolymer chemicals. They are available in monofilament and braided form and provide wound support for 3 weeks to 6 months, depending on the material. They are easily absorbed by the body after breakdown. These materials are pliable and easy to handle, even in the braided form. Most are coated for ease of handling and to reduce friction.

Polymer sutures are dyed to make them easier to see on the surgical field. However, they are also available in their natural color for superficial use. Absorbable synthetic sutures are used in most types of tissue and cause little tissue reaction compared to surgical gut. Polymers are used in their dry state.

BIOPOLYMER Absorbable biopolymer suture is manufactured through patented recombinant DNA technology (Tepha, Lexington, Mass.). The applications of biopolymer are similar to those for synthetic polymers, but biopolymer has 50% greater tensile strength and is biocompatible with body tissue. The suture is moderately easy to handle.

For more information on this new technology, see the manufacturer's website at http://www.tepha.com.

Non absorbable Suture

SILK Silk suture is derived from fibers produced by the silkworm. It has a long history of use. The most famous advance in suturing invented by Halstead involved the use of very fine silk sutures placed in close approximation. Silk is soft and pliable and has excellent tensile strength. It is available in braided or twisted form. Silk strands are coated to prevent wicking. Silk handles exceptionally well, and the knots remain secure and flat. Silk suture is used in most deep tissues, especially in intestinal, vascular, ophthalmic, and neurosurgical procedures. Dermal silk is used to close the skin in areas where the incision is subjected to excessive strain. Virgin silk is used mainly for ophthalmological procedures because of its pliability and performance in eye tissue. Silk begins to break down after about 1 year and usually is absent from tissue after 2 years.

NYLON Nylon was the first synthetic suture material available (1940) and is still widely used. It is available in braided or monofilament strands. The most outstanding feature of nylon is that is causes little or no tissue reaction and passes very easily through delicate tissues of the eye or blood vessels. Also, nylon has a very high tensile strength. However, in larger sizes it is stiff, difficult to handle, and may cut through tissue. Nylon suture loses its tensile strength over time. It is used when long-term strength is not required and is available in black, blue, green, and clear colors in braided or monofilament strands, coated or uncoated.

POLYESTER Polyester fiber suture is extremely strong, easy to handle, and relatively inert in tissue. It is braided and is available coated or uncoated. The coated form is widely used for cardiovascular surgery, especially when grafts are used, because of its strength-to-size ratio. Polyester suture is green, blue, or white.

POLYPROPYLENE Polypropylene is an extremely inert monofilament suture. Its smooth surface makes it popular for plastic, ophthalmic, and vascular surgery. Because of its high tensile strength, it is used for retention sutures, particularly in abdominal wall closure. Polypropylene knots are flat and do not tend to back out when placed properly. It is somewhat difficult to handle in larger sizes. It is available in a wide variety of sizes, can be used when infection is present, and can be left in place for extended periods. It is clear or blue in color.

STAINLESS STEEL Stainless steel is the strongest of all suture materials. It is widely used in the approximation of bone and other connective tissue. Surgical stainless steel suture has no significant inflammatory properties. It is available in monofilament and twisted form.

Stainless steel suture requires special handling. It kinks easily, and the ends are needle-sharp. The suture ends can puncture gloves, drapes, and other soft materials. Stainless steel suture is dispensed from the package as long, precut strands. The strands have considerable spring, and the ends must be handled carefully to control them. They must be kept straight and delivered without kinks or bends, which can tear through tissue as the strand is drawn through.

To prepare steel suture lengths, carefully remove a single strand from the package just before use. Place a hemostat on one end to maintain control. If the strand is to be threaded through a needle, thread the strand 1 or 2 inches (2½ to 5 cm) from the end and put a twist at the eye to secure the strand in place. Use a needle holder or wire holder to make the twist. Never use suture scissors to cut stainless steel wire. Always use wire scissors designated for this purpose.

Bits of stainless steel wire must be removed from the field and collected in a container during surgery. These are sharp items that can cause injury and must be treated as sharps on the surgical field.

SELECTION OF SUTURE

The selection of suture and needle for a particular tissue is based on the tissue type, the age and medical condition of the patient, and the healing prognosis. Surgeons have a large selection of suture materials, needle sizes and types, and specialty products designed for specific surgical needs. The surgeon's choice depends on these specific requirements, on practice and experience with previously used suture materials, and on tradition. People tend to use materials with which they are familiar. Many new materials have been introduced in the past few decades. Some show definite advantages over previously used materials, but with few exceptions, substances that have been used for many years, such as silk and nylon, remain in use with good results.

Variables for Suture Selection

- *Critical nature of the tissue:* Sutures placed in critical tissue or areas of the body such as the heart, blood vessels, and certain structures of the respiratory tract require nonabsorbable suture.
- *Healing time:* Absorbable suture can be used on *noncritical* tissue that heals very quickly. Examples are the mouth and other mucosal tissue, subcutaneous tissue, and epithelial tissue.
- *Required strength during healing:* Some tissues (usually connective tissues) are under high stress in the body. These areas require non absorbable suture or suture in the larger sizes (size 0 and up). Examples are abdominal fascia, tendon, and ligament.
- *Requirement for little or no scar formation:* A successful surgical outcome sometimes depends on almost complete absence of scarring. In some locations of the body, any scarring or granulation tissue around knots can result in a decrease or loss of function. Structures of the hand such as tendon and nerve repair require very inert (causing little or no tissue reaction) suture materials. Internal structures of the eye also require very inert suture materials. The suture must pass through the tissue with no resistance or tissue fraying, even at the microscopic level. In general, monofilament sutures are more inert than multifilament. Stainless steel (reserved for connective tissue), nylon, and polypropylene are the most inert.
- *Urinary tract:* Suture knots or remnants that might come in contact with urine or kidney filtrate can become the source of stones or other mineral deposition. For this reason, absorbable sutures are used in these tissues.
- *Risk of infection:* Some surgical procedures carry a high risk of infection either because of their classification (see earlier

discussion) or because of the patient's condition. In these cases a strong suture line with resistance to absorption is needed. A non absorbable suture or absorbable suture with long absorption time may be used. Wounds that are actively infected are not sutured.

- *Skin:* Selection of skin suture is based on many different variables. Any breakdown of skin can result in infection, but skin is also exposed to many small injuries by penetration, bruising, abrasion, and contact with heat and cold. At the same time, patients usually want the skin to heal with minimal scarring or other disfigurement. The selection of skin sutures or staples depends on a balance of requirements.
- *Cosmetic closure:* A cosmetic closure is one that has the least negative effect on the patient's body image. Naturally, skin closure of the face and other exposed areas of the body is the focus of cosmetic closure. Sutures selected for cosmetic closure are inert and usually monofilament to cause the least tissue injury as the suture is drawn through.

Table 22-3 lists tissue types and sutures associated with them to assist in learning.

SURGICAL NEEDLES

Surgical needles are made from high quality steel alloy or titanium. The combination of metals used in the manufacturing process renders the needles strong and inert. Needles are available in several types, according to their *eye* (the area where suture is threaded or attached), shape or curvature, and point style. Surgical needles have three distinct parts: the point, the body, and the eye.

NEEDLE EYE

The eye of the needle provides the attachment for the suture. Three types of needle eyes are available: the closed eye, the French eye (also called a *split* or *spring eye*), and the atraumatic (swaged) suture (Figure 22-7). The conventional closed eye needle resembles a sewing needle, and the eye hole is round, rectangular, or square. French eye needles have two eyes that are connected by a slit from the top through the eyes, with ridges that hold the sutures in place.

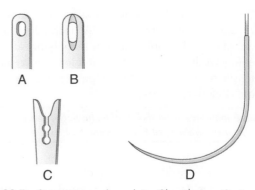

Figure 22-7 **Suture eyes. A** and **B**, Closed eye. **C**, French eye. **D**, Atraumatic eye. *(Redrawn from Phillips N: Berry and Kohn's operating room technique, ed 10, St Louis, 2004, Mosby.)*

Table 22-3 Suture Types, Characteristics, and Applications

Generic Name	Trade Names	Available Coating	Size	Mono filament or multifilament	Indication	Handling Quality	Contraindication	Postoperative Strength >50%
Non absorbable Suture								
Silk	Perma-hand Sofsilk Mersilk	Silicone Wax	5 to 8-0	Multi	General Cardiovascular Ophthalmological Neurological	Superior	Known allergy	70% at 14 days
Nylon	Dermalon Ethilon Monosof Supramid	—	2 to 11-0	Mono	Ophthalmological Plastic Cardiovascular Microsurgery	Excellent	Where permanent retention is necessary	81% at 1 year
Nylon braided	Bralon Supramid Extra Surgilon	Silicone	2 to 7-0	Multi	Ophthalmological Cardiovascular Neurological	Excellent		
Polypropylene	Prolene Deklene II Pronova Surgipro	—	2 to 10-0	Mono	Plastic surgery Ophthalmological Neurological Cardiovascular	Fair	None	70% at 14 days Significant strength at 2 years
Polyester	Ti-Cron Ethibond Mersilene Surgidac Cottony II Polydek Tevdek	Silicone Polybutylate None None None PTFE	5 to 8-0	Multi	General Cardiovascular	Excellent	None	No significant loss of tensile strength in tissue
Polybutester	Vascufil Monofil Novafil	Vascufil polymer	2 to 10-0	Mono	General Ophthalmological Cardiovascular	Excellent	Neural Microsurgery	No significant loss of tensile strength in tissue
UHMWPE (ultrahigh-molecular-weight polyethylene)	Force Fiber Hi Fi Magnumwire Twinfix	None	5 to 5-0	Multi	Cardiovascular Allograft Orthopedic	Excellent		No significant loss of tensile strength in tissue
Stainless steel	Stainless steel	—	10 to 12-0	Mono Multi	Orthopedic Sternal Tendon Ligament Retention	Difficult to handle	Known allergy Where radiotransparency is necessary	Permanent
Stainless steel coated with PTFE	Flexon	PTFE		Twisted	For temporary cardiac pacing	Good	Known allergy	
Expanded PTFE (ePTFE)	Gore-Tex	—	0 to 7-0	Mono	Cardiovascular Oral surgery General	Excellent	Known allergy	Permanent

Continued

Table 22-3 Suture Types, Characteristics, and Applications—cont'd

Generic Name	Trade Names	Available Coating	Size	Mono filament or multifilament	Indication	Handling Quality	Contraindication	Postoperative Strength >50%
Absorbable Suture								
Natural collagen	Chromic gut	Chromium salt	2 to 7-0	Mono	Mucosa Superficial blood vessels	Fair	Cardiovascular Ophthalmological Presence of infection	10 to 14 days absorption
	Plain gut	None			Mucosa			5 to 10 days absorption
Polydioxanone (PDS II)	PDS II	—	2 to 6-0	Mono	Gynecological Plastic Colon Pediatric cardiovascular Ophthalmological	Good	Adult cardiovascular Microsurgery Neural	14 days
PDS antibacterial	PDS Plus	Triclosan						
PDS barbed	V-loc	None	0	Mono with unidirectional barbs	Gynecological Intestine			
Polyglycolide (PGL)	Dexon S Polysorb	Calcium stearoyl lactylate Caprolactone copolymer		Multi	General Ophthalmologic	Excellent	Cardiovascular Neural	14 days
Polyglytone 621	Caprosyn	None	2 to 6-0	Mono	General soft tissue and ligation	Good	Cardiovascular Neural Microsurgery Ophthalmological	60% at 5 days
Polyglyconate	Maxon	—	1 to 7-0	Mono	Pediatric Cardiovascular	Excellent	Adult cardiovascular Ophthalmological Microsurgery Neural	65% at 3 weeks
Polyglactin 910 (PGL)	Vicryl	Polyglactin 370, calcium stearate	3 to 9-0	Multi	General soft tissue ligation Ophthalmologic	Excellent	Cardiovascular Neural	14 days
PGL	Vicryl Plus	Triclosan		Multi			Ophthalmological	
Poliglecaprone 25 PGLC	Monocryl	—	1 to 6-0	Mono	Subcuticular closure Soft tissue	Superior	Cardiovascular Neurological Microsurgery Ophthalmological	7 days
Poly(hydroxybutyrate) suture produced by recombinant DNA technology	Tephaflex	None	2 to 5-0	Mono	General soft tissue and ligation		Cardiovascular Neural Microsurgery Ophthalmological	

B & S, Brown and Sharp gauge; *PTFE,* polytetrafluoroethylene (Teflon).

Few surgeons use eyed needles. However, the surgical technologist must be familiar with their use. Eyed needles are identified by their shape and by the type of eye. Threading and passing eyed needles in rapid succession are skills that require practice. When the needle is threaded, the suture must be passed from the inside of the needle curve to the outside. The short end should extend approximately 4 inches (10 cm) from the eye. Both ends must be prevented from adhering to the shank of the needle holder. When the surgeon receives the suture, both the short and long ends must be free.

SWAGED (ATRAUMATIC) SUTURE

Most commercial needles are now manufactured with the suture preattached. This is called a swaged or atraumatic suture. The suture is inserted into the eye end of the needle, and the area is crimped and sealed. This produces a nearly seamless connection between the needle and the suture and also allows faster suturing with minimal tissue trauma.

The French eye (or spring eye) needle was used before swaged sutures became available, and some surgeons still prefer them. When the spring eye needle is threaded, the end of the suture is pressed down over the top of the spring, which causes it to snap into the eye (Figure 22-8). The suture should not be pulled through the eye after it is in place, because this strips the suture and may break it.

A detachable suture (Figure 22-9) is one in which the suture can be detached from the needle by pulling it straight back from the **swage**. These are referred to by their proprietary names, such as *De-tach* and *Control-release*.

A *double-armed suture* is one with a needle swaged to each end. This type of suture is used for circular tissue, such as in ophthalmic surgery, or for hollow structures, such as blood vessels or the intestine (Figure 22-10).

NEEDLE SHAPE

Needles are available in a number of different shapes to conform to their use. The curvature of a needle relates to the body and radius of the needle. The curve is measured as a circumferential fraction in a complete circle. Curvature designations are $\frac{1}{4}$, $\frac{3}{8}$, $\frac{1}{2}$, and $\frac{5}{8}$. For example, a $\frac{1}{2}$-curve needle is exactly one half the circumference of a circle.

In general, deep tissue in a confined space requires a more extreme curve. The curved needle allows the surgeon to dip beneath the surface of the tissue and retrieve the point as it emerges. The shape and characteristics of a needle are shown in Figure 22-11.

NEEDLE SIZE

Needle size is measured by the diameter of the shaft and the dimension from tip to eye. Historically, suture needles were identified by their curvature and name. These names are seldom used, and many have been replaced by common manufacturer codes or shape.

NEEDLE POINT

Many different types of needle points are available (Figure 22-12). However, they all are variations of the three basic types:

- Blunt
- Tapered
- Cutting

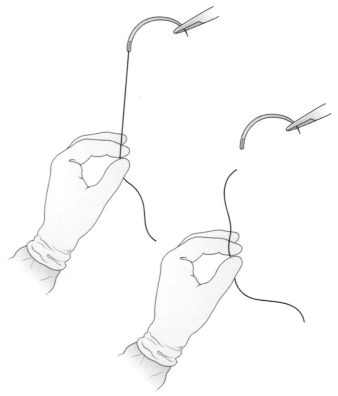

Figure 22-9   Detachable swaged suture.

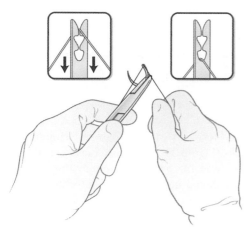

Figure 22-8   Technique for mounting suture on a French eye needle. *(Redrawn from Phillips N: Berry and Kohn's operating room technique, ed 10, St Louis, 2004, Mosby.)*

Figure 22-10   Double-armed suture used for anastomosis or suturing of circular incisions (e.g., the eye) or in gastrointestinal and vascular surgery.

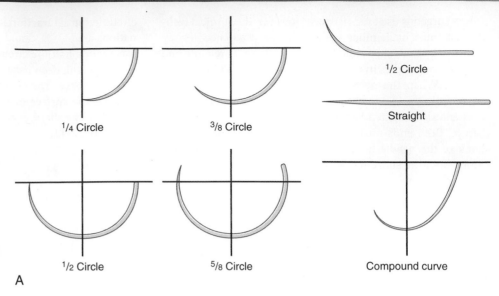

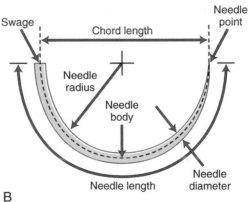

Figure 22-11 A, Needle shape and curvature. **B**, Characteristics of the needle.

The *blunt needle* is a round shaft with a blunt tip. It pushes tissue aside as it moves through it. It does not puncture the tissue, but rather slides between tissue fibers. It is the least traumatic and safest needle point. The blunt needle traditionally has been used only for suturing friable tissues and organs that are soft and spongy, such as the liver, spleen, and kidneys. The blunt needle now is advocated for general suture use because it significantly reduces the risk of needlestick injury and transmission of blood-borne diseases.

The **tapered needle** has a round body that tapers to a sharp point. It punctures tissue, making an opening for the body of the needle to follow. Its primary use is for suturing soft tissue, such as muscle, subcutaneous fat, peritoneum, dura, and gastrointestinal, genitourinary, biliary, and vascular tissue.

The cutting needle has a cutting edge along its shaft. A needle with the cutting edge on the inside of the curve is called a *conventional cutting needle*. A needle with the cutting edge on the outside or lower edge of the curve is called a *reverse cutting needle*.

Cutting needles are used on fibrous connective tissue, such as the skin, joint capsule, and tendon. The conventional cutting needle has a triangular shaft. Its cutting edge is on the inside curve of the needle; as the needle is drawn through tissue, the curve tends to slice tissue in an upward direction. The reverse cutting needle solves this problem by locating the cutting edge

on the outside of the curve, away from the direction of tension during suturing. It is stronger than the conventional cutting needle and produces minimal scarring.

The taper cut needle has a reverse cutting edge at the tip and a round body. The point of the needle is tapered. Taper cut needles are used for suturing dense fibrous connective tissue, such as the fascia, tendon, and periosteum.

Spatula needles are side-cutting needles with a flat surface on the top and the bottom. These are used in ophthalmic surgery to separate corneal and scleral tissue.

SUTURE STORAGE, PACKAGING, AND DISPENSING

STORAGE

Sutures are stored in individual boxes containing multiple suture packs (Figure 22-13). Suture racks may be kept in substerile areas and in closed cabinets in the operating room. Suture carts should not be brought into the operating room, where they can become contaminated with blood and body fluids. At the start of surgery, only the minimum number needed is opened. The surgical technologist anticipates the need for additional sutures as the case progresses and requests them in time.

POINT/BODY SHAPE	APPLICATION
Conventional cutting Point Body	Skin, sternum
Reverse cutting Point Body	Fascia, ligament, nasal cavity, oral mucosa, pharynx, skin, tendon sheath
Precision point cutting Point Body	Skin (plastic or cosmetic)
PC PRIME needle Point Body	Skin (plastic or cosmetic)
MICRO-POINT reverse cutting needle Point Body	Eye
Side-cutting spatula Point Body	Eye (primary application), microsurgery, ophthalmic (reconstructive)
CS ULTIMA ophthalmic needle Point Body	Eye (primary application)
Taper Point Body	Aponeurosis, biliary tract, dura, fascia, gastrointestinal tract, laparoscopy, muscle, myocardium, nerve, peritoneum, pleura, subcutaneous fat, urogenital tract, vessels, valve
TAPERCUT surgical needle Point Body	Bronchus, calcified tissue, fascia, laparoscopy, ligament, nasal cavity, oral cavity, ovary, perichondrium, periosteum, pharynx, sternum, tendon, trachea, uterus, valve, vessels (sclerotic)
Blunt Point Body	Blunt dissection (friable tissue), cervix (ligating incompetent cervix), fascia, intestine, kidney, liver, spleen

Figure 22-12 **Needle points and shapes.** *(From* Wound closure manual, *Somerville, NJ, 1999, Ethicon Inc.)*

PACKAGING

Suture manufacturers have developed innovative methods of packaging that are important to surgeons, surgical technologists, and nurses.

The following are important features of a packaging system:

- *Product protection:* The package must maintain sterility and protect sutures and needles from damage during storage and dispensing.
- *Efficient dispensing:* The design of the packaging system must ensure that the suture can be withdrawn rapidly and smoothly without tangling or knotting.
- *Selection:* Package labeling should be easy to associate with a specific suture. Rapid selection is desirable.
- *Minimal packaging:* A packaging system that produces minimal waste is desirable. Excessive wrapping and packaging are time-consuming to dispose of and create clutter on the surgical field.
- *Environmentally responsible:* Packaging should reflect an effort to promote the use of biodegradable materials.

READING A SUTURE LABEL

Sutures packages contain information that the surgical technologist needs to know when selecting suture. In Figure 22-14, note the name, size, and color of the suture, type and size of the needle (when applicable), lot number, and expiration date.

PRESENTATION

Suture presentation varies among suture manufacturers. However, the products themselves are standard.

- *Suture-needle combination:* One suture-needle combination is provided per pack (Figure 22-15).
- *Multiple suture strands:* One suture package contains multiple precut strands of suture (Figure 22-16).
- *Suture reel:* A spool of suture material is wound into a round reel.
- *Multiple suture-needle combinations:* One package contains multiple suture-needle combinations in detachable format (Figure 22-17).
- *Double-armed suture:* One pack contains a single suture strand with a needle attached at each end.

SUTURING TECHNIQUES

The primary use of sutures is to repair or construct tissue. The process of suturing that results in holding two tissue edges together is called *approximation*. Suture is also used to tie, or **ligate,** bleeding vessels. Sutures are tied using special techniques to ensure that the knots are secure. Each loop of the knot is referred to as a **throw**. When requesting a suture-needle during a procedure, the surgeon may refer to it as a stitch.

The surgical technologist must learn to anticipate the need for sutures and pass them in the accepted manner. The general principles and technique for each use of suture can be applied to all surgeries.

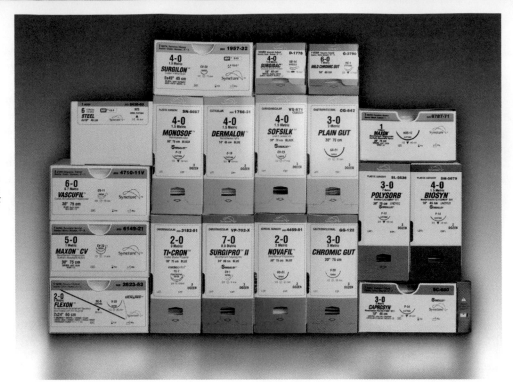

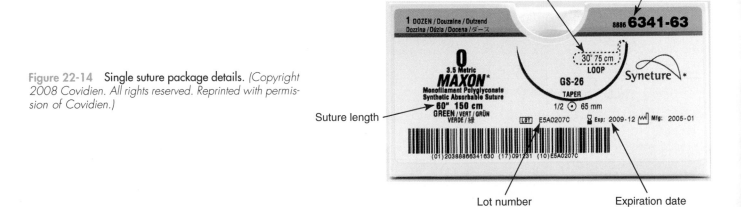

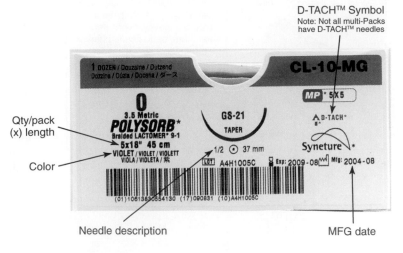

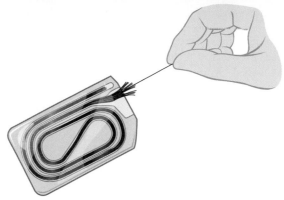

Figure 22-16 Race track packaging for single suture strands.

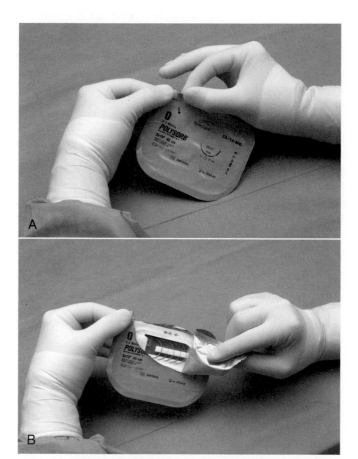

Figure 22-17 Multiple detachable needles in a single pack. *(Copyright 2008 Covidien. All rights reserved. Reprinted with permission of Covidien.)*

A suture technique is the method and pattern of the suture through the tissue. Two general types of suturing technique are used, continuous and interrupted.

CONTINUOUS SUTURE

The continuous or **running suture** has a knot at the beginning and one at the end. It is composed of one continuous strand of suture. The needle is alternated from one side of the tissue edge to the other (Figure 22-18). This suture technique is rapid and uses relatively little suture material. A disadvantage is that

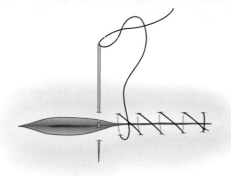

Figure 22-18 Continuous (running) suture.

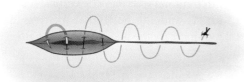

Figure 22-19 Subcuticular suture.

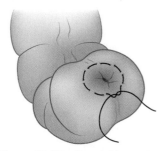

Figure 22-20 Purse-string suture.

if one point along the suture breaks during healing, the entire strand may pull out. Compared with interrupted sutures, a running suture is easier to place but is not as strong.

Subcuticular Suture

The subcuticular or buried suture is a type of running suture, used for cosmetic closure and in pediatric patients. The needle is placed within the dermis from side to side (Figure 22-19). This technique brings the skin edges together in close approximation, and no suture material is visible from the outside. The technique produces a very fine scar or no scar.

Purse-String Suture

The *purse-string suture* is a special continuous suture technique for closing the end of a tubular structure (lumen), such as the appendix, its most common application. In this technique, one end of the suture is anchored and stitches are placed around the periphery of the open lumen. The suture then is drawn tight around the neck of the lumen and tied (Figure 22-20).

Locking Suture

The locking stitch provides added strength to a running suture line. As the needle is passed through each side of the wound edges, it is passed underneath one loop. This equalizes the tension between each loop of the suture and provides increased hemostasis on the wound edges. A newer "self-locking" or *barbed* or quill suture contains intermittent projections that grip tissue in one direction, not allowing the suture to back out. This technology takes the place of locking sutures where applicable.

INTERRUPTED SUTURE TECHNIQUE

Interrupted sutures are individually placed, knotted, and cut (Figure 22-21). The finished suture line is very strong, because the tension of the wound edges is distributed over many anchor points. Many interrupted stitches produce a secure suture line with minimal scarring. The vertical mattress suture (Figure 22-22, *A*) and the horizontal mattress suture (see Figure 22-22, *B*) increase the incision line strength even more.

SPECIALTY USES OF SUTURE

RETENTION SUTURES

Retention sutures are a type of interrupted technique used to provide additional support to wound edges in abdominal surgery. In this technique, heavy sutures are placed though all the tissue layers of the body wall several centimeters from the primary suture line and perpendicular to the incision. As each suture is drawn tight, it pulls the edges of the incision into approximation without cutting into the tissue. Plastic or rubber *bolsters*, or small lengths of tubing, are threaded through the suture to prevent it from cutting into the patient's skin (Figure 22-23).

SUTURE LIGATURE

A suture ligature is used to ligate a large bleeding vessel. The purpose of the technique is to prevent the ligature from sliding off the vessel. A needle-suture combination is used. The surgeon passes the needle through the midsection of the vessel and adds an additional wrap around the outside. The needle is removed, and the ligature is tied snugly. Many surgeons do not cut the suture ends, but rather place a clamp on them (tagging the suture) until they are certain that no bleeding will occur. A suture ligature may be referred to as a *stick tie* (Figure 22-24).

ORTHOPEDIC ANCHORING DEVICES

Surgical repair of the joint capsule often requires sutures to stabilize tendon and muscle. A number of innovative devices have been developed in recent years to meet the increasing demand for long-lasting, stable reattachment mechanisms. Most systems use a biosynthetic anchor with a heavy composite suture such as a polyethylene core jacketed with polyester *(FiberWire)* or polydioxanone-polyethylene jacketed with caprolactone and glycolide *(Orthocord).* The anchoring device is attached to the suture, which can be drawn through the joint using a special shuttle instrument. Anchoring systems require their own instrumentation, and each device a has specific commercial name and method for placement. Refer to Chapter 31 for illustrations of anchoring devices.

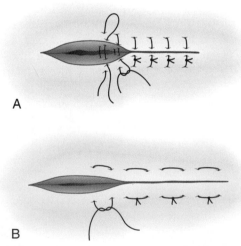

A

B

Figure 22-22 **A,** Vertical mattress sutures. **B,** Horizontal mattress sutures.

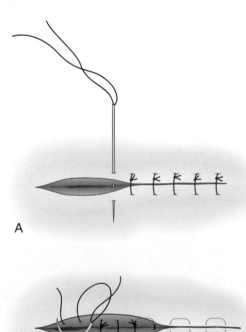

A

B

Figure 22-21 **A,** Interrupted sutures (superficial). **B,** Deep interrupted sutures in two layers.

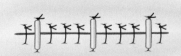

Figure 22-23 Retention sutures.

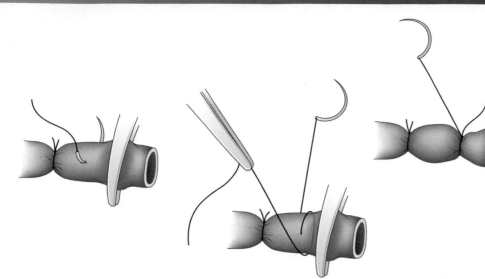

Figure 22-24 Use of the suture ligature on a vessel.

SUTURE HANDLING TECHNIQUES

One of the primary skills in surgical technology is the preparation and passing of sutures. Surgeons are accustomed to receiving sutures from the scrub in a prescribed manner for safety and efficiency of movement.

SAFETY

1. Suture needles are hazardous on the sterile field. They can cause injury and increase the risk of blood-borne contamination.
2. Good technique in handling sutures prevents their loss in the surgical wound. Lost items are a safety hazard and increase operative time and team stress.
3. Inappropriate tissue-needle combinations can cause unnecessary trauma to tissue.
4. Proper preparation of sutures increases their potential to facilitate uncomplicated healing.

NEEDLESTICK INJURY ON THE FIELD

If a needlestick injury occurs during surgery, the Centers for Disease Control and Prevention recommends immediate medical care. Although immediate attention may not be possible, the wound site should be washed with antiseptic soap and care sought as soon as possible. Appropriate steps can be taken to mitigate the risk of blood-borne disease, including postexposure prophylactic drugs and testing for infectious disease.

EFFICIENCY OF MOVEMENT

1. An efficient process for passing sutures reduces operative time.
2. Sutures are very expensive. Conservative use lowers the total cost to patients and facilities.
3. Poor technique in preparing sutures can result in waste, because sutures break, disengage from the needle, and are lost on the sterile field.

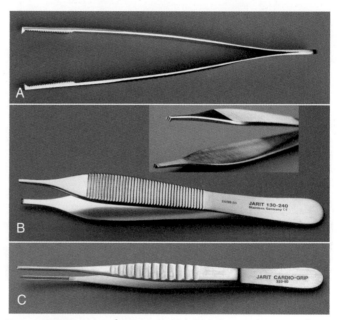

Figure 22-25 **Tissue forceps. A,** Toothed forceps for general use. **B,** Adson forceps for skin. **C,** DeBakey forceps for vascular tissue. (Courtesy Jarit Instruments, Hawthorne, NY.)

SUTURING INSTRUMENTS

Curved suture needles are mounted on a needle holder (also called a *needle driver*) for use. Select a needle holder that is the correct length for the depth of the wound and the correct weight (heavy or delicate). The jaws of the needle holder must be selected according to the delicacy of the needle. Needle holders used in general surgery have diamond or carbon steel inserts over the portion that holds the needle. This prevents the needle from slipping or rotating. The type and size of the needle holder are adjusted to the size of the needle.

The surgeon nearly always uses tissue forceps to stabilize the tissue while suturing. The scrub selects the forceps by length, weight, and type of tip according to the tissue to be sutured. The general categories of tip are smooth and toothed (Figure 22-25). The most delicate needle holders are

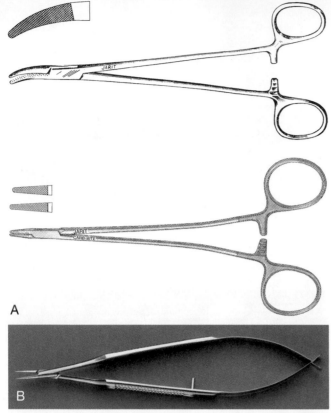

A

B

Figure 22-26 Needle holders. A, Standard needle holders. **B,** Needle holder for delicate tissue. *(Courtesy Jarit Instruments, Hawthorne, NY.)*

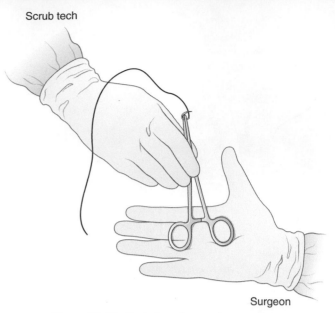

Scrub tech

Surgeon

Figure 22-27 Technique for passing a suture.

those used in microsurgery and ear and ophthalmic surgery (Figure 22-26).

- *Smooth forceps* are used on mucous membrane organ tissue (e.g., the spleen and kidneys) and on any tissue that bleeds easily.
- *Toothed forceps* are used on connective tissue, including the skin.
- *Vascular forceps* are specially designed with a scored insert at the working tip; this prevents puncturing of the blood vessel but provides sufficient friction to hold.

TECHNIQUE FOR PASSING SUTURES

Mount the needle about 0.5 mm from the end of the swaged section. Do not clamp the swage, because this weakens it and places the needle holder too far back for correct balance. Drape the suture end over the back of your hand before you pass it. This prevents it from becoming caught in the surgeon's hand as he or she receives the suture. The "armed" needle holder must be passed so that the surgeon does not have to reposition it in the hand or look up from the surgical site. It must be oriented correctly (Figure 22-27).

The position of the needle holder in relation to the suture needle depends on:

- Whether the surgeon is right-handed or left-handed
- Whether the surgeon stands opposite the scrub or next to the scrub
- Whether the suture is requested as "back-handed"

Regardless of where the surgeon stands in relation to the scrub, the needle must always be positioned so that it does not have to be repositioned for use. A left-handed surgeon sutures by driving the needle into the tissue in a counterclockwise direction. A right-handed surgeon drives the needle clockwise. *An exception to this is the back-handed suture, in which the direction is reversed.*

One method of learning the correct orientation of the mounted needle holder is to practice the movements with another person as if you were the one suturing. Work with a colleague and position yourself as the surgeon would be. The logic of presenting the suture in correct spatial orientation will be immediately apparent. Orienting the suture needle so it points to the surgeon's chin may also be helpful for some learners.

PASSING MULTIPLE SUTURES

Since the adoption of swaged needles in surgery, the technique of rapid-sequence threading has been replaced by multiple needle-suture packs. The manner in which the needle is packaged often determines how quickly and safely sutures can be passed to the surgeon. More paper and many more needles are generated than in the past, increasing the risk of a lost or retained needle and increased expense.

To prevent needle injury and keep pace with the surgeon, follow these guidelines:

1. Keep suture packs organized. Know where each type of suture is. As soon as a free needle is returned, immediately place it on the magnetic board or sharps holder.
2. Sutures are passed on an exchange basis. Have a loaded needle prepared at all times.
3. Load the needle holder before removing the entire needle-suture from its package.
4. Do not use the sponge bucket for suture wrappers. A needle may be lost among the sponges, and it is extra work for the circulator to pick out the wrappers.

SUTURE TIES

Suture strands are available in precut or full-length strands ranging from 12 to 60 inches (30 cm to 1.5 m). The scrub must cut full-length sutures according to the surgeon's requirements. The following technique is used to cut full-length suture into thirds:

1. Remove the coiled suture from its package. Place the coil over one hand and pull the free end slowly to uncoil the strand.
2. Grasp each end of the strand and pull the center into thirds (Figure 22-28).

Continuous reels or rolls of suture are also used for repeated blood vessel ligation. The surgeon holds the reel and uses the amount needed. The reels contain 54 inches (135 cm) of suture material. When suture reels are used, the entire reel is passed (placed in the surgeon's palm). The surgeon usually replaces the reel in the Mayo tray after use, or the technologist can retrieve it from the surgical field after use.

A suture may be passed around a vessel or duct with a clamp. This type of tie is passed by securing one end of the suture to the end of the clamp. The clamp is passed in the normal manner, but the suture length should be draped over the scrub's hand in the same way a mounted needle is passed. If this type of tie is needed during a procedure, the surgeon may ask for a **tie on a passer** or simply a tie. The scrub is expected to assess whether a passer is required. Commonly a right angle or long curved clamp is used to pass a tie. When mounting a tie, insert the tip of the suture into the nose (tip) of the clamp (Figure 22-29).

Double-armed sutures are used on circular or tubular suture lines. When a double-armed suture is passed, only one needle is mounted on the needle holder. The surgical technologist must take care that the unsecured needle does not snag on drapes or other items on the surgical field.

HOW TO CUT SUTURES

Occasionally the surgeon asks the surgical technologist to cut suture ends when tying a knot. When sutures are cut, the ends must be short to reduce the amount of foreign material in the wound, but long enough that the knot does not untie. When the suture is cut too short, the knot may actually be cut. If this happens, the surgeon replaces the suture with another.

The proper technique for cutting sutures is as follows:

1. Use only sharp suture scissors; never use tissue scissors on suture material.
2. To cut the suture, open the scissors slightly. Use the tip of the scissors to cut.
3. Hold the scissors as shown in Figure 22-30.

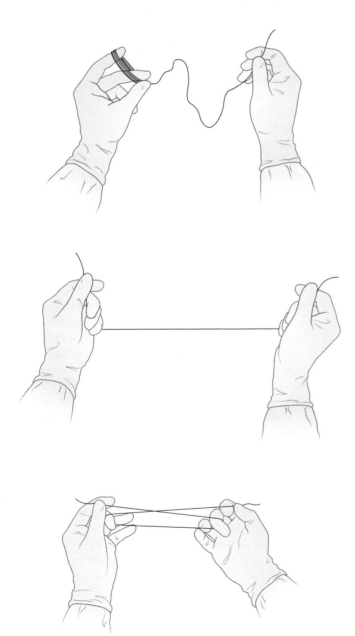

Figure 22-28 Dividing long suture into thirds. *(Redrawn from Phillips N: Berry and Kohn's operating room technique, ed 10, St Louis, 2004, Mosby.)*

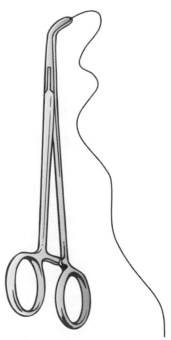

Figure 22-29 Suture tie on a passer. *(Redrawn from Phillips N: Berry and Kohn's operating room technique, ed 10, St Louis, 2004, Mosby.)*

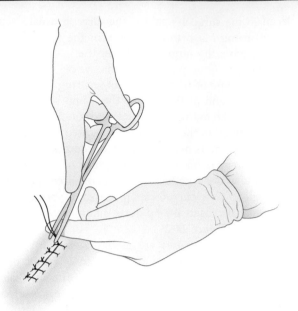

Figure 22-30 **Cutting sutures.** Note the use of the ring finger through the ring handle. This provides the best control.

4. Place your index finger over the top of the scissors to steady the blades. Turn the scissors at a 45-degree angle. This creates a small "whisker." Cut the suture ends while keeping the scissors at an angle.
5. When cutting sutures and performing other tasks at the same time, it is convenient to "palm" the scissors in one hand (Figure 22-31).
6. Remove any cut suture ends from the wound area to prevent them from falling into the wound.

SUTURE REMOVAL

When the surgeon needs to remove old (deep) sutures from a previous surgery, the knots usually are embedded in scar tissue and may be difficult to grasp and cut. A straight, fine-tipped hemostat works best for pulling out old sutures. The scrub should provide a towel into which the extracted suture pieces can be deposited so that they do not drop back into the wound.

TISSUE IMPLANTS

Tissue implants are used to replace or augment the patient's own tissue. Tissue loss can be caused by a number of conditions and incidents, including trauma or injury, congenital deformity, surgical excision and resection, and any number of degenerative diseases. This loss of tissue can create a significant defect in the anatomy. Many of these tissues may be replaced or substituted with biological dressing, implanted materials, or synthetic prosthetic materials. Tissue grafts usually are obtained from a registered tissue bank (central location in the health care facility or community) unless the tissue is from the patient's body. In this case, it may be used immediately or stored in the health care facility.

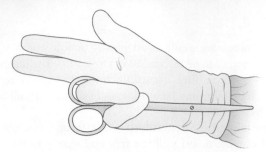

Figure 22-31   Palming the suture scissors.

IMPORTANT TERMS

Allograft: A tissue graft derived from human tissue. Allografts are tested for infectious disease and infection before distribution from the tissue bank.

Autologous autograft: Tissue obtained from the patient's body and implanted in another site, such as a bone graft taken from the hip for implantation in the spine.

Bovine graft: Tissue graft of beef origin.

Epithelialization: The migration of epithelial cells into the wound during healing.

Implant: Any type of tissue replacement or device placed in the body.

Porcine graft: Graft taken from pig tissue.

Wound cover: Tissue used to cover large defects in skin, usually a result of burns, trauma, or infection. Wound cover materials may be used temporary until healing occurs.

Xenograft: A graft derived from animal or synthetic source.

GRAFTS

Skin Grafts

Skin grafts are used to replace skin that has been destroyed by disease or injury. The skin is a critical barrier against infection and fluid loss. A skin substitute is needed to protect deep tissues from injury and contamination. Traditionally, skin grafts were taken only from the patient's own body, because these were the most successful. Now, other biological materials are available that can provide excellent protection against infection while reducing scarring and preventing fluid loss. Some grafting materials also aid the formation of granulation tissue in wounds. (The surgical techniques used in skin grafting are discussed fully in Chapter 30.)

Porcine Dermis

Pig skin is used to temporarily cover a full-thickness injury. The graft does not develop vascularization. After 1 to 2 weeks, the graft sloughs. Porcine grafts are available in sheets and rolls and may be frozen, fresh, or dried. Some grafts are soaked in iodophor, and these should not be used on patients allergic to Betadine.

Amniotic Membrane

Amniotic membrane from human placentas can be used as a biological dressing for burns, skin ulcers, and infected wounds.

This type of graft may also be used to cover spina bifida defects and in corneal surgery. The placenta has two layers or membranes: the *amnion*, which is used primarily in partial-thickness wounds, and the *chorion*, which is used primarily in full-thickness wounds. The amnion may be used fresh, frozen, or dried. Both membranes may be obtained from a tissue bank.

Engineered Skin Substitutes

Engineered skin substitutes (artificial skin) were created because of the lack of available human skin to cover large defects and wounds. All artificial skin has an outer layer that creates a barrier to infection, and many products include a dermal element that guides the cell during epithelialization. In addition to providing a barrier to infection, artificial skin reduces the severe pain associated with frequent dressing changes. It also decreases the risk of scar **contracture**.

Biobrane is a biosynthetic dressing made of a silicone film in which a nylon fabric is partially embedded. The matrix encourages blood clotting between the fibers, resulting in good contact until new skin growth takes place. Biobrane is used in clean burn wounds that do not require surgical excision (partial-thickness burns) and as a protective covering over a meshed autograft. It is not used in chronic wounds because it lacks antimicrobial properties.

TransCyte is a temporary skin substitute derived from human fibroblasts (cells that secrete collagen matrix material). It is frozen so that no cellular metabolic activity remains; however, essential structural proteins are intact. TransCyte typically is used as a temporary skin dressing before autografting over clean partial-thickness burns or for surgically excised, full-thickness, and deep partial-thickness burns.

Integra Bilayer Matrix Wound Dressing is an immediate wound cover for partial- and full-thickness soft tissue injuries and chronic wounds. It is composed of a semipermeable polysiloxane (silicone) layer that acts like epidermis. It controls fluid loss and provides a flexible, adherent covering that resists shearing and tearing. The structure is a porous matrix of bovine collagen and glycosaminoglycan (similar to the structure of a cell wall). This creates a bed for cellular and capillary growth.

Integra Dermal Regeneration Template is an alternative to allografting. It is the only approved skin substitute that regenerates the dermis. The template is positioned on the skin, and a 0.05-inch epidermal autograft is performed. The template must be protected against shearing and displacement. Both Integra products are contraindicated in the presence of infection.

Cultured epithelial autograft *(Epicel)* (Genzyme, Cambridge, Mass.) is an epidermal replacement generated from a biopsy of skin taken from the patient. Keratinocytes are duplicated in 2 to 3 weeks.

Foreskin grafts are obtained from neonates and used as a temporary skin barrier in the treatment of noninfected skin ulcers. *Apligraf* has two layers, a human-derived epidermis and bovine collagen dermis. The epidermis provides a barrier while the dermal layer heals. Apligraf is gradually replaced by host cells, which eliminates the need for additional split-thickness skin grafting.

Bone Graft

Bone grafts are used for structural support and to stimulate new bone growth in a defect caused by trauma or a congenital anomaly. Two types of bone are used for grafting, cancellous bone and cortical bone. Cancellous bone is porous, and tissue fluid can reach deep into it, allowing most of the bone cells to live. Cortical bone is very rigid and strong. It typically is used to repair skeletal defects because of its strength. Cortical bone is fixed into position with metal sutures or plates and screws. Many types of bone grafts can be done:

- *Autologous grafts:* Grafts made from the patient's body.
- *Allogeneic grafts:* Grafts made from nonliving cadaver bone.
- *Composite grafts:* Grafts made of a combination of cadaver bone, morcellated allograft bone, and marrow.
- *Demineralized bone matrix (DBM):* A processed material made from collagen, protein, and growth factors. It is used as granules, chips, putty, or gel.
- *Ceramic materials:* These provide structural support only.
- *Graft composites:* Grafts that contain combinations of DBM and marrow, ceramic-collagen, and ceramic-autograft-collagen combinations.

Umbilical Cord

Human umbilical cord is used in vascular surgery to replace an artery when saphenous autografting is not feasible.

SYNTHETIC IMPLANTS

Most tissue implants are derived from synthetic or biopolymer materials. Examples include artificial heart valves, pacemakers, and artificial joints. Implants are regulated by the FDA and are approved as medical devices after rigorous testing. Implants must meet certain criteria for a successful surgical outcome. They must be:

- Compatible with body tissue.
- Available as a sterile product or able to withstand a sterilization process.
- Proven safe and nonpathogenic.
- Able to provide adequate tissue coverage and vascularization around the implant.
- Able to provide adequate stability for the intended use.

The process for sterilizing implants is discussed in Chapter 11.

METALS

Stainless steel, Vitallium, titanium, and other alloys have been used in the manufacture of orthopedic implants for many years. The materials are strong, resilient, and inert. Polyetheretherketone (PEEK) polymer reinforces the implant and prevents leakage and wear.

METHYLMETHACRYLATE

Methylmethacrylate is a synthetic bone cement used to secure prosthetic implants into bone and for remodeling during cranioplasty. Bone cement is mixed on the sterile field using two components, methylmethacrylate powder and a volatile liquid. Because the fumes created by the chemical mixture are toxic, the cement must be mixed in a special closed container (refer to Chapter 31 for details). The manufacturer's recommendations for proper mixing and safety precautions should be followed.

RESORBABLE IMPLANTS

Synthetic polymer implants composed of polylactic acid (PLA) polymer currently are used in orthopedic and maxillofacial surgery. The newer generation of biopolymers manufactured using recombinant deoxyribonucleic acid (DNA) technology also has been approved for surgical use, including implants.

POLYETHYLENE

Porous polyethylene implants are often used in facial reconstruction. The porous nature of the implant allows for both soft tissue and vascular ingrowth. As collagen grows into the implant, the framework of the implant becomes stronger.

SILICONE

Silicone and Silastic are two very common implant materials. They are relatively inert and durable. Implants are available in many forms, including gel, sponge, film, tubing, liquid, and sheets. These implants should not be handled with bare hands, and care should be taken to ensure that they do not pick up lint or dust, because any foreign material can cause an inflammatory reaction around the implant.

WOVEN SYNTHETICS

Vascular grafts are made from a number of woven synthetic materials. These include Dacron, polytetrafluoroethylene (PTFE), and polyester.

WOUND DRAINAGE

PURPOSE

The presence of fluid in a surgical wound can delay healing and cause infection. Fluid sometimes accumulates as part of the inflammatory process or as a result of oozing from small capillaries. The accumulation of **serosanguineous fluid** (blood and serum) becomes a medium for microbial growth. To prevent this, a wound drain is inserted in selected cases before closure.

All but very simple drainage systems require a reservoir to collect the fluid. This prevents the spread of infection and allows measurement and analysis to determine the progress of healing. Drains are placed in the wound before complete closure or through a separate incision through the body wall near the main incision (sometimes called a "stab wound"). The surgical technologist should be familiar with common drainage systems. Drainage reservoirs must always be kept lower than the patient's wound site to prevent backflow of the drainage fluid. Strict aseptic technique and universal precautions

must be used when attaching and detaching connection tubes and when emptying contents. The amount and description of the contents must be documented in the patient chart whenever a drain is emptied.

PASSIVE DRAIN

A passive drain creates a passage from the tissue inside the wound to the outside of the body. These are used when drainage is minimal. The *Penrose* drain is a simple tubular length of nonlatex material similar to surgical glove material. Before closing, the surgeon places the drain loosely in the wound and secures it with sutures. A gauze dressing is placed over the drain to collect fluid from the wound.

NOTE: *An older technique of placing a sponge inside the drain to collect fluid (commonly called a "cigarette drain") is no longer practiced because this system increases the risk of wound infection.*

A gravity drain is used in wounds or hollow structures that produce significant amounts of fluid but do not require suction for removal. Examples of gravity drainage are the *T-tube, Pezzer,* Malecot, and Foley catheters. The T-tube is used specifically for bile duct drainage and is connected to a bile bag by a length of clear tubing. The *Foley catheter* and *Malecot* drain provide continuous drainage after genitourinary surgery. Various other types of ureteral drainage tubes may also be used after surgery of the kidney or ureter; these are discussed Chapter 26. Wound drains such as the Pezzer, Malecot, mushroom, and Penrose are usually placed in the wound by positioning the proximal end with a blunt nosed forcep such as a Mayo or Pean clamp. One or two nonabsorbable sutures may be used to secure the drain to the body wall if necessary.

SUCTION DRAINS

A suction drain pulls serum and blood from the wound by a negative-pressure device. A tube is placed in the center of the wound and connected to a one-way valve in the drain reservoir. Air is evacuated from the container by squeezing it to activate the negative pressure, and the wound tubing is attached to the deflated reservoir. As the reservoir returns to its normal shape, it withdraws fluid from the wound in the same way a bulb syringe is used to pull fluid. Two common suction drains are the Hemovac (Figure 22-32) and the Jackson-Pratt (Figure 22-33).

WATER-SEALED DRAINAGE SYSTEM

A water-sealed drainage system is used to pull fluid or air from the thoracic cavity after thoracic surgery or trauma to the thorax. The thoracic cavity is normally under negative pressure. The difference between atmospheric pressure and thoracic pressure allows the lungs to expand easily. Loss of negative pressure causes the lung to collapse. After surgery or a penetrating injury to the chest wall, negative pressure must be restored. The underwater drainage system performs this task.

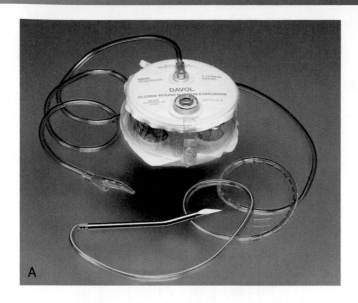

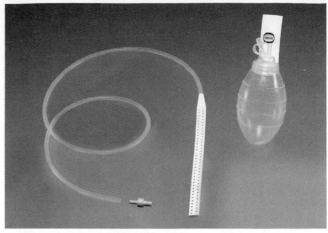

Figure 22-33 **Jackson-Pratt suction-reservoir drain.** The perforated tubing is placed inside the surgical wound, and the distal end is connected to the hand suction device. *(From Rothrock JC: Alexander's care of the patient in surgery, ed 13, St Louis, 2007, Mosby.)*

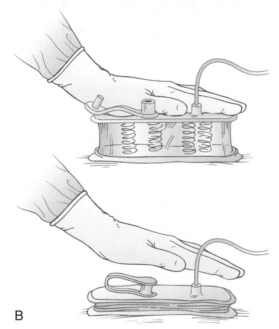

Figure 22-32 **A,** Hemovac suction drain. The proximal end of the drain tubing is placed in the open surgical wound. The distal end is attached to the metal trocar. This is used to make a tunnel for the tubing. **B,** The tubing is connected to the reservoir. After wound closure, the reservoir is compressed, and the tab is closed creating suction within the wound and drawing fluid out. *(A from Rothrock JC: Alexander's care of the patient in surgery, ed 13, St Louis, 2007, Mosby; B redrawn from Phillips N: Berry and Kohn's operating room technique, ed 10, St Louis, 2004, Mosby.)*

The drainage system has three separate water chambers sealed in a plastic unit. One or more chest drainage tubes are placed in the thorax and connected to the drainage system. When suction is applied to one of the chambers, air or fluid is pulled into the collection system. Each of the remaining chambers contains a small amount of water, which prevents the loss of negative pressure in the thoracic cavity (Figure 22-34).

When any drainage system is in use, the collection unit must remain below the level of the insertion tube. This

prevents fluids from reentering the drainage space. Chest drainage systems must never be allowed to back up into the thorax, because this can cause immediate collapse of a lung. When a patient with an underwater chest drainage system is transferred, the system must be kept upright. If the collection system falls over, it should be righted and checked for cracks. Make sure all tubes and connections are tight. If any doubt exists about the integrity of the system, seek help immediately.

STOMA POUCH

A stoma pouch or bag is used to collect body fluids following stoma surgery in which an artificial orifice to the outside of the body is created surgically. The stoma site progresses through a period of remodeling during healing. However, in the first days following surgery, the objective of the pouch is to provide a leak-proof system to collect fluid while maintaining a healthy wound around the stoma opening.

DRESSINGS

FUNCTIONS

Sterile wound dressings are placed over the incision site at the close of surgery. Many types of wound dressings are available, each with a specific purpose. For example, dressings:

- Prevent environmental contamination of the incision
- Collect exudate from the wound
- Provide mechanical support of the operative site
- Prevent the accumulation of necrotic tissue
- Provide continuous contact with an antiseptic or antibacterial agent

Elaborate dressings have multiple components. In most cases, the initial layer comes in direct contact with the wound. Additional dressings are added to protect and support the operative site.

DRESSING MATERIALS

Materials in direct contact with the surgical wound usually have a nonstick surface. Telfa and various petroleum-based products, or bacteriostatic agents (e.g., povidone and bismuth) are impregnated into gauze to prevent it from sticking when the dressing is removed.

Flat dressings generally are made with loose gauze fabric. Absorbent gauze "fluffs" can be used to cushion the wound site and provide extra protection. Absorbent dressings are layered over the primary dressing and designed to isolate wound exudate. The *ABD* (abdominal) pad is a large absorbent dressing used to cover draining wounds (Figure 22-35, *A*).

Rolled dressing materials are used for wrapping a limb. They may be plain gauze or an elasticized material (see Figure 22-35, *B*). Kling gauze is very pliable and soft and can be molded over a limb to provide uniform coverage. Elastic roller bandage is used when compression is needed. *Elastoplast* roller bandage is a highly adherent dressing that provides compression and mild support to the wound. *Tube stockinet* is a thin, sock like sleeve that fits over the limb to protect a gauze bandage or provide protection under a plaster cast.

Gauze packing is used in a cavity, such as the nose or an open wound. It is available in a long, thin strip and packaged in a bottle or similar container. This type of dressing usually is removed early in the recovery period, because it can rapidly become a source of infection.

Ointments and other medicines are not usually applied over a surgical wound. However, the dressing itself may be impregnated with a bacteriostatic agent (Figure 22-35, *C*). Narrow gauze strips used are used for this purpose (see Figure 22-35, *D*).

Adhesive tape is needed for most dressings. Tape is used to secure a flat dressing. Paper or "silk" tape is lightweight and has minimal adhesive properties. Plastic tape is pliable and has more adhesive strength. Cloth tape is seldom used for surgical wounds because it is difficult and painful to remove. Commercially available dressings that resemble a large Band-Aid (gauze surrounded by silk or paper adhesive) are also available. This type of dressing may be referred to as an Owens dressing. Liquid or spray skin adhesives such as benzoin and Mastisol are used to increase the sticking ability of tapes and adhesive dressings.

Steri-Strips are used to approximate small incisions and protect the wound. These are used in minor surgery and for minor wounds (Figure 22-36). A small amount of biological adhesive, such as benzoin liquid or spray, may be applied to the skin for extra adhesion before the strips are applied. In some minor wounds, Steri-Strips serve as a dressing because they protect the incision line.

A simple occlusive film dressing *(OpSite)* is one that prevents most environmental exposure. The film is semipermeable to air but prevents direct contact with the incision site. Film dressing is contraindicated for use in deep cavity wounds normally used on superficial wounds, burns, and abrasions.

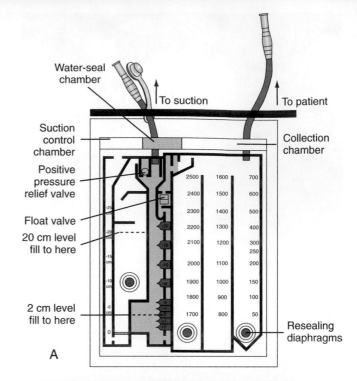

A

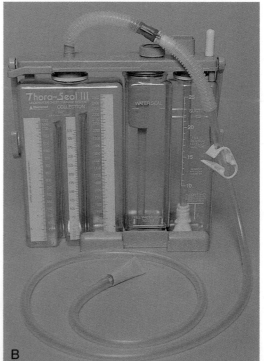

B

Figure 22-34   Underwater sealed chest drainage. A, Schematic of disposable chest suction system. The collection chamber receives drainage from the chest cavity. The middle chamber is the water seal which allows air to leave the pleural space and prevents air from entering. The left chamber is connected to suction exert pulling pressure from the pleural cavity. **B,** Photo of drainage system. (**A** *from Lew SM, Heitkemper MM, Kirksen SE:* Medical-surgical nursing: assessment and management of clinical problems, *ed 6, St Louis, 2004, Mosby;* **B** *from Elkin MK, Perry AG, Potter PA:* Nursing interventions and clinical skills, *ed 3, St Louis, 2004, Mosby.)*

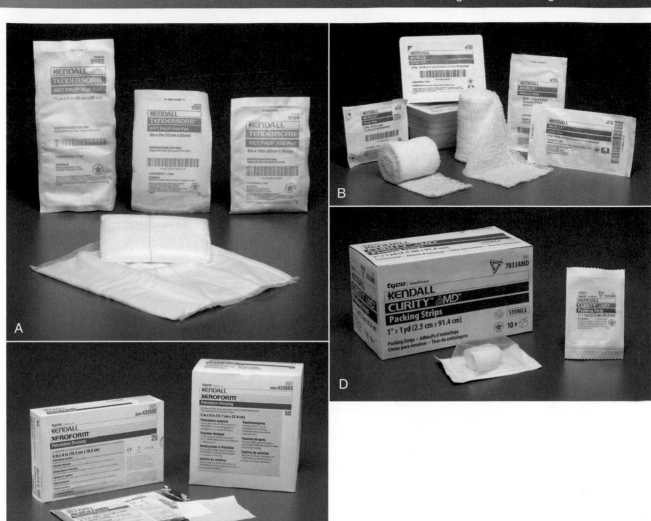

Figure 22-35   **A**, ABD pad used for draining wounds. **B**, Rolled dressing material. **C**, Dressings with antibacterial agents. **D**, Gauze strips. *(Copyright 2008 Covidien. All rights reserved. Reprinted with permission of Covidien.)*

SIMPLE AND COMPOSITE DRESSINGS

FLAT DRESSING

The most common and simplest type of surgical wound dressing is a thin, nonstick pad covered by one or two layers of flat gauze secured with tape. Additional layers of gauze or ABD pad are used if the surgeon anticipates drainage. If a mechanical drain has been inserted into the wound, layers of absorbent gauze are placed around the drain. An ABD pad may be placed over this and secured with tape.

PRESSURE DRESSING

A pressure dressing most often is used over a skin graft. The graft must remain in close contact with the underlying tissue to retain its vitality and become integrated into the new site. Slight pressure on the graft site prevents serous fluid from lifting the skin graft away from the recipient site. A stent dressing is a type of pressure dressing in which gauze or other material is molded into a thick pad that fits the graft area. Sutures are placed around the graft site. The long suture ends are then tied over the pad to secure it in place (Figure 22-37).

SUPPORT DRESSING

Supportive dressings are used to prevent or limit movement of the surgical wound during healing. Orthopedic procedures often require the use of supportive dressings and appliances. Thick cotton covered with stretch gauze is used for soft support. Hard casting materials are used when complete immobility is required. (Casting and other orthopedic techniques are discussed in Chapter 31.)

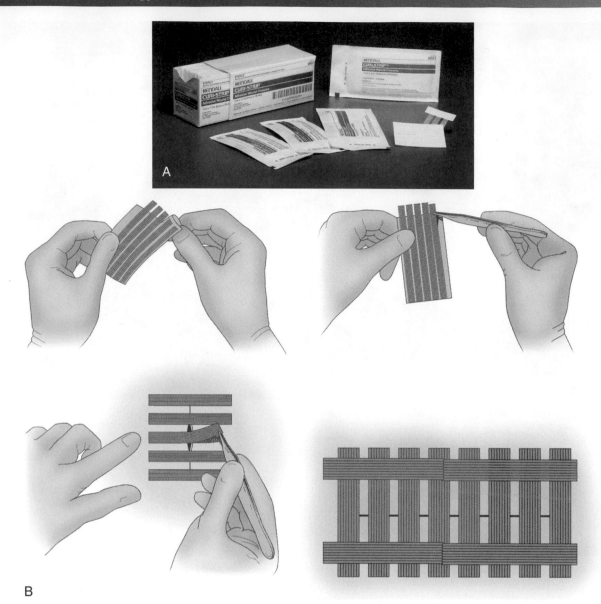

Figure 22-36 **A,** Skin closure strips packaged. **B,** Skin closure strips in use. (**A** *copyright 2008 Covidien. All rights reserved. Reprinted with permission of Covidien. Covidien, Mansfield, Mass;* **B** *from Rothrock JC: Alexander's care of the patient in surgery, ed 13, 2007, Mosby.*)

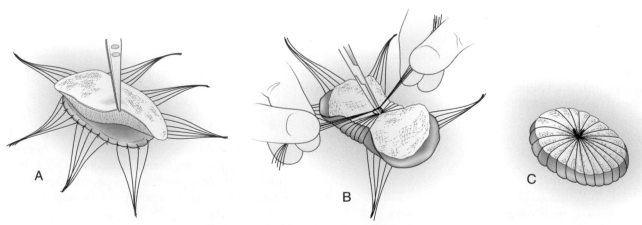

Figure 22-37 Stent dressing used to cover a skin graft.

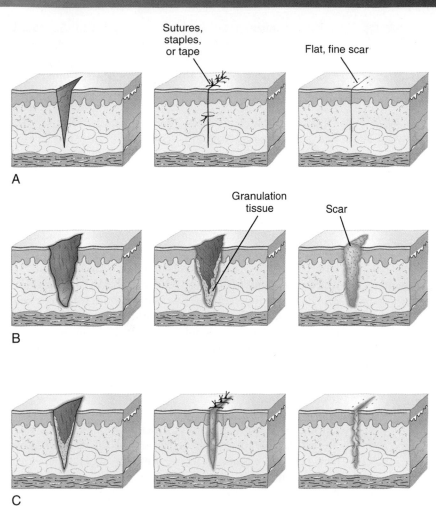

Sutures, staples, or tape

Flat, fine scar

A

Granulation tissue

Scar

B

C

Figure 22-38 Process of wound healing. A, Healing by first intention. Wound edges are brought together with sutures, staples or tape. **B,** Healing by second intention. The wound is left open because of infection that would quickly dissolve suture materials and cause further tissue reaction. The wound heals from the bottom up by continuous laying of granulation tissue. **C,** Healing by third intention. Infection is no longer present in a previously open wound, which is closed now with sutures.

WOUND HEALING AND COMPLICATIONS

CLASSIFICATION OF WOUNDS

The wound healing process (Figure 22-38) is classified according to whether it is clean or contaminated, sutured or left open. Surgical wounds are classified by the potential risk for infection (Box 22-2).

A surgical wound that is sutured together heals by **primary intention**. This means that the cut tissue edges are in direct contact.

A wound that is not sutured must heal by *secondary intention*. This type of wound heals from the base. The healing process involves filling the tissue gap with granulation tissue. It is much slower, and the resulting scar can be quite large compared with primary intention closure. Sometimes a skin graft is necessary because the wound is too large to heal without risk of contamination and infection. Wounds that are infected or grossly contaminated (e.g., those caused by a traumatic injury) also require secondary intention healing.

Third intention healing, or delayed closure, is a process in which an infected or a contaminated wound is treated and the wound space is packed to prevent serum accumulation and to protect it against environmental exposure. When sufficient granulation tissue has filled in the wound, it is sutured.

PROCESS OF WOUND HEALING

Two types of tissue repair occur naturally. Parenchymal tissue heals by replication of special cells. Parenchymal cells are found in epithelial tissue, such as the mucous membranes, fallopian tubes, vagina, gastrointestinal tract, and urinary tract. Bone marrow cells are also parenchymal cells. Other cells, such as those found in the liver, also multiply, but division stops once growth and development are complete. These tissues are referred to as *stable cells*.

The permanent cells of the body do not regenerate or divide when they are injured. Permanent cells make up muscles (including heart muscle) and nerves. Tissues that cannot regenerate or repair themselves are replaced by connective tissue after injury. This connective tissue is commonly called *scar tissue*. Scar tissue has few of the characteristics of the original tissue. It has none of the special functions of the permanent cells, such as nerve transmission or secretion. It simply fills the gap left by the injury. The process of tissue repair involves the growth and modeling of scar tissue.

Box 22-2 Wound Classification

Clean Wound (1% to 5% Risk of Postoperative Infection)

Example
Total hip replacement, vitrectomy, nerve resection.

Characteristics
Uninfected.
  Clean.
  No inflammation.
  Closed primarily (all tissue layers sutured closed).
  Respiratory, gastrointestinal, genital, and uninfected urinary tracts were not entered.
  May contain closed drainage system.

Clean-Contaminated Wound (3% to 7% Risk of Postoperative Infection)

Example
Cystoscopy, gastric bypass, and removal of oral lesions.

Characteristics
Respiratory, gastrointestinal, genital, or urinary tracts were entered without unusual contamination.
  No evidence of infection or major break in aseptic technique.
  Includes surgery of the biliary tract, appendix, vagina, and oropharynx.

Contaminated Wound (10% to 17% Risk of Postoperative Infection)

Example
Removal of perforated appendix, removal of metal fragments related to an explosion.

Characteristics
Open, fresh, accidental wound.
  Major break in aseptic technique occurred during the surgical procedure.
  Gross spillage from the gastrointestinal tract occurred.
  Presence of acute, nonpurulent inflammation.

Dirty or Infected Wound (>27% Risk of Postoperative Infection)

Example
Incision and drainage of an abscess.

Characteristics
Old traumatic wounds with devitalized tissue.
  Existing clinical infection.
  Perforated viscera.

PHASES OF HEALING

The healing process, which involves the growth of new cells and replacement with connective tissue, is divided into three primary phases: the inflammatory phase, the proliferative phase, and remodeling. Under normal healing conditions, these phases progress naturally from the moment of injury until the wound is healed.

Inflammatory Phase

The inflammatory phase of healing begins as soon as tissue is injured. The natural process of hemostasis described previously begins the healing process. Inflammation, platelet aggregation, and the formation of a scab are followed by the cellular phase.

During inflammation, phagocytes migrate to the wound site and digest excess fibrin, bacteria, and cell fragments, a process that usually takes 3 to 4 days. The phagocytes are replaced by macrophages, which remain in the wound for a much longer period. Macrophages attract fibroblasts and release growth factors, which initiate the proliferation of epithelial cells and the growth of new blood vessels. During this period, tissue debris is continually removed by the macrophages.

Proliferative Phase

The proliferative phase begins about day 4 or 5 and continues for approximately 2 weeks.

During this phase, fibroblasts synthesize *collagen* and other cell matrices. These form the ground substance of the new tissue, providing support and strength. This new tissue is called *granulation tissue.* Epithelial cells begin to form at the edges of the wound and migrate to the middle, forming a new wound surface. When sufficient epithelial cells have filled in the wound, the scab sloughs away, leaving the new layer. Wound strength increases steadily, and sutures are removed at the end of this phase.

Remodeling

The last stage of wound repair begins after about 3 weeks. During the remodeling phase, which lasts 22 days to 1 year, the collagen is continually replaced and absorbed in stress areas. As the wound heals, it contracts slightly. However, large wounds (e.g., those caused by a burn injury on the back, buttocks, or posterior neck) contract as they heal. Contracted tissue prevents mobility and causes cosmetic defects. The contracture can be released surgically or prevented with physical therapy and the use of specialized dressings during healing. When the proliferation of collagen is excessive, the scar is called a *keloid.* Keloids most commonly develop in individuals of African descent.

CONDITIONS THAT AFFECT WOUND HEALING

Complications can occur at any time in the wound healing process but usually are evident in the first week after surgery. Wound complications can occur at the surface incision or in deep tissue, resulting in delayed healing or breakdown of the wound.

Immune System

The body's ability to heal depends on the immune response. Radiotherapy and other types of cancer therapy lower immune resistance, retard healing, and increase the risk of postoperative infection.

Chronic Disease

Diabetes, endocrine disease, and vascular disease are examples of chronic diseases that affect the healing process. A patient with a chronic disease is physiologically stressed before surgery. Tissues may be weakened, and cellular metabolism may be compromised.

Nutrition

During healing, the body uses extra nutrients in the form of protein for repair and carbohydrates for cellular energy. These must be continuously available throughout the healing process. A debilitated or nutritionally depleted patient may not have the reserves for this extra metabolic activity. Extensive burns and trauma require particularly high levels of nutrients for healing.

Obesity

An obese patient is at high risk for surgical complications. Added tension on the surgical site can result in incisional failure. Adipose tissue has a poor blood supply, which decreases vascularity to the wound site and prevents the cellular oxygenation and nutrition necessary for healing. The poor ventilation and respiratory deficiency common to obese patients also contribute to wound complications.

Age

The mechanisms of healing tend to become impaired as a person ages. The blood supply to tissues is reduced, which decreases oxygenation of the cells. Metabolism generally is slowed, and this affects the body's ability to regenerate tissue and build the collagen necessary for healing. Increased physiological stress can predispose an older patient to infection or other complications.

Surgical Technique

The surgical technique affects the health status of wound tissues. Rough handling or failure to irrigate tissues adequately during surgery can result in tissue breakdown in the postoperative period. Retractors that bruise and macerate tissue can cause healing complications at the wound's edges. These can lead to *tissue edema* (fluid accumulation in interstitial spaces) and inflammation of the peritoneal layer. Inflammation causes the release of serosanguineous fluid, which becomes a medium for infection. Tissue layers must be approximated in anatomical position to prevent *dead space,* where serum can accumulate. Excessive stress on suture points can tear and bruise tissue and is very uncomfortable for the patient. All these factors contribute to postsurgical complications.

WOUND COMPLICATIONS

SURGICAL SITE INFECTION

Postoperative (surgical site) infection can occur at any time in the healing process but is more likely in the first week. The first signs of infection are excess inflammation and serous discharge from the wound. At this stage, medical and nursing personnel take immediate action to halt the process of infection.

A variety of debriding agents and dressings, in addition to meticulous care of the wound, contribute to treating a surgical site infection. However, if the infection threatens to become systemic, the patient is prescribed antibiotics and may require aggressive wound care. This includes continuous wound irrigation, **debridement** (removal of dead tissue), and holistic care to improve the patient's nutritional status. Sometimes a sinus tract forms at the site of the infection. This is a small open space through which exudate from the wound seeps through the tissue. This tract develops a lining that must be surgically removed to allow the tissue to close over and heal. Wound drainage is an important factor in the healing of an infected wound. Closed suction drainage may be required to flush the wound of bacteria, pus, and tissue debris. Infections that penetrate the body wall (abdominal wall, thoracic cavity) can become life-threatening as vital organs are involved. At this level, the patient may require critical care and must face a very long and difficult recovery period.

SEROMA AND HEMATOMA

A *seroma* is a collection of serous fluid that develops in the wound during healing. This is caused by tissue trauma incurred during the surgery. The seroma acts as a physical barrier between the wound's edges and prevents healing. A **hematoma** is a collection of blood that forms in a surgical wound because of incomplete hemostasis during surgery. In addition to the dangers arising from an unsecured blood vessel, a hematoma increases the risk of wound infection. With both seromas and hematomas, reentry of the wound may be required to resolve the problem.

DEHISCENCE

Tissue breakdown at the wound margins is called **dehiscence**. Inflammation is evident, and some serous fluid or pus may be present. Dehiscence can occur at the skin margins or may extend to deeper tissue layers. Complex infected wounds can take weeks or months to heal. A complication of infection is fistula formation. A **fistula** is a tract that leads from the point of infection to a point of eruption outside the body. One or more fistulas may form.

If infection is present, the dressing routine may be altered. A moist dressing sometimes is applied and allowed to dry between dressing changes. The dry dressing pulls away dead tissue and exudate. Many types of dressings are used in the treatment of wounds (Table 22-4).

Wound breakdown can lead to abdominal wall defects that require surgery. Scars formed after wound breakdown have little strength compared to healthy tissue, and the anatomical planes are disrupted. This can lead to a hernia or rupture in the body wall under the intact skin.

EVISCERATION

Evisceration is dehiscence with protrusion of the abdominal contents outside the wound. Although rare, evisceration requires immediate action to replace and hydrate the extruded tissues and prevent necrosis. Abdominal evisceration can involve a portion of the bowel or omentum. If the dehiscence is small, the viscera may slide through the defect or become trapped by it, resulting in necrosis.

Table 22-4 Dressings and Specialty Wound Care Products

Name	Other Names	Type	Description	Uses
Surgical Dressings				
Sterile gauze square	Gauze sponge Flat dressing Gauze dressing "Flat" "Topper"	Flat surgical dressing	Lightweight gauze folded into squares; sterile	For an uncomplicated surgical incision with no drainage. Used in combination with nonadherent layer and surgical tape.
Telfa pad	Telfa	Nonadherent flat fabric pad	Square of compact, felted material with an outer covering of Telfa; used for its nonstick properties.	Clean surgical wound. Also used in surgery for care of specimens.
Clear Telfa	Clear Telfa	Nonadherent flat wound covering	Single-layer clear Telfa	Used to cover delicate incisions when a nonadherent surface is required (e.g., burns, skin grafts).
Gauze fluff	Fluffs "Bulky dressing" Kerlix fluff	Diamond weave, flat wound dressing folded many times	Diamond weave, crimped, soft gauze square of synthetic material folded into squares; can be unfolded and "fluffed" to increase loft	Used to provide soft padding and drainage in simple draining wounds or in delicate surgical repair (e.g., hand surgery).
Transparent film dressing	Film; also various brand names	Film dressing	Single-layer clear adhesive square	Used primarily for intravenous (IV) sites; also used for donor skin graft sites, ulcers.
Cotton sponge	Dermacea Cotton prep sponge	100% cotton flat sponge	Flat gauze sponge with wide "crimped" diamond weave; 100% cotton for lint-free use	For lint-free prepping and wound packing.
ABD pad	Combine dressing "Bulky dressing" ABD	Nonwoven, padded dressing	Oversize square pad; nonwoven material is contained in a lightweight, smooth outer covering that may be water-repellent	Used for draining wounds when absorption is required.
Vaseline gauze	Petrolatum gauze	Impregnated nonadherent gauze	Gauze strip impregnated with Vaseline or similar petrolatum substance	Used to cover delicate incisions where tearing of tissue would disrupt repair (e.g., hand, face, minor burns, skin graft, circumcision).
Xeroform gauze	Xeroform dressing	Impregnated nonadherent gauze	Gauze strip or square impregnated with 3% bismuth tribromophenate	Used as for other nonadherent dressings; has bacteriostatic properties*; promotes moisture.
Webril	Webril Rolled cast padding	Rolled bandage; nonsterile	Soft felted 100% cotton	Used under pneumatic tourniquet and casts for padding and protection.
Roll gauze	Rolled gauze Roller gauze Bandage Rolled bandage	Sterile rolled gauze bandage	Gauze bandage roll, small to medium-size weave made of synthetic or 100% cotton; molds easily to shape	Used to overwrap surgical wound on a limb. Also used in conjunction with flat dressings and other padded dressings.
Kerlix rolled gauze; soft roll	Kerlix Kerlix roll Kerlix roller gauze	Sterile rolled gauze bandage	Crimped, rolled gauze bandage with a wide diamond weave	As for *roll gauze*. Diamond weave permits ease of conforming around limb.
Gauze packing	Adaptic Packing strips Gauze packing	Gauze packing material	Narrow, fine-weave gauze in a continuous strip; may be impregnated with a bacteriostatic agent* or petrolatum	Used for packing sinus structures, fistula tracts, or wounds healing by third intention. Single long strip allows incremental placement in the wound.

Table 22-4	Dressings and Specialty Wound Care Products—cont'd			
Name	**Other Names**	**Type**	**Description**	**Uses**
Compression bandage	Stretch bandage Ace wrap Elastic bandage Coban	Nonsterile rolled compression bandage	Elasticized roller bandage can be supplied as lightweight stretch gauze or heavier stretch cloth; secured with clips or tape or may be self-adhering	Used as a pressure dressing for limbs. Used over a gauze dressing or other type of dressing in direct contact with surgical wound.
Specialty Wound Care				
Hydrocolloid	Hydrocolloid; also known by brand names	Hydrocolloid occlusive gel dressing	Contains gel-forming agents in a foam or film; self-adhesive and occlusive; adheres to wet or dry wound	Used in clean, granulating wounds with little drainage. Promotes healing by providing moisture and barrier to bacterial invasion. Also, absorbs moisture. May be used in conjunction with sterile maggot therapy.
Intersorb mesh	Intersorb	Wide mesh burn dressing	Layered, wide mesh gauze made of 100% cotton for lint-free surface	Used as a specialty dressing for burns.
Hydrogel gauze	Hydrogen dressing	Hydrogel-impregnated dressing	Gauze square or strips impregnated with Hydrogel	Hydrogel provides moisture in the wound and supports natural lysis and absorption of necrotic tissue. Can be conformed to fit the wound.
Moist gauze	Sodium chloride dressing Wet-to-dry dressing Wet dressing	Wet-to-dry dressing	Saline-moistened, loosely woven gauze squares	Used to pack the wound and mechanically debride tissue. When gauze packing has dried, it is removed, pulling away necrotic or devitalized tissue.
Foam dressing	Foam	Padded, nonadherent dressing	Soft foam material covered with smooth, nonadherent coating	Used to cushion and protect chronic wounds and absorb exudate. Commonly used for pressure sores.
Alginates	Alginate dressing	Protective gel dressing	Gel dressing made from seaweed that is highly absorbent and biodegradable; rinses easily with saline solution	Used in deep wounds, fistulas, venous and diabetic ulcers, burns and pressure ulcers. Provides moisture and enhances epithelialization.

*Antibiotic ointments (e.g., "triple antibiotic") are no longer recommended for use on surgical wounds. Bacteriostatic agents are preferred, and these are indicated only in selected cases.

ADHESIONS

An **adhesion** is a band of scar tissue between the abdominal or pelvic organs and the peritoneum. Adhesions usually are associated with infection or multiple abdominal surgeries. Adhesions can cause pain and discomfort. They also increase the risk of injury to organs during surgery.

KEY CONCEPTS

- An uncomplicated surgical outcome is influenced by management of the wound during surgery. This includes maintaining the sterile field, gentle handling of tissues, keeping tissues irrigated, appropriate use of instruments and sutures, and maintaining hemostasis. Tissue viability is promoted by good technique, whereas poor surgical technique results in tissue bruising and edema, avoidable hemorrhage, and high risk of infection.
- The surgical technologist participates and assists in many roles associated with wound management. Some tasks require direct assistance such as retracting tissue, sponging, and irrigation whereas others need indirect assistance such as preparing sutures, assembling surgical devices, and maintaining the sterile field.
- Tissue retraction is necessary to provide exposure to anatomical structures within the wound. The surgical technologist is often required to retract delicate tissues or organs that can be easily injured though poor technique. Important points of technique are applying the correct amount of tension on tissue without causing injury and

maintaining consistent traction on tissue to prevent slippage of the retractor.

- The Halstead principles of surgery were developed more than 100 years ago by the famous surgeon William Halstead. These principles revolutionized the way surgery was conducted and his teachings on surgical wound management are still considered to be essential in surgical practice.
- The principles and practice of wound management are based on the care and handling of tissues in a way that minimizes tissue damage, promotes healing, and prevents postoperative wound complications.
- Hemostasis is an essential element of wound management. Techniques used to control bleeding in the surgical wound include the use of the electrosurgery unit to coagulate bleeders, biochemical and mechanical hemostats, clamping (occluding) a blood vessel, and tissue ligation with sutures. Blood replacement or fluid resuscitation is required when the techniques of hemostasis are inadequate to maintain the level of circulating blood.
- Surgical sponges are used for absorbing fluids in the surgical wound, for dissecting tissue, for cushioning tissue during retraction, and for packing—applying pressure to bleeding tissue. Surgical sponges are available in specific sizes and configurations. Specific techniques are used to prevent the loss of a sponge in the surgical wound.
- Learning the many types of suture materials and suture-needle combinations is a gradual process that can evolve as new materials are developed. The selection of a specific type and size of suture to be used in a surgical procedure is the surgeon's responsibility. The technologist's role is to deliver the required suture at the required time in the procedure.
- A universal system is used to indicate a suture's size, regardless of the type of material or configuration. The system relates to the diameter of the suture strand.
- Specific suture types and sizes are associated with the strength and type of tissue in which they will be used, the suturing technique, and the classification of the wound. Surgeons generally know what kind of suture they will require before surgery. This information will be listed along with the tissue type and layer associated with it. The surgical technologist is responsible for recognizing the tissue type and layer, and then providing the correct suture at the correct time in the procedure.
- Surgical needles are identified by thickness and shape of the shaft, degree of curvature, and type of point. Many combinations of these elements are possible. The surgical technologist is generally required to prepare specific needle and suture combinations as indicated on the surgeon's preference card, and make them available at the appropriate time.
- Suture is packaged in a way that facilitates rapid delivery in a tangle-proof system. The system varies by manufacturer and according to the type of suture.
- The use of a specific suturing technique depends on the type of tissue, strength of the closure required, condition of the patient, and wound classification. This information

is related to the amount of suture required for a surgical case, and the role of the surgical technologist in cutting the sutures.

- Sharps injuries increase the risk of blood-borne infection in health care workers. Specific techniques are used to prevent injury during surgery. These include confining sharps to a magnetic sharps pad or other sharps device, passing sutures on a "one given-one received basis," and disposing of sharps in a designated container after surgery.
- A variety of implant materials is used in reconstructive surgery, repair, and replacement procedures. These include synthetic (manmade), metal, and those derived from animal or human tissue. Engineered and biosynthetic materials that are incorporated into the patient's own tissue during the healing process are also used.
- A wound drainage system draws fluid from within the surgical wound in the postoperative phase. This is done mechanically using a suction device or passively by gravity drainage. The release of fluid from the interstitial spaces and cells occurs as a part of the inflammatory process. This process is initiated by trauma or the mechanics of the surgery itself. Accumulated fluid in the surgical wound retards healing because it prevents contact between tissue edges during healing.
- A water-sealed drainage system is used following thoracic surgery to reestablish normal negative pressure in the chest cavity, which allows lung expansion.
- The surgical technologist is responsible for preparation of and assistance in applying wound dressings. The type and material used in the wound dressing are normally stated on the surgeon's preference card.
- Dressings protect the incision site, acting as a barrier to environmental contamination. A dressing may also provide external support following orthopedic procedures.
- The physiological process of healing is influenced by many factors that the surgical technologist should understand as part of wound management.
- Surgical wound complications in the healing period are associated with the patient's general medical condition, age, and surgical technique.

REVIEW QUESTIONS

1. Explain how suture is sized.
2. Name four types of surgical needles.
3. How are sutures regulated in the United States?
4. What is the function of a double-armed suture?
5. What is the purpose of a suture ligature?
6. Define *allograft*, *autograft*, *xenograft*, *autologous*, and *allogeneic*.
7. List the functions of a dressing.
8. What is the purpose of a surgical drain?
9. Explain negative pressure in the thoracic cavity and how water-sealed drainage is used to restore this after surgery.
10. What is dehiscence? How is it different from evisceration?

CASE STUDIES

Case 1

The surgeon asks you for a size 2-0 silk suture. After you have given the surgeon the suture, you realize that you have mistakenly passed a 3-0 suture. The surgeon has already inserted the suture and is about to tie it. What will you do?

Case 2

You placed a package of surgical gut in a basin to rinse it and make it more pliable. You forgot that the suture was in the basin, and now it is very limp and waterlogged. Is it safe to use?

Case 3

While you are passing a double-armed suture, the free needle snags on the drapes and breaks. What is the next step?

Case 4

You have been working on a vascular case for 3 hours. You are completely out of ties. When should you have requested more ties? After you receive the ties from the circulator, you cannot take the time to place them under the Mayo stand towel. Now you have three packages of ties in three different sizes. The ties are mixed up on top of the Mayo stand in no particular order. What problems can this cause, and how should you have prevented this problem?

Case 5

At the close of the case, the surgeon's assistant leaves to attend to another patient. The surgeon asks you to cut sutures for him. When you cut the first suture, you slice through the knot and the suture comes out. What is the next step?

REFERENCES

Centers for Disease Control and Prevention: *Surgical site infection (SSI) toolkit, Activity C: ELC prevention collaboratives*, 2009. Accessed September 21, 2011, at http://www.cdc.gov/HAI/pdfs/toolkits/SSI_toolkit021710SIBT_revised.pdf.

U.S. Food and Drug Administration: *Medical devices, products and medical procedures, recently approved clearances*. Accessed September 21, 2011, at http://www.fda.gov/MedicalDevices/ProductsandMedicalProcedures/DeviceApprovalsandClearances/Recently-ApprovedDevices/default.htm.

BIBLIOGRAPHY

Autosuture, IncSurgical staplersAccessed June 15, 2008, athttp://www.autosuture.com

Porth C: *Pathophysiology concepts of altered health states*, ed 6, Philadelphia, 2002, Lippincott Williams & Wilkins.

Thibodeau G, Patton K: *Anatomy and physiology*, ed 6, St Louis, 2007, Elsevier/Saunders.

Wood FM, Kolybaba ML, Allen P: The use of cultured epithelial autograft in the treatment of major burn injuries: a critical review of the literature, *Burns* 32:395, 2006.

General Surgery

CHAPTER OUTLINE

LEARNING OBJECTIVES

After studying this section the reader will be able to:

1. Identify the anatomical regions and structures of the abdominal wall
2. Discuss specific elements of case planning for abdominal wall hernias including instruments and repair materials
3. Describe basic pathology related to abdominal wall weakness
4. Describe common procedures used to correct abdominal wall hernias
5. Identify key anatomical structures of the gastrointestinal system
6. Discuss common diagnostic procedures of the gastrointestinal system
7. Discuss the basic pathology of the gastrointestinal system
8. Discuss specific elements of case planning for gastrointestinal surgery
9. Describe common techniques used in gastrointestinal surgery including anastomosis and bowel technique
10. Discuss common surgical procedures of the gastrointestinal system.
11. Identify key anatomical structures of the biliary system, liver, pancreas, and spleen
12. Discuss common diagnostic procedures of the liver, biliary system, pancreas, and spleen
13. Discuss specific elements of case planning for surgery of the liver, biliary system, pancreas, and spleen
14. Describe common surgical procedures of the liver, biliary system, pancreas, and spleen
15. Identify key anatomical structures of the breast
16. Discuss surgical treatment of breast cancer
17. Describe specific elements of case planning for breast surgery
18. List and describe common surgical procedures of the breast

TERMINOLOGY

THE ABDOMEN

Abdominal peritoneum: The serous membrane lining the walls of the abdominal cavity. The retroperitoneum is the posterior aspect. In surgical discussions, abdominal usually refers to the anterior aspect.

Direct inguinal hernia: A hernia that results from weakness in the inguinal floor.

Evisceration: Protrusion of the viscera outside the body as a result of trauma or wound disruption.

Fistula: An abnormal tract or passage leading from one organ to another or from an organ to the skin; usually caused by infection.

Hernia: A protrusion of tissue under the skin through a weakened area of the body wall.

Incarcerated hernia: Herniated tissue that is trapped in an abdominal wall defect. Incarcerated tissue requires emergency surgery to prevent ischemia and tissue necrosis.

Incisional hernia: The postoperative herniation of tissue into the tissue layers around an abdominal incision. This may occur in the immediate postoperative period or later, after the incision has healed.

Indirect inguinal hernia: A hernia that protrudes into the membranous sac of the spermatic cord. This condition usually is due to a congenital defect in the abdominal wall.

Linea alba: A strip of avascular tissue that follows the midline and extends from the pubis to the xiphoid process.

McBurney incision: An incision in which the oblique right muscle is manually split to allow removal of the appendix.

TERMINOLOGY (cont.)

Reduce: To replace or push herniated tissue back into its normal anatomical position.

Strangulated hernia: A hernia in which abdominal tissue has become trapped between the layers of an abdominal wall defect. The strangulated tissue usually becomes swollen as a result of venous congestion. Lack of blood supply can lead to tissue necrosis.

Ventral hernia: A weakness in the abdominal wall, usually resulting in protrusion of abdominal viscera against the peritoneum and abdominal fascia.

Viscera: The organs or tissue of the abdominal cavity.

GASTROINTESTINAL SURGERY

Anastomosis: A surgical procedure in which two hollow structures are joined .

Billroth I procedure: A gastroduodenostomy, or surgical anastomosis, of the stomach and the duodenum.

Billroth II procedure: A gastrojejunostomy, or surgical anastomosis, of the stomach and the jejunum.

Bowel technique: A method of preventing cross-contamination between the bowel contents and the abdominal cavity.

Esophageal varices: Distended veins of the esophagus, caused by advanced liver disease. The condition occurs as a result of portal vein obstruction arising from fibrosis of the liver. Esophageal varices may bleed profusely.

Exploratory laparotomy: A laparotomy performed to examine the abdominal cavity when less invasive measures fail to confirm a diagnosis.

Gastrostomy: A surgical opening through the stomach wall connecting to the outside of the body or another hollow anatomical structure.

Laparotomy: A procedure in which the abdominal cavity is surgically opened. The techniques used for laparotomy are used for all open surgical procedures of the abdomen.

Morbid obesity: A condition in which the patient's body mass index (BMI) is 40 or higher, and the individual is at least 100 pounds (45 kg) over the ideal weight despite aggressive attempts to lose weight.

Nasogastric (NG) tube: A flexible tube inserted through the nose and advanced into the stomach. The NG tube is used to decompress the stomach or to provide a means of feeding the patient liquid nutrients and medication.

-ostomy: A suffix that refers to an opening between two hollow organs; for example, gastroduodenostomy, a surgical procedure that joins the stomach and duodenum.

Ostomy: A technique in which a new opening is made between a tubular structure such as the intestine or ureter and the outside of the body or another hollow structure or organ.

Stoma: An opening created in a hollow organ and sutured to the skin to drain the organ's contents (e.g., an intestinal or ureteral stoma). A stoma may be a temporary or permanent method of bypass.

Stoma appliance: A two- or three-piece medical device used to collect drainage from a stoma. The appliance is attached to the patient's skin and completely covers the stoma. This allows free drainage into a collection device or bag.

BILIARY SYSTEM, LIVER, PANCREAS, AND SPLEEN

Cirrhosis: A disease of the liver in which the tissue hardens and the venous drainage becomes blocked. It usually is caused by chronic alcoholism but may result from other disease conditions.

Friable: A descriptive term for tissue that means fragile and easily torn, and may bleed profusely. Some disease states produce friable tissue. The liver and spleen normally are friable.

Lobectomy: Surgical removal of one or more anatomical sections of the liver.

Segmental resection: Anatomical resection of the liver in which segments divided by specific blood vessels and biliary ducts are removed.

BREAST SURGERY

Body image: In psychology, the way a person sees himself or herself through the eyes of others. A negative body image can severely affect a patient's sense of identity and social and personal interactions.

Hook wire: A device used to pinpoint the exact location of a nonpalpable mass detected during a mammogram; also referred to as a hook needle. A fine wire is inserted into the mass during the examination, and the tissue around the needle is removed for pathological examination and definitive diagnosis.

Mastectomy: A procedure in which breast tissue, including the skin, areola, and nipple, is removed, but the lymph nodes are not removed; also called a simple mastectomy.

Modified radical mastectomy: A procedure in which the entire breast, nipple, and areolar region are removed. The lymph nodes also are usually removed.

Sentinel lymph node biopsy (SLNB): A procedure in which one or more lymph nodes are removed to determine whether a tumor has metastasized. Other lymph nodes may be removed periodically to determine whether metastasis has occurred.

Skin flap: A flap that is created by incising the skin and cutting it away from the underlying tissue to which it is attached. The flap can be increased in size or "raised" as it is enlarged by dissection.

Subcutaneous mastectomy: A procedure in which the breast is removed, but the skin, nipple, and areola are left intact; also called a lumpectomy.

Technetium-99: A radioactive substance used to identify sentinel lymph nodes.

Wire localization: A biopsy procedure in which a hook wire is inserted under fluoroscopy into tissue suspected of being cancerous. The tissue surrounding the hook wire is removed.

INTRODUCTION

General surgery encompasses procedures of the abdomen and noncosmetic procedures of the breast. The organs and organ systems involved include the following:

- Abdominal wall
- Gastrointestinal (GI) system
- Biliary system (the gallbladder and associated structures)
- Spleen
- Pancreas

- Hepatic system
- Breast

Although these regional systems remain in the category of general surgery, the trend increasingly is toward specialization. This is particularly true for bariatrics (the medical and surgical treatment of morbid obesity) and breast and GI surgery.

General surgery also may include superficial procedures, which rarely extend deeper than the subcutaneous tissue, such as excision of common skin lesions (e.g., lipomas, sebaceous cysts) and other minor lesions.

SECTION I: THE ABDOMEN

STRUCTURE AND REGIONS OF THE ABDOMEN

The body is divided into semiclosed compartments, or cavities, that contain specific anatomical structures and organs (Figure 23-1, Table 23-1). The cavities are separated by membrane, muscle, and other connective tissue. The *abdominal cavity* contains the abdominal **viscera** (organs). The *pelvic cavity* contains structures of the reproductive, genitourinary, and lower GI systems. The *retroperitoneal cavity* contains the kidneys, adrenal glands, and ureters. The anterior abdominal cavity is separated from the retroperitoneal cavity by the posterior abdominal peritoneum.

The abdomen is divided into four major sections, or landmarks, called *quadrants* (Figure 23-2). Quadrants are often mentioned as the general location of a medical finding or anatomical structure. For example, a medical report may state, "The patient presented with tenderness in the right upper quadrant." The quadrants are named by location:

- Right upper quadrant (RUQ)
- Left upper quadrant (LUQ)
- Right lower quadrant (RLQ)
- Left lower quadrant (LLQ)

The abdomen is divided into nine regions by an imaginary grid made by two vertical and two horizontal lines (Figure 23-3):

- Left and right rib
- Left and right flank

Figure 23-1 **The major body cavities.** (See Table 23-1 for the organs contained in individual cavities.) *(From Thibodeau G, Patton K: Anatomy and physiology, ed 6, St Louis, 2007, Mosby.)*

Table 23-1	Organs of the Ventral Body Cavities
Body Cavity	**Organs**
Thoracic Cavity	
Right pleural cavity	Right lung
Mediastinum	Heart
	Trachea
	Right and left bronchi
	Esophagus
	Thymus gland
	Aortic arch and thoracic aorta
	Venae cavae
	Lymph nodes and thoracic duct
Left pleural cavity	Left lung
Abdominal Cavity	
Right upper quadrant	Liver
	Gallbladder
	Colon
	Portions of the small intestine
Left upper quadrant	Stomach
	Pancreas
	Spleen
	Colon
	Portions of the small intestine
	Kidneys
	Adrenal glands
	Descending aorta
	Ureters
Pelvic cavity	Ureters
	Uterus and adnexa (female)
	Prostate gland (male)
	Urethra
	Urinary bladder
	Sigmoid colon
	Rectum

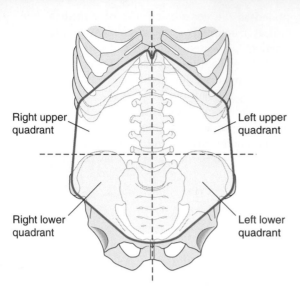

Figure 23-2   The quadrants of the abdomen and associated organs. *(From Garden O, Bradbury A, Forsythe J, Parks R: Principles and practice of surgery, ed 5, Edinburgh, 2007, Churchill Livingstone/ Elsevier.)*

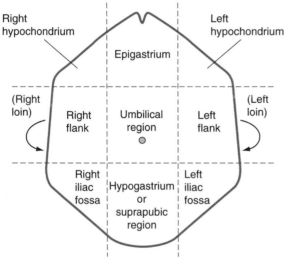

Figure 23-3   The nine regions of the abdomen. *(From Garden O, Bradbury A, Forsythe J, Parks R: Principles and practice of surgery, ed 5, Edinburgh, 2007, Churchill Livingstone/Elsevier.)*

- Left and right inguinal area
- Epigastric region: upper abdomen
- Umbilical region: area near the umbilicus
- Hypogastric region: lower abdomen

TISSUE LAYERS

The abdominal wall encloses the ventral (front) part of the abdominal cavity and extends from the diaphragm to the pubis. It is composed of distinct tissue layers, which support the abdominal organs. These layers are:

- Skin
- Subcutaneous fatty tissue (often called "sub-cu")
- Fascia
- Muscle
- Peritoneum

The fatty and skin layers are contiguous; the muscles cross each other and attach at different levels in the fascia. The *subcutaneous* layer lies directly under the skin. It is composed of lobulated adipose (fat), which varies in thickness from $\frac{1}{4}$ inch (0.63 cm) to more than 8 inches (20 cm).

The muscles and fascia of the abdominal wall protect the abdominal viscera. They move the upper body in flexion and rotation. The muscles also assist in respiration and in "bearing down" during defecation and childbirth. Two longitudinal rectus muscles attach from the pubis to the fifth, sixth, and seventh *costal* (rib) cartilages. Lateral to the rectus muscles are the three flanking muscles: the transverse external oblique, internal oblique, and transverse abdominis muscles. The muscle groups are interrupted by tendons and surrounded by deep fascia, subserous fascia, and the abdominal peritoneum. The rectus sheath is a broad fascial layer that extends across the abdomen without interruption. The rectus muscles are attached to the rectus sheath close to the midline, or **linea alba**, which extends the full length of the midline (Figure 23-4).

The **abdominal peritoneum** (also called the *parietal peritoneum*) is a strong serous membrane that lines the abdominal cavity. The peritoneum protects the viscera in the abdomen and secretes serous fluid, which lubricates the abdominal structures, allowing them to slide over each other easily. Sections of peritoneum fold back to connect the abdominal organs. The *mesentery* is an extension of the peritoneum that attaches to the posterior abdominal wall and fans out to cover the small intestine. The *greater omentum* is another extension of the serous membrane covering the stomach, duodenum, and part of the colon. These extensions are often referred to as *peritoneal reflections.*

INGUINAL REGION

The muscles, ligaments, and fasciae of the inguinal and femoral (groin) regions are more complex than those of the central and upper abdomen. A basic understanding of the tissue layers can best be acquired by studying the illustrations included here.

As the fascial layers continue into the pelvis, they pass in front of the two rectus muscles. Here the inguinal canal splits between the muscle layers near the inguinal ligament. The inguinal canal originates at an opening in the transversalis fascia at the deep inguinal ring and continues to the superficial inguinal ring. The *Hesselbach triangle* is the area bounded by the rectus abdominis muscle, the inguinal ligament, and the inferior epigastric vessels. This is the area associated with an inguinal hernia (Figure 23-5). The space is larger in the male than in the female, which corresponds to the higher incidence of inguinal hernias in males.

The spermatic cord in the male follows the inguinal canal and contains the following structures:

- Spermatic fascia
- Cremaster muscle
- Genitofemoral nerve
- Ductus deferens
- Lymph vessels
- Testicular vein and artery

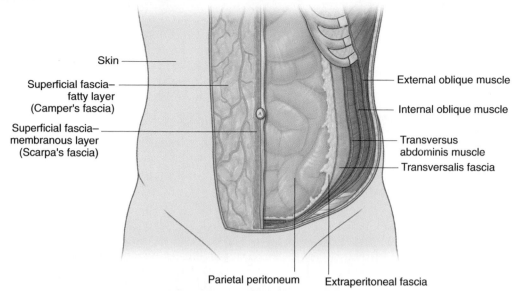

Figure 23-4 **The layers of the abdominal wall.** *(From Drake R, Vogel W, Mitchell A: Gray's anatomy for students, Edinburgh, 2004, Churchill Livingstone.)*

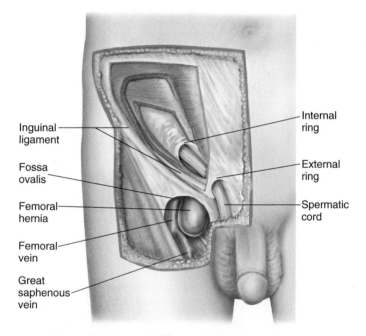

Figure 23-5 **The anatomy of the inguinal region.** *(From Seidel HM, Ball JW, Dains JE, Benedict GW: Mosby's guide to physical examination, ed 5, St Louis, 2002, Mosby.)*

ABDOMINAL INCISIONS

Abdominal incisions are named according to their anatomical location (Figure 23-6 and Table 23-2). Surgical technologists should become familiar with the following traditional incisions and the abdominal structures associated with them while keeping in mind that other region-specific incisions will be encountered in practice:

- Midline incision
- Paramedian incision
- Subcostal incision
- Flank incision
- Inguinal incision
- McBurney incision
- Rocky Davis
- Midabdominal transverse
- Lower transverse incision (Pfannenstiel)

ABDOMINAL WALL HERNIAS

The most common pathology of the abdominal wall is a **hernia**. This is a protrusion of tissue through a defect or weakness in the abdominal wall. The weakness may be caused by a congenital anomaly, previous surgery, or injury. Hernias most often occur in the inguinal and femoral regions. A hernia may also occur along the linea alba, umbilicus, or previous abdominal incision.

A hernia may require urgent surgical treatment when it causes pain or if the herniated tissue becomes trapped or strangulated by the surrounding tissue; this is called an **incarcerated** or **strangulated hernia**. This deprives the herniated tissue of its blood supply and may lead to necrosis. Table 23-3 lists common types of abdominal wall hernias.

CASE PLANNING

Surgery for repair of a hernia may be performed in the outpatient setting. Most patients arrive the day of surgery and can be discharged on the same day. Both open and minimally invasive surgical techniques are used.

The patient is placed in the supine position for procedures of the abdominal wall. Few procedures require a laparotomy. A retention Foley catheter may be inserted before surgery to decompress the bladder during repair of an inguinal or a femoral hernia. General or spinal anesthesia commonly is used.

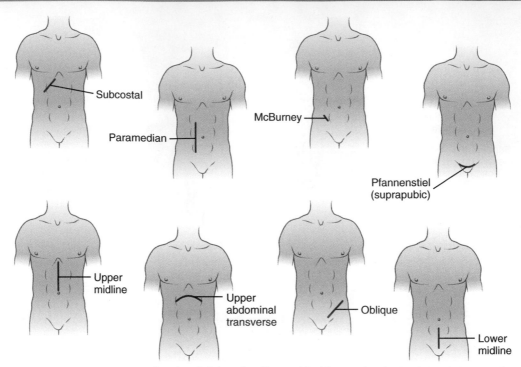

Figure 23-6 **Incisions used in the abdominal wall.** *(Modified from Rothrock JC: Alexander's care of the patient in surgery, ed 12, St Louis, 2003, Mosby.)*

Table **23-2** | **Types of Abdominal Incisions**

Incision	Tissue Layers	Exposure	Details
Midline (upper and lower)	Skin Subcutaneous fat Fascia (linea alba) Abdominal peritoneum	Lower esophagus Stomach Small intestine Liver Biliary system Spleen Pancreas Proximal colon	A midline incision is made through the skin, subcutaneous fat, and the linea alba. This is the center of the fascial layer to which the rectus muscles attach; it is also an avascular area of the rectus sheath.
Paramedian (upper and lower)	Skin Subcutaneous fat Anterior rectus muscles Rectus fascia Abdominal peritoneum	*Right:* Biliary system Pancreas *Left:* Spleen Sigmoid colon	This is a muscle-splitting incision. It is less painful than a subcostal muscle-cutting incision for access to the upper quadrants.
Subcostal	Skin Subcutaneous fat Rectus muscles Fascia Abdominal peritoneum	*Right:* Biliary system Spleen *Bilateral* (chevron): Liver transplantation.	This incision follows the lower rib margin in a semicurved shape; it is painful postoperatively.
McBurney	Skin Subcutaneous fat Fascia Oblique and transversalis muscles Abdominal peritoneum	Appendix	This incision is made on the right side, at an oblique angle, in the flank below the umbilicus; it is a muscle-splitting incision and offers only limited exposure.
Inguinal (oblique)	Skin Subcutaneous fat Fascia Muscle Ligaments Peritoneum	Muscles and fascia of the inguinal abdominal wall Spermatic cord Inguinal ring Abdominal ring Inferior epigastric artery and vein	This incision is used to gain access to the inguinal region for hernia repair; it also may be used for internal access to the spermatic cord.
Lower transverse abdominal (Pfannenstiel)	Skin Subcutaneous fat Rectus fascia Rectus muscles	Uterus Adnexa Bladder Access for cesarean section	This incision follows the natural skin folds to achieve cosmetic closure; it is very strong and offers good exposure to the pelvic contents.

Table 23-3	**Hernias of the Abdominal Wall**	
Condition	**Description**	**Considerations**
Incisional hernia	Protrusion of abdominal tissue through one or more abdominal layers. This results from a previous abdominal incision that failed to heal completely or later broke down because of obesity, infection, or disease.	May require mesh reinforcement to bridge and strengthen the tissue edges.
Strangulated hernia Incarcerated hernia	Tissue protruding from the hernia may become swollen and squeezed. This may result in local ischemia or other complications.	Strangulated hernia is an emergency condition requiring surgery to release the tissue and prevent ischemia and necrosis.
Indirect inguinal hernia	A hernia in which abdominal viscera slides into the inguinal canal from the deep inguinal ring. Herniated tissue may extend through the superficial ring in the spermatic cord into the scrotum or labia.	Usually caused by a congenital weakness in the inguinal ring. Surgery may be necessary.
Direct inguinal hernia	Protrusion of abdominal or inguinal tissue directly through the transversalis fascia	The condition is usually acquired in older men.
Femoral hernia	A hernia arising from a weakness in the transversalis fascia below the inguinal ligament.	Occurs mainly in women and may require surgery to prevent tissue incarceration.
Umbilical hernia	Abdominal wall defect occurring in the linea alba at the umbilical ring seen in infants and adults.	Rarely requires surgery. Incarceration is more common in obese adults.
Spigelian hernia	Rare hernia occurring between the transverse abdominis and rectus muscles.	Rarely diagnosed but seen occasionally during surgery for other reasons.

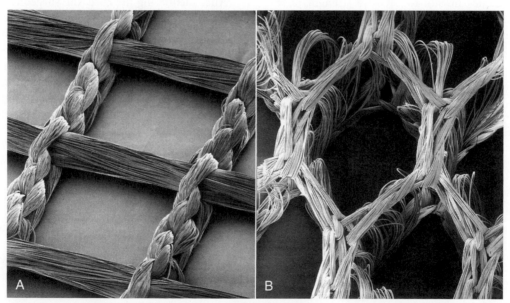

Figure 23-7 **A** and **B,** Magnified view of mesh material. Newly formed tissue infiltrates through the weave to provide a strong bridge between layers of the abdominal wall. *(Copyright © 2008 Covidien. All rights reserved. Reprinted with the permission of Covidien.)*

A laparotomy set is used for procedures involving the abdominal wall. Braided synthetic sutures and surgical mesh commonly are used to repair defects in the fascia. Monofilament suture may also be used. Most surgeons use a tapered needle, although surgical staples may also be used. Infected abdominal wounds generally are not closed beyond the fascial layer. However, heavy monofilament synthetic retention sutures may be placed behind the line of incision.

Surgical mesh is used for most hernia repairs (Figure 23-7). Biosynthetic mesh is made of synthetic material similar to

suture (e.g., Prolene, Dacron, and Mersilene). The principle of mesh repair is to provide a bridge of strong material over the abdominal wall weakness and release tension on the tissue edges during repair and healing. During the remodeling phase of healing, scar tissue fills the spaces of the mesh in the same way that mesh fabric is used to hold new plant growth in bare soil.

Mesh is available in sheets or patches that are fitted at the edge of the defect (Figure 23-8). A patch usually is measured and cut during surgery, although precut patches are available.

Figure 23-8   Fabric mesh for hernia repair showing the actual size relationship of threads to open space. *(Copyright © 2008 Covidien. All rights reserved. Reprinted with permission of Covidien.)*

Sutures used on hernia repair are usually the softer, more pliable synthetics or silk to increase strength of the weakened abdominal wall and to ensure that the tissues stay in approximation during the entire healing period. The strength of the repair depends on the abdominal fascia closure, with or without the use of a synthetic patch. Polyester silk, surgical staples, and the newer biosynthetic sutures are often used. The strength of the closure is increased using interrupted rather than running sutures for the fascia layer. Absorbable synthetic sutures size 3-0 can be used on the hernia sac, which is composed of more delicate peritoneal tissue.

SURGICAL PROCEDURES

OPEN REPAIR OF AN INDIRECT INGUINAL HERNIA

Surgical Goal

Open repair of an indirect inguinal hernia is performed to restore strength to the inguinal floor and prevent the abdominal viscera from entering the inguinal canal.

Pathology

An abdominal wall defect is an actual tear, an enlarged opening, or a weakened area in the abdominal wall. Defects can be congenital or acquired later in life. An **indirect inguinal hernia** results in protrusion of the abdominal viscera into the inguinal canal from the deep inguinal ring. In males, the herniated tissue can extend through the superficial ring, within the spermatic cord, and into the scrotum. In females, the tissue can protrude into the labia. In both genders, the tissue can produce a bulge. Figure 23-9 shows the steps involved in the repair of an indirect inguinal hernia in a male.

TECHNIQUE

1 A right or left inguinal incision is made.
2 The layers of the abdominal wall are incised, and the edges are retracted.
3 The spermatic cord is dissected from preperitoneal fat and other surrounding tissue.
4 The spermatic cord is retracted with a small Penrose drain.
5 The hernia sac is dissected from the cord and opened. The contents are pushed back into the abdomen.
6 The hernia sac is ligated with ties or a purse-string suture.
7 A synthetic mesh patch is sutured into place over the defect.
8 The abdominal wall is closed.

Discussion

The patient is placed in the supine position, prepped, and draped for a lower abdominal incision. The surgeon incises the skin over the groin using the skin knife. Both sharp and blunt dissection are used to separate the tissue layers and expose the hernia. Several hemostats can be placed on the edges of the fascia to retract it and expose the spermatic cord.

After identifying the cord, the surgeon carefully separates it from the hernia sac. Blunt dissection with a dry sponge is used to tease tissue from the surface of the cord. A small Penrose drain is used to retract the spermatic vessels and vas deferens (spermatic cord). The scrub should moisten the drain in saline before passing it to the surgeon. Dissection is continued to the level of the defect in the abdominal wall. The surgeon then uses Metzenbaum scissors to dissect the hernia sac away from the cord.

The hernia sac is opened, and the edges are grasped with hemostats. Using a finger or a dissector sponge mounted on forceps, the surgeon then pushes the contents of the sac back into the abdomen. If the defect is very small, it can be ligated. For large sacs, a purse-string suture of 2-0 synthetic absorbable material is placed around the neck of the sac. The excess neck tissue above the suture is cut away and removed as a specimen. An alternative method is to invert the sac and imbricate (fold under) the edges with sutures.

If mesh is used to reinforce the defect, it is trimmed to match the size of the floor of the inguinal canal, and a small hole is made to allow the spermatic cord to emerge in its normal anatomical position. Precut mesh patches are also available. The edges of the mesh are secured with synthetic sutures or staples. The incision is then closed in multiple layers as follows:

1. *Fascia:* 2-0 nonabsorbable or absorbable synthetic sutures
2. *Subcutaneous tissue:* 2-0 or 3-0 absorbable sutures
3. *Skin:* Staples or 3-0 or 4-0 nonabsorbable sutures

LAPAROSCOPIC REPAIR OF A DIRECT INGUINAL HERNIA

Two techniques are currently used for the laparoscopic approach to a direct inguinal hernia:

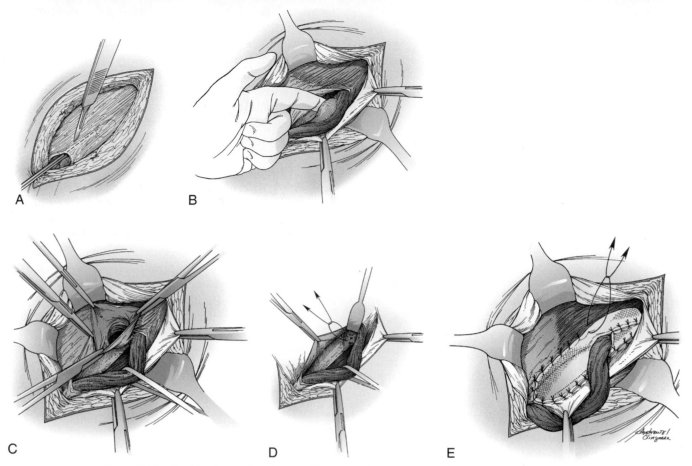

Figure 23-9 **Repair of an indirect inguinal hernia. A,** The aponeurosis (fascia) of the external oblique muscle is incised. **B,** The hernia sac is bluntly dissected from the spermatic cord. **C,** The hernia sac is opened, and the edges are retracted with hemostats. Note the Penrose drain retracting the spermatic cord. **D,** The sac is ligated. **E,** Mesh is placed across the defect and sutured in place. *(Modified from Moody FG: Atlas of ambulatory surgery, St Louis, 1999, Mosby.)*

- Transabdominal preperitoneal (TAPP) laparoscopy
- Total extraperitoneal (TEP) surgery

In the TAPP approach, a pneumoperitoneum is created and the inguinal canal is entered via the abdominal cavity. In the TEP approach, instead of a pneumoperitoneum, the preperitoneal space is inflated with a balloon dissector, which expands the tissue planes (Figure 23-10).

Surgical Goal

Laparoscopic direct hernia repair is the preferred technique to **reduce** herniated tissue and strengthen the inguinal floor. This procedure is less traumatic than open surgery and allows the patient to return to normal activity more quickly.

Pathology

A **direct inguinal hernia** arises from a defect behind the superficial inguinal ring in the inguinal floor, through the transversalis fascia. The defect is defined by an area called the Hesselbach triangle, which is bounded by the conjoint tendon, inguinal ligament, and inferior epigastric vessels. This is an acquired hernia that occurs most often in older men. Unlike with an indirect hernia, the protruding tissue rarely descends into the scrotum. The defect gradually becomes larger with age or obesity. Increased intraabdominal pressure ("bearing down") with heavy lifting or pulling can precipitate a large, painful direct hernia.

TECHNIQUE

TAPP Procedure

1 Pneumoperitoneum is established, and trocars are inserted into the abdomen.
2 A transverse incision is made above the direct hernia space.
3 The weakened area in the pelvic floor is reinforced with mesh.
4 The peritoneum is closed.
5 Pneumoperitoneum is released, and the port incisions are closed.

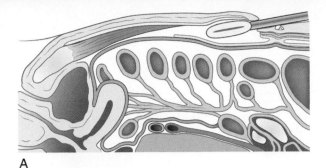

A

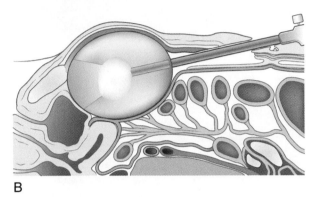

B

Figure 23-10 Repair of an inguinal hernia using a balloon expander. **A,** The expander is inserted into the extraperitoneal space. **B,** The balloon is expanded and the space maintained.

TECHNIQUE

TEP Procedure

1 A periumbilical incision is made through the rectus sheath.
2 Tissues are dissected manually and then retracted.
3 A balloon tissue expander is introduced.
4 The preperitoneal space is inflated, and the expander is removed.
5 A balloon trocar is inserted to seal the space.
6 Two additional 5-mm ports are created.
7 The direct or indirect hernia is reduced, and polypropylene mesh is secured over the defect.
8 The wounds are closed as for a transabdominal preperitoneal (TAPP) procedure.

Discussion

TRANSABDOMINAL PREPERITONEAL LAPAROSCOPY For TAPP laparoscopy, pneumoperitoneum is established and 5-mm ports are placed in the umbilicus and iliac regions. The laparoscope is inserted through the umbilical port.

The surgeon identifies the hernia and then grasps the hernia sac with endoscopic forceps or a grasper. A transverse (horizontal) incision is made in the peritoneum above the direct space with scissors, an electrosurgical unit (ESU), or an ultrasonic dissector. The peritoneum is retracted with right angle retractors to expose the pelvic floor. Surgical mesh is introduced through the largest port. Surgical staples are used to attach the mesh to the Cooper ligament and to close the peritoneum. The pneumoperitoneum is released, and the

fascial and skin layers are closed with 2-0 sutures or skin staples.

The technique for exposing a direct hernia is the same as for an indirect hernia. The hernia sac is incised or dissected from the spermatic cord with blunt dissection. Unlike in open surgical repairs, the sac is not ligated. Biosynthetic mesh is placed over the defect and stapled into place as for an indirect hernia. The pneumoperitoneum is released and the wounds are closed with synthetic absorbable sutures and skin staples.

TOTAL EXTRAPERITONEAL SURGERY For TEP surgery, the preparation of the patient is the same as for a TAPP procedure. However, pneumoperitoneum is not used in the TEP approach. Instead, the surgeon makes a small incision lateral to the midline, exposing the rectus muscle sheath. This opening is expanded with digital dissection. A balloon expander is inserted into the incision and inflated with air or normal saline. The balloon dissector is removed, and the space is maintained with gas insufflation.

Specially designed ports are available to seal the preperitoneal space. Two 5-mm trocars are inserted into the preperitoneal space. When all trocars are in place, the hernia is repaired as described previously.

OPEN REPAIR OF A FEMORAL HERNIA

Surgical Goal

Open repair of a femoral hernia is performed to reduce abdominal tissue (usually intestine) that has entered the femoral canal. The abdominal wall defect is closed to prevent recurrence.

Pathology

A femoral hernia arises from a defect in the transversalis fascia inferior to the inguinal ligament. The femoral ligament, artery, and nerve pass through the femoral canal, which is usually tight enough to prevent abdominal viscera from entering this space. Multiple childbirth, obesity, and inherent weakness in the abdominal wall can create a weakness in the fascia that can allow herniation of abdominal tissue into the canal. It most often occurs in women, rarely in men.

TECHNIQUE

1 The groin is incised on the affected side.
2 The hernia sac is identified and opened.
3 The sac is ligated and removed.
4 Synthetic mesh is secured over the defect.
5 The wound is closed in layers as for an inguinal hernia.

Discussion

The surgeon incises the groin and uses the ESU to extend the incision and control bleeding. Right angle retractors are placed at each end of the wound. When the fascial layer has been incised, the outer membrane of the sac is elevated with curved hemostats and a small incision is made with the knife or ESU. The incision then can be opened fully, allowing exploration of the sac. The contents of the sac are reduced.

The sac is then closed. The edges are grasped with small hemostats, and a purse-string suture is placed at the neck. The edges are trimmed and removed from the field as specimens, and the purse-string suture is then tightened. At this point, mesh may be sutured in place over the defect. All tissue layers are closed as described previously.

REPAIR OF AN INCISIONAL OR VENTRAL HERNIA

Surgical Goal

The goal of ventral hernia repair is to remove a weak or infected scar in the abdominal wall and remodel the tissue with mesh bridge. Scar tissue lacks the organized blood supply of normal tissue and heals more slowly than normal tissue. Mesh may be used to repair a noninfected ventral hernia.

An **incisional hernia** sometimes develops if the wound becomes infected during the healing period. In advanced infection, a fistula may develop in the scar tissue. A **fistula** is a tract or tunnel through the tissue that develops a lining of epithelium. This is the same process that occurs in decorative body piercing (pierced ears or other skin). The constant drainage of pus prevents the fistula from healing, whereas newly injured tissue heals because fibrin and collagen cells at the site of injury join and weld the tissue together. Therefore, the goal of fistula surgery is to remove the entire tract and its skin cells so that the newly "injured" tissue edges heal normally.

Pathology

A **ventral hernia** refers to any hernia occurring in the abdominal wall, excluding the groin or inguinal area. A ventral hernia often occurs as a result of previous abdominal surgery and is sometimes referred to as an incisional hernia. Abdominal wall weakness and herniation can be caused by

- Obesity with inherent weakness in the abdominal wall
- Previous or concurrent infection at the surgical site
- Extensive strain on the incision, often related to obesity
- Poor tissue healing as a result of metabolic disease, such as diabetes or alcoholism
- Repeat operations in the same location

If the tissue is infected at the time of primary closure, normal healing is delayed. When the incision does heal, the edges are not well integrated into the peripheral tissue, and the area becomes weak. Obesity or excessive strain on the incisional line pulls the weak tissue apart. As the incision line becomes weaker, the abdominal viscera are pushed through the defect. Small tracts containing fat and scar tissue are painful and can lead to further infection or strangulation. The bands of tissue are removed to prevent a recurring hernia.

If the abdominal wall ruptures (or is torn through trauma), the viscera can protrude outside the body. This condition is called an **evisceration**.

TECHNIQUE

1 The abdominal scar is removed and the edges of the previous incision are trimmed.
2 Old sutures are removed.
3 Abdominal adhesions are separated from the viscera and the interior abdominal wall.
4 Synthetic mesh is secured over the abdominal defect.
5 All layers of the abdominal wall are closed.

NOTE: If the wound and tissue edges are infected, the peritoneum and fascia can be closed and the remaining layers left to heal by secondary intention, from the base of the wound to the surface.

Discussion

To begin the surgery, the surgeon places several Allis clamps on the abdominal scar. These are used to apply countertraction on the scar while it is incised, first with a skin knife and then with the ESU. The scrub retains the scar as a specimen.

Sutures from previous surgery are removed with a straight hemostat and scissors or knife. A folded towel placed near the incision is convenient for the surgeon to wipe the suture remnants from the hemostat.

After the sutures have been removed, the surgeon may attempt to reestablish normal tissue planes by trimming and reducing superficial fascia and fatty tissue. The surgeon remodels the edges of the incision, which usually are ragged and poorly defined. In most cases it is not necessary to perform a laparotomy to repair an incisional hernia unless adhesions (scar tissue that binds the abdominal viscera) must be released or the hernia originates from the abdominal peritoneum. Generally only the fascia requires reinforcement and repair.

Once the wound edges have been trimmed and the tissue layers clearly defined, the incision can be closed. A mesh bridge often is sutured or stapled across the edges of the deep fascia. The tissue layers are then closed with interrupted sutures and skin staples. Tension on the wound can be relieved by using a heavy continuous suture (e.g., polydioxanone suture) through all layers or by using retention sutures with bolsters as discussed in Chapter 22.

UMBILICAL HERNIA REPAIR

Surgical Goal

Umbilical hernia repair is performed to repair an abdominal wall defect in the periumbilical region.

Pathology

An umbilical hernia is the result of a defect in the linea alba at the umbilical ring. This hernia is most common in children and usually disappears spontaneously by age 2. In adults, the hernia appears more frequently in individuals with a high BMI. The sac of an umbilical hernia frequently has a small base, which increases the risk of tissue strangulation.

TECHNIQUE

1 A periumbilical incision is made.
2 The linea alba defect is identified.
3 The defect is dissected free of any tissue and the musculo-fascial margins are identified.
4 The defect is repaired with sutures or mesh.
5 The wound is closed.

Discussion

See discussion of the repair of a ventral hernia.

SPIGELIAN HERNIA REPAIR

Surgical Goal

Spigelian hernia repair is performed to reduce the protrusion of a peritoneal sac, preperitoneal fat, or other abdominal viscera through a defect in the abdominal wall called the *spigelian zone.*

Pathology

The spigelian zone is the area of muscle attachment between the transverse abdominis muscle and the lateral edge of the rectus muscle. Spigelian hernias are very rare and occur mainly in individuals over age 60. The condition often is discovered during surgery for other reasons.

TECHNIQUE

1 A skin incision is made.
2 The hernia sac is identified and resected.
3 The contents of the sac are reduced into the peritoneal cavity.
4 The defect is repaired as for an inguinal hernia.

Discussion

The patient is placed in the supine position. A skin incision is made 0.8 inch (2 cm) above the symphysis pubis and extended through the external and internal oblique muscles and the transversalis muscle. The hernia sac is identified. The sac's contents are examined closely for ischemia, the sac is resected, and the contents are reduced into the peritoneal cavity. The defect is repaired using the same techniques as for inguinal and ventral hernias. During resection and reduction, the surgeon must identify a direct or an indirect hernia. During repair, the hernia between the muscle layers is incorporated into the suture line. Biosynthetic mesh may be required for support of larger defects.

SECTION II: GASTROINTESTINAL SURGERY

SURGICAL ANATOMY

ESOPHAGUS AND STOMACH

The esophagus is a tubular structure that extends from the pharynx to the stomach. Food travels along its length by a combination of voluntary and involuntary muscle action called paristalsis. Reverse peristalsis results in regurgitation of the stomach contents. The esophagus enters the abdominal cavity at the level of the diaphragm. In the adult, it measures approximately 10 inches (25 cm).

The stomach is located just under the diaphragm in the left upper abdomen. The three contiguous anatomical sections of the stomach are the *fundus* (upper portion), the *body* (midsection), and the *antrum* (distal or lower portion).

The wall of the stomach contains an outer serosa, two inner layers of smooth (involuntary) muscles, and a submucosal lining which lies in folds called *rugae.* The submucosa secretes hydrochoric acid and pepsin for the breakdown of proteins and carbohydrates which is aided by the mechanical action of the muscle layers. A mucous barrier is also secreted to prevent damage to the stomach tissue itself by these chemicals. Two orifices (openings) and associated sphincters provide continuity between the esophagus and the duodenum. These are the *cardia,* which communicates with the esophagus, and the *pylorus,* which opens into the duodenum. Only a few molecules (which include alcohol and some simple carbohydrates) are absorbed by the stomach.

A sheet of connective and vascular tissue, called *omentum,* attaches to the greater and lesser curvatures of the stomach and covers the intestinal folds and provides warmth and protection to the viscera. This peritoneal sheet also contains fat lobules, and may form outpockets which can become diseased. Whenever a portion of the stomach is removed or remodeled, the omentum must be divided from its attachments.

SMALL INTESTINE

The small intestine is the proximal portion of the intestinal tract. It extends from the pylorus of the stomach to the proximal end of the large intestine and contains three anatomical sections known as the duodenum, ileum, and jejunum. The individual tissue layers of the digestive tube are similar to the stomach and are the inner mucosa, submucosa muscle, and serosa. In order for the body to utilize ingested food, it must be broken down into component parts and absorbed through the intestinal wall. This complex physiological process involves many different enzymes and hormones. Digestion and absorption of fats, proteins, carbohydrates, and other soluble molecules such as vitamins, takes place in the small intestine which also secretes mucous, enzymes, hormones, and serous fluid.

The duodenum is approximately 8 to 10 inches (20 to 25 cm) long. It receives *chyme* (liquefied food broken down by the stomach). The pancreatic duct (*duct of Wirsung*) and the common bile duct from the liver drain digestive enzymes into this section of the intestine.

The jejunum is approximately 9 feet (2.7 m) long. It connects with the ileum, which is approximately 13.5 feet (4 m) long. These sections are suspended from the abdominal wall by a sheet of vascular tissue called the *mesentery,* which supplies blood and lymph to the lower sections of the small intestine. During resection of the jejunum or the ileum, the mesentery must be clamped and divided from the intestine.

The tissue layers of the small intestine are similar to those of the stomach and large intestine. The inner surface of the small intestine has small fingerlike projections called *villi,* which increase the surface area of the intestinal lumen and contain blood and lymphatic vessels. The small intestine terminates at the *cecum,* the first portion of the large intestine.

LARGE INTESTINE (COLON)

The large intestine extends from the distal ileum to the rectum and is divided into five distinct sections: the ascending colon, the transverse colon, the descending colon, the sigmoid colon, and the rectum. The colon measures about 5 feet (1.5 m) in the adult. The long axis of the colon forms a series of puckers called hautra which are formed by contraction of a longitudinal band of muscle called the teniae coli.

As mentioned previously, the first section of the large intestine is a blind pouch called the *cecum.* The terminal end of the cecum has a slender tube, called the *vermiform appendix,* which has no function and can become infected. The ascending colon extends upward behind the right lobe of the liver. The transverse colon then crosses the abdomen to the left, below the stomach. The descending colon extends downward on the left side of the abdomen and terminates at the sigmoid colon, which lies in the pelvic cavity. The sigmoid colon terminates at the rectum.

The primary functions of the large intestine are absorption of water and electrolytes, and formation of fecal waste. Essential resident bacteria in the colon decompose undigested substances and produce gaseous waste as a product of fermentation. They also produce vitamin K and certain B vitamins which are absorbed into the body.

RECTUM AND ANUS

The distal 4 to 5 inches (10 to 12.5 cm) of the intestine is the *rectum,* which terminates at the *anal canal.* This section is lined with folded tissue. Two muscular sphincters in the anal canal control the release of feces to the outside of the body (called *defecation*). The internal sphincter is composed of involuntary (smooth) muscle. The external sphincter is under voluntary control (striated muscle). The opening of the anal canal is called the *anus.*

Figure 23-11 illustrates the sections of the GI system.

DIAGNOSTIC PROCEDURES

The presence of GI disease is confirmed primarily by imaging studies, blood and metabolic studies, and physical examination. Endoscopy (described later) often is performed before open or laparoscopic surgery. Biopsy and visual examination of the inner surface of the intestine and stomach are performed to rule out or confirm carcinoma and provide tissue for further tests. Contrast studies performed under fluoroscopy frequently are done to outline the GI structures. Other important imaging tools are magnetic resonance imaging (MRI), ultrasound, and computed tomography (CT).

CASE PLANNING

During laparotomy and laparoscopy, patients are at high risk for hypothermia. Therefore, thermoregulation is a high priority for patient safety during all abdominal procedures. A forced-air warming system is used. Irrigation solutions are maintained in a solution warmer. Exposure of the patient is kept to a minimum in the perioperative period, and the patient is covered with warm blankets before and after surgery. Compression stockings or a sequential compression device is used during all lengthy laparotomy procedures to prevent deep vein thrombosis.

The patient is placed in the supine position for most laparoscopic and open surgery of the GI system. Exceptions are procedures that require perineal access, such as abdominoperineal resection. In these cases, the low lithotomy position may be used. The patient's arms are placed on arm boards. The operating table is tilted into normal or reverse Trendelenburg position, depending on the anatomical exposure required during the procedure.

Patients undergoing surgery for morbid obesity require particular attention to safety during positioning. The operating table must be able to accommodate up to 800 pounds (360 kg). Extensions must be well padded, and great care must be taken in transferring the patient between the stretcher and the operating table.

INSTRUMENTS

A basic laparotomy set is used for GI surgery. A separate GI set with clamps and grasping instruments is added; the clamps and graspers must be atraumatic and nonpenetrating (Figure 23-12). Vascular clamps may be required. Long instruments may be added, depending on the size of the patient.

Sharp dissection is performed with Metzenbaum scissors, the ESU, ultrasound shears (Harmonic system), or a high-frequency coagulator (LigaSure).

Babcock clamps are used to grasp intestinal tissue. Smooth or vascular forceps are used for suturing the mucosal layers. Resection of the bowel or stomach is performed with atraumatic clamps or with surgical stapling instruments. Atraumatic clamps do not close tightly over the tissue; rather, they leave a small amount of space to prevent crushing. Long intestinal clamps may be covered with soft rubber tubing to provide a snug seal on the tissue; these are generally referred to as *rubber-shod clamps.* Although they are not commonly used, some facilities may include them in a GI set.

When the bowel, omentum, and mesentery have been exposed, a Poole suction tip should be available. This tip has numerous openings, which prevent excess suction pressure on delicate tissue.

Surgical stapling instruments frequently are used in resection and anastomosis. These include systems that apply both linear and circumferential rows of staples.

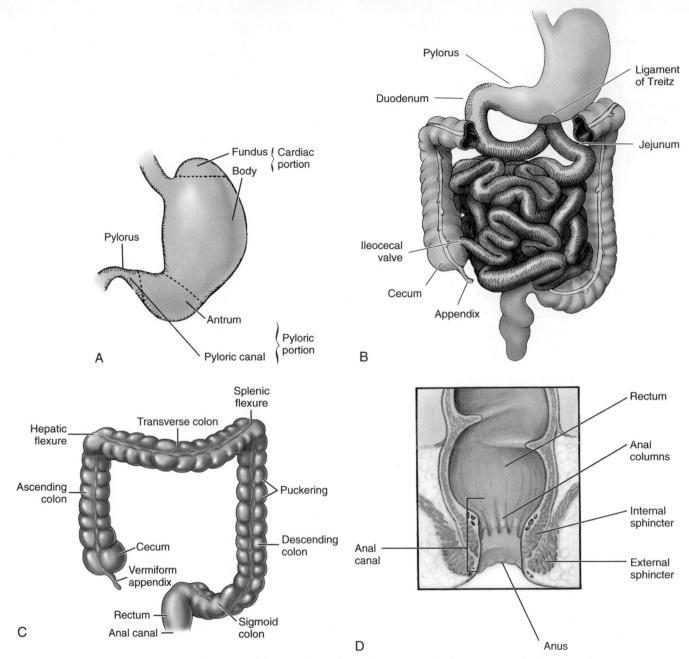

Figure 23-11   **A,** The regions of the stomach. **B,** The small intestine. **C,** The large intestine. **D,** The sigmoid colon, rectum, and anal canal. (*A and B modified from Rothrock JC: Alexander's care of the patient in surgery, ed 12, St Louis, 2003, Mosby; C modified from Herlihy B, Maebius NK: The human body in health and illness, ed 2, Philadelphia, 2003, WB Saunders; and D modified from Applegate EJ: The anatomy and physiology learning system, ed 2, Philadelphia, 2000, WB Saunders.)*

EQUIPMENT AND SUPPLIES

Special equipment that might be required during GI surgery includes the following:

- High-frequency (HF) vessel-sealing system (e.g., LigaSure)
- Ultrasound scalpel
- Vessel loops for large vessel dissection
- Ultrasound probe
- Bowel bag (a plastic bag used to enclose the bowel during open surgery to prevent tissue dehydration)
- Temporary ostomy bag

SUTURES

GI procedures require sutures or surgical staples for resection and anastomosis of the bowel, mesentery, and omentum. Suture closure usually is performed in two or three layers. Fine absorbable sutures (3-0 or 4-0) on a taper needle are used to close the mucosa and submucosa. The outer serosal layer can be closed with fine interrupted silk or synthetic material on a taper needle. Large vessels and vascular bundles are ligated with sutures, surgical clips, or a vessel-sealing instrument (e.g., LigaSure). Large vessels of the omentum and mesentery often are secured with 0 or 2-0 suture ties.

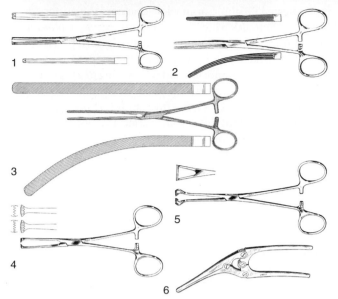

Figure 23-12 Gastrointestinal clamps. *1,* Allen clamp; *2,* Bainbridge clamp; *3,* Doyen clamp; *4,* Allis clamp; *5,* Babcock clamp; *6,* Payr clamp. *(Courtesy Jarit Instruments, Hawthorne, NY.)*

TECHNIQUES IN GASTROINTESTINAL SURGERY

Special techniques are common to most GI procedures. A surgical vocabulary has been developed that describes these (Table 23-4).

The GI system is a continuous "tube" attached to the abdominal and pelvic wall by a complex system of vascular membranes. These attachments limit the mobility of sections in the abdominal cavity and help prevent obstruction, especially in the intestine. To remodel a section of intestine or stomach, the surgeon must free up portions of these attachments (mesentery and omentum). This involves a technique of clamping the tissue, cutting it, and maintaining hemostasis. This called *mobilizing* the section (bowel or stomach).

The traditional method of mobilization involves clamping a section, ligating it with suture, and then incising it. Electrosurgery commonly has been used to coagulate bleeders and to incise the tissue. However, newer energy modalities have replaced some of the traditional techniques. Ultrasonic technology is used to cut and coagulate tissue simultaneously.

Table 23-4 Surgical Techniques Used for the Gastrointestinal System

Term or Technique	Definition	Example
Resection (*verb:* resect)	A procedure in which a section of an organ is cut apart or removed.	A portion of the intestine is removed. If one of the free ends is surgically closed as a blind end, it is called a *stump.*
Anastomosis (*verb:* anastomose)	A procedure in which two hollow organs are joined surgically.	Placing sutures around the circumference of the two cut edges can join two hollow structures. This applies to portions of the gastrointestinal (GI) system and other hollow systems, such as blood vessels and organ ducts.
Division (*verb:* divide)	In surgery, a procedure in which one section of tissue is cut away from another. This differs from *resection,* in which a portion of the organ is removed.	Recall that the small intestine is attached to the mesentery, a loose connective tissue containing many major blood vessels. When a section of small intestine is removed, the mesentery must be divided from the intestine to free up the section.
Cross-clamp	To place one or more clamps at a right angle to a tube or vessel.	The "cross" simply refers to the angle of the clamp in relation to the organ or tissue.
Double-clamp	To place two clamps over a section of tissue to prevent bleeding when the tissue is severed.	Double-clamping is performed before a tissue that might bleed profusely is divided or cut. In the case of GI structures, a section of intestine or stomach must be double-clamped before it is cut. This prevents hemorrhage and the release of fluids from the intestine or stomach.
Mobilization (*verb:* mobilize)	The freeing up of tissue from its attachments before anastomosis or resection.	No tissues in the body are free-floating. Blood and lymph vessels, connective tissue, and membranes nourish and protect tissue. To remove tissue or to reconstruct the anatomy, the tissue must be removed from its normal attachments. Mobilization requires dissection or division.
Clamp and divide	To both double-clamp and divide tissue. Because the purpose of the clamps is to prevent bleeding, the tissue inside the jaws of the clamp must be sealed with the electrosurgical unit (ESU) or with suture ties. If surgical stapling instruments are used, the instrument clamps, staples, and cuts the tissue in one process.	During mobilization of the intestine, the surgeon repeatedly applies two hemostatic clamps, divides the tissue, and seals the tissue with the ESU or ties the cut ends. For the scrub, the tools needed are: • Two hemostats (e.g., Kelly, Mayo, Crile) • ESU or tissue scissors • Two ties (if the ESU is not used) • Suture scissors (if ties are used)

Vessel-sealing systems are used to coagulate tissue bundles and blood vessels. Surgical stapling devices are commonly used in GI surgery and often replace the clamping, cutting, and suturing techniques required in resection and mobilization.

ANASTOMOSIS

Anastomosis is the joining of two hollow structures by sutures, staples, or a combination of both. In GI surgery, anastomosis can be performed between any structures of the system. The suffix **-ostomy** means anastomosis. For example, a gastroduodenostomy is an anastomosis between the stomach and duodenum. A duodenoduodenostomy is the removal of a section of duodenum and rejoining of the two limbs, or open ends of the duodenum. Ileostomy refers to an opening made between the ileum and the outside abdominal wall for drainage.

Anastomosis was historically performed using a technique in which two or even three layers of sutures were placed in a circumference around the two hollow structures in order to join them. Stomach or intestinal clamps were used to bring the two structures together while suturing took place. This technique is still used today, although surgical staples are used more frequently. These techniques are illustrated and described later in the surgical procedures sections. No matter which technique is used to perform an anastomosis, efforts are made to prevent spillage of the GI contents into the wound and maintain aseptic technique.

BOWEL TECHNIQUE

In all procedures involving the intestine, special precautions are taken to prevent contamination of instruments and supplies by the bowel contents; this is known as the **bowel technique**. During this procedure instruments and supplies used while the bowel is open are kept separate from all other sterile items. Contaminated supplies are confined to the Mayo stand and a designated basin. Instruments on the back table are kept "clean" (uncontaminated), and no items are exchanged between the back table and the Mayo stand while the bowel is open. After closure of the bowel, all contaminated instruments and supplies are removed from the field and Mayo stand.

Before the abdomen is closed, the surgical team dons fresh gloves (and possibly also fresh gowns, depending on the facility's protocol). Fresh sterile drapes are placed over those used during the first part of the procedure. Fresh sterile sponges, sutures, ESU instruments, and suction tips are opened for use during closure. Many scrubs set up a separate closure stand with the needed suture materials and instruments. The contaminated Mayo stand must be removed from the field.

SURGICAL PROCEDURES

DIAGNOSTIC AND OPERATIVE ENDOSCOPY

Perioperative Considerations

Endoscopy is an outpatient procedure, and the surgery is performed with the patient under sedation. This can be provided in a dedicated GI clinic or in a location near the postoperative care unit. High-risk patients who require extensive physiological monitoring may require an anesthesia care provider and an extended recovery. In all cases, physiological monitoring includes cardiac monitoring and monitoring of oxygen saturation, respiratory function, blood pressure, and level of consciousness. Although not usually painful, endoscopy can be uncomfortable. With light or moderate sedation, patients are able to respond to commands, and the airway is maintained without artificial support.

Preparation for endoscopy includes a period of fasting or dietary restriction, depending on the extent and type of endoscopic procedure. Upper GI studies require limitations on oral intake. Lower GI endoscopy requires dietary restrictions and an enema, which the patient can self-administer the day before the procedure.

NOTE: A complete discussion of the technology, handling, and reprocessing of fiberoptic endoscopes is presented in Chapter 24.

Gastrointestinal endoscopy is performed for the following purposes:

- To establish or confirm a diagnosis by direct visualization and biopsy
- To perform selected surgical procedures (restricted to surgery in which bleeding is minimal and the risk for technical complications is low)
- To allow postoperative inspection of the surgical site from within the lumen of the GI tract and for screening

ESOPHAGODUODENOSCOPY

Esophagoduodenoscopy (EGD) is diagnostic endoscopy of the esophagus, stomach, and proximal duodenum. Specific goals are:

- Direct diagnostic observation of the inside of the esophagus and duodenum, with biopsy.
- Treatment of varices (varices are prone to frequent bleeding and sometimes require emergency treatment).
- Sclerotherapy of **esophageal varices** (a method of reducing varices by injecting a sclerosing agent directly into the vein to shrink it).
- Polyp removal (polyps are small, benign mucosal outgrowths in the lumen of the esophagus).
- Endoscopic **gastrostomy** for insertion of a feeding tube.
- Placement of a stent for an esophageal stricture.

TECHNIQUE

1 The patient is positioned and sedated.
2 The endoscope is coated with water-soluble gel.
3 The endoscope is inserted into the mouth.
4 The scope is advanced and the tissues are examined.
5 Instruments are passed through the scope at the head of the endoscope.
6 Specimens are withdrawn and retained by the scrub.

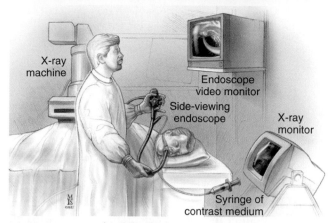

X-ray machine

Endoscope video monitor

Side-viewing endoscope

X-ray monitor

Syringe of contrast medium

Figure 23-13 Esophagoduodenostomy with endoscopic retrograde pancreaticoduodenoscopy. (Artwork is reproduced, with permission, from the Johns Hopkins Gastroenterology and Hepatology Resource Center. www.hopkins-gi.org, copyright 2008, Johns Hopkins University. All rights reserved.)

Discussion

Before the procedure, the scrub should ensure that the endoscope, video equipment, and data storage devices are in working order and ready for use.

The patient is sedated and placed in the lateral position. A small amount of lubricating gel is put on the tip of the scope, and a bite block is inserted into the patient's mouth. Anesthetic spray is applied to the pharynx.

The insertion tube (the distal end of the endoscope) is advanced slowly, and the tissues are examined. Real-time digital imaging is performed to view the anatomy (Figure 23-13). If biopsy samples are taken, the scrub passes biopsy instruments to the surgeon and helps thread the tip into the instrument port. A number of procedures may be initiated at this point.

- *Injection of esophageal varices:* The scrub prepares the sclerosing agent, which is injected through the endoscope after needle placement in the varicosity.
- *Varicocele banding:* A special banding system is passed through the endoscope and the varicosity is ligated.
- *Esophageal dilation:* Graduated dilators are introduced over a guidewire under fluoroscopy after endoscopic examination.
- *Insertion of an esophageal stent:* A self-expanding esophageal stent may be inserted to dilate and hold open a stricture caused by tumor. The stent is preloaded into an insertion device, which is threaded to the level of the stricture and released. It remains in place as a palliative measure.
- *Endoscopic laser therapy:* A neodymium-yttrium-aluminum garnet (Nd:YAG) laser may be used to debulk an esophageal tumor.

The scrub assists the surgeon by guiding long instruments into the endoscope and receiving them as they are withdrawn. Care must be taken to ensure that all specimens are immediately placed in the liquid specimen container, as directed by the surgeon. The specimen is cleaned from the biopsy forceps

with a sterile hypodermic needle or by swishing the tip in the specimen cup liquid.

If laser surgery is planned, all safety precautions are observed to prevent patient fires or burns (see Chapter 18).

At the close of the procedure, the scrub helps ensure that the patient is comfortable. Specimens are carefully labeled and recorded. Endoscopic equipment is cleaned and prepared for critical decontamination according to facility policy.

Postoperative considerations include monitoring for effective gag reflex, pain, and complete recovery from sedative drugs. The patient is taken to the postoperative recovery unit or a designated area of the outpatient area for observation and monitoring before discharge to home.

COLONOSCOPY

Colonoscopy, or "lower GI" endoscopy, is endoscopy of the large intestine. The procedure is used for diagnostic purposes and for minor surgery, such as:

- Removal of polyps
- Biopsy or removal of lesions that do not require resection
- Coagulation of small bleeding diverticula
- Laser treatment of small tumors
- Routine screening for colon cancer

Combined colonoscopy and laparoscopic surgery may be used during resection of the lower GI system.

TECHNIQUE

1 The patient may or may not be sedated, depending on the procedure.
2 The patient is placed in the left lateral position.
3 The scope is lubricated and slowly advanced into the colon.
4 The colon is inflated with air to increase visualization of the tissues.
5 The colon is examined and the intended procedure is performed.
6 The scope is withdrawn.

Discussion

Colonoscopy requires sedation of the patient. The procedure can be uncomfortable and embarrassing for the patient. The scrub should offer support throughout the procedure. The technique used to obtain biopsy samples and for other minor procedures is similar to EGD.

The patient is placed in the left lateral position. The individual should be covered with warm blankets, and only the lower back and buttocks should be exposed. A small protective drape can be placed over the pelvis to prevent soiling of bed linens.

The scope is lubricated with water-soluble gel and gently inserted into the anus. It is then advanced slowly. When the proximal colon is in view, the surgeon begins to withdraw the scope slowly while examining the mucosa. Air may be instilled into the colon with a pump attachment. This may cause the patient some discomfort, and the scrub should offer reassurance. As the scope is withdrawn, the length of the colon is examined for lesions and abnormalities. Digital photographs of any suspect tissue are taken. Suction and irrigation are controlled at the scope head. The scrub should make sure the irrigation reservoir remains full by refilling it as needed.

Cupped or brush biopsy forceps are guided through the scope. As tissue is withdrawn from the endoscope, the scrub receives the forceps and maintains control on the tip to ensure that the specimen is not lost. The specimen can be removed from the tip with a hypodermic needle or by swishing the tip in the specimen cup.

Postoperative considerations include observation for pain or bleeding and sensitivity to any medications given during the procedure. The patient is released from the outpatient department soon after the procedure.

SIGMOIDOSCOPY

Sigmoidoscopy is performed to examine tissue and/or obtain a biopsy specimen of the sigmoid colon and rectum. The patient is placed in the prone or lithotomy position, and the scope is introduced. Biopsy tissue can be obtained or rectal polyps can be removed with cup biopsy forceps.

LAPAROTOMY

Surgical Goal

A **laparotomy** is open surgery of the abdominal cavity for access to the abdominal organs. A laparotomy that is performed to confirm a diagnosis or to detect a specific pathological condition is called an **exploratory laparotomy**.

TECHNIQUE

Opening the Abdomen

1 An incision is made through all layers of the abdominal wall.
2 The contents of the abdominal cavity are explored.
3 The edges of the wound are covered with moist laparotomy sponges and a self-retaining retractor is put in place.
4 The intended procedure is performed.
5 The wound is irrigated and drains are inserted.
6 The abdominal layers are closed and dressings are applied.

Discussion

The patient is placed in the supine position, prepped, and draped for a midline incision. When draping is completed, the scrub moves the Mayo stand up to the field below the wound site. The scrub may stand opposite the surgeon, with the Mayo stand positioned at the level of the patient's knees. This gives the surgeon room to work while allowing the exchange of instruments on the sterile field. The ESU and suction tubing are secured to the top drape. Two dry laparotomy sponges are placed on the field. When suction, the ESU pencil, and sponges are in place on the field, the skin incision is made. The skin knife is then removed from the field.

The skin incision exposes the subcutaneous layer that lies just under the skin. This layer usually is incised with the ESU. Large bleeding vessels can be clamped with Kelly or Crile hemostats and ligated with fine suture ties or coagulated with the ESU (Figure 23-14).

The incision is carried through to the next layer, the fascia. At this level, the scrub should have small Richardson or U.S. retractors available for the assistant. The surgeon incises the layer with the scalpel deep knife or ESU and extends the incision as needed with the ESU or curved Mayo scissors. If the

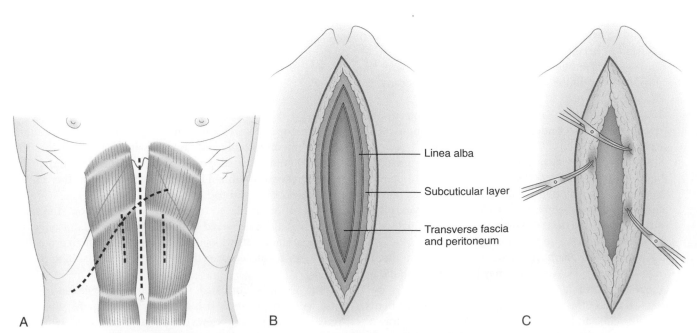

Figure 23-14 Laparotomy incision. **A,** Anatomical location of upper abdomen incisions. **B,** Skin and subcutaneous layers. **C,** Clamps on vessels in the subcutaneous layer.

Linea alba

Subcuticular layer

Transverse fascia and peritoneum

A   B   C incision is not on the midline, the muscle layers are separated manually. The abdominal peritoneum is then visible. The scrub prepares several moist lap sponges and a self-retaining retractor.

All loose 4 × 4 sponges must be removed from the surgical field and only laparotomy sponges used. Any 4 × 4 sponges must be mounted on sponge forceps while the abdomen is open.

The peritoneum is lifted with hemostats, and a small incision is made with the deep knife or Metzenbaum scissors. The incision is carried deeper with scissors or the ESU.

The abdominal contents are then exposed. From this point on, only saline-moistened sponges are used. The scrub passes the moistened sponges to the surgeon, who covers the tissue edges to protect them from the self-retaining retractor. The self-retaining abdominal retractor is now placed in position by the surgeon and assistant. At this time, the surgeon explores the abdominal cavity for evidence of disease. When the area of disease has been located, the surgeon packs the abdominal contents away from the diseased area with several moistened lap sponges. A specific surgical procedure then can be initiated.

During the procedure, the scrub has the following duties:
- Keep the surgical field clear of instruments not in use.
- Keep the ESU tip free of tissue debris and in its holster.
- Exchange soiled sponges for clean ones.
- Keep loose items (e.g., needles, small dissecting sponges, suture wrappers) off the Mayo stand. Small dissecting sponges go on the field or Mayo tray only when mounted on the appropriate clamp. Needles must be mounted on a needle holder.
- Protect the field from contamination.
- Anticipate the needs of the surgeon.
- Receive and properly maintain any specimens.
- Notify the surgeon of any break in aseptic technique.
- Participate in sponge and item counts at the appropriate time.

CLOSURE After irrigation, the surgeon and assistant remove all sponges and instruments from the abdomen, the first count is initiated. The incision then is closed in layers. The choice of suture materials (absorbable, nonabsorbable, synthetic, or natural fiber) depends on the amount of tension on the incision, the wound classification, the size of the patient, and the surgeon's preference. The first count is done before the peritoneum is closed.

When all sponges and instruments have been removed from the abdomen, the surgeon's assistant grasps the edges of the peritoneum with several hemostats. The peritoneum usually is closed with a continuous suture using 0 or 2-0 absorbable suture with a taper needle. The fascia may be sutured with the peritoneum as a single layer, and a variety of materials, both synthetic and nonsynthetic, may be used. Nonsynthetic materials currently are favored for their strength and lack of reactivity in tissue. If the fascial layer is closed separately, 2-0 suture most often is used in patients who are not obese.

During closure of the fascia, the assistant retracts the skin and subcutaneous layer with U.S. or Richardson retractors.

Toothed tissue forceps are used during closure of the abdominal wall.

Retention sutures may be placed before peritoneal closure in patients who are at risk of wound dehiscence. Size 0 or 1 retention sutures are placed approximately 1.2 inches (3 cm) behind the incision line, catching all layers of the abdominal wall. The suture is threaded through a short length of flexible tubing (bolster) before the knots are tied. This distributes the tension evenly along the retention suture and prevents it from tearing through the tissue (see Chapter 22).

The subcutaneous layer is closed with interrupted sutures of 3-0 Dexon, Vicryl, or chromic gut. Fine tapered needles are used. Skin closure often is performed with staples. Alternative methods, such as subcuticular or fine interrupted sutures, may be used in selected patients for a cosmetic closure. If staples are used, the assistant pulls the tissue edges together with two Adson skin forceps while the surgeon places the staples across the incision. At the completion of skin closure, the scrub or surgeon places the dressings over the wound. The drapes are then removed, and tape is applied to the dressings by the circulator or surgeon.

EXCISION OF AN ESOPHAGEAL DIVERTICULUM (OPEN PROCEDURE)

Surgical Goal

In excision of an esophageal diverticulum, the esophageal diverticulum is removed and the wall of the esophagus is strengthened to prevent recurrence.

Pathology

A pharyngoesophageal diverticulum (sometimes called a *Zenker diverticulum*) is mucosa and submucosa that have herniated through the cricopharyngeal muscles. The condition, which occurs in patients older than 60, causes food particles to become temporarily trapped.

TECHNIQUE

1 The patient is placed in the supine position with the head and neck turned and hyperextended to the patient's right.
2 An incision is made over the defect.
3 The diverticulum is dissected from the surrounding tissue.
4 The sac is ligated and the stump is invaginated into the pharyngeal wall.
5 The pharyngeal muscle opening is closed with interrupted 2-0 absorbable sutures. The skin is closed with 4-0 absorbable, subcuticular sutures.

Discussion

The patient is placed in the supine position with a shoulder roll under the affected side to hyperextend the neck. An incision is made over the area of the defect, usually extending from the inner border of the sternocleidomastoid muscle from the level of the hyoid bone to a point (0.8 inch [2 cm]) above the clavicle. The incision is carried through the skin and fine subcutaneous tissue. Bleeders are controlled with the ESU or fine suture ties. A thyroid spring retractor may be used to retain the superficial tissues. A small incision is made in the muscle with the ESU. The edges are then pulled aside with small right angle retractors. The trachea is retracted separately, and the base of the diverticulum is dissected free. Dissection is performed with the ESU, smooth tissue forceps, and Metzenbaum scissors.

The diverticulum is grasped with a Babcock clamp and dissected free. When the base of the diverticulum is free of attachments, it may be resected with a right angle surgical stapler (for sacs larger than 1.2 inches [3 cm]) or ligated at the base with 2-0 absorbable synthetic sutures. If sutured, the stump of the sac is incorporated into the muscle fibers with fine sutures.

The wound is closed in layers with 3-0 absorbable sutures. The skin can be closed with surgical staples or nonabsorbable interrupted 4-0 sutures.

Patients may require overnight observation in the hospital for postoperative bleeding or edema. A brief period of fasting may be required.

TRANSABDOMINAL REPAIR OF A HIATAL HERNIA

Surgical Goal

Nissen fundoplication commonly is performed to treat *gastroesophageal reflux disease (GERD)*. In this procedure, the upper stomach is wrapped around the esophagus below the hiatus to act as a sphincter. This prevents back flow of the stomach contents into the esophagus.

Pathology

The gastric contents normally are prevented from entering the esophagus by the lower esophageal sphincter, which has sufficient pressure to prevent the backflow of stomach contents into the esophagus. Loss of pressure or tone in the lower esophageal sphincter allows the highly acidic stomach contents to wash into the esophagus, causing erosion of the esophageal mucosa. GERD causes pain, esophageal erosion, and respiratory irritation and can lead to esophageal cancer.

TECHNIQUE

1 Pneumoperitoneum is established, and trocars are placed in the abdomen.
2 The liver is retracted upward.
3 The stomach is mobilized.
4 The phrenoesophageal membrane and crura are dissected free.
5 The lower esophagus is mobilized.
6 The hiatal hernia is repaired with sutures.
7 The upper portion of the fundus is wrapped around the distal esophagus and sutured in place.
8 The wound is irrigated.
9 The cannulas are removed, and pneumoperitoneum is released.
10 The trocar wounds are closed.

Discussion

Pneumoperitoneum is established and three 5-mm trocars are placed. The liver is retracted upward to expose the lower esophagus as it passes through the diaphragm. A liver retractor or atraumatic forceps is used to lift the liver. Some surgeons wrap a Penrose drain around the stomach for retraction. The assistant may retract the stomach, which can then be divided from the omentum. A Harmonic scalpel frequently is used for dissection and coagulation.

The phrenoesophageal membrane and ligament, which adhere to the esophagus under the liver, then are divided with the Harmonic scalpel or fine scissors. This exposes the crura. If the patient has a hiatal hernia, it is repaired at this stage of the procedure. A gastric bougie is inserted orally by the anesthesia care provider, and the hiatus is sutured together with three or four nonabsorbable synthetic sutures. The bougie is then withdrawn.

FUNDOPLICATION First, the surgeon must mobilize the upper stomach from its attachments to the omentum. The short gastric vessels are legated. The mobilized portion then is grasped with an atraumatic forceps and wrapped around the esophagus. The anesthesia care provider passes a gastric bougie (flexible tube) through the esophagus and into the stomach to gauge the diameter of the gastric sleeve. With the tube in place, the stomach wrap is secured with interrupted sutures through the seromuscular layers of the esophagus and stomach.

The sleeve is approximated with several interrupted sutures. Ethibond or a similar synthetic braided suture material is used for fundoplication. The gastric tube is then removed, and the gastric fold is inspected to ensure adequate constriction.

All cannulas are removed, the pneumoperitoneum is released, and the wounds are closed with absorbable sutures and skin staples or sutures (Figure 23-15).

Patients who have had a laparoscopic procedure usually are discharged the same day as surgery. After a brief postoperative period, patients are normally symptom-free.

VAGOTOMY

Surgical Goal

Vagotomy is performed to reduce gastric enzymes by severing the nerves that control their release.

Pathology

Vagotomy is selective occlusion of portions of the vagus nerve as it branches over the stomach. This interrupts nerve transmission and reduces acidic secretions. Selective disruption of the vagus nerve traditionally has been used to control the release of stomach acid and treat peptic ulcer disease. Current knowledge about the mechanism of peptic ulcer and the relationship between ulcers and *Helicobacter pylori* as a causative factor has significantly reduced the number of vagotomy procedures. If the procedure is performed through a small laparotomy incision or by laparoscopy, the nerve is ligated with surgical metal clips at one or more locations as it branches

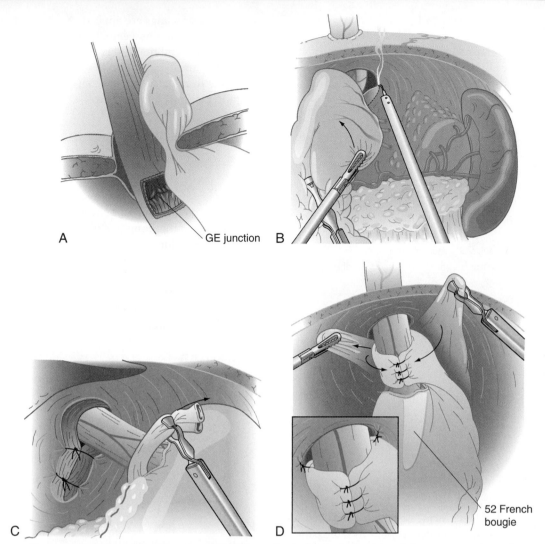

Figure 23-15 Transhiatal hernia repair (*Nissen fundoplication*). **A,** View of the gastroesophageal junction, with a portion of the stomach protruding through the hiatus. **B,** The crura are dissected to expose the hiatus. **C,** Sutures are placed through the crura to close the defect. **D,** Fundoplication (wrapping) of the stomach around the distal esophagus. An esophageal catheter (bougie) is inserted. *(From Townsend CM: Sabiston textbook of surgery, ed 17, Philadelphia, 2001, WB Saunders.)*

from the esophagus. This procedure is performed in conjunction with gastric resection.

TECHNIQUE

1 A laparotomy is performed.
2 The esophagus is mobilized.
3 The left (posterior) and right (anterior) vagus nerves are resected.
4 The wound is closed.

Discussion

The abdomen already has been entered for gastric resection. The assistant retracts the liver upward using a Weinberg or wide Deaver retractor. Long Metzenbaum scissors and long fine tissue forceps are used to divide the esophagus from the attached peritoneal membrane. When the esophagus has been exposed, the surgeon retracts it using a long Penrose drain.

The surgeon retracts a portion of the vagus nerve with a long nerve hook. Two long right angle clamps are placed across the nerve, which is divided, and the segment is passed off the field as a specimen. The right and left specimens are kept separate for pathological examination. The severed edges of the nerve are then clamped with ligation clips or ligatures. The procedure is repeated on the other side of the esophagus.

The wound is closed in layers as for gastric resection.

PERCUTANEOUS ENDOSCOPIC GASTROSTOMY

Surgical Goal

Percutaneous endoscopic gastrostomy (PEG) is a common method of providing access to the stomach through a flexible tube inserted through the abdominal wall.

Pathology

A gastrostomy tube is inserted to provide feeding for patients who are unable to eat normally because of disease or trauma. Patients who require continuous gastric decompression after surgery are also candidates for insertion of a PEG tube.

TECHNIQUE

1 A small (4- to 5-mm) upper midline or left upper paramedian incision is made through all layers of the abdominal wall. The anterior fundus of the stomach is picked up with two more atraumatic grasping clamps (Babcock or Allis clamps). Traction sutures may be inserted through the stomach wall to replace the clamps.
2 A purse-string suture is placed in the stomach wall at the location where the tube will be inserted.
3 The stomach is perforated with the electrosurgical unit (ESU) within the purse-string suture.
4 The stomach contents are immediately suctioned.
5 Small bleeding vessels in the stomach mucosa are coagulated with the ESU.
6 The stomach catheter is inserted into the perforation, the purse-string suture is tied, and a second purse-string suture is placed around the catheter.
7 The abdominal wall is secured to the stomach wall with sutures.
8 A second incision is made in the abdominal wall and the catheter tip is brought out through this incision.
9 The catheter is secured to the skin and dressings are applied.

Discussion

Open gastrostomy often is performed at the patient's bedside or in the interventional radiology department with the patient under conscious sedation. The PEG kit, which is prepackaged, includes the gastrostomy tube and accessories.

The surgeon enters the abdomen through a short left upper paramedian incision. The assistant retracts the wound edges with right angle retractors while the surgeon identifies and grasps the stomach with two Babcock or Allis clamps. The surgeon brings a portion of the stomach into view through the incision.

If used, traction sutures are placed at this time. Two separate nonabsorbable sutures are placed through the stomach wall, and the ends are used for traction. When traction sutures are used, the clamps are removed.

A purse-string suture is placed through all layers of the stomach where the tube will be inserted. The surgeon makes a small perforation in the center of the purse-string suture with the ESU. The scrub should have suction immediately available as soon as the gastric incision is made to prevent the spillage of gastric contents.

The feeding tube is then placed through the perforation, and the purse-string suture is tied. A second purse-string suture may be placed for added strength. The stomach is then sutured to the abdominal wall at the entry site.

The catheter tip is grasped with a large clamp, such as a Péan clamp, and pulled to the outside of the body through a second small incision. The tube is secured to the skin with

sutures and dressings are applied. A gastrostomy is shown in Figure 23-16. Patients generally tolerate insertion of a PEG tube very well, and many are relieved to have an alternative to nasogastric intubation. The PEG tube is flushed before and after use. Residual stomach contents may be measured by aspiration with a 50-mL syringe.

PARTIAL GASTRECTOMY, BILLROTH I AND II (OPEN PROCEDURE)

Surgical Goal

In a partial gastrectomy, a diseased portion of the stomach is removed. The remaining portion is anastomosed to the duodenum or the jejunum.

Pathology

Partial gastrectomy usually is performed to treat gastric carcinoma, benign tumor, or chronic ulceration in which there is high risk of carcinoma.

TECHNIQUE

1 A laparotomy is performed through an upper right or midline incision.
2 The stomach is mobilized from the omentum.
3 The gastrohepatic ligament is identified and divided.
4 The duodenum or jejunum is mobilized from the omentum.
5 The intestine is cross-clamped with two intestinal clamps and the tissue is divided into two sections.
6 The intestinal stump is closed.
7 The stomach is double-clamped and divided. The open stomach edges are sutured or stapled together.
8 The stomach is anastomosed to the duodenum or jejunum.
9 The abdomen is irrigated and closed in layers.

Discussion

Partial (subtotal) gastrectomy requires reconstruction of the stomach to maintain continuity of the GI tract. The method and location of anastomosis depend on the extent and type of pathology, the patient's overall condition and age, and the surgeon's preferred technique. The gastric pouch (the remainder of the stomach after resection) can be attached to the small intestine, or the divided end of the intestine can be attached directly into the stomach.

A laparotomy is performed through an upper midline incision. The surgeon examines the abdominal contents to determine the extent of disease and to select a site for anastomosis. The exact lines of resection are determined and the stomach is mobilized from the ligaments, vessels, and omentum. The scrub should be prepared with many Mayo, Crile, or Kelly clamps, vessel clips, and suture ties. Suture ligatures are used on the major vessels of the stomach and omentum.

For the mobilization of the stomach, Allis or Babcock clamps are used to hold traction on the stomach while the omentum is divided from the greater curvature. After double-clamping the segments of omentum, the surgeon divides the tissue with dissecting scissors, the ESU, or an HF vessel-sealing

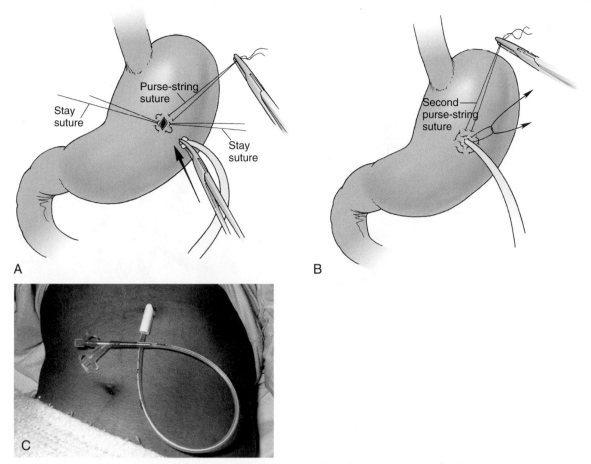

Figure 23-16 **A,** Gastrostomy. A purse-string suture is placed in the stomach wall with traction sutures. The tube is inserted through a small incision. **B,** The suture is tightened. **C,** The gastrostomy tube in place. *(**B** from Moody FG: Atlas of ambulatory surgery, St Louis, 1999, Mosby; **C** from Garden O, Bradbury A, Forsythe J, Parks R: Principles and practice of surgery, ed 5, Edinburgh, 2007, Churchill Livingstone/Elsevier.)*

system. The lesser curvature of the stomach is mobilized with the same technique.

When mobilization is completed, the surgeon places two intestinal cross clamps (Kocher or Allen type) side by side across the duodenum (**Billroth I procedure**) or the jejunum (**Billroth II procedure**). An incision is then made between the two clamps. The duodenal or jejunal stump is closed with a stapling instrument or fine sutures. The stomach is cross-clamped and divided.

Hand-suturing and surgical stapling are the two techniques commonly used to join the stomach with the intestine. Although stapling instruments are commonly used, the scrub should also be familiar with the traditional two-layer suture closure. Stapling procedures involving the stomach and small intestine are discussed in the next section.

HAND SUTURE TECHNIQUE FOR GASTROINTESTINAL ANASTOMOSIS The intestine and stomach are made up of separate tissue layers, the outer serosa, smooth muscle, submucosa, and mucosa. Two suture lines are used to create the anastomosis. The inner suture catches the mucosa, submucosa, and muscle layers. The outer serosal layers of both structures are joined

separately. Absorbable suture can be used for the inner closure and absorbable or nonabsorbable sutures for the serosa.

To begin the anastomosis, the surgeon brings the cross-clamped sections close together. A traction suture is placed at each end. An outer row of sutures is placed, joining the two structures. Next, the surgeon makes two incisions, one on each side of the suture line. This exposes the inner lumen of the intestine (or stomach). The surgeon brings the inner layers together with continuous running or interrupted sutures. Finally, the outer layer is completed circumferentially with interrupted sutures. The double layer of sutures prevents leakage.

Stapling instruments have largely replaced traditional suturing techniques in GI anastomosis. If stapling instruments are preferred, the gastrointestinal anastomosis (GIA) and thoracoabdominal (TA) linear staplers are used to resect the stomach and intestine (see Chapter 12).

GI technique is observed, and any instruments or sponges in contact with the open tract are removed from the field. These are not used on the closed GI tract.

Before the surgical wound is closed, the abdomen is irrigated with antibacterial solution. A Penrose drain may be

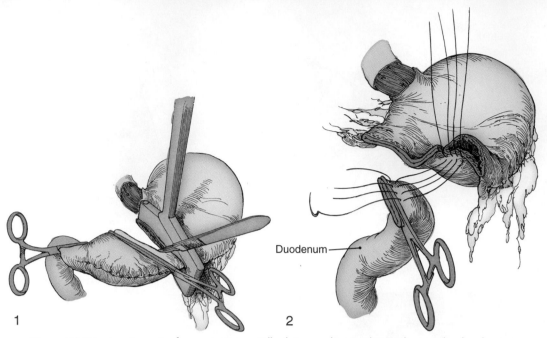

Figure 23-17   Anastomosis after gastrectomy: Billroth I procedure (end-to-end gastroduodenal anastomosis). *(From Economou SG, Economou TS: Atlas of surgical technique, ed 2, Philadelphia, 1996, WB Saunders.)*

placed in the abdomen, and a PEG tube may be inserted for gastric decompression. If this is required, it is inserted before closure.

See Figures 23-17 and 23-18 for illustrations of Billroth I and Billroth II procedures.

After gastrectomy, patients may require continuous gastric decompression with a **nasogastric (NG) tube** or, for longer postoperative care, with a PEG tube. Patients are followed closely for signs of peritonitis.

LAPAROSCOPIC BAND GASTROPLASTY FOR MORBID OBESITY

Surgical Goal

Band gastroplasty is performed for the treatment of morbid obesity. Nutritional intake is restricted by creating a small pouch in the proximal stomach. Food passes slowly into the stomach while creating a feeling of fullness.

The pouch is created by encircling the upper stomach with an inflatable band. The inner part of the band connects with a tube and saline reservoir implanted in the body wall. This allows the band to be filled from an external port embedded in the subcutaneous tissue. Tension on the band is adjusted by adding or removing saline and thereby regulating the flow of food out of the pouch and into the stomach. Several different types of bands are available. The most commonly used is the Lap-Band, described here, although the more traditional Roux-en-Y procedure is also performed by some surgeons.

Pathology

Morbid obesity is a condition in which the patient's body mass index (BMI) is at least 40. The BMI is a ratio of the weight and height calculated by a specific formula: (weight in pounds × 703)/(height in inches)². Obesity is an endemic health problem in the United States. It contributes to cardiovascular disease, cancers of the breast and large intestine, diabetes, stroke, urinary stress incontinence, and depression. Approximately 400,000 people die annually as a result of obesity in the United States. Society often regards morbid obesity as a moral failure in the patient, and there is strong social stigma associated with the disease.

Prospective patients are screened and usually are required to attempt conservative weight loss measures before surgical intervention. Criteria include:

- Motivation and commitment to weight loss
- Abstinence from alcohol and tobacco
- Absence of psychological factors that could hinder a successful outcome

Bariatric surgery has a long history of attempts to restrict food intake or cause poor nutrient absorption. Early radical gastric bypass procedures resulted in severe malabsorption and multiple medical problems related to nutrient deficiency. Other techniques, such as vertical band gastroplasty, have been abandoned because of failure to achieve the medical goal (patients alter their eating habits to include high-calorie liquids) or stenosis (narrowing) of the stomach outlet.

Adjustable gastric binding does not result in malabsorption, it is reversible, and it can be performed as minimally invasive surgery. Postoperatively the patient experiences rapid satiety after eating a small amount of food, which passes

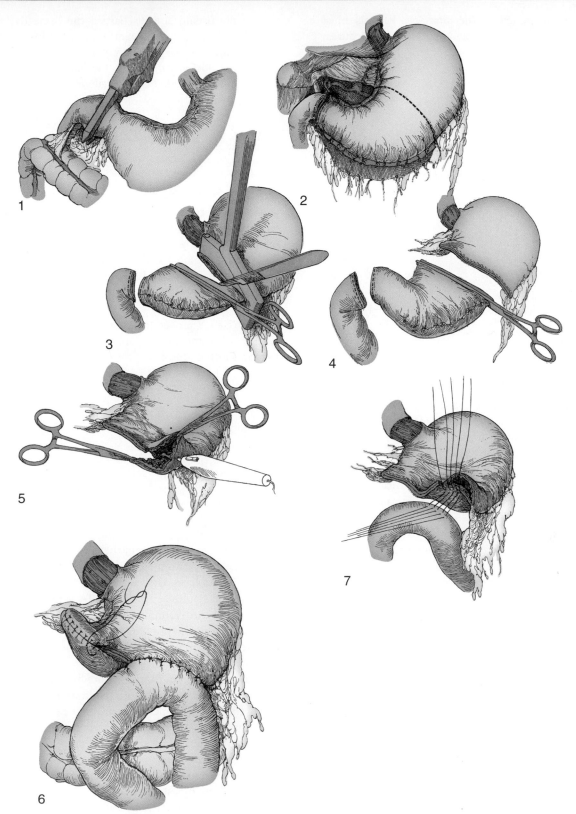

Figure 23-18 Billroth II procedure (end-to-side gastrojejunostomy). *(From Economou SG, Economou TS: Atlas of surgical technique, ed 2, Philadelphia, 1996, WB Saunders.)*

slowly from the pouch to the stomach. Patients must be screened preoperatively for suitability for the procedure.

TECHNIQUE

1 Pneumoperitoneum is established and trocars are placed through the abdominal wall.
2 The laparoscope and retracting and dissecting instruments are inserted.
3 The liver is retracted.
4 The peritoneum is divided between the top of the spleen and the esophagus.
5 A tunnel is created around the proximal stomach to accommodate the band.
6 The band is placed around the proximal stomach and secured.
7 The gastric wall is folded over the band and sutured in place.
8 The saline port and tubing are implanted and tested.
9 The wounds are closed.

Discussion

An operating table that can support up to 800 pounds (360 kg) must be available. Extensions and side attachments, including a footboard, are essential for patient safety. Long instruments (e.g., trocars) are required in most cases. A 15-mm trocar is required for insertion of the band. Two or three 5- or 10-mm trocars are also required.

Pneumoperitoneum is established and trocars are placed at the xiphoid, umbilicus, and subcostal areas. The surgeon retracts the liver upward and uses an ESU hook or a Cavitron Ultrasonic Surgical Aspirator (CUSA) to separate or clear a space between the stomach and the omentum. Fatty tissue is also dissected away from the stomach.

A path for the band is created near the crura (the muscular junction between the stomach and the esophagus). This is done with a blunt dissector or forceps.

The scrub prepares the band by testing it for leaks. This is done by flushing it with normal saline. After flushing, 5 mL of saline is left in the band and tubing. The scrub should place a small knot at the distal end of the tubing or use a clamp to prevent saline from leaking from the tube.

The tube is inserted into the abdomen and fitted around the upper stomach.

To prevent the band from sliding up or down, it is secured to the fundus. A portion of the gastric wall is folded over the band and secured with several silk or Ethibond sutures. The tubing is brought out through the 15-mm trocar, and all the trocars are removed.

A trocar site is enlarged and carried to the fascia with sharp dissection. Heavy sutures are then placed in the fascia (Figure 23-19).

The tubing is cut, and saline is allowed to flow. The distal end is connected to the port, and the preplaced sutures are threaded through the port. The port and excess tubing are placed in the abdomen. The fascial sutures are then tied, and the abdominal incisions are closed and dressed with Steri-Strips.

Patients usually are discharged the same day they have laparoscopic surgery. The band is adjusted by injecting additional saline into the port percutaneously under fluoroscopy. In the first postoperative year, the band is adjusted three to four times; thereafter, it is adjusted yearly to ensure continued weight control.

ROUX-EN-Y GASTRIC BYPASS

Surgical Goal

The Roux-en-Y procedure is performed to bypass the distal stomach and reestablish continuity from the stomach to the jejunum. In this procedure, a large portion of the stomach is bypassed and a gastric pouch is created. The anastomosis between the pouch and the jejunum substantially reduces the amount of food absorbed by the body.

Pathology

The Roux-en-Y procedure traditionally has been used to treat gastric ulcers and gastric carcinoma. It currently is also used to treat morbid obesity.

TECHNIQUE

1 The abdomen is entered.
2 The gastric pouch is created.
3 The jejunum is transected.
4 A gastrojejunostomy is created.
5 A jejunojejunostomy (Roux-en-Y anastomosis) is performed.
6 The wound is closed.

Discussion

After entering the abdomen, the surgeon makes a small hole in the lesser omentum at the level of the proposed partition. The TA-90 stapler is placed across the stomach at the partition site, and the staples are fired. A GIA stapler is used to close and transect the jejunum.

To create a new opening between the jejunum and the stomach, the surgeon makes two stab wounds to accommodate the forks of the GIA stapler. The stapler is inserted into the stab wounds, and the staples are fired. Silk sutures may be used to close the stab wounds. The Roux-en-Y (jejunojejunostomy) anastomosis is performed with the GIA instrument. The common opening between the two portions of jejunum is then closed with the TA-55 stapler. The wound is irrigated and closed in routine fashion (Figure 23-20).

Weight loss is more rapid after Roux-en-Y surgery than with band gastroplasty. Patients who did not have the procedure for morbid obesity are followed carefully for adequate nutritional intake.

TRANSHIATAL ESOPHAGECTOMY

Adenocarcinoma and squamous cell carcinoma are the most common types of esophageal cancer. These cancers are treated surgically with esophagectomy in the early stage of the disease.

Transhiatal esophagectomy is performed through combined cervical and upper midline incisions. The esophagus is

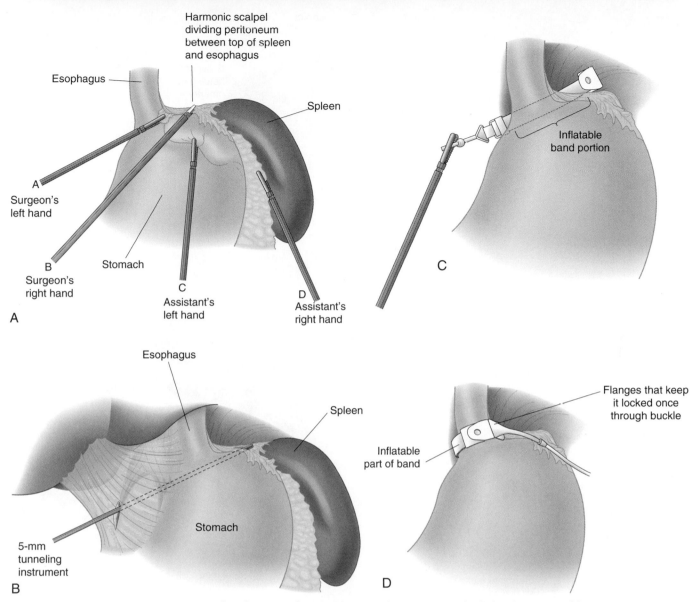

Harmonic scalpel dividing peritoneum between top of spleen and esophagus

Esophagus

Spleen

A
Surgeon's left hand

B
Surgeon's right hand

Stomach

C
Assistant's left hand

D
Assistant's right hand

A

Inflatable band portion

C

Esophagus

Spleen

Stomach

5-mm tunneling instrument

B

Flanges that keep it locked once through buckle

Inflatable part of band

D

Figure 23-19   Gastric banding procedure. **A,** The visceral peritoneum is divided at the antrum of the stomach (angle of His). **B,** A tunneling instrument is placed behind the stomach. **C,** An inflatable band is inserted through the tunnel. **D,** The band is locked in place. *(From Townsend CM: Sabiston textbook of surgery, ed 17, Philadelphia, 2001, WB Saunders.)*

mobilized to the hiatus through the cervical incision, and the stomach is mobilized through the abdominal incision. The stomach is then brought upward, and an anastomosis is formed with the proximal esophagus. This approach is used to avoid a thoracotomy.

SEGMENTAL RESECTION OF THE SMALL INTESTINE

Surgical Goal

Resection of the small intestine is removal of a section followed by surgical anastomosis to maintain continuity of the intestinal tract.

Pathology

Resection of the small intestine is performed to treat obstruction, disease, or carcinoma.

Intestinal obstruction is a general term that encompasses a number of mechanical pathological conditions that can block the intestine and require emergency surgery. Obstruction can lead to perforation, necrosis resulting from ischemia, and peritonitis. The most common obstruction pathological conditions include:

- *Strangulation* of a loop of bowel by a defect in the abdominal wall (hernia).
- *Volvulus:* Twisting of the bowel on itself.
- *Intussusception:* Telescoping of the intestine (this occurs mainly in children and results in ischemia and necrosis of the bowel).

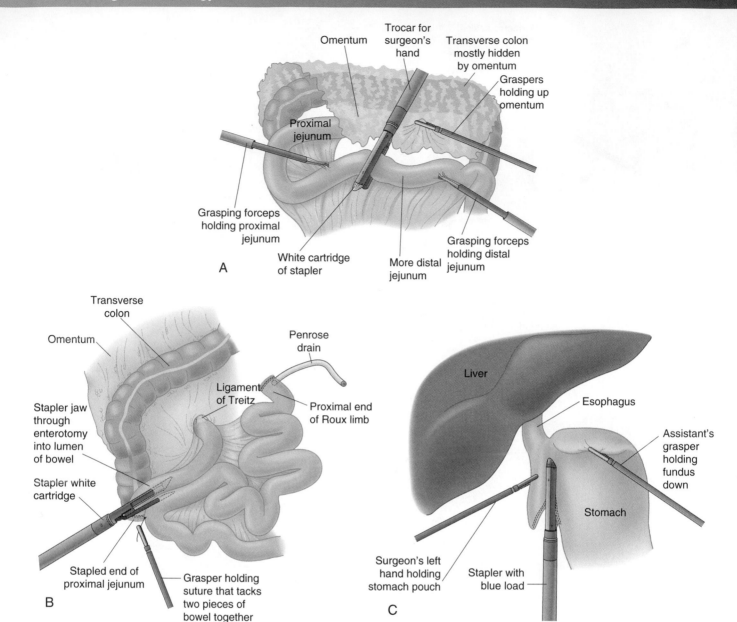

Figure 23-20 **Roux-en-Y gastric bypass. A,** The jejunum is divided with a surgical stapler. **B,** The stapler is placed for a side-to-side anastomosis. **C,** The gastric pouch is created. *(From Townsend CM: Sabiston textbook of surgery, ed 17, Philadelphia, 2001, WB Saunders.)*

- *Paralytic ileus:* Paralysis of the ileum; this occurs most often as a postoperative complication or as a result of pelvic or back injury and peritonitis.

A *peptic ulcer* may lead to perforation of the duodenum and requires surgery to prevent peritonitis. A small ulcer may be repaired, or a short segmental resection may be required.

TECHNIQUE

1. A laparotomy is performed through a midline incision.
2. The diseased tissue is identified.
3. The segment is mobilized.
4. The intestine is cross-clamped and the intestine is divided into two sections.
5. A surgical stapling device can be used to resect the intestine, or the intestine can be divided and anastomosed with sutures.
6. The wound is closed in layers.

Discussion

The abdomen is entered through a midline incision. The abdomen is explored for disease and the intestine inspected. The intestine is mobilized from the omentum along the site of resection with Metzenbaum scissors, an ESU, or a vessel-sealing system. Larger mesenteric arteries are secured with surgical clips or suture ligatures.

Two methods of resection and anastomosis are used in current practice—surgical stapling and the more traditional method of resection and anastomosis by suturing.

The bowel is cross-clamped with two intestinal clamps placed close together at each incision site in the bowel. The intestine is then incised between the clamps, and the diseased portion of intestine is removed as a specimen.

Resection and anastomosis can be performed using several techniques.

- *End-to-end:* The two intestinal "limbs" are sutured together circumferentially.
- *Side-to-end:* One limb is sutured closed, and the other is implanted in a longitudinal incision in the other limb.
- *Side-to-side:* Longitudinal incisions are made in each limb, and these are joined together.

When surgical stapling techniques are used, the site of bowel resection is identified and the peritoneal covering of the mesentery is incised on each side using the ESU or Metzenbaum scissors. The mesenteric vessels are dissected free, clamped, divided, and ligated with size 3-0 sutures (silk has been traditionally used for this part of the procedure, although other nonabsorbable materials are now replacing silk in some institutions). Alternatively, large vascular staples can be used for ligation. Additional ligatures are often placed adjacent to the staples to ensure hemostasis.

The bowel is transected with a GIA-60 stapler and noncrushing intestinal clamps are placed at each end of the stapled sections. The ends of the bowel can then be stapled or sutured by hand.

A layered suture anastomosis is performed by aligning the two ends of the intestine and rotating them outward. The inner layer is closed with continuous or interrupted stitches of absorbable sutures (e.g., chromic or Vicryl), and the outer serosa is closed with interrupted 3-0 or 4-0 sutures (e.g., Vicryl or silk).

The mucosa is closed with continuous or interrupted absorbable sutures. The serosal layer can be sutured with interrupted absorbable or nonabsorbable sutures (Figure 23-21). The mesentery is repaired with interrupted absorbable sutures. The wound is irrigated, all bleeders are controlled, and the incision is closed in layers.

REMOVAL OF MECKEL'S DIVERTICULUM

Meckel's diverticulum occurs at the distal ileum. Surgical removal prevents ulceration and perforation. The condition arises from a congenital remnant of the umbilical duct. This procedure follows the technique of minor resection of the small intestine.

RESECTION OF THE COLON

Surgical Goal
In resection of the colon, a section of the large intestine is removed and its continuity is restored by anastomosis or brought to the outside of the body as a colostomy.

Pathology
Resection of the colon is performed for treatment of carcinoma or ulcerative colitis or perforated or recurrent diverticula of the colon.

TECHNIQUE

1 The abdomen is entered.
2 The diseased portion of the bowel is identified and isolated.
3 The bowel is cross-clamped and divided.
4 An end-to-end anastomosis is performed.
5 The wound is closed.

Discussion
The abdomen is entered through a midline incision. The surgeon explores loops of intestine to identify the portion to be removed. A wide margin of intestine on each side of the lesion also is removed if the lesion is cancerous. This often includes the distal ileum.

The intestine is mobilized from the mesentery with Metzenbaum scissors, an ESU, or a vessel-sealing system. Larger mesenteric arteries are secured with surgical clips or suture ligatures.

When the colon is isolated, the selected segment is double-clamped at each end with intestinal clamps. The bowel is then divided between each set of clamps and passed off the field in a basin. At this point, the bowel is open and the risk of wound contamination exists. To help prevent this, the surgeon may place two lap sponges around the base of the intestinal stumps to isolate them.

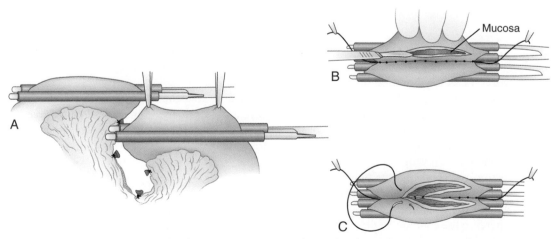

Figure 23-21 **Anastomosis of the small intestine (end-to-end technique).** Surgical staples are most commonly used, but some surgeons may prefer to use sutures. **A,** The clamped intestinal stumps are aligned. **B,** The mucosa is sutured. **C,** The muscle and serosal layers are sutured.

NOTE: *Resection and anastomosis may be done with a surgical stapling device. If sutures are used for anastomosis, the first layer of interrupted sutures is placed in the serosa. Fine silk or synthetic absorbable suture release (De-tach) needles are commonly used. The scrub should take care to place returned needles on a magnetic needle board or other such device as soon as the surgeon discards the needle. These needles are very small and may be easily lost in the rapid exchange between the surgeon and the scrub. The first and last sutures of the initial suture layer are left long to be used in traction.*

After making double incisions in the bowel, the surgeon places a second layer of interrupted chromic gut 3-0 sutures swaged to a fine GI needle. The surgeon continues the interrupted sutures until the two intestinal lumens are joined. The intestinal clamps are removed, and a final reinforcing suture layer is placed.

NOTE: *If resection and anastomosis are performed using surgical stapling techniques, the procedure for mobilizing omentum is the same as described earlier. The area of site of bowel transection is selected and a small opening made in the mesentery using the ESU or Metzenbaum scissors. The ileum is then transected using a GIA-60 stapler. The colon is also transected after the stapler has been reloaded. The peritoneal covering of the mesentery is clamped, divided, and ligated in the area of the anastomosis. The anastomosis is performed by bringing the two limbs of the bowel in alignment and placing stay sutures at each end of the staple lines. Two openings are made in the bowel stumps to insert the forks of the GIA-60 instrument, and one fork is positioned inside each bowel lumen. The GIA-60 is closed and fired, completing the anastomosis. The staple line is inspected and may be reinforced with sutures as needed. The TA-55 stapler is used to close the common opening, which may also be sutured.*

The final step in the procedure is closure of the mesentery. Interrupted 3-0 sutures of silk or chromic gut are used.

Bowel technique is now performed as described previously. After contaminated instruments and supplies have been removed from the field and sterile drapes positioned around the wound, the team dons fresh gowns and gloves. The wound is irrigated (in some operating rooms this is done before the changeover) and closed in routine fashion.

GASTROINTESTINAL STOMA

An **ostomy** is a procedure in which a portion of the intestine is divided and the open end is secured to the skin, draining the bowel contents outside the body. The opening is then called a **stoma**. A disposable ostomy pouch is used to collect intestinal fluid; this is a **stoma appliance**. The appliance system consists of an adherent skin wafer with an opening for the stoma and a collection reservoir that fits tightly into the skin wafer. The patient drains the collection reservoir as needed and changes it every few days. The appliance fits tightly over the stoma and adheres to the contours of the body to limit leakage and odor. After the disruption of the GI tract, the remaining part of the intestinal system becomes nonfunctional for digestion but is left intact. A small intestine stoma

of the ileum is called an *ileostomy,* and a stoma of the large intestine is called a *colostomy* (Figure 23-22).

Before surgery, the surgeon and the ostomy nurse discuss the exact location of the ostomy, considering the patient's lifestyle and age and protection of the ostomy from the belt line. The site is drawn on the skin before surgery as a reference for the surgeon.

The location of an ostomy depends on the section of the intestine to be removed. An *end colostomy* is formed when the proximal end of the resected intestine is brought through the abdominal wall and sutured in place as described previously. A *double colostomy*, commonly called a loop colostomy, is one in which both sections of cut bowel are brought out through the abdominal wall. The double colostomy allows the bowel to remain nonfunctional for a period of healing. The two ends then are reconnected as a separate surgery.

A *loop colostomy* does not require resection and anastomosis. A loop of bowel is brought out and held in place with an appliance that prevents the loop from slipping back into the abdomen.

The patient's psychological and physical adjustments to an ostomy procedure depend on many factors. Body image at the time of surgery, developmental age, level of debilitation before the procedure, and family and professional support affect the patient's ability to accept the change.

Stoma care requires qualified patient teaching by a certified ostomy specialist. Patients require a period of adaptation while learning to care for the ostomy. The stoma nursing team provides psychological and social support, as well as technical assistance with stoma fit, cleansing, and emptying procedures.

For further information on the extensive postoperative care and nursing considerations, see the United Ostomy Associations of America website at http://www.uoaa.org.

Postoperative considerations for all colostomy patients include routine monitoring after the use of general anesthesia, with special attention to fluid and electrolyte balance. The ostomy site is monitored closely for ischemia, retraction, or prolapse.

LOOP COLOSTOMY

Surgical Goal

For a loop colostomy, a loop of large intestine is brought out through a small abdominal incision, sutured to the skin, and opened. The resulting colostomy serves as a temporary bypass for the evacuation of bowel contents.

Pathology

A colostomy is performed to give the bowel a rest after colon resection. The procedure also may be performed in the treatment of inflammatory disease or obstruction of the colon. The loop colostomy is closed when fecal diversion is no longer needed.

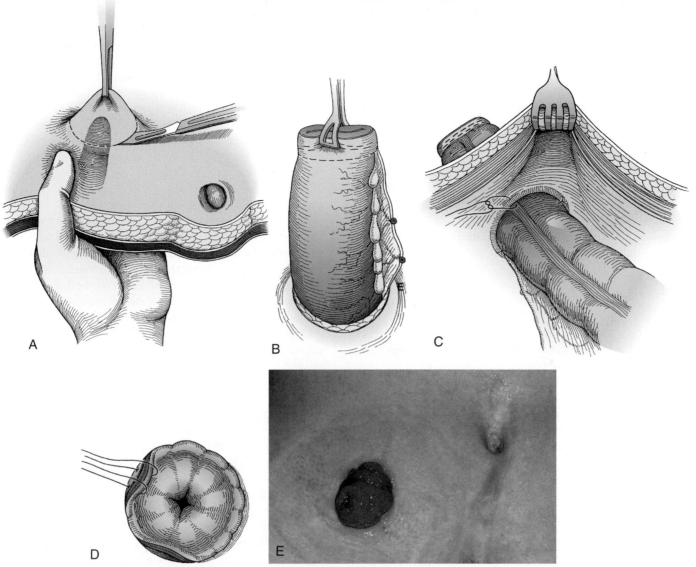

Figure 23-22 Colostomy. A, A disc of tissue is removed from the body wall. **B,** The intestinal stump is brought through the opening in the skin. **C,** The bowel may be sutured on the internal side. **D,** The bowel is everted and sutured to the skin. **E,** The healed stoma. *(D modified from Bauer JJ: Colorectal surgery illustrated, St Louis, 1993, Mosby; E from Garden O, Bradbury A, Forsythe J, Parks R: Principles and practice of surgery, ed 5, Edinburgh, 2007, Churchill Livingstone/Elsevier.)*

TECHNIQUE

Opening

1 The abdomen is entered.
2 A small portion of the transverse colon is mobilized.
3 The mobilized bowel is brought out through the incision.
4 For a loop colostomy, a butterfly anchor or rod is inserted under the loop and anchored.
5 The wound is closed.
6 The loop is incised 24 to 48 hours after the procedure.

Closing

1 The skin edges around the colostomy are incised.
2 Dissection is carried to the peritoneum.
3 The colostomy edges are trimmed and sutured together.
4 The loop is allowed to retract into the abdomen.
5 The wound is closed.

Discussion

OPENING The abdomen is entered through a short transverse median or upper paramedian incision. The assistant retracts the abdominal wall with a right angle retractor. Babcock clamps are used to grasp the loop of transverse colon.

The surgeon divides the bowel from its attachments to the omentum with Metzenbaum scissors and an ESU. An avascular area of the omentum is chosen for the mobilization. However, if blood vessels are encountered, these are clamped and ligated with fine sutures, surgical clips, or a vessel-sealing system.

When mobilization is complete, the loop of intestine is brought out of the abdomen, and a butterfly anchor or plastic colostomy rod is placed under the loop to prevent it from retracting into the abdomen. If a butterfly anchor is used, it is anchored through the needle ports with sutures. The wound then is closed in standard fashion around the loop.

CLOSING THE STOMA After the patient has been prepped and draped, a gauze sponge is placed at the opening of the colostomy. This prevents gross contamination of the wound by fecal material. The surgeon then incises the skin around the edges of the colostomy. The incision is carried through the subcutaneous and fascial layers. The peritoneum is dissected free of the colostomy with Metzenbaum scissors. To prevent contamination of the peritoneal cavity, the colostomy is surrounded with one or two lap sponges. The surgeon then trims the skin from the edges of the colostomy.

The surgeon closes the colostomy by inserting two layers of suture through the colostomy edges. The first layer is closed with running or interrupted 3-0 absorbable sutures swaged to a fine needle. A second layer of interrupted 3-0 or 4-0 silk sutures is placed over the first suture line. The bowel then is allowed to slide back into position in the peritoneal cavity, and the wound is closed in routine fashion.

PARTIAL COLECTOMY

Surgical Goal

A partial colectomy is performed to remove a section of diseased colon and restore continuity to the intestine.

Pathology

A colectomy is removal of part or all of the large intestine. The colon is removed to treat carcinoma, ulcerative colitis, diverticulitis, and intestinal obstruction.

TECHNIQUE

1 A laparotomy is performed through a midline or left paramedian incision.
2 The colon is divided from retroperitoneal structures.
3 The mesentery between the duodenum and the right colon is dissected.
4 The omentum is divided.
5 The remaining mesentery, colon, and distal ileum are dissected free.
6 Atraumatic clamps are placed across the bowel at each end of the area to be resected.
7 An end-to-end anastomosis is made between the right colon and the proximal ileum.

Colostomy
8 An incision is made through the abdominal wall at the ostomy site.
9 The proximal end of the resected colon is brought through the abdominal wall and sutured in place.
10 The intestinal stump is closed.
11 The wound is closed in layers.

Discussion

Colectomy is the general term applied to removal of the large intestine. A specific term is used to identify the section that is resected (e.g., *transverse colectomy*). *Colectomy* can refer to complete removal or segmental resection. In this description, the sigmoid colon and rectum are not removed.

The surgeon performs a laparotomy through a midline or paramedian incision. If a colostomy is planned, the paramedian incision on the opposite side of the ostomy often is preferred to separate the stoma from the surgical incision and prevent contamination of the incision site. The area of resection is completely mobilized as described previously. Atraumatic Babcock and Allis clamps are used to grasp the bowel. Systematic dissection of the mesentery, major arteries, and peritoneal reflections is performed until all attachments are eliminated. An anastomosis then is performed as described previously.

COLOSTOMY If a colostomy is performed, the distal intestinal stump is closed in two or three layers. Surgical staples or sutures are used. The surgeon creates the stoma by making a circular incision through the skin and abdominal wall at the stoma site. The incision is carried to the peritoneum, and the proximal stump is brought through the abdominal wall. Small right angle retractors are used to retract the wound edges. The bowel edges are then everted, and two layers of fine absorbable or silk sutures are placed; the deeper layer penetrates the full thickness of the severed ileum and a more superficial layer is placed at the level of the skin. The epidermis itself is not sutured to the stoma.

Bowel technique is initiated as described previously. The wound is irrigated with antibacterial solution before closure. An ostomy bag may be fitted temporarily over the stoma.

Related Procedures

ILEOTRANSVERSE COLOSTOMY An ileotransverse colostomy is the removal of a portion of the ileum and transverse colon with side-to-side anastomosis of the ileum and colon.

Patients are particularly monitored for signs of infection and of fluid and electrolyte imbalance related to loss of large sections of tissue. The stoma site is checked regularly for any signs of ischemia. The stoma is not fully functional for a number of days after surgery and may require suctioning. The stoma nurse consultant participates in postoperative care of the site and in patient support. As the stoma heals, changes are made in the type and configuration of the ostomy appliance.

ABDOMINOPERINEAL RESECTION

Surgical Goal

In abdominoperineal resection, the anus, rectum, and sigmoid colon are removed en bloc through combined abdominal and perineal incisions. The abdominal approach includes resection of the upper colon. A separate perineal exposure is used to mobilize the anus, rectum, and sigmoid colon, allowing removal of the specimen. The normal anatomy of the rectum is shown in Figure 23-23, *A*.

Pathology

Abdominoperineal resection is the complete removal of the rectum and anus with pelvic dissection and removal of a portion of the colon for the treatment of cancer of the rectum.

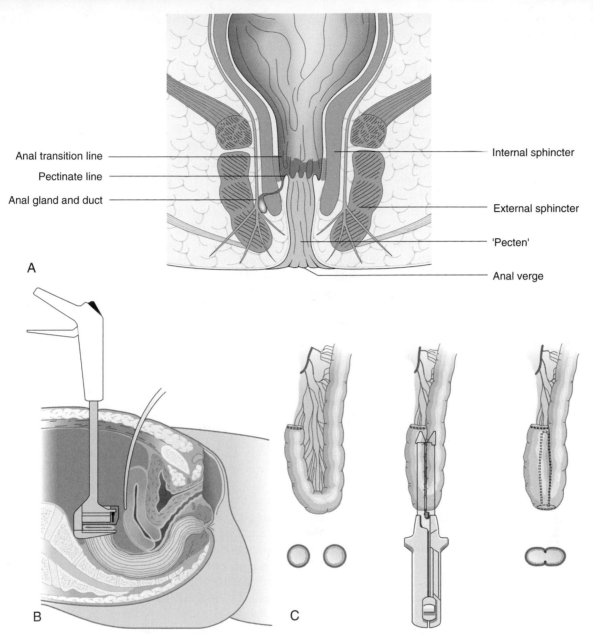

Anal transition line

Pectinate line

Anal gland and duct

Internal sphincter

External sphincter

'Pecten'

Anal verge

A

B

C

Figure 23-23 **A,** The normal anatomy of the anorectal canal. **B,** The thoracoabdominal stapler is used to close the rectal stump after resection of the abdominal colon. **C,** The gastrointestinal anastomosis stapler is used to form an anal pouch from the ileum. The end-to-end anastomosis stapler is used to bring the stapled ileal pouch into position. It can then be hand-sutured in place. (**A** from Garden O, Bradbury A, Forsythe J, Parks R: Principles and practice of surgery, ed 5, Edinburgh 2007, Churchill Livingstone/Elsevier; **C** from Townsend CM: Sabiston textbook of surgery, ed 17, Philadelphia, 2001, WB Saunders.)

TECHNIQUE

1 The abdomen is entered.
2 The lesion is located and the bowel is mobilized.
3 The colon is divided in an area proximal to the lesion.
4 A colostomy is performed and the abdomen is closed.
5 The lower sigmoid colon, rectum, and anus are mobilized and removed.
6 The perineal incision is closed.

Discussion

Abdominoperineal resection requires two incisions and two anatomical approaches or surgical sites. The two surgical fields (one pelvic and one perineal) can be performed as one continuous procedure or two simultaneous procedures, with one team operating on the pelvic portion and a second on the perineal field. Two setups are needed for either technique. Two scrubs are needed for simultaneous procedures.

When the operation is performed with two teams working simultaneously, the patient is placed in the lithotomy position. Because the abdominal team has restricted space in which to work, the scrub on this team must stand slightly behind the assistant rather than in the usual position (standing next to the assistant). The scrub must take special care to prevent contamination while working in this awkward position.

During simultaneous procedures, the scrub on the lower team stands next to the surgeon, as for vaginal procedures. The surgeon usually performs the procedure while sitting. Both scrubs must remember that usually only one circulator is available to assist both teams. The scrubs should anticipate needed equipment before the procedure begins. This prevents confusion when the two surgical teams are working with one circulator between them. The procedure is discussed here as if performed by one team.

The surgeon enters the abdomen through a long midline incision. The surgeon then examines the colon and determines the line of resection. Mobilization of the colon includes isolation of the mesenteric tissue and omentum that contain diseased lymph nodes. The surgeon frees the colon from its attachments by double-clamping the tissue with Mayo clamps. The tissue between the clamps is divided with Metzenbaum scissors or an ESU, and the sections are ligated with silk, Vicryl, or Dexon ties. As mobilization continues, longer instruments are needed. The scrub must have an ample supply of Péan clamps, long right angle clamps, and small sponge dissectors. Large blood vessels are clamped with right angle or Péan clamps and ligated with suture ligatures. The scrub should have one or two suture ligatures ready at all times during the dissection.

Mobilization of the colon proceeds to the level of the levator muscles. At this point the abdominal dissection may be halted if the remaining dissection cannot be performed through the pelvic approach. The surgeon places two intestinal clamps across the bowel at the proximal end of the mobilized area. The proximal end of the divided bowel may be ligated temporarily with heavy sutures. To provide continuity of the bowel, an anastomosis is created between the descending colon and the rectum using the EEA circular stapler. To reconstruct the pelvic floor, the surgeon may suture a portion of the omentum to it.

To prepare a site for the colostomy, the surgeon incises a small circle in the abdomen using the skin knife and carries the incision through the abdominal wall with the ESU. The small disc of tissue is then passed to the scrub as a specimen. The proximal end of the bowel is brought through the circular incision and temporarily clamped in place while the abdominal incision is closed in routine fashion.

To create the colostomy, the surgeon everts the edges of the bowel stoma and sutures the edges of the skin using interrupted sutures of absorbable 3-0 suture on a fine cutting needle.

Surgery from the perineal end begins as the surgeon places a heavy silk purse-string suture through the anus to occlude it. The perineum is incised, and rectal dissection is performed with the ESU and scissors. Large bleeding vessels are double-clamped and ligated with silk or Dexon. As the incision becomes deeper, Péan clamps are used to grasp the bowel attachments, as described in the abdominal portion of the procedure.

Dissection is continued until the surgeon reaches the previously mobilized area of the bowel. The entire specimen is delivered through the perineal incision. The surgeon then irrigates the wound. Interrupted sutures are used to close the

tissue planes and avoid "dead space," which can lead to infection. One or two Penrose drains or a suction drain is placed in the wound, which is then closed with size 0 chromic gut, Vicryl, or Dexon. The skin is approximated with the surgeon's choice of nonabsorbable material and dressed with a bulky abdominal pad and gauze sponges. Illustrations for the procedure are shown in Figure 23-23, *B* and *C*.

Related Procedure

PROCTOCOLECTOMY WITH AN ILEAL POUCH Proctocolectomy with an ileal pouch involves the creation of an ileal pouch and anal anastomosis to provide fecal continuity and conserve the sphincter.

Radical surgery in which large portions of tissue are removed requires meticulous critical care observation and methodologies. This care begins in the postanesthesia care unit (PACU) and continues well into the postoperative recovery after the patient has been discharged to the intensive care unit or ward. Detailed care plans, which include hemostasis, fluid and electrolyte balance, thermoregulation, and monitoring for infection, are implemented by members of the critical care nursing and medical staffs.

APPENDECTOMY (OPEN TECHNIQUE)

Surgical Goal

An appendectomy is the removal of the appendix, a blind, narrow, elongated pouch that is attached to the cecum (Figure 23-24).

Pathology

The appendix is removed during acute infection to prevent rupture and treat peritonitis. The procedure may be performed as a prophylactic (preventive) measure when surgery is performed in the abdomen for other reasons. The procedure then is called an *incidental appendectomy.*

TECHNIQUE

1 The abdomen is entered.
2 The appendix is isolated from the mesoappendix.
3 The appendix is ligated and removed.
4 A purse-string suture is placed around the stump of the appendix.
5 The wound is closed.

Discussion

There are two approaches to appendectomy—open and laparoscopic technique. Open technique is used in cases where perforation has occurred, there is significant risk of perforation, or an abdominal mass has been discovered during preoperative assessment. Laparoscopic technique is indicated for most other cases. Both approaches are described in the following sections.

The abdomen is entered through a **McBurney incision**. The muscle layers are manually separated and the peritoneum entered. The assistant retracts the wound edges with a right

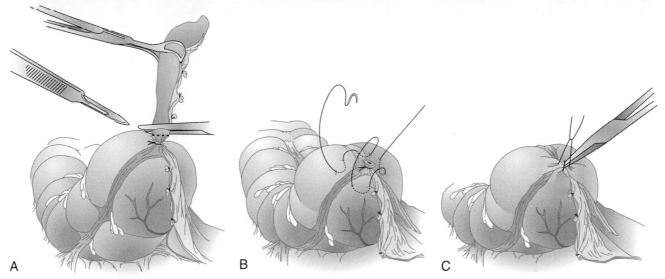

Figure 23-24 **Classic open appendectomy. A,** The appendix is divided from the cecum after ligation. **B,** A purse-string suture is placed around the stump. **C,** The stump is buried and the purse-string suture is closed. (*C from Ortega JM, Ricardo AE: Surgery of the appendix and colon. In Moody FG: Atlas of ambulatory surgery, Philadelphia, 1999, WB Saunders.*)

angle retractor. The surgeon then grasps the appendix with Babcock clamps and delivers it into the wound site.

The appendix is isolated from its attachments (mesoappendix) to the bowel with Metzenbaum scissors and the ESU. Portions are ligated with free ties of 3-0 nonabsorbable suture until the appendix is completely mobilized.

A Babcock clamp is placed on the body of the appendix, which the assistant elevates. The surgeon then places a straight Kelly clamp at the base to compress the tissue. A ligature of 3-0 nonabsorbable suture is tied over the compressed base. The assistant then places a straight Kelly clamp above the knot.

A purse-string suture is placed around the base, and the suture ends are left long. The appendix now can be removed. The scrub should place a small basin on the field. A lap sponge is placed around the base of the appendix. The surgeon severs the appendix with the deep knife and places it along with the specimen into the basin, which is now contaminated and removed from the field.

The assistant buries the appendix stump in the cecum while the surgeon ties the purse-string suture. The wound is irrigated with warm saline solution, and the abdomen is closed in routine fashion.

POSTOPERATIVE CONSIDERATIONS Routine postoperative care is provided in the PACU. Particular attention is given to signs of infection related to possible spillage of bowel contents during the procedure. Pediatric patients generally recover very quickly from appendectomy.

APPENDECTOMY (LAPAROSCOPIC TECHNIQUE)

Surgical Goal

The appendix commonly is removed using a laparoscopic technique (Figure 23-25).

TECHNIQUE

1. Pneumoperitoneum is established.
2. Trocars are placed.
3. The appendix is divided from the mesoappendix.
4. A ligature is placed at the base of the appendix.
5. The appendix is severed and removed through a 10-mm cannula.
6. The appendix stump is sealed.
7. Pneumoperitoneum is released and the trocars are removed.
8. The wounds are closed.

Discussion

Pneumoperitoneum is established and a 10-mm trocar is placed near the umbilicus. In cases of acute appendicitis, a second, larger trocar is inserted into the midline below the suprapubic line. A third port is placed in the upper right quadrant.

The patient is placed in the Trendelenburg position. The surgeon then locates the appendix by systematically moving aside the large intestine with an atraumatic endoscopic grasper, such as a Babcock clamp, until the cecum is found.

After inspecting the abdominal cavity, the surgeon mobilizes the appendix. The tip of the appendix is retracted upward to produce traction. The mesoappendix is divided with scissors or the ESU and ligated with vessel clips or a surgical stapler.

After the appendix has been mobilized, it can be amputated from the cecum. Two ties are placed around the appendix between the lines of amputation, one at the base of the appendix and the other just above it. The appendix then is transected with the ESU, scissors, or GIA surgical stapler. The specimen is brought out through the 10-mm port using a specimen retrieval bag.

The stump of the appendix may be inverted and a purse-string suture placed at the base. This is done to contain the

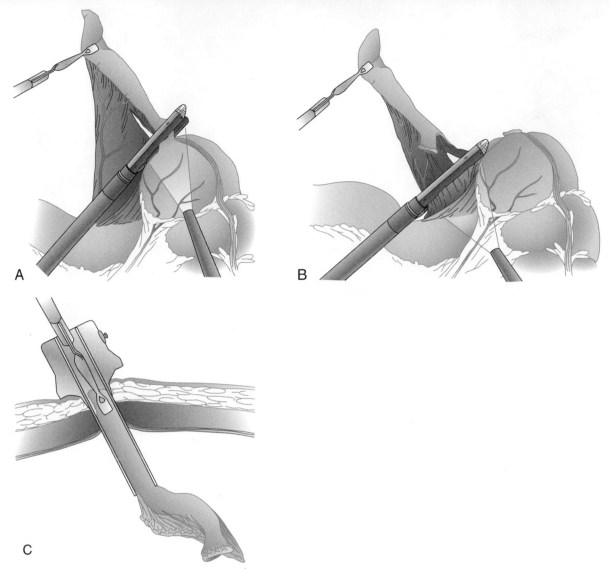

Figure 23-25 Laparoscopic appendectomy. **A,** The appendix is amputated with the gastrointestinal anastomosis stapler. **B,** The mesoappendix is divided. **C,** The appendix is brought out of the abdomen through one of the operative ports. (**C** from Moody FG: Atlas of ambulatory surgery, Philadelphia, 1999, WB Saunders.)

stump and prevent contamination of the abdominal cavity. If signs of contamination are noted, the surgeon takes a culture swab from the free fluid in the abdomen.

The wound is irrigated with antibacterial solution and the pneumoperitoneum is released. A soft rubber drain may be placed if the risk of postoperative infection or excessive drainage exists.

HEMORRHOIDECTOMY

Surgical Goal

Hemorrhoids are removed for pain management and to prevent bleeding and infection.

Pathology

The venous plexus of the anal canal may become congested or distended, causing pain, bleeding, and prolapse outside the anal canal. Venous distention most often is caused by pregnancy and obesity. A genetic predisposition may also influence the incidence in certain individuals. People whose occupations require constant sitting or standing are also at high risk for symptomatic hemorrhoids. Stage IV hemorrhoids remain outside the anal canal, causing frequent bleeding and severe pain. These are treated surgically.

Discussion

Hemorrhoidectomy most often is performed using one of the following methods:

- Ligation with an elastic ring to constrict and shrink the vein
- Laser treatment
- Removal with the ultrasound scalpel

These procedures may be performed in the outpatient setting with the patient receiving a local anesthetic; only in rare cases is hospitalization required. The application of elastic

O rings currently is the most common procedure. The patient is placed in the prone or lithotomy position. The buttocks may be taped to expose the anus, which is dilated to allow access to the base of the hemorrhoids. The hemorrhoid is grasped with the McGivney ligator or a similar device, which discharges a Silastic O ring over the vein. No dressings are applied.

EXCISION OF A PILONIDAL CYST

Surgical Goal

Excision of a pilonidal cyst is performed to remove a pilonidal cyst.

Pathology

A pilonidal cyst is a congenital defect in which epithelial tissue develops below the surface of the skin in the area of the sacrum and coccyx. The cyst is removed when it causes recurrent infection in the area. A *sinus tract* (a channel leading to an abscess) often is present.

TECHNIQUE

1 The extent of the fistula is determined.
2 The tract is incised around its circumference.

Discussion

If a sinus tract is present, the surgeon begins the procedure by inserting a probe into the tract. The probe identifies the exact location of the sinus and the cyst itself. The surgeon may want to inject dye into the sinus tract. If so, the scrub should have a blunt needle, syringe, and methylene blue dye available.

The area around the sinus is incised with the skin knife. The scrub must retract the skin with rake retractors as the surgeon deepens the incision. Using the ESU or a deep knife, the surgeon incises the subcutaneous layer. The incised tissue mass then is grasped with a Kocher or an Allis clamp for traction. The dissection continues until the sacrum is exposed and the en bloc tissue can be removed. Bleeding vessels are controlled with the ESU or ties of 3-0 Vicryl, Dexon, or gut.

The wound may be left open to heal. In this case, it is packed with iodophor gauze. Primary closure is performed if no infection is present at the site of the wound. The subcutaneous tissue is closed with 3-0 absorbable suture. The skin is closed with interrupted nonabsorbent sutures.

EXCISION OF AN ANORECTAL FISTULA

Surgical Goal

A fistula is excised to promote approximation of tissue edges and close the tract.

Pathology

A fistula is a tract or tunnel in normal or infected tissue. The tract remains open because of the constant drainage of pus or

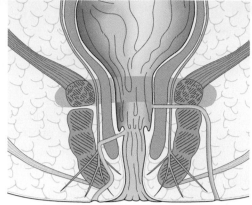

Low intersphincteric fistula   Trans-sphincteric fistula

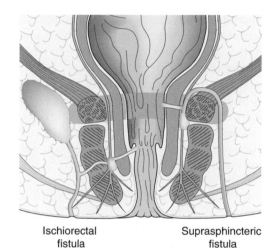

Ischiorectal fistula   Suprasphincteric fistula

Figure 23-26 **An anal fistula involving the sphincter.** *(From Garden O, Bradbury A, Forsythe J, Parks R: Principles and practice of surgery, ed 5, Edinburgh, 2007, Churchill Livingstone/Elsevier.)*

because the tissue lining the tract does not contain cells that normally initiate wound healing. Circumferential excision of the tract removes scar tissue and promotes closure and healing. An anal or rectal fistula often arises from an infected fissure in the anal sphincter (Figure 23-26).

Discussion

The patient is placed in the prone position, and the buttocks are taped to expose the anus. The surgeon dilates the rectum and inserts a rectal retractor. A malleable probe is then inserted into the fistula to determine its depth. When the extent of the fistula has been determined, the surgeon makes a circular incision around the fistula where it communicates with the skin. The incision is carried along the length of the fistula with the ESU. The incised tissue is removed as a specimen.

The wound is not sutured; rather, it is dressed with iodophor plain packing.

SECTION III: SURGERY OF THE BILIARY SYSTEM, LIVER, PANCREAS, AND SPLEEN

SURGICAL ANATOMY

LIVER

The liver, gallbladder, spleen, and pancreas are located in the midabdominal cavity. The spleen lies in the upper left quadrant, beneath the diaphragm and posterior to the stomach. The liver occupies most of the upper right abdominal space and a portion of the left upper quadrant.

The liver is a large vascular organ that aids digestion and the filtration of toxic substances from the body. It has many vital functions in the body including carbohydrate, fat, and protein metabolism, the storage of glycogen and synthesis of glucose, and the storage of vitamins and minerals. The liver also is responsible for the synthesis of clotting factors, immune factors, and plasma proteins. It also filters toxins and bacteria from the blood and metabolizes drugs. It is divided into two major sections, or lobes, the right lobe and the left lobe, which are separated by the falciform ligament. These sections are identified by the *bifurcation* (Y-shaped division of a hollow anatomical structure) of the portal vein with right and left bile ducts. The vascular supply of the liver is derived from the hepatic artery and the hepatic portal vein. The liver is drained by the hepatic veins, which connect to the inferior vena cava.

The two lobes of the liver are further divided into eight subsections, according to their blood supply. The blood supply to each section is carried in a pedicle containing a bile duct, a hepatic artery, and a branch of the portal vein. Because each section is connected to its own pedicle, resection of an entire lobe requires dissection of the pedicle from the lobe and secure ligation of the pedicle, including the specific portion of the hepatic vein.

The liver is encapsulated by a thick fibrous sheath called the *Glisson capsule*. Fibrous sheaths also cover and protect the blood vessels and biliary ducts. These sheaths are continuous with the abdominal peritoneum and must be carefully dissected and mobilized before liver resection or anastomosis of the biliary system to another abdominal structure.

The anterior surface of the liver, which is in contact with the diaphragm, is referred to as the *right* and *left subphrenic spaces*. The *subhepatic space* lies between the peritoneal covering on the liver and the right kidney. These spaces are clinically significant. The subphrenic spaces are common sites of abscesses, and the subhepatic space can trap intestinal contents after a rupture of the appendix and become infected.

BILIARY SYSTEM

The biliary system includes the gallbladder, hepatic ducts, common bile duct, and cystic duct. The gallbladder is a small sac located under the right lobe (ventral side) of the liver. It is composed of smooth muscle and has an inner surface of absorptive cells.

The function of the biliary system is to produce, store, and release *bile*, which is composed of bile salts, pigments, cholesterol, lecithin, mucin (a glycoprotein), and other organic substances. Bile is necessary for the breakdown of cholesterol and helps stimulate peristalsis in the small intestine during digestion. It is formed in the liver and stored in the gallbladder.

Bile formed in the liver is released from the right and left hepatic ducts. These ducts converge to form the common hepatic duct. From the common hepatic duct, bile flows into the gallbladder through the cystic duct. When food enters the stomach, the gallbladder contracts, releasing stored bile into the common bile duct. Bile then enters the duodenum through an opening called the *ampulla of Vater*. This opening into the duodenum is shared by the pancreatic duct, which allows the release of pancreatic enzymes. The release of both bile and pancreatic enzymes is controlled by a sphincter at the ampulla called the *sphincter of Oddi*.

The hepatic and biliary anatomy is shown in Figure 23-27.

PANCREAS

The pancreas is an elongated lobulated gland that lies inferior to the liver, behind the stomach. This organ has two landmarks, the head and the tail. The head, which is the broader portion of the gland, lies in the curve of the duodenum and is connected to the duodenal portion of the small intestine. The pancreatic duct (duct of Wirsung), which is the central duct of the pancreas, communicates with the duodenum at the ampulla of Vater, a location shared with the common bile duct. The tail of the pancreas lies near the hilus of the spleen. The pancreas produces insulin and glucagon, which are necessary for digestion of carbohydrates. Insulin and glucagon are synthesized in a specific regions of the pancreas called the *Islets of Langerhans*. Insulin is synthesized and secreted directly into the blood stream by alpha cells while glucagon is synthesized and released by beta cells. Delta cells in the pancreas produce *somatostatin* which controls the rate of nutrient absorption from the intestine. Gamma cells in the pancreas secrete *pancreatic polypeptide* which reduces appetite. The pancreas also produces enzymes such as trypsin, chymotrypsin, carboxypeptidase, and elastase which are necessary for protein digestion.

SPLEEN

The spleen is a kidney-shaped organ that is extremely vascular and relatively soft. It lies under the diaphragm in the left upper abdomen (Figure 23-28). This organ destroys aged red blood cells, stores blood, filters microorganisms from the blood, and plays a major role in the immune system of the body. Because of its vascularity and location, vehicular and sports accidents often cause traumatic injury of the spleen. The spleen can be removed safely, without harming the body's ability to function, and this procedure is indicated whenever splenic hemorrhage becomes life-threatening. This is because hemorrhage is difficult to control without clamping the splenic arteries, and removal has little or no long-term medical consequences for most patients.

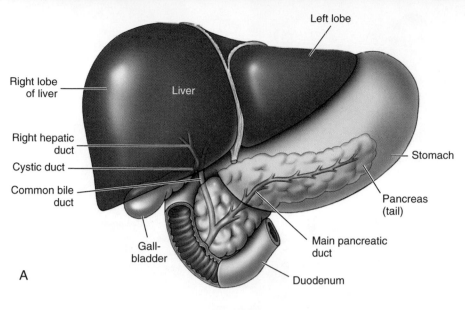

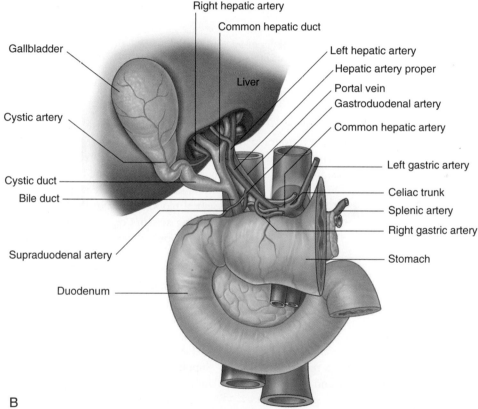

Figure 23-27 **A,** The biliary and hepatic anatomy. Note the position of the spleen and the main pancreatic duct (duct of Wirsung). **B,** Details of the biliary system. (**A** *modified from Herlihy B, Maebius NK: The human body in health and illness, ed 2, Philadelphia, 2003, WB Saunders;* **B** *from Drake R, Vogl W, Mitchell A: Gray's anatomy for students, Edinburgh, 2004, Churchill Livingstone.*)

DIAGNOSTIC PROCEDURES

Diseases of the liver, biliary system, pancreas, and spleen have direct consequences on metabolism, digestion, production of blood cells, and blood clotting. The symptoms of disease often are dramatic, and the diagnostic process is initiated when a patient presents with symptoms of pain, jaundice, diabetic pathology, or generalized weakness.

Blood tests can detect substances normally filtered by the liver and pancreas. Liver function tests measure liver enzymes and other chemicals. The liver is responsible for hundreds of physiological processes in the body. Specific blood tests are performed according to the presenting symptoms.

Imaging studies, including those that use contrast media, are done to outline organs and observe the movement of bile through the biliary system. Pancreatic imaging is used

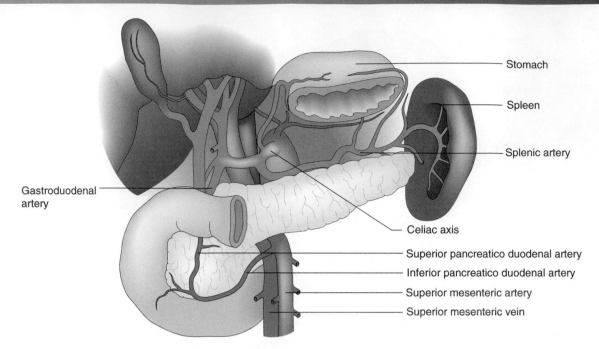

Stomach

Spleen

Splenic artery

Gastroduodenal artery

Celiac axis

Superior pancreatico duodenal artery

Inferior pancreatico duodenal artery

Superior mesenteric artery

Superior mesenteric vein

Figure 23-28   Anatomical relationship of the spleen and arterial system. *(From Garden O, Bradbury A, Forsythe J, Parks R: Principles and practice of surgery, ed 5, Edinburgh, 2007, Churchill Livingstone/ Elsevier.)*

to detect stones and tumors and the ducts may also be revealed if a contrast medium is used. Endoscopic retrograde pancreaticoduodenoscopy is performed to explore the ducts visually and for simple endoscopic procedures.

CASE PLANNING

INSTRUMENTS

Procedures of the liver, biliary system, pancreas, and spleen require basic laparotomy instruments. Vascular instruments are needed for major resection procedures and for major hepatic surgery.

Because these accessory organs contain many ducts and blood vessels, right angle clamps should be available with all procedures. These clamps allow the surgeon to reach underneath and around the blood vessels, ducts, and connective tissue attachments of the organs.

Procedures of the biliary system and pancreas, including choledochoscopy and endoscopic retrograde cholangiopancreatography (ERCP), sometimes require intraoperative use of flexible fiberoptic endoscopes. These scopes are inserted into the small ducts of the accessory organs to locate stones, tumors, or benign lesions.

SPECIAL EQUIPMENT AND SUPPLIES

The organs of the hepatic system and spleen are **friable** (delicate), and any tear or rupture can result in profuse bleeding that sometimes is difficult to control. Therefore, hemostasis is a major technical concern during surgery of the liver or spleen. Hemostatic techniques must include individual blood

vessels and capillary bleeding. The ultrasonic scalpel and ESU may be used to cut and coagulate the tissue. *Skeletonization* (the removal of parenchyma and other connective tissues around a structure) of the hepatic and biliary system requires meticulous care to prevent hemorrhage and to preserve the essential blood supply to the organs. This is performed with dissecting scissors or an ultrasonic system. Vessel loops and surgical clips frequently are used to retract and ligate vessels. An HF vessel-sealing system (e.g., LigaSure) also is used.

Hemostatic agents used in surgery include the following:

- Microfibrillar collagen (Avitene, Instat)
- Oxidized cellulose (Surgicel)
- Topical thrombin
- Absorbable gelatin (Gelfoam)
- Fibrin hemostatic tissue adhesive

Supplies required for intraoperative cholangiography include:

- Contrast medium (Diazotrite)
- Injectable saline
- 50- and 30-mL syringes
- Stopcock and 3-way syringe adapter
- Cholangiocatheter

SURGICAL PROCEDURES

ENDOSCOPIC RETROGRADE CHOLANGIOPANCREATOGRAPHY

Selected patients can benefit from endoscopic procedures, such as ERCP, before biliary, hepatic, and pancreatic surgery. The procedure is performed in the outpatient setting in the interventional radiology department, and conscious sedation is used. The endoscope is inserted through the upper GI tract and guided into the duodenum and ampulla of Vater. A contrast medium is injected into the biliary and pancreatic ducts. Biopsy samples may be taken from the ducts and stones removed (see the section on EGD).

LAPAROSCOPIC CHOLECYSTECTOMY

Two common diseases of the biliary system are *cholelithiasis* (the presence of gallstones) and *cholecystitis* (inflammation of the gallbladder). The main components of gallstones are cholesterol and bilirubin. High blood cholesterol and obesity contribute to the formation of gallstones, which can lead to blockage of the bile ducts. Obstruction increases the concentration of bile and results in swelling, pain, and infection. Obstructive jaundice occurs in biliary disease. Bilirubin, a normal byproduct of the breakdown of hemoglobin, is absorbed into normal bile. Biliary obstruction causes increased serum levels of bilirubin, resulting in toxicity.

TECHNIQUE

Cholecystectomy

1 Pneumoperitoneum is established and trocars are placed in the abdomen.
2 The gallbladder is retracted upward with a grasper.
3 The cystic duct, cystic artery, and common bile duct are dissected free.
4 The cystic duct and artery are occluded.

Intraoperative Choledochoscopy

5 An incision is made into the cystic duct.
6 The cystic duct is dilated.
7 The choledochoscope or ureteroscope is inserted and stones are removed with a stone basket.
8 A second set of radiographs may be taken.

Completion of Cholecystectomy

9 The gallbladder is dissected from the underside of the liver with the electrosurgical unit (ESU) probe, hook, or scissors.
10 A grasper is used to remove the gallbladder from the abdomen through a 10-mm trocar site.
11 The abdominal cavity is irrigated.
12 A T-tube may be inserted for continuous postoperative drainage.
13 Individual trocar wounds are closed.
14 If used, the T-tube is attached to a drainage bag.

Discussion

Laparoscopic cholecystectomy now is commonly performed as an ambulatory procedure with rapid recovery. In the past, *common bile duct exploration (CBDE)* was performed during cholecystectomy. CBDE now is frequently performed before surgery as an endoscopic procedure.

The patient is placed in the supine position, and the abdomen is prepped and draped for a laparoscopy. In this procedure, four trocars are placed: an umbilical 10-mm trocar, an additional 10-mm trocar at the midline, and two 5-mm trocars at the axillary line. This procedure usually requires a 30-degree telescope to view the gallbladder, which lies high in the abdominal cavity.

The laparoscope is inserted through a 10-mm port. A straight locking grasper is inserted through one axillary trocar and used to apply upward traction on the gallbladder. The assistant maintains retraction on the gallbladder. The patient then may be repositioned into the reverse Trendelenburg position as the dissection continues. An additional grasper may be placed on the gallbladder.

The cystic duct and artery are exposed. Sharp dissection with scissors, an additional grasper, and an ESU hook may be used to separate the cystic duct and artery. After the cystic duct and artery have been isolated, surgical clips are used to ligate both structures. An additional clip may be placed over the cystic duct at the base of the gallbladder. The duct and artery are then divided. Operative cholangiography usually is performed at this stage of the procedure.

COMMON BILE DUCT EXPLORATION Intraoperative CBDE and stone removal have been largely replaced by preoperative endoscopic procedures in which stones are removed before surgery. However, this part of the procedure is performed in some health care facilities.

If stones are present, the surgeon extends the exploration by dilating the cystic duct with a balloon catheter. This is done by threading a guidewire through the cystic duct and into the common duct. The balloon catheter is inserted over the guidewire and slowly inflated with saline solution. The surgeon can remove single stones by slowly withdrawing the catheter. Common duct stones also can be flushed out with a high-pressure irrigation device. Any stones that fall into the abdominal cavity are retrieved with an endoscopic grasper. Stones also may be retrieved through the fiberoptic choledochoscope or ureteroscope as described in the following section.

INTRAOPERATIVE CHOLEDOCHOSCOPY If a choledochoscopy is to be performed, an additional camera and monitor must be available. A small incision is made in the common bile duct, and the fiberoptic choledochoscope or ureteroscope can be inserted over the guidewire. Stones are retrieved with a stone basket.

The scrub receives all stones in a dry container. Any stones that are inadvertently dropped into the abdominal cavity are retrieved with grasping forceps. When all stones have been removed, a second cholangiogram may be taken.

Completion of Cholecystectomy

The gallbladder is dissected free of the underside of the liver (liver bed). Upward traction is maintained, because this puts some tension on the gallbladder and the tissue plane directly underneath and facilitates dissection. The surgeon uses the ESU hook, scissors, or Harmonic shears to separate the connecting tissues and free the gallbladder from the liver completely. A large grasper is inserted into the 10-mm subxiphoid (uppermost) port. The smaller graspers are used to "hand" the gallbladder to the larger grasper. The gallbladder is then extracted through the 10-mm trocar.

The scrub should receive the gallbladder in a small basin, taking care not to allow its contents to spill onto the surgical field.

A T-tube may be inserted at this time to produce continuous postoperative drainage of the common bile duct. The limbs of the T-tube are trimmed, and the tube is inserted through the uppermost trocar. The limbs of the tube are threaded into the common bile duct, and the long end is pulled through the trocar. The common bile duct is closed with endoscopic sutures. The abdominal cavity then is irrigated, and each trocar incision is closed with absorbable sutures and skin staples. The T-tube is secured to a drainage bag.

CHOLECYSTECTOMY AND OPERATIVE CHOLANGIOGRAPHY (OPEN TECHNIQUE)

Surgical Goal

A *cholecystectomy* is the removal of a diseased gallbladder. *Operative cholangiography* comprises imaging studies in which a contrast medium is injected into the biliary ducts to detect gallstones or a stricture.

Operative cholangiography is seldom performed, because significant evidence indicates that it does not improve the patient's outcome, and it increases the risk of injury to the common bile duct. In current practice, preoperative retrograde endoscopy is used to detect stones and for lithotomy. Laparoscopic surgery is the preferred technique for cholecystectomy.

TECHNIQUE

1 The abdomen is entered through an upper midline or right subcostal incision.
2 The liver is retracted, exposing the gallbladder.
3 The gallbladder is grasped for retraction and manipulation.
4 The gallbladder is drained of bile.
5 The bile ducts are identified and isolated.
6 The cystic artery is ligated.
7 The cystic duct is clamped.
8 The gallbladder is mobilized from the liver bed.
9 Cholangiography is performed.
10 Stones are removed.
11 A T-tube may be inserted.
12 The wound is closed.

Discussion

Open cholecystectomy and CBDE have been replaced almost completely by laparoscopic techniques. A small number of patients require open surgery.

The abdomen is incised and a self-retaining retractor is put in position. A Deaver or Harrington retractor is used to retract the liver and expose the gallbladder. Hemostasis is maintained with the ESU. If the gallbladder is distended with bile, the surgeon may drain it with a trocar fitted to the suction tubing

or with a large-bore needle and syringe. After the trocar has been withdrawn, a Mayo clamp is used to seal the hole.

To start the dissection of the gallbladder, ducts, and vessels, a Péan or similar clamp is placed across the body of the gallbladder, which then is retracted upward. The peritoneal membrane, which covers the cystic duct, artery, and common bile duct, is incised with a scalpel or Metzenbaum scissors. The dissection is continued with scissors, fine-toothed forceps, and small sponge dissectors. When the cystic artery has been fully exposed, it is occluded with right angle clamps and ligated with vessel clips.

Dissection and ligation of bleeding vessels is completed with scissors and right angle clamps until the cystic and common bile ducts are exposed and dissected free. Operative cholangiography is performed at this stage of the procedure.

Operative Cholangiography

To begin operative cholangiography, the surgeon places two traction sutures of 3-0 silk through the wall of the cystic duct. An incision then is made between the sutures with a # 11 scalpel blade or Potts scissors.

The scrub should have a cholangiocatheter, contrast medium, stopcock, and 30- or 50-mL syringe available. The contrast medium is prepared before the cholangiography:

1. The circulator distributes the contrast medium and injectable saline to the scrub. The contrast medium is diluted according to the surgeon's order. At least 30 mL of contrast medium solution should be prepared. The solution is aspirated into the syringe, which is attached to a stopcock and cholangiocatheter.
2. All air bubbles are removed from both the syringe and the catheter (these appear as solid white spots on radiographs and can be interpreted as stones).
3. The scrub places a clamp across the catheter near its tip to prevent air from backing up into the syringe. The syringe, cholangiocatheter, and its attaching clamp are then passed to the surgeon.

The surgeon threads the tips of the cholangiocatheter through the incision in the cystic duct and advances it into the common bile duct. The catheter may be secured with a suture tie or vessel clip. All instruments and radiopaque sponges must be removed from the field, and a sterile drape is placed over the sterile field and the incision.

The C-arm then is brought into position, and the surgeon injects the contrast medium. Stones are removed under fluoroscopy. A balloon biliary catheter often is used to remove stones. The catheter probe is advanced beyond the level of the stone, the balloon is inflated, and the catheter is withdrawn, bringing the stones with it. Stones are also removed with gallbladder dilators, scoops, or a stone basket catheter. As the stones are removed, the scrub receives them as specimens.

CLOSURE When all stones have been removed, the cystic duct is ligated and the gallbladder is removed. The liver bed may be closed with fine absorbable sutures. If postoperative drainage is required, a T-tube is inserted into the common duct at this time. The ductal incision then is closed with 3-0 or 4-0 absorbable sutures on a fine tapered needle. The long end of the T-tube is brought out of the wound and later attached to a collection bag. Penrose drains are inserted into the abdominal cavity, and the ends are brought through a stab wound near the main incision. The wound is irrigated with warm saline solution and closed in layers.

CHOLEDOCHODUODENOSTOMY AND CHOLEDOCHOJEJUNOSTOMY

Choledochoduodenostomy (anastomosis between the common bile duct and duodenum) and choledochojejunostomy (anastomosis between the common bile duct and jejunum) are rarely performed in modern surgical practice. Endoscopic stone retrieval now is the gold standard for the treatment of obstruction of the distal common bile duct (CBD), an indication for bypass of the CBD.

SPLENECTOMY

Surgical Goal

The spleen is removed surgically to stop hemorrhage caused by trauma or to treat disease.

Pathology

The spleen is vulnerable to rupture and extensive hemorrhage as a result of abdominal trauma. Splenic tissue is delicate and easily torn and has a rich vascular system. Its location in the abdomen makes it vulnerable to injury caused by the steering wheel in a motor vehicle accident. Injury during a contact sport is another common cause of splenic rupture.

The spleen also is removed to treat selected immune and blood disorders and cancer.

Elective laparoscopic splenectomy may be performed for certain diseases of the spleen, except trauma or an enlarged organ. The laparosocopic technique follows similar instrumentation and abdominal access as that described in laparoscopic cholecystectomy.

TECHNIQUE

1 A laparotomy is performed.
2 Blood and clots are immediately removed from the abdomen.
3 The splenic artery and vein are digitally compressed to control bleeding.
4 An intestinal or a vascular clamp is placed across the major vessels.
5 The extent of injury is assessed.
6 If total splenectomy is to be performed, the splenic artery and vein are cross-clamped, occluded, and divided.
7 The lienorenal ligament is divided by sharp dissection.
8 The peritoneum is dissected from the spleen with sharp and blunt dissection.
9 The gastric vessels are divided, clamped, and ligated.
10 The gastrosplenic ligament is divided.
11 A suction drain is placed in the wound.
12 Hemostasis is secured and the wound is closed in layers.

Discussion

Severe splenic trauma may be a life-threatening condition that requires immediate operative intervention. However, more conservative treatment is adequate for low-grade trauma cases. CT scanning and ultrasound are now used to grade splenic injury. Conservative nonsurgical therapy is adequate for injuries that do not affect hemodynamic stability. Because multiple injuries may be involved in traumatic accidents, there is no definitive method of determining the exact cause of instability. In these cases, emergency surgery is indicated when systolic pressure falls below 90 mm Hg with no response to intravascular resuscitation.

In preparation for the surgery, the scrub should have a major laparotomy set, vascular clamps, and kidney pedicle clamps, depending on the surgeon's preference.

The type of sutures is specified. They usually include silk or synthetic nonabsorbable sutures to ligate the splenic artery and vein and the gastrosplenic vessels. Surgical clips are used throughout the procedure to secure small bleeders as they are encountered during the dissection.

Remember that during emergency surgery for acute hemorrhage of any kind, four major requirements must be met to stop the bleeding:
1. *Access:* The surgeon must have access to the hemorrhage site. This starts with a rapid laparotomy.
2. *Visualization* (ability to see structures directly): Retraction, either manual or self-retaining, must be established quickly. Suction must be available immediately to clear blood and clots. The scrub may be required to assist in suctioning and evacuating blood clots while passing other needed instruments.
3. *Good lighting:* Excellent lighting is required to locate and stop the hemorrhage. This is the collaborative duty of the scrub and the circulator. Remember to angle the surgical light toward the proximal end of the wound.
4. *Clamps:* Clamps are required to occlude the bleeding vessels. The scrub must have vascular, pedicle, and other hemostatic clamps immediately available on the field.

Two suctions must be available as soon as the abdomen is opened. These are used to evacuate the blood and clots from the abdomen so that the splenic vessels can be located and manually compressed. The scrub should have a large basin available to evacuate and remove large blood clots from the abdominal cavity as soon as the abdomen is opened. Laparotomy sponges are used in rapid succession as the bleeding is controlled.

The surgeon's assistant evacuates the blood clots and places a self-retaining retractor while the surgeon locates the splenic artery and vein. Even though the procedure moves quickly, safety techniques are still observed. The scrub must watch the wound, have equipment available, and use methodical, smooth movements in assisting.

A blood recovery system (e.g., Cell Saver) may be used immediately to replace blood. As soon as the splenic vessels are located, they are clamped with a pedicle or vascular clamp. When the vascular supply to the spleen has been controlled, the wound can be more carefully cleared of blood and the extent of damage ascertained. The splenic artery and vein may be ligated at this time. Heavy silk or synthetic suture ligatures are used to secure the vessels. Two or more ligatures may be used.

The wound is explored for other areas of trauma. The abdominal retractors may be repositioned at this time. Sharp and blunt dissection with Metzenbaum scissors and sponge dissectors are used to separate the lienorenal ligament from the body of the spleen. The gastric vessels are clamped or clipped and divided in the usual manner. The gastrosplenic ligament is then separated with Metzenbaum scissors, and the spleen is delivered from the wound.

If the spleen is to be repaired rather than removed, absorbable sutures are used to oversew the tear. Hemostatic agents (e.g., Gelfoam, Avitene, or Surgicel) are used to coagulate areas of capillary bleeding.

The surgeon examines the abdominal cavity again to ensure that all hemorrhage has been controlled and to locate any other areas of abdominal trauma. The wound then is irrigated with antibacterial solution. One or more drains are placed in the vicinity of the splenic pedicle, and the wound is closed in layers.

PANCREATICODUODENECTOMY (WHIPPLE PROCEDURE)

Surgical Goal

In the Whipple procedure, the head of the pancreas and duodenum and a portion of the jejunum, distal stomach, and distal section of the common bile duct are removed. The biliary system, pancreatic system, and GI tract are reconstructed.

Pathology

The Whipple procedure is performed for curative or palliative treatment of pancreatic cancer.

TECHNIQUE

1 A laparotomy is performed through a bilateral or inverted V (bilateral subcostal) incision.
2 The duodenum is mobilized with blunt and sharp dissection. All vessels in the area of the proposed anastomosis are double-clamped, ligated, and divided.
3 The gastrocolic ligament and omentum are mobilized as in step 2.
4 The distal stomach is mobilized and transected.
5 The common bile duct is clamped and separated from the duodenum.
6 Vascular attachments to the jejunum are divided.
7 The jejunum is cross-clamped and divided.
8 The pancreas is transected.
9 The specimen is removed.
10 The GI, biliary, and pancreatic systems are reconstructed.

Discussion

Pancreaticoduodenectomy is a radical operation that requires 5 to 8 hours to complete. Because the procedure includes

elements of pancreatic, biliary, intestinal, and gastric procedures, the scrub should prepare all instruments normally used in these specialties. Most are included in a major laparotomy set. Vascular instruments should be added to the sterile setup in case vessel repair is required. Extra suction and two ESU sets sometimes are needed. Long instruments and wide retractors (e.g., wide Deaver and Harrington retractors) should also be available. Right angle clamps are used throughout the procedure.

Much of the procedure includes meticulous dissection, management of bleeding, and anastomosis. The surgeon's preferred sutures are made available but should be distributed to the sterile field economically. Additional sutures and other equipment, such as sponges, vessel loops, and scalpel blades, should be held in reserve. Extra surgical towels and half-sheet drapes should be available to keep the operative site orderly and clean. The risk of infection increases with the duration of the procedure. Recall that increased handling of instruments and equipment also increases the risk of contamination.

Sterile irrigation and water to soak instruments must be kept fresh during a long procedure. The scrub should attempt to keep instruments clean and free of tissue debris. Extra gloves for the team should be readily available but not opened onto the sterile field.

To understand the techniques used in this procedure, the surgical technologist should review procedures learned previously. These resection procedures are performed in succession, and the essential ducts and hollow organs are reconnected to restore function. The reconstruction phase of the procedure can be performed with surgical staples, sutures, or a combination of the two techniques. Variations on the Whipple procedure can be done, and the exact resection depends on the pathological condition. The procedure commonly includes resection of the head of the pancreas, distal portion of the stomach, duodenum, gallbladder, and common bile duct. Reconstruction procedures include:

- Gastric resection and gastrojejunostomy (in some procedures the stomach is not resected)
- Intestinal resection and anastomosis
- Choledochojejunostomy or choledochoduodenostomy
- Pancreatojejunostomy

Table 23-5 describes the areas of resection.

The patient is placed in the supine position, prepped from the nipple line to midthigh, and draped for a laparotomy. The abdomen is entered through a long midline incision. The surgeon explores the bowel and other organs for evidence of metastasis and extension of the tumor. This will determine if resection is achievable. The wound is packed with moistened lap sponges, and a self-retaining retractor is placed in the usual manner. Accessory retractors or a self-retaining retractor fitted with attachments (Thompson or Bookwalter) is used.

The procedure begins with mobilization of the duodenum, which is attached to the peritoneal reflection (an extension of the abdominal peritoneum). The surgeon separates loose connective tissue from the duodenum with the ESU. The lower

Table 23-5	Reconstruction Using the Whipple Procedure
Normal Anatomical Structure	**Postreconstruction Configuration**
The duodenum is continuous from the distal stomach to the jejunum.	The duodenum and a portion of the jejunum are removed. A portion of the proximal jejunum is removed.
The distal stomach is continuous with the duodenum.	The gastric omentum attachments are divided and the distal (lower) third of the stomach is removed. The remaining gastric section is attached to the jejunum with a side-to-side technique.
The common bile duct is an extension of the common hepatic duct and communicates directly into the duodenum at the ampulla of Vater.	The common bile duct is divided just below the Y-junction of the cystic and hepatic ducts. The common bile duct is anastomosed to the jejunum with an end-to-side technique.
The pancreatic duct communicates with the duodenum at the ampulla of Vater.	The head of the pancreas is removed and the remaining portion is anastomosed to the jejunum with an end-to-end or side-to-side technique.

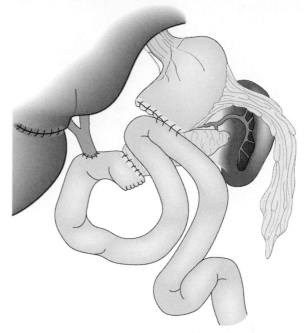

Figure 23-29 **Whipple procedure anastomoses.** *(From Garden O, Bradbury A, Forsythe J, Parks R: Principles and practice of surgery, ed 5, Edinburgh, 2007, Churchill Livingstone/Elsevier.)*

third of the stomach is separated from the omentum in the proposed area of resection.

The stomach then is resected from the jejunum and the two structures. A side-to-side anastomosis is performed. The surgeon performs this step using a surgical stapling instrument or by clamping the stomach with Payr or Allen clamps and performing a traditional two-layer closure. Absorbable and silk 2-0 and 3-0 sutures are used for the anastomosis.

The duodenum is retracted, and the common bile duct is exposed and divided. The common bile duct is anastomosed to the jejunum. Anastomosis of the GI tract is performed as described in Table 23-5. The cystic duct is attached to the jejunum (choledochojejunostomy) later in the procedure. The junction of the duodenum and jejunum (duodenojejunal flexure) is divided.

The pancreas is resected with both sharp and blunt dissection. The pancreatic duct must be identified and preserved for attachment to the jejunum. When all bleeding has been controlled and attachments have been divided between the accessory organs, the specimen is removed. The scrub should receive it in a basin.

Reconstruction of the GI tract continues with an end-to-end pancreatojejunostomy. An end-to-side, single-layer choledochojejunostomy is then performed. Individual sponge and needle counts must be performed before the anastomosis of the stomach and intestine.

After the reconstruction is complete, the surgeon irrigates the wound with antibacterial solution and inspects each anastomosis for leakage. When hemostasis has been completely secured, one or more abdominal drains are placed in the abdomen. The wound is then closed. Figure 23-29 shows the completed anastomoses.

After radical surgery, the patient recovers in the PACU and may be taken to the intensive care unit (ICU) for observation. Complex physiological monitoring is performed throughout the initial phases of postoperative recovery. As normal homeostasis returns, the patient is still monitored for metabolic and renal function, infection, and fluid and electrolyte balance.

LAPAROSCOPIC DISTAL PANCREATECTOMY

Surgical Goal

In a laparoscopic distal pancreatectomy, a portion of the tail of the pancreas is removed for palliative treatment of a malignant tumor or to remove a benign lesion. Splenectomy may be performed during the procedure.

Pathology

Cancer of the pancreas usually is well advanced at the time of diagnosis. The survival rate is less than 3% in 5 years. Alcoholism and biliary reflux are common causes of pancreatitis that lead to pancreatic adenocarcinoma. Pancreatic resection may be performed if the tumor is localized in one area. Partial pancreatectomy offers palliative treatment for metastasis.

TECHNIQUE

1 Pneumoperitoneum is established.
2 Four abdominal ports are created.
3 The gastric arteries and branches are ligated.
4 The splenocolic ligament is incised.
5 The spleen is mobilized.
6 The pancreas is retracted upward.
7 The splenic artery and vein are exposed and ligated.
8 A linear surgical stapler is used to transect the tail of the pancreas.
9 The specimen is removed with a specimen retrieval bag.
10 A 15-mm port is extended by at least 2 mm.
11 The spleen is divided into sections and brought out of the abdominal cavity through the retrieval bag.
12 An abdominal drain is placed.
13 Trocars are removed and pneumoperitoneum is released.
14 The wounds are closed.

Discussion

Pneumoperitoneum is established, and four trocars are placed in the abdomen. A 12-mm port is placed above the umbilicus for the laparoscope. A 15-mm port is inserted below the left costal margin, and a 5-mm port is placed at the left costal margin. The fourth port is inserted into the subxiphoid area.

After examining the abdominal cavity, the surgeon incises the gastrocolic ligament using blunt dissection or a Harmonic scalpel. This creates access to the gastric arteries and branches. These vessels are ligated with surgical clips and divided or coagulated with the ESU. The splenocolic ligament and peritoneal attachment to the spleen are then incised.

The pancreas is freed from the retroperitoneum and elevated with an atraumatic retractor to gain access to the splenic vein and artery. These are clamped and divided. When the spleen has been freed from its vascular attachments, the surgeon must *transect* the pancreas with a linear stapler (e.g., the GIA II). Bleeding from the severed surface of the pancreas is controlled with the ESU. The pancreas is placed in a specimen retrieval bag and removed. The spleen then is divided into small pieces and delivered from the wound through the 15-mm port.

A small abdominal drain may be placed in the wound, which is then irrigated. All instruments are removed from the abdomen, and the pneumoperitoneum is released.

Individual ports are sutured with absorbable sutures and skin staples.

SEGMENTAL RESECTION OF THE LIVER

Surgical Goal

Hepatic resection is performed to remove a portion of the liver to treat a benign or malignant tumor. Segmental resection or lobectomy is the usual approach for tumor removal. **Segmental resection** involves the removal of one or more of the nine liver segments. **Lobectomy** is the removal of one or more of the major lobes of the liver: the right lobe, the left lobe, or the entire right lobe and a portion of the left (called *right hepatic trisegmentectomy*).

Pathology

The most common indication for liver resection is a malignant liver tumor. The tumor may be primary (the original source of the cancer) or metastatic (cancer that has spread from another location in the body). The most common type of liver tumor is metastatic, especially those that arise from primary tumors in which the blood supply is drained by the portal vein. Primary liver tumors are rare. Cancer of the liver usually is well advanced by the time it is diagnosed. Less common indications for liver resection include parasitic disease, infection, and laceration or trauma of the liver.

TECHNIQUE

1 A laparotomy is performed through a subcostal, median, or paramedian incision. The surgeon explores the abdominal cavity to evaluate the extent and location of diseased tissue. Intraoperative ultrasound may be used to identify segments associated with the diseased tissue.
2 Moist laparotomy sponges are used to pack the abdominal viscera away from the liver. Additional laparotomy sponges are placed between the diaphragm and the liver.
3 A self-retaining retractor is placed in the abdomen.
4 The abdominal cavity is examined for evidence of disease.
5 The pedicle segment is identified and individual vessels and ducts (bile duct, hepatic artery, and portal vein branch) are dissected free.
6 Ultrasound may be used or methylene blue dye may be injected into the pedicle to stain the segment and identify the exact anatomical boundaries.
7 The pedicle structures are clamped and ligated.
8 The liver segment is resected.
9 Hemostasis is secured.
10 An abdominal drain is placed in the wound.
11 The wound is closed in layers.

Discussion

Liver resection follows diagnostic studies, including percutaneous needle biopsy performed under MRI or ultrasound guidance in an outpatient setting.

A laparotomy is performed through a right subcostal, midline, or paramedian incision. After entering the abdomen, the surgeon examines the liver and adjacent viscera. This may be done before or after a self-retaining retractor is placed in the wound. Because of the size of the liver and the wide exposure required, a self-retaining retractor with accessory attachments often is used. Before placing the retractor, the surgeon places moist laparotomy sponges over accessory organs surrounding the liver and between the liver and the diaphragm.

One of the areas in which sponges often are retained is the *subphrenic area* (under the diaphragm). The scrub counts all sponges placed in the wound, taking special care to note those placed in this area of the abdomen.

After all retractors have been placed, the surgeon examines the diseased segment. A sterile ultrasound Doppler probe may be needed to determine the segmental location of the tumor.

Removal of liver segments requires identification and dissection of veins, arteries, and ducts that branch into each segment. The scrub must watch the field and observe the progress of the dissection, passing the appropriate instruments to the surgeon as needed.

To begin the resection, the surgeon dissects the attachments between the liver and abdominal wall, such as the falciform ligament. To perform a segmental resection, the surgeon must locate the correct segment pedicle. These two steps of the procedure are performed with the standard dissecting instruments. The surgeon may need to place an additional retractor at the top of the incision to displace the liver upward. A Harrington retractor or wide Deaver retractor may be used here. The surgeon protects the liver with a moist laparotomy sponge and uses the hand to expose the ligaments that attach the liver to the posterior wall of the abdomen. The ultrasonic scalpel and aspirator (CUSA) may be used to expose the pedicle where it branches into the parenchyma.

At this stage, the surgeon must identify the exact borders of the segment. If multiple segments are to be removed, all ligament attachments are transected during the procedure. A common method is to begin dissection at the pedicle (at the hilum of the liver) and follow the structures into the parenchyma, using the ultrasonic scalpel or ESU to resect the liver tissue. If this approach is used, the surgeon temporarily stops the vascular supply to the segment by applying vascular clamps across the vessels that supply that segment. This prevents excess bleeding during the dissection.

An alternative method is to first identify the pedicle structures and then inject methylene blue dye into the pedicle. The methylene blue dye enters the pedicle structures and stains the segment that includes the tumor. If this technique is used, the scrub should have methylene blue dye, a 10-mL syringe, and the surgeon's preferred needle for injection. A small Silastic catheter may be attached to the hub of the needle and syringe.

When the portal (branches of the portal vein) and pedicle structures and appropriate segment have been identified, the pedicle structures are individually clamped, ligated, and transected. The pedicle and portal structures are ligated with silk, synthetic nonabsorbable suture, or surgical staples.

The liver segment can be resected at this point. The surgeon scores the segment using the ESU. Complete resection is performed with the ESU, CUSA, or Harmonic scalpel or by finger fracture (the surgeon uses the hand to "break" the parenchyma along the lines of resection). At the completion of the resection, the liver bed and raw surfaces must be free of hemorrhage. The argon beam coagulator and ESU typically are used to secure hemostasis. An abdominal drain (e.g., Jackson-Pratt or Penrose drain) is placed in the wound, which is closed in layers as for a laparotomy.

LIVER TRANSPLANTATION

Surgical Goal

The goal of transplantation is to replace a diseased liver with a donor organ.

Pathology

In adults, liver transplantation is performed in selected patients for conditions that result in end-stage liver disease, such as **cirrhosis** not related to bile stasis, autoimmune disorder, or neoplasms.

Transplantation Considerations

Transplantation is a joint effort that involves the organ procurement agency and the host hospital. (Refer to Chapter 16.) The procedures for both donor and recipient are complex. Protocols for the technical as well as the medicolegal aspects of the process require many individuals and professional coordination. The basic considerations and technical points are presented here as a basis for advanced practice.

The donor procedure involves multiple organ procurement from a *heart-beating donor* as described in Chapter 16. The procedure is carried out by the procurement agency under the supervision of a transplant coordinator. The liver is removed with all accessory arteries, including the celiac artery, portal vein, vena cava, and common bile duct. After procurement, the liver is transported to the recipient facility by the procurement agency. The time between organ procurement and transplantation usually is about 10 hours.

The setup for transplantation requires extensive patient care equipment, similar to that required for cardiac surgery. This equipment includes devices for complex physiological monitoring, patient warming, a blood warmer, cold slush basins, physiological fluids, and a crash cart (defibrillator and emergency drugs).

Liver transplantation is a complex procedure that requires advanced surgical nursing and technology.

TECHNIQUE

Recipient Procedure

1 Midline and bilateral subcostal incisions are made.
2 The liver is mobilized with sharp and blunt dissection.
3 The vena cava is mobilized.
4 The hepatic artery, portal vein, and common bile duct are mobilized and clamped.
5 The liver is removed.
6 The donor liver is positioned in the right upper quadrant.
7 The vena cava and portal vein are anastomosed from the recipient to the donor liver.
8 Clamps on the vena cava and portal vein are released to allow the flow of blood.
9 Bleeding is controlled and the anastomosis sites are monitored for leakage.
10 When hemostasis is achieved and the blood supply to the liver has been measured, the hepatic artery is anastomosed to the donor artery.
11 The common bile duct is anastomosed to the duodenum or jejunum
12 The wound and all incision sites are examined carefully for leakage and liver perfusion is checked.
13 The wound is irrigated and drains are placed.
14 The incision is closed.

SECTION IV: BREAST SURGERY

SURGICAL ANATOMY

The breasts lie within the fascia of the anterior chest wall from the second to the sixth ribs. The breast is composed of glandular, connective, and fat tissue contained within extensions of fibrous ligaments that radiate from the nipple to the periphery of the breast. Membranes or septal ligaments separate each of these radial sections. Each breast has about 15 to 25 separate sections. The glandular tissue forms clusters or small lobes, which are interspersed with alveoli that contain the secretory cells that form milk (Figure 23-30).

The intralobar ducts communicate from the glandular lobes. These ducts lead to the lactiferous ducts and reservoir and then open at the nipple. The nipple contains glandular, vascular, nerve, and epithelial tissue and is centered in the *areola,* a circular area of darkened skin. Small nodes in the areola contain sebaceous glands. Estrogen and progesterone, secreted cyclically and during pregnancy, cause the areola to darken.

Breast tissue changes with development of the individual, hormonal changes, pregnancy status, and nutritional state.

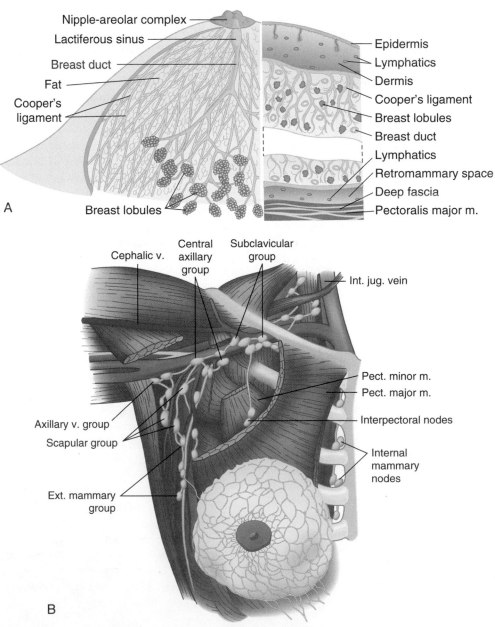

Figure 23-30   A, Breast anatomy. The cutaway on the right illustrates the tissue layers. The breast is supported by deep fascia and muscle. **B,** The axillary anatomy, showing lymph node drainage and the vascular supply. *(From Donegan WL, Spratt JS: Cancer of the breast, Philadelphia, 1988, WB Saunders.)*

The release of breast milk and other secretions from the nipple is controlled by complex hormonal changes.

The upper thoracic lymph drains to the axillary lymph nodes. This is an important anatomical feature, because cancer staging and diagnostic surgery often require biopsy of one or more axillary lymph nodes. The type and extent of change in the lymph nodes is a primary determinant of the disease outcome and survival rate.

BREAST CANCER

Most noncosmetic surgical procedures of the breast are performed for the treatment of cancer. Breast cancer diagnosis and treatment is a surgical specialty that has advanced greatly in the past two decades. Procedures that were common 10 years ago may never be performed in most clinical facilities. However, the psychological and social consequences of a cancer diagnosis have not changed. This aspect of patient care remains a critical concern of those caring for a patient undergoing breast surgery.

Breast cancer is the leading cause of death in women age 20 to 59 in the United States. Improvements in diagnostic technology and aggressive public health campaigns in the United States have increased the reported number of cases of cancer in the last 10 years. This is due to early detection. Invasive ductal carcinoma is the most common type of breast cancer. Risk factors include a family history of breast cancer, benign breast disease, and hormonal conditions that result in early menarche and late menopause. Breast cancer in men accounts for 0.8% of all breast cancers. The annual mortality rate for male breast cancer averages 400, compared with 400,000 in women.

Cancer *staging* is used to determine the possible outcome and options for treatment. However, the final decision rests with the patient, in consultation with the primary health care specialist, surgeon, and oncologist. (See Chapter 7 for a description of the cancer staging process.)

Breast cancer treatment has changed radically over the past 20 years, with a tendency toward less radical surgery. Early detection combined with improved chemotherapy and radiological treatment now provide an equal or better outcome compared to the radical mastectomy performed routinely several decades ago.

A range of procedures is available for surgical management of a breast tumor. These include:

- *Needle aspiration biopsy,* which usually is performed in the physician's office to confirm a cystic mass.
- *Fine-needle insertion* into the suspect mass, with immediate surgical excision and frozen section. This is followed by breast-conserving surgery (*lumpectomy* or segmental resection), with or without lymph node excision.
- *Sentinel node detection and biopsy* followed by breast-conserving surgery and axillary node dissection.
- *Breast-conserving procedures,* such as lumpectomy and segmental resection.
- *Mastectomy (preplanned)* for advanced metastatic cancer or as a prophylactic procedure in high-risk patients.

Breast-conserving surgery with sentinel node biopsy is now the choice of most oncologists unless the cancer is advanced at the time of presentation. The prognosis is influenced more by the extent of lymph node involvement than by the size of the breast tumor.

Table 23-6 describes diagnostic procedures of the breast.

Table **23-6**	**Diagnostic Procedures of the Breast**	
Type	**Description**	**Considerations**
Breast self-examination (BSE)	Women and men are taught how to perform BSE by a primary care professional. The procedure for BSE involves systematic palpation of the breast and axillary region and visual examination, starting at age 20.	The patient should be instructed by a qualified health professional who can answer questions and make sure the patient understands the procedure and its importance.
Clinical examination	The clinical examination involves palpation and visual examination of the breasts by a qualified health professional.	Women in their 20s and 30s should have a clinical examination every 3 years.
Mammography	A mammography is a radiological examination of the breasts for detection of masses or other lesions.	Mammography is the only screening method effective for the detection of nonpalpable lesions. A yearly mammogram is recommended for women age 40 or older.
Fine-needle aspiration	A fine-gauge needle is inserted into a suspect breast mass and tissue (cells and fluid) is withdrawn for examination and diagnosis.	This procedure may be performed in the physician's office.
Stereotactic biopsy	The patient lies prone on the mammography table with the breast isolated. A computer-assisted needle is guided into the suspect mass and a core sample is withdrawn.	This procedure is less invasive than surgical biopsy. Stereotactic technology provides accurate placement of the needle and has a 96% accuracy for detecting cancer.

CASE PLANNING

PSYCHOLOGICAL CONSIDERATIONS

For most women, the breast reflects reproductive ability and **body image** and secures feminine identity. Surgery of the breast threatens these images and can produce anxiety and depression. Increased public awareness of breast cancer and advanced technology for early detection have increased women's ability to take an active part in breast health. Breast tumors also can occur in men, but the incidence is very low.

Although early detection is an important advance in breast medicine, the prospect of surgery remains an emotional and difficult issue for the patient. The patient's need for emotional support requires health care professionals to listen to the patient and support and acknowledge her feelings. The clinician's most important role in providing support is to provide a calm presence and to convey respect for the patient's feelings.

Reconstructive breast surgery may be done immediately after a mastectomy or as a separate procedure at a later date. The patient may enter a deep grieving period after such radical surgery. Psychological support at this time is critical in restoring the patient's positive self-image.

POSITION AND DRAPING

Breast surgery is performed with the patient in the supine position. A pad may be placed under the affected side at the level of the back to elevate the affected area. The affected arm is prepped and draped free in most cases, except for a simple lumpectomy without axillary node dissection.

If the arm is draped free, an arm board is used, as in limb surgery. This allows the surgeon to manipulate the arm for exposure to the axilla at various angles. Care must be taken not to allow the arm to drop off the arm board during surgery.

INSTRUMENTS AND SUPPLIES

Surgery of the breast requires general surgery instruments and a plastic surgery set. Senn, vein, and other small retractors are needed for breast biopsy. Surgical clips, absorbable and nonabsorbable sutures, and an ESU are used for hemostasis. Vessel loops are needed for retraction of deep veins, arteries, and nerves. Wound drains include the Jackson-Pratt, Hemovac, and simpler gravity drains, such as the Penrose drain. The ESU is used extensively in radical breast surgery. The surgeon may require a nerve stimulator to differentiate blood vessels from small nerves during dissection of the chest wall and axilla.

SURGICAL PROCEDURES

WIRE LOCALIZATION AND BREAST BIOPSY

Surgical Goal

Wire localization is the insertion of a fine wire into a breast mass during fluoroscopy. This device may be referred to as a hook wire or hook needle. The wire is taped in place, and surgical biopsy is performed at the site of the wire. This is a specific technique used to identify the site of a suspected mass, whereas needle biopsy is used to withdraw a small amount of fluid and cells for pathological analysis.

TECHNIQUE

1. During mammography, the patient is prepped and a local anesthetic is administered in the area of the mass.
2. A **hook wire** assembly is inserted into the mass.
3. The wire is secured to the patient's skin with tape.
4. The patient is transferred to the operating room.
5. Additional prep solution may be applied gently around the site of the needle.
6. The patient is draped for an excisional biopsy of the breast.
7. The needle is located and an elliptical incision is made that includes the needle and a margin of skin.
8. The incision is continued through the subcutaneous and breast tissue, including a 1- to 2-cm margin. Small rake retractors are placed in the wound edge.
9. The needle and tissue are removed and the tissue is examined by the pathologist for clear margins.
10. If the tissue is malignant or if the tumor margins are not clear of cancer cells, a more extensive procedure may be initiated, or the surgery may be deferred for 24 hours.
11. The breast tissue is closed with 3-0 absorbable suture.
12. The skin is closed with sterile adhesive strips.

Discussion

The patient is admitted for surgery immediately after placement of a hook needle during mammography or ultrasound. After administration of an anesthetic, the breast is gently prepped to avoid dislodging the needle. A fenestrated body drape is then applied. Care must be taken not to displace the needle during the draping.

The surgeon begins the procedure by making an elliptical skin incision around the hook wire. The surgeon then uses Metzenbaum scissors to increase the depth of the incision. Senn retractors or small rakes are placed at the wound edges. Scissors rather than an ESU are used to complete the dissection to avoid distorting the margins of the mass. Allis clamps may be used to grasp the tissue during dissection. The specimen, with identification needle intact, is delivered to the pathologist for examination. If the margins of the specimen are *not* clear of tumor, additional tissue is removed and examined. When the margins include a clear area of 0.4 to 0.8 inch (1 to 2 cm), the wound is closed.

The excision site is irrigated with warm saline and closed with several subcutaneous interrupted sutures of absorbable synthetic material. The skin usually is closed with sterile strips or subcuticular sutures.

SENTINAL LYMPH NODE BIOPSY

Surgical Goal

The procedure for **sentinel lymph node biopsy (SLNB)** involves injection of isosulfan blue dye, radioactive material (**technetium-99**), or both directly into the breast mass or nearby. Both materials may be used to track the lymph nodes visually (dye) and by gamma ray emission (technetium-99). The technetium then is tracked with a device similar to a Geiger counter.

If radioactive material is used, it may be injected 2 hours or longer before surgery in the nuclear medicine department. Isosulfan is injected at the time of surgery to provide greater visibility of the nodes. Surgery for node excision then follows.

NOTE: *Isosulfan blue may cause anaphylactic shock in some patients. When used in conjunction with SLNB, the patient is monitored carefully throughout the procedure. A crash cart must be immediately available in these cases.*

Pathology

Sentinel lymph nodes are usually located at the proximal axillary lymph chain. A metastatic tumor in the breast drains (theoretically) first to these nodes. Excision of the sentinel nodes is an alternative procedure to axillary lymph node dissection, in which 10 or more nodes are removed for preventive treatment. Sentinel node excision may be appropriate only in selected patients with a low risk of metastasis.

TECHNIQUE

1 The breast mass or biopsy site from previous surgery is injected with technetium-99.
2 A gamma ray–detecting probe is used to determine which lymph nodes are affected.
3 The affected nodes are marked with a dye pen.
4 The patient is prepped and draped for excisional biopsy.
5 Isosulfan is injected into or near the breast mass.
6 The sentinel nodes are removed.

Discussion

Excisional biopsy of sentinel nodes follows the techniques used for superficial axillary exploration. Only nodes identified by gamma ray emission are removed by superficial surgery. This may precede excision of the breast mass. The scrub must provide a separate container for each node and ensure that they are identified appropriately.

BREAST-CONSERVING SURGERY FOR A MASS (LUMPECTOMY, SEGMENTAL MASTECTOMY)

Surgical Goal

A breast mass is removed to confirm a diagnosis or to treat malignancy. The mass is excised, ensuring that the margins are completely free of cancer cells. Axillary dissection to remove a group of lymph nodes or removal of selective sentinel lymph nodes may be performed during the same procedure. Analysis of the mass by frozen section is done during surgery; this determines the extent of the excision discussed and planned with the patient before surgery. Figure 23-31 shows the possible incisions for an excision procedure.

In a skin-sparing (subcutaneous) mastectomy, the overlying skin tissue, the areola, and the nipple are not removed. An implant may be placed immediately after the procedure.

Pathology

Both malignant and some benign breast neoplasms generally present as a mass that is visible with imaging studies or that can be detected by palpation. A mass smaller than 0.4 inch (1 cm) usually is not palpable and is detected with routine mammography or other imaging techniques. Gynecomastia, which is excess breast tissue in the male, is caused by a hormonal imbalance and usually is treated medically. Mastectomy may be required if the condition does not respond to medical treatment.

TECHNIQUE

1 An incision is made at the border of the areola or directly over the tumor mass.
2 The mass is grasped with one or more Allis clamps and excised using sharp dissection.
3 Hemostasis is maintained with fine sutures or an electrosurgical unit (ESU) needle.
4 The specimen may be marked with sutures for orientation and then removed for pathological examination.
5 After the pathology report is received, the wound is extended to include a greater portion of the breast.
6 Sentinel lymph node biopsy may be performed through a separate incision.
7 The wound is irrigated.
8 Drains are placed in the wound.
9 The wound is closed.

Discussion

The skin incision is made along skin lines drawn preoperatively. This incision is carried through the subcutaneous and breast tissue with Metzenbaum or Mayo scissors. Small bleeders are coagulated with a needle point ESU tip. A spatula ESU tip generally is not used for en bloc removal of a suspect mass, because this may obliterate the tissue margins and obscure a diagnosis.

The surgeon grasps the subcutaneous and breast tissue with two or more Allis clamps. The scrub should have retractors available as the incision is extended to deep tissue. Small rake or Senn retractors can be used for shallow retraction, and right angle retractors (small Richardson or Deaver retractors) are needed for deeper excision. Hemostasis is maintained with fine absorbable sutures and electrosurgical needle.

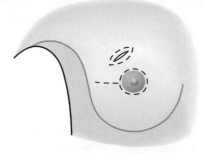

Lateral extension can increase axillary exposure

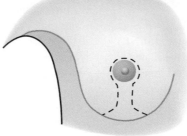
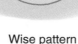

Wise pattern

Figure 23-31 **Incisions for a skin-sparing biopsy.** *(From Townsend CM: Sabiston textbook of surgery, ed 17, Philadelphia, 2001, WB Saunders.)*

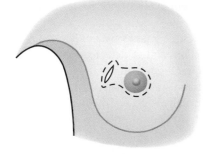
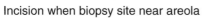

Incision when biopsy site near areola

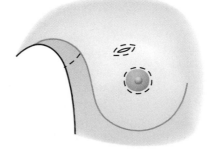

Incision when biopsy site remote from areola with axillary incision for lymphadenectomy

As the excision is extended, 4 × 4 sponges should be removed from the field and replaced with laparotomy sponges. A 4 × 4 sponge can be easily lost inside the breast wound, especially if the excision is deep.

The specimen is removed in one piece. The surgeon may place one or more sutures on the periphery for identification of the margins. These must be carefully preserved. The breast wound may be closed at this time, or closure may be delayed until axillary dissection is completed.

AXILLARY DISSECTION Axillary lymph nodes, which drain the breast, can include cancer cells from a malignant tumor. To gain access to the axillary nodes, the surgeon makes an incision just below the upper axillary fold. This tissue plane includes the subcutaneous and fascia layers. The lower flap is tapered toward the chest wall.

After the flaps have been created, right angle retractors are placed along the edges. The pectoralis muscles are then retracted to expose the axillary vein and its small branches. These are clamped and divided. The axillary vein is ligated with silk sutures. Small branches may require fine suture ligation or surgical clips. The surgeon continues to dissect the axillary tissue to expose the two major nerves in this area (thoracic and intercostobrachial nerves). These nerves must be preserved during node dissection. Vessel loops are placed under the nerves with a right angle clamp. Axillary tissue containing the nodes is then dissected away from the underlying muscle.

Before closing the axilla, the surgeon may place a Jackson-Pratt or Penrose drain in the wound. If a closed suction drain

is used, the end is brought out through a small stab incision near the main incision. The drain is secured with one or two nonabsorbable sutures. The wounds are closed in two layers. The axilla and subcutaneous breast tissue are closed with interrupted absorbable sutures. The skin is closed with running subcuticular sutures of the surgeon's choice.

MASTECTOMY

Surgical Goal

The goal of **mastectomy** is to remove the entire breast. The extent of axillary dissection depends on the cancer stage and other factors:

- In a total (or simple) mastectomy, the entire breast is removed. The axillary lymph nodes are not removed, and the muscles of the chest wall are preserved.
- In a **modified radical mastectomy**, the entire breast is removed, and complete axillary dissection with excision of nodes is performed.
- In a **radical mastectomy** (rarely performed) the entire breast, all axillary nodes, and the chest wall muscles are removed.

Pathology

Subcutaneous mastectomy is performed for primary tumors with clear margins.

TECHNIQUE

1 The skin and subcutaneous tissue are incised in an elliptical pattern.
2 The skin flaps are raised to the previously marked areas and retracted with skin hooks.
3 Lateral edges of the flaps are carried to the edge of the latissimus dorsi muscle.
4 Large perforating blood vessels are ligated and secured.
5 The breast and deep fascia are dissected away from the pectoralis muscle.
6 The specimen is dissected free from the lateral chest wall and axilla.
7 Intercostal arteries and veins are ligated and divided.
8 The axillary flap is raised, preserving the axillary vein and nerves.
9 The axillary tissues are further dissected from the surrounding muscles and ligaments.
10 The specimen is removed.
11 Hemostasis is maintained.
12 Two suction drains are placed in the wound.
13 The ends of the pectoralis minor muscle are sutured together.
14 The flaps are closed with skin staples, subcuticular suture, and sterile adhesive strips.
15 A soft bulky dressing is placed over the wound.

Discussion

Historically, a radical mastectomy (i.e., removal of the breast and chest wall muscles and fascia, as well as complete axillary excision) was the only treatment available for a malignant breast mass. This procedure now is rarely performed. Radical mastectomy has been modified, and it is indicated only for late presentation of chest wall metastasis arising from a primary breast tumor.

To begin the procedure, the surgeon marks both the incision and the extent of the skin flaps. Incising the skin and creating a space between the skin and the underlying tissue creates a **skin flap**. This is called *raising a skin flap*. In this procedure, the skin flaps include subcutaneous tissue. The superior and anterior flaps are extended to the previously marked lines on the skin. Skin hooks are used to elevate the flaps and extend the dissection.

The surgeon uses sharp dissection to carry the flaps deeper to the edge of the latissimus dorsi muscle. The scrub should have two ESU units available so that one can be cleaned while the other is in use. As large blood vessels are encountered, they are ligated with surgical clips and divided or clamped and secured with silk ties. The surgeon separates the breast and fascial tissue from the pectoralis major muscle. The skin flaps are retracted gently to preserve their blood supply and to prevent bruising and ischemia at the edges.

Axillary dissection is a continuous part of this procedure. Rake or Richardson retractors are placed over the axillary edge of the incision. Blunt rakes are preferred to prevent puncturing the skin in this area. An additional right angle retractor or narrow Deaver or Richardson retractor may be needed for the medial side of the incision.

Tributaries of the axillary vein are exposed and cross-clamped with right angle clamps; they are then divided, and clipped or ligated. For level III node dissection, the surgeon must sever the pectoralis minor muscle with the ESU. Retraction of the pectoralis muscles with right angle retractors exposes the axillary tissues. The specimen is dissected from the chest wall and muscles. The apex may be marked with a suture for pathological identification.

The surgeon then may pass the specimen to the scrub, who receives it in a small basin. Before closing the wound, the surgeon places two suction drains in the axilla and brings the ends out at the lateral chest wall. The ends of the pectoralis minor muscle are sutured together with absorbable sutures.

The wound is irrigated with antibacterial solution and closed in layers. Absorbable subcutaneous sutures are placed. The skin is closed with a running subcuticular suture or skin staples, depending on the surgeon's preference.

KEY CONCEPTS

- The surgical technologist must be able to identify abdominal wall structures aid in selecting the correct instruments, suture materials, and surgical devices used in abdominal wall repair and in other general surgery procedures involving the abdomen.
- Pathology related to structural weakness of the abdominal wall contributes to the surgeon's overall strategy for repair, which in turn contributes to the surgical technologist's case planning and implementation.
- The surgical technologist's familiarity with common procedures of the abdominal wall contributes to successful preparation before and anticipation during the surgery.
- Knowledge of key anatomical structures and pathology of the gastrointestinal system contributes to the surgical technologist's ability to anticipate the need for instruments, sutures, and other equipment during the surgical procedure.
- Bowel technique used during intestinal surgery is used to prevent postoperative infection and is a skill in which the surgical technologist is proficient. Other special techniques used in GI surgery include anastamosis of major structures.
- Knowledge of key anatomical structures and procedures of the liver, biliary system, pancreas, and spleen are necessary for case planning and anticipation of the surgeon's needs during a surgical procedure.
- An awareness of breast anatomy and tissue structure is important to selecting the correct instrument during surgery.
- Basic pathology of the breast contributes to the surgical technologist's care of the patient and to case planning.

REVIEW QUESTIONS

Section I: Abdominal Wall Surgery

1. Discuss the importance of knowing the names of the abdominal regions.
2. What is the significance of the linea alba?

3. What are the primary tissues of the abdominal wall?
4. Name five abdominal incisions and the organs associated with them.
5. What is the principle involved in hernia repair with biosynthetic mesh?
6. What is the difference between a direct inguinal hernia and an indirect inguinal hernia?
7. Describe an incarcerated hernia. What causes this condition?
8. Describe how you would dress an infected incisional hernia. List the supplies needed and briefly state why you would use them.

Section II: Gastrointestinal Surgery

1. Why are compression stockings used during lengthy procedures?
2. Describe bowel technique and why it is used.
3. When a patient is positioned for bariatric surgery, what special safety precautions are practiced?
4. What is the principle of Nissen fundoplication surgery?
5. Study the bowel instruments listed in this chapter. What are the common design features of grasping and clamping instruments?
6. Define *anastomosis, resection,* and *mobilization.* List several instruments used in these techniques.
7. What is a bowel obstruction?
8. What is a stoma?

Section III: Surgery of the Biliary System, Liver, Pancreas, and Spleen

1. Why is the spleen removed rather than repaired after severe trauma?
2. Why do esophageal varices form in advanced cirrhosis?
3. What structure drains bile after a cholecystectomy?
4. What procedure has replaced operative cholangiography in modern surgical practice?
5. What are the surgical priorities in emergency surgery for a ruptured spleen?

6. Review and explain the preparation of Avitene, Surgicel, and Gelfoam for use in a surgical wound.
7. Which handheld retractors might be used to retract the liver during gallbladder surgery?
8. Why is it dangerous for bile to spill into the abdominal cavity during gallbladder surgery?

Section IV: Breast Surgery

1. Why do women have more options for breast cancer surgery now than they did 20 years ago?
2. What is BSE?
3. What is the difference between needle aspiration and stereotactic biopsy?
4. Why is dye used during sentinel node biopsy?
5. Why is the arm of the affected side draped free during many breast procedures?
6. Describe how you would handle and maintain a breast biopsy sample for frozen section.
7. What is the principle of sentinel node biopsy?
8. What retractors should be available for tissue-sparing mastectomy?
9. Why is the ESU not used for dissection of a breast tumor?

BIBLIOGRAPHY

Bland KI, Copeland EM: *The breast: comprehensive management of benign and malignant disorders,* ed 3, Philadelphia, 2004, WB Saunders.

Murray SS, McKinney ES, Gorrie TM: *Foundations of maternal-newborn nursing,* ed 3, Philadelphia, 2002, WB Saunders.

Porth CM, Kunert MP: *Pathophysiology: concepts of altered health states,* ed 6, Philadelphia, 2002, Lippincott Williams & Williams.

Rothrock JC: *Alexander's care of the patient in surgery,* ed 13, St Louis, 2007, Mosby.

Thibodeau G, Patton K: *Anatomy and physiology,* ed 6, St Louis, 2007, Mosby.

Townsend C: *Sabiston textbook of surgery,* ed 17, Philadelphia, 2004, WB Saunders.

Minimally Invasive Endoscopic and Robotic-Assisted Surgery

24

CHAPTER OUTLINE

LEARNING OBJECTIVES

After studying this chapter the reader will be able to:

1. Discuss the advantages and constraints of minimally invasive surgery (MIS)
2. Describe the preparation of the patient for MIS
3. Describe the function of each component of the imaging equipment used in MIS
4. Discuss the care of a rigid endoscope
5. Describe the surgical technique used for insufflation in laparoscopy
6. List the risks associated with insufflation
7. Describe the trocar-cannula system used in all MIS
8. Describe the specific electrosurgical risks of direct and capacitive coupling
9. Describe the structure and function of a flexible endoscope
10. Discuss the proper protocol for processing rigid and flexible endoscopes
11. Describe the principles of robotic surgery
12. Discuss the concept of cartesian geometry as it applies to robot design
13. Describe robotic movements and classification
14. Discuss training resources for robotic surgery
15. List the three main components of robotic surgery and describe their function
16. Identify possible methods of decontaminating and reprocessing robotic instruments
17. Describe the roles of team members during robotic surgery

TERMINOLOGY

Active electrode monitoring (AEM): A method of reducing the risk of patient burns during monopolar electrosurgery. AEM systems stop the electrical current whenever resistance is high anywhere in the circuit.

Arthroscopy: Endoscopic surgery of a joint.

Auxiliary water channel: A channel in the flexible endoscope used to deliver irrigation fluid at the tip.

Biopsy channel: A channel that extends the full length of a flexible endoscope and is used to retrieve biopsy tissue.

Camera control unit (CCU): The main control source for the video camera. The unit captures video signals from the camera head and processes them for display on the image system.

Cannula: In minimally invasive surgery, a cannula is a slender tube inserted through the body wall that is used to receive and stabilize telescopic instruments.

Capacitive coupling: In minimally invasive surgery, the unintended transmission of electricity from the active electrode to an adjacent conductive pathway, sometimes resulting in a patient burn.

Control head: The proximal section of a flexible endoscope where the controls are located.

Diagnostic endoscopy: A diagnostic procedure in which a long, flexible, fiberoptic tube is inserted into a body cavity for viewing and diagnosis.

Digital output recorder: During video-assisted surgery, digital signals are captured from the video camera and transmitted to an image system. The digital output recorder processes these signals.

Direct coupling: In minimally invasive surgery, the transmission of electricity directly from one conductive path to another, such as from the active electrode to a conductive instrument.

Docking: In robotic surgery, the process of positioning the robotic instruments in the exact location over the patient so that instruments can be safely attached to their ports in the body cavity.

Elevator channel: A channel that extends the full length of a flexible endoscope and receives biopsy forceps or other instruments.

TERMINOLOGY (cont.)

Endocoupler: A device that connects the endoscope to the camera.

Extracorporeal: A term meaning "outside the body." In minimally invasive surgery, it refers to a technique for placing sutures in which the knots are formed outside the body and then tightened after they have been introduced into the surgical wound.

Gain: In electronics, the intensity of the signal.

Haptic feedback: Tactile feedback, conveyed from tissue to the hand when a hand instrument is used. Robotic instruments do not provide any tactile feedback.

High definition (HD): A type of video format. The clarity of the image is based on the number of signals (pixels) emitted by the camera. HD format has a 16:9 aspect ratio, which is 7 times greater than standard definition.

Imaging system: The combined components of the endoscopic system, which create the image captured in the focal view of the endoscope.

Insertion tube: The long, narrow portion of the flexible endoscope that is inserted into the body.

Instrument channel: A channel that extends the full length of a flexible endoscope and receives instruments during flexible endoscopy.

Insufflation: In minimally invasive surgery, inflation of the abdominal or thoracic cavity with carbon dioxide gas.

Intracorporeal: A term meaning "inside the body." In minimally invasive surgery, it refers to a suture technique in which sutures are knotted and secured inside the patient.

Intravasation: The unintended absorption of irrigation fluids into the body.

Knot pusher: A device used to secure suture knots during minimally invasive surgery.

Ligation loop: A commercially prepared suture loop used to secure structures during minimally invasive surgery.

Light cable: The fiberoptic light cable that transmits light from the source to the endoscopic instrument; sometimes called a *light guide.*

Light source: A device that controls and emits light for endoscopic procedures.

Master controllers: In robotic surgery, the nonsterile hand controls that manipulate surgical instruments.

Optical angle: The angle at which light is transmitted at the distal end of a fiberoptic or video endoscope.

Pixel: An element in each silicon chip contained within a device that produces electronic images such as those seen on a surgical image system used in minimally invasive surgery.

Pneumoperitoneum: An abdomen insufflated or distended with carbon dioxide gas during laparoscopy.

Resectoscope: A surgical endoscope that has the capability of morcellation, or tissue fragmentation.

Robot: A mechanical device that can be programmed to perform tasks.

Standard definition (SD): A type of video format. The clarity of an image is based on the number of signals (pixels) emitted by the camera. A standard definition format displays 640 × 480 pixels in a rectangular image.

Stereoscopic viewer: In robotic surgery, the binocular lens system of the surgeon console.

Telesurgery: A type of robotic surgery in which surgery is performed from a nearby location through computer-mediated instruments. In telesurgery, no direct physical contact with the instruments occurs.

Veress needle: A spring-loaded needle used to deliver carbon dioxide gas during insufflation.

Video cable: In video-assisted endoscopy, the cable that transmits digital data from the camera head to the camera control unit and from the image system to the output recorder.

Video printer: A device that stores and prints output data viewed through the video endoscope.

White balance: A procedure for adjusting the light color of the video camera to other components of the system.

INTRODUCTION

Endoscopic or minimally invasive surgery is performed by inserting instruments into the body through small narrow incisions or a natural body orifice. Although this technique has been available for several decades, the advances in biotechnology of the past 10 years have enabled this surgical technique to be used in many surgical specialties.

Two types of endoscopic systems are discussed in this chapter:

- **Minimally invasive surgery (MIS)** is performed using a rigid lensed telescope and long instruments, which are introduced into small incisions at the operative site. In this technique, the operative space may be enlarged with fluid or carbon dioxide. The goal of the minimally invasive technique is primarily surgical rather than diagnostic (Figure 24-1).

- **Diagnostic endoscopy** and operative endoscopy usually are performed with a flexible, semirigid, or rigid endoscope that is inserted into a natural orifice in the body. The lens system, channels for introducing small instruments, and light system are contained in one long tube. Flexible endoscopy is used to assess the regional anatomy, to obtain tissue biopsies, and to perform minor surgical procedures (Figure 24-2). The rigid endoscope is used to perform a surgical assessment and operative procedures, such as transurethral resection of the prostate and transcervical resection of a uterine fibroid tumor.

Terminology in the field of MIS and endoscopy is evolving along with the rapid technological advances in systems and instruments. In general, the term *telescopic instruments* refers to the rigid lensed instrument used in MIS. The term *endoscope* is used to describe the flexible lensed instrument that is

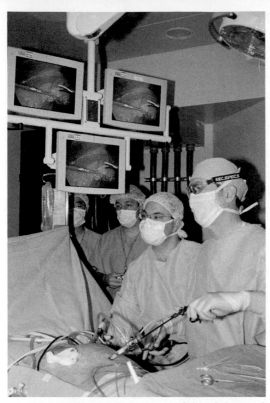

Figure 24-1 Minimally invasive surgery of the abdomen (laparoscopy). A lensed telescope with camera and long instruments are introduced into small incisions. The camera image is projected to a central monitor. (©2012 Photo courtesy of KARL STORZ Endoscopy-America, Inc.)

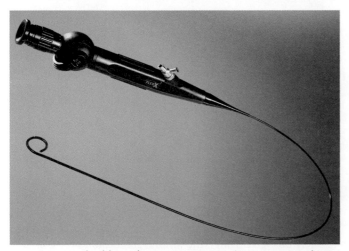

Figure 24-2 Flexible endoscopy. (©2012 Photo courtesy of KARL STORZ Endoscopy-America, Inc.)

passed through a natural orifice for assessment or surgery of a hollow organ, duct, or vessel.

SECTION I: MINIMALLY INVASIVE SURGERY

PRINCIPLES OF MINIMALLY INVASIVE SURGERY

Minimally invasive surgery is a technique in which telescopic (long, narrow) instruments are introduced into the body

through one or more small incisions in which a narrow tube called a **cannula** has been inserted. The cannula is inserted through the body wall with the aid of a sharp trocar, which fits inside the cannula and is slightly advanced beyond the tip of the cannula. This is referred to as a trocar-cannula system. Some systems use a blunt obturator in place of the trocar. The trocar or obturator punctures the body wall and leads the cannula into position. The trocar or obturator is then withdrawn, leaving only the cannula, which remains in place throughout the surgery and receives the telescopic surgical instruments. The cannula in place is referred to as a **port**. The cannulas protect the body wall and also maintain a seal between the inside of the body and the outside environment. To perform surgery inside the body, the surgeon inserts a slender optical telescope through one of the cannulas. The image seen through the endoscope is projected and enlarged onto one or more flat screen image systems. Surgery is performed by adjusting the endoscope to obtain different views and by manipulating the telescopic instruments as they appear on the screen. The components of the system include the telescope, fiberoptic light source and cables, image system, data capturing system, and data output recorder. These are explained later in the chapter.

Advanced optical and digital technology has expanded the use of minimally invasive techniques to many surgical specialties. The principles of MIS are the same across all specialties. Common techniques are discussed briefly in this chapter and in more detail in the chapters on surgical procedures. Box 24-1 lists commonly performed minimally invasive surgical procedures by specialty.

MIS requires telescopic instruments that are inserted through one or more small incisions directly or through a cannula. Because the operative site is not exposed through an incision in the skin, an imaging system is required in all types of endoscopy and MIS. Electronic digital technology is used for transmitting images from the telescope to the image system.

Exposure (ability to see the anatomy) of the surgical site differs according to the specialty. Because the instruments are located within tightly enclosed tissue planes or spaces, a method of expanding the space is needed to safely operate. During laparoscopy, the abdominal cavity is filled with carbon dioxide, which balloons the body wall outward. This process is called **insufflation**. In **arthroscopy** (MIS of the joint spaces), the anatomical space is filled with irrigation fluid. Hollow organs, such as the bladder, are filled with saline or other isotonic fluids during endoscopy. In some anatomical regions, such as the inguinal area, a balloon dissector may be used to separate dense tissue planes without causing trauma.

All MIS procedures require electrosurgery or other energies, such as high-frequency cutting and coagulation devices, for hemostasis and tissue dissection. Electrosurgical techniques and the risks associated with them are described in this chapter and in Chapter 18.

TYPES OF MIS

Five basic types of MIS are now commonly used. With the advent of microchip technology in surgical devices, newer

Box **24-1** Common Minimally Invasive Surgery Procedures by Specialty

General Surgery and Gastroenterology
Adrenalectomy
Appendectomy
Esophagectomy
Gallbladder procedures
Gastrectomy
Gastric reflux procedures
Hernia repair
Intestinal resection
Lymph node biopsy
Pancreatectomy
Parathyroidectomy
Pyloromyotomy
Splenectomy

Gynecology
Excision of fibroids
Exploratory laparotomy
Hysterectomy
Ovarian cystectomy
Radical hysterectomy for uterine cancer
Removal of fibroids
Repair of vesicle vaginal fistula
Tubal ligation
Uterine artery embolization for fibroids

Orthopedic Surgery
Ablation of bone tumor
Arthroscopy
Carpel tunnel release
Endoscopic spine surgery
Fracture of the pelvis
Periarticular and intraarticular fractures of the extremities
Rotator cuff repair
Shoulder instability repair
Spinal decompression
Spinal fixation
Total hip replacement

Unicompartmental knee replacement
Vertebroplasty

Thoracic Surgery
Fundoplication for gastroesophageal reflux
Lung procedures
Myotomy for achalasia
Repair of hiatal hernia
Thoracic sympathectomy

Cardiac Procedures
Atrial septal defect
Coronary artery bypass graft (CABG)
Mitral and tricuspid valve procedures
CABG (off pump)
Patent foramen ovale

Otorhinolaryngology
Removal of nasal and sinus tumors
Sentinel lymph node biopsy for head and neck tumors
Sinus surgery
Transcatheter laser treatment of vascular malformations
Transoral laser resection of peripharyngeal/laryngeal tumors

Vascular Surgery
Ablation of varicose veins
Balloon angioplasty and carotid stenting
Renal and peripheral artery stenting
Repair of abdominal and thoracic aortic aneurysms

Urology
Cystic decortication
Diagnosis and removal of kidney stones
Endoscopic exploration of the urinary tract
Endoscopic tumor biopsy
Nephrectomy
Prostatectomy
Pyeloplasty
Treatment for strictures and tumors of the urinary tract

categories of MIS have emerged and those that have been used for the last few decades have been greatly improved in technology, patient safety, and surgical outcome. The multiple port technique is still the most common technique for gaining access to the surgical site. There are now several important categories of MIS with which the technologist should be familiar.

Multiple-Incision MIS
This is the traditional method and the one most commonly used for MIS. One port receives the camera and up to four others are placed for surgical instruments.

Single-Incision Laparoscopic Surgery
Single-incision laparoscopic surgery (SILS) is one of the newer techniques in MIS, although it was used in tubal ligation procedures in the 1970s. It is also known as *single-port access* (SPA) and *one-port umbilical surgery* (OPUS). In this

technique, a single small incision is made at the base of the umbilicus, and a large-bore flexible port with three subports is placed in the abdominal wall. Because the tissue layers at the umbilicus are relatively uncomplicated, the single port can be safely pushed through the umbilical incision, where it stays during the procedure. Instruments and camera are threaded through the instrument ports as needed. The disadvantage of this system is the tight working space on the field. The technique has been safely used for gastric, intestinal, gallbladder, and other uncomplicated procedures.

Video-Assisted Thoracoscopic Surgery
Video-assisted thoracoscopic surgery (VATS) is not a new technique, but because of its ability to enter smaller spaces of the body, its use has expanded to include pathology not only of the thoracic cavity but also of the anterior thoracic and lumbar spine. The indications for VATS are the same as for thoracotomy, but recovery is much faster, with

less postoperative pain and a shorter hospital stay. VATS allows entry into the chest cavity without sacrificing a rib and rib spreading, both of which are extremely painful postoperatively.

Natural Orifice Transluminal Endoscopic Surgery

The natural orifice transluminal endoscopic surgery (NOTES) technique is relatively new. It involves endoscopic entry of the body through a natural orifice and then making an incision within the body to gain further access to the pathology. Current techniques are under development for transvaginal and transgastric procedures. The technique has some advantages over traditional endoscopic procedures as patients seek better cosmetic results with less risk for postoperative infection.

Robotic Surgery

Robotic surgery, which is discussed later in the chapter, incorporates the multiple-port system with robotic technology in which the surgeon operates from a nonsterile console to perform the surgery, after the ports have been placed and the camera and instruments are connected to the robotic interface. The camera and surgical instruments are controlled from the console. The surgical assistant and scrub engage the sterile instruments into the robotic interface as needed while the surgeon remains at the console to perform the surgery. At the completion of the procedure, the instruments are withdrawn from their ports, and the surgeon resumes a sterile role to close the incisions.

ADVANTAGES AND DISADVANTAGES OF MINIMALLY INVASIVE SURGERY

ADVANTAGES

MIS has many advantages over open surgery. Powerful high quality optical systems allow the surgeon to perform delicate procedures while viewing the surgical site on a video monitor, which enlarges the field of view and allows all members of the team to see the operative area. Telescopic instruments used in MIS are very small and capable of powerful hemostatic and cutting modalities. Most of these instruments can perform the same tasks as standard instruments. Open surgery generally requires a longer healing time than MIS because of the increased tissue trauma involved in entering the operative site. Patients undergoing MIS are able to resume normal activities sooner, and the hospital stay is shorter. Many types of MIS are performed in the outpatient setting, which is convenient and often less costly.

In summary, the advantages are:
- Reduced tissue trauma
- Less blood loss
- Less pain
- Faster recovery and return to normal activities
- Can be done as outpatient surgery in many cases
- Reduced postoperative pain
- Increased patient satisfaction
- Less costly

DISADVANTAGES

Not all patients are suitable for MIS. Patients who have undergone previous abdominal procedures have a high risk of *abdominal adhesions* (scarring of organs that causes adherence to the peritoneal wall). This presents a risk of perforation as the trocar and cannula are advanced through the body wall. Other risks are related to the technology and the patient's medical condition coming into surgery. Two areas of particular concern are the use of gas to create a pneumoperitoneum and the fluid distention of body cavities, necessary in specific types of surgery. These are discussed in detail later in the chapter. Unintentional perforation of abdominal viscera is the most common complication in abdominal laparoscopic surgery. Other significant risks are equipment failure and thermal injury related to the use of electrosurgery, laser, and ultrasound technologies.

The technique used in MIS requires long delicate instruments. Consequently, leverage is reduced, and the tactile feedback is different from that with standard instruments. Endoscopic instruments are limited in their range of motion (except those used in robotic surgeries, which are multidirectional). Withdrawing and inserting them into body cavities is sometimes awkward. The operating space is very small, which reduces maneuverability and may lengthen the duration of a procedure.

The image seen through the telescope is projected onto an image system. Although the technologies used in MIS provide high resolution and excellent color, they are subject to distortion from either an error in the electronic system or mechanical problems with the instruments. As with all medical devices, personnel must be familiar with the equipment used in MIS, including how it works and what to do in case of failure. A disadvantage of MIS is the need for advanced and continuous training for all perioperative staff members. Surgical technologists need to be current on advances in the technology to provide the safest environment for the patient.

In summary, the limitations of MIS are:
- Highly advanced technological features require steep learning curves for new perioperative staff members, including surgeons.
- Vision system errors and failures can result in sudden surgical complications.
- MIS instruments and equipment are expensive to lease, purchase, and maintain.
- Instruments have limited range of motion.
- Some procedures take longer than open surgery.
- The operative site is projected as a two-dimensional picture rather than the natural three-dimensional view of the eye.

PREOPERATIVE PREPARATION AND PATIENT SAFETY

Patients undergoing endoscopic MIS are prepared according to the anatomical location of the surgery. Preoperative preparation for an MIS procedure follows the same or similar protocols as open surgery, with additional attention to risks associated with MIS technology.

PATIENT POSITIONING

The positions used for MIS procedures depend on the surgical site and the patient's physiological condition. In general, patient positioning for MIS is identical to that for open surgery. However, some MIS procedures require a steep pitch in the operating table—into Trendelenburg or reverse Trendelenburg. Extreme positions used to displace the abdominal viscera can increase risks associated with pressure such as nerve and vascular damage and hypotension.

- *Upper abdomen or lower esophagus:* The patient is placed in reverse Trendelenburg position to displace abdominal viscera. A padded footboard is used to prevent the patient from sliding downward. Changes in table position intraoperatively require immediate attention to patient safety. The scrub must adjust the Mayo stand and any other overhead tables to ensure that the new position does not create pressure points between the patient and the underside of the Mayo tray.
- *Pelvic or lower abdominal procedures:* The patient is placed in the Trendelenburg position. This can compromise the patient's lung capacity and cause hypotension from increased pressure on the vena cava. A gynecological patient is placed in the lithotomy position, which exposes the patient to risks associated with popliteal nerve and vessel injury. In steep Trendelenburg position, there is a danger of the patient sliding toward the head of the table. In the past, shoulder braces were routinely used to prevent this. However, shoulder braces can cause significant injury and are used only when necessary with careful attention to pressure on the brachial plexus.
- *Thoracoscopy and nephroscopy:* Procedures of the lungs, bronchi, and upper urinary tract are performed with the patient in the lateral position.
- *Laryngoscopy, bronchoscopy, esophagoscopy, and mediastinoscopy:* Procedures of the upper airway, upper gastrointestinal tract, and mediastinum are performed with the patient in the supine position, although a conscious patient undergoing bronchoscopy may be placed in the Fowler position.

SKIN PREP AND DRAPING

The skin prep and draping techniques used for minimally invasive procedures allow for the possibility of conversion to an open case. This is particularly true for laparoscopic, retroperitoneal, and thoracoscopic surgery, which are more likely to be converted than other types of surgery. Draping is extended to match the prep area needed for an open incision, as discussed in Chapter 20. An indwelling urinary catheter is usually placed before laparoscopy (MIS of the abdomen or pelvic cavity) and in other selected cases according to the patient's condition.

MAINTAINING PATIENT NORMOTHERMIA

The use of carbon dioxide and fluid technology for distention of body cavities presents a risk of hypothermia. Carbon dioxide rapidly cools as it fills the abdominal space, and this can significantly lower the patient's core temperature. Fluid distention used in other body cavities such as the bladder, uterus, and joint spaces may have the same effect. Carbon dioxide pumps are equipped with a warming feature, which must be monitored carefully. Fluids for distention are warmed before instillation. Normal means for maintaining core temperature are also employed during MIS. These include the use of warm air blankets, limiting body exposure to a minimum, and attention to physiological monitoring.

ENDOSCOPIC SETUP

During surgery, the scrub should keep endoscopic instruments in a rack on the instrument table. This maintains them safely and helps the scrub identify them quickly. Always separate endoscopic instruments to protect them from damage by heavier equipment. Telescopes in particular should be maintained on a towel or other soft surface to prevent them from rolling off the table. If a warm water thermos is used for prewarming, it should be kept in an area of the instrument table where it will not be jarred or knocked over.

Nonpenetrating clamps must be used to secure cords and tubing to drapes. This prevents damage to fiberoptic and camera cables. Always allow sufficient slack on cord attachments and be alert to changes in table position, which can cause cords to be dragged.

Cable and cord connections differ according to the type of endoscopic equipment used. *The scrub should be familiar with the facility's equipment before participating as a solo scrub.* A dry run of equipment is a necessary part of learning endoscopic and MIS procedures.

When passing an instrument to the surgeon, always orient the instrument so that the working tip points downward. The scrub may help position the instrument into a cannula. In robotic-assisted MIS, the scrub helps lock the instrument into the robotic arm.

During MIS, the room lights usually are dimmed or powered off. One of the operating lights should be positioned over the instrument table to help the scrub identify and prepare instruments and supplies. This prevents errors and accidents.

CONVERSION TO AN OPEN CASE

Any minimally invasive procedure has the potential to become an open case. In MIS involving body cavities (e.g., laparoscopy and pelvic and thoracic surgery), preparations are made to include the possibility of *open surgery.* Operative permits are signed with this consideration, and any equipment needed to convert to an open case must be prepared and made immediately available. Some surgeries are scheduled and planned to include both MIS and open stages.

Regardless of whether the conversion is an emergency, it is performed very rapidly. Preoperative planning reduces the risk of accident. When the MIS procedure is planned, the scrub and circulator consult the surgeon's preference card for an open procedure. Sterile supplies are collected and located where they can be retrieved and opened within minutes of the decision to convert to an open case. Accidents with equipment occur when personnel rush through the procedure without previous planning.

During conversion to an open case, the scrub must communicate directly with the circulator to make sure all cords and tubing are free. Camera cords and fiberoptic cables must be protected from injury during the conversion to an open case. These can become tangled in the drapes or fall to the floor when disconnected. Deliberate and purposeful actions help protect equipment during the conversion.

Instruments are quickly exchanged and endoscopic instruments carefully put aside. Standard operating instruments are delivered to the surgical table, and the scrub prepares for immediate incision while receiving other equipment from the circulator. Suction, electrosurgical instruments, and sharps are delivered first so that the open procedure can begin without delay. Sponges, instruments, and sharps are counted as distributed as in all cases.

TECHNIQUES AND EQUIPMENT USED IN MINIMALLY INVASIVE SURGERY

Equipment used in MIS, including robotics, requires a high level of technical knowledge and attention to detail. The devices are complex and require planning and preparation before use. The surgical technologist may be responsible for troubleshooting and setup of the imaging equipment. Responsibility for devices used in insufflation, fluid distention, and continuous irrigation may be shared with the registered nurse circulator and anesthesia care provider. Unless the operating room uses a designated integrated suite in which all components such as the imaging system, electrosurgical, and other power units are stationary or built into the room system, these must be carefully arranged so that cords and connecting cables are protected from damage and moisture. The specific arrangement of equipment must provide a safe environment and adhere to principles of aseptic technique. Safety features and precautions related to equipment are presented here. These must be adapted to individual operating room systems.

IMAGING SYSTEM

Endoscopic MIS is dependent on the collective functioning of the imaging components (Figure 24-3). A malfunction in any one component affects the others and may reduce patient safety. The components of the **imaging system** include:

- Light source
- Light cable
- Surgical telescope (or endoscope)
- Camera head
- Camera control unit (CCU)

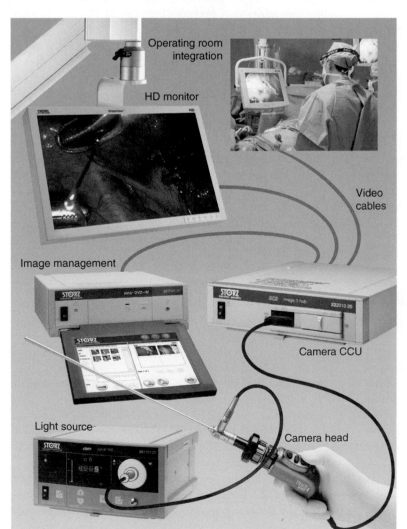

Figure 24-3 **Imaging components used in minimally invasive surgery.** Imaging begins with the telescope; the xenon light source is connected to the endoscope by a fiberoptic cable. The camera head reads the images and transmits them to the camera control unit (CCU). From there the images are transmitted to an image management unit, which can produce digital files of the images. The CCU also transmits digital images to the high-definition (HD) monitor, which is necessary to view the operative field. Further imaging is provided to other monitors or information systems through an integrated operating room system. (©2012 Photo courtesy of KARL STORZ Endoscopy-America, Inc.)

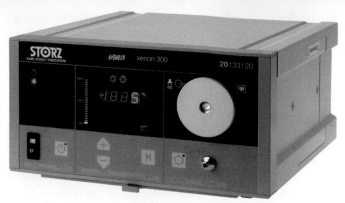

Figure 24-4 Fiberoptic light source. The xenon light source provides light to the telescope via a fiberoptic cable. (©2012 Photo courtesy of KARL STORZ Endoscopy-America, Inc.)

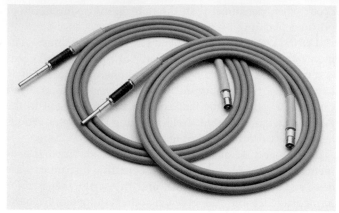

Figure 24-5 Fiberoptic cable connecting the light source to the endoscope. (©2012 Photo courtesy of KARL STORZ Endoscopy-America, Inc.)

- Video cables
- Monitor screen
- Image management system

Light Source and Fiberoptic Cable

The **light source** transmits light to the fiberoptic **light cable** and telescope (Figure 24-4). The light source control panel is used to adjust the modes and light intensity. The light is transmitted from bulbs, which are fitted inside the unit. The control panel permits variable adjustments in light intensity, and an infrared filtering system allows the use of lower wattage bulbs. The automatic mode of the light source controls the brightness of the image. However, if more light is required, the **gain** (the signal intensity) is increased rather than the light intensity.

High-resolution video endoscopy requires very intense white light. Xenon lamps therefore are preferred. Many types and models of light sources are available, but most are similar in design and operation.

The light emitted from the telescope is cool as long as the light cable is attached to the telescope. *Light rays emitted from the end of the cable when it is detached from the telescope are extremely hot.* The lighted end of a cable can ignite drapes, sponges, and other materials, especially in the presence of flammable or ignitable liquids such as alcohol.

NOTE: *Always turn the light source to its lowest or standby mode before disconnecting it from the telescope or light cable.*

The fiberoptic light cable (Figure 24-5) transmits light from the light source to the camera head or telescope. The cable is composed of many thousands of glass or plastic fibers, which are aligned in parallel longitudinal bundles. These fiberoptic bundles are delicate and easily broken by sharp impact or overflexing of the cable. The fiberoptic cable is securely attached to the light source on the control panel. Because cables of one manufacturer or model are often used with a different model light source, an adaptor may be needed at the connecting point. Adaptors must be available and in place before surgery.

CARE AND SAFETY OF CABLES The care of fiberoptic cables is illustrated in Figure 24-6.

- Handle fiberoptic cables gently. When storing or transporting the cable, coil it loosely. Do not hang the cable; instead, store it in a flat position.
- Do not allow the cable to strike a hard surface. This can cause the fiberoptic bundles to fracture. Internal fractures are not visible from the outside.
- Inspect cables for exterior damage before using them.
- Power off the light source before connecting or disconnecting the cable. This prevents inadvertent contact between the beam and ignitable materials.
- Do not handle light source bulbs with bare skin. Skin oils can reduce the life span of the bulb.
- Attach the light cable with care. The cable may require an adaptor to fit the light source.
- Keep bulb replacements for the power source on hand. Xenon light sources have bulbs that have a finite life, and replacements must be immediately available during surgery.
- Clean and reprocess the cable according to the manufacturer's directions.

Rigid Telescope

The telescope contains the serial lens system, which captures the images illuminated at the tip. Light is transmitted to the telescope through the fiberoptic cable, which attaches near the *eyepiece* (Figure 24-7).

The optical features and dimensions of the telescopes are:
- **Optical angle**: The direction in which lenses are focused on the image. This is measured in degrees, usually 0, 30, 45, and 70 degrees.
- *Diameter*: The diameter of the telescope shaft, measured in millimeters (mm).
- *Length*: The length of the telescope shaft, measured in millimeters.

GUIDELINES FOR HANDLING TELESCOPES Telescopes are delicate and expensive. Malfunction or damage to the instrument can cause patient injury and increased surgical time.

The surgical technologist is responsible for handling and maintaining the telescope in a manner that prevents these errors. The following recommendations are guidelines only.

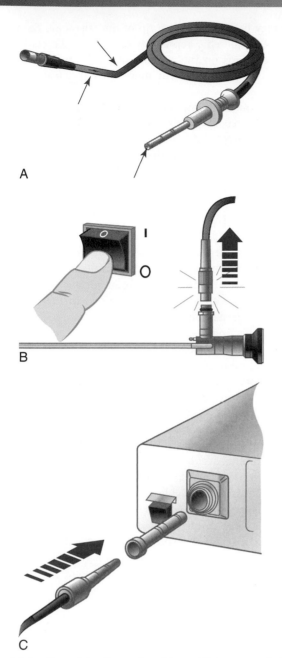

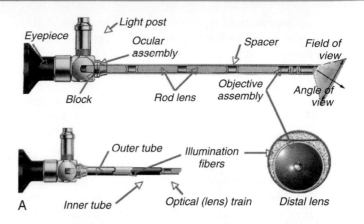

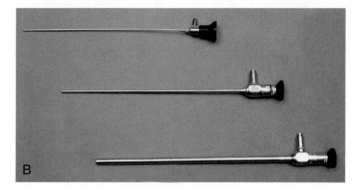

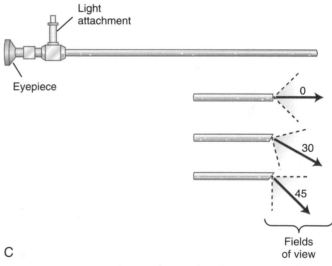

Figure 24-6 Care of the fiberoptic cable and light source. **A,** Fiberoptic light cable: Do not use a cable that is damaged. Look for cuts, nicks, and indentations in the insulation. Make sure the appropriate adaptor tip is used. **B,** Power off the light source. Make sure the power switch is OFF before connecting or disconnecting the light cable. **C,** Cable adaptor and plug. Make sure the proper adaptor is used when attaching the cable plug to the power source. *(Courtesy Olympus America, Center Valley, Pa.)*

Figure 24-7 **A,** Inner lenses of a rigid endoscope. **B,** Endoscope length: 2 mm, 5 mm, and 10 mm. **C,** Lens angles are available at 0 degrees, 30 degrees, and 45 degrees. *(**A** ©2012 Photo courtesy of KARL STORZ Endoscopy-America, Inc.; **B** from Goldberg JM, Falcone T: Atlas of endoscopic techniques in gynecology, Philadelphia, 2001, WB Saunders; and **C** redrawn from Phillips N: Berry and Kohn's operating room technique, ed 10, St Louis, 2004, Mosby.)*

The manufacturer's manual should be consulted for specific detailed care.

- *Always hold the telescope by its head (heavier) end, never by the tip or shaft.* When the telescope is held by the lighter end, the weight of the headpiece can bend the shaft and damage the instrument.
- *Take care to prevent scratches or dents in the shaft of the telescope.* Contact with heavy instruments or sharps can easily damage the delicate optical system and insulation.

- *Use only lint-free, soft material to wipe the telescope.* Some woven materials can cause minute scratches on the lens and surface of the instrument. These can lead to blurring and distortion of the transmitted image. Do not allow oils to come in contact with the lens surface.
- *Never assume that the telescope has been checked for damage by others.* Everyone who handles endoscopic

equipment, from reprocessing to end user stage, has an equal responsibility to ensure the integrity of the instruments. It is the particular duty of the scrub to deliver a safe, properly working telescope to the surgeon (Figure 24-8).

- *Prevent lens fogging during surgery.* When the telescope is introduced into the body, the temperature difference creates fogging on the telescope lens. To prevent fogging, the telescope may be maintained in a warm water bath before use. Defogging agents may also be used on the lens before use. Be sure to dry the lens to before handing it to the surgeon to ensure that there is no distortion resulting from defogging. During surgery, check the lens for a clear view by visually looking through it.

Video Camera

The video camera receives visual data from the telescope and allows the surgeon to view structures without looking directly into the telescope. Modern surgical video cameras contain one or three solid-state silicon chips, which produce electrical signals that are amplified and displayed on a digital monitor. Three-chip cameras produce natural color images, which is important to the identification of pathology. Video chips are located in the camera head, or, in some newer models,

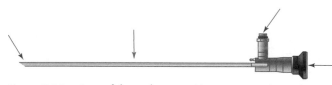

Figure 24-8 Care of the endoscope. Always inspect the endoscope for any nicks or dents. The shaft must be straight to prevent damage to the internal lenses on insertion. *(Courtesy © Olympus, America, Inc.)*

they may be located at the tip of the telescope. Each silicon element in the chip represents one **pixel**. The clarity of the image depends on the number of pixels (signals) or silicon units the chip contains. The more units, the clearer the image appears.

Image quality is derived from the quality of the optics, the lighting source, and the electronic capabilities of the system. The circuit used in video endoscopy is called a *charge-coupled device* (CCD). This allows the electrical charges (signals) to be converted into pixels or picture elements. These are related to colors, and each pixel is stored and recovered separately. Some CCD systems can support more than 65,000 colors. Systems that process a higher number of pixels have excellent resolution, even when lighting is very dim.

The video format is the manner in which a video signal transmits information. Individual cameras can use specific formats, and this information is important to the camera's compatibility with other components in the system. Always check the compatibility of the camera with the video system when connecting them.

An important aspect of the video format is the horizontal-to-vertical ratio of the pixels. This contributes to the clarity and resolution of objects transmitted to the monitor. The **standard definition (SD)** format has an aspect ratio of 4:3, which represents 640×480 pixels per vertical line. The **high definition (HD)** format has a 16:9 aspect ratio, which is 7 times greater than SD.

COMPONENTS OF THE CAMERA HEAD Numerous styles of camera heads are available, but most have common components (Figure 24-9). The telescope mount or coupler connects to the telescope through a coupler, lever, or slide control. The *focus ring* clarifies the endoscopic image. The camera head

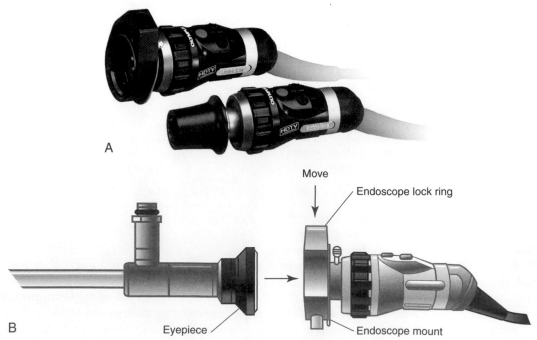

Figure 24-9 A, Camera heads. Note the couplers, which connect the camera to the endoscope. **B,** Camera head with endocoupler. *(Courtesy © Olympus, America, Inc.)*

may have other options, such as white balancing and VCR controls. The **endocoupler** connects the camera to the telescope and is specific to the type of camera and scope in use. Some telescopes allow direct viewing without a coupler. Options for viewing the surgical site include monitor only or a combination of viewing through the telescope with projection to a monitor.

CARE OF THE CAMERA HEAD The camera head is delicate and must be handled with care. Always follow the manufacturer's instructions for assembly, reprocessing, and compatibility with other components of the vision system. Following some basic guidelines can help prolong the life of the camera and prevent breakdown during surgery:

- Hold the camera firmly when transporting it.
- When connecting and disconnecting the camera head, make sure the lock ring is disengaged. Also make sure the camera is firmly attached to the lock ring after engaging.
- When connecting the eyepiece, make sure it is firmly engaged. Never try to force or twist these connections together. They should connect smoothly and easily.
- Connect the camera and video plug only when the system is powered off. Do not disengage these plugs with power on.
- When connecting the camera head to the camera control center, do not bend or twist the camera cable. All connections must be dry before connection.
- Disconnect the camera cable by grasping the plug, not the cable.
- After connecting the camera head to the telescope and camera control unit, make sure the light is clearly emitted and is not flickering.
- Focus adjustment is made before surgery. Do not repeatedly turn the camera head, because this can cause damage. Make sure the mount is locked during focusing.

WHITE BALANCE All cameras must be white-balanced before each procedure. This is a procedure to adjust the light color to the other components in the system. To white-balance the camera, connect the light cable to the telescope and power up the light on high (or according to the manufacturer's specification). Direct the lens of the telescope at a solid white object (it is preferable to avoid using porous or woven material, such as a surgical sponge, because this can cause shadows on the image). The **white balance** usually is registered automatically by the light source.

Camera Control Unit

The **camera control unit (CCU)** is the receptacle (socket) for the camera. It contains the controls for light intensity, white balance, and resolution (Figure 24-10). It also receives connections to the power mains and video output remote control. The unit captures video signals from the camera head and processes them for display on the monitor. A computer keyboard may be used in controlling the video display and other functions. The CCU should be able to convert SD to HD signals or vice versa so that images from one format can be viewed by another.

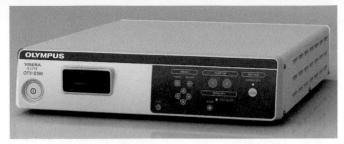

Figure 24-10 Camera control unit. *(Courtesy © Olympus, America, Inc.)*

Video Cables

The **video cable** transmits digital data from the camera head to the CCU and from the monitor to the output recorder. These high quality cables use fiberoptic systems, which are necessary for HD signals. Like all fiberoptic cables, the video cable can be easily damaged by rough handling or misuse, and the same care given to light cables should be applied to the video cable.

The video cables are patched into the system at the back of the CCU and have dedicated receptacles, which are clearly marked.

Digital Output Recorder

During video-assisted surgery, digital signals are captured from the video camera and transmitted to a monitor. The **digital output recorder** processes these signals. Data can also be transmitted to remote locations and input from other imaging processes integrated into the camera output.

The output recorder communicates with other components of the video system (camera, camera processor, and remote control) through cable connections. Integrated systems require specific knowledge about the compatibility of these devices and their connections.

The **video printer** records and stores images transmitted through the image system. Photographic images can be reproduced as paper or on a video disc. Newer systems use digital image technology with a standard personal computer (PC) card adapter. Moving or still images can be saved, catalogued, and recovered with greater storage capacity and transmission with a PC or other digital transmission system (Figure 24-11).

Monitor

The video monitor shows a projected image of the surgical site in real time. The monitor most commonly used is the flat panel (liquid crystal display [LCD]) monitor. New HD systems are displayed in a wide screen format. Although the image captured by the endoscopic video is circular, the wide screen covers the entire image by increasing the horizontal field of view and reducing the vertical field. This results in a full-screen image.

The monitor's resolution must be matched to the camera's capabilities to provide the clearest view. The 16:9 ratio monitor is best for displaying HD signals. Because the human eye has a wider horizontal view than vertical view, images displayed on the 16:9 monitor are more natural looking and less fatiguing for the eyes during surgery.

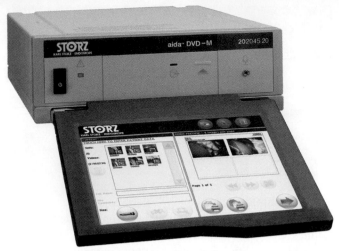

Figure 24-11   The digital output recorder processes signals from the video camera and produces printed or stored images. The recorder interfaces with other components through cable connections. (©2012 Photo courtesy of KARL STORZ Endoscopy-America, Inc.)

Equipment Cart

The equipment cart (also called a *tower*) provides shelves for safe storage and transportation of video equipment. Carts are designed to provide power strips with dedicated receptacles for video components (Figure 24-12). Carts allow equipment to be moved safely and efficiently. An alternative design for equipment is suspension by overhead booms, which are commonly built into integrated operating rooms.

Specialty Telescopes

Specialty telescopes are designed to fit the anatomical and technical needs of surgical specialties, such as abdominal, orthopedic, thoracic, and gynecological surgery. Design features include length, diameter, channels for continuous irrigation, and electrosurgical capability.

A **resectoscope** is a rigid telescope contained within a cutting and coagulating instrument; it is used in the sectional removal (resection) of tissue. The resectoscope commonly is used in genitourinary and gynecological surgery to remove tumors of the bladder and uterus and to resect the prostate. The resectoscope is fitted with a cutting tip that uses laser or electrosurgical energy to remove tissue. (Resectoscopic techniques are described in Chapters 25 and 26.)

Common specialty rigid telescopes include the following:
- *Laparoscope:* Abdominal and pelvic surgery
- *Arthroscope:* Joint surgery
- *Hysteroscope:* Surgery of the uterus
- *Thoracoscope:* Thoracic surgery
- *Nephroscope:* Kidney surgery
- *Cystourethroscope:* Surgery of the bladder and associated structures

Figure 24-13 shows common specialty telescopes and resectoscopes.

TROCAR-CANNULA SYSTEM

A trocar and cannula system is used to create ports or channels through the body wall for insertion of MIS instruments.

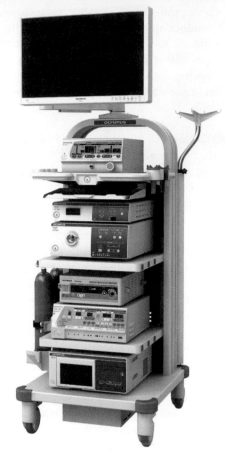

Figure 24-12   Equipment cart with monitor. (Courtesy © Olympus, America, Inc.)

This system is most commonly used during laparoscopic abdominal surgery and thoracic MIS. The trocar is a solid rod with a tapered or sharp end that fits inside the hollow tube cannula. The trocar and cannula are assembled by the surgical technologist before insertion into the patient. When assembled, the point of the trocar protrudes slightly beyond the end of the cannula (Figure 24-14). To insert the trocar and cannula, the surgeon makes a small incision in the body wall and advances the unit through the tissue. When the trocar is in the correct position, the surgeon withdraws it, leaving the hollow cannula in place. The cannula then receives endoscopic instruments.

Features

Trocar-cannula systems can be disposable, reusable, or reposable. Single-use trocars are commonly used, and bladeless trocars are also available. Cannulas are available in the following ranges:

1. Pediatric: 5 to 8 mm
2. Adult: 5 to 10 mm
3. Large and special purpose (e.g., specimen retrieval): 10 to 15 mm

It is important that the cannula remain stable during surgery. Therefore, all cannulas are designed to provide a snug interface and a system for retention in surrounding tissue.

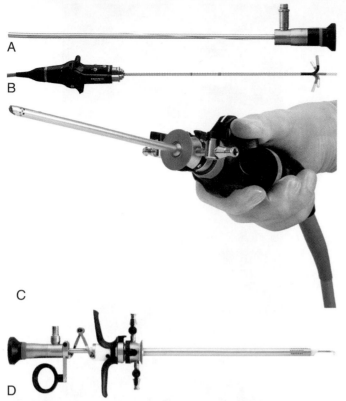

Figure 24-13 **Endoscopes and resectoscopes. A,** Rigid laparoscope. **B,** Deflectable tip video laparoscope. **C,** Arthroscope. **D,** Resectoscope. *(Courtesy © Olympus, America, Inc.)*

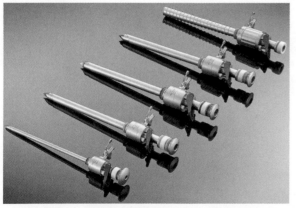

Figure 24-14 **Trocar-cannula systems.** The unit is inserted into a body cavity and the trocar is withdrawn. The cannula remains in place to receive instruments during surgery. *(©2012 Photo courtesy of KARL STORZ Endoscopy-America, Inc.)*

To prevent injury on insertion and provide a seal once they are in place, trocar-cannula systems have the following features:

- An expanding or dilating tip that provides a seal between the cannula and tissue
- Blunt trocar tips, which do not penetrate tissue but push it aside during entry
- Threaded trocar design to help guide the trocar on insertion

- Perforations or flanges to permit anchor sutures at the proximal end of the cannula
- Fabric or foam interface between the cannula and the body wall
- Optical trocars, which allow the passage of the viewing telescope as the cannula is advanced

Many cannula systems have a reducer ring at the proximal end. This allows a smaller diameter instrument to be passed through a larger cannula. Variable diameter seals are also available.

Trocar Placement

Abdominal surgery usually requires at least three trocars unless SILS surgery is being performed. These are placed according to the type of surgery to be performed. The video telescope usually is placed near the midline, approximately 10 inches (25 cm) above the pubic symphysis. This allows a broad view of the abdominal and pelvic contents. Other trocars are placed at strategic positions at the right or left of the midline. A ruler may be used to measure the exact location of the trocar insertion points.

TISSUE EXPANSION TECHNIQUES

MIS is performed in a small space with restricted visualization of the surgical anatomy. This can lead to inadvertent injury to tissues outside the focal area of the telescope. Various methods are used to expand tissue planes atraumatically and create space at the surgical site:

- *Insufflation* of the abdominal cavity, which expands the abdominal wall and allows clear viewing of the abdominal viscera
- *Continuous irrigation* or fluid distention of a cavity or joint space
- *Balloon expansion* of tissue planes, such as the preperitoneal space and inguinal area

Insufflation

Insufflation is a process in which the abdominal and sometimes the thoracic cavity are filled with carbon dioxide (CO_2) gas. This provides a clear view of the anatomy and permits safe entry of the rigid telescope and other instruments during the procedure. CO_2 gas is used because it is nontoxic, readily absorbed by the body, and nonflammable. The CO_2 gas is warmed before insufflation. This maintains the patient's core temperature and prevents fogging of the telescope lens.

Carbon dioxide is delivered to the patient from a tank reservoir via clear tubing. The *insufflation unit* is the control console for delivering the correct amount, temperature, and pressure of CO_2.

SAFETY FEATURES OF THE INSUFFLATION UNIT

- High-flow and low-flow pressure control settings
- Effective leakage compensation
- Gas-warming capacity (expanding CO_2 gas is rapidly cooling)
- Fluid sensor and filter guard to prevent infectious bacteria from entering the system and being shunted into the patient

- Audible and visual warning signals to indicate when pressure exceeds the programmed amount.

To create a **pneumoperitoneum**, the surgeon inflates the abdomen with CO_2 through a large-bore needle called a **Veress needle** or other similar device. Before the Veress needle is used, the technologist should check its spring action. The spring is designed to retract the needle when resistance is met at the tip; this alerts the surgeon to possible obstruction during placement.

Before inserting the needle into the abdominal cavity, the surgeon places a penetrating clamp on each side of the umbilicus. The clamps are used to lift the abdominal wall upward, creating a space between it and the viscera. The surgeon makes a small stab incision in the superficial tissues at the umbilicus. The needle is then pushed through the abdominal wall at an angle to prevent injury of structures below.

A saline test often is done to verify the position of the Veress needle in the abdominal cavity. A 10-mL syringe filled with normal saline is attached to the hub of the Veress needle. If needle placement is correct, the saline drains by negative pressure into the abdominal cavity. After position verification, the insufflation tubing is attached to the needle (Figure 24-15).

NOTE: *Before it is attached, the tubing is flushed with CO_2 gas to purge any air from the tube and prevent air embolism.*

The control console is adjusted to deliver a steady level of gas through the tubing. The pressure usually is maintained at 12 to 18 mm Hg.

The risks and precautions associated with pneumoperitoneum are listed in Box 24-2. Many of these are the responsibility of the professional nursing staff. However, the surgical technologist must be aware of the risks to ensure the patient's safety at all times.

Continuous Irrigation and Fluid Distention

Continuous irrigation is a technique used in arthroscopic MIS, hysteroscopy, and cystoscopy. Fluid is instilled into a body cavity or space to expand it and provide continuous flushing of small tissue fragments and blood generated during tissue remodeling. These can obscure the view of the telescope.

The choice of fluid used for continuous irrigation depends on the electrosurgical instruments used in the procedure. Older electrosurgical systems require nonconductive solutions such as glycine, sorbitol, or mannitol. Some newer systems may be safely used with isotonic saline irrigation. The risk of electrical conduction and fluid balance depend on the choice of solutions. The surgical technologist must ensure that the correct solution is used, according to the electrode manufacturer's guideline.

RISKS When a body cavity or organ is filled with fluid during surgery, the risk exists that it will be absorbed into the vascular system; this is called **intravasation**. Injury is caused when the pressure of the irrigation fluid exceeds a safe level, causing fluid to enter the vascular system, thereby increasing blood pressure or causing electrolyte imbalance. The circulating

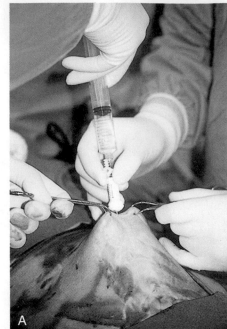

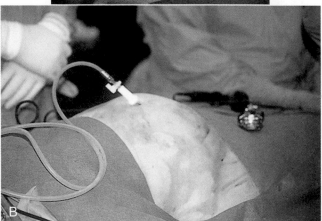

Figure 24-15 Insufflation of the abdomen for laparoscopy. **A,** The Veress needle has been inserted in the abdominal cavity. A syringe is attached to the hub of the needle to check for negative pressure. **B,** The insufflation tubing is attached to the Veress needle and carbon dioxide is allowed to flow into the abdomen. *(From Nagle GM: Genitourinary surgery, St. Louis, 1997, Mosby.)*

nurse and surgeon monitor fluid pressure during fluid distention procedures. Fluid is instilled by a pump or by a gravity system in which irrigation liquid flows into and out of the space through sterile tubing (Figure 24-16). An automated pump system is advantageous for controlling and maintaining a specific pressure, because as the pressure reaches a specified level, fluid is released from the cavity, preventing injury. The circulating nurse and scrubbed surgical technologist share responsibility for keeping track of the amount of fluid used and the amount of runoff during the procedure.

Balloon Dissection

Many balloon dissection devices are available that can create anatomical space in tissue planes. The *balloon dissector* is used in reconstructive plastic surgery and in vascular and abdominal wall procedures. These devices have a telescopic tube with

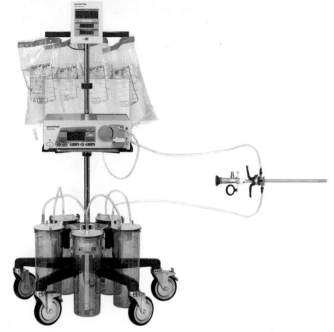

Figure 24-16 **Continuous irrigation for use during minimally invasive surgery.** Fluid is controlled by a pressure monitor, which should be used when the resectoscope is used (shown). *(Courtesy © Olympus, America, Inc.)*

an elastic balloon at the tip or long axis of the tube. The tube is inserted into the tissue plane, and the balloon is inflated with air. This pushes the surrounding tissues aside without causing trauma and provides an anatomical space for the telescope and other instruments (Figure 24-17).

SPECIMEN RETRIEVAL

Morcellation

For tissue specimens or remnants to be retrieved from the body during MIS, they must be small enough to fit through the cannula opening. Large specimens and dense tissue are reduced to small pieces by a process called *morcellation*. The morcellator reduces tissue to pulp, which can be suctioned from the wound.

A tissue *shaver* commonly is used in endoscopic nasal and orthopedic procedures. In endoscopic nasal sinus surgery, it is used to remove masses, polyps, and redundant tissue from the endothelial surface. The shaver suctions soft tissue into the cutting channel, where a spiral burr shaves it into small pieces. In orthopedic and neurosurgery, soft tissue, cartilage, and small bone fragments may also be reduced using this technique.

Large tissue specimens are retrieved through the abdominal wall through a retractable tissue bag inserted into a large port (cannula). The surgeon captures the organ into the bag and retracts the open portion to secure the contents. The bag then is withdrawn through the port. For extremely large specimens, an 18-mm port may be required for extraction.

In some procedures, particularly during natural orifice endoscopic procedures, specimens may be withdrawn through a body orifice, such as the vagina in gynecologic endoscopic procedures.

ENERGY SOURCES USED IN MINIMALLY INVASIVE SURGERY

Energy sources used for tissue coagulation and cutting were introduced in Chapter 18. Electrosurgery, ultrasonic devices, and lasers are used routinely in minimally invasive procedures. The use of these devices in a closed space (within a body cavity or hollow organ) increases the possibility of injury, because although the operative site is accessible through the ports, "blind" spots exist outside the immediate view of the endoscopic camera. Burns may not be noticed or diagnosed until the signs and symptoms of burned or perforated viscera develop, leading to infection and peritonitis. Also, the limited working space for instruments inside body cavities and spaces increases the technical difficulty in using extremely powerful cutting and coagulation instruments. Instrument collisions

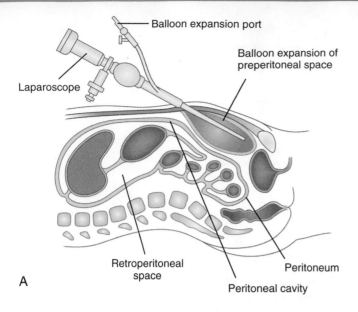

A

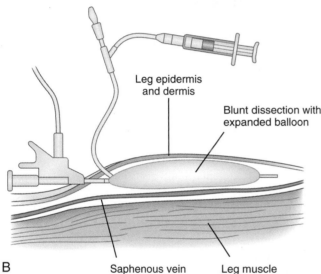

B

Figure 24-17 **Balloon expansion.** A balloon expander may be used to create a space for the insertion of minimally invasive instruments. **A,** Expansion of the preperitoneal space, commonly performed in hernia repair. **B,** Balloon expansion for removal of the saphenous vein for transplantation. *(Redrawn from Rothrock JC: Alexander's care of the patient in surgery, ed 12, St Louis, 2003, Mosby.)*

and inadvertent tissue contact with the device can result in severe injury to the patient.

Electrosurgery and Risks

Specific risks are associated with electrosurgical techniques used during MIS. The risk may be greater when monopolar instruments are used. The following are known to cause patient injury. The surgical technologist is responsible for checking all instruments and other devices before they are passed to the surgeon for use.

INSULATION FAILURE All MIS instruments are insulated with materials that do not conduct electricity. However, insulation can be damaged, and poor quality manufacturing may produce

an inferior instrument that is dangerous to use. Insulation failure can lead to patient burns when stray electrosurgical energy seeks a circuit and jumps to an alternative conductive path (i.e., the break in insulation).

DIRECT AND CAPACITIVE COUPLING In **direct coupling**, the active electrode comes in contact with another instrument capable of conducting electricity, causing the tissue in contact with the instrument to be burned. This effect is used deliberately when the surgeon grasps tissue with a conductive clamp and then touches the active electrode to the clamp. This transmits electrosurgical energy through the clamp and into tissue within the grasp of the instrument.

Unintentional direct coupling is a different matter. Electrosurgical energy can be transmitted from the tip of the active electrode to nearby instruments when they are accidentally touched or are close to each other, causing accidental burns.

Capacitive coupling occurs when stray electrical current is transmitted from an electrosurgical instrument or other conductive material to tissue, even though no break in the insulation may be apparent. Stray current, the cause of capacitive coupling, can be caused by a number of instrument configurations:

- The active electrode is threaded through a metal cannula.
- The active electrode is an integral part of the operating laparoscope.
- The active electrode is threaded through a metal suction-irrigation tube.

In these cases, as mentioned previously, the stray current causes the problem. In MIS, the tubular cannula or the housing of a telescope can act as a capacitor. A *capacitor* is a point in an electrical circuit where energy is built up or stored between insulators. Energy from the active electrode can travel through the cannula or other capacitive areas near the electrode. With a metal cannula, the energy is dispersed over a wide area and may not cause a problem. However, plastic cannula anchors can insulate the cannula from the body wall. In this configuration, electricity passes down the cannula and can cause a burn on contact with deep body tissue.

RISK REDUCTION AND PREVENTION The risk of patient burns from electrosurgery and MIS can be reduced or eliminated. All perioperative personnel must be alert to potential risks and take an active role in preventing injury.

- The most effective means of preventing burns is **active electrode monitoring (AEM),** a system in which the instruments are self-monitoring during use (e.g., AEM products [Encision, Boulder, Colo.]).
- Continually check instruments and surgical telescopes for damage, especially along the insulated areas and shafts.
- All-metal cannulas are the safest type. Never use hybrid cannulas (those constructed of plastic and metal).
- A continual need to increase the power setting may indicate a problem in the system. Check first before continuing to increase the power.
- Reprocess all instruments, including telescopes, according to the manufacturer's specifications to prevent damage, which can lead to patient injury.

- Always follow established hospital guidelines for handling and setting up endoscopic and minimally invasive equipment.
- Do not place electrical cords and fiberoptic cables across traffic areas in the operating room.
- Do not allow kinks and knots to develop; any cord that appears damaged must be immediately removed from service.
- Never allow electrical cords to come in contact with wet surfaces.

Ultrasonic Energy

Ultrasonic technology is used during MIS for coagulation and cutting (see Chapter 18). Ultrasonic energy coagulates tissue by creating a cool coagulum at the cellular level. No electrical energy and very little heat are involved. Ultrasonic systems include the SonoSurg (Olympus America, Center Valley, Pa.) and Harmonic scalpel (Ethicon, Johnson & Johnson, New Brunswick, NJ).

High-Frequency Bipolar Electrosurgery

High-frequency bipolar electrosurgery is used to coagulate and cut through tissue. Bipolar energy can be an effective method of hemostasis when the combination of low power and high frequency is used. High-frequency energy is transmitted from a power source unit connected to the specialty instruments by a cord, similar to monopolar electrosurgery. Some power sources are capable of producing both bipolar and monopolar energy. However, high-frequency units use a separate, dedicated power source. The PK technology system (ACMI, Southborough, Mass.) is an example of this type of high-frequency/low-temperature instrumentation. A hook probe most commonly is used to simultaneously cut and coagulate tissue. Scissors and grasping instruments are also available. PK technology is also used in the Intuitive robotic system (described later in this chapter).

Laser

Laser technology is used in conjunction with some types of minimally invasive and endoscopic surgery. In these procedures, the lasing fiber is introduced through the cannula or flexible telescope and applied to tissue. Advances in digital technology have greatly increased the precision and efficacy of laser endoscopy. However, the hazards related to a small working space and blind areas out of view of the camera also apply to laser surgery. All precautions and safety measures presented in Chapter 18 apply to laser use in all types of MIS and endoscopic surgery.

NOTE: *Refer to Chapter 18 for a complete discussion of laser surgery, including patient and user safety.*

SURGICAL INSTRUMENTS IN MINIMALLY INVASIVE SURGERY

Instrument Design

Endoscopic instruments are designed to perform a precise surgical task in a confined space. The handles and fulcrums are located at some distance from the working end. Hinges, springs, and valves are very small, and the success of the surgery depends on the efficiency of the mechanical design. A rotational design, such as that used in robotic surgery, allows the tip of the instrument to swivel in an arc, increasing the maneuverability of the instruments.

Instruments are supplied in reusable, disposable, and reposable types (only critical components, such as the tips, are disposable). The grip mechanism on endoscopic instruments is important to the ergonomics and precision of the tool. Long procedures require continued delicate control. This is enhanced by comfortable handles and good balance between the tips and handles.

The most common handle design is a transaxial type, which has two finger rings at a 90-degree angle to the long axis of the instrument. Because of the short fulcrum and flexibility of the instruments, the amount of applied force is greatly reduced in an endoscopic instrument. Examples of telescopic instruments are shown in Figures 24-18 through 24-20.

Retractors

Many retractor designs are available, but each uses the same principle as open surgery retractors. Because of the limited operating space, retractors extend from the tip of the shaft and flare out or curve at various angles. A probe (rod or hook) is often used to manipulate and retract tissue.

Scissors

Endoscopic scissors are available in straight, curved, and hooked configurations. In open surgery, dissection of tissue planes and cutting frequently are performed with scissors; in endoscopic procedures, they often are also performed using electrosurgery or ultrasonic shears.

Forceps

As are their open surgery counterparts, grasping instruments, including clamps and forceps, are commonly used in MIS. Some provide atraumatic grasping, whereas others penetrate the tissue. The working tips of endoscopic graspers match those of graspers for open surgery.

Suction and Irrigation Tips

Irrigation is used throughout the endoscopic procedure to keep the focal lens area clear of small bits of tissue and debris. These can fill the field and obscure the view because of the degree of magnification in the lens system. If hemorrhage occurs, the surgeon has no way to locate the bleeding vessel without pinpoint suction. The scrub should have irrigation and suction available at all times during the procedure. Irrigation is delivered through a single irrigation tip or a combination suction-irrigation system.

Hemostatic Clips and Staples

The surgical clip appliers used in open surgery have counterparts in MIS. Disposable delivery systems are the most reliable, and these are commonly used for approximating tissue and resection. Clips are used in place of suture ligatures to

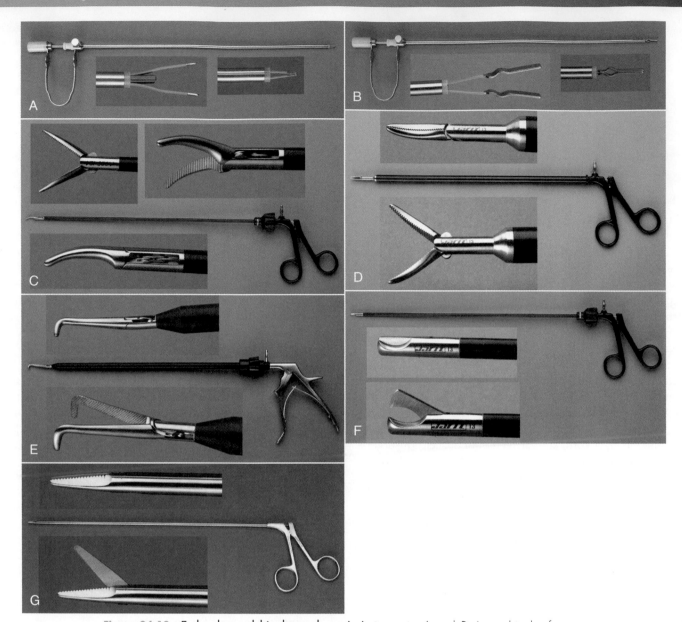

Figure 24-18 Endopolar and bipolar endoscopic instruments. **A** and **B**, Large bipolar forceps. **C**, Maryland forceps. **D**, Maryland dissecting forceps. **E**, Mixter forceps. **F**, Hook scissors. **G**, Jarit Supercut scissors. *(Courtesy Jarit Instruments, Hawthorne, NY.)*

occlude blood vessels or other types of hollow structures, such as the bile ducts. A disposable clip applier can deliver multiple clips in succession without reloading.

Stapling instruments are routinely used in open surgery (see Chapter 12). Endoscopic stapling instruments are most commonly used in laparoscopic surgery and VATS.

Sutures and Ligation Devices

Ligation in endoscopic procedures is performed with many different devices and techniques. Electrosurgical and ultrasound modalities have replaced traditional sutures in many procedures. However, needles and sutures remain in use. Various instruments have been designed to tie knots, snug knots, and suture tissue within a confined space. Three types of methods are commonly used: the extracorporeal technique,

the intracorporeal technique, and the pretied surgical loop. The pretied loop and Surgiwip (Covidien, Norwalk, Conn.) devices are shown in Figure 24-21.

In the **extracorporeal** suture technique, the knot is tied outside the body cavity and then pushed into place with a **knot pusher** using the following technique: A swaged suture-needle combination is grasped with a needle holder and passed through the endoscopic cannula to the inside of the body. The needle is pushed through the tissue with the aid of an additional grasping instrument via a separate cannula. The suture-needle combination is withdrawn, and the needle removed outside the wound. The knots can then be formed without tightening outside the body and introduced back into the body via the cannula. They are then tightened with the knot pusher.

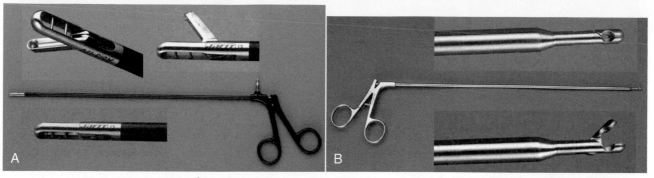

Figure 24-19 **Biopsy forceps. A,** Biopsy punch. **B,** Microbiopsy forceps. *(Courtesy Jarit Instruments, Hawthorne, NY.)*

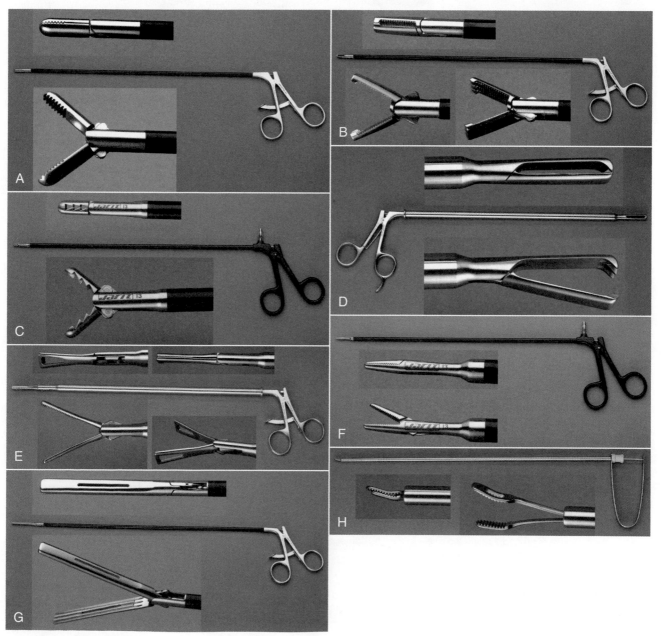

Figure 24-20 **Endoscopic graspers. A,** Grasper with ratchet. **B,** Allis grasper. **C,** Bipolar toothed grasper. **D,** Claw grasper and extracting forceps. **E,** Duval tip. **F,** Bipolar micrograsper. **G,** DeBakey forceps. **H,** Atraumatic forceps. *(Courtesy Jarit Instruments, Hawthorne, NY.)*

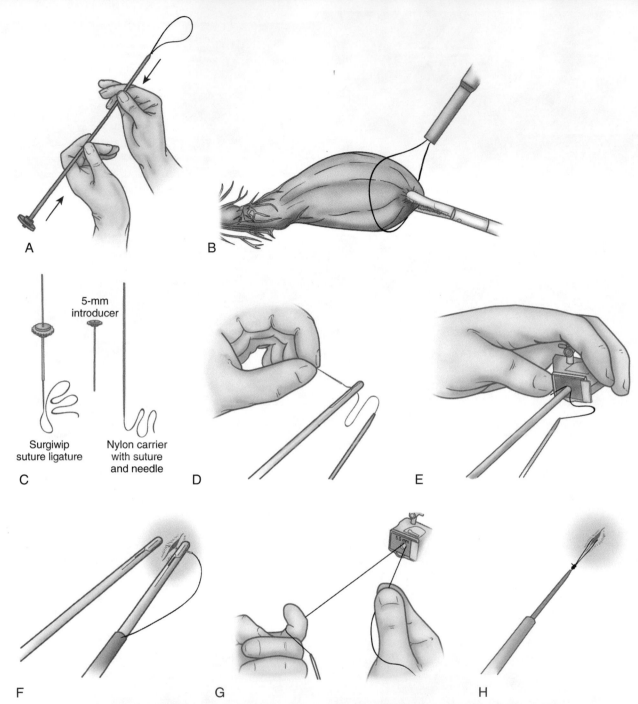

Figure 24-21 **Endoscopic suture devices.** **A,** Commercially prepared pretied loop. **B,** The pretied loop is used to snare and ligate a structure, such as the gallbladder. **C,** Surgiwip components. **D,** The suture is grasped with a needle holder. **E,** Suture is introduced through the abdominal port (cannula). **F,** Suturing the tissue. **G,** The end is brought back through the port and tied outside the body. **H,** The knot is pushed through the cannula with the carrier and secured in tissue. *(From Rothrock JC: Alexander's care of the patient in surgery, ed 13, St. Louis, 2007, Mosby.)*

In the **intracorporeal** technique, the suture is knotted and tightened inside the body with two grasping instruments inserted into two separate cannula ports.

The suture or pretied **ligation loop** such as the Surgiwip is used when a tissue structure requires ligation rather than suturing. A loop of suture contained in a carrier, similar to a snare, is delivered through the laparoscope and looped around the tissue, such as the appendix. The loop then is tightened, the suture ends cut, and the carrier removed.

CARE OF INSTRUMENTS USED FOR MINIMALLY INVASIVE SURGERY

The care of telescopes and other MIS instruments requires particular attention to the delicate nature of the instruments and the potential for patient injury. Equipment used in MIS represents a significant cost to the facility. Inferior instruments must never be used, and the chain of care starts before surgery and continues throughout the intraoperative and postoperative reprocessing periods.

Inspection

WHEN TO INSPECT INSTRUMENTS

- Before use
- During surgery
- After the procedure
- Immediately after decontamination
- Before disinfection and sterilization

WHAT TO LOOK FOR

- Working ability (mechanical function)
- Surface defects
- Overall integrity (components are positioned correctly and connections are tight)
- Cleanliness (instruments must be free of debris and body fluids before use during surgery)

Check the working motion of the instrument. As with standard instruments, scissors must mesh smoothly. Grasping instruments are used heavily in endoscopic procedures and subject to wear. Make sure the jaws are even and meet in exact alignment at the tips. Any instrument with a spring mechanism must compress easily and return to neutral position smoothly. Check hinge pins and other mechanical attachments to make sure they are secure. Check for straightness. Sight the shanks and shafts of the instrument while rotating it to make sure no bends are present. Inspect sharp instruments, such as reusable trocars and Veress needles, for burrs or dullness. Remove damaged sharps from service.

Carefully examine the surface of all instruments for defects such as scratches, dents, or nicks (Figure 24-22, *A*). The long shafts of instruments are particularly vulnerable to defects from normal wear. Loss of integrity to the instrument insulation creates a risk for patient burns. Never deliver a damaged instrument to the sterile field.

Pay particular attention to the lens system, coupling fittings, and shaft (see Figure 24-22, *B*). Inspect the distal lens and eyepiece for debris by observing them under indirect light. Look for scratches, chips, and fingerprints.

Look through the eyepiece to check for lens clarity. Rotate the telescope shaft to check all surfaces. If any obstruction appears, the lens may be damaged. Fogging may be caused by moisture trapped between the lens and seal, an indication of leakage. Check for straightness by observing the telescope end to end.

Electrosurgical instruments must be checked to make sure no breaks in the insulation are present. Even a small defect may transmit stray current and cause an unintentional burn (see Figure 24-22, *C*).

Intraoperative Care

During surgery, instruments should be kept as clean as possible. Use a damp sponge to wipe the tips and instrument shafts. Suction tips should be flushed frequently to prevent clogging. Use only sterile water to clean instruments because it is hemolytic and does not erode instruments.

As instruments are used, replace them in a specific location on the instrument table or in a specialized instrument rack. Do not stack endoscopic instruments in a basin, because this can damage them. An orderly instrument table protects and preserves instruments.

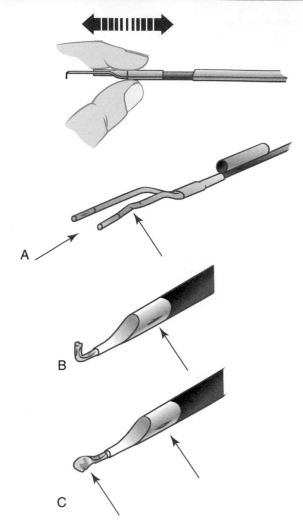

Figure 24-22 Care of endoscopic instruments. A, Examine the surface of the telescope. **B,** Pay particular attention to the lens system, couplings, and shaft. **C,** Electrosurgical instruments must be inspected to ensure that there are no breaks in the insulation. *(Courtesy Olympus, America, Inc.)*

The rigid telescope should be protected by placing it on a lint-free towel or in a warm water bath when not in use. Do not allow the lens to come in contact with oil. Keep the tip and shaft away from sharp objects and heavy instruments. To prevent the telescope from dropping from the sterile field, make sure cables and tubing are slack. Disconnect cables and tubing when transferring the instruments from the operative field to the instrument table.

When surgery is complete, endoscopic instruments are processed according to the manufacturer's guidelines and hospital policy. All instruments must pass through a cleaning and terminal decontamination or sterilization process immediately after use.

FLEXIBLE ENDOSCOPY

PRINCIPLES

Flexible (and semirigid) endoscopy is a method of viewing the inside of body passages and hollow organs, such as the gastrointestinal system, urinary bladder, uterus, nasal sinuses, bronchial tree, and larynx. During flexible endoscopy, the surgical endoscope is introduced through a natural opening in the body, such as the mouth, nose, or cervix. The scope is carefully advanced, and the interior tissues are examined with video-assisted technology or directly through the instrument's lens system. The surgeon can remove tissue for biopsy or take cell brushings through the flexible endoscope. Diagnosis is also made by visual examination of the tissues as they appear on the monitor at the time of the procedure.

The flexible endoscope most often is used for examination, visual exploration, and biopsy. Some procedures and specialties use a semirigid scope, which is a hybrid form of the rigid endoscope discussed later in the chapter.

EQUIPMENT USED IN FLEXIBLE ENDOSCOPY

Flexible Endoscope

The flexible endoscope has two main sections, the head and the insertion tube (Figure 24-23). The endoscope **control head** connects with the digital camera, optical system control handles, suction, and irrigation. Endoscopes that do not have a video camera also have an eyepiece on the control head. The fiberoptic light cable inserts into the control head to provide illumination. The control head also has the dials that operate the flexing mechanism at the distal end of the tube. The **insertion tube** is the component of the endoscope that enters the patient's body. The interior of the insertion tube contains the fiberoptic light channel, which terminates at the tip of the instrument.

Inside the endoscope are the optical components and channels for irrigation, air, and instruments. The **instrument channel** receives biopsy forceps, brushes, and other instruments used to remove tissue specimens. This channel is the largest one. The **biopsy channel** port is located near the junction of the control head and the insertion tube.

Some endoscopes may have an **auxiliary water channel** and an **elevator channel**. The water channel is used to clear blood and tissue debris from the lens. The elevator channel is used to manipulate instruments and remove tissue specimens. An air channel is used to insufflate the lumen of the gastrointestinal tract to create space in the same way as in a pneumoperitoneum. The tip of the insertion tube is operated at the control head to obtain rotational views of the anatomy within the focal area of the lens.

Imaging System

The vision system of the flexible endoscope is very similar to that used for MIS. A camera control unit and digital output recorder perform the same functions outlined previously. Video output is viewed on the LCD or plasma monitor, as in rigid endoscopy.

MIS may be assisted with a flexible endoscope for increased visibility of the anatomy. In these procedures, the flexible

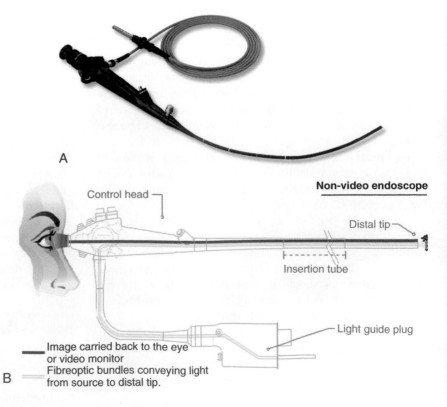

Figure 24-23 **A,** Fiberoptic gastroscope. **B,** Schematic of endoscope design. *(Courtesy Olympus America, Center Valley, Pa.)*

Non-video endoscope

Control head

Distal tip

Insertion tube

Light guide plug

Image carried back to the eye or video monitor

Fibreoptic bundles conveying light from source to distal tip.

endoscope is managed by a separate team performing MIS through the rigid endoscope. Combined procedures of the abdomen and gastrointestinal tract are enhanced with the use of both technologies.

TECHNIQUE

Flexible endoscopy usually is performed in an outpatient setting. The procedures are relatively short compared with MIS or open surgery. Ambulatory outpatients usually are discharged as soon as they have recovered from the effects of sedation.

After the patient has been sedated and positioned, the endoscopist introduces the insertion tube, examining tissue and recording digital or camera images. Biopsies are taken with the aid of forceps, graspers, or biopsy brushes.

The surgeon is assisted by the scrub, who helps position the patient and prepares equipment and instruments. During the procedure, the scrub maintains suction and irrigation devices and helps place biopsy instruments into the endoscope. The scrub also receives specimens as they are withdrawn from the endoscope and properly preserves and documents them.

The scrub may also provide direct patient care in all phases of the procedure.

REPROCESSING ENDOSCOPES AND INSTRUMENTS

Disassembly and proper reassembly is critical to safe reprocessing (cleaning, disinfection, sterilization). Reprocessing is discussed in this chapter rather than in Chapter 11, which covers disinfection and sterilization, so that the student can easily refer to discussions and definitions of instrument components in this chapter.

PROTOCOLS AND STANDARDS

The endoscope is a complex instrument with channels, valves, spring fittings, and stopcocks. The endoscope and other instruments often come in contact with areas of the body that have a high level of bioburden. Debris can become trapped in the mechanisms and harbor infectious material. For these reasons, a systematic cleaning process that follows an established protocol is necessary to ensure the patient's safety.

Hospital policy for reprocessing endoscopes follows guidelines established by the Occupational Safety and Health Administration (OSHA), an agency of the U.S. Department of Labor, and every manufacturer of surgical endoscopes provides detailed instructions on the specific care of its equipment. A general overview of reprocessing is presented here.

PRECLEANING OF RIGID ENDOSCOPES

All immersible instruments and rigid endoscopes must be precleaned immediately after use in surgery. Endoscopes and accessories should be disassembled according to the manufacturer's instructions. Manual cleaning removes much of the tissue and body fluid trapped in crevices and fittings. This is done with enzymatic cleaner, a clean cloth, and a soft brush. Endoscopic instruments can be soaked briefly in an enzymatic detergent bath before precleaning.

Guidelines for Precleaning Instruments

1. Instruments are best transported in a covered container from the point of use to the cleaning area. They can be transported wet or dry. However, immediate soaking (transport in a wet bath) aids more complete cleaning. Do not soak instruments for longer than 1 hour or as directed by the instrument manufacturer.
2. Before cleaning instruments, make sure to open all stopcocks, ports, and channels.
3. Separate the telescopes from other instruments for individual processing.
4. Follow the manufacturer's instructions for a compatible enzymatic bath. Do not exceed the recommended water temperature.
5. While cleaning, look for defects in the surface of the instrument. Look for any sign that the instrument housing and insulation are damaged. Remember that even small nicks or scratches can create a pathway for stray electricity and cause burns.
6. Use a long brush to clean the inside of tubes and lumens. Irrigate these with large amounts of enzymatic fluid. Reusable brushes must be terminally disinfected and sterilized between uses.
7. Clean air and water channels with forced air or as recommended by the manufacturer.
8. Do not submerge or allow any fluid to enter electrical connections or units! These should be wiped clean with an approved surface disinfectant.
9. Flush all ports with enzymatic solution and make sure all surfaces have been cleaned. Some types of stopcocks may be disassembled for cleaning. Always verify before attempting disassembly.
10. After cleaning, rinse all surfaces and channels of the instruments with deionized or sterile water. Make sure that every part of the instrument is rinsed to remove detergent and debris loosened during cleaning.
11. Drain the instruments and dry them.

Precleaning Optical Parts and Lenses

Disassemble the adapter from the light cable. Then proceed as follows:

1. If the endoscope has an eyepiece cap, remove it.
2. Clean the lens surface with a lint-free cloth and ethanol or isopropanol, or as directed by the manufacturer.
3. When cleaning lenses and optical surfaces, take care not to abrade or scrape the lenses. Do not use a brush to clean the optical surfaces.
4. Check the lenses of the endoscope. Look for any cloudiness or discoloration. Cloudiness is a sign of leakage. If you suspect the lens fitting has leaked, remove it from service after decontamination and sterilization according to manufacturer's specifications.

Ultrasonic cleaning is commonly used for stainless steel instruments. However, many instruments are not approved for this type of system, and the process may damage them. Always read and follow the manufacturer's written protocol regarding ultrasound cleaning. For endoscopic equipment that can be cleaned in this fashion, use caution when processing the instruments in the ultrasound cleaner.

FLEXIBLE ENDOSCOPE REPROCESSING

Flexible endoscopes are particularly difficult to clean. The ports and long tube channels trap debris, and determining how much has been removed during cleaning is difficult. An automatic reprocessor therefore is used. Several manufacturers have developed enclosed reprocessing machines that terminally disinfect the system as long as precleaning has been properly performed. Always read and follow the manufacturer's instructions when using this type of system, because failure to do so may result in serious injury.

Before disinfection in an automatic reprocessor, several steps must be carried out to ensure patient safety.

1. Precleaning is performed as soon as possible after the procedure. The insertion tube is thoroughly cleaned with detergent solution. Detergent solution then is flushed through the air-water and auxiliary channels and removed with air suction.
2. The endoscope must be leak-tested after precleaning. This is done to prevent water from entering the system during the remaining steps of reprocessing. The manufacturer's instructions for leak testing must be followed, and the leak testing equipment used must be compatible with the individual endoscope.
3. After the leak test, the endoscope is cleaned manually. This is done by submerging the instrument in detergent solution and cleaning all surfaces with a soft cloth. A suction pump and syringe are used to flush detergent through the instrument channels and ports, and a soft brush is inserted to clean any debris.
4. After detergent cleaning, complete rinsing is necessary to remove all traces of detergent and debris.
5. All water is removed from the instrument's channels and exterior. The endoscope may then be processed in an automated endoscope reprocessor according to the manufacturer's specifications.

DISINFECTION AND STERILIZATION

After instruments have been thoroughly cleaned, they must be disinfected. High level disinfection kills 100% of *Mycobacterium tuberculosis*. The process of disinfection is specified by the manufacturer of the equipment.

Sterilization methods for endoscopic instruments vary with the type of equipment and the manufacturer's specifications. Instruments used in sterile areas of the body, including the vascular system, require sterilization before reuse. Some equipment, including cameras, may be steam-sterilized, whereas others require ethylene oxide gas or other methods. Equipment that is sterilized by a method other than that specified by the manufacturer may be damaged, and this can increase the risk of patient injury.

SECTION II: ROBOTIC SURGERY

PRINCIPLES OF ROBOTIC SURGERY

A **robot** is a mechanical device that can be programmed to perform tasks. Robotic surgery combines the techniques of MIS with computer-guided instruments that are controlled remotely through a nonsterile interface system.

ROBOTIC MOVEMENT

The overall design of the surgical robotic system provides movements that closely resemble the coordinated actions of the human body, particularly the shoulders, arms, and hands. The robotic arm, which is an extension of the control unit, has degrees of "freedom" that allow pivoting, turning, and flexing motions. These motions are enabled by articulated (jointed) sections of the arm and instruments.

In robotic engineering, cartesian coordinate geometry is used to design and replicate these movements. In the cartesian system of geometry, the robotic arm moves in particular spatial dimensions—vertical, horizontal, and pivotal. The degree of rotation is the ability to turn, or *pivot* (perform rotational turns), on a 360-degree axis. The vertical and horizontal axes allow the arm to move up, down, side to side, and back and forth.

CLASSIFICATION OF ROBOTS

OSHA has published classifications of industrial robots. In this system, robots are classified according to their design and "reaching space" or *working envelope,* which is the actual space in which they move. The design configuration of the robot determines the types of movements it can perform. The robotic design allows pivoting, vertical, horizontal, and circular movements. Joints or articulations on a robotic arm provide many of these movements.

The robot's movement within its working envelope is controlled from a distance or through its sensing devices. These sensing devices react to the environment and respond according to the preprogrammed commands. A servo-controlled robot responds through its sensors. A non–servo-controlled robot has no sensing or feedback ability. The movement of these robots is through physical stops and switches, which are triggered by the presence of a physical barrier such as a wall or object in the path of the robot.

DA VINCI SURGICAL SYSTEM

The da Vinci surgical system (Intuitive Surgical, Sunnyvale, Calif) is used in many specialties and currently is the only system marketed for telesurgery—surgery performed through a type of videoconferencing in which the surgeons and operating room setup are located at one audiovisual terminal, and a trainer or group of students is able to watch at another. The da Vinci system enhances the surgeon's skills by scaling down and refining hand movements as the surgeon manipulates the instruments through the computer-mediated robotic system.

During robotic-assisted MIS, trocars and cannulas are inserted at strategic anatomical locations at the operative site. The telescopic instruments and rigid endoscope are threaded through the cannulas, and surgery is performed through the cannulas. In robotic **telesurgery**, instruments are inserted manually or with electronic assistance but are controlled through a remote nonsterile console near the sterile field. The term *telepresence* describes the surgeon's virtual interface with the surgical anatomy. The computer-mediated instruments have the same flexion and rotational ability as the human hand. However, instead of being directly manipulated, they are controlled by the surgeon through the remote console.

The surgeon sits at the nonsterile console a few feet from the patient. The surgical field is viewed on a three-dimensional console screen, and the surgeon operates the instruments and camera by manipulating the hand and foot controllers of the console. The controllers simulate the hand-eye and instrument coordination of open surgery, but there is no direct physical contact between the controllers and the instruments. This system is called a *telechir* in robotic terminology.

The images transmitted by the digital endoscopic camera are refined and highly magnified on both the console screen and the image system screen. The images can be manipulated (sized, rotated, and integrated with other imaging data) and recorded as permanent or real-time data.

Robotic systems have tremendous accuracy, but they also are very complex; like all medical technologies, they present a risk of malfunction and failure. Many of the skills and much of the knowledge acquired during robotics training is dedicated to preventing or minimizing the effects of malfunction. The purpose of this discussion is to provide an overview of the robotics system and to highlight safety considerations. Perioperative staff members learn how to operate the robotic system and deliver safe patient care through the manufacturer's training program and other resources available through their facility's robotics coordinator and in-service instructors.

ADVANTAGES AND DISADVANTAGES OF ROBOTIC SURGERY

When comparing robot with human capabilities, it is important to remember that robots cannot replace the human ability to make judgments or to make sense of and use qualitative information for the patient's benefit.

Because telesurgery surgery is always used in conjunction with minimally invasive techniques, robotics is compared with traditional MIS.

ADVANTAGES

- *Robotic endoscopic images are three dimensional.* Standard endoscopes transmit a two-dimensional view. During robotic surgery, the endoscopic image is captured and processed by the stereoscopic viewer of the surgeon's console. This view closely approximates what the eye would perceive during open surgery. The advantages over the

two-dimensional view are greater depth perception and increased precision.

- *Tremor and movement scaling are reduced.* The robotic system scales the surgeon's hand movements so that the effects of tremor are greatly reduced or removed. Hand tremor prevents safe and accurate movements in delicate surgery. This innovation allows surgeons to perform procedures that were seldom performed in the past.
- *Robotic instruments closely replicate human movement.* Standard endoscopic instruments have limited range of movement. This is because the surgeon's hand operates the instrument outside the channel of the endoscopic cannulas. Instruments used in robotic surgery can rotate in a full circle (called the degree of freedom) and perform many more pivoting movements compared with standard MIS techniques. These movements more accurately replicate the range of movement in the human hand and wrist than those of standard endoscopic equipment. The exact movements are described relative to three axes of movement. *Yaw* allows the instrument to move toward the left or right in space as it moves on the vertical axis. *Pitch* is movement of the instrument tip up or down. *Roll* is the side-to-side movement of the instrument on a horizontal axis.

DISADVANTAGES

- *The robotic system is expensive and uses valuable resources.* The robotic system requires a substantial investment both in money and time spent learning, coordinating, and managing the system. Robotic instruments cost thousands of dollars and must be discarded after limited use. These instruments contain electronic components and expensive raw materials that may never be recycled or recovered. Hospitals may never regain the initial cost of implementing a robotic system, and the relative human need for such systems is still the subject of debate.
- *Robotic systems require a specialist on-site coordinator.* Even though ample training opportunities are available for perioperative staff, the complexity of the system requires an on-site robotics coordinator. This individual receives extensive training in the operation and safety of the system and usually is responsible for training and orienting staff members new to the system. This requires planning and time allocation, as well as advanced management skills. Staff shortages can make this a disadvantage for startup and continuing education.
- *Surgeons must be trained to operate at the nonsterile console.* Training for robotics surgery is readily available. However, surgeons must relearn techniques as they apply to remote instrument manipulation. Among the new skills that surgeons must learn is the loss of **haptic feedback**. This is the tactile sensation, or "feel," of the instruments during surgery. During robotic telesurgery, the surgeon must rely on vision alone while manipulating the hand and foot controllers. There is no feedback on the tension of an instrument or the feel of a suture knot on tissue. With time, these techniques can be mastered. However, a

steep learning curve usually is required while the surgeon learns to operate without "touch" sensation on the tissues and instruments.

TRAINING FOR ROBOTICS

The robotic telesurgery system is complex and requires special training for all members of the surgical team. Training for the da Vinci system is available from the manufacturer at various teaching locations. During training, surgeons and other perioperative professionals have the opportunity for hands-on learning as well as didactic lectures on the system and how it works.

ROBOTIC TRAINING TOPICS AND METHODS

- System preparation and management
- Inanimate labs and skills development
- Surgical procedure training at various institutions using robotic systems already in use at those hospitals
- Dry runs on setup and procedure
- Troubleshooting the equipment
- Video podcast and live teaching through the Internet

The surgical technologist should have access to both off-site and on-site learning opportunities. In addition to the manufacturer's training, other resources are available:

- In-service programs provided by the robotics nurse manager/supervisor
- In-service with visiting specialists, including the manufacturer's trainers
- Observation in scrub and circulating roles
- Dry runs
- Practice under direct supervision
- Continuous mentoring and feedback

As robotics technology is modified and refined, technologists must continue to advance their skills and knowledge. Opportunities outside the perioperative environment, including conferences and special training programs, are excellent resources for continuing education. Information on these resources is available from the robotics in-service coordinator and through the manufacturer of the system.

SURGICAL SPECIALTIES AND ROBOTICS

Robotic-assisted MIS is performed in a variety of specialties. Because robotics is a rapidly evolving technology, new procedures are in development. The examples below are the most common:

- Orthopedic surgery: Joint replacement procedures
- Cardiothoracic surgery: Valve repair, lung resection
- General surgery: Gastrointestinal resection, biliary surgery, removal of tumors
- Gynecological surgery: Hysterectomy, myomectomy, sacrocolpopexy
- Urological surgery: Prostatectomy, cystectomy
- Neurosurgery: Tumor resection

COMPONENTS OF THE ROBOTIC SYSTEM: STRUCTURE AND PURPOSE

The da Vinci system is commonly used in the United States and is described in this chapter. *This discussion is not intended to replace the formal training required to operate the system safely.* Specific information on the troubleshooting of components and the care and handling of instruments and other delicate parts is readily available in formal training provided by the manufacturer.

Three main components make up the robotic system (Figure 24-24):

- The surgeon's console
- The patient cart
- The imaging (vision) system

The components are connected by cables, which relay information needed to operate the system and provide immediate feedback from one component to another. In this way, each component "talks" to the others so that commands given at any point can be immediately integrated into the system. The components have their own override features to prevent errors.

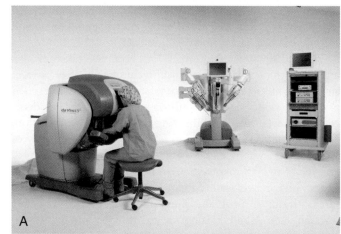

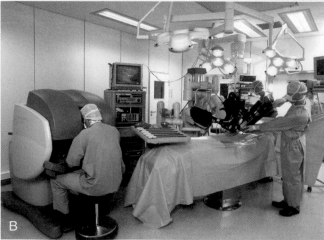

Figure 24-24 **A,** Components of the robotic system. *Left to right:* Surgeon's console, patient cart, image system. **B,** Operating room setup for robotic surgery. Note that the surgeon controls the instruments remotely while seated at the nonsterile console. *(Courtesy Intuitive Surgical, Inc., 2007.)*

PATIENT CART

The patient cart (in practice referred to as "the arms" or "the robot") consists of a central column, vertical arms with movable joints, and a large base that contains a motor drive. A digital touch screen is located on the central column. Robotic arms convey the instruments and camera to the endoscopic cannulas. The cart is part of the sterile field, and each arm is individually draped before it is positioned over the sterile field.

BASE AND POWER DRIVE

The cart is driven and steered by a manual or power drive motor, which is operated from the back of the cart base, similar to a portable radiograph machine. A set of switches and a throttle are used to operate the motor drive. In the da Vinci system, these controls are located near the drive handles. Feedback information about the throttle and power status is clearly visible to the operator, who is positioned at the back of

the unit. In the event of a power failure, manual controls are used to move and position the cart safely.

SETUP JOINTS

Movable *setup joints* extend directly from the central column and are used to change the position of the component arms, which hold the instruments. An electronic clutch system powers the movement of the joints. Feedback on their position and status is provided through light-emitting diode (LED) signals. The setup joints are movable in both the vertical and horizontal directions.

PATIENT CART ARMS

The patient cart arms move around a remote center on the patient cart. The remote center is a fixed location that facilitates optimum alignment and positioning of the cart arms.

The da Vinci system has two or three instrument arms and one camera arm (Figure 24-25). The arms function as the

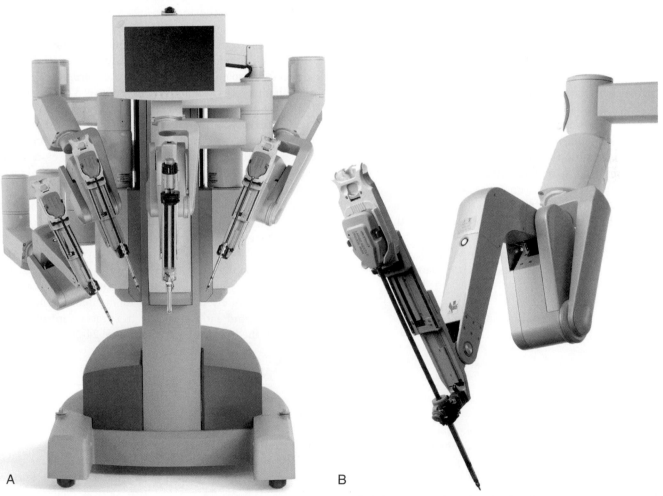

A   B

Figure 24-25 **A,** Close-up of the patient cart (also called the *arms* or the *robot*) for the da Vinci robotic surgical system, showing three instrument arms. The touch screen image system is at the top of the patient cart. **B,** The underside of the instrument arm showing the instrument in place. Instruments are changed as needed by guiding them into the arm. A digital clutch system locks the instrument in place. *(Courtesy Intuitive Surgical, Inc., 2007.)*

instrument "holders," and they interface with the surgeon's console. The arms have a wide range of motion to assist in correct alignment of instruments and the cannulas into which they are inserted. The instrument and camera arms are moved with the aid of an electronic clutch system, which allows the instruments to pivot at the cannula ports.

Although the instruments are controlled by the surgeon at the nonsterile console, the surgical assistant and scrub assist in loading them into the instrument arms. Just as in standard MIS, the scrub also maintains the sterile robotic instruments and passes them to the field as needed.

MONITOR

The monitor, or touch screen, receives electronic signals from the camera head and controller and transmits them as digital output. The monitor can also display output from other forms of diagnostic imaging, such as ultrasound and magnetic resonance imaging. These images are controlled and positioned at the surgeon's console and can also be manipulated on the draped touch screen by scrubbed personnel.

DA VINCI INSTRUMENTS

INSTRUMENT DESIGN AND TYPE

The da Vinci instruments are complex, computer-programmed tools. The programmed movements of the tips and articulated joints of the patient cart arms are controlled by the system's software. The instruments are loaded into the patient cart arms as needed during surgery. This task is performed by the surgical assistant and qualified scrub. Instruments are designed with a limited life span. Each insertion into the patient represents one "use" of the instrument. After the instruments have reached their maximum number of uses (the average is about 10 uses), they must be discarded. At the time of this writing, each instrument costs about $2,500.

The da Vinci instruments provide full rotational tips with flexion on all axes. A variety of instrument types is available.

Classification of Robotic Instruments
- Scissors
- Grasper
- Knife
- Probe
- Needle holder
- Ultrasonic energy instruments
- Electrosurgical instruments (monopolar and bipolar)
  Examples of these instruments are shown in Figure 24-26.

REPROCESSING

As mentioned, instruments in the da Vinci system have a predetermined life span based on the number of actual uses or procedures. The instruments are sterilized between patients until they reach their predetermined life span (approximately 10 uses). Instrument heads and electronic components are cleaned, disinfected, and sterilized according to specific protocols. The surgical technologist or nurse should consult the manufacturer for detailed information and training in the care of robotic instruments. This ensures that the methodology is safe and update with any changes in technology, a likely occurrence in this rapidly evolving area of robotic biotechnology.

Online Resources for Reprocessing
da Vinci provides an excellent online resource for reprocessing its equipment. Before using this system, the surgical staff should attend training with the da Vinci specialist, who can explain how the preprocessing systems work, which chemicals are allowed, and which are not.

To access the online procedure manual, go to http:// www.myendosite.com/manuals/Intuitive.pdf or search "intuitive instruments reprocessing."

SURGEON'S CONSOLE

The surgeon's console contains the remote nonsterile controls. In standard MIS, the surgeon is a scrubbed member of the team. In robotic-assisted surgery, the surgeon is not scrubbed; he or she sits at the console and manipulates the instruments and other equipment using hand and foot controllers. The surgeon's console is placed outside the sterile field but close enough for effective communication between the surgeon and other members of the team.

The **stereoscopic viewer** provides three-dimensional images of the surgical site (Figure 24-27). Digital images are transmitted to the viewer from the endoscope. Before surgery, the surgeon makes adjustments to the seating, optical viewer, and intercom while his or her head is outside the viewer. The system is engaged when the surgeon places the head in the viewer. The screen displays icons that are status indicators for all components and diagnostic imaging. The intercom controls are also located in the viewer. The control pads of the console allow the surgeon to control the interface between components of the system. The **master controllers** and foot switch panel allow the surgeon to manipulate the surgical instruments and endoscope. Electrosurgery controls are also located in the foot switch panel (Figure 24-28).

VISION SYSTEM

Components

The vision components of the robotic system provide a high quality image of the surgical site. The digital image is picked up from the endoscope and transmitted through the camera control unit to the display and monitor on the surgeon's console. The endoscope has two optical channels, which project a three-dimensional image on the monitor and console screen.

The components of the da Vinci robotic vision system include:
- Endoscope

- Camera and camera cable assembly
- Camera control unit
- Illuminator (light source)
- Video processing unit
- Image system (touch screen)
- Stereo viewer

Components of the robotic vision system are comparable to the high quality digital vision systems used in MIS. The da Vinci system uses adaptors and connecting cables that are compatible with its system. HD or SD systems are available.

Endoscopes are available with straight or angled tips and in various sizes. The most commonly used are 5 mm and 12 mm. The camera and camera cable are attached to the endoscope at the sterile field and are available in HD or SD format. The endoscope assembly contains the cable, CCD, camera body, sterile adaptor, and telescope.

The touch screen, CCU, focus controller, and illuminator are part of the vision cart. The cart also has shelves and storage compartments for accessory equipment such as gas tanks and adaptors.

SETUP AND SEQUENCE FOR ROBOTIC SURGERY

ROOM SETUP

Robotic surgery requires that components be positioned in a way that optimizes safety and communication among team members during the intraoperative phase. The robotic components should be positioned according to the type of surgery and the configuration of nonmovable equipment in the room (Figure 24-29). All component cables must lie flat on the floor and in alignment. When the components are positioned, the following must be considered:

- Traffic into, out of, and around the operating room can dictate where the components are placed. Remember that the sterile field includes the patient and operating table, instrument tables, and draped equipment, including the patient cart. Position the equipment in a manner that protects the field from contamination by personnel moving about the room and nonsterile equipment. The patient cart

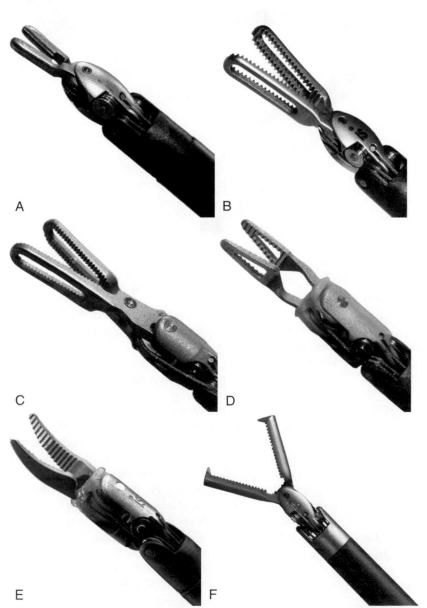

Figure 24-26 **A,** DeBakey forceps. **B,** Cadière forceps. **C,** Prograsp forceps. **D,** Precise bipolar forceps. **E,** Maryland bipolar forceps. **F,** Toothed forceps.

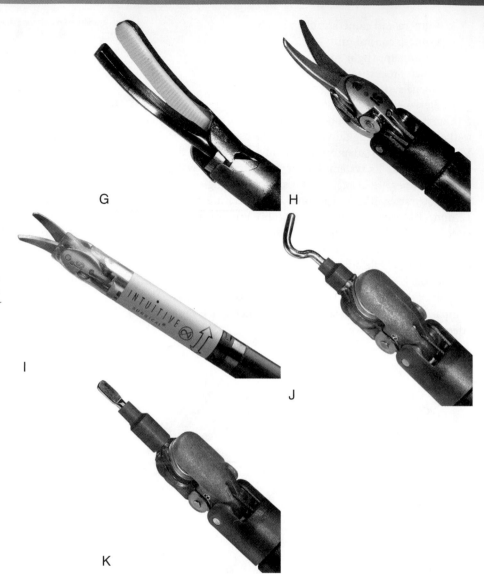

Figure 24-26, cont'd   G, Harmonic shears. **H**, Curved scissors. **I**, Fine dissecting scissors. **J**, Cautery hook. **K**, Cautery spatula. *(Courtesy Intuitive Surgical, Inc., 2007.)*

(robot) must not be placed near the patient's head, because this would interfere with anesthesia activities and also presents a safety problem.

- Robotic components are connected by dedicated cables. Position the equipment in a way that facilitates safe connections. Do not suspend cables or drape them over equipment. Dedicated power receptacles are recommended for each component, which must be within reach of the receptacle.
- Communication is critical during robotic-assisted surgery. Make sure the surgeon can see and talk to the surgical assistant. Remember that the surgeon is seated at the surgeon's console, and this component is stationed outside the sterile field.
- The patient cart, on which the instrument arms are mounted, is part of the sterile field. It is positioned directly over the patient in the proper location for the type of surgery to be performed (e.g., laparoscopic, urogenital, or thoracic procedure). It is positioned after it has been draped and the instrument cannulas have been placed.

SEQUENCE OF OPERATION

The operative setup must be preplanned so that anesthesia time is not used for tasks that can and should take place before surgery. The robotic system requires many adjustments and selections of options. Documentation of these adjustments and information pertaining to the surgeon's preference must be available before every setup.

Before surgery, the surgeon adjusts the components of the console so that the seat and optical viewer are at the correct position. All other options regarding instrument selection and manipulation are made at this time. Nonsterile connections, except those required after the patient cart is in its sterile position, can be made before surgery. This includes setting the correct location of the patient arms with respect to the central column (**docking**). System connections include main power, system cables, auxiliary devices, video patch, and recording unit. All nonsterile equipment is checked to ensure that adaptors and cables are available and ready for operation.

During the sterile setup, the scrub assembles the sterile portion of the vision system and sets up the instruments in

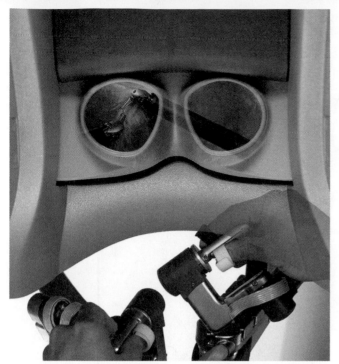

Figure 24-27 Surgical site through the three-dimensional viewer. Instruments are controlled with the master controllers (hand devices) and foot switches. *(Courtesy Intuitive Surgical, Inc., 2007.)*

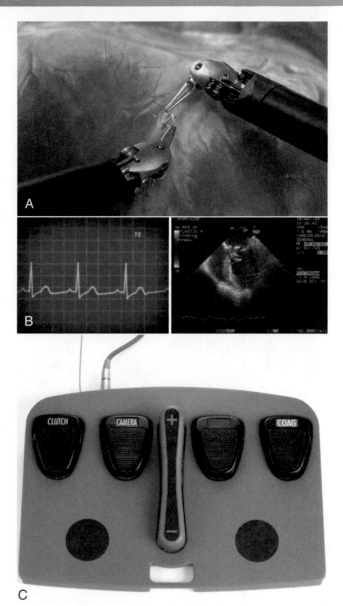

Figure 24-28 **A,** Surgeon's view through the three-dimensional viewer. **B,** Patient monitoring and diagnostic images are transmitted in real time to the surgeon's console. **C,** Foot controls. Note that the electrosurgical unit is also controlled by a foot switch. *(Courtesy Intuitive Surgical, Inc., 2007.)*

order of use. Drapes for the patient cart and camera are prepared in proper sequence. Before the patient is brought into the operating room suite, the robotic camera lens must be calibrated for white balance and focus.

As previously mentioned, the robotic cart is brought to the sterile field after the patient prep, draping, and placement of cannulas for surgery. The patient cart and arms and the camera cable are draped during the routine sterile setup or just before use. The cart is then protected from contamination until it is brought into position.

Before docking, nonsterile personnel must position the patient arm remote center at the correct distance from the cart tower to allow the instruments complete range of motion. After this is done, the cart can be docked. This procedure requires two people, one to position the cart physically and the other to provide instructions at the sterile field.

Once the sterile patient cart is in position, the robotic arms are moved using clutch bottoms, positioned over the trocars, and locked onto them. This completes the docking, and robotic surgery can proceed.

SPECIAL ROLES OF THE SURGICAL TEAM

SURGEON

The surgeon participates as both a sterile and nonsterile team member. At the start of the case, the surgeon performs sterile techniques to place the trocars. He or she then breaks scrub to operate from the surgeon's console. The surgeon returns to the sterile field (after scrubbing, regowning, and gloving) near

the close of the procedure to remove the trocars and close the incisions. The surgeon directs the flow of the procedure and is responsible for coordinating the activities of everyone on the team.

SURGICAL ASSISTANT

The surgical assistant is a scrubbed team member. In robotic surgery, the assistant performs other specific tasks at the sterile field. These include exchanging instruments on the sterile robotic arms and managing any instruments that are outside the control of the robotic system. For example, in gynecological surgery, the first or second assistant controls the uterine manipulator. The assistant works closely with the scrub to

Da Vinc Surgical System in a General Procedure Setting

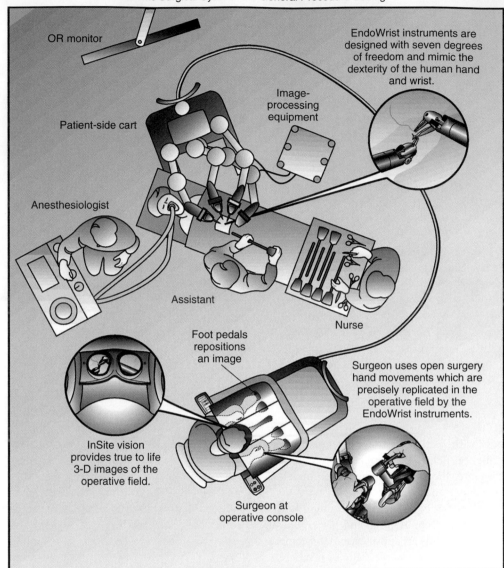

OR monitor

EndoWrist instruments are designed with seven degrees of freedom and mimic the dexterity of the human hand and wrist.

Image-processing equipment

Patient-side cart

Anesthesiologist

Assistant

Nurse

Foot pedals repositions an image

Surgeon uses open surgery hand movements which are precisely replicated in the operative field by the EndoWrist instruments.

InSite vision provides true to life 3-D images of the operative field.

Surgeon at operative console

Figure 24-29 Room setup for robotic-assisted surgery. *(Courtesy Intuitive Surgical, Inc., 2007.)*

maintain a clean, safe operative field. Instrument exchanges and management of the sterile robotic components is the dual responsibility of the surgical assistant and the scrub.

SURGICAL TECHNOLOGIST

During surgery, the scrub performs routine tasks associated with all procedures at all stages, preoperative, intraoperative, and postoperative. Tasks specific to robotics are mainly associated with preparation of the equipment, adjustments, and instrument exchange.

In addition to working closely with the surgeon's assistant, the scrub maintains the robotic instruments during surgery and assists or directs the draping procedures. After the cannulas have been placed, the scrub may direct the positioning of the patient cart. The scrub is familiar with the operation of all electronic and vision components, assisting in registration and white and black balance.

As instruments are exchanged into the robotic arms, the scrub interprets the LED signals indicating the status of the instruments and protects them during insertion. The scrub may be required to operate the clutch system that operates the instrument arms while the instruments are outside the patient's body. The scrub also must be familiar with the touch screen options and assists in sterile adjustments at the monitor.

At the close of surgery, the scrub assists in retraction of the instrument and patient cart arms after the instruments have been withdrawn from the cannulas. At this point, the robotic system is disengaged and routine closure is performed. In the postoperative stage, the scrub prepares the instruments and equipment for cleaning and decontamination and assists the circulator in shutdown and stowing of the robotic system.

CIRCULATOR AND ROBOTICS COORDINATOR

The circulating nurse, surgical technologist, and nonsterile personnel perform all routine tasks required for safe patient care. The robotics coordinator circulates or directs other scrubbed and nonsterile staff during surgery. In robotic surgery, the circulator is required to maintain a safe environment while troubleshooting the system. This individual must be familiar with the operation of the system's components and assists in positioning, registration, and distribution of supplies and equipment. Two circulators can share the nonsterile duties of both patient care and assistance with the robotic system. The certified surgical technologist (CST) coordinator manages the technological aspects of robotic safety and ensures that equipment and instruments are properly managed and stored. This individual may also coordinate the robotics system with its commercial and educational representative and ensure that safety standards are implemented.

KEY CONCEPTS

- Operative MIS involves less tissue trauma and postoperative pain and a shorter recovery time compared with open surgery.
- MIS patients must be carefully screened, because not all patients are good candidates.
- MIS involves complex electronic and imaging systems. All team members must study the technologies involved and remain current with new developments in the specialty.
- The operative principle of MIS is that surgery is performed on internal organs from outside the body using telescopic instruments and an operative telescope, which projects the surgical site onto a monitor.
- The components of the MIS imaging system must be compatible.
- Risks associated with MIS include complications resulting from insufflation, extravasation, and unsafe electrosurgical technique.
- Preoperative preparation of the patient for MIS is the same as for open surgery, because there is always the possibility that the case will convert to an open procedure if an emergency arises.
- MIS is performed in a dimmed operating room to enhance viewing on the video monitor. A dedicated light must be positioned over the instrument table to prevent accidents and errors.
- MIS instruments are extremely delicate and expensive. Care and handling require attention to detail and knowledge of instrument design.
- MIS is practiced in nearly every surgical specialty. The most common applications are in abdominal, gynecological, orthopedic, thoracic, and genitourinary surgery.
- Reprocessing of MIS instruments is performed according to the manufacturer's instructions. Most instruments can be steam-sterilized but require careful cleaning and decontamination before sterilization.

- Because MIS is performed in limited anatomical spaces, various techniques are used to open these tissue planes. Insufflation and fluid expansion are the two most common methods.
- Electrosurgery during MIS can increase the risk of patient burns because the instruments are not always under direct vision of the lensed telescope. Extra caution and vigilance are necessary to prevent patient injury.
- During flexible endoscopy, a flexible tube is inserted into a body cavity for diagnostic assessment, biopsy, and minor surgery.
- The rigid endoscope is used for resection of tumors and more complex surgery of the genitourinary tract and in gynecological procedures.
- Flexible endoscopes are available for many surgical specialties.
- Reprocessing of the flexible endoscope is a primary issue in infection control. This is because the endoscopes are used in semicritical areas of the body and may have a heavy bioburden.
- The protocol for reprocessing of endoscopes is established by health care organizations, guided by safety and accrediting agencies.
- Surgical robotics is a method of performing telesurgery. This is surgery performed from a remote location through the medium of a programmable machine.
- In the United States, only one surgical robotics system, the da Vinci system, has been approved for use in telesurgery.
- Robotic surgery requires extensive training and a considerable investment by the health care institution.
- The da Vinci system does not replace the surgeon and is always used in conjunction with MIS techniques.
- The main advantages of telesurgery are that it scales down the surgeon's hand movements to remove any tremor and greatly magnifies the surgical site.
- At this time, there are no conclusive studies to show that robotic procedures provide better overall patient outcomes than those obtained with traditional minimally invasive procedures.

REVIEW QUESTIONS

1. What patients would not be good candidates for minimally invasive laparoscopic surgery?
2. Explain how abdominal adhesions can cause injury during MIS.
3. Explain how the view of the surgical site is transmitted to the monitor during endoscopic surgery.
4. What would the effect be on a fiberoptic light if some of the fibers were broken?
5. In what ways are the physical aspects of minimally invasive instruments different from standard instruments used in open surgery?
6. What do you think might be the reasons for converting from an endoscopic surgery to open surgery?
7. What are the physiological risks to the patient during insufflation?

8. Compare the risks of stainless steel trocars and plastic or nonconductive trocars.
9. Explain the difference between capacitative coupling and direct coupling.
10. What is the role of the surgical technologist in preventing patient burns during the use of electrosurgery in MIS?
11. What are the advantages of robotic surgery?
12. What are some of the resources available for learning the techniques of robotic surgery?
13. Why is room setup so important during robotic surgery?
14. What role does the technologist have in patient safety during robotic surgery?

CASE STUDIES

Case 1

The risk of inadvertent thermal injury (burns) to abdominal viscera during minimally invasive surgery of the abdomen (laparoscopy) can be prevented by using risk reduction measures. Some of these measures are under the direct control of the scrubbed surgical technologist. Using your knowledge of electrosurgery, outline a risk reduction plan. Use a time-related structure for the plan (preoperative, intraoperative, and postoperative). Use material learned in this chapter and Chapter 18 to formulate the plan.

Case 2

A patient is undergoing hysteroscopy with ablation of uterine fibroid tissue using monopolar electrosurgery. An error has occurred in selection of the uterine distention fluid, and the patient has symptoms of fluid overload (hypervolemia) with severe hypertension. Explain the process of intravasation and how this error could have been prevented. Why does intravasation occur?

Case 3

Flexible endoscopy is often performed as a diagnostic procedure in outpatient clinics. A surgical technologist may assist during the procedure and in care of the endoscopic equipment and instruments. He or she may also be required to provide direct care to the patient in positioning, transporting, and taking vital signs. Based on your current knowledge of communication skills, patient moving and handling, and care of high-technology equipment used in endoscopy, describe which aspects of this role might be difficult for you personally. In your self-evaluation, explain what you might do to increase your knowledge base and skills.

BIBLIOGRAPHY

American Society for Gastrointestinal Endoscopy: Multi-society guideline for reprocessing flexible gastrointestinal endoscopes, *Gastrointestinal Endoscopy* 62:1, 2003.

Association of periOperative Registered Nurses (AORN): *Standards, recommended practices and guidelines, 2007 edition*, Denver, 2007, AORN.

Brown University: *Robotic surgery*. Accessed January 16, 2009, at http://biomed.brown.edu/Courses/B11082105Groups/04/index.html.

Catalone B, Koos G: Flexible endoscopes avoiding reprocessing errors critical for infection prevention and control, *Managing Infection Control* 80, June 2005, Accessed January 16, 2009, at http://www.olympusamerica.com/msg_section/files/mic0605p74.pdf.

Catalone C, Fickenscher K: Emerging technologies in the OR and their effect on perioperative professionals, *AORN Journal* 86:958, 2007.

Francis P: The evolution of robotics in surgery and implementing a perioperative robotics nurse specialist role, *AORN Journal* 83:629, 2006.

Intuitive Surgical: *da Vinci S surgical system interactive training tool: facilitator's guide*, Sunnyvale, Calif, 2005, Intuitive Surgical.

Intuitive Surgical: *da Vinci surgical system user's manual*, Sunnyvale, Calif, 2007, Intuitive Surgical.

Khraim F: The wider scope of video-assisted thoracoscopic surgery, *AORN Journal* 85:1199, 2007.

Olympus America: *Reprocessing Olympus GI endoscopes*. Training video 140/160/180 series, Center Valley, Pa, Olympus America. Accessed January 16, 2009, at http//www.olympusamerica.com/msg_section/cds/cds_videos.asp.

Rigdon J: Robotic-assisted laparoscopic radical prostatectomy, *AORN Journal* 84:759, 2006.

Talamini M, Hanly E: Technology in the operating suite, *Journal of the American Medical Association* 293:863, 2005.

U.S. Department of Labor: *OSHA technical manual: industrial and robot system safety*. Accessed November 29, 2007, at http://www.osha.gov/dts/shta/otm/otm_iv_4.html.

Vangie D: Advancing patient safety in laparoscopy: the active electrode monitoring system, *Patient Safety & Quality Healthcare* May/June 2005. Accessed January 16, 2009, at http://www.psqh.com/jayjune05/aems.html.

Gynecological and Obstetrical Surgery

25

CHAPTER OUTLINE

LEARNING OBJECTIVES

After studying this chapter the reader will be able to:

1. Identify key anatomical structures of the female reproductive system
2. Discuss common diagnostic procedures of the female reproductive system
3. Discuss specific elements of case planning for gynecological and obstetrical surgery
4. Discuss surgical techniques used in gynecological and reproductive surgery
5. List and describe common gynecological and obstetrical procedures

TERMINOLOGY

GYNECOLOGICAL AND REPRODUCTIVE TERMINOLOGY

Ablate: To remove or destroy tissue.

Adnexa: A collective term for the ovaries, fallopian tubes, and their connective and vascular attachments.

Coitus: Sexual intercourse.

Colposcopy: Microscopic examination of the cervix.

Cystocele: A herniation of the bladder into the vaginal wall.

Dermoid cyst: A mass arising from the germ layers of the embryo that contains tissue remnants, including hair and teeth.

Electrolytic media: Fluids that contain electrolytes and therefore can transmit an electrical current.

Episiotomy: A perineal incision made during the second stage of labor to prevent the tearing of tissue.

Fibroid: See Leiomyoma.

Hyperplasia: An excessive proliferation of tissue.

Incomplete abortion: Expulsion of the fetus with retained placenta before 20 weeks' gestation.

Intravasation: The absorption of the fluid into the vascular system, leading to increased blood pressure and possible death related to fluid overload. This occurs during surgery when distention fluid used during endoscopic procedures is absorbed through large blood vessels in the bladder or uterus.

LEEP: Loop electrode excision procedure. In this technique, an electrosurgical loop is used to remove a core of tissue from the cervical canal.

Leiomyoma: A fibrous, benign tumor of the uterus that usually arises from the myometrium.

Menarche: The onset of menstruation, menses.

Menorrhagia: Excessive bleeding during menses.

Missed abortion: An abortion in which the products of conception are no longer viable but are retained in the uterus.

Obturator: A blunt-nosed instrument that is inserted through the sheath of a rigid endoscope or hysteroscope to protect the tissue as the instrument is advanced.

Papanicolaou (Pap) test: A diagnostic test in which epithelial cells are taken from the endocervical canal and examined for abnormalities that can lead to cervical cancer.

Parturition: Birth.

Perineum: The anatomical area between the posterior vestibule and the anus.

PID: Pelvic inflammatory disease. PID is caused by a sexually transmitted disease or some other source of infection. It causes scarring of the fallopian tubes and adhesions in the abdominal and pelvic cavity.

Transcervical: Literally, "through the cervix." In surgery, a transcervical approach means that surgery is performed by passing instruments through the cervix.

OBSTETRICAL TERMINOLOGY

Amniotic fluid: Fluid around the fetus in the uterus.

Amniotic membranes: Two membranes that encase the fetus, amniotic fluid, and placenta during pregnancy.

APGAR score: Method of assessing neonate according to respiratory rate, color, reflex response, heart rate, and body tone.

TERMINOLOGY (cont.)

Birth canal: The maternal pelvis and soft structures through which the baby passes during birth.

Breech presentation: Presentation of the baby in which the buttocks or feet deliver first.

Cerclage: A procedure in which a suture ligature is placed around the cervix to prevent spontaneous abortion.

Cord prolapse: Complication of pregnancy in which the umbilical cord emerges from the uterus during labor and may be compressed against the maternal pelvis or the vagina. This can cause obstructed blood supply to the fetus.

Eclampsia: A seizure during pregnancy, usually as a result of pregnancy-induced hypertension.

Ectopic pregnancy: Implantation of the fertilized ovum outside the uterus.

Epidural: A type of anesthesia in which the anesthetic is delivered through a small tube into the epidural space of the spinal cord relieve pain in labor.

Fetal demise: Death of the fetus.

Gestational age: The age of the fetus as measured in the number of weeks from conception.

Hemorrhage: Continuous bleeding from a pathological cause.

Incompetent cervix: A condition in which previous cervical injury results in repeated spontaneous abortions.

Labor: The process of regular contraction of the uterine muscle that results in birth.

Meconium: A nearly sterile fecal waste that accumulates while the fetus is in the uterus. It is passed within the first few days after birth.

Normal spontaneous vaginal delivery (NSVD): A normal delivery of the fetus, without the need for medical intervention. The normal birth process.

Nuchal cord: A complication of pregnancy in which the umbilical cord is wrapped around the neck of the fetus. This may lead to obstructed blood flow to the fetus.

Placenta: The organ that transfers selected nutrients to the fetus during pregnancy.

Placental abruption: Premature separation of the placenta from the uterine wall after 20 weeks' gestation and before the fetus is delivered.

Placenta previa: A complication of pregnancy in which the placenta implants completely or partly over the cervical os. In this position, the placenta begins to bleed as it separates from the cervix during labor.

Prenatal: The period of pregnancy before birth.

Presentation: Refers to the part of the baby that descends into the birth canal first.

Suprapubic pressure: Pressure that is applied downward on the patient's abdomen just above the pubic bone.

Uterus: The muscular organ that holds the fetus and the placenta during pregnancy.

INTRODUCTION

Obstetrical and gynecological surgery is a combined medical-surgical specialty. Gynecology focuses on the treatment and prevention of diseases affecting the female reproductive system. Fertility medicine combines gynecology and endocrinology to achieve and maintain pregnancy. Obstetrics relates to the process of pregnancy and birth (**parturition**).

In addition to providing routine surgical assistance in gynecological procedures, surgical technologists are employed in the obstetrical department or free-standing childbirth center. This specialty requires a high level of knowledge not only about anatomy and physiology, but also about important psychosocial factors that influence the process of childbirth. Normal childbirth is included in this chapter as an introduction to this specialty.

SECTION I: GYNECOLOGICAL AND REPRODUCTIVE SURGERY

SURGICAL ANATOMY

UTERUS

The uterus and associated organs of the female reproductive system are located in the anterior female pelvic cavity. The uterus is roughly pear-shaped, approximately 3 inches (7.5 cm) long and 2 inches (5 cm) deep. It houses and protects the fetus during pregnancy. It is composed of thick muscular tissue and is suspended in the pelvic cavity by ligaments that completely enclose the organ (Figure 25-1). Two fallopian tubes communicate directly with the interior of the uterus at each lateral "horn" of the uterus. The superior (upper) portion of the uterus, which lies above the insertion of the fallopian tubes, is called the *fundus*. The middle portion is called the *body,* and the lower portion is the *cervix* (Figure 25-2). The uterus normally tilts forward in the pelvic cavity, with the fundus closest to the anterior abdominal wall. However, variations occur and usually are not significant. The cervix is approximately 0.8 to 1.2 inches (2 to 3 cm) long and communicates directly with the vagina through a small orifice called the *external os*. During labor and childbirth, the os dilates as the cervix thins (*effaces*) to provide an opening for the fetus to emerge.

Structure

The endometrium, which lines the uterus, changes under hormonal influence and with pregnancy. It is continuous with the lining of the fallopian tubes and the vagina. The myometrium is a thick muscular layer that is continuous with the muscles of the vagina and the fallopian tubes. The myometrium contracts during childbirth and menses. The perimetrium, or outer serous layer of the uterus, is a reflection (folding back) of the abdominal peritoneum over the bladder. This forms a pouch called the *cul-de-sac;* the fold is called the *bladder flap*.

The *cervix* is the lower neck of the uterus. It extends into the vaginal vault. The opening of the cervix is called the *cervical os*. The os is dilated for **transcervical** procedures; it also dilates naturally under hormonal influence during childbirth. The os has two anatomical sections, the external os and the internal opening. These two openings communicate by means of a short canal.

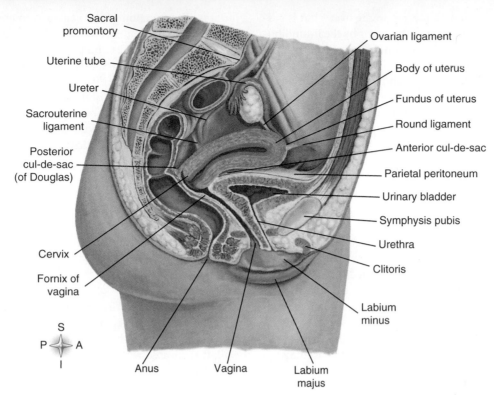

Figure 25-1 **The pelvic cavity.** Note the position of the urinary structures in relation to the uterus. *(From Thibodeau G, Patton K: Anatomy and physiology, ed 6, St Louis, 2007, Mosby.)*

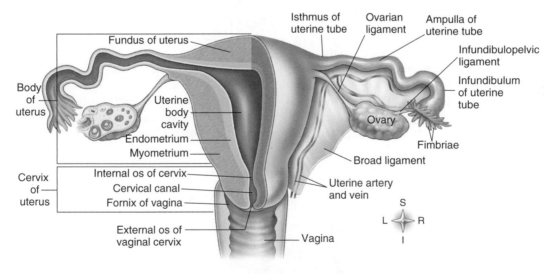

Figure 25-2 **The uterus and adnexa.** *(From Thibodeau G, Patton K: Anatomy and physiology, ed 6, St Louis, 2007, Mosby.)*

Uterine Ligaments

The uterine ligaments sometimes are difficult to picture and understand. The broad ligaments suspend the uterus from the pelvic wall. Above the broad ligaments, near the fallopian tubes, lie the round ligaments, which help suspend the uterus anteriorly. The cardinal ligaments lie below the broad ligaments and provide the primary support for the uterus. The uterosacral ligaments curve along the bottom of the uterus and attach it to the sacrum.

FALLOPIAN TUBES

The two fallopian tubes attach directly to the uterus, one on each side. Each fallopian tube has four sections: the *interstitial section,* which connects to the uterus; the narrow *isthmus* in the midportion; the *ampulla,* which is the widened portion of the tube; and the *infundibulum,* the terminal end of the tube. The *fimbriae* are small projections that extend from the end of the tube. These direct the ovum toward the infundibulum during ovulation. The fallopian tube is very narrow

(3 to 5 mm wide). It is not connected to the ovary, but is suspended from the upper margin of the pelvis by the infundibulopelvic ligament. The lower margin is suspended by the mesosalpinx. Surgery of the fallopian tube usually requires dissection of the mesosalpinx, which frees the tube from its attachments. The fallopian tube, the ovaries, and their ligaments are collectively called the **adnexa**.

OVARIES

The ovaries secrete the female hormones. They lie on each side of the uterus in the upper portion of the pelvic cavity. The ovaries are suspended by the mesovarium, peritoneal tissue attached to the uterus by ovarian ligaments. The ovary is oval and approximately 1.5 inches (3.75 cm) long. Each ovary contains approximately 1 million eggs, which are present at birth.

The fibrous outer layer of the ovary, called the *cortex*, contains follicles that hold ova in different stages of maturity. The inner core of the ovary, the *medulla*, is composed of connective and vascular tissue. Vesicles in the medulla hold the immature ova, which are stimulated to mature after puberty. The development and release of the ova are influenced by the pituitary gland, which stimulates the gonadotropic hormones luteinizing hormone (LH) and follicle-stimulating hormone (FSH). Ova remain in hormone-secreting follicles and develop in stages until they are released from the ovary. A complete cycle is called the *ovarian cycle.*

VAGINA

The vagina, or vaginal vault, is a muscular passageway that shares a thick fibrous wall with the rectum on the posterior side and the bladder on the anterior side. The vagina extends from the vestibule, or introitus (opening to the outside of the body), to the uterine cervix, which protrudes at the upper vagina. The recessed areas around the cervix are referred to as *fornices.* The function of the vagina is to enable sexual intercourse (**coitus**) and delivery of the fetus during childbirth.

The vaginal lining is composed of thick connective tissue covered with epithelium. The lining has numerous folds, called *rugae*, which can distend during childbirth. The tone, lubrication, and elasticity of the vaginal mucosa are influenced by the level of female sex hormones, especially estrogen. After menopause (cessation of ovulation), a decrease in hormonal levels results in loss of elasticity, changes in the vaginal pH, and dryness.

VULVA

The structures that together make up the external genitalia are called the *vulva* (Figure 25-3).

MONS PUBIS

The mons pubis is a raised mound of tissue that protects the symphysis pubis. It is covered with skin and contains connective and fatty tissue that is continuous with the lower pelvic wall. It is covered with somewhat coarse hair that develops at puberty.

LABIA MAJORA

The labia majora are two external folds of adipose tissue that envelop the perineal area. They are extensions of the anterior mons pubis. They encircle the vestibule and protect the external genitalia.

LABIA MINORA

The labia minora are bisectional (composed of two sections) and lie directly beneath the labia majora. The two sections come together anteriorly, where they are attached by the

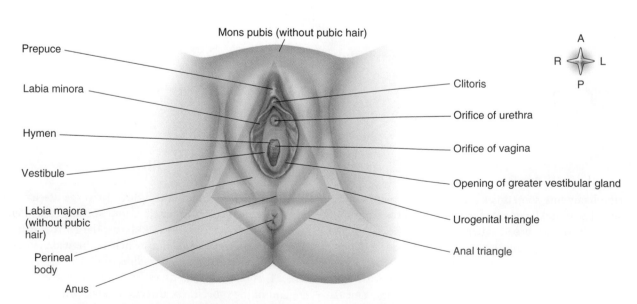

Figure 25-3   Structures of the vulva. *(From Thibodeau G, Patton K: Anatomy and physiology, ed 6, St Louis, 2007, Mosby.)*

frenulum. Anteriorly, they meet just in front of the clitoris to form the prepuce (hood) and are continuous with the vaginal mucosa.

CLITORIS

The clitoris is a highly vascular organ that contains sensitive erectile tissue. It projects slightly from the anterior folds of the labia minora. A fold of skin, called the *prepuce* or hood, covers the clitoris and is formed by the superior juncture of the labia minora. The clitoris, which is protected by the folds of the labia majora, becomes engorged and highly sensitive during sexual excitation.

VESTIBULE

The term *vestibule* refers collectively to all the structures located within the labia minora. The vestibular glands collectively include the *Skene* glands (paraurethral glands) and the Bartholin glands. The Skene glands are two small, paired glands that lie beneath the floor of the urethra, which terminates at the urethral meatus within the vestibule. The Bartholin glands lie on both sides of the vestibule and secrete mucus during sexual intercourse. These glands are homologous to the bulbourethral glands in the male.

HYMEN

The hymen is a thin vascular fold of tissue that attaches around the entrance of the vagina. The hymen separates the vagina from the vestibule. In the young female, the membrane is usually but not always intact. The membrane generally is torn during coitus and then remains as a notched membrane, which may be further reduced during childbearing.

PERINEUM

The **perineum** is located between the posterior vaginal wall and the anus. Incision into the perineum exposes the strong connective tissue and muscles of the pelvic floor. The perineum may be incised during the second stage of labor to prevent tearing when the baby's head emerges through the birth canal. This is referred to as an **episiotomy.**

OVARIAN (MENSTRUAL) CYCLE

The ovarian cycle is characterized by hormonal and physical changes that occur regularly from **menarche** (the onset of menstrual periods) until menopause (cessation of natural childbearing). The cycle is controlled by a complex feedback system involving hormones of the pituitary, hypothalamus, and ovaries. The ovarian cycle is approximately 28 days long, with normal variation. The cycle occurs in distinct phases:

1. *Follicular phase:* This phase lasts from day 1 to day 14. In this phase, the levels of FSH and LH rise, and a small number of graafian follicles containing the immature ova begin to develop. The fastest growing follicle secretes estrogen, which blocks FSH and stops continued development of the other follicles. When more than one follicle reaches maturity simultaneously, a multiple pregnancy can occur.

2. *Ovulatory phase:* This phase begins approximately 14 days from the start of the cycle and lasts from 16 to 32 hours. The estrogen level falls, and progesterone is secreted by the follicle (the corpus luteum [CL]). This causes the release of the ovum, which leaves a small, blister-like structure on the surface of the ovary. The ovum is picked up by the fimbriae of the fallopian tubes to enable fertilization.

3. *Luteal phase:* The luteal phase begins approximately on day 16 and lasts approximately 12 days. After ovulation, the corpus luteum secretes estrogen and progesterone. This triggers changes in the endometrium in preparation for implantation of a fertilized ovum. If fertilization does not occur, the FSH and LH levels fall, the CL regresses, and the endometrial lining is shed (menstruation occurs).

DIAGNOSTIC PROCEDURES

PATIENT HISTORY AND PHYSICAL EXAMINATION

Diagnosis of a gynecological condition begins with a history and physical examination. These are completed well before any surgical decisions are made. The physical examination includes a complete review of systems with a manual internal (vaginal) examination. Information for the evidence-based medical assessment is derived from the following:

- *Menstrual history:* The year of menarche, the start of menopause, and the history of any diseases or abnormal menstruation. It also includes the duration and amount of monthly flow, characteristics of blood (clots and size), pain, or other symptoms.
- *Obstetrical history:* The number of pregnancies (called *gravity*) and the course of each pregnancy; the number of successful pregnancies, fetal deaths, and full-term and premature births at 24 weeks or more gestation (called *parity*); and the number of hours in labor and the weights of infants at birth.
- *Use of contraceptives:* The type used, whether the patient feels confident with that technology, and whether barrier protection was used against sexually transmitted diseases (STDs).
- *History of previous infection:* The type of infection, treatment, and possible or known exposure to the human immunodeficiency virus (HIV).
- *Signs and symptoms:* Abnormal bleeding, such as postcoital bleeding, spotting between periods, **menorrhagia** (excessive bleeding during menstruation), and dyspareunia (painful intercourse); abdominal or genital pain, vaginal discharge, color, odor, and amount; signs of prolapse or uterine hernia (e.g., pressure on the vaginal wall and irritation).
- *Current medications and allergies:* Current over-the-counter (OTC) medicines, prescription drugs, current or past allergies, and history of substance abuse.
- *Family history:* Family members with cancer, gynecological disease, obstetrical problems, fetal demise, or fetal abnormalities.

- *Social history:* Living situation, stability in the family unit, physical or emotional abuse in the social or family environment, and access to social support.

PREOPERATIVE MALIGNANCY SCREENING

Preoperative testing for malignancy involves a combination of tests, which may include routine blood tests and a serum CA-125 test (tumor marker blood test). These combined assessment tools provide substantial data for estimating the risk of malignancy before surgical intervention. Laparoscopy provides a further means of assessment.

IMAGING TECHNIQUES

Ultrasound and Sonohysterography

Pelvic or transvaginal ultrasound is commonly used to assess the reproductive system and the stages of pregnancy. Ultrasound is also used during pregnancy to detect fetal abnormalities, gender, and gestational age.

A newer technique, called *sonohysterography,* provides greater clarity of ultrasonic images. In this process, normal saline, lactated Ringer solution, or 1.5% glycine is injected into the uterine cavity through a small transcervical catheter before ultrasound testing. This procedure is replacing hysterosalpingography, because it is safer, is painless, and does not require exposure to radiation.

Hysterosalpingography

In hysterosalpingography, a radiological contrast medium is injected into the uterus and fallopian tubes. Fluoroscopy is then used to visualize the uterus and tubes. The procedure is performed under light sedation.

Magnetic Resonance Imaging

Magnetic resonance imaging (MRI) is a more precise tool for diagnosis than ultrasonography or sonohysterography. MRI reveals the exact location and size of tumors. It can determine the extent of tumor invasion into the myometrium. Congenital anomalies in the reproductive track are extremely clear with MRI, and the images assist preoperative planning for reconstructive surgery.

CERVICAL AND ENDOMETRIAL BIOPSY

The **Papanicolaou (Pap) test** is used to screen for cervical cancer. Superficial endocervical (epithelial) cells are collected from the internal cervical os with a delicate plastic "brush." The brush then is swirled in a prep solution, which is used to prepare a series of microscope slides. Abnormal epithelial cells can indicate early-stage cancer or precancerous tissue changes.

Culture of the endocervical and vaginal environment is performed to isolate specific nonresident organisms such as chlamydia, herpes, and *Trichomonas vaginalis.* A test for beta-hemolytic streptococci also is done during pregnancy. Screening for the human papilloma virus (HPV) can be performed during routine cervical cancer screening. Evidence of abnormal epithelial cells or a positive test result for high-risk HPV strains is followed by **colposcopy,** which is the microscopic examination and biopsy of the cervix. During colposcopy, the cervix is painted with acetic acid, which causes preinvasive cells to appear white. These areas are biopsied with forceps.

CONE BIOPSY OF THE CERVIX

Epithelial carcinoma of the cervix or severe dysplasia (abnormal cells) may be treated with cone biopsy. This involves the removal of a circumferential core of tissue around the cervical canal. The cone biopsy encompasses the abnormal cells for a conclusive diagnosis of invasive carcinoma. Conization most often is performed using a local anesthetic and an electrosurgical loop filament. The technique is referred to as a *loop electrosurgical excision* procedure **(LEEP).** A LEEP can be done during colposcopy in the outpatient setting. Laser energy may also used to perform conization.

HYSTEROSCOPY

During hysteroscopy, a semirigid or rigid hysteroscope is used to examine the interior of the uterus and to perform selected operative procedures. The uterus is filled with a clear fluid to increase visibility (see discussion of hysteroscopy later in the chapter).

PSYCHOSOCIAL CONSIDERATIONS

Psychosocial considerations for the obstetrical or gynecological patient concern reproductive ability and social, cultural, family, and community expectations. In many women, body image and identity are closely linked with the patient's ability to reproduce and to care for her children.

The patient's developmental age is an important aspect of clinical care. Younger patients often associate genital surgery with extreme violations of privacy and social taboos. In the perioperative experience, the child is encouraged to yield to examination and touch that she has been culturally and socially trained to resist. Exposure of and focus on the genitals can create feelings of embarrassment, confusion, fear, and uncertainty, all of which require great tact, patience, and empathy on the part of the caregiver. Respect for the patient's modesty is an obvious prerequisite in all cases. Each step of the surgical preparation should be explained to the patient in terms she can understand. Reassurance from the primary caregiver before surgery can ease the fear of surgery.

Patients of childbearing age can be very fearful of reproductive surgery, seeing it as a threat to their reproductive ability. Other patients may feel relieved that long-term medical problems will be resolved. Surgery may also hold the promise of reproductive ability, and patients undergoing procedures to restore reproductive function can experience emotional fluctuations of hope and worry.

Cancer surgery creates feelings of fear and grief. Women of childbearing age may be particularly vulnerable to grieving and depression related to the loss of reproductive ability.

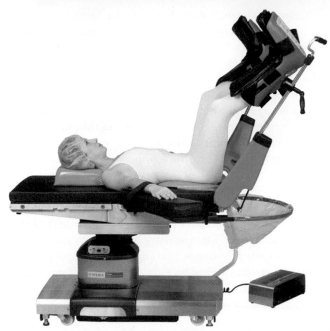

Figure 25-4 Lithotomy position for transvaginal or transcervical procedures. (© 2008 by STERIS Corporation. All rights reserved.)

CASE PLANNING

POSITIONING

Most gynecological procedures are performed with the patient in the supine or lithotomy position (Figure 25-4). Patient safety considerations for the lithotomy position are fully discussed in Chapter 19. Critical safety considerations for the lithotomy position are as follows:

1. Protect the patient's modesty and dignity at all times, even when the patient is anesthetized.
2. All patients must wear antiembolism stockings or a sequential pressure device.
3. When the patient is placed in the lithotomy position, raise both legs simultaneously and slowly into the stirrups—this requires two people. No exceptions can be made.
4. When raising the legs into the stirrups, make sure the hips are slightly externally rotated. At no time should the knees or hips be allowed to drop laterally, because this can dislocate the knees or avulse the hip joint.
5. Raise or lower the patient's legs only after the anesthesia care provider has advised that it is safe. Placing the patient in the lithotomy position may cause changes in blood pressure.
6. When operating the lower table break, make sure the patient's hands are not near the break.
7. When lowering the legs from the stirrups, follow the same procedure as for raising them: two people are required, and the move must be performed slowly to prevent injury.

TEAM POSITIONING

The surgeon may operate from either side of the patient during open procedures. During abdominal procedures, a right-handed surgeon stands at the patient's left side. This allows the best access to the pelvis. The scrub should stand to the patient's right unless otherwise directed. During laparoscopic procedures, the patient is placed in the low lithotomy position, and one assistant is positioned at the foot of the table. A pregnant patient usually is positioned in a modified left lateral position to prevent hypotension from pressure on the vena cava by the fetus.

During vaginal procedures, the scrub is in an awkward position, with the back table placed at the foot of the patient, behind the surgeon or at the side. This requires the scrub either to reach across the front of the surgeon and assistants or pass equipment between them. Neither option is entirely satisfactory; the scrub must take care to prevent contamination of the field in either position.

SKIN PREP AND DRAPING

Gynecological procedures are performed with the patient in the supine or lithotomy position. Skin prepping usually includes both abdominal and vaginal prep with insertion of a Foley catheter. A uterine manipulator (internal cervical retractor) is inserted after the vaginal prep for selected laparoscopic procedures.

The order of prepping for a combined abdominal-vaginal prep is as follows:
1. The perineal prep is performed first. The rationale for this is to prevent possible contamination of the abdomen from splashed droplets during the perineal prep.
2. Always prepare the two sites sequentially, *not simultaneously.*
3. A separate prep kit and gloves are required for each site.

Chapter 20 presents a complete discussion of the surgical skin prep.

INSTRUMENTS

Tissue of the reproductive system varies from extremely delicate to very strong and fibrous. Procedures of the fallopian tubes require atraumatic graspers and delicate dissecting instruments. A bipolar electrosurgical unit (ESU) is used rather than a monopolar type, which produces more heat and is less precise. Microinstruments are used to anastomose the fallopian tubes.

The fibrous ligaments that surround the uterus are capable of suspending the pregnant uterus and several quarts of amniotic fluid for many months. These tissues are richly supplied with large blood vessels, which require tight, strong clamps that do not slip during surgery. The uterus itself is composed of strong, thick muscle fibers that require heavy dissecting scissors and toothed or grooved clamps (e.g., Heaney or Kocher clamps) for resection. Laparoscopic instruments are specialized for reproductive structures; they include Babcock or other atraumatic forceps, Harmonic shears, a monopolar hook dissector, graspers, and a vessel-sealing system.

Figures 25-5 through 25-7 show common gynecological instruments. Open gynecological procedures of the pelvic cavity require a general surgery setup with uterine clamps,

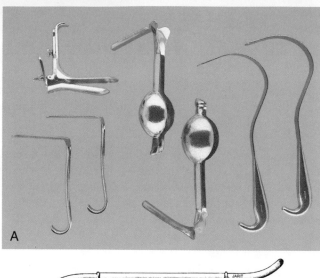

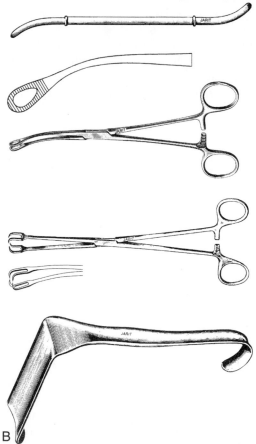

Figure 25-5   Vaginal instruments. **A,** Speculums and retractors. **B,** *Top to bottom:* Hanks cervical dilator, sponge forceps, cervical tenaculum, Sims retractor. *(A from Tighe SM: Instrumentation for the operating room, ed 6, St Louis, 1999, Mosby; B courtesy Jarit Instruments, Hawthorne, NY.)*

plus additional atraumatic clamps (e.g., Babcock forceps and vascular forceps) for handling the fallopian tubes, ovaries, and bowel. Long instruments are needed for patients who are deep-bodied and for deep pelvic procedures. Harmonic shears and a high-frequency (HF) vessel-sealing system often are used during uterine surgery. Hysterectomy and resection of uterine neoplasms often are performed with a combination of cutting and coagulating techniques.

Transvaginal pelvic procedures require vaginal speculums and long instruments, including uterine clamps and heavy dissecting scissors. Instruments can easily slip off the surgical field onto the floor during transvaginal surgery. Unlike in abdominal surgery, in which the surgical field is flat and contiguous with the instrument tables, during vaginal procedures there is an open gap between the patient (the operative site) and the sterile instrument table. Because of this, various clips, pockets, and instrument holders and magnetic pads are attached to the lithotomy drape to prevent instruments from dropping to the floor. These are helpful, but it is best to have extra sterile instruments (especially forceps and dissecting scissors) and ESU pencils available.

Transcervical procedures require graduated cervical dilators, uterine sounds, forceps, sharp and smooth curettes, and an ample supply of sponges. Suction and a monopolar ESU or HF bipolar electrosurgical unit are needed for all procedures. A variety of active electrode tips are required for selected procedures, such as endometrial ablation or removal of intrauterine lesions.

Procedures of the external genitalia require small (7- to 9-inch [17.5- to 22.5-cm]) plastic surgery instruments, as well as regular dissecting scissors, fine-tipped hemostats, forceps, ESU, and 4 × 4 sponges. Fine scalpel blades (e.g., #15 and #11) are also used.

EQUIPMENT AND SUPPLIES

Equipment for obstetrical and gynecological surgery is divided into categories by type and approach to the procedure. Most abdominal procedures are performed using minimally invasive techniques. Laparoscopic equipment includes appropriate-sized telescopes, trocars, imaging equipment, and carbon dioxide insufflation unit. (This technology is described fully in Chapter 24, which describes minimally invasive surgery and techniques used during basic laparoscopy.)

Transvaginal access to the uterine cavity requires a hysteroscope and components, such as tubing, imaging equipment, and distention fluid pump. Other specialty equipment that might be needed during hysteroscopy includes cutting loops, a suction curette, or a vaporization electrode.

DRUGS

A variety of drugs are used during reproductive diagnosis, surgery, and labor. Many reproductive drugs are available to control fertility, hormonal dysfunction, and diseases of the reproductive system. Relatively few are used in the intraoperative period or during labor. (Anesthetics and pain medications are discussed in Chapter 14.) Other drugs not classified specifically for use in obstetrical or gynecological surgery may be administered for conditions that arise during labor and delivery (e.g., hypotensive drugs or electrolyte replacement fluids).

Dyes and Stains

Colored dyes are used to identify and trace anatomical structures during assessment. Methylene blue dye is used during hysterosalpingography to verify the patency of the fallopian

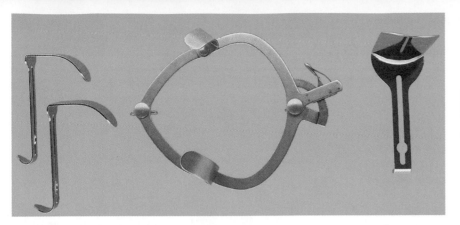

Figure 25-6 Pelvic retractors. O'Sullivan-O'Connor retractor with bladder blade. *(From Tighe SM: Instrumentation for the operating room, ed 6, St Louis, 2003, Mosby.)*

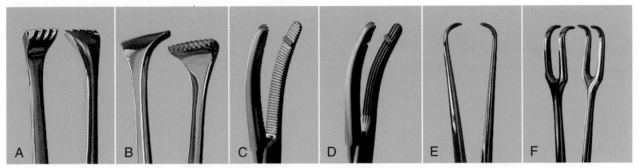

Figure 25-7 Uterine tissue clamps. A, Allis clamp. **B,** Allis-Adair clamp. **C** and **D,** Heaney clamps. **E,** Single-toothed tenaculum. **F,** Double-toothed tenaculum. *(From Tighe SM: Instrumentation for the operating room, ed 6, St Louis, 2003, Mosby.)*

tubes. Acetic acid (Monsel solution) is used during colposcopy to reveal areas of abnormal cervical tissue. Lugol solution is also used during colposcopy for staining the cervix during the Schiller test.

Vasoconstrictors

The drug vasopressin (Pitressin) causes construction of blood vessels when injected. This drug, which is used for emergency cardiac response, may be injected into the uterus during hysterectomy or into a benign uterine tumor to prevent bleeding during removal.

Uterotropic Drugs

Drugs that enhance uterine contractility are given during labor and after cesarean section and abortion. Oxytocin (Pitocin) is administered after delivery of the fetus and placenta to prevent postpartum hemorrhage. The drug Pitressin must not be confused with Pitocin. Methylergonovine (Methergine) is an ergot alkaline that is administered after abortion to enhance uterine contractions and control uterine bleeding.

SUTURES

Gynecological surgery involves many types of tissue. The following sutures are commonly used:

- *Uterine ligaments and vessels:* Absorbable synthetic 0 to 2-0 taper needle
- *Bladder reflection:* Absorbable synthetic 2-0 to 3-0 small taper needle
- *Ovary:* Absorbable synthetic 3-0 to 4-0 small taper needle
- *Fallopian tube repair or anastomosis:* Inert monofilament or braided 5-0 to 7-0
- *Vaginal vault:* Absorbable synthetic 2-0 to 3-0 medium curved needle
- *Plastic procedures of the vulva:* Nylon, Prolene, or other monofilament, 3-0, 4-0; $\frac{3}{8}$ circle cutting needle

SURGICAL TECHNIQUES IN GYNECOLOGICAL AND REPRODUCTIVE SURGERY

LAPAROSCOPY

Many abdominal procedures of the reproductive system are performed as laparoscopic surgery. Chapter 24 presents a complete description of minimally invasive surgery techniques, including equipment, approach, special safety considerations, and perioperative patient care. The scrub should be familiar with these before approaching the gynecological specialty. A general review of techniques includes:

1. The laparoscope (its use and handling)
2. Imaging systems used in laparoscopy (components and how to use them)
3. Instruments (their use and care)

4. Carbon dioxide (CO_2) insufflation (techniques and patient safety)
5. Safe use of a monopolar and an HF bipolar ESU in laparoscopy
6. Use of vessel-sealing systems (e.g., LigaSure)
7. Ultrasonic cutting and coagulating systems (e.g., SonoSurg, Harmonic shears)

The principles of laparoscopic surgery apply to the pelvic and combined vaginal-pelvic procedures discussed in this chapter. During laparoscopic pelvic surgery, the uterus is retracted with a uterine manipulator. This instrument is placed through the cervical os after the complete abdominal and vaginal prep and immediately before surgery. The handpiece of the manipulator is accessible outside the perineum, where it is handled (usually by the assistant) under the guidance of the surgeon.

ABDOMINAL PROCEDURES

LAPAROSCOPY: GENERAL TECHNIQUE

Surgical Goal

Many abdominal and pelvic procedures now can be performed using minimally invasive techniques. (Chapter 24 presents a complete discussion of the techniques and equipment used in laparoscopy.) Table 25-1 shows instruments that are specific to gynecological laparoscopic procedures.

Pathology

Gynecological surgery now is routinely performed laparoscopically for medical conditions that previously required laparotomy. These include procedures of the ovaries, fallopian tubes, and uterus.

TECHNIQUE

1 Vaginal and abdominal preps are performed.
2 A Foley retention catheter is inserted into the bladder.
3 Dilation and curettage may be performed.
4 A uterine manipulator is inserted into the cervix.
5 The patient is draped for exposure to the perineum and pelvis.
6 Pneumoperitoneum is established, and the laparoscope is introduced into the abdomen (Figure 25-8).
7 Additional trocars are placed, depending on the surgical objectives.
8 The uterus, adnexa, and abdominal wall are examined.
9 A specific procedure is performed.
10 The trocars are removed and pneumoperitoneum is released.
11 If a uterine manipulator has been used, it is removed, and the cervix is inspected for injury.
12 The perineum is dressed with a pad.

Discussion

The abdomen, perineum, and vagina are prepped for a combined procedure. A dilation and curettage (D & C) often is

Table 25-1 | Laparoscopic Gynecological Instruments

Instrument	Use
10-mm Allis clamp	Grasping the myometrium, large myomas, and large ovarian cysts after drainage Removing specimens from the abdominal cavity
Hook scissors	Cutting through very dense tissue
Metzenbaum scissors with monopolar capability	Dissection Cutting Simultaneous coagulation and cutting
Bowel grasper	Manipulation of the bowel Retraction
Monopolar hook	Incising and coagulating
Biopsy forceps	Removing peritoneal or ovarian specimens
Maryland dissector	Blunt dissection
Standard grasper	Tissue handling Manipulation
Suction-irrigation probe with Poole sleeve. The probe connects to a handle with trumpet valves for separate suction and irrigation. Irrigation is introduced through a plastic tube connected to irrigation fluid.	Hydrodissection Aspiration of fluids and clots Irrigation
Aspiration needle (14 gauge)	Withdrawal of fluid from cysts
Alligator grasper	Grasping myoma tissue Retrieving specimens

performed in conjunction with a laparoscopy (discussed later). After the D & C, a uterine manipulator is inserted into the cervix. The manipulator provides a means of retracting the uterus from the perineum while laparoscopy is ongoing. Once the manipulator is in place, the patient can be draped using routine techniques.

To start the procedure, the surgeon elevates the abdominal wall manually by inserting two sharp towel clips on either side of the umbilicus. This lifts the wall away from the retroperitoneal vessels. A nick is made in the periumbilical region with the scalpel. A Veress needle then is inserted into the periumbilical incision, and saline is injected into the needle port. Negative pressure in the abdomen pulls the saline into the abdomen. This demonstrates that the needle has cleared any viscera or vessels. The needle is attached to insufflation tubing to start a controlled pneumoperitoneum. An alternative technique is to insert the trocars without using the Veress needle. The first port is used to receive the laparoscope. Secondary trocars are inserted as needed.

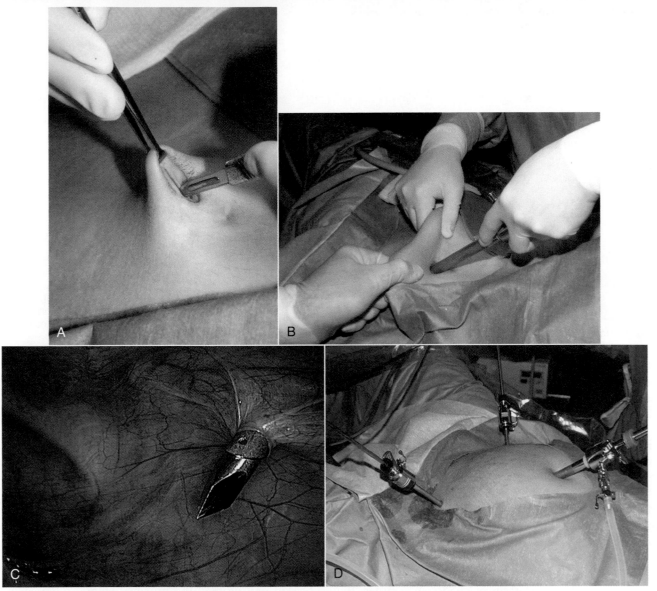

Figure 25-8 Laparoscopy. A, Vertical infraumbilical incision. **B,** A trocar is inserted through the incision. **C,** The trocar is inserted under direct vision of the telescope. **D,** Three ports are placed in the abdomen. Note the insufflation tube (*lower right*). *(From Goldberg JM, Falcone T: Atlas of endoscopic techniques in gynecology, Philadelphia, 2001, WB Saunders.)*

NOTE: *The dangers and risks of pneumoperitoneum are thoroughly described in Chapter 24. The scrub must review these safety features before participating in a laparoscopic procedure.*

When the surgery is complete, the trocars are removed. The pneumoperitoneum is released, and the umbilical port is removed. Trocar sites are closed with fine absorbable suture on a cutting needle. The sites may be dressed with Steri-Strips.

After laparoscopy, patients are closely observed for signs of embolism, infarct, and hemorrhage in the immediate postoperative period. Patients experience shoulder pain for several days postoperatively as a result of the pneumoperitoneum and referred pain from the diaphragm.

LAPAROSCOPIC TUBAL LIGATION

Surgical Goal
Tubal ligation is performed to block the passage of ova through the tube and prevent implantation in the uterus. Tube-sparing techniques may be performed to facilitate reversal.

Pathology
The fallopian tube receives the female ovum after its release from the ovary. The ovum is moved along the tube, is fertilized there, and eventually implants in the uterine lining. Surgical blockage prevents implantation (pregnancy) and development of a fetus.

Many techniques for tubal ligation have been developed. The most popular are application of Silastic bands and clips.

TECHNIQUE

1 Pneumoperitoneum is established.
2 *Coagulation:* Using a single laparoscopic port with an operating channel, the surgeon can use bipolar forceps to coagulate the fallopian tube.
3 After coagulation, the fallopian tube may be transected.
4 *Falope ring method:* A loop of the fallopian tube is drawn into a ring applicator. A Silastic **O** ring is released over the loop, and the loop is then released. The ring causes necrosis of the loop.
5 *Filshie clip:* A clip is applied over the fallopian tube.
6 The ports are withdrawn and the wounds are closed.

Discussion

Tubal ligation was the first procedure to be performed with the laparoscope. Three methods commonly used are described in the following sections. The patient is placed in the low lithotomy position and prepped for abdominoperineal access. The uterine manipulator is inserted before surgery. One or two trocars are placed in the abdomen after pneumoperitoneum has been established. The assistant may retract the uterus using the uterine manipulator; this brings the tubes into laparoscopic view. Atraumatic forceps (e.g., Babcock forceps) are used to elevate the tubes, which are then occluded by one of the three methods discussed next. The trocars are withdrawn, and the pneumoperitoneum is released. The trocar sites are closed with synthetic absorbable suture and Steri-Strips or skin staples. The uterine manipulator is carefully withdrawn.

TRANSECTION AND COAGULATION The fallopian tube is grasped with a Babcock forceps or endoscopic grasper. The HF bipolar unit is used to sever the tube and coagulate the free ends.

FALOPE RING For the Falope ring method, the scrub loads a small Silastic **O** ring into a ring applicator. The surgeon inserts the applicator into the trocar site and withdraws a loop of the fallopian tube into the applicator. The Silastic ring is ejected over the loop, which is then released back into the pelvis (Figure 25-9). The loop causes local ischemia and eventual necrosis of the loop of tissue.

FILSHIE CLIP For the Filshie clip procedure, the Filshie applicator is inserted through the single port. The clip is applied over the fallopian tube and clamped in place (Figure 25-10). After the procedure, instruments are withdrawn and the pneumoperitoneum is released. One or two deep sutures are inserted and the skin is closed.

Open tubal ligation through a minilaparotomy incision or after cesarean section may be performed with the Irving or Pomeroy technique. In this procedure, the fallopian tube is

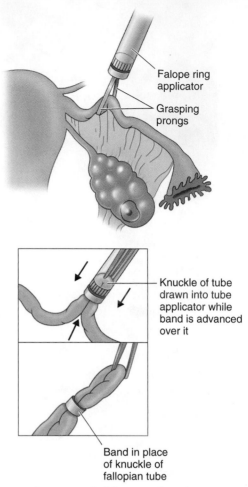

Figure 25-9 Falope ring tubal ligation. The Silastic ring applicator is used to grasp the tube, retract it, and apply the **O** ring. *(From Falcone T, Hurd W: Clinical reproductive medicine and surgery, Philadelphia, 2007, Mosby.)*

severed and ligated. The proximal stump is buried in the uterine serosa with several absorbable sutures. The Irving technique is shown in Figure 25-11.

LAPAROSCOPIC MANAGEMENT OF AN OVARIAN MASS

Surgical Goal

Exploratory laparoscopy is performed to confirm the pathology of an ovarian mass. Preoperative evaluation of a mass is routine in all procedures. Ovarian cysts are removed to determine their pathology and for cancer staging, as explained in Chapter 7. *Oophorectomy* (removal of the ovary) or ovarian cystectomy (removal of an ovarian cyst) may be performed during laparoscopy. The scrub should also be prepared for transition to an open case.

Pathology

FUNCTIONAL OVARIAN CYST Normally during the ovarian cycle, several ovarian follicles begin to mature. The dominant

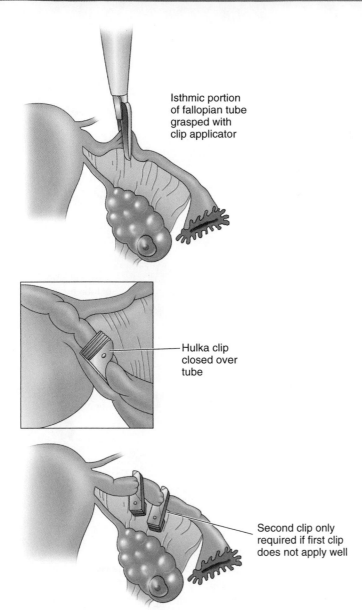

Isthmic portion
of fallopian tube
grasped with
clip applicator

Hulka clip
closed over
tube

Second clip only
required if first clip
does not apply well

Figure 25-10 **Filshie clip method of tubal ligation.** *(From Falcone T, Hurd W: Clinical reproductive medicine and surgery, Philadelphia, 2007, Mosby.)*

follicle continues to form, whereas the others rupture spontaneously; these are referred to as *functional ovarian cysts.* Occasionally these form benign fluid- or blood-filled cysts, which regress normally. Polycystic ovary syndrome (PCOS) is diagnosed in women with persistent multiple cystic follicles. The condition is associated with obesity, diabetes, or other forms of insulin resistance. Persistent cysts may be removed surgically.

TERATOMA A teratoma (also called a **dermoid cyst**) is a common ovarian tumor that arises from one of the germ layers of the developing embryo. The tumor persists throughout development and may contain hair, teeth, sebaceous

material, and skin, which are normal components of the germ layer. A teratoma may be malignant but seldom causes symptoms. Most are found incidentally during ultrasound or surgery for other reasons.

BENIGN AND MALIGNANT OVARIAN TUMOR Benign ovarian tumors include cystadenomas and mucinous cystadenomas. These tumors are rarely malignant, but they can become quite large, requiring removal of the ovary.

The three types of primary ovarian malignancy are epithelial cancer (90% of cases), germ cell cancer, and gonadal stroma. Ovarian cancer is among the most lethal cancers. Metastasis generally occurs before a diagnosis is made. Exploratory laparotomy or laparoscopy is required for definitive diagnosis with staging. Cytological washing with tumor debulking may provide palliative treatment.

TECHNIQUE

1 Pneumoperitoneum is established.
2 The abdomen is explored, and surgical staging is performed.
3 A cyst is identified, and the outer membrane (cortex) is incised.
4 The edge of the cyst cortex is grasped, and the dissection is started.
5 The cortex is everted, and dissection is continued until the cyst is completely mobilized.
6 The cyst or mass is brought out of the abdomen through a retrieval bag or vaginal incision.
7 The surgeon examines the cystic bed and controls bleeding with the electrosurgical unit (ESU).
8 If the cyst ruptures, the abdomen is irrigated with copious amounts of lactated Ringer solution.

Discussion

Laparoscopic management of ovarian cysts depends on the size and type of cyst and the risk of malignancy. Spillage of a potentially malignant cyst is always avoided to prevent the spread of cancerous cells (seeding). A large cyst can be removed through a specimen retrieval bag and a 10-mm trocar port.

The patient is placed in the low lithotomy position, prepped, and draped for a laparoscopic procedure. After pneumoperitoneum has been established, the surgeon examines the abdominal contents. Cancer staging and pelvic washing may be performed at this point. Pelvic washing provides a medium for the collection of cells, which can be evaluated postoperatively. For pelvic washing, 50 to 100 mL of normal saline is introduced into the abdomen, and the fluid is then aspirated and retained as a specimen.

To remove a cyst, the surgeon incises the cortex (outer covering) of the cyst without rupturing it. The incision is made with fine scissors or the ESU pencil. The cortex is removed using blunt dissection. An atraumatic grasper may be used at

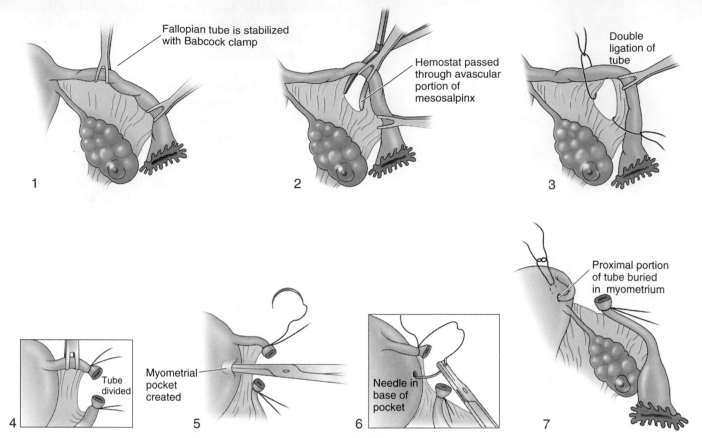

Figure 25-11   Classic Irving technique of open tubal ligation. *(From Falcone T, Hurd W: Clinical reproductive medicine and surgery, Philadelphia, 2007, Mosby.)*

this point to facilitate removal. A suction-irrigator may be used to separate the cyst from the cortex. Bleeders are controlled with the bipolar ESU.

The specimen is protected from rupture and placed in a specimen retrieval bag. The bag is delivered through a 10-mm trocar port, with the bag opening advanced ahead of the specimen. The cyst contents can then be safely aspirated (Figure 25-12). If the specimen is too large for retraction, it can be reduced with a morcellator and the pieces can be brought out through the bag opening. An alternative method of removing large specimens is to make an incision in the uterine cul-de-sac and deliver the cyst through the vagina. The peritoneal reflection (bladder flap) is then repaired with absorbable sutures.

A teratoma is removed intact by sharp dissection and extracted through a specimen retrieval bag using the technique described previously. If rupture occurs, the abdominal cavity is thoroughly irrigated with normal saline. A frozen section may be performed at the time of laparoscopy to determine the need for more radical surgery.

In some cases, complete removal of the ovary may be indicated after laparoscopic assessment and staging. The technique used requires dissection of the ovarian ligaments. This is performed with the ultrasonic scalpel, fine dissecting scissors, and probe. Ovarian vessels are occluded with fine staples,

the bipolar ESU, a vessel-sealing system, or absorbable ligature loops. Once the ligaments have been released and bleeding controlled, the ovary can be withdrawn from the abdominal cavity through a large port and specimen retrieval bag. The ports are removed, and the pneumoperitoneum is released. Individual wounds are closed with absorbable sutures and skin staples.

MICROSURGICAL TUBAL ANASTOMOSIS

Surgical Goal

Tubal anastomosis is performed to restore continuity to the fallopian tube to reverse tubal ligation or to treat another condition.

Pathology

Obstruction of the fallopian tube frequently occurs as a result of an infection that spreads from the lower genital tract to the uterus, fallopian tubes, and ovaries. According to the Centers for Disease Control and Prevention (CDC), approximately 1 million women per year acquire pelvic inflammatory disease (**PID**) as a result of genital tract infections. Of these, 100,000 women become infertile and 150 die.[1] The causal organism usually is *Chlamydia trachomatis* or *Neisseria gonorrhoeae*,

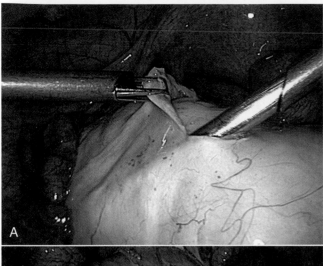
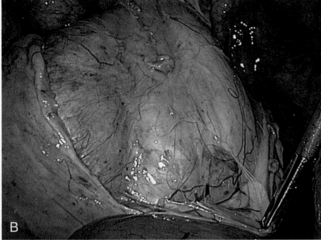
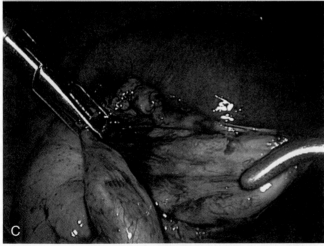

Figure 25-12 **Removal of an ovarian cyst. A,** The cyst wall is dissected with a hydrodissector. **B,** Dissection of the cyst wall is nearly complete. **C,** The body of the cyst is grasped and removed from the ovary. *(From Goldberg JM, Falcone T: Atlas of endoscopic techniques in gynecology, Philadelphia, 2001, WB Saunders.)*

which cause scarring and loss of fertility. Reconstruction and tubal anastomosis are performed to restore function after infection or to reverse a previous tubal ligation. The following technique is used to reconstruct the fallopian tube with occlusion at the uterine junction.

TECHNIQUE

1 A pelvic laparotomy is performed.
2 The proximal fallopian tube is excised.
3 The proximal tube is transected until patency can be demonstrated with indigo carmine dye.
4 The distal tube is transected and tested as in step 3.
5 Stay sutures are inserted to bring the two tube segments into exact alignment.
6 An inner layer of sutures is placed circumferentially in the tube.
7 The tubal serosa is anastomosed.
8 The mesosalpinx is sutured together.
9 The tube is again infused with dye to confirm patency.

Discussion

Surgery to restore **patency** (an unobstructed passageway) to the fallopian tube is performed with the operating microscope. The procedure frequently is performed laparoscopically.

The exact technique required for tubal anastomosis depends on the pathological condition. If the tube is diseased or if the two segments to be joined differ greatly in size, the procedure becomes more complex because the larger segment must be reduced to fit the smaller end.

The patient is placed in the low lithotomy position for access to the cervix and intrauterine cavity during surgery. The abdomen is entered through a transverse pelvic incision. A self-retaining O'Connor or O'Sullivan retractor is placed in the wound, and the bowel is packed away from the uterus with moist laparotomy sponges. The patient may be placed in a slight Trendelenburg position to allow gravitational displacement of the abdominal organs.

The surgeon retracts the uterus with a tenaculum and locates the fallopian tube, mesosalpinx, ureter, and uterine ligaments. Before beginning the procedure, the surgeon may inject the fundus of the myometrium with vasopressin to control hemorrhage. Continuous irrigation may be used to locate microscopic bleeders. A solution of glycine or lactated Ringer solution is used.

The proximal end of the occluded area is grasped with toothed forces, and the serosa of the tube is incised with an ESU needle. The incision is carried through the tube with the microdissecting rod. Small bleeders are controlled with the microbipolar forceps.

The tube then is fully transected with iris scissors or some other fine-tipped, sharp scissors. The proximal side is lifted, and the peritoneal serosa is excised at the uterine body. This incision is carried deeper with scissors. If patency is not evident, the dissection is repeated proximally.

Indigo carmine or methylene blue dye is instilled transcervically to establish patency of the tube where it communicates with the uterus.

The distal segment of the tube is then dissected from the mesosalpinx, and the outer (peritoneal) tissue of the tube is incised with the bipolar ESU. The segment is divided with iris scissors or other fine-tipped, sharp scissors, using the same technique as for the proximal segment. The surgeon then irrigates the distal segment with indigo carmine dye using a Stangel cannula. The appearance of the dye at the severed end indicates patency.

The two segments are then anastomosed. Stay sutures are placed and tagged with fine, small hemostats. Nylon or polypropylene 8-0 or 9-0 suture with a tapered needle are used for the anastomosis. A two-layered anastomosis is performed. If the uterine myometrium has been incised, it is repaired with 6-0 sutures.

The serosa and mesosalpinx of the tube are closed with interrupted 8-0 sutures. Indigo carmine dye is instilled into the tube to confirm that it is patent. The abdominal wound is irrigated and closed in layers.

Microsurgical tubal anastomosis is shown in Figure 25-13.

LAPAROSCOPIC-ASSISTED VAGINAL HYSTERECTOMY

Surgical Goal

Laparoscopic-assisted vaginal hysterectomy (LAVH) is the removal of the uterus by a combined laparoscopic and vaginal approach. It is the most common approach to hysterectomy. The uterine ligaments, adhesions, and any other attachments are released through the abdominal portion of the procedure. The vaginal cul-de-sac is opened, and the specimen is removed vaginally.

Pathology

The LAVH approach for hysterectomy can be performed for early-stage uterine malignancy, benign tumors, or endometriosis. *Endometriosis* is a disease in which endometrial tissue develops anywhere outside the uterus, most often on the abdominal viscera. The tissue remains responsive to hormonal changes and causes pain, bleeding, and scarring. Conservative treatment focuses on pain management and hormone therapy. Surgery may be necessary to remove endometrial tissue. The cause of endometriosis is unknown.

TECHNIQUE

1 The patient is placed in a low lithotomy position, prepped, and draped for a combined abdominal-vaginal approach.
2 Pneumoperitoneum is established, and three or four trocars are placed.
3 The pelvic cavity is assessed for disease and anatomical anomalies.
4 The uterine ligaments are divided.
5 The bladder is dissected from the uterus.
6 The uterine arteries may be dissected at this stage or deferred to the vaginal portion of the procedure.
7 The posterior cul-de-sac is incised.
8 Surgery is shifted to the vaginal approach.
9 The uterine vessels are ligated, and the specimen removed vaginally.
10 The vaginal cuff is oversewn and laparoscopic incisions closed.

Discussion

LAVH requires two setups, one for the laparoscopic portion and one for the vaginal approach. The procedure is routinely performed with traditional minimally invasive techniques (described here) or using the da Vinci robotic system. The principle techniques are the same for both procedures. Refer to Chapter 24 for a discussion of basic robotic techniques. The setup for the vaginal approach includes a vaginal hysterectomy set, ESU, and sutures for ligation and bladder flap closure. Synthetic sutures (0 and 2-0) should be available. Long forceps (e.g., Russian or toothed forceps) are needed for closing the bladder flap. Sponge forceps and 4 × 4 sponges are used until the bladder flap is closed.

The patient is placed in the lithotomy position, prepped, and draped for a combined abdominal-perineal approach. Pneumoperitoneum is established, and three or four trocars are placed in the lower abdominal cavity. The pelvis is examined carefully to determine the extent of disease. Adhesions are released with the bipolar ESU during exploration to open up the pelvic space for thorough exploration and to prepare for uterine dissection.

The scrub should have Harmonic shears, a vessel-sealing system, suction, and irrigation available during exploration. Endoscopic instruments (e.g., uterine clamps, probe, HF bipolar ESU, and monopolar ESU) should be available. Preformed suture ligatures may be required if the uterine vessels are secured by the laparoscopic approach.

The surgeon divides the uterine ligaments and incises the uterovesical peritoneum. If the uterine arteries are to be divided at this stage, this is performed by ligation with heavy synthetic sutures, a radiofrequency vessel-sealing system (see Chapter 18), or surgical staples. The vessel bundles are then severed to free the uterus. Note that it is more common for the vessels to be ligated from the vaginal incision. Before shifting to the vaginal portion of the procedure, the surgeon incises the posterior cul-de-sac, creating communication between the pelvic cavity and the proximal vaginal vault.

The surgeon then shifts to the vaginal approach. The uterine vessels are ligated and severed, and the specimen is delivered through the cul-de-sac. Small bleeders are controlled with the ESU, and the bladder flap is closed with running suture of 2-0 or 3-0 absorbable synthetic material.

The laparoscope and trocars are removed, the pneumoperitoneum is released, and the abdominal incisions are closed with absorbable suture.

NOTE: *A laparoscopic hysterectomy is performed using the steps just described, except that the procedure is completed laparoscopically. The uterus is removed through a large trocar and specimen retrieval bag.*

TOTAL ABDOMINAL HYSTERECTOMY

Surgical Goal

In a total abdominal hysterectomy (TAH), the uterus is surgically removed through a pelvic incision.

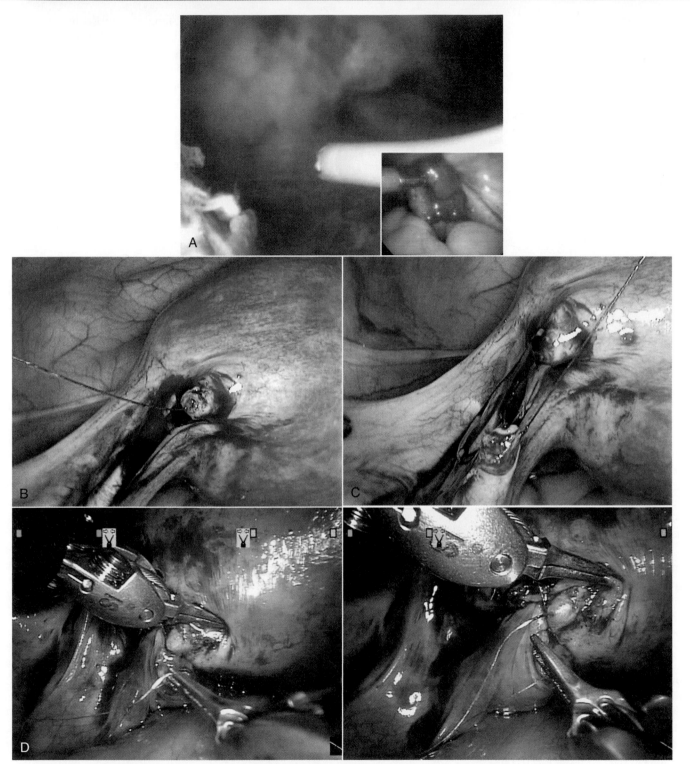

Figure 25-13 **Microsurgical tubal anastomosis. A,** The fallopian tube has been infused with methylene blue dye and incised sagittally. This creates an anastomosis site free of adhesions. **B,** Traction sutures are placed on the outer edge of the tube. **C,** The tubal portions are approximated. **D,** Anastomosis is performed with the da Vinci robotic system. *(From Falcone T, Hurd W: Clinical reproductive medicine and surgery, Philadelphia, 2007, Mosby.)*

Pathology

In the past, open abdominal hysterectomy was the only method available for removal of the uterus. Laparoscopic hysterectomy now is commonly performed. However, open hysterectomy remains an option for selected patients for the treatment of endometrial cancer, endometriosis, large fibroid tumors, abnormal uterine bleeding, and uterine prolapse. TAH includes removal of the uterus and cervix. Unrelated to cervical cancer, endometrial cancer is associated with obesity and high levels of circulating estrogen. All stages of endometrial cancer may also require lymph node excision with internal or external radiation therapy.

TECHNIQUE

1 The abdomen is entered through a transverse pelvic incision.
2 The round ligament is clamped, divided, and ligated.
3 The incision is carried anteriorly to the peritoneal bladder reflection.
4 The bladder is dissected from the lower uterine segment, creating a bladder flap.
5 Dissection of the uterine ligaments and arteries is carried to the vaginal cuff.
6 The cervix is incised circumferentially and amputated from the vaginal cuff.
7 The uterus is removed, and the specimen is passed from the surgical field.
8 The vaginal cuff is grasped with clamps and sutured.
9 The previously dissected bladder flap is reattached.
10 The abdominal wound is irrigated and closed in layers.

Discussion

The patient is placed in the supine position. After a routine abdominal and vaginal prep, a Foley catheter is inserted for continuous urinary drainage. A lower midline or Pfannenstiel incision can be used for a hysterectomy. The incision traverses the lower abdomen approximately 3 to 4 inches (7.5 to 10 cm) above the symphysis pubis.

To begin the surgery, the surgeon makes a transverse skin incision and extends it through the subcutaneous tissue with the ESU. The next layer, the fascia, is entered with the scalpel, and the incision is lengthened with curved Mayo scissors. The surgeon then grasps one edge of the fascial margin with two or more Kocher clamps. Using blunt dissection, the surgeon separates the fascia from the underlying muscle.

This procedure is repeated on the lower fascial margin. The muscle layer is then divided manually. The peritoneum is incised with the scalpel, and the incision is lengthened with Metzenbaum scissors. A self-retaining retractor (e.g., O'Sullivan, O'Connor, or Balfour retractor) is placed in the wound. The surgeon packs the bowel away from the uterus with moist lap sponges.

The surgeon isolates the uterus by severing it from the uterine ligaments, ovaries, and fallopian tubes. Beginning with the round ligaments, the surgeon double-clamps, divides, and ligates each attachment with suture ligatures. Heaney, Heaney-Ballentine, or Masterson forceps usually are used for this part of the procedure. The scrub should have at least four of these clamps available on the Mayo stand.

Absorbable suture is used to ligate the ligaments. Chromic gut or absorbable synthetic suture on large tapered needles is used. To divide the ligaments, the surgeon uses curved Mayo scissors or the scalpel. Long instruments should be available if the patient has a deep pelvis.

The surgeon mobilizes the uterus to the level of the bladder. At this point, the bladder is continuous with the uterus; both organs are attached by a peritoneal covering. Using Metzenbaum scissors and long tissue forceps, the surgeon separates the two structures by dissecting the peritoneal covering away from the bladder. When the bladder has been separated from the uterus, mobilization is continued.

At the level of the cervix, long Allis or Kocher clamps are placed around the edge of the cervix, and it is divided from the vagina. The surgeon uses long scissors or the long scalpel to divide the tissue. This maneuver completely frees the uterus, which is passed to the scrub. All instruments that have come in contact with the cervix or vagina must be kept separate from the rest of the setup. The specimen and isolated instruments should be received in a basin.

To close the wound, the surgeon first closes the vaginal vault where it was separated from the cervix. Absorbable sutures of the same type used on the uterine ligaments are used. The muscular layer of the vagina is closed with figure-of-eight sutures. After closing the vagina, the surgeon uses 2-0 or 3-0 suture on a small tapered needle to reattach the bladder flap.

The abdominal wound is irrigated with warm saline and checked for bleeders. To close the abdomen, the surgeon grasps the edges of the peritoneum with several Mayo clamps. The peritoneum is closed with running suture of size 0 absorbable suture swaged to a tapered needle. The muscle tissue may be loosely approximated with three or four interrupted absorbable sutures. The fascial layer is closed with a wide variety of sutures, absorbable or nonabsorbable, usually size 0 or 2-0. The subcutaneous tissue usually is approximated with 3-0 interrupted absorbable sutures. The skin is closed with staples or subcuticular running suture.

The process of an abdominal hysterectomy is shown in Figure 25-14.

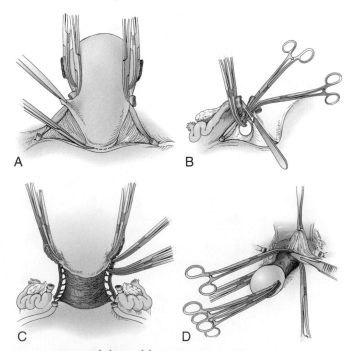

Figure 25-14 Abdominal hysterectomy. **A,** The anterior ligaments have been clamped, cut, and tied, allowing access to the broad ligament. Size 0 absorbable sutures are used for ligation. **B,** The fallopian tube and ovarian ligament are clamped and divided. Heavy suture ligatures are placed through the vascular bundles. **C,** The uterine vessels are clamped and divided at the level of the cervix. **D,** The uterus can now be completely divided. The peritoneal closure is made with interrupted or running sutures of absorbable synthetic material. *(Modified from Gershenson DM, DeCherney AH, Curry SL, Brubaker LC: Operative gynecology, ed 2, Philadelphia, 2001, WB Saunders.)*

RADICAL HYSTERECTOMY

Surgical Goal

A radical hysterectomy involves dissection and wide removal of the uterus, tubes, ovaries, supporting ligaments, upper vagina, and pelvic lymph node chains.

Pathology

A radical hysterectomy is performed to treat pelvic malignancy. Endometrial cancer is the most common type of cancer in the female reproductive tract. It occurs most often in women 55 to 65 years of age and rarely in those younger than 40. Risk factors for endometrial cancer include endometrial **hyperplasia** (excess proliferation of tissue) related to prolonged estrogen stimulation, obesity, diabetes mellitus, hypertension, or PCOS. It is a slow-growing cancer, and painless bleeding is the primary symptom. The diagnosis is made by dilation and curettage (D & C).

TECHNIQUE

1 The abdomen is opened through a lower midline incision.

2 The retroperitoneal space is entered, and retractors are placed.

3 The round and infundibulopelvic ligaments are clamped and ligated.

4 The ureter is identified and retracted with a vein retractor.

5 The iliac artery, obturator fossa, and ureter are dissected of lymph and connective tissue.

6 A lymph gland dissection is performed bilaterally.

7 The uterine artery and vein are clamped, cut, and double-ligated.

8 The peritoneal reflection of the bladder is dissected from the cervix and vagina.

9 The cul-de-sac is opened, and the uterosacral and cardinal ligaments are resected and ligated.

10 The upper vagina is mobilized, and the paraurethral tissues are removed.

11 The upper vagina is cross-clamped and divided, and the specimen is removed.

12 The vagina is closed with running locked suture.

13 The pelvic incision is closed.

14 Sump or gravity drains may be placed in the wound.

15 The abdominal wound is closed in layers and dressed.

16 Vaginal packing may be used.

17 A perineal pad is placed.

Discussion

In a radical hysterectomy, the uterus, tubes, and ovaries, together with most of the parametrial tissues and the upper portion of the vagina, are removed. The ureters are dissected from the paracervical structures so that the ligaments supporting the uterus and vagina can be removed, leaving the uterus intact. The procedure is similar in technical aspects to pelvic exenteration (described later). The scrub should be prepared for extensive dissection and resection of pelvic structures. The dissection progresses from the pelvis to the upper vagina.

The patient is prepared for a lengthy surgery. Compression stockings or a sequential compression device is applied before surgery. A warm air mattress is prepared, and the temperature and fittings are carefully monitored throughout the procedure. A Foley retention catheter is inserted before surgery, and the urinary output is assessed during the perioperative period. Blood loss is calculated by weighing sponges and measuring suction waste compared with irrigation solution used intraoperatively.

The patient is placed in the low lithotomy position and prepped for access to the abdomen and perineum. A vaginal prep is performed before the abdominal prep, according to standard aseptic practice.

Long dissecting instruments (e.g., right angle clamps, long Metzenbaum scissors, toothed forceps, and long curved hemostats) are used intermittently with the ESU. Suture ligatures of size 0 and 2-0 synthetic absorbable material are needed to secure large vessels during dissection. As the dissection progresses, individual lymph nodes may be dissected and removed. The scrub should keep these separate and according to the surgeon's orders.

Deep pelvic procedures require particular attention to sponge and instrument counts, because items can easily be lost in the wound. In addition to routine counts, the scrub should keep track of lap sponges placed in the wound. Throughout a long procedure, the scrub should maintain a clean work space and ensure that instrument tips are free of tissue debris. A basin of water used for maintaining instruments intraoperatively must be kept fresh.

A midline abdominal incision is made, and the tissue layers are divided in the usual manner. An O'Sullivan, O'Connor, or similar self-retaining retractor is positioned. The abdomen is packed with moist laparotomy sponges, and the retroperitoneum is incised. Handheld right angle retractors may be used at this stage. Tissue planes are then developed around the bladder, rectum, uterine ligaments, and ureters. The peritoneal reflection of the bladder is incised with long Metzenbaum scissors or the ESU. Vein retractors or narrow Penrose drains may be requested to retract the ureters once they are isolated. The large vessels of the uterus are resected and ligated. A vessel-sealing system may be used to secure hemostasis. The uterosacral ligaments are then transected along the sacrum in the space between the posterior vagina and the rectum. Posterior and lateral dissection continues to the level of the upper vagina, which frees the specimen. The scrub should have a basin available in the field to receive the specimen.

Wound closure includes the vaginal cuff, retroperitoneum, peritoneum, and abdominal wall. The wound is irrigated, and hemostasis is secured as layers are closed. A count is performed before each layer is sutured.

The vaginal cuff (proximal vagina) is closed with size 0 synthetic absorbable suture. The retroperitoneum is sutured with 2-0 suture of the same material. The abdominal wall is then routinely closed. A suprapubic catheter may be put in place to ensure urinary function. A Penrose or sump drain may be inserted before the abdomen is closed, and the wound is dressed with gauze squares.

After radical abdominal or pelvic surgery, the patient is closely monitored for urinary output, hemorrhage, and infection. The patient may recover in the postanesthesia care unit, or she may be taken directly to the intensive care unit, depending on her physiological status at the close of surgery.

PELVIC EXENTERATION

Surgical Goal

Pelvic exenteration is performed to treat metastatic cancer. It involves the complete removal of the rectum, the distal sigmoid colon, the urinary bladder and distal ureters, and the internal iliac vessels and their lateral branches. All pelvic reproductive organs and lymph nodes, as well as the entire pelvic floor, pelvic peritoneum, levator muscles, and perineum, are removed. A partial anterior or posterior exenteration can be performed, depending on the origin and extent of the cancer.

Pathology

Pelvic exenteration is performed for metastatic carcinoma of the cervix, endometrium, ovary, or vagina when conservative treatments have failed.

Discussion

Total pelvic exenteration is performed only after all other treatment options have failed. The procedure involves resection and reconstruction of all organs of the pelvic cavity. (These procedures are discussed separately in relevant chapters; resection of the bowel and bladder are described in Chapters 23 and 26.) Surgical preparation of the patient requires strict attention to physiological monitoring and homeostasis. The relative length of the surgery adds some technical difficulty for the scrub and circulating team. Care of the patient requires constant monitoring, and the technical needs for supplying ample sutures, sponges, and other items are demanding. The scrub must take care to keep an orderly setup, paying attention to setting priorities. Meticulous dissection, anastomosis, and hemostasis are performed throughout the procedure. (Refer to the techniques and patient care described under Radical Hysterectomy.)

TECHNIQUE

1. The patient should be positioned with lithotomy stirrups and prepped for an abdominal/perianal approach. This position allows access without disruptive positioning changes.
2. A long midline incision is made from the symphysis pubis to the umbilicus, and the abdomen is opened.
3. A second incision is made within the perineum and encircling the vestibule and anus.
4. The peritoneal cavity is explored for metastasis to the liver, the nodes of the celiac axis, the superior mesenteric artery, and the para-aortic tissues.
5. The pelvis is explored for lymph node involvement. If negative findings are noted, retractors are placed and the small bowel is packed with moist lap sponges.
6. The sigmoid mesocolon is mobilized and sectioned with intestinal clamps, a scalpel, or a stapling device.

7. The proximal end of the sigmoid mesocolon is exteriorized through the left side of the abdomen; an intestinal clamp is left across the lumen for later use, when the permanent colostomy is secured to the skin.
8. The remaining sigmoid mesentery is clamped, cut, and ligated down to and including the superior hemorrhoid vessels. Long instruments and sutures are used to reach the deep pelvic sutures.
9. The distal sigmoid colon is closed with inverting suture. The sigmoid colon and rectum are mobilized from the sacrococcygeal area by blunt and sharp dissection.
10. The lateral pelvic peritoneum is cut, and all vessels and ligaments are clamped, cut, and double-ligated.
11. The bladder is separated from the symphysis pubis down to the urethra.
12. The ureters are identified and divided; the proximal ends are left open for urinary drainage, and the distal ends are ligated.
13. The hypogastric artery, internal iliac vein, and superior and inferior gluteal vessels are exposed, clamped, double-ligated, and cut. The external iliac vein is retracted to allow evacuation of the obturator fossa contents, leaving the obturator nerve intact. Care must be taken to preserve the sacral plexus and sciatic nerve.
14. The internal pudendal vessels are identified, isolated, ligated with transfixion sutures, and cut. The remaining soft tissue attachments are clamped and cut. These steps are performed on the opposite sides of the patient.
15. A deep elliptical perineal incision is made.
16. The rectal coccygeal and lateral attachments of the levator muscles are severed.
17. The paravesical and paravaginal tissues are resected from the periosteum of the symphysis pubis and pubic rami.
18. The specimen is removed.
19. Hemostasis is secured, and the wound is closed in layers.
20. Abdominal hemostasis is secured.
21. The anastomosis is made between the ileal segment and the ureters.
22. An external ileal stoma is placed on the right side of the abdomen.
23. A gastrostomy tube is placed in the stomach.
24. The abdominal wound is closed in layers.
25. A colostomy is created.
26. The wounds are dressed, and drainage devices are applied to the colostomy and ileostomy stomas.

TRANSCERVICAL PROCEDURES

HYSTEROSCOPY

Principles

During hysteroscopy, a fiberoptic hysteroscope is inserted through the cervix and into the uterus. This technique is used to assess the uterine cavity endocervix and the lower uterine segment and for selected operative procedures. Operative hysteroscopy is indicated for intrauterine pathology, such as polyps, leiomyoma, adhesions, and septal defects of the uterus. To obtain a clear view of the uterine wall, the surgeon distends the uterine cavity with fluid. This allows small blood clots and other tissue debris to be removed and maintains a clear view. Distention fluid enters through the hysteroscope via a monitored pump system. Waste fluid is released as fresh fluid enters, which provides continuous irrigation.

Examination, biopsy, and surgical procedures are performed through the hysteroscope and operating channels in the same way that cystoscopic surgery is performed through the bladder. Biopsy and resection using a variety of energy technologies (e.g., laser, HF bipolar electricity, and automated ablation) can be performed through the hysteroscope.

Uterine Distention

As mentioned, during hysteroscopy the uterine cavity must be distended. In the past, carbon dioxide gas or viscous fluid (Dextran 70) was used. *These methods are no longer considered safe.* Uterine insufflation with CO_2 poses the risk of death from gas embolism, because high-pressure, low-volume gas is forced into open vessels during an operative procedure. CO_2 insufflation is used only when no operative procedures are planned. When CO_2 is used, the Trendelenburg position is not used, because it increases the risk of embolism.

Dextran 70 was commonly used as a distention fluid in the past because its high viscosity created a crystal clear field and prevented leakage during surgery. *This distention fluid is rarely used today.* The primary reason is the risk of fluid intravasation, toxicity, and allergic reaction. **Intravasation** is absorption of the fluid into the vascular system, leading to increased blood pressure and possible death related to fluid overload. A toxic reaction to Dextran 70 can lead to disseminated intravascular coagulopathy, in which the body's clotting mechanism is greatly diminished. This may result in death from microvascular hemorrhage.

SAFE UTERINE DISTENTION Low-viscosity fluids have largely replaced CO_2 and Dextran 70 as a means of uterine distention. An isotonic solution, such as normal saline, is used for all procedures *except those that require monopolar electrosurgery.*

NOTE: *Use of monopolar electrosurgery during hysteroscopy requires the use of a hypotonic, nonelectrolytic distention fluid. This is because the flow of current must travel directly from the point of contact (the active electrode) to the inactive electrode (the patient grounding pad) and back to the ESU control unit.*

If electrolytic solutions are used with the monopolar circuit, electricity would be dispersed throughout the fluid and might cause patient burns.

Intravasation and fluid overload are always risks during uterine distention. Hypotonic fluids create an additional risk of death from severe *hyponatremia* (low serum sodium level). Meticulous monitoring of fluid is required throughout a hysteroscopy. The scrubbed and circulating teams are jointly responsible for tracking the amount used and the rate of flow during a procedure. Recovered fluid (that which is released from the uterine cavity as waste during the procedure) is constantly computed against fluid instilled to determine the potential amount absorbed by the body. If fluid overload occurs during surgery, the procedure may be terminated immediately and the patient treated.

Hysteroscope

The hysteroscope may be rigid or semirigid. A rigid scope incorporates a 12- to 30-degree angled lens at the distal tip. A 0-degree lens is also available, although less seldom used. The main components of the instrument are the sheath and operating channels. The operative scope has a large sheath to permit insertion of instruments and a channel for instilling the distention medium.

The hysteroscope is inserted into the uterus with the sheath in place. The main operating channel receives the telescope, and side channels, controlled by stopcocks, receive accessory instruments. The main channel is fitted with rubber gaskets that prevent the backflow of distention fluid. Both double-channel and single-channel sheaths are available. Some models have separate channels for the telescope and the liquid medium used to flush fluid and debris from the uterus while operating at the same time (Figure 25-15).

Imaging System

Fiberoptic light is used to illuminate the surgical site during hysteroscopy. Equipment includes a standard fiberoptic light cable and xenon light source. The digital imaging system, which is similar to the laparoscope, has video components, including a monitor, video cable, and image management system. (Chapter 24 presents a complete discussion of digital imaging.)

Operating Instruments

Most hysteroscopic procedures require 3-mm instruments, although 2-mm accessories are available for very fine tissue dissection. Standard instruments including scissors, graspers, biopsy forceps, ESU, and laser fibers are commonly used. A variety of tips are available for HF bipolar and standard monopolar ESU. These include the ball tip, spring tip, needle, and loop electrodes used for removing polyps and dense tumors.

Flexible instruments can be fitted into the deflector bridge. A suction cannula and flexible catheter are used to remove blood clots, debris, blood, and mucus and to inject the liquid medium. Rigid and semirigid instruments are inserted directly into the sheath.

Resectoscope

The intrauterine resectoscope is used to remove polyps, subcutaneous leiomyomas, and uterine adhesions.

The resectoscope has a 0- or 12-degree telescope inserted into a separate sheath. A spring-loaded handle retracts and exposes the loop-shaped electrode tip, which shaves and coagulates tissue when activated. As tissue is removed from the uterine wall, it remains free-floating in the liquid medium until it is flushed from the uterine cavity. The advantage of the loop resectoscope is that it can both shave and coagulate tissue bit by bit, so that bleeding can be easily controlled.

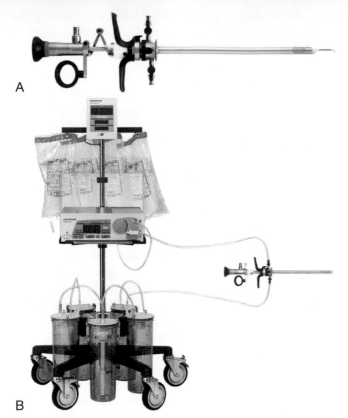

Figure 25-15   A, A resectoscope is used for therapeutic hysteroscopy. Note the cutting-coagulation loop on the distal end. **B,** A fluid distention system for use with the resectoscope. Note that the fluid pressure is regulated to prevent intravasation and subsequent fluid overload, which may cause serious patient injury. *(Courtesy Gyrus ACMI, Inc., Southborough, Mass.)*

The resectoscope is constructed with an outer sheath that allows fluid outflow and an inner sheath for continuous irrigation. Specimens are morcellated and retrieved through the distention fluid.

HYSTEROSCOPIC ENDOMETRIAL ABLATION

Surgical Goal

The goal of endometrial ablation is the destruction and scarification of the endometrium to render it nonfunctional.

Pathology

The endometrium, which lines the uterine cavity, is made up of two layers. The functional layer lies over the basal layer and proliferates during the endometrial cycle under hormonal influence. It is sloughed off during menstruation and is replaced throughout the endometrial cycle. Abnormally heavy menses (menorrhagia) can result in anemia and abdominal pain.

NOTE: *The term* dysfunctional uterine bleeding *has been replaced by the more precise term* abnormal uterine bleeding *(AUB).*

Women who no longer want to become pregnant and have attempted conservative treatment for excessive menstrual bleeding are offered endometrial ablation after conservative treatment has failed. Destruction of the endometrium prevents or reduces menses and is not reversible. The procedure is only performed in women who do not want a future pregnancy. The endometrial tissue is destroyed by the procedure, thereby making normal implantation impossible.

Current gynecological practice offers a number of safe, effective methods of endometrial ablation. Common procedures are roller ball ablation (electrocoagulation) and global (reaching all areas of the endometrium) endometrial ablation using an intrauterine device. Cryoablation and radiofrequency ablation are also available. Laser ablation is no longer routinely offered because of complications and injury. Other techniques have proven to be effective and less expensive without the risks associated with laser surgery.

TECHNIQUE

Roller Ball Ablation

1 The patient is prepared for hysteroscopy.
2 The cervix is dilated.
3 A dilation and curettage is performed.
4 The endometrium is assessed for pathology with the hysteroscope.
5 The resectoscope with roller ball electrode is reinserted into the cervix.
6 Nonelectrolytic distention fluid is infused into the uterine cavity for use with a monopolar electrosurgical unit (ESU).
7 A roller ball electrode is used to ablate the endometrium.
8 The endometrium is again assessed.
9 The resectoscope is withdrawn.

TECHNIQUE

Global Endometrial Ablation

1 Hysteroscopy is performed after cervical dilation.
2 The balloon ablation device is inserted into the uterine cavity and activated.
3 The uterine cavity is again assessed by hysteroscopy.

Discussion

The patient is placed in the lithotomy position, and a vaginal prep is performed. Hysteroscopic examination is performed before and after the ablations. Any lesions, such as polyps or other growths, are removed before ablation to ensure separate pathological assessment. A D & C often is performed before ablation to rule out endometrial cancer. Fluid distention of the uterus depends on the type of ablation planned. Monopolar electrosurgical instruments require *nonelectrolytic media* (e.g., glycine, mannitol, and sorbitol) for distention. Bipolar HF electrosurgery requires **electrolytic media**, such as normal saline.

Roller ball ablation is performed with a ball tip electrode and resectoscope. This is an electrosurgical procedure and therefore requires all safety precautions associated with electrosurgery. After assessing the uterus with the hysteroscope, the surgeon systematically applies a 3-mm roller ball tip to coagulate and desiccate the endometrial tissue. The surgeon begins with the lower uterine segments and proceeds to the cornual region.

In global endometrial ablation, most of the endometrial surface is affected by the ablation method. Global ablation procedures are "blind" (i.e., they are not done under direct visualization of the hysteroscope or resectoscope). A variety of methods can be used for global ablation:

- The NovaSure system consists of a radiofrequency controller, disposable ablater, CO_2 canister, desiccant, and operating system. This system delivers radiofrequency energy through the device, which is inserted into the uterine cavity. It measures impedance while delivering the energy to **ablate** the tissue. The device automatically stops when impedance reaches a dangerous level.
- The ThermaChoice UBT system includes a silicone balloon catheter with impeller, umbilical cable, and controller, which monitors temperature and pressure. The balloon is inserted and filled with 5% dextrose in water. As the balloon is distended, it begins a warming cycle that reaches 188.6° F (87° C). At this temperature, the endometrium is destroyed within 8 minutes. Safety features of the system prevent overheating and overdistention.
- The Hydro ThermAblator uses a 0.9% sodium chloride solution and a rigid hysteroscope. A D & C is performed, and a rigid scope then is used to fill the uterine cavity with saline. The temperature is automatically raised and measured. The active ablation phase reaches 176° F (80° C) and remains at that temperature for 10 minutes. A cool down period is then initiated, and the flushing phase is completed. The device is then withdrawn.
- HerOption Uterine Cryoablation uses a cryotherapy probe and compressed gas to achieve temperatures below 32° F (0° C) to freeze the endometrium. The procedure is carried out under direct ultrasonographic guidance. The probe is activated sequentially and followed by a short heating cycle.

Most methods of endometrial ablation are performed in an outpatient setting, and the patient is allowed to return home the same day. Severe cramping and watery discharge are expected for several days postoperatively. Patients are provided home care instructions on the danger signs of uterine perforation and infection. Few women experience complete amenorrhea after the procedure, and repeat treatment may be required.

MYOMECTOMY

Surgical Goal

Myomectomy is the removal of a benign leiomyoma **(fibroid)** of the myometrium to control bleeding and prevent pressure on other structures in the pelvis. Submucosal myomas can be removed with the resectoscope.

Pathology

A **leiomyoma** is a benign, smooth muscle tumor of the uterus (Figure 25-16). These tumors may cause abnormal uterine bleeding and lead to anemia, or they may impinge on adjacent structures, causing pain or dysfunction.

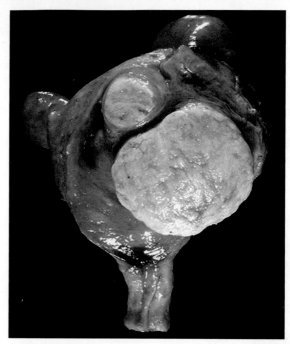

Figure 25-16 **A large myoma specimen.** *(From Canby C: Problem based anatomy, St Louis, 2007, WB Saunders.)*

TECHNIQUE

1 The patient is prepared for hysteroscopy as described previously.
2 After cervical dilation, a double-sheath resectoscope is inserted.
3 The uterine cavity is irrigated and infused with distention fluid.
4 A resectoscope loop is used to shave and coagulate tumor tissue.
5 The outer sheath is removed to flush out the sectioned tumor pieces. Alternatively, the cervix may be further dilated and sponge forceps used to remove pieces of tumor.
6 The myoma is reduced until it is level with the endometrium.

Discussion

The patient is placed in the lithotomy position, prepped, and draped as for endometrial ablation.

The procedure begins as the surgeon dilates the cervix and inserts the resectoscope sheath with or without an **obturator**, which is a blunt-tipped rod that is advanced ahead of the sheath to protect the tissue from injury. If used, the obturator is removed after insertion of the sheath.

A resectoscope with a 0-degree or fore-oblique telescope is inserted into the cervix. The resectoscope is surrounded by an 8- or 9-mm sheath, which has an insulated tip to prevent contact between the active electrode and the outer sheath. The outer sheath provides inflow of the distention fluid. A bridge attachment allows entry of the electrodes.

As mentioned, the resectoscope has a spring-loaded handle that operates the active electrode loop. The surgeon removes sections or slices of tissue by repeatedly looping a small portion of tissue and drawing it into the resectoscope. This cuts and coagulates the tissue and releases it into the uterine cavity, where it is flushed out through the resectoscope sheath.

Bleeding can also be controlled by the ball electrode attachment of the resectoscope. The surgeon flushes irrigation fluid and tissue by removing the outer sheath and allowing the fluid to drop into the perineal drape.

The procedure is complete when the tumor is level with the endometrium. All specimen pieces must be retrieved and collected for pathological examination.

LOOP ELECTRODE EXCISION PROCEDURE

Surgical Goal

In the loop electrode excision procedure, a core of tissue is removed from the endocervix to remove cancerous or precancerous tissue.

Pathology

Squamous cell carcinoma of the cervix is the most common and easily treated cancer of the reproductive tract with early diagnosis. It is almost always associated with HPV types 16, 18, 31, and 33. A diagnosis is made after a positive Pap test with atypical cells is followed by colposcopy and tissue biopsy. During colposcopy, the cervix is examined microscopically with the aid of acetic acid (Lugol solution). The acid causes the atypical cells to turn white, allowing clear identification and removal. If a biopsy shows invasion of atypical or precancerous cells, LEEP is indicated.

TECHNIQUE

1 The surgeon grasps the cervix with a single-toothed tenaculum.
2 A local anesthetic is injected into the cervical canal.
3 A loop electrode is used to remove tissue from the cervix.
4 A ball electrode is used to control bleeding.

Discussion

The patient is placed in the lithotomy position, prepped, and draped for a vaginal procedure. The surgeon infuses the cervix with a local anesthetic. The anterior lip of the cervix is grasped with a tenaculum. A disposable loop electrode is then used to make a circumferential incision around the os. The specimen is removed for pathological examination. The loop electrode is then replaced with a ball coagulator, which is used to coagulate the area of the excision. The cervical cone tissue is sectioned and examined carefully for the depth of cellular invasion. This determines the need for more radical surgery.

DILATION AND CURETTAGE

Surgical Goal

In dilation and curettage, sharp and smooth curettes are used to remove the surface of the endometrium through a transvaginal approach.

Pathology

A D & C may be performed for diagnostic purposes, to terminate a pregnancy, or to treat abnormal uterine bleeding.

TECHNIQUE

1 The uterine depth is measured with a uterine sound.
2 The cervix is dilated with graduated dilators.
3 Curettes are used to remove endometrial tissue.

Discussion

The patient is placed in the lithotomy position. The bladder may be emptied with a straight catheter. The patient is then prepped and draped for a vaginal procedure. The surgeon stands or sits at the foot of the operating table. The scrub should stand next to the surgeon. To begin the procedure, the surgeon places an Auvard speculum in the vagina. The surgeon then grasps the anterior lip of the cervix with a tenaculum and retracts it slightly forward and downward.

A uterine sound is inserted into the cervix to measure its depth and position. This prevents accidental perforation during the procedure. The surgeon dilates the cervix with a Hagar, Pratt, or Hank uterine dilator.

After cervical dilation, the surgeon places a Telfa dressing on the posterior edge of the vagina. The uterus is then gently curetted, and the specimen is collected on the Telfa. The technologist should have several types and sizes of curettes available, including smooth, sharp, and serrated. When curettage is complete, the Telfa is removed and passed to the scrub. Both the Telfa and specimen are placed in a container for pathological examination.

TERMINATION OF PREGNANCY (ABORTION)

Surgical Goal

Abortion is the termination of a viable pregnancy. The remains of a fetus are surgically removed from the uterus after fetal death.

Discussion

Termination of a pregnancy may be advised for medical reasons, or a woman may undergo elective abortion according to the restrictions of gestational age and the age of the mother, which vary according to state law. Medical abortion is performed when the pregnancy endangers the health or life of the mother, when the fetus is likely to die, or when a pregnancy is the result of rape or incest. The reasons for elective abortion are defined by the woman. Surgical abortion by suction or extraction is performed between 4 and 24 weeks' gestation. A D & C may be performed at 4 to 12 weeks' gestation. Most surgical abortions are performed at 12 to 14 weeks' gestation. Preoperative counseling is provided in all cases. Terms related to spontaneous abortion are defined in Table 25-2.

The patient is placed in the lithotomy position and prepped for a vaginal procedure. Sedation and cervical block anesthesia or local infiltration of the cervix is administered. A D & C is performed as described previously, and the suction probe used to remove the contents of the uterus. The contents are documented as *products of conception* and retained as a tissue

Table 25-2	Types of Spontaneous (Noninduced) Abortion
Complete abortion	Expulsion of all products of conception. Surgical intervention is not necessary.
Incomplete abortion	The products of conception have been expelled but the placenta retained. Medical intervention may be necessary to control hemorrhage.
Inevitable abortion	The cervix is dilated and there is rupture of the membranes or vaginal bleeding. The products of conception have not been expelled.
Missed abortion	Undiagnosed and undetected embryonic or fetal demise (death); the products of conception are not expelled.
Septic abortion	Severe uterine infection associated with abortion.
Threatened abortion	Uterine bleeding without cervical dilation occurring before 20 weeks' gestation.

specimen. Complications of surgical abortion include perforation of the uterus and incomplete removal of the uterine contents, which can result in bleeding or infection.

TRANSVAGINAL AND VULVAR PROCEDURES

VAGINAL HYSTERECTOMY

Surgical Goal

For a vaginal hysterectomy, a transcervical approach is used to remove the uterus.

Pathology
See Total Abdominal Hysterectomy.

TECHNIQUE

1 A circumferential incision is made in the vaginal mucosa at the base of the cervix.
2 The surgeon partly mobilizes the uterus by sequentially incising and ligating the uterine ligaments.
3 The peritoneal reflection of the bladder (bladder flap) is dissected from the uterus.
4 The uterus is completely mobilized and removed.
5 The bladder flap is reconstructed.
6 The peritoneum is closed.
7 The deep vaginal incision is closed.

Discussion

Transvaginal hysterectomy is selected as an approach in selected patients in whom surgical access is adequate to perform surgery safely, and in those who are suitable for outpatient surgery or early discharge. The transvaginal approach is less painful and provides early return to normal activities unless there are postoperative complications.

The patient is placed in the lithotomy position, prepped, and draped for a vaginal procedure. A pocket drape should be attached to the perineal drape. The bladder is drained with a straight catheter during the prep.

The surgeon grasps the cervix with a uterine tenaculum. Using the scalpel or curved Mayo scissors, the surgeon makes a circumferential incision around the cervix, separating the vaginal mucosa and fascia from the body of the cervix. This incision exposes the first set of ligaments, which are double-clamped, divided, and ligated with suture ligatures of size 0 synthetic absorbable material on a tapered needle.

The posterior peritoneum is elevated with toothed tissue forceps and incised with the scalpel or scissors. With the peritoneal cavity open, the surgeon removes the peritoneal reflection of the bladder from the uterus using Metzenbaum scissors. The assistant retracts the bladder upward with a Sims or Heaney retractor. The scrub must have long tissue forceps and long dissecting scissors available because the mobilization is carried deep into the pelvis.

Mobilization of the uterus continues until it is completely free. The uterus then is removed as a specimen. Before closing the peritoneum, the surgeon closes the bladder flap with running suture of 2-0 absorbable synthetic material on a small curved needle. The peritoneum is then closed with running absorbable suture. A perineal pad is placed over the perineum to absorb any drainage from the wound.

REPAIR OF A CYSTOCELE AND RECTOCELE (ANTERIOR-POSTERIOR REPAIR)

Surgical Goal

Herniated tissue of the anterior and posterior vagina is reduced, and the vaginal walls are reconstructed.

Pathology
A **cystocele** (herniation of the bladder) and a *rectocele* (herniation of the rectum) occur when the musculature and connective tissues become weakened and prolapse against the anterior and posterior vaginal walls. The most common cause is pregnancy. The pelvic floor provides support to the intestinal and genitourinary structures, especially during pregnancy, when gravity pulls the fetus downward and stretches the ligaments and muscles. Repair and reconstruction of the supportive structure restores normal function and relieves discomfort and pain.

TECHNIQUE

1 The anterior vaginal mucosa is incised.
2 The surgeon grasps the incision edges with Allis clamps.
3 Blunt and sharp dissection are used to create a tissue plane between the vaginal mucosa and the submucosal connective tissue.
4 The dissection is continued to the bladder neck.
5 The vaginal wall is reconstructed with sutures.
6 The posterior vaginal wall is incised, and steps 2 and 3 are repeated.
7 The tissue plane is continued to the rectum.
8 Sutures are placed across the rectal musculature to reconstruct the pelvic floor.
9 The vaginal mucosa is sutured closed.

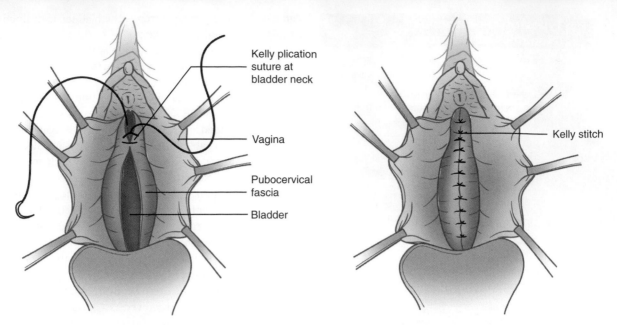

Figure 25-17   **Cystocele repair.** Allis clamps are placed on the periphery of redundant tissue, and the vaginal wall is strengthened with interrupted sutures. *(From Seidel HM et al: Mosby's guide to physical examination, ed 5, St Louis, Mosby.)*

Discussion

ANTERIOR REPAIR The patient is placed in the lithotomy position, prepped, and draped for a vaginal procedure. The patient also is catheterized.

The surgeon inserts a weighted speculum into the vaginal outlet. The cervix is grasped with a tenaculum and retracted. Using the scalpel or curved Mayo scissors, the surgeon makes an incision in the anterior vaginal wall. The edges of the incision are grasped with several Allis clamps. These are fanned out to distend the tissue edges and delineate the plane between the mucosa and the connective tissue underneath.

With the tissue planes exposed, the surgeon uses a 4 × 4 sponge to push the connective tissue off the mucosa. This technique of blunt dissection effectively separates the two tissue layers and creates a flap (the vaginal mucosa) with a minimum of bleeding. The technologist should have ample sponges available. As the sponge becomes moist, its surface becomes smooth, and the sponge is less effective for dissection. The curved Mayo scissors are used alternately with sponges to continue the dissection to the level of the bladder.

During this portion of the procedure, the assistant or scrub may be required to retract the superior vaginal vault upward with a lateral (Heaney) right angle retractor. This elevates the roof of the vagina and exposes the dissection plane.

NOTE: *During retraction, the scrub should exert gentle, even pressure on the retractor to prevent bruising and hematoma in the vaginal mucosa.*

When the dissection has reached the bladder neck, several sutures of size 0 chromic gut or synthetic absorbable sutures are placed through the fascia and pulled laterally. This tightens

the tissue and prevents the bladder from bulging. The edge of the vaginal mucosa is measured over the repair, and the edges are trimmed. The mucosa is then approximated with running or interrupted sutures of absorbable material, usually of the same size as that used on the bladder repair.

POSTERIOR REPAIR To begin the posterior repair, the surgeon places two Allis clamps in the posterior vaginal wall and makes a small transverse incision between them. The assistant provides traction on the clamp as described in the anterior repair. The techniques used in anterior repair are repeated to the level of the rectum. The levator muscles and fascia then are brought together and tightened with absorbable interrupted sutures, and the vaginal mucosa is repaired. A self-retaining catheter may be inserted. Figure 25-17 shows the repair of a cystocele.

VAGINOPLASTY

Surgical Goal

Vaginoplasty is performed to create a functional vagina (neovagina) to facilitate sexual intercourse. Several different procedures currently are performed to achieve the surgical goal. The following procedure uses a vaginal mold and skin graft. Alternatives include peritoneal skin flap grafts or combination tissue grafts.

Pathology

A congenital abnormality of the müllerian ducts during fetal development can result in the absence of the vagina or uterus, a condition referred to as *müllerian agenesis*. Other defects occur with this anomaly, but the absence of the vagina and uterus is the most common presentation. Patients usually are diagnosed during puberty because the onset of menarche is delayed. The external genitalia and hormonal levels are normal. Although normal childbirth is not possible, patients may undergo in vitro fertilization and surrogate pregnancy. The cause of müllerian agenesis is unknown.

TECHNIQUE

1 A split-thickness skin graft is obtained.

2 The graft is fitted around a vaginal mold.

3 An incision is made through the vaginal vestibule.

4 Subcutaneous connective tissue is dissected.

5 A vaginal space is created for the mold.

6 The mold and graft are fitted in the vaginal space, and the labia are sutured.

7 Approximately 1 week after surgery, the initial mold is removed.

8 A removable mold is used during the 6-month postoperative period.

Discussion

Before surgery, the patient is counseled to provide her with information about reproductive alternatives and to ensure that she understands the procedure and postoperative therapy. As mentioned, most patients are diagnosed during adolescence, and this developmental period is distinguished by a search for identity and strong peer approval. It is important for perioperative personnel to understand the emotional impact of the diagnosis and procedure and to offer appropriate support to the patient.

During the first stage of the procedure, a split-thickness skin graft is taken from the buttocks or thigh. The buttocks are a preferred site because of scarring. If the buttocks area is used, the patient is placed in the prone position. The area is prepped and draped. A sponge soaked in epinephrine solution may be applied to the graft site to produce local vasoconstriction. Mineral oil then is applied to the site, and a dermatome is used to remove the split-thickness graft. (This procedure is discussed fully in Chapter 30.) The donor site may be dressed with an Opsite. The patient may then be placed in the supine position for the vaginoplasty. The perineum, thighs, and abdomen are prepped, and a Foley catheter is inserted.

A small draped table may be useful for preparation of the graft. A dermatome, square basin, forceps, sponges, and vaginal mold should be available before the graft is taken. Immediately after harvesting, the skin graft is placed through a skin mesher. This removes blood clots and allows serous fluid to escape from the graft. The graft is then placed around the mold. The scrub should place the transplant in a square basin and place it in a protected area of the prep or back table. The graft is covered with sponges moistened with saline.

A perineal incision is made between the rectum and the urethra. The ESU is used to coagulate small bleeders. The scrub should have Hagar dilators available, according to the surgeon's preference. A tunnel is then made through the subcutaneous tissue with digital separation or dilators. Meticulous hemostasis is necessary to ensure uniform contact between the graft and the tunneled opening.

After the tunnel is created and hemostasis has been secured, the graft transplant is fitted in the opening and secured with several fine absorbent sutures. The labia are approximated with several 2-0 or 3-0 sutures of synthetic material on a cutting needle. The wound is dressed with absorbent gauze. This concludes the first stage of the procedure. The patient remains on bed rest during this period.

Approximately 1 week after the first procedure, the patient is returned to the operating room so that the vaginal mold can be removed. The patient is placed in the lithotomy position, and a perineal prep is performed. The surgeon may remove the sutures during the skin prep, and the used instruments must be removed from the field completely.

The mold is carefully removed and placed in a small sterile basin. The neovagina is then irrigated with warm saline and assessed for any signs of inflammation, infection, or blood clots. A soft adjustable mold is then fitted carefully into the space. The mold is not sutured.

Postoperative Considerations

The soft mold remains in place intermittently for the next 3 months after surgery; it is removed during defecation and urination to prevent expulsion. Approximately 6 months is required for complete healing and normal function. Complications, including infection, fistula, and constriction, may occur during the initial postoperative period. The steps of a vaginoplasty are shown in Figure 25-18.

REPAIR OF A VESICOVAGINAL FISTULA

Surgical Goal

A vesicovaginal fistula is a small, hollow tract that connects the bladder to the vagina. Fistulous tracts can be caused by infection or trauma. Chronic fistulous tracts are lined with epithelial tissue, which prevents the tract from closing. The surgical goal is to incise the length of the tract and remove this tissue. The fascial layer that separates the bladder from the vagina is approximated. Healing then can occur normally, and urine is prevented from draining into the vagina.

Pathology

A vesicovaginal fistula may be caused by a traumatic penetrating injury, infection, radiation therapy that thins and weakens the pelvic structures, vaginal birth, or chronic inflammation. Urine drains into the vagina, causing irritation and incontinence. The fistula may extend into the urethra. The repair may be approached through pelvic laparotomy or vaginally. A pelvic approach is required when the tract occurs in the proximal vaginal vault. A vaginal exposure is described here.

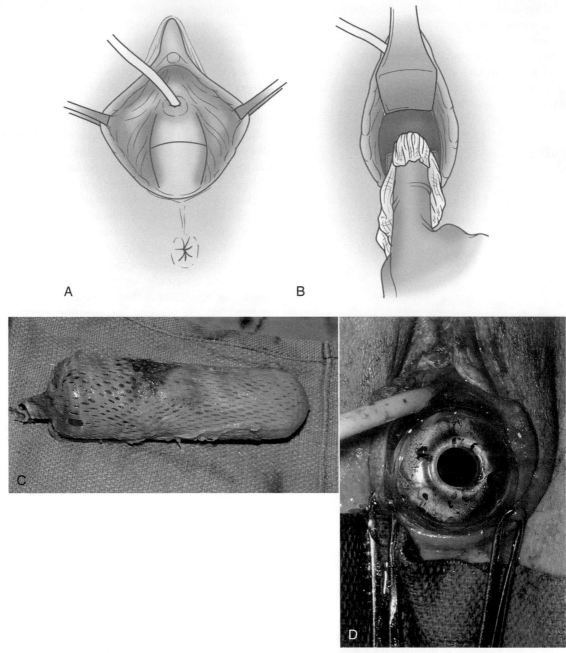

Figure 25-18   Vaginoplasty. A, A transverse incision is made in the vaginal vestibule. **B,** Blunt dissection is used to make a space for the vaginal implant. **C,** A skin graft covers the Plexiglas mold. **D,** The graft and implant in place. The implant is removed after the graft has integrated into the neovagina. *(B from Rothrock J: Alexander's care of the patient in surgery, ed 7, St Louis, 2007, Mosby; C and D from Falcone T, Hurd W: Clinical reproductive medicine and surgery, Philadelphia, 2007, Mosby.)*

TECHNIQUE

1 The surgeon grasps the edge of the tract with two or more Allis clamps.

2 A metal probe may be placed in the fistula to identify its course. Diagnostic procedures, including instillation of a contrast medium, may have preceded the surgery. Films obtained from the procedure show the route of the fistula.

3 The tissue around the fistula is sharply dissected.

4 A tissue plane is created between the bladder and the fistula with sharp and blunt dissection.

5 The mucosa is inverted, and sutures are placed through the smooth muscular layer and mucosa.

6 An internal layer of sutures is placed in the bladder.

7 The edges of the vaginal wall are repaired.

8 An indwelling Foley catheter is placed.

Discussion

The patient is placed in the lithotomy position, prepped, and draped for a perineal incision. The surgeon places an Auvard or Sims retractor in the vagina to expose the fistula. A malleable probe is inserted into the fistula. The surgeon then uses dissecting scissors to make a circular incision around the probe and fistula. The surgeon carries this incision the full length of the fistula with dissecting scissors until the anterior bladder wall is exposed. Two lateral retractors may be placed in the vagina for better exposure. The surgeon creates a tissue plane between the bladder and the fistula with sponge dissectors or by sharp dissection.

When the bladder mucosa and smooth muscle layer have been exposed, the surgeon inverts the bladder tissue layers and approximates the edges with double-layer, interrupted 3-0 sutures of absorbable material. The vaginal wall is repaired with size 0 or 2-0 sutures. A Foley catheter may be inserted into the bladder at the close of the procedure.

REPAIR OF RECTOVAGINAL FISTULA

Surgical Goal

A rectovaginal fistula is a tract between the rectum and the vagina. Surgical repair closes the defect and prevents fecal material from draining into the vagina. A number of different procedures have been developed for repair of rectovaginal fistulas, including patch grafts (allograft or porcine), flap grafts, and advancement grafts. In simple cases, the fistula is excised and the resulting tissue edges approximated with sutures.

Pathology

A rectovaginal fistula may be caused by vaginal or rectal trauma, childbirth, Crohn disease, radiation therapy, chronic inflammation, or infection. A fistulous tract allows fecal material to drain into the vagina, causing infection, emotional distress, and social isolation.

TECHNIQUE

1 The fistula is exposed.
2 A tissue plane is created around the defect.
3 The vaginal wall is incised, exposing the deep layers of the rectum.
4 The plane is carried to the rectal outlet.
5 The fistula is completely excised and removed.
6 The levator muscle, mucosal defect, and vaginal wall are repaired.
7 A Foley catheter is inserted.

Discussion

The patient is placed in the lithotomy position for a vaginal approach, whereas the jacknife position is preferred for a rectal approach. Routine prepping and draping is performed according to the required position.

To begin the procedure for a vaginal approach, the surgeon places a weighted retractor in the vagina. A malleable probe is then used to define the extent of the fistula. The assistant grasps the posterior wall of the vagina with Allis clamps to produce traction across the fistula. A circular incision is then made around the fistula with the scalpel or dissecting scissors. Toothed tissue forceps are used to pick up the edge of the tissue as it is incised. Metzenbaum scissors are used to follow the tract and create a tissue plane between the tract and the deep tissue.

The vaginal wall is then grasped and incised with scissors, exposing the wall of the rectum. The surgeon incises the tissue around fistula along its length. If necessary, the perineal floor may require suture reinforcement to restore strength to the muscles. Interrupted sutures of synthetic absorbable material are used. Sutures are placed until the defect is closed and the repair is secure. A Foley catheter is placed at the close of the procedure.

More complex procedures are required for fistulas that are located in the distal anus or those that are subject to chronic infection. A diverting stoma may be required for selected patients during the healing period.

REMOVAL OF A CYSTIC BARTHOLIN GLAND

Surgical Goal

The procedure for removal of a cystic Bartholin gland removes a cyst and the associated Bartholin gland to prevent recurrence of the cyst and infection.

Pathology

The Bartholin glands are a common site of cyst formation. The cyst may become infected, and in such cases, surgical removal is indicated. Infection of a Bartholin gland is extremely painful, and many patients arrive for surgery in distress.

TECHNIQUE

1 The labia minora are retracted and secured to the skin.
2 The mucosa overlying the cyst is incised.
3 The cyst and sometimes the gland are removed.
4 The wound edges are secured open with small sutures.

Discussion

The patient is placed in the lithotomy position, prepped, and draped for a perineal incision.

The surgeon may begin the procedure by securing the labia minora laterally with sutures or small skin staples. A curved incision is then made in the mucosa over the cystic gland. The incision is lengthened with Metzenbaum scissors. Small bleeders are coagulated with the ESU.

The gland and the cyst may be removed together, or the cyst may be dissected away from the gland with dissecting scissors. The wound edges are secured open with sutures to allow secondary closure, as in marsupialization. This procedure is illustrated in Figure 25-19.

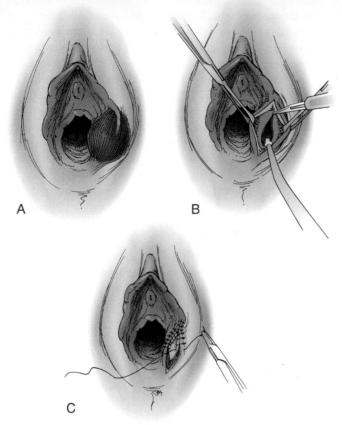

Figure 25-19   Bartholin gland cyst. **A,** An infected Bartholin gland may become cystic. **B,** An incision is made over the skin and wall of the cyst. **C,** The cyst wall may be everted and sutured to the skin to prevent recurrence. *(Modified from Gershenson DM, DeCherney AH, Curry SL, Brubaker LC: Operative gynecology, ed 2, Philadelphia, 2001, WB Saunders.)*

VULVECTOMY

Surgical Goal

Vulvectomy is surgical excision of the labia, clitoris, and inguinal and pelvic lymph nodes and is performed to treat cancer of the vulva.

Pathology

Cancer of the vulva represents about 5% of all genitourinary carcinomas. It is more common among women older than 60. Most invasive carcinoma that involves the lymph nodes is seen in this age group. Local vulvar cancer (vulvar intraepithelial neoplasm) appears to be associated with some strains of HPV.

Discussion

Vulvectomy may be performed as a simple or radical procedure. In the past, simple vulvectomy was performed to remove only the lesion itself and a margin surrounding it. This procedure is rarely performed now because of the disfiguring results and increased incidence of cancer in younger patients. *Skinning vulvectomy,* in which only the skin of the vulva is removed, usually by laser surgery, is the preferred procedure for noninvasive lesions. *Labioplasty* refers to reconstruction or reduction of the labia. Reduction may be performed for hypertrophy of the labia which can occur as a result of multiple childbirths. In this case, a predetermined margin of the labia is removed by sharp dissection. Radical vulvectomy (described next) is a complex procedure involving groin exploration, lymph node removal, and wide resection of the lesion and adjacent tissue.

The patient is placed in the lithotomy position, prepped, and draped for lower abdominal and perineal incisions. Instruments and equipment used in the perineal portion of the procedure are kept separate from those for the groin procedure. Two setups may be created to isolate the perineal equipment. Gloves and gowns are changed for the groin procedure, according to the surgeon's directions.

The surgeon begins the procedure by making a large elliptical incision around the vulva. The incision encompasses the labia minora, labia majora, and clitoris. A second incision is made superior to the urethral orifice and encompasses the vagina. The surgeon grasps the skin edges of the incision with Allis clamps and carries dissection through the subcutaneous and connective tissues of the vulva. The assistant provides traction on the tissue edges while the surgeon incises and coagulates the tissue, creating a block of tissue that will be removed.

Large bleeding vessels are clamped with small hemostats and ligated with fine absorbable sutures or coagulated with the ESU. The vulva is removed en bloc when the dissection and mobilization are complete. The specimen is isolated from the setup that will be used on the groin dissection.

The assistant next inserts a right angle retractor into the superior portion of the vagina. A Heaney lateral retractor is typically used. The surgeon then incises the posterior vaginal mucosa and uses interrupted sutures of absorbable material, size 0 or 2-0, to strengthen the connective tissues of the posterior pelvic floor. The mucosal incisions are closed with size 2-0 or 0 absorbable sutures. If the excision is narrow, the skin edges may be directly closed. Several subcutaneous sutures may be needed to prevent an open pocket between the tissue layers. The skin is closed with interrupted monofilament synthetic sutures.

The groin excision is carried out through bilateral inguinal incisions. After incising the skin, the surgeon extends the incision to the inguinal chain. Exposure to these lymph nodes follows a dissection similar to that of inguinal hernia. Lymph nodes are located within the connective tissue. The surgeon removes the nodes individually using sharp dissection and controls bleeding with the ESU and suture ties of absorbable material.

Wound closure is carefully performed to prevent seroma in the postoperative period. Penrose drains may be placed in the inguinal incisions. The wounds are closed in layers to obliterate "dead space" where fluid might collect. Interrupted sutures of 2-0 and 3-0 absorbable material are used to close deep tissue layers. The skin is closed with surgical staples and dressed with bulky gauze fluffs and an abdominal pad.

SECTION II: OPERATIVE OBSTETRICAL PROCEDURES

INTRODUCTION

Birth is a physiological process that seldom requires interventions for a healthy mother. Mother and fetus are linked during pregnancy as the mother's body accommodates to the growing fetus. Healthy mothers usually provide a nourishing environment that produces a healthy baby. The placenta plays a major role in the fetus' health by allowing essential nutrients to pass from the mother's blood to the baby. Failure of the placenta to function, for any reason, can be life-threatening to the fetus. Many medical and obstetrical problems are identified before birth. Unexpected problems that arise during **labor**, at birth, or after birth can present as emergencies that threaten the life of the mother or the baby. Surgical technologists may be asked to assist in a variety of roles during emergency situations.

STAGES OF PREGNANCY

Development of the embryo and fetus occurs when the ovum is fertilized by sperm, which normally occurs in the fallopian tube. The combination of chromosomal material from each completes the fertilization process. The egg passes through early embryonic development as it moves into the **uterus** and implants in the endometrium, about 10 days after fertilization. As the embryo grows, distinct developmental changes occur. The embryonic stage ends at week 8, and the fetal period begins.

During development, fetal circulation begins shortly after conception. Changes in the endometrial cells provide nourishment and protection for the fetus. The **placenta** is a thick organ that adheres to the uterus on the maternal side. The fetal side contains large vessels within the structure's smooth membranes. The umbilical cord, which attaches to the placenta, contains the umbilical artery and vein and communicates directly with fetal circulation.

Fetal membranes surround the growing fetus and are filled with **amniotic fluid**. The two membranes, the *chorion* and the *amnion*, are very close together. The amnion is continuous with the umbilical cord. The fluid-filled sack in which the fetus develops protects it against physical injury and also maintains thermoregulation. The watery environment allows the fetus to move and develop without restriction (Figure 25-20).

Average normal gestation occurs over 40 weeks and is marked by predictable growth patterns that can be measured by ultrasound. **Prenatal** assessment is performed throughout gestation to ensure that fetal development progresses normally and to detect complications early. Abdominal ultrasound is routinely used to assess pregnancy (Figure 25-21).

COMPLICATIONS OF PREGNANCY

PLACENTAL ABRUPTION

The placenta is the organ that acts as a filter from mother to baby; it allows nutrients to pass from the mother's blood to the fetus and carries away waste products. It is essential to the life of the fetus during the entire pregnancy. The placenta attaches to the uterine wall and grows during pregnancy to accommodate the fetus' needs. **Placental abruption** is a premature separation of the placenta from the uterine wall after 20 weeks' gestation and before the fetus is delivered (Figure 25-22). A variety of conditions can cause abruption, such as abdominal trauma, abnormalities of the uterus, a short umbilical cord, and hypertension. Abruption of the placenta from the uterine wall can be partial or complete. Abruption of the placenta presents as vaginal bleeding and sometimes concealed bleeding. The fetus has a good chance of surviving if half of the placenta remains attached to the uterus. **Fetal demise** results if the entire placenta separates from the uterus. If this happens during labor, fetal distress is evident during monitoring of the fetal heart. The woman may experience increased abdominal tenderness and back pain. If delivery is not imminent, a cesarean section is necessary.

PLACENTA PREVIA

During normal labor, the baby's head is pushed toward the cervix, and the cervix begins to thin. Eventually the cervix dilates to about 10 cm, thins out, and becomes part of the lower uterus. Normally the placenta implants on the uterine wall, far from the uterine opening (cervix). The location of the placenta usually is identified on routine ultrasound scans in the prenatal period. **Placenta previa** occurs when the placenta implants completely or partly over the cervical os (Figure 25-23). In this position, the placenta begins to bleed as it separates from the cervix during labor. The amount of bleeding is greater when the placenta covers the cervix completely. Sudden **hemorrhage** is life-threatening to both mother and fetus. An immediate cesarean section is necessary to prevent fetal death and maternal hemorrhage. Often hemorrhage can be prevented if a cesarean section is performed before labor begins.

PREGNANCY-INDUCED HYPERTENSION

Pregnancy-induced hypertension (PIH) is diagnosed as high blood pressure that occurs only during pregnancy after 20 weeks' gestation. PIH may be mild and monitored but not treated, or it may be severe and affect other systems, such as

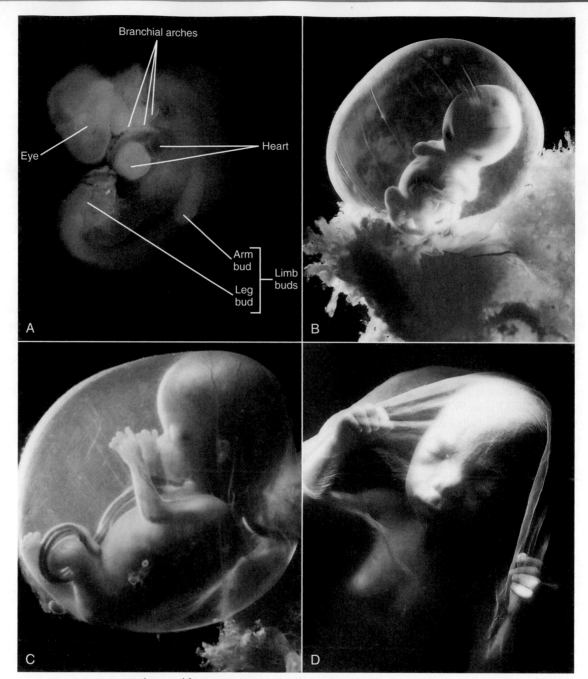

Figure 25-20   Embryonic life. **A,** 35 days. **B,** 49 days. **C,** 12 weeks. **D,** 16 weeks. *(From Thibodeau G, Patton K: Anatomy and physiology, ed 6, St Louis, 2007, Mosby.)*

the kidneys (proteinuria), liver (elevated liver enzymes), and blood (low platelets). It also can lead to maternal seizures (**eclampsia**). This disease process is also referred to as *toxemia* and *preeclampsia*. It usually occurs in the first pregnancy, but its cause is unknown. Hypertension can constrict blood flow to the placenta and fetus, resulting in a small fetus and placenta. If this occurs or if symptoms worsen, labor is induced artificially with drugs. During the induction, the mother may receive medicines intravenously to reduce the risk of seizures, although this is rare if the mother is receiving preventive medication. If a seizure occurs, it usually lasts 60 seconds or less, but it may be life-threatening to the fetus and mother. Airway maintenance is of primary importance during a

seizure; therefore, airways usually are within easy reach in each labor room. Once the mother's condition has stabilized after a seizure, a cesarean section can be performed.

NUCHAL CORD

An umbilical cord wrapped one or more times around the baby's neck is called a **nuchal cord**. This usually occurs with an active fetus in the early months of pregnancy, when there is plenty of room for the fetus to move. A nuchal cord is seldom diagnosed before labor, but it may be suspected if the baby's heart rate decreases markedly during contractions. If the nuchal cord is tight, blood flow through it will be

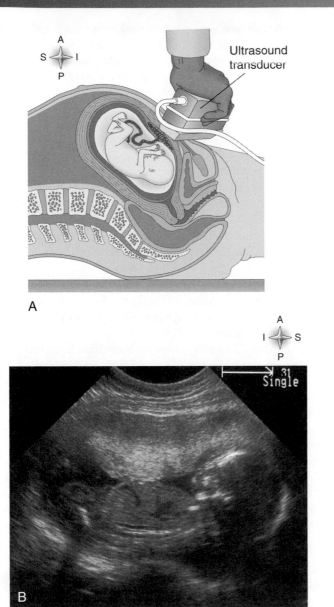

Figure 25-21 **A,** Ultrasound assessment of the fetus. **B,** Sonogram of the fetus. *(From Thibodeau G, Patton K: Anatomy and physiology, ed 6, St Louis, 2007, Mosby.)*

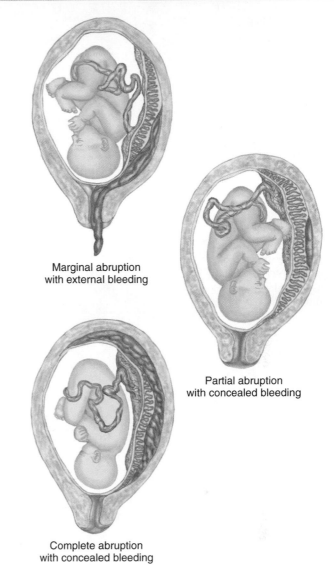

Marginal abruption with external bleeding

Partial abruption with concealed bleeding

Complete abruption with concealed bleeding

Figure 25-22 **Placental abruption.** *(From Murray SS, McKinney ES: Foundations of maternal-newborn nursing, ed 4, Philadelphia, 2006, WB Saunders.)*

constricted during contractions as the baby moves downward, causing the heart rate to slow markedly. After this, the heart rate may return to a normal range. Usually babies recover from this labor stress and are born with the cord around the neck. However, if the fetal heart rate continues to decrease markedly with every contraction and takes longer to recover to a normal rate, the baby may become too stressed to deliver vaginally. A cesarean section may be an option if delivery is still hours away. If the baby is delivered with a nuchal cord, it usually is not a problem to slip the cord over the head or, alternatively, clamp and cut it before the body is born.

LACK OF LABOR PROGRESS

During labor, the baby is expected to make steady progress through the **birth canal**, maneuvering into appropriate positions that provide the best fit for the baby's head and the maternal pelvis. Various problems can occur to impede this process. These include weak contractions, a fetal head that is not flexed sufficiently or is tilted to the side, or a fetal head that is too large to fit through a narrow maternal pelvis. Some positions of the baby's head require more room in the pelvis (e.g., babies who are "face up"). If diagnosed early in labor, maternal position changes or manual manipulations on the fetal head may help rotate the baby into a better position for descending through the birth canal. If this fails or if the baby is too large (or the mother's pelvis is too small), then progress is impeded and a cesarean section is needed.

CORD PROLAPSE

During pregnancy, membranes extending from the edge of the placenta encase the fetus as it moves in a water-filled environment as described previously. Normally, the amniotic sac remains intact until labor. When the **amniotic membranes**

Marginal

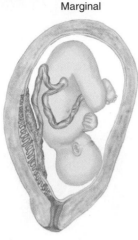

Placenta is implanted
in lower uterus but its
lower border is >3 cm
from internal cervical os.

Total

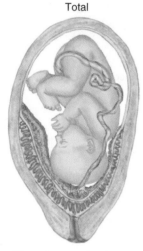

Placenta completely covers
internal cervical os.

Partial

Lower border of placenta
is within 3 cm of internal
cervical os but does not
fully cover it.

Figure 25-23 **Placenta previa.** *(From Murray SS, McKinney ES: Foundations of maternal-newborn nursing, ed 4, Philadelphia, 2006, WB Saunders.)*

break spontaneously or artificially, the amniotic fluid flows out of the vagina. If the fetal head is not low in the birth canal and the membranes rupture, there is a chance the umbilical cord may be swept in front of the baby's head with the flow of water and may lodge in the vagina or even outside the vagina. When the cord precedes the head, **cord prolapse** has occurred. This rarely happens before labor begins but can persist during labor. This condition is more likely with a breech **presentation** or an excess of amniotic fluid. When the cord precedes the baby in the birth canal, it can be compressed by the baby's head as it presses against the cervix and maternal pelvis. This reduces or stops the flow of oxygen to the baby. This condition requires an emergency cesarean section. In rare cases, the birth may occur vaginally if the cord prolapses suddenly along with the amniotic sac. The baby's head then follows with the next contraction. The nurse, midwife, or physician who

discovers this problem puts counterpressure on the baby's head at the vaginal outlet to reduce cord pressure while the woman is quickly moved to the operating room. In case of a pending emergency, the operating room staff is notified and a setup prepared. However, there may be little time between the diagnosis of cord prolapse and the start of surgery.

BREECH PRESENTATION

A **breech presentation** occurs when the baby's feet, knees, or buttocks enter the birth canal before the head. This can be a difficult, long labor that stresses the baby and the mother. It usually is diagnosed before labor, but it may be missed. If this position is known in the prenatal period, attempts can be made to change the position so that the head presents first. Before 38 weeks' gestation, the woman can try positions at home to rotate the baby. If these fail, she is likely to be scheduled for a procedure to rotate the fetus. This is called a *version*. If attempts to change the baby's position fail, a cesarean section is scheduled. Few physicians or nurse-midwives conduct planned breech deliveries. Most breech deliveries are unplanned, are imminent, or occur with a twin birth. If the fetus is not too large and contractions are consistent and strong, breech birth is possible. Dangers include a compressed umbilical cord, cord prolapse, and impinged fetal arms or head. Both physicians and nurse-midwives learn maneuvers to facilitate the breech birth, and extra hands may be called for to keep the baby's head flexed (**suprapubic pressure**), to position the bed or the mother, and to resuscitate the baby. Breech babies often are stressed and present with thick **meconium** at birth. Ideally, a good pediatric team is present to attend the birth, but if a delay occurs, assistance for suctioning the baby's airway may be requested.

DIAGNOSTIC TESTS

Pregnancy test: The pregnancy test detects the hormone human chorionic gonadotropin (hCG) either in the blood or the urine. hCG can be quantified in a blood test to assess whether the level is increasing at the expected rate in the first trimester. A pregnancy is confirmed most often by ultrasound or detection of a fetal heartbeat.

Ultrasound scans: Ultrasound is routinely used for a variety of tasks in pregnancy. It is useful for assessing fetal age if the last menses is unknown. Transvaginal ultrasound in the first trimester can determine the **gestational age** within 3 to 5 days. A diagnostic ultrasound performed at 18 weeks may be useful for identifying some types of fetal defects and confirming the gestational age. Ultrasound is commonly used in pregnancy for checking fetal growth, amniotic fluid volume, fetal position, and the location of the placenta.

Routine blood and urine tests: Routine blood and urine tests include tests that may affect the health of the present baby or of subsequent babies. These tests include:

- *Maternal blood type, Rh, and antibody screen:* These tests are important in the event transfusion is needed after hemorrhage. A negative Rh factor in the mother may induce her to make antibodies against her baby if she is exposed to the baby's Rh-positive blood (at birth or if bleeding during pregnancy). If the mother is Rh positive, she receives anti-D immunoglobulin at 28 weeks' gestation and again postpartum if her baby is Rh positive. This prevents the formation of antibodies against future Rh-positive babies during gestation. The antibody screen also confirms the presence of antibodies to other blood types.

- *RPR (rapid plasma reagin) syphilis antibody test:* Syphilis is a sexually transmitted infection that can be passed to the baby during pregnancy. It causes a variety of defects or miscarriage, depending on the maternal stage of the disease.
- *Rubella antibody testing:* Rubella can cause severe defects or miscarriage if contracted by the mother in the first 16 weeks of pregnancy.
- *Human immunodeficiency virus and acquired immunodeficiency syndrome (HIV/AIDS) screening:* HIV infection and AIDS can be transmitted to the baby during pregnancy or birth, or through breast milk.
- *Hepatitis B:* This disease can be transmitted to the baby during pregnancy or through breast milk and may cause liver cancer if left untreated in the newborn.
- *Screening for gonorrhea and chlamydia:* These diseases can be passed to the baby during its passage through the birth canal, resulting in respiratory or eye infections and blindness if left untreated after birth. The diagnosis is made by cytological examination of a cervical smear or by a urine test.
- *Complete blood count (CBC):* This test is performed to diagnose anemia, insufficient platelets, or an increased white blood cell count indicating infection.
- *Cervical cancer screening (Pap smear):* The Pap smear is routinely done during prenatal care. It detects abnormal cells and HPV, which can cause cervical cancer.
- *Maternal serum screen:* This blood test is done at 16 to 18 weeks' gestation to screen for three or four biochemical markers in the maternal blood that indicate the baby's risk for Down syndrome, spina bifida, and trisomy 18. If the test is positive, the woman may decide to undergo amniocentesis to confirm the diagnosis.
- *Urine culture:* This culture is routinely done on the first prenatal visit to detect a urinary tract infection. Asymptomatic urinary tract infection may occur during pregnancy, and an untreated infection can lead to pyelonephritis (kidney infection) and preterm labor.

NORMAL VAGINAL DELIVERY

As mentioned, the birth of a term baby is a normal event that seldom requires intervention. The event is called a **normal spontaneous vaginal delivery (NSVD)**. The birth usually occurs in a labor room with the mother's friends or relatives present as support. In many locations, the mother can chose her position for birth, especially if she is not medicated and able to position herself. More often, she may have an **epidural** to relieve pain that may prolong the pushing phase of labor.

As the baby's head emerges, the tissues around the vagina and perineum stretch. The period for this stretching is longer if this is the mother's first vaginal birth, and lacerations of the vagina, perineum, or labia may result. If the fetal heart rate remains below 100 beats per minute and the baby's head is near but not immediately delivering, the physician or nurse-midwife may incise the perineum to provide a wider opening and hasten delivery. This is called an *episiotomy,* and it requires sutures following delivery. Once the baby is born and has been dried, and the umbilical cord has been cut, the physician or nurse-midwife inspects the perineum for lacerations or extension of the episiotomy.

The placenta usually is delivered within 20 minutes after birth and may be assisted by gentle cord traction, the administration of an oxytocic drug, a maternal squatting position, or breast feeding. After delivery of the placenta, the perineum is repaired. Lacerations or extensions of the episiotomy rarely go through the entire vaginal tissue to the rectal mucosa (fourth-degree laceration) or into the rectal sphincter (third-degree laceration). It is very common to repair a laceration that involves the muscles between the vagina and rectum (second-degree laceration) or a laceration of the vaginal mucosa (first-degree laceration). Lacerations along the side of the vagina occur less often. Repairs are done with 3-0 absorbable suture (polyglycolic acid or chromic on a tapered needle) except for rectal mucosal and labial repairs, which are done with 4-0 absorbable suture.

The scrub should have a basic vaginal set and general surgery instruments. Right angle retractors (e.g., Heaney or Sims lateral retractors) should be included. A simple closure kit includes Allis and Kelly or Crile clamps. Curved Heaney and Metzenbaum scissors, needle holders, Adson forceps, or single-toothed tissue forceps may be used for skin and subcutaneous repairs.

IMMEDIATE POSTPARTUM CARE

Postpartum care includes monitoring the status of the mother and baby during this immediate transition. During the first 2 hours, the mother's blood pressure, pulse, and respirations are assessed every 15 minutes and her temperature is taken hourly. During this time, the nurse also checks her bleeding by giving a firm uterine massage. A firm uterus means that the muscles of the uterus are tight, squeezing the small blood vessels that fed the placenta during pregnancy and thus minimizing bleeding. The mother may receive intravenous medication to increase uterine tone, which prevents postpartum bleeding.

If the mother received an epidural anesthetic, she is monitored for return of sensation and ability to mobilize. Full mobility and ability to urinate is expected within 1 hour after discontinuation of the anesthetic. As soon as she is able, she may eat and drink normally.

NEWBORN CARE

The baby usually is dried and stimulated immediately after birth. If all is normal, and the mother agrees, the baby can remain on her abdomen. The baby is assessed according to the American Pediatric Gross Assessment Record, commonly known as the **APGAR score.** This includes the following assessment parameters:

- Respiratory rate
- Color
- Reflex response
- Heart rate
- Body tone at 1 and 5 minutes after birth

A score of 2, 1, or 0 is given for each parameter. A score of 7 to 10 is considered normal; a score of 4 to 6 indicates mild to moderate depression; and a score of 0 to 3 indicates severe depression. It is important that the baby maintain a temperature of about 98.6° F (37° C). This can be done by drying the baby and providing a warm environment (e.g., a baby warmer or skin-to-skin contact with the mother or father while keeping the baby covered). Respirations, heart rate, and temperature are monitored every 15 minutes in the first hour or two. The baby is most alert in the first hour after birth and eager to suck. Breast feeding during this time has many benefits, such as augmenting uterine contractions and facilitating bonding between mother and baby. The baby's weight and length can be obtained once the baby is warm and stable.

The immediate postpartum period is an important time for both mother and baby as they transition into a new phase of life. Each health care facility has a set of guidelines for care. The mother's and father's preferences also should be taken into consideration. Hospital personnel can provide a supportive, calm, and private environment to assist the family while gathering critical assessments of the status of mother and baby.

OBSTETRICAL PROCEDURES

CESAREAN DELIVERY

Surgical Goal

A cesarean section (commonly called a *C-section*) is the surgical removal of the fetus through the abdomen.

Pathology

A cesarean section is medically necessary when the mother's life is in jeopardy and for obstetrical conditions that would result in fetal death. Some of these conditions are:

- Transverse, breech, or other malpresentation of the fetus
- Prolapsed umbilical cord
- Ruptured placenta (placental abruption)
- Delivery of the placenta ahead of the fetus (placenta previa)
- Active genital herpes infection
- Previous cesarean section
- Cephalopelvic disproportion (the fetus cannot be delivered through the pelvis because of its shape)
- Failure to progress
- Prolapsed cord
- Toxemia
- Diabetes

TECHNIQUE

1. A low transverse or midline incision is made to the level of the rectus muscles.
2. The muscles are separated manually.
3. The peritoneum is elevated with two hemostats, and a small hole is made between the clamps.
4. The peritoneum is divided with scissors.
5. Large bleeders are clamped but not ligated or coagulated.
6. The peritoneal reflection of the bladder (bladder flap) is divided from the uterus with Metzenbaum scissors.
7. A bladder retractor is placed on the lower edge of the incision, and the bladder is displaced downward.
8. A small transverse incision is made in the uterus with the scalpel.
9. The scrub brings the suction without metal tip, bulb syringe, and bandage scissors near the wound.
10. The uterine incision is extended with the bandage scissors.
11. Amniotic fluid is quickly suctioned from the open uterus.
12. The assistant applies pressure to the upper abdomen while the surgeon rotates the baby's head into view.
13. The baby's nose and mouth are immediately suctioned with the bulb syringe or a separate suction catheter (e.g., DeLee suction catheter).
14. The baby is removed from the uterus.
15. The umbilical cord is double-clamped and cut with bandage scissors. One clamp is released slightly to fill two blood collection tubes.
16. The baby is handed over to the infant resuscitation team for care.
17. The placenta is delivered, and the remaining fluid and blood are suctioned from the wound.
18. The uterus is closed in layers.
19. The abdomen is closed in layers.

Discussion

A cesarean section can be scheduled, or it may be done as an emergency procedure. If the procedure is scheduled (e.g., a repeat C-section), a spinal or an epidural anesthetic is administered and a regular setup can be done.

An emergency delivery occurs very quickly. If a general anesthetic is given, time is extremely critical to prevent fetal anesthesia and to correct the condition that caused the emergency. In emergency surgery, several instruments are used to start the procedure and safely deliver the baby. In many cases, lack of time may prevent a normal setup.

In emergency cases, fetal monitoring may be in place when the patient arrives, along with trained staff from the obstetrics unit. A newborn resuscitation unit is brought in along with respiratory resuscitation equipment and emergency drugs. A suction line from the operating room must be dedicated to the resuscitation unit.

The patient is placed in the supine position with a small wedge pad under the right hip to prevent aortocaval compression by the fetus. Such compression can cause hypotension of the mother due to decreased return blood flow to the heart, and this may cause fetal hypoxia.

A Foley catheter is normally already in place. The patient is fully prepped and draped before anesthesia is started. However, physiological monitoring is initiated as soon as the patient enters the operating room suite.

As soon as the technologist has performed hand antisepsis and donned gown and gloves, the following items, which are adequate to deliver the baby, should be prepared:

1. Laparotomy drape
2. Scalpel
3. Lap sponges
4. Mayo clamps (four to six)
5. Metzenbaum scissors
6. Bladder retractor (DeLee or the bladder blade from a Balfour retractor)
7. Hemostats (e.g., Kelly or Crile clamps)
8. Bandage scissors
9. Suction tubing (two)
10. Bulb syringe

The surgeon enters the abdomen through a midline or Pfannenstiel incision. The incision is carried to the muscles, which are divided by hand. Bleeders are clamped but are not ligated or coagulated, to save time, unless the hemostats obstruct the surgeon's view or are in the way. Before entering the peritoneum, the surgeon elevates it with two Mayo clamps. The surgeon then makes a small incision between the clamps.

The peritoneal incision is lengthened with Metzenbaum or Mayo scissors. The peritoneal reflection of the bladder then must be separated from the uterus. This is done with Metzenbaum scissors and blunt dissection. When the bladder flap has been removed, a bladder retractor is placed over the lower edge of the incision and the bladder is retracted downward, away from the uterus.

Just before the uterus is entered, the scrub must bring the suction tubing (without a tip), bulb syringe, bandage scissors, and scalpel to the surgical field. The surgeon makes a small incision in the uterus and deepens it with the bandage scissors. The blunt tip of the bandage scissors prevents injury to the fetus.

The scrub must remove the scalpel from the field immediately to prevent injury to the baby or a team member.

As soon as the uterus is opened, the scrub places the tip of the suction tubing at the edge of the incision to aspirate amniotic fluid. The assistant applies pressure to the upper abdomen while the surgeon grasps the baby's head and delivers it from the uterus. The bulb syringe is used immediately to suction the baby's nose and mouth. A second suction should be available, and a flexible suction catheter attached to clear the baby's airway.

Extra laparotomy sponges should be available. The surgeon delivers the baby from the uterus and places the infant on the mother's abdomen. The surgeon clamps the umbilical cord with two Mayo clamps and severs it with bandage scissors. The scrub must have two blood specimen containers in hand to receive cord blood. The surgeon releases one of the Mayo clamps slightly to fill the containers. The scrub caps these and passes them to the circulator.

The baby is handed to the resuscitation team and placed in the warming unit. The baby is again suctioned and dried, oxygen is administered as needed, and the baby is assessed. The infant then may be taken to the nursery or intensive care unit.

As the baby is handed over to the resuscitation team, attention again must be directed to the mother. The scrub places a large basin on the field to receive the placenta, which is delivered from the uterus.

The surgeon grasps the edges of the uterus with sponge forceps, Duval lung clamps, or Collin tongue clamps. These are atraumatic clamps that prevent maceration of the uterine incision during closure.

A count is required before the uterus is closed.

The uterine incision is closed with (two) two-layer size 0 running absorbable suture. The surgeon then may attend to any bleeders, which are coagulated with the ESU or ligated with suture ties. When the wound is clean and dry, the remaining layers are closed.

NOTE: in the past some surgeons used an intramyometrial injection of oxytocin (directly into the uterine muscle) to control postpartum hemorrhage. However, this practice has been found to have no advantage over intravenous oxytocin routinely administered in the postpartum stage.[2]

The bladder flap is closed with a running suture of 2-0 or 3-0 absorbable suture on a taper needle. The remaining layers are closed in routine fashion, and the wound is dressed with sterile dressings. A cesarean section is shown in Figure 25-24.

SURGICAL TREATMENT OF AN ECTOPIC PREGNANCY

Surgical Goal

In an **ectopic pregnancy**, the fertilized egg implants outside the uterus. The fallopian tube is a common site of ectopic implantation. Tubal rupture requires emergency surgery to control hemorrhage. The surgical goal is to control bleeding and remove the embryo. A laparoscopic or an open approach may be used, depending on the patient's condition and the surgeon's choice.

Pathology

Ectopic pregnancy occurs most often in the fallopian tube (tubal pregnancy). Risk factors include a previous history of PID, smoking (reduces tubal motility), previous tubal surgery, and a history of STD infection. Tubal rupture, hemorrhage, and hypovolemic shock can be rapidly fatal. Early tubal pregnancy may be treated with methotrexate, which causes embryonic death. As mentioned, the surgery may be performed laparoscopically or through open surgery. An open approach is discussed in the next section, although techniques are similar for both types of surgery.

Discussion

Two approaches may be utilized in the surgical treatment of an ectopic pregnancy: salpingectomy (complete removal of the

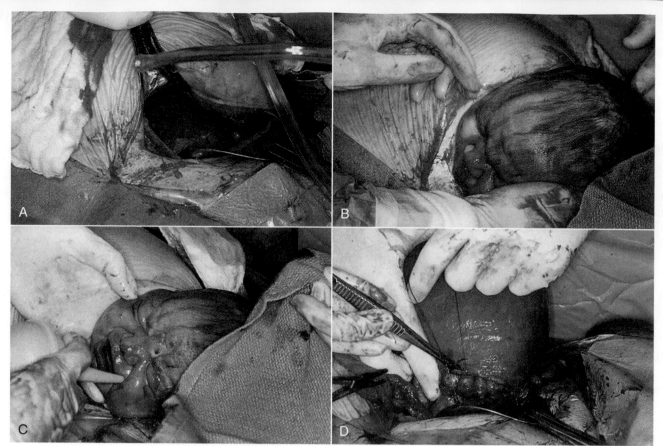

Figure 25-24 **Cesarean section. A,** The uterus is entered through a transverse incision. **B,** The fetal head is brought through the incision. **C,** Suction is used to clear the airways. **D,** Heavy sutures are used to close the uterus. *(From Murray SS, McKinney ES: Foundations of maternal-newborn nursing, ed 4, Philadelphia, 2006, WB Saunders.)*

affected fallopian tube) and salpingostomy (removal of the tubal contents with preservation of the tube.

The patient is placed in the supine position, prepped, and draped for a laparotomy. A Pfannenstiel incision is used to open the pelvic cavity. If the ectopic pregnancy has already ruptured, the scrub must be prepared for surgical hemorrhaging. The scrub should have suction and irrigation immediately available. Clots are removed manually, and the source of the bleeding is identified as quickly as possible. A basin should be placed on the field to receive the blood clots. A self-retaining retractor may or may not be inserted during this stage of the procedure. When the bleeding has been controlled, the embryo (or tube and embryo) can be removed. In all approaches, the scrub should have an ample supply of Mayo and Crile clamps available. Suture ligatures of fine absorbable synthetic material or surgical staples may also be required soon after the start of the procedure.

SALPINGECTOMY To control the bleeding, the surgeon may cross-clamp the fallopian tube and mesosalpinx with Mayo or Crile clamps. The tube then is resected with the HF bipolar ESU. Suture ligatures may also be used. (In laparoscopic surgery, Harmonic shears, staples, or pretied ligatures are used.)

SALPINGOSTOMY Tube-preserving surgery requires incision of the tube and removal of the embryo, with irrigation and suction. Reconstruction of the tube is done at the time of surgery or deferred until a later date. The tube is grasped with Babcock forceps, and a small incision is made with a scalpel, needle electrode, or ultrasonic scalpel. The embryo is removed using irrigation and fine forceps. The ESU is used sparingly to prevent scarring. The tube is irrigated and may be left to heal by secondary intention.

The surgery is complete after the wound has been irrigated and carefully examined for any bleeding. The wound is then closed in layers. The skin is closed with staples or subcuticular suture and Steri-Strips (Figure 25-25).

SURGICAL TREATMENT OF CERVICAL INSUFFICIENCY

Surgical Goal

Recurrent spontaneous abortion occurs when the cervix dilates spontaneously during the second or third trimester. Surgical intervention to prevent spontaneous abortion may be performed before or during pregnancy. In transabdominal **cerclage** (TAC) and transvaginal cerclage (TVC), a synthetic

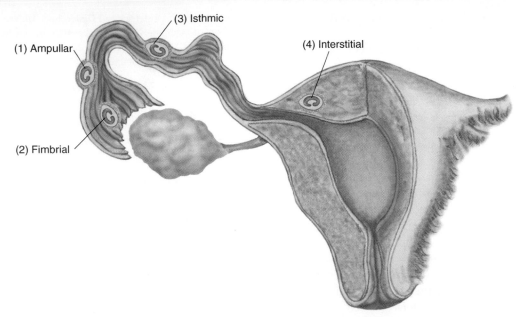

(1) Ampullar

(2) Fimbrial

(3) Isthmic

(4) Interstitial

Figure 25-25   **Ectopic pregnancy.** *(From Murray SS, McKinney ES: Foundations of maternal-newborn nursing, ed 4, Philadelphia, 2006, WB Saunders.)*

band or sutures may be placed around the cervix to prevent dilation.

Pathology

The cause of **incompetent cervix** has not been identified. It may be associated with cervical trauma, including conization of the cervix, laceration, and previous cerclage. *Cerclage remains controversial, because the data are insufficient to prove that the procedure is effective.* The American Congress of Obstetricians and Gynecologists (ACOG) recommends cerclage only for patients with a history of three or four previous unexplained spontaneous abortions. ACOG further states that the procedure should be limited to pregnancies in which fetal viability has been achieved. *This is because of the fetal morbidity and fetal mortality associated with the procedures.*[3]

Traditional treatment for early spontaneous abortion historically led to the development of various types of cerclage. The Shirodkar and McDonald procedures are just two of many types of cerclage in which a suture was placed around or through the cervix. These procedures have been modified many times over the decades, and cerclage is now identified by terms that are more exact. The proper terms are transabdominal, high transvaginal, or low transvaginal cerclage. The procedures are seldom performed because of the risks stated previously.

In TVC, a synthetic band is placed around the proximal cervix through a vaginal approach. In TAC, sutures are placed at the internal cervical os, which is approached through an abdominal incision. Delivery by cesarean section is required after TAC.

TAC is performed through a short suprapubic incision. The ureterovesical fold is incised and retracted, and a tunnel is made through the paracervical tissue. Several sutures of heavy Mersilene are then placed at the internal cervical os. The ureterovesical fold is closed with running suture of size 0 or 2-0

absorbent synthetic suture, and the pelvic incision is closed in layers.

TVC is performed with the patient in the lithotomy position. The cervix is retracted with sponge forceps, and a circumferential incision is made at the highest (proximal) point of the cervix. A narrow strip of Mersilene tape is then placed around the cervix, and the paracervical tissue is closed with interrupted 2-0 or 3-0 synthetic absorbable sutures.

KEY CONCEPTS

- Knowledge of key anatomical structures and pathology of the female reproductive system contributes to the surgical technologist's ability to anticipate the need for instruments, sutures, and other equipment during the surgical procedure.
- Key diagnostic procedures in gynecology are important to patient care and may also involve a surgical procedure.
- Specific surgical techniques used in gynecological surgery include laparoscopy and hysteroscopy.
- Familiarity with specific gynecological and obstetrical procedures is necessary for accurate case planning and participation in the scrub role.

REVIEW QUESTIONS

1. What is the rationale for performing the perineal prep ahead of the abdominal prep in combined access procedures?
2. Discuss uterine distention solutions used for high-frequency bipolar surgery and monopolar surgery. What is the rationale for using nonelectrolytic versus electrolytic solutions in each case?
3. Why does the uterine distention fluid have to be closely monitored during hysteroscopy?

4. List the risks of the lithotomy position and the precautions needed to prevent injury.

5. Review the imaging system components for laparoscopy found in Chapter 24. List the components and their basic use.

6. What is the risk of allowing an ovarian cyst to rupture into the pelvic cavity during surgery?

7. Babcock clamps usually are required for any surgery of the fallopian tubes. Why wouldn't a Kocher clamp be used instead?

8. During laparoscopy and removal of tissue, such as a morcellated tumor or an ovarian cyst, a specimen retrieval bag is used to remove the specimen from the abdomen. What size trocar is needed when a specimen retrieval bag is used?

9. Radical abdominal and pelvic procedures, such as pelvic exenteration and the Whipple procedure, are performed much less often now than they were several years ago. What do you think are the reasons for this?

10. Consider a situation in which you are called to scrub for an emergency cesarean section. What is the minimum instrumentation and equipment you should have ready when the mother is brought into the operating room? Assume that your instrument tray is open and the Mayo stand is draped, but you have no instruments on the Mayo stand. The surgeon is ready to start; you have approximately 3 minutes to prepare for abdominal entry and removal of the baby.

REFERENCES

1. Centers for Disease Control and Prevention: *Sexually transmitted diseases surveillance, 2007, Chlamydia.* Accessed January 16, 2009, at http://www.cdc.gov/std/stats07/chlamydia.htm.

2. Department of Obstetrics and Gynecology, University of Colorado School of Medicine: 37th Vail Obstetrics and Gynecology Conference. Vail, Colo, February 20–25, 2011.

3. Ressel G: Practice guidelines: ACOG releases bulletin on managing cervical insufficiency, *American Family Physician* 69:436, 2004.

BIBLIOGRAPHY

Baggish MS, Barbot J, Valle RF: *Diagnostic and operative hysteroscopy: a text and atlas*, ed 2, St Louis, 1999, Mosby.

Economou SG, Economou TS: *Atlas of surgical technique*, ed 2, Philadelphia, 1996, WB Saunders.

Falcone T, Hurd W: *Clinical reproductive medicine and surgery*, Philadelphia, 2007, Mosby.

Gershenson DM, DeCherney AH, Curry SL, Brubaker LC: *Operative gynecology*, ed 2, Philadelphia, 2001, WB Saunders.

Goldberg JM, Falcone T: *Atlas of endoscopic techniques in gynecology*, Philadelphia, 2001, WB Saunders.

Greibel C, Halvorsen J, Golemon T, Day A: Management of spontaneous abortion, *American Family Physician* 72:1243, 2005.

Hunt RB: *Text and atlas of female infertility surgery*, ed 3, St Louis, 1999, Mosby.

Moody FG: *Atlas of ambulatory surgery*, St Louis, 1999, Mosby.

Murray SS, McKinney ES, Gorrie TM: *Foundations of maternal-newborn nursing*, ed 3, Philadelphia, 2002, WB Saunders.

Porth CM: *Pathophysiology: concepts of altered health states*, ed 7, Philadelphia, 2004, Lippincott Williams & Williams.

Raz S: *Atlas of transvaginal surgery*, ed 2, Philadelphia, 2002, WB Saunders.

Genitourinary Surgery

CHAPTER OUTLINE

LEARNING OBJECTIVES

After studying this chapter the reader will be able to:

1. Identify key anatomical structures of the genitourinary system
2. Discuss common diagnostic tests and procedures of the genitourinary system
3. Discuss specific elements of case planning for genitourinary surgery
4. Describe common pathology of the genitourinary system
5. List and describe common genitourinary procedures

TERMINOLOGY

Arteriovenous fistula (or AV shunt): Surgically created vascular access for patients undergoing hemodialysis.

Calculi: Stones caused by the precipitation of minerals, such as calcium, and other substances from the urine or kidney filtrate.

Epispadias: A rare congenital abnormality in which the opening of the urethra is on the dorsum of the penis. This anomaly does not usually occur in isolation but is part of a more complex set of defects of the urogenital system.

Extracorporeal shock wave lithotripsy (ESWL): A procedure in which ultrasonic sound waves are used to pulverize kidney or gallbladder stones.

Foley catheter: A retention catheter with an expandable balloon at the distal end.

Glomerular filtration rate (GFR): An indication of kidney function in which serum creatinine (normally filtered by the kidney) is measured.

Indwelling catheter: A urethral or ureteral catheter that is left in place.

Intravasation: The absorption of irrigation fluids into the vascular system, which causes fluid overload and can result in cardiac arrest.

Meatotomy: A procedure in which a small incision is made in the urethral meatus to relieve a stricture. A topical anesthetic is used.

Nonelectrolytic: Nonconductive; nonelectrolytic solutions must be used for bladder distention or continuous irrigation whenever the electrosurgical unit (ESU) is used.

Percutaneous: A term for a procedure that is performed "through the skin." For example, in percutaneous nephroscopy, the nephroscope is inserted into the kidney through a skin incision.

Reflux: Flow of a body fluid in the direction opposite its normal path. Urinary reflux is backward flow of urine into the ureter or kidney.

Resectoscope: A cutting instrument used to remove and coagulate tissue piece by piece. It is used in conjunction with endoscopic procedures to remove tumors or other tissue, such as the prostate or endometrium.

Retrograde pyelography: Imaging studies of the renal pelvis in which a contrast medium is instilled through a transurethral catheter. *Retrograde* refers to flow, which is opposite the normal direction.

Specific gravity: The ratio of the density of a fluid compared to water. The specific gravity of urine is an important diagnostic tool.

Staghorn stone: A large, jagged kidney stone that forms in the renal pelvis.

Stent: A supportive catheter that is placed in a duct or tube to allow fluids to pass through while the duct heals.

Straight catheter: A urinary catheter used for one-time drainage of the bladder. It may be called a "red Robinson" or simply a "Robinson" catheter.

Suprapubic catheter: A bladder catheter inserted through the skin in the suprapubic area of the abdomen.

Tamponade: An instrument or other device that puts pressure on tissue, usually to stop bleeding.

Torsion: Twisting of an organ or a structure on itself. Torsion may cause local ischemia and necrosis.

Transurethral: Surgical access through the urethral orifice. The term also may describe an instrument that enters the bladder through the urethral meatus.

INTRODUCTION

Genitourinary (GU) surgery includes procedures of the urethra, bladder, ureters, and kidneys. It also includes surgery of the male reproductive system (i.e., the testicles, penis, and accessory structures). Three common approaches are used in GU surgery:

- *Transurethral surgery:* Surgery is performed through a flexible or rigid fiberoptic endoscope inserted through the external urethra. This provides direct visualization and access to the lower urinary tract, including the urethra, bladder, prostate gland, and ureters.
- *Open surgery:* Surgery that is performed through an open incision in the abdomen (including the retroperitoneum) or flank. Many procedures that were performed with the open technique can now be performed using minimally invasive techniques.
- *Minimally invasive surgery:* Closed procedures that are performed using **percutaneous** (through the skin) endoscopic techniques, such as laparotomy and nephrotomy.

NOTE: *GU procedures performed exclusively on newborns or infants are described in Chapter 35.*

SURGICAL ANATOMY

RETROPERITONEAL CAVITY

The *retroperitoneal cavity* (also referred to as the retroperitoneal *space*) lies posterior to (behind) the peritoneal cavity. Unlike the viscera of the abdominal cavity, the organs in this space are embedded in dense muscle, fascia, and fatty tissue. These connective tissues support the structures and protect them from injury. The retroperitoneal space is covered on the anterior side by the *retroperitoneum*, a serous (fluid-producing) membrane. Surgical access to the organs in the retroperitoneum is gained through the abdominal peritoneum, the flank, or the back.

KIDNEY

The kidneys are the primary organs for filtration of the blood. Two kidneys normally are located in the retroperitoneal cavity at the level of the 12th thoracic vertebra (Figure 26-1). The right kidney usually sits lower than the left. The kidneys are supported by dense fascia and fatty tissue.

Two main tissue layers make up the kidney: the outer layer, the *cortex*; and the inner layer, the *medulla*. The cortex is covered with strong fibrous tissue and contains portions of the microscopic tubules that filter the blood. The medulla is composed of 8 to 12 large collecting areas called the *renal pyramids*.

A notched area on the medial side of each kidney is called the *hilum*. The ureter, renal artery, and vein emerge from this area. At this point the ureter opens into the *renal pelvis* of the kidney, which branches into sections called *renal calyces* (Figure 26-2).

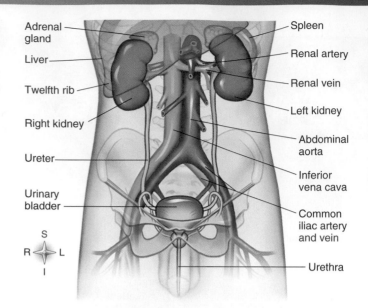

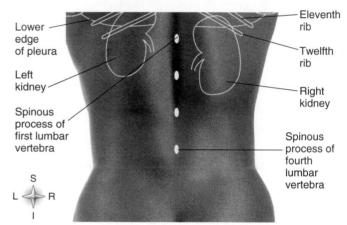

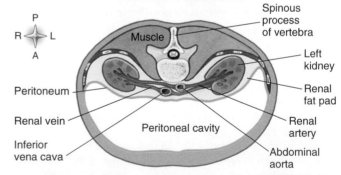

Figure 26-1   The kidneys, ureters, and associated blood vessels lie in the retroperitoneal cavity. *(From Abrahams P, Hutchings RT, Marks SC: McKinn's color atlas of human anatomy, ed 4, St Louis, 1999, Mosby.)*

Nephron

Although the kidney appears as a dense, continuous tissue, the microscopic structure is extremely complex. Each kidney has about 1 million filtering units, called *nephrons*. Each nephron communicates directly with the vascular system through a capillary structure called the *glomerulus*. The glomerulus is composed of a vast system of microscopic tubules that communicate directly with the capillaries to filter the blood. The capillary network of each nephron is contained within a space

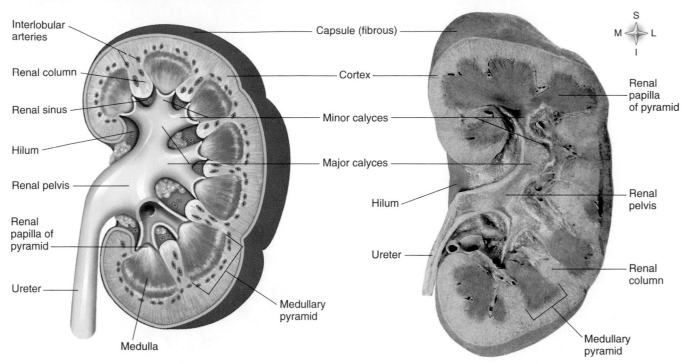

Figure 26-2 The kidney, showing the layers, pyramids and collecting tubules, and ureter. *(From Brundage DJ: Renal disorders, St Louis, 1992, Mosby.)*

called the *Bowman capsule* (Figure 26-3). This structure is closely related to the nephron tubules where filtering takes place. The juxtaglomerular cells in the Bowman capsule release *renin* which is necessary for regulation of blood pressure.

Blood flows into the capillary network through the efferent arteriole of the glomerulus. As the blood circulates through the microscopic capillaries, fluid (glomerular filtrate) moves selectively into the Bowman capsule. Proteins and cells remain in the blood, but other substances cross the arterial membrane and enter the capsule. The filtrate then moves into the nephron tubules. The glomerulus can filter about 125 mL per minute. This is referred to as the **glomerular filtration rate (GFR)**.

THE FORMATION OF URINE Filtrate is continually refined as it moves through the tubules. Each renal tubule has a parallel capillary. Substances are selectively moved from the blood into the tubules (a process called *secretion*) and from the tubules into the blood (called *absorption*) according to osmolality (solutes contained in the fluid) and membrane permeability. This is why diseases of the circulatory system, such as hypertension or arteriosclerosis, can affect the kidneys and damage this delicate transport system.

As filtrate moves through the tubules, electrolytes, nonorganic salts, and water, which the body needs to maintain homeostasis, are absorbed from the filtrate back into the circulatory system. The tubule system is divided into specific regions, which filter certain substances. These regions are called the *proximal tubule*, the *loop of Henle*, and the *distal convoluted tubule*.

Note that some diuretics are called "potassium-sparing" drugs. This type of diuretic prevents excessive loss of potassium across the capillary membrane, which is an undesirable side effect of many diuretics.

From the renal tubules, the filtrate enters the *renal calyces* (sing., *calyx*) and renal pelvis, which communicates directly with the *ureters*. The ureters are the collecting and transport areas for filtrate. Each ureter carries filtrate into the bladder. Once it enters the bladder, the filtrate is referred to as *urine*. Urine is excreted from the body through the *urethra*. Filtrate and urine are sterile throughout the length of the system; they become *potentially* contaminated by the environment in the periurethral areas, such as the distal urethral orifice (Figure 26-4).

Kidney Stones

Kidney stones (**calculi**) are formed by the precipitation of specific salts from filtrate that becomes supersaturated. Stones can become lodged in the kidney itself or can migrate into the ureters. Stones rarely form in the bladder. The crystalline structure of stones is jagged and sharp, and they cause nearly unbearable pain and nausea in the patient. Most small stones pass through the urinary tract without treatment. However, stones in the upper urinary tract can cause obstruction and anuria (decreased or no urinary output), kidney abscess, and sepsis. Renal calculi can therefore be considered a medical emergency.

Kidney stones may be seen in many different diseases, including hyperparathyroidism, increased absorption of calcium in the intestine, chronic urinary tract infection, high protein intake, and the use of some drugs. Specific stone types are associated with each condition.

Calculi may be removed surgically or reduced with **extracorporeal shock wave lithotripsy (ESWL)**. A specific patient criterion for ESWL is individuals in whom spontaneous passage of a stone might present a danger to themselves or

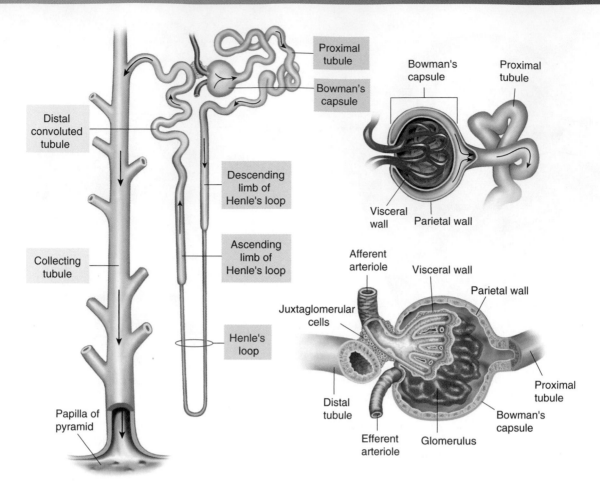

Figure 26-3   The nephron and Bowman capsule. *(From Brundage DJ: Renal disorders, St Louis, 1992, Mosby.)*

others (e.g., pilots, physicians); also, only specific types of stones are suitable for this type of treatment.

ADRENAL GLANDS

The *adrenal glands* are paired organs that lie on the medial side of the upper kidney. The gland has two layers, the outer cortex and the inner medulla. The adrenal glands secrete glucocorticoids, mineralcorticoids, and adrenal sex hormones. Blood is supplied to each gland by the aorta and branches of the renal and inferior phrenic arteries. The adrenal glands are important in the production of norepinephrine and epinephrine, which are necessary for functioning of the autonomic nervous system.

URETERS

In adults, each ureter is about 12 inches (30 cm) long and about 5 mm in diameter. The ureter is a three-layered tubular structure; it has an outer fibrous layer, a middle muscular layer, and an inner mucosal layer. Urine moves along the ureter by *peristalsis*, which is the segmental contraction and relaxation of the ureter's muscular layer.

Each ureter enters the bladder at the *ureterovesical junction*, which is located in the lower bladder.

BLADDER

The urinary bladder lies behind the symphysis pubis in the pelvic cavity. The wall of the bladder is composed of four tissue layers: the outer serosa, the muscular layer, the submucosa, and the inner mucosa. The distal portion of the bladder is called the *trigone*. This triangular region has both superficial and deep muscle layers. The superficial layer extends into the bladder neck of the female and into the proximal portion of the urethra in the male. The trigone has three corners that correspond with the two ureteral openings and one urethral opening (Figure 26-5).

Urine is excreted from the bladder by the process of *micturition* (urination), which is activated by sphincter muscles in the bladder neck. These muscles are controlled by the autonomic nervous system, which maintains retention or release of urine.

URETHRA

Female

The *urethra* communicates with the lower bladder to enable excretion of urine from the body. In the female, it leaves the bladder at the trigone and is embedded in the levator muscles of the pelvic floor. The urethral opening, the *meatus*, is located

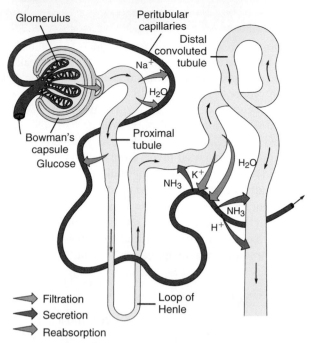

Figure 26-4   **Urine formation.** As filtrate moves through the tubules, electrolytes, salts, and water are absorbed from the filtrate back into the circulatory system. The tubule system is divided into specific regions, which filter certain substances. These regions are called the *proximal tubule*, the *loop of Henle*, and the *distal convoluted tubule*. (*From Thibodeau G, Patton K:* Anatomy and physiology, *ed 6, St Louis, 2007, Mosby.*)

on the midline of the labia near the clitoris. The proximal urethra is composed primarily of smooth muscle tissue. The periurethral muscles on the pelvic floor support the distal urethra and aid in sphincter control. Two small, mucus-secreting glands (the *Skene glands*) are located on each side of the urethra just inside the meatus.

Male

The male urethra exits the bladder and continues to the end of the penis, terminating at the urethral meatus. The male urethra is divided into several distinct parts. The *prostatic urethra* begins at the bladder neck and passes through the center of the prostate gland, which surrounds the urethra distal to the bladder. The midportion is called the *membranous urethra*. The distal, or *cavernous, urethra* is the distal end, which extends the length of the penis.

REPRODUCTIVE STRUCTURES OF THE MALE

SCROTUM AND TESTICLES

The *scrotum* is a layered tissue sac that encases the testicles. The skin of the scrotum contains numerous folds, or *rugae*, and is continuous with the perineum. The inner layer of the scrotum is composed of fascia and dartos muscle. In cold environments, the dartos retracts the testicles closer to the body; it relaxes when the ambient temperature is warm. This

temperature regulation system protects the *spermatozoa* (male reproductive cells) produced by the testicles.

The testicles are enclosed within a fibrous membrane called the *tunica vaginalis*. A septum in the scrotum separates the two testicles. The internal structure of the testicle is composed of tightly coiled tubules and ducts that produce sperm. The smallest units of this ductal system are the *seminiferous tubules*. Testosterone, the primary male sex hormone, is produced in these tubules, which communicate with the larger efferent ductules, epididymis, and vas deferens. The vas deferens exits the testicle at the superior end and joins the ejaculatory structures of the pelvis.

EPIDIDYMIS

The *epididymis* is a convoluted duct that secretes seminal fluid, the liquid substance that gives sperm mobility through the male reproductive tract.

VAS DEFERENS

The *vas deferens* joins the epididymis with the ejaculatory duct. It passes through the inguinal canal in the abdominal wall at the level of the internal ring. At this level, it lies inside the spermatic cord, a strong tubular structure that includes nerves, blood vessels, and lymphatic tissue. The vas deferens continues across the bladder and ureter, where it meets the opening of the seminal vesicle and forms the ejaculatory duct. The paired ejaculatory ducts traverse the prostate gland and terminate at the urethra.

SEMINAL VESICLES

The seminal vesicles are paired structures situated close to the ejaculatory duct at the proximal end. These vesicles (saclike structures) secrete approximately 60% of the semen (the ejaculatory fluid containing sperm).

PROSTATE GLAND

The *prostate gland* surrounds the urethra and secretes an alkaline fluid that contributes to seminal fluid. The gland is divided into six lobes covered by a fibrous *prostatic capsule*. The function of the prostate is production of some components of seminal fluid.

BULBOURETHRAL GLANDS

The bulbourethral glands (also called *Cowper glands*) are paired structures that lie just below the prostate on each side of the urethra. These glands secrete mucus, which contributes to the total volume of the semen.

PENIS

The penis is suspended at the pubic arch by fascia. The body of the penis is composed of several columns of tissue. Two dorsal columns, called the *corpora cavernosa* (sing., corpus cavernosum) are composed of spongy vascular tissue necessary for functional erection of the penis. The columns are separated by a septum and bound together by a fibrous sheath. A third tissue column, called the *corpus spongiosum*, encloses the urethra. The distal portion of the corpus spongiosum forms the *glans penis*, which is covered by skin called the *prepuce* or *foreskin*. During *circumcision*, the foreskin is removed. The *corona* is the recessed tract at the base of the glans.

Figure 26-6 illustrates the male reproductive system.

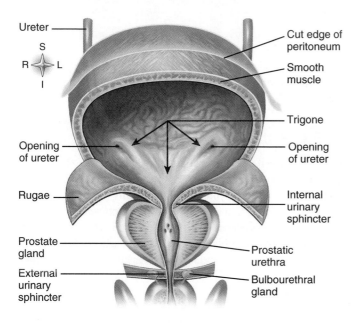

Figure 26-5   Structures and tissue layers of the bladder in the male. Note the position of the prostate gland which surrounds the prostatic segment of the urethra. *(From Thibodeau G, Patton K: Anatomy and physiology, ed 6, St Louis, 2007, Mosby.)*

KIDNEY DIALYSIS

The kidneys normally remove waste products from the blood. Without this function, the body becomes quickly weakened by toxins produced during normal metabolism. Kidney dialysis is a procedure that performs this function in patients with chronic and end-stage renal disease. The two types of kidney dialysis are *hemodialysis* and *peritoneal dialysis*. Dialysis is performed regularly, or it can be done as an emergency procedure to remove ingested toxins from the blood that otherwise would lead to immediate kidney failure. Patients receiving dialysis treatment have a restricted lifestyle and frequently are facing a poor disease outcome. The extreme shortage of donor kidneys and the rigorous dialysis schedule, which determines the patient's quality of life, often lead to depression, which is particularly common in hemodialysis patients.

HEMODIALYSIS

During hemodialysis, the blood is shunted into a heparinized hemodialysis machine, where it passes through a series of membranes and a dialyzing solution that filters waste and then returns the blood to the body. Blood leaves the body through an artery and is returned through a vein. Electrolytes and other substances can be added to the blood during dialysis as needed. The process normally takes about 3 hours and is performed three or four times a week in a dialysis clinic or at home.

For access to the vascular system, an **arteriovenous fistula** (or **AV shunt**) is created surgically. In this procedure, a major vein and artery (usually the radial) are anastomosed, or an artificial graft is implanted to connect the artery and vein. The fistula or AV shunt is used to access the vascular system during dialysis. Hemodialysis patients are extremely careful of their AV access sites and need to take precautions to prevent injury

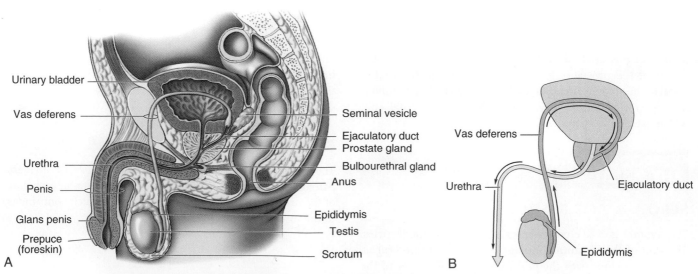

Figure 26-6   The male reproductive system. **A,** Cross section of the pelvic cavity and male reproductive organs. **B,** Schematic showing the path of the ejaculatory duct, vas deferens, and urethra. *(From Herlihy B, Maebius NK: The human body in health and disease, ed 2, Philadelphia, 2003, WB Saunders.)*

at the site. (The procedure for an AV shunt or a fistula is performed by a vascular surgeon and is described in detail in Chapter 32.)

PERITONEAL DIALYSIS

During peritoneal dialysis, a Silastic tube is implanted in the suprapubic peritoneal space. Dialysis solution is instilled into the catheter. The solution remains in the peritoneal cavity and slowly extracts metabolic wastes using the peritoneum as an osmotic filter. The fluid then is removed. The total dwell time may be 4 to 6 hours, and the entire process can be performed by the patient.

DIAGNOSTIC TESTS

The primary function of the urinary system is to filter metabolic waste from the blood. Therefore many laboratory tests in GU disease focus on the presence or absence of substances found in the blood and urine. Imaging tests are performed to outline the structures of the GU system, to observe its function, and to detect tumors. Structural pathology of the genitourinary system is diagnosed through cystoscopic examination, CT scanning, and enhanced imagery. Figure 26-7 illustrates some of the common pathologies of this type. A more detailed table of pathology is found in Appendix D.

URINALYSIS

In a healthy adult, the kidneys produce about 3.2 pints (1.5 L) of urine per day. The main components of urine are water (95%) and solutes (5%). Urinalysis is performed to detect specific substances, both normal and abnormal, in the urine. Filtrate can be sampled from any location in the upper urinary tract. This is often necessary to detect abnormalities caused by disease in a specific location within the kidney or ureter. Urine is obtained directly through a catheter inserted into the bladder or by collection as it passes from the body; the latter may be a single sample or the amount collected over 24 hours.

Simple urinalysis provides basic information about substances such as the blood, glucose, and white blood cells. The physical characteristics of urine are also important. Odor, color, density, and clarity have specific clinical significance, which can help confirm disease. Microscopic examination reveals the presence of blood cells, cell fragments, and other metabolic substances. Infection of the bladder or other locations in the urinary tract may be detected by the presence of protein or blood cells in the urine. A simple dipstick test can be used for screening purposes, and urine culture and sensitivity (discussed in Chapter 7) may be performed to confirm a diagnosis and determine the appropriate antimicrobial therapy.

The presence of protein in the urine is an important diagnostic sign. Albumin is a primary protein component of the blood. Normally, the glomerulus allows very little protein to cross the capillary system and into the filtrate. Therefore albumin in the urine may be a sign of glomerulus disease. Specific tests for urine albumin are routinely performed when kidney disease is suspected.

The **specific gravity** (the ratio of the density of urine compared to water) is an important indicator of the concentration of solutes in the urine. Dissolved solutes are present after filtration in the kidney. Therefore, the specific gravity provides important information about the hydration of the body and also the kidney's ability to maintain fluid balance. The specific gravity is measured with a calibrated hydrometer or urinometer.

BLOOD TESTS

The presence or absence of specific substances in the blood reveals kidney function. Expected values of chemicals and metabolic products in the blood shift in kidney disease. An increase in certain substances can mean that harmful waste products are not filtered out of the blood; other tests and clinical studies must be performed to arrive at a proper diagnosis.

Glomerular Filtration Rate

The serum creatinine or **glomerular filtration rate (GFR)** measures the rate of creatinine clearance from the blood. Creatine is a metabolic by-product of muscle metabolism that normally is filtered by the kidney tubules. However, it is not reabsorbed. The GFR is measured as the amount of creatinine filtered per minute. This is an important test of kidney function. Blood creatinine begins to rise when the GFR is about 50% of normal.

Blood Urea Nitrogen

Measurement of the blood urea nitrogen (BUN) is a test that assesses the elimination of urea from the liver. Urea is a waste product formed in the liver as a product of protein metabolism. Normally it is cleared by the kidneys. The blood urea value may indicate renal failure, but it is also influenced by protein intake, age, and hydration.

TISSUE BIOPSY

Biopsy samples of the kidney, bladder wall, or other tissues of the GU tract are removed for microscopic pathological testing.

IMAGING STUDIES

Imaging studies provide the basis of diagnosis for both functional and physiological disease. Imaging provides a permanent record of the shape, location, and density of structures. Selected studies also can detect stones or malformation of the tubes and ducts of the urinary system. The following imaging studies are commonly used:

- *Computed tomography (CT):* CT is the preferred method for imaging tumors of the kidney. Noncontrast helical CT is used to diagnose calculi.
- *Fluoroscopy:* C-arm fluoroscopy (real-time radiography) is used in many imaging studies.
- *Intravenous urography:* This process involves radiographic studies using a contrast medium, which is injected intravenously to obtain serial radiographs of the renal pelvis and

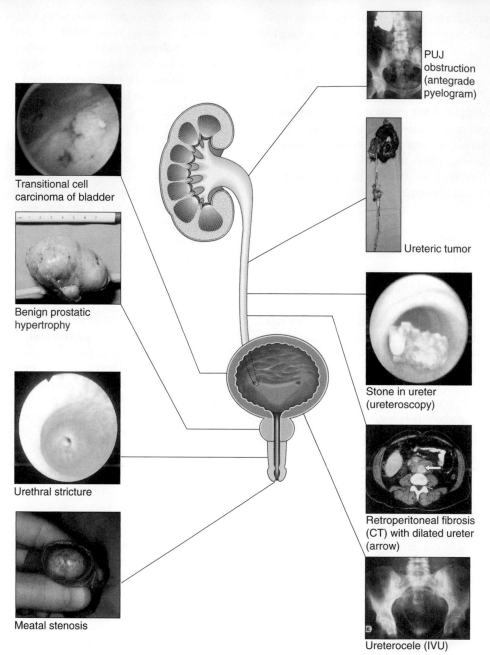

Transitional cell
carcinoma of bladder

Benign prostatic
hypertrophy

Urethral stricture

Meatal stenosis

PUJ
obstruction
(antegrade
pyelogram)

Ureteric tumor

Stone in ureter
(ureteroscopy)

Retroperitoneal fibrosis
(CT) with dilated ureter
(arrow)

Ureterocele (IVU)

Figure 26-7   Genitourinary pathology. *IVU,* Intravenous urogram; *PUJ,* pelviureteric junction. *(From Garden O, Bradbury A, Forsythe J, Parks R: Principles and practice of surgery, ed 5, Edinburgh, 2007, Churchill Livingstone)*

calyces. The rate of emptying and the size of the ureters are also measured.

- *KUB:* This is a radiograph of the kidney, ureters, and bladder. A KUB may be used to outline structures of the urinary system, including any stones larger than 2 mm. However, CT is now preferred for stone imaging, because stones of all types are visible, and even small stones can be seen.
- *Micturating cystourethrogram (MCU):* This study provides images of the bladder (cystography) while it is emptying. A contrast medium is instilled into the bladder via a catheter, and images are obtained during urination.

- *Magnetic resonance imaging (MRI):* MRI provides an extremely detailed assessment and is commonly used in the diagnosis of tumors.
- *Nuclear imaging:* Radioisotope scanning is used in GU studies to detect metastasis arising from a primary tumor of the prostate.
- *Retrograde ureteropyelography:* Retrograde injections are made using a catheter inserted into the ureter. A contrast medium is instilled into the catheter and viewed with fluoroscopy.
- *Ultrasonography:* Ultrasound is one of the first-line imaging techniques used in GU medicine. It is used in the

assessment of patients who are unsuitable for CT or other forms of radiographic exposure.

CASE PLANNING

POSITIONING

A number of patient positions are used in GU surgery, depending on the type of surgery and the techniques to be used. Rigid cystoscopy and ureteroscopy are always performed with the patient in the lithotomy position, although the supine position may be used for flexible cystoscopy. The supine position is used for open abdominal approaches to the bladder and for laparoscopic surgery of the prostate. The lateral position is the most common open approach for a flank incision, which provides exposure of the kidney and ureters. The prone position may be used for endoscopic nephroscopy. Prepping and draping routines follow standard procedures, as discussed in Chapter 20.

INSTRUMENTS FOR OPEN GENITOURINARY PROCEDURES

Open GU procedures require specialty and general surgery instruments. The ureters are extremely delicate and require atraumatic clamps, such as Babcock clamps. Right-angle and Schnitz (tonsil) clamps frequently are used to occlude vessels and for blunt dissection. Vessel loops made of Silastic or cotton are commonly used to retract blood vessels.

Kidney procedures may require kidney pedicle clamps, which have right-angle jaws for reaching around the back of the pedicle. Vascular clamps are required for procedures involving the renal arteries or whenever temporary interruption of the kidney's blood supply is necessary. Fine-tipped needle holders are needed for both kidney and ureteral procedures, because the sutures are fine and the needles are very small.

Most prostate procedures are now performed using minimally invasive surgery (MIS). However, if open surgery is required, prostate retractors and grasping clamps are required, as are right-angle clamps and general surgery instruments. Instruments for open GU surgery are shown in Figures 26-8 and 26-9.

Surgery of the vas deferens and repair of penile anomalies require plastic surgery or microsurgical instruments. MIS instruments (Figure 26-10) are used in percutaneous nephroscopy, laparoscopy, and transurethral (cystoscopic) surgery.

ENDOSCOPIC INSTRUMENTS

Rigid Cystoscope

A rigid *cystoscope* is passed through the urethral meatus for diagnostic or operative procedures. The cystoscope is the precursor to the modern cystourethroscope. In this text, the term *cystoscope* is used to describe the modern transurethral scope. However, the surgical technologist should understand that the current scopes have more advanced technological and surgical capabilities than the cystoscope used in the past.

The optical system of the scope provides a number of angles of vision. The *direct forward scope* (0 degrees) is useful for viewing the urethra and for use with the *urethrotome* (an instrument used in sharp dissection of the urethra). A 45- or 30-degree scope is used for viewing the entire bladder and for insertion of the ureteral catheters. The cystoscope has many components for performing diagnostic and surgical procedures. The instrument is the optical portion of the scope. It contains the lenses, which magnify the target image.

The *Brown-Buerger* cystoscope ranges in size from 14 to 26 French (Fr). The most common size for adults is 21 Fr. This scope has two sheaths to accommodate a ureteral catheter and accessory instruments. The *McCarthy panendoscope* ranges in size from 14 to 30 Fr. This scope is used with a fore-oblique telescope. The *Wappler* cystoscope combines the functions of the Brown-Buerger and McCarthy scopes. The sheath size ranges from 17 to 24 Fr. The scope accepts suction and irrigation accessories, and a ureteral scope can be passed through it.

Sheath

The sheath is a hollow tube that serves as a passageway for the instruments used during cystoscopy and resection. The telescope is inserted into the sheath before it is passed into the urethra. The sheath allows the use of operative accessories, instruments, suction, and irrigation. The sheath has attachments that accept the instruments and irrigation tubing. The tip may be beveled or oblique. The main operating channel receives the telescope, and side channels, controlled by stopcocks, accept the accessory instruments. A *bridge* attaches to the head of the scope and accepts accessory tools.

Obturator

Before the sheath is placed inside the urethra, a blunt, round-tipped *obturator* is placed inside the sheath. The obturator tip advances ahead of the sheath and protects the wall of the urethra from abrasion during insertion. The obturator may be straight or deflecting (able to be turned to the side).

Resectoscope

A **resectoscope** is a transurethral electrosurgical instrument used to remove small fragments of tissue. It consists of an endoscope, sheath, obturator, and electrosurgical loop, which cuts and coagulates target tissue inside the bladder. The handle of the resectoscope contains a spring mechanism that operates the retractable loop (active electrode) at the tip. During resection surgery, the instrument is inserted through the urethra and bladder to remove tumors or resect the prostate or other tissue in the bladder space. The loop is applied to tissue and retracts it into the instrument, simultaneously cutting and coagulating it.

Resectoscopes vary by operating mechanism. Most use a spring mechanism described previously. The most common type is the Iglesias resectoscope. The resectoscope uses electrosurgical energy to excise tissue from the bladder, urethra, or prostate. The sheath usually is a size 24 to 28 Fr and is made of fiberglass to prevent a short circuit and patient burns. The working element of the resectoscope, which is inserted through the sheath, has a channel for a telescope and cutting electrode.

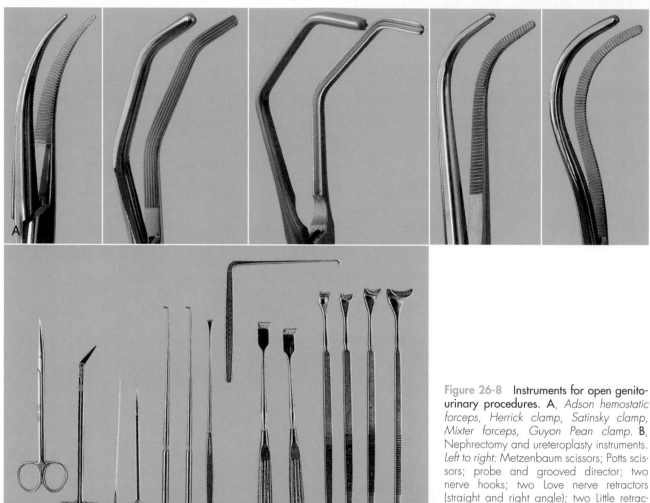

Figure 26-8 Instruments for open genito-urinary procedures. **A,** *Adson hemostatic forceps, Herrick clamp, Satinsky clamp, Mixter forceps, Guyon Pean clamp.* **B,** Nephrectomy and ureteroplasty instruments. *Left to right:* Metzenbaum scissors; Potts scissors; probe and grooved director; two nerve hooks; two Love nerve retractors (straight and right angle); two Little retractors; four vein retractors. *(From Tighe SM: Instrumentation for the operating room, ed 7, St Louis, 2007, Mosby.)*

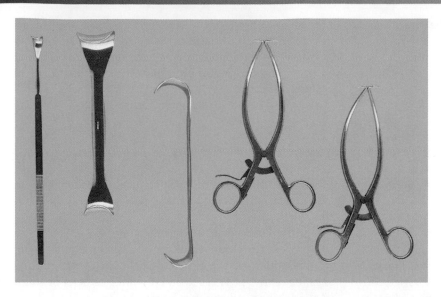

Figure 26-9 Prostatectomy instruments. *Left to right.* Vein retractor; Goulet retractor (two views); Gelpi retractors. *(From Tighe SM: Instrumentation for the operating room, ed 6, St Louis, 2003, Mosby.)*

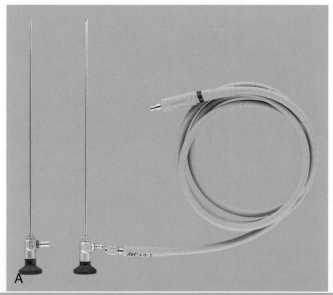

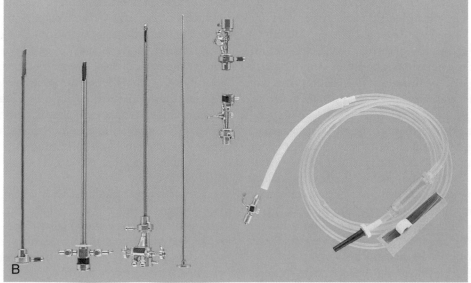

Figure 26-10 Endoscopic instruments. **A,** Cystourethroscope. **B,** Cystoscope and light guide; cystoscope sheath; deflector; obturator; bridges; fluid tubing. *(From Tighe SM: Instrumentation for the operating room, ed 6, St Louis, 2003, Mosby.)*

The cutting electrode cuts and coagulates the tissue. As with other electrosurgical (ESU) systems, a variety of tips are available. The loop electrode is commonly used during resection procedures. Figure 26-11 shows a resectoscope and accessories.

Imaging System

The imaging system used in GU endoscopy is the same as for other endoscopes (see Chapter 24). A fiberoptic light or liquid cable connects the cystoscope to the fiberoptic xenon light source. Other components of the imaging system are fully discussed in Chapter 24.

URINARY CATHETERS

A catheter is a hollow tube made of a flexible, synthetic material, such as Silicone or Teflon-coated rubber. A variety of ureteral and urethral catheters may be used during GU procedures. The lumen, or bore, of the catheter is measured in French, and sizes range from 7 to 26 Fr. Catheters are designated by number, and as the number of a catheter decreases, the lumen diameter also decreases. The catheters most commonly used are in the range of 16 to 18 Fr. Retention catheters also have a retention balloon size, which is measured in cubic milliliters.

Urinary catheters are used for a variety of purposes, including:

- Short-term urinary drainage
- Continuous urinary drainage
- Bladder irrigation
- Hemostasis and evacuation of blood clots
- Continuity of the urethra or ureters

Urethral Catheters

Two common types of catheters are the **indwelling catheter**, or Foley catheter, which has a balloon or flange at the proximal tip, and the **straight catheter** (also called a *Robinson* catheter), which is used for temporary bladder drainage.

The **Foley catheter** is available in a variety of types and balloon sizes. The three-way balloon catheter is used for intermittent or continuous bladder irrigation. A large, 30-mL balloon catheter is used postoperatively as a **tamponade** (used to apply pressure against a tissue or opening). This type is used after transurethral resection of the prostate to control bleeding.

The Foley catheter is the most common type of urinary catheter. It is retained in the bladder by an inflatable balloon at the end of the catheter. Sizes 8 through 30 Fr with a retention balloon of 5 to 30 mL are available. The smaller balloon is used for simple retention, and the larger balloon is used postoperatively to maintain hemostasis, as described previously. After it is placed in the bladder, the balloon is inflated with sterile water. The larger balloons may be inflated to as much as 120 mL for greater hemostatic efficiency.

The *Phillips* catheter is straight but differs from the straight catheter in that one end has a screw tip designed to accept a filiform (a small catheter advanced through a urethral stricture). The filiform has a smaller diameter than the catheter and is easily manipulated in the urethra.

The *coudé* catheter may be straight or may be a Foley retention type. This type of catheter has a firm rubber tip or beak that is used to facilitate its passage through a false urethral passage or past anatomical prominences in the urethra or in an enlarged prostate.

Urethral catheters are shown in Figure 26-12.

Ureteral Catheters

Assorted ureteral catheters are used for both open and closed procedures. General uses are:

- To provide a method of instilling a contrast medium into the ureter and kidney for **retrograde pyelography** radiographic studies.
- To provide immediate drainage of a ureter.
- To provide temporary drainage of a ureter after a procedure. In this case, the catheter may be left in place during healing. This type is called an indwelling catheter or **stent**. An indwelling catheter may be attached to a calibrated collection system to measure output.
- To keep the ureter open to allow a stone to pass.
- To bypass a stone or tumor.
- To block the ureteral opening during radiographic studies.
- To identify a structure during open procedures.
- To obtain urine specimens or renal washings from the kidney.

Ureteral catheters are radiopaque and have graduated marks so that the surgeon can see how deeply the catheter is inserted.

The Braasch bulb or cone-tip catheter is used to occlude the ureteral orifice during imaging studies when a contrast medium is injected during retrograde pyelography.

Other commonly used catheters are the whistle-tip, round-tip, spiral-tip, and olive-tip catheters (Figure 26-13).

Ureteral Stent

A ureteral stent is a particular type of ureteral catheter. It is a thin, flexible tube usually constructed of woven Dacron or polyurethane, that is threaded into the ureter temporarily or for a defined period to help urine drain from the kidney to the bladder or to an external collection system. A ureteral stent is placed in the ureter to provide continuous flow of urine to the bladder. Ureteral stents may be used in patients with an active kidney infection or with diseased bladders (e.g., as a result of cancer or radiation therapy). Alternatively, ureteral stents may be used during or after urinary tract surgical procedures to provide a mold around which healing can occur, to divert the urinary flow away from areas of leakage, to manipulate kidney stones or prevent stone migration before treatment, or to make the ureters more easily identifiable during difficult surgical procedures.

The stent may remain in place for the short term (days to weeks) or for the long term (weeks to months). The size, shape, and material of the ureteral stent to be used depend on the patient's anatomy and the reason the stent is required. Most stents are 5 to 12 inches (12 to 30 cm) long and have a diameter of 1.5 to 6 mm.

Several types of stents are used. They can be made of durable and biocompatible silicone, polyurethane, or some other copolymer. The stent may have a collar, a double-J configuration, a pigtail, or a coil to minimize migration into the renal pelvis

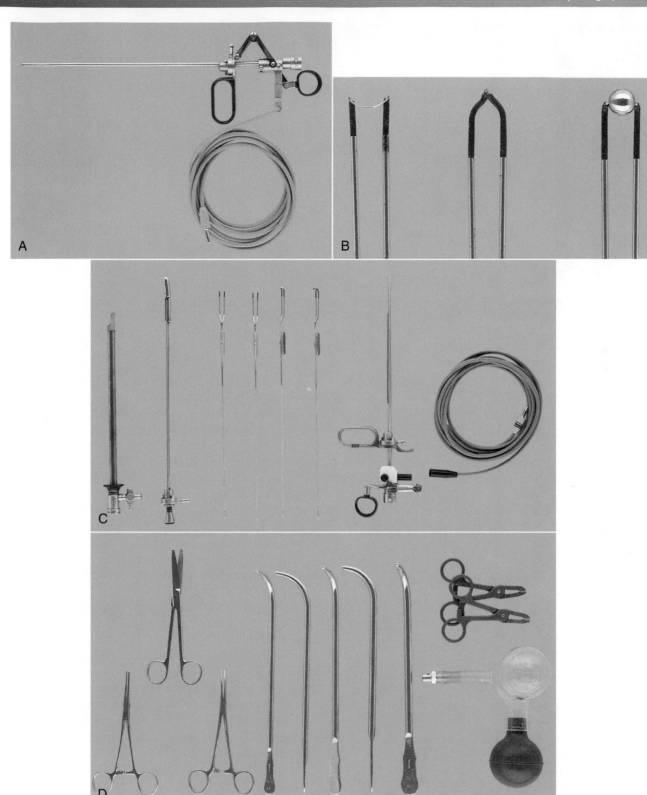

Figure 26-11 **A,** Resectoscope. **B,** Cutting tips. **C,** *Left to right:* Resecting sheath; deflecting sheath; resection loops with resectoscope and power cord. **D,** *Top left:* Mayo dissecting scissors. *Bottom left to right:* Crile hemostats; Van Buren urethral sounds; Ellik evacuator.

Continued

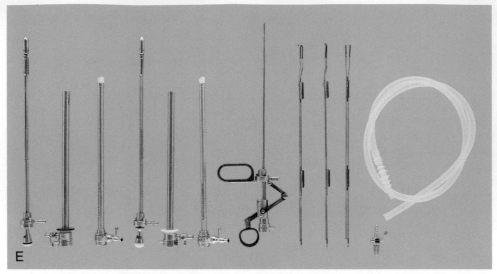

Figure 26-11, cont'd **E,** *Left to right:* Resectoscope, working elements and electrodes. *(From Tighe SM: Instrumentation for the operating room, ed 6, St Louis, 2003, Mosby.)*

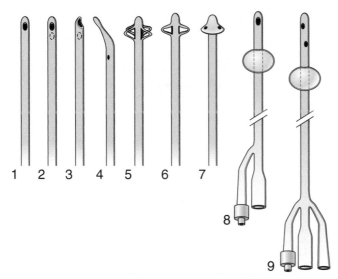

Figure 26-12 **Urinary catheters.** *1,* Conical-tip catheter. *2,* Robinson catheter. *3,* Whistle-tip urethral catheter. *4,* Coudé olive-tip catheter. *5* and *6,* Malecot catheter. *7,* Pezzer catheter. *8,* Foley retention catheter. *9,* Three-way irrigation catheter. *(Modified from Walsh PC, Retik AB, Vaughan ED, et al: Campbell's urology, ed 8, Philadelphia, 2002, WB Saunders.)*

or bladder. During cystoscopy, the stent is passed through the cystoscope and over a guidewire into the ureter, where it remains fixed for internal urinary drainage. As described for ureteral catheters, some types of stents are used to identify ureters and provide external drainage intraoperatively.

The indwelling pigtail catheter is a type of J-stent; this refers to its ability to maintain the form and shape of the ureter. The catheter maintains patency in the ureter to allow a stone or urine to pass. During insertion, a guidewire is placed in the lumen of the catheter, which gives it some stiffness while guiding the catheter. Once the catheter is in place, the wire is removed, and the distal end forms a J or slight spiral, which holds it in place. The distal end may be sutured to the patient's skin to allow for a noninvasive removal. This type of catheter is also used during ESWL.

EQUIPMENT

Electrosurgical Unit

Electrosurgery is used in both open and transurethral procedures. As in other specialties, electrosurgery in GU surgery is delivered through many types of instruments. The most common ESU devices are the "pencil" and the bipolar cutting and coagulation instruments. The resectoscope, discussed in Chapter 24, is used in transurethral procedures and in the presence of continuous irrigation. Safety hazards are associated with the use of electrosurgical equipment in the presence of fluids. The cystoscopy assistant must understand these principles (see Continuous and Intermittent Irrigation, later).

The grounding plate may be placed on the patient's thigh or waist. It must be placed over a fleshy area and never over a bony prominence. The ESU should be placed on the lowest setting, which is increased gradually as directed by the urologist.

Microscope

An operative microscope is used during fine reconstructive surgery, laser ablation, and vaporization of lesions. The use and care of the operating microscope are described in Chapter 27.

Laser

The neodymium/yttrium-aluminum-garnet (Nd:YAG), carbon dioxide (CO_2), tunable dye, and argon lasers typically are used in GU surgery. Certain aspects of laser use are discussed in particular procedures in this chapter, but the reader should review all safety precautions discussed in Chapter 18.

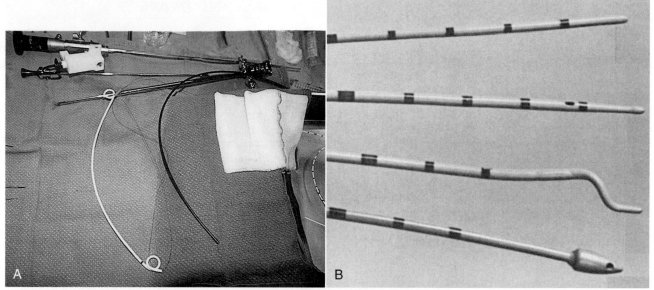

Figure 26-13 **A,** Ureteral catheters and stents. **B,** Ureteral catheters. *Top to bottom:* Round tip, olive tip, spiral tip, and conical or bulb tip. *(A from Nagle GM: Genitourinary surgery: perioperative nursing series, St Louis, 1997, Mosby; B from Walsh PC, Retik AB, Vaughan ED, et al: Campbell's urology, ed 8, Philadelphia, 2002, WB Saunders.)*

TECHNIQUES IN TRANSURETHRAL SURGERY

Most procedures of the kidneys, ureters, bladder, and urethra are performed with a flexible or rigid endoscope. Two techniques are commonly used:

- *Cystoscopy:* A rigid or flexible cystoscope is used for transurethral assessment and procedures of the lower GU tract, including the urethra, bladder, and prostate gland.
- *Ureteroscopy:* A rigid or flexible ureteroscope is inserted through the urethra and advanced into the renal pelvis and ureter. Surgery is performed through the lumen of the scope.

Although cystoscopy is considered a clean-contaminated procedure, most facilities ensure that all equipment is sterile to prevent cross-contamination. (Chapter 24 presents a discussion of endoscopic reprocessing, both sterile and clean-contaminated.)

CYSTOSCOPY ROOM

Transurethral procedures take place in a specialized cystoscopy ("cysto") room. This dedicated surgical suite has all the equipment needed to perform diagnostic or therapeutic procedures.

The cystoscopy table has accommodations for continuous drainage, intraoperative fluoroscopy, and radiography. The cystoscopy table differs from the standard operating table in that it is designed to maintain the patient in the lithotomy position, receive radiograph cassettes, and allow for drainage of irrigation fluid. The stirrups of the table are adjustable and removable, and radiograph cassettes are placed in a hollow space built into the table. Irrigation fluid is directed into a drainage tray at the foot of the table. The tray is covered with

a wire mesh plate that can be sterilized for resection procedures when tissue specimens are evacuated with the irrigation solution.

More extensive and modern cystoscopy rooms include digital data recording and equipment for video-assisted transurethral and ureteroscopy surgery.

CYSTOSCOPY ASSISTANT

Most facilities employ a *cystoscopy (cysto) assistant.* This is a trained surgical technologist or nurse whose main duty is to work in this specialty. Other perioperative staff in the department may have little clinical time in the cystoscopy room and thus would not have the opportunity to learn about the specialty. The system is efficient as long as the cysto assistant is available at all times. However, if this person is absent, other staff members must take the individual's place. A written protocol should be available for all staff members.

The cysto assistant performs duties as a scrub and circulator. After donning sterile gloves, the assistant sets up the instrument table and all other sterile equipment. The urologist usually does not require a scrub; therefore, after setting up the supplies, the assistant removes his or her gloves and functions as a circulator during the case.

During a cystoscopic procedure, the circulator has the following responsibilities:

1. Remain in the room at all times unless otherwise directed by the urologist.
2. Connect the nonsterile ends of the power cables or suction tubing.
3. Open sterile supplies for the urologist as needed.
4. Replace irrigation bottles as they empty and note the number of bottles used.

5. Receive any specimens from the urologist and label them properly.

6. Monitor the patient's vital signs every 15 minutes if a local anesthetic is used during the procedure.

After a cystoscopic procedure, the circulator has the following responsibilities:

1. Assist in transferring the patient from the cystoscopy table to the gurney and accompany the urologist or anesthesiologist to the postanesthesia care unit.

2. Transfer any tissue or fluid specimens to the designated area and record them in the specimen log.

3. Put away nonsterile supplies used during the procedure.

4. Transfer soiled equipment to the workroom and carry out proper terminal sterilization or decontamination of the equipment.

5. The surgical technologist may be responsible for maintaining a current inventory of surgical supplies and for communicating with manufacturers' representatives.

POSITIONING

The patient is placed in the lithotomy or the supine position, depending on the type of endoscopy to be performed. Rigid endoscopy requires the lithotomy position, whereas the supine position can be used for flexible endoscopy. Patient safety in the cysto room is the same as for other procedures. However, many cysto patients are older which requires extra care to prevent overabduction of the hips or rapid changes in position. Patients are helped to the cystoscopy table from the gurney and given clear but gentle direction during the transfer.

All patients are moved gently and with consideration for their individual physical ability. The cystoscopy stirrups are a modified (lower) version of those used commonly in open procedures involving the genital and perianal areas.

The lithotomy position is embarrassing for most patients. However, perioperative personnel help the patient by making the position as comfortable as possible. The patient's dignity should be protected, and the patient must not be exposed unless necessary. Talking to the patient often eases apprehension, and preparatory steps for the procedure should be explained in straightforward terms.

Temperatures in the cysto room are kept quite low, and safety procedures to maintain patient thermoregulation must be maintained. Warm blankets should be available as soon as the patient enters the room, and the patient's comfort should be maintained throughout the procedure

When the patient is positioned for cystoscopic procedures, the buttocks must be in line with or just over the table break with the legs supported by knee crutches or stirrups. Assistants must become familiar with the type of stirrup used in their facility. Stirrups must be padded correctly to prevent pressure on the peroneal nerve. Knee crutches are commonly used in many facilities. These place weight on the popliteal space (behind the knee) and can damage the nerves and blood vessels in this area. Ample padding, with the weight of the knee equally distributed, helps prevent injury. Foam or gel padding provides the safest cushioning.

PREPPING AND DRAPING

Skin prep for cystoscopic procedures includes the entire perineum, external genitalia, and pubis. A perineal drape with a waterproof shield is used for procedures that require continuous bladder irrigation.

INTRAOPERATIVE IMAGING

Intraoperative imaging techniques, including radiography and fluoroscopy, are commonly used during cystoscopy. The cystoscopy table is specially constructed to accommodate the C-arm, and most operating rooms now have permanent radiographic capability in the GU cystoscopy room.

Digital imaging of the operative site during endoscopy is performed through the camera head of the flexible endoscope. Imaging systems used in endoscopic GU surgery are similar to those used in other specialties. The components include the following:

- Light source and fiberoptic cable
- Camera head (endoscopes)
- Camera control unit
- Video cables
- Digital output recorder
- Monitor
- Equipment cart

These components are discussed in detail in Chapter 24.

CONTINUOUS AND INTERMITTENT IRRIGATION

During cystoscopic procedures, the bladder is distended with fluid to enhance visualization of the internal structures. Continuous irrigation flushes blood and tissue debris from the focal site during a procedure.

*NOTE: Whenever electrosurgical instruments are used, the irrigation fluid must be **nonelectrolytic** (containing no electrolytes). These fluids cannot transmit or disperse electricity.*

The electrosurgical instruments are used "underwater" within the distention and irrigation fluid. Electrolytic solutions, which *do* contain electrolytes, cause electrical current to disperse throughout the fluid. This reduces the ESU's ability to cut and coagulate. The distention solutions most commonly used during electrosurgery are *sorbitol* and *glycine*.

Sterile distilled water may be used during assessment of the bladder and retrograde pyelography, which do not require electrosurgery.

Absorption of irrigation fluid (**intravasation**) may result in vascular overload. The assistant must accurately monitor the amount of fluid used and collected as runoff during a procedure to assess the amount absorbed.

Continuous irrigation is provided in 1-L and 3-L airtight plastic bags and closed-unit tubing. A pumping unit regulates the amount of flow. Pressure is regulated by a combination pump and pressure regulator or by gravity flow. The assistant is responsible for ensuring a continuous flow of fluid during the procedure.

The solutions used in surgery are stored in a fluid warmer. The warmer must be carefully maintained and checked frequently to ensure that the temperature is safe. Fluid warmers may contribute to increased hemorrhage, because the warm water suppresses or delays the body's natural clotting mechanism. Bladder spasm or *hypothermia* may occur when cold irrigation solutions are used. The assistant must verify the surgeon's orders for the solution type and temperature before a procedure.

ANESTHESIA

Most patients receive a local or topical anesthetic for diagnostic cystoscopy. In males, a local anesthetic in solution may be instilled into the bladder or penis. For females, cotton-tipped applicators are dipped in an anesthetic and inserted into the urethral meatus. Lidocaine gel (1% or 2%) typically is used for this purpose. Monitored sedation or a spinal or general anesthetic may be used for complex procedures.

TRANSURETHRAL (CYSTOSCOPIC) PROCEDURES

CYSTOSCOPY

Description

Cystoscopy is surgery of the distal GU system performed with an operative cystourethroscope. Basic cystoscopy for visual assessment is performed at the start of any transurethral procedure.

TECHNIQUE

1 The patient is placed in the supine position on the urology table. Low lithotomy stirrups or knee crutches are used to abduct and externally rotate the patient's legs.
2 The patient is prepped and draped for a perineal procedure.
3 A topical anesthetic or water-soluble anesthetic solution is instilled into the urethra.
4 Urethral dilation is performed as needed.
5 The sheath and telescope or obturator are lubricated and inserted into the urethra.
6 The obturator is removed.
7 The bladder is filled with a distention medium.
8 The surgeon examines the urethra and bladder from all angles.
9 Diagnostic and operative procedures are performed.

Discussion

The components of the basic setup for cystoscopy are listed in Box 26-1. The bladder is emptied with a straight catheter, and a sterile urine specimen is obtained. A rigid cystoscope is lubricated with water-soluble or lidocaine gel and inserted into the urethra (Figure 26-14).

The continuous irrigation fluid is instilled. The obturator is then removed, and any residual urine is collected in the

Box **26-1** Basic Setup for Cystoscopy
Cystoscopy pack (gowns, towels, drapes)
Sterile gloves
Cystourethroscope
Cystoscopy irrigation tubing
Albarrán bridge
Catheter adapters
Lateral and fore-oblique telescope
Electrosurgical unit
Bugbee electrodes
Penile clamp
Luer-Lok stopcock
Water-soluble lubrication gel
Irrigation solution
Fiberoptic light source
Small prep basin with sponges
Specimen containers
Lead aprons
Laser units (if required)
Syringes
Assorted catheters

specimen container. The urethra and bladder are examined. When this process is complete, the instruments are removed and the solution is drained from the bladder.

URETHRAL DILATION AND URETHROTOMY

Surgical Goal

In urethral dilation and urethrotomy, the urethra is dilated to relieve a stricture. Phillips filiforms and followers, graduated sounds (dilators), or balloon dilators may be used for this purpose. A **urethrotomy** is a small incision made in the internal urethra to release scar tissue or other stricture. Instruments used for dilation are shown in Figure 26-15.

Pathology

Urethral stricture other than that caused by an enlarged prostate gland may be caused by scarring from a previous trauma, by infection of the urethra, or by a congenital anomaly. If dilation is ineffective, a urethrotomy is performed.

Discussion

Dilation and urethrotomy precede routine diagnostic cystoscopy. Stricture of the urethra is a common condition in GU disease, and dilation of the urethral stricture may be performed as an isolated procedure. Urethral dilation often is necessary to allow instruments to pass through the urethra during surgery.

Many types of dilators are available. Filiforms are very small rods with a threaded distal end. The threaded portion accepts all sizes of followers, which are larger dilators in graduated sizes. Van Buren sounds are graduated metal rods. All sounds are first lubricated and then introduced slowly to avoid lacerating the urethra.

Urethrotomy is performed with the urethrotome, which is inserted to the point of stricture under direct visualization. A small incision is made into the structure, and a urethral

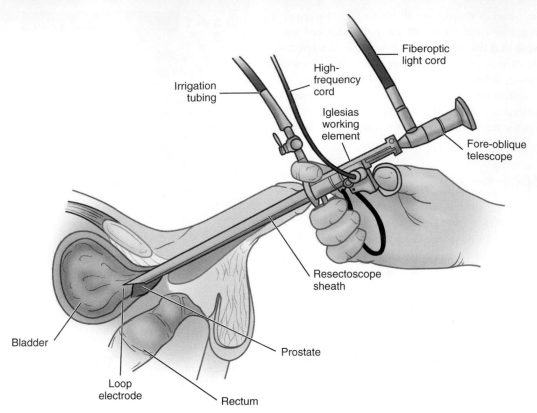

Figure 26-14   Cystourethroscope during operative cystoscopy. Note the connections for irrigation, high-frequency electrosurgery, and fiberoptic light. *(From Rothrock J: Alexander's care of the patient in surgery, ed 17, Philadelphia, 2007, Mosby.)*

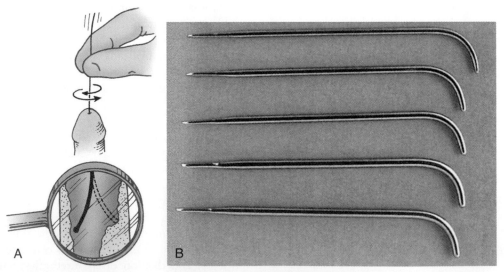

Figure 26-15   A, Use of a coudé catheter to release a urethral stricture. **B,** Urethral sounds. *(A From Rothrock J: Alexander's care of the patient in surgery, ed 17, Philadelphia, 2007, Mosby; B from Tighe SM: Instrumentation for the operating room, ed 7, St Louis, 2007, Mosby.)*

catheter is inserted. The catheter is left in place during the initial healing period (3 to 5 days after surgery).

A related procedure is a **meatotomy** (meatoplasty), in which a small incision is made in the urethral meatus to relieve a stricture. As a stand-alone procedure, a meatotomy is performed on pediatric patients to release scar tissue. Infection or previous dilation of the urethral meatus can result in scarring and partial obstruction. A topical anesthetic

is applied, and fine scissors are used to make a very small incision in the meatus. Healing occurs by secondary intention.

Tissue Biopsy

Tissue biopsy is performed with cup forceps or with a flat wire basket commonly used for ureteroscopic assessments. A cell biopsy can be taken from the bladder with the cytology brush. After the specimen is retrieved on the brush, the technologist agitates the brush gently in normal saline to release the cells from the brush.

Bleeding and edema of the urethra are the most common complications of cystoscopic procedures. Urinary retention may occur as a result of pain or swelling. However, it generally is self-limiting and resolves spontaneously.

MANAGEMENT OF CALCULI

Surgical Goal

Calculi are removed from the ureter and urethra to relieve pain and restore continuity to the urinary tract.

Pathology

Renal stones are crystalline minerals and salts that precipitate from urine. The exact cause is unknown. They are the most common cause of urinary tract obstruction. The jagged structure of urinary calculi causes excruciating pain. Many types of calculi can occur, and each is composed of a different substance. Stones cause obstruction, pain, and infection and damage the urinary tract. Most calculi occur in the kidneys; they seldom form in the bladder.

Discussion

Bladder calculi, which do not pass through the urethra unaided, may be managed in several ways. Small stones may be grasped with stone-grasping forceps. A lithotrite is a specialized instrument that grasps and crushes the stone.

After routine cystoscopic assessment, the surgeon introduces the lithotrite into the scope. Under direct vision, the stone is crushed, and small pieces are flushed out of the bladder with an Ellik evacuator. Bleeders are coagulated with the Bugbee active electrode. Bladder stones must be retained in a dry container for pathological assessment.

TRANSURETHRAL RESECTION OF THE PROSTATE

Surgical Goal

In transurethral resection of the prostate (TURP), the prostate is removed with a resectoscope inserted through the urethra.

Pathology

Enlargement of the prostate generally is related to infection, a benign tumor, or malignancy. *Benign prostatic hyperplasia* is nonmalignant enlargement of the prostate gland, which can occur in men older than 40. The prostate enlarges in two ways. In one type of growth, cells multiply around the urethra, causing obstruction. In the other type of growth, or middle lobe prostate growth, cells grow into the urethra and the bladder outlet area. Obstructive disease may cause **reflux** (backward flow) of urine, infection, and difficulty voiding. Benign prostatic hyperplasia is commonly treated by resection.

TECHNIQUE

1 The patient is positioned and prepped for a perineal procedure.
2 The bladder and bladder neck are assessed.
3 The urethra is dilated.
4 The resectoscope is inserted into the urethra.
5 The prostate is resected systematically.
6 Fragments are flushed from the bladder and collected as specimens.
7 The resectoscope is withdrawn, and a 30-mL Foley catheter is inserted.

Discussion

The patient is placed in the lithotomy position. A routine cystoscopy is performed with a 30-degree lens to evaluate the bladder and other structures. During resection, continuous irrigation or bladder distention with a nonelectrolytic solution (e.g., sorbitol or glycine) is used to maintain a clear surgical field and to evacuate small pieces of tissue.

Continuous irrigation permits clear visualization during resection. The resectoscope is constructed with an outer sheath that allows fluid to flow out of the instrument. Irrigation fluid must be maintained. As mentioned, a solution warmer is used to prevent hypothermia.

The surgeon lubricates the cystoscope and inserts it into the urethra. The obturator then can be removed, allowing the bladder to drain. The cysto assistant should be prepared to collect urine from this sample, because it will be submitted for analysis. Irrigation fluid is then instilled into the bladder. The bladder is assessed, and the cystoscope is removed.

The urethra is then dilated with van Buren sounds. The resectoscope is inserted, and resection begins at the middle and lateral lobes and continues in a systematic pattern. The small pieces of tissue that are released into the irrigation fluid may be evacuated with an Ellik evacuator or a Toomey syringe. The technologist must retain all pieces of specimen for pathological examination in a small basin.

After resection, a three-way Foley catheter is inserted, and the bladder is irrigated to ensure adequate flow and hemostasis. The catheter remains in place for 12 to 24 hours.

NOTE: *Transurethral resection of a bladder tumor is performed in the same manner as TURP.*

Other minimally invasive techniques used in prostatectomy include laser and transurethral needle ablation using ultrasound. TURP is illustrated in Figure 26-16.

After a TURP procedure, the patient may remain catheterized for several days to facilitate irrigation of the bladder. Possible postoperative complications include:

- Incontinence
- Impotence
- Infertility
- Passage of semen into the bladder instead of the urethra (retrograde ejaculation)
- Urethral stricture

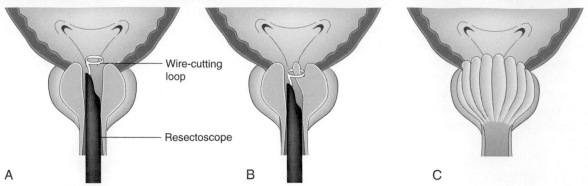

Figure 26-16 **A,** Transurethral resection of the prostate (TURP). An electrosurgical cutting loop is inserted through the urethra. **B,** The cutting loop is drawn back along the resectoscope sheath, cutting and coagulating the hypertrophied prostate. **C,** Prostatic capsule with prostate removed. *(From Garden O, Bradbury A, Forsythe J, Parks R: Principles and practice of surgery, ed 5, Edinburgh, 2007, Churchill Livingstone.)*

FLEXIBLE AND RIGID URETEROSCOPY

Transurethral ureteroscopy is performed with a flexible or rigid ureteroscope. Ureteroscopy commonly is performed for the following:

- Diagnosis of congenital anomalies, disease, or trauma of the ureters and renal pelvis
- Management of renal calculi
- Tissue biopsy from the ureter or renal pelvis
- Management of ureteral stricture

A flexible ureteroscope ranges in size from 6.9 to 9 Fr. The flexible tip allows the scope to be positioned in the renal pelvis and advanced into the calyces. The ureteroscope has working channels for the insertion of instruments, suction, and irrigation.

A rigid ureteroscope is designed to accept accessory instruments, and the scope also has designated channels for suction, irrigation, and a telescope. A small-diameter, semirigid ureteroscope is narrower than 7.5 Fr. This allows dilation of the tip under direct vision. Rigid and flexible scopes often are used in the same surgery, each providing functions necessary to the procedure. For example, the rigid scope is used to dilate the lower ureter to allow passage of the flexible scope. The rigid scope is also used to implant catheters and stents (Figure 26-17). Instruments required for a ureteroscopy are listed in Box 26-2.

Irrigation

Irrigation fluid can be delivered through a pump or manually through the channel used for the working instruments. Sterile saline is used for most procedures that do not require the ESU. Sorbitol or glycine is used when electrosurgery is required. A contrast medium may be added to the irrigation fluid for a fluoroscopic examination.

Use of the Ureteroscope

The flexible ureteroscope is inserted with the aid of a guidewire made of Teflon-coated stainless steel. The guidewire is passed through the scope and advanced into the ureter and renal pelvis under fluoroscopy. The ureteroscope is then advanced over the wire. The ureter may be dilated with a balloon dilator.

After the scope is positioned in the renal pelvis, the flexible tip can be deflected to enter the renal calyces. Accessory instruments are threaded into the working channels to perform various types of procedures as described earlier.

Biopsy

Tissue biopsy is performed with cup forceps or with a flat wire basket. Cell biopsy can be taken with the cytology brush. After the specimen is retrieved on the brush, the technologist agitates the brush gently in a prepared specimen container holding normal saline to release the cells from the brush.

Tumor Removal

Tumors can be removed by fulguration using the ESU or the holmium:YAG laser. Tumor tissue may also be removed in small increments using a resectoscope. In this case, tissue specimens must be retrieved and collected for pathological examination. (Chapter 18 presents a complete discussion of laser use and safety.)

Treatment for Calculi

The ureteroscope is used to remove or destroy stones in the renal pelvis or ureter. A rigid ureteroscope is inserted after the guidewire. Laser energy is delivered through a small quartz fiber (filament) to fragment the stone. An accessory such as a wire prong grasper or basket then can be used to extract fragments through the endoscope.

In flexible ureteroscopy, two guidewires are required. The first is a safety guidewire, and the second is used to facilitate insertion of the endoscope.

SURGERY OF THE MALE EXTERNAL GENITALIA

CIRCUMCISION (ADULT)

Surgical Goal

Circumcision is the removal of the prepuce (foreskin), which is done to improve hygiene and for cultural and religious reasons.

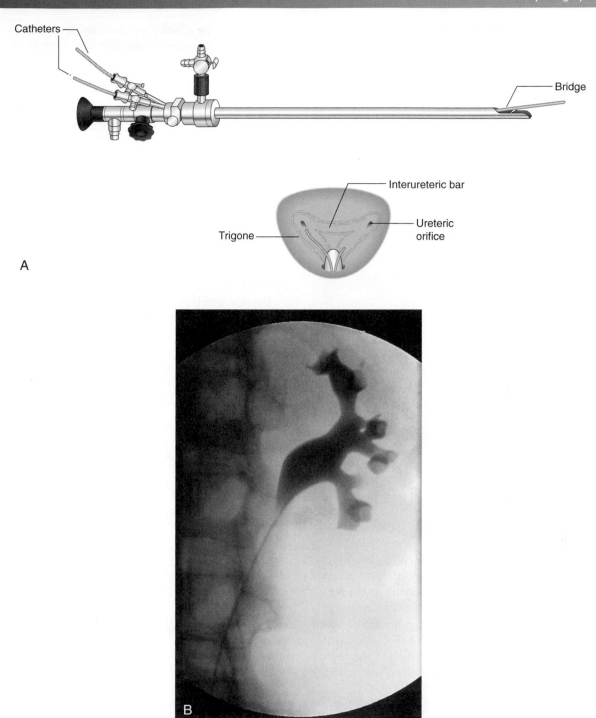

Figure 26-17   **A**, Cystourethroscope with bridge for insertion of urethral catheters. **B**, Retrograde ureteropyelogram. The catheter is passed into the renal pelvis, and contrast medium is injected. *(From Garden O, Bradbury A, Forsythe J, Parks R: Principles and practice of surgery, ed 5, Edinburgh, 2007, Churchill Livingstone.)*

Pathology

An uncircumcised male may develop a number of conditions that affect the glans and foreskin. Skin detritus can become trapped between the foreskin and glans, leading to infection and scarring. In these conditions the foreskin cannot be retracted from the glans (phimosis), or it adheres to the base of the glans and cannot be returned to its normal anatomical position (paraphimosis).

Some evidence indicates that uncircumcised males may be at risk for penile cancer related to repeated infection or exposure to human papilloma virus (see Chapter 9). In general, circumcision is widely practiced. It may be a cultural practice, or it may be related to the perception that penile hygiene is enhanced by circumcision. Circumcision for adherence to religious tradition is practiced in the Jewish faith.

Box **26-2** Ureteroscopy Instruments
Ureteroscope
Guidewires
Cystoscope
Saline for irrigation
Connectors and tubing
Three-way stopcock
Syringes (20 and 50 mL)
Contrast media
Lithotripter (as needed)
Grasper
Stone basket
Double-lumen catheter
Ureteral dilators
Active fulgurating electrode
Luer-Lok connectors
Specimen containers

TECHNIQUE

1 The foreskin is measured and marked.
2 The foreskin is pulled down over the glans with straight hemostats.
3 A dorsal incision is made in the skin and carried circumferentially.
4 The foreskin may be sutured to the corona and dressings applied.

Discussion

The patient is placed in the supine position, prepped, and draped with a small fenestrated sheet. The coronal ridge is outlined with a skin scribe to identify the incision. The surgeon places several Kelly, Crile, or mosquito hemostats on the edge of the prepuce. A longitudinal incision is made on the dorsal side of the foreskin with fine dissecting scissors. The incision is carried circumferentially around the prepuce, and small bleeders are controlled with the ESU.

The surgeon then sutures the wound edges to the corona with 4-0 or 5-0 interrupted absorbable sutures. The wound is dressed with petrolatum gauze.

Postoperative Considerations

Complications after circumcision are rare. However, bleeding and infection may occur. Infection is prevented with routine wound care and maintaining cleanliness of the site.

CHORDEE REPAIR

Surgical Goal

During chordee repair, constrictive penile tissue is released, allowing the penis to assume a normal (anatomical) position.

Pathology

Chordee is a congenital downward curvature of the penis caused by a band of connective tissue between the urethral opening and the glans. Chordee can be caused by a short urethra, fibrous tissues connecting the urethral opening, or both.

Discussion

A chordee may be surgically repaired any time after 6 months of age. The goals of surgery are to improve the appearance and function of the penis.

If the chordee is the result of skin tightening, the physician may shorten the dorsal foreskin and remove any fibrous tissue causing the curvature. If associated with hypospadias, chordee is corrected at the time of the hypospadias repair.

The patient is placed in the supine position and prepped and draped for a perineal procedure. A traction suture of 5-0 silk is placed through the glans. The planes on the shaft of the penis are dissected to the fascial layer.

The skin overlying the distal urethra is dissected free of its attachments to the urethra and the distal shaft. A 26-gauge butterfly needle is then inserted into the penile corpora, and normal saline is injected. This demonstrates any fibrous bands, which are dissected and released with fine tissue scissors. On completion of the release, the tissue is closed with 4-0 or 5-0 absorbable suture.

HYPOSPADIAS REPAIR

Surgical Goal

Hypospadias results in shortening of the urethra. The meatus can appear along the penile shaft or at the base of the scrotum.

Pathology

Hypospadias is a common congenital anomaly involving incomplete development of the distal urethra. This results in ventral shortening of the penis during erection and nonanatomical location of the urethral meatus. The defect has doubled in both incidence and severity in the past 15 years, with no apparent reason for the increase.

Discussion

Many procedures have been developed to treat hypospadias. The exact approach depends on the severity of the defect. Simple repair of the penis is performed in an outpatient setting, usually in one procedure. The principle of the technique is reconstruction of the urethra using a graft from the foreskin or buccal skin (the inside of the mouth). The urethra is thus extended, and the penile tissue is reconstructed around it. A urethral catheter is left in place during the initial postoperative period.

NOTE: **Epispadias** is a very rare condition in which the urethral meatus is located on the top side of the penis. This defect is associated with exstrophy of the bladder and other developmental defects of the pelvis and GU system.

Figure 26-18 illustrates a procedure for hypospadias.

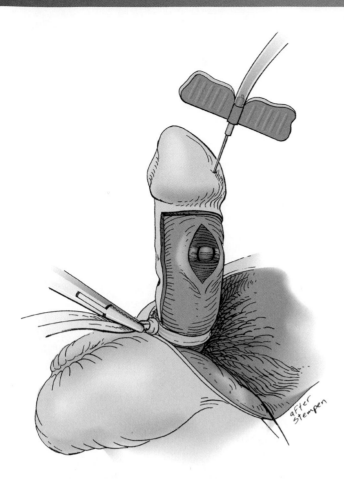

Figure 26-18 **Hypospadias.** *(From Walsh PC, Retik AB, Vaughan ED, et al: Campbell's urology, ed 8, Philadelphia, 2002, WB Saunders.)*

PENECTOMY

Surgical Goal

Penectomy is partial or complete amputation of the penis for the treatment of cancer of the glans penis. An important goal of the surgery is to preserve voiding and erectile function whenever possible.

Pathology

Squamous cell carcinoma of the penis is a *rare* disease, especially in Western countries where most males are circumcised (1,250 reported cases in 2010). The disease rarely affects uncircumcised men and can occur anywhere on the penis but is most frequently found on the glans and foreskin.

Discussion

Early-stage squamous cell carcinoma of the penis can be treated conservatively with local excision of the affected tissue without penectomy. Partial penectomy in which only the glans is removed is more common for late-stage cancer. The psychological effects of penectomy are severe, and all attempts are made toward conservative surgical treatment. In many patients, circumcision is adequate. The following description describes partial penectomy, which is the most common procedure for invasive squamous cell carcinoma.

The patient is placed in the supine or lithotomy position, and the external genitalia including a wide margin prepped and draped. The skin incision may be marked to extend over 2 cm of the lesion. The dissection may be performed using the Mohs technique, described in Chapter 30. In this procedure, the tumor margins are identified and the tissue specimen examined as a frozen section. The excisional margin is then increased until the edges are no longer positive for cancerous cells. More commonly, amputation is performed to at least 2 cm proximal to the tumor. During excision, the tumor is covered using a surgical glove to prevent seeding of cancer cells to the operative site. Some surgeons place a tourniquet at the base of the penis. A Foley catheter is inserted before the skin incision to isolate the urethra during the procedure, or it may be inserted during dissection.

The circumferential skin incision is made using a #15 surgical blade. Small Allis or mosquito clamps may be used to grasp the incised skin edges for traction. The penile skin is retracted proximally to enable further dissection of the tissue planes. The incision is carried to the level of the Buck fascia. The Buck fascia is then incised laterally to create a new dissection plane. This may be performed with fine plastic scissors such as tenotomy scissors or other fine tissue scissors. Peanut sponge dissectors should be available to dissect the tissue between the tunica albuginea and the neurovascular tissue. Hemostasis is controlled using fine mosquito forceps and size 4-0 suture ties to ligate the penile vessels.

The sharp tissue dissection is carried through the two corpora structures to the urethra circumferentially, leaving an addition 1 cm of skin that will be used to cover the defect.

The urethra is isolated to extend approximately 1 cm from the two corpora and then divided. The specimen is thus freed and passed to the surgical technologist.

The defects in the corpora are closed using interrupted horizontal mattress sutures, usually of 2-0 or 3-0 polydioxanone on a small curved needle. In order to form the urethostomy, the urethra is splayed on one side. The skin is then sutured to form a YV-plasty with the urethra everted over the opening. The urethra is secured to the skin using size 4-0 interrupted absorbable sutures. The operative stages are shown in Figure 26-19. If only the glans is to be removed, the skin flap can be brought over the defect using a buttonhole technique to form the urethostomy. In this case a small hole is made in the skin flap to accommodate the urethra, which is secured to the skin as in the YV-plasty.

The wound is dressed can be dressed using xeroform gauze strips over the incision site covered with plain gauze and Coban dressing. The Foley catheter remains in place for 3 to 5 days.

INSERTION OF A PENILE IMPLANT

Surgical Goal

A penile implant is surgically placed to treat impotence caused by organic disease. Two types of implants are available, a semirigid implant and an inflatable reservoir implant.

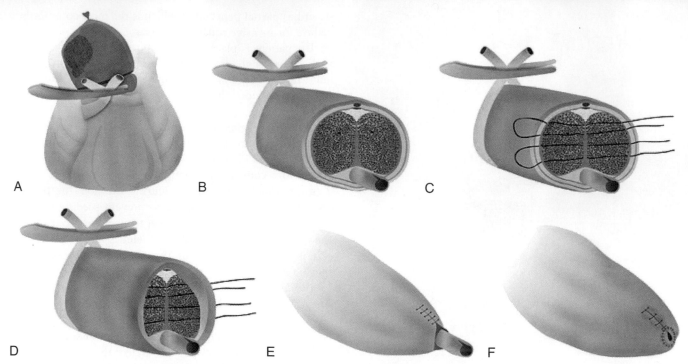

Figure 26-19   Penectomy. A, Tourniquet is placed. An impermeable dressing covers the glans and prevent seeding of cancer cells. **B,** A circumferential incision is made to the level of the dartos fascia with urethral catheter in place. **C,** Mattress sutures are placed. **D,** The skin is retracted laterally to provide a tension free closure. **E,** A Y-V plasty is performed around the urethra. **F,** Attachment of the urethra to skin using 4-0 sutures. (*From Greenbert R: Surgical management of carcinoma of the penis, Urologic clinics of North America 37:3, 2010, Saunders.*)

Pathology

A malfunction in the erectile system of the penis most often is caused by neurological disease, diabetes, vascular disease, or a psychological problem. Patients for whom no organic cause can be found are carefully screened for this procedure.

TECHNIQUE

1. A small incision is made at the base of the scrotum.
2. The tunica is incised to expose the corpus layer.
3. An implant inserter is positioned into the corporal tunnel, and the implant is put in place. This is repeated on each side of the penis.
4. A pocket is created in the scrotum for the pump.
5. A tunnel is made through the external ring to accommodate the reservoir.
6. The transversalis fascia is incised, and the reservoir is positioned.
7. The cylinders and pump are connected and tested.
8. The incisions are closed.

Discussion

Many types of inflatable penile implants are available. Each manufacturer provides detailed instructions on the tools and techniques used to place the implant. The technique described here uses an inflatable pump manufactured by American Medical Systems.

This surgery has three parts and the system has three components. The cylinders are placed in the corpora cavernosa of the penis and can be inflated by the patient. The pump is placed surgically in the scrotum, and the reservoir, which contains the cylinder medium, is placed in the inguinal area.

The three-piece prosthesis has a fluid-filled reservoir that is placed into the abdominal wall. The pump release valve is located in the scrotum and the two inflatable cylinders are located inside the penis.

The patient is placed in the supine or lithotomy position, prepped, and draped for a scrotal approach. The scrotum is incised, and the corpora cavernosa are exposed. The prosthesis cylinder is loaded onto a Furlow inserter and placed into the penile shaft. The pump is implanted in the scrotum, and the reservoir is inserted through the inguinal ring. Once the reservoir has been placed and inflated and the tubing has been connected, the device is tested in inflation and deflation. The incision is closed with a subcuticular suture and a supportive dressing is applied. The procedure is shown in Figure 26-20.

VARICOCELECTOMY

Surgical Goal

Varicocelectomy is ligation of the veins of the testes to reduce venous backflow of blood into the internal spermatic veins. It is done to improve spermatogenesis.

Pathology

A varicocele is a vascular abnormality in which the pampiniform venous plexus (veins of the spermatic cord) of the scrotum is dilated. The venous plexus can become twisted and dilated in the same manner as varicosity in the legs. The condition is associated with infertility, resulting in poor semen quality and sperm production. Varicocele may result in atrophy of the testis and is usually treated in adults.

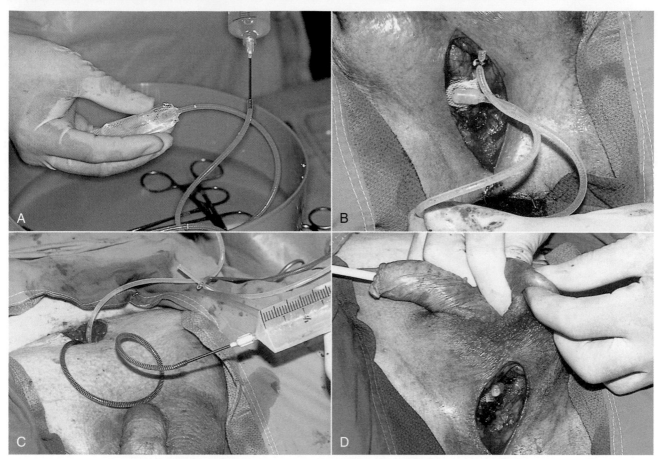

Figure 26-20 Penile implant. A, Preparation of the reservoir. **B,** Placement of the reservoir and cuff in the perineal incision. **C,** The reservoir and pump are filled with Hypaque to the appropriate volume. **D,** The pump is tested. *(Courtesy American Medical Systems, Minnetonka, Minn.)*

TECHNIQUE

1 An incision is made in the inguinal region below the external ring.
2 The fascia is divided, and the spermatic cord is isolated.
3 Varicose veins and tributaries are ligated with clips.
4 The incision is closed.

Discussion

Techniques for varicocelectomy include retroperitoneal, inguinal, and subinguinal varicocele repairs with and without magnification, laparoscopic repair, and percutaneous varicocelectomy with radiographic embolization of the internal spermatic veins.

A 0.8- to 1.2-inch (2- to 3-cm) incision is made inferior to the level of the external ring. The incision is carried to the fascia. The spermatic cord is identified and then bluntly mobilized and grasped with a Babcock clamp. The cord is lifted to the level of the incision, and a Penrose drain is placed around it. At this stage the operating microscope may be introduced.

The spermatic fascia is incised and the testicular artery and veins identified. The veins are ligated with vessel clips or fine nonabsorbable suture.

Once all external spermatic veins have been divided, the cord is returned to the scrotum. The incision is closed with a 5-0 Monocryl subcuticular closure and reinforced with Steri-Strips.

HYDROCELECTOMY

Surgical Goal

A hydrocele is a benign, fluid-filled sac that develops in the anterior testis. It is drained and removed to prevent rupture and hemorrhage.

Pathology

A hydrocele may arise from trauma, infection, or tumor, or as a result of peritoneal dialysis. It also may occur as a congenital condition related to failure of the internal ring to close in fetal life.

TECHNIQUE

1 An incision is made in the scrotum over the hydrocele.
2 The hydrocele sac is brought out of the scrotum.
3 The sac is incised and emptied.
4 The incision is closed.

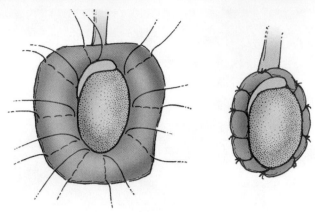

Figure 26-21   Hydrocele. The tunica vaginalis has been folded on itself and sutured in place to prevent recurrence. *(From Rothrock J: Alexander's care of the patient in surgery, ed 17, St Louis, 2007, Mosby.)*

Discussion

The patient is placed in the supine position and prepped for a scrotal incision. The surgeon makes a small incision in the scrotum using the ESU. The hydrocele is delivered from the scrotum without rupturing it, and the ESU is used to make a small incision in the sac membrane. The scrub should have suction immediately available to drain the sac, which is excised and removed. An alternative technique is to open the sac, evert the edges, and suture them to the surface of the testicle (Figure 26-21). The surgeon may insert a small Penrose drain in the wound, which then is closed in two layers with fine absorbable sutures. A bulky gauze dressing is applied.

Swelling and bleeding may occur in the immediate postoperative period.

ORCHIECTOMY

Surgical Goal

Orchiectomy is the surgical removal of one or both testicles.

Pathology

Removal of one testicle most often is performed in cases of testicular carcinoma or **torsion** (twisting of the testis, resulting in ischemia and necrosis). Rotation of the testicle is related to a congenital anomaly or occurs as a result of vigorous activity in young males. Torsion is a medical emergency, because the testicular blood vessels may be occluded, resulting in ischemia and necrosis of the testicle. Bilateral orchiectomy may be performed to control metastatic carcinoma of the prostate.

TECHNIQUE

1 An incision is made in the scrotum.
2 The testicle is mobilized using sharp and blunt dissection.
3 The spermatic vessels and vas deferens are clamped and divided.
4 The vascular structures and vas deferens are ligated.
5 The scrotum is closed.

Discussion

Testicular cancer usually arises from the germ (reproductive) cells of the male. It represents 1% of all cancers, but it is the most common cancer among young men. Early screening and vigorous public health campaigns have lowered the incidence in the past several decades.

Torsion of the testicle is rotation of the testicle around its proximal attachments. This causes interruption or complete cessation of the blood supply to the testicle, resulting in partial or complete necrosis of the organ. The cause of torsion is related to a combination of weak (scrotal) fascial attachment and vigorous exercise. Orchiectomy is performed only when the testicle cannot be saved.

Orchiectomy can be performed using local anesthesia with sedation or with general anesthesia. The patient is placed in the supine position, prepped, and draped for a scrotal incision.

The surgeon makes a 1- to 1.2-inch (2.5- to 3-cm) midline incision into the anterior scrotal wall with a #15 blade. Using sponges and manual dissection, the surgeon separates the testicle from the fascia and subcutaneous tissue. This technique exposes the tunica vaginalis. The surgeon then delivers the testicle from the scrotal sac. Bleeders are controlled with the ESU.

The spermatic cord is identified, and the vas deferens is separated, doubled-clamped, cut, and ligated with 2-0 Vicryl ties. The testicular artery and veins are cross-clamped with Kelly or Mayo clamps. The tissue vessels are divided with the ESU and ligated with size 0 absorbable synthetic suture ligatures.

The spermatic cord is replaced in anatomical position, and the septal layers are closed with a 3-0 Vicryl running suture. The wound is closed with an interrupted or subcuticular suture on a fine cutting needle. Antibiotic ointment may be applied to the incision. Dressing consists of gauze fluffs and a scrotal support. Testicular prosthetics may be inserted at the time of surgery or in a subsequent procedure.

Complications following orchiectomy may include those expected following cessation of testosterone production. These include loss of libido, fatigue, and tenderness of the breasts. Patients are prescribed testosterone postoperatively to prevent these symptoms. However, testosterone therapy may increase the risk of osteoporosis.

Patients undergoing orchiectomy require counseling both preoperatively and postoperatively. Loss of reproductive functions can result in depression, especially for young men.

VASECTOMY

Surgical Goal

Elective sterilization is performed by removing a section of the vas deferens and sealing the free ends. This prevents the movement of sperm through the ejaculatory ducts.

TECHNIQUE

1 The scrotum is incised.
2 The vas deferens is isolated.
3 The duct is cross-clamped, and a section is removed.
4 The ends of the severed duct are coagulated.
5 The incision is closed.

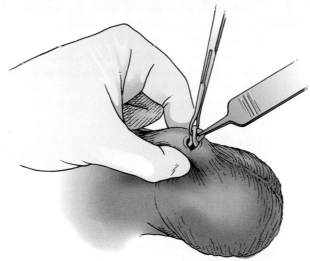

Figure 26-22 **Vasectomy.** The vas deferens is grasped with Babcock forceps through a scrotal incision. *(From Walsh PC, Retik AB, Vaughan ED, et al: Campbell's urology, ed 8, Philadelphia, 2002, WB Saunders.)*

Discussion

The patient is placed in the supine position, prepped, and draped for a scrotal incision. A local anesthetic (e.g., 1% or 2% lidocaine) is injected at the raphe with a 26- to 27-gauge needle.

The surgeon makes a small (0.4-inch [1-cm]) incision in the proximal scrotum over the vas deferens. Blunt and sharp dissection are used to isolate the vas tubule. Small bleeders are coagulated with the needle-point ESU.

The duct is cross-clamped, leaving a short section between the clamps. This surgeon transects and removes this section. The two severed ends of the vas deferens are coagulated with the ESU. The scrotum is closed with fine interrupted absorbable sutures. A bulky gauze dressing is applied.

The procedure for a vasectomy is illustrated in Figure 26-22.

VASOVASECTOMY (REVERSAL OF A VASECTOMY)

Surgical Goal

Vasovasostomy is the surgical anastomosis of the vas deferens to restore continuity after vasectomy.

Pathology

Approximately 35,000 men per year undergo a vasectomy reversal in the United States. Anastomosis of the vas deferens is performed to restore fertility.

TECHNIQUE

1 An incision is made over the vasectomy site.
2 The vas deferens is identified.
3 The operative microscope is brought to the field.
4 The ends of the vas deferens are prepared for anastomosis.
5 The anastomosis is performed.
6 The incision is closed.

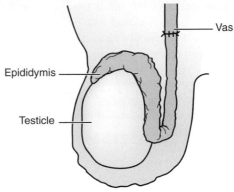

Figure 26-23 **Reversal of a vasectomy.** *(From Phillips N: Berry and Kohn's operating room technique, ed 10, St Louis, 2004, Mosby.)*

Discussion

The patient is placed in the supine position and prepped for a groin incision. A vasovasostomy may be performed using a local block, epidural, spinal, or general anesthetic. The operating microscope is used for the anastomosis once the initial incision has been made.

A vertical scrotal incision is made directly over the site of the vasectomy, and the vas deferens is mobilized above and below the vasectomy site. The vas deferens is incised with a scalpel below and above the vasectomy site to provide clean edges for the anastomosis. A small amount of seminal fluid is expressed. This is preserved as a specimen to determine whether live sperm are present. The surgery continues even if the results are negative. The distal end of the vas is resected until a normal lumen is visible.

The two ends are placed closely together and held in place with an approximator clip. A two-layer anastomosis is used to close the duct. Anchoring sutures of 9-0 nylon suture are first placed through the muscular layer of the cut ends. The inner layer of the duct is identified, and an anastomosis is performed with 10-0 nylon suture. The second layer is anastomosed with 9-0 nonabsorbable interrupted sutures. The wound is closed in two layers with 3-0 and 4-0 absorbable suture.

Patients are monitored for postoperative swelling and possible hemorrhage. Severe injury to the spermatic artery during the procedure may lead to an atrophic testicle, although this is a rare complication. Reversal of a vasectomy is shown in Figure 26-23.

IMPLANTATION OF TESTICULAR PROTHESIS

Surgical Goal

Testicular prostheses are implanted after orchiectomy. A suprapubic approach is used to prevent postoperative infection.

Discussion

A 1.6- to 2-inch (4- to 5-cm) horizontal incision is made over the pubic symphysis. The ESU is used to extend the incision through the fascial layer. The spermatic cord is exposed and retracted with a Penrose drain. The testicular prosthesis is placed into the scrotal sac after hemostasis has been secured.

A purse-string suture of 3-0 silk is used to close the neck of the scrotum. The fascia is closed with 3-0 Vicryl, and the skin is closed with a 4-0 subcuticular suture. Steri-Strips and a gauze dressing are applied to the incision site.

SURGERY OF THE BLADDER AND URETERS

SUPRAPUBIC CYSTOSTOMY

Surgical Goal

Cystostomy is the insertion of a **suprapubic catheter** into the bladder for drainage. The catheter is inserted through a percutaneous or open approach.

Pathology

A suprapubic catheter is implanted to divert urine from the bladder directly to the outside of the body, bypassing the urethra. This done following surgery that requires urinary diversion (urethral or bladder surgery) and to eliminate the need for long-term urethral catheterization, which may lead to a urinary tract infection.

TECHNIQUE

Open Procedure
1 A suprapubic incision is made.
2 The space of Retzius is entered.
3 The catheter is positioned in the bladder.
4 The bladder and wound are closed.

Discussion

The patient is placed in the supine position, prepped, and draped for a suprapubic incision. The incision passes through the skin, fatty subcutaneous layer, fascia, and muscle fibers. The peritoneal cavity is not entered, because the area lying between the bladder and the symphysis pubis (the space of Retzius, which is the operative site) is bounded superiorly (at the top) by the abdominal peritoneum. Because the muscle fibers are quite vascular and contain many large veins, the technologist should have an ample supply of lap sponges available. The surgeon makes the incision with the scalpel and carries it through to the bladder with the ESU or dissecting scissors.

The surgeon places two Allis clamps on the bladder wall and makes a small incision between the clamps. A purse-string suture then is placed around the bladder incision, and the catheter is threaded into the bladder. A Malecot, Pezzer, or proprietary percutaneous catheter is used. The purse-string suture is tied snugly around the catheter, and the bladder incision is closed with size 0 or 2-0 interrupted sutures of chromic gut swaged to a tapered needle. The suprapubic incision then is closed in layers.

Percutaneous Approach

In an alternative method of suprapubic drainage, a Silastic catheter is placed in the bladder through a stab wound in the skin made over and through the bladder wall. A Cystocath catheter is commonly used. To insert the catheter, the surgeon uses a #11 knife blade to make the small stab incision. The Cystocath kit comes complete with a trocar and cannula, which are thrust through the stab incision. The trocar then is removed, and the catheter is inserted through the cannula. The surgeon removes the cannula and places a Silastic disc over the catheter and attaches it to the patient's skin with surgical adhesive. The wound is neither sutured nor dressed.

CYSTECTOMY

Surgical Goal

Cystectomy is the total or partial removal of the bladder. This procedure is performed most often to treat bladder cancer.

Pathology

Bladder cancer is the second most common cancer of the GU system (prostate cancer has the highest incidence). It arises most frequently from the transitional cells. The diagnosis is made by cystoscopy, which includes cytological brushing or bladder washing to collect cells for pathological assessment.

Total cystectomy is indicated for small invasive tumors that penetrate the bladder wall. A more conservative partial cystectomy may be performed when cancer staging reveals no lymph node metastasis. After a cystectomy, a false bladder may be constructed using a portion of the ileum (see Ileal Conduit).

TECHNIQUE

1 A lower midline incision is made and carried to the bladder.
2 The bladder is dissected, and major vessels are controlled.
3 The bladder is elevated to expose the cul-de-sac and peritoneum.
4 The bladder is dissected from the rectal wall.
5 The bladder pedicles are clamped and divided.
6 The broad ligament is incised, and the posterior vaginal wall, bladder neck, and proximal urethra are mobilized.
7 Males: The prostate and prostatic ligaments are mobilized and divided.
8 The urethra is cross-clamped and divided. The specimen is removed en bloc.
9 A urinary diversion procedure is initiated.

Discussion

If the patient is a male, prostatic instruments are required. A major laparotomy set is used for all cases. The scrub should have vessel loops, umbilical tapes, and a narrow, long Penrose drain available for retraction.

The patient is placed in the supine or low lithotomy position and prepped for a lower midline incision. A Foley catheter is inserted.

To begin the surgery, the surgeon makes a lower midline incision. The urachus (the fibromuscular attachment at the umbilicus) is clamped and divided. A self-retaining retractor (typically a Bookwalter retractor) is placed in the wound, and the bowel is packed away from the bladder with moist laparotomy sponges. If a lateral approach to the bladder is used, the duodenum and colon are packed to one side. The ureters are dissected and then transected from the bladder to increase mobilization.

The bladder is elevated, and each side (lateral pedicle) of the bladder is dissected separately. The internal iliac artery is identified, ligated, and divided. Branches also are ligated. Right-angle clamps often are used to pass suture ties under vessels during the dissection. The scrub should have a variety of sizes available. Heavy silk sutures or vascular clips typically are used to occlude the vessels. In the male, the vas deferens is divided with the urethra.

The bladder is retracted upward, and the peritoneum is incised. The anterior rectal wall is dissected free from the bladder. This exposes the seminal vesicles and prostate in the male, or the posterior vaginal wall in the female. The lateral pedicles of the bladder are mobilized, divided, and ligated with silk sutures or surgical clips. In the female, the broad ligament is excised to the level of the ovary and fallopian tubes. The surgeon separates the posterior vaginal wall from the bladder using blunt dissection. The vaginal vault is closed after the excision.

The anterior dissection continues with dissection of the prostate away from the pubis. The ESU is used frequently to control small vessels that communicate with the prostate. The ESU tip must be kept clean. During the later stages of the dissection, the ESU is used often.

The urethra is isolated with a vessel loop or umbilical tape, clamped, and divided. The remaining fascial attachments are released and the specimen is removed. A urinary diversion surgery is initiated. After a cystectomy, an ileal conduit or similar neobladder is created.

ILEAL CONDUIT

Surgical Goal
In an ileal conduit procedure, a functional bladder is constructed with a loop of bowel that is brought out of the abdominal wall. A stoma is created for urine drainage. This procedure has been widely successful for urinary diversion.

Pathology
Urinary diversion away from the bladder is performed before or after a radical cystectomy, in which the bladder and surrounding tissue have been removed as a treatment for cancer.

TECHNIQUE

1 The bowel is mobilized to free a section of ileum.
2 The ileum is transected, and the proximal ileal segment and mesentery are closed.
3 The distal and proximal sections of the ileum are anastomosed.
4 The ureters are implanted into the ileal pouch.
5 A stoma is created in the abdomen.
6 A suction drain is placed in the incision, which is closed in layers.

Discussion
Many of the techniques used in this procedure are discussed as part of the bowel procedure (see Chapter 23). In preparation for the procedure, the scrub should have gastrointestinal and long instruments available.

The patient is placed in the supine position, and a Foley catheter is inserted. The patient then is prepped and draped for an abdominal incision (usually a low midline incision). To begin the procedure, the surgeon enters the abdomen and retroperitoneal cavity. A large self-retaining retractor is placed in the wound. A portion of the large intestine and adjoining ileum is mobilized, as for a bowel resection.

A linear stapling instrument may be used to resect the proximal limb of the ileum. The two severed ileal limbs are then anastomosed. When traditional suturing methods are used, four intestinal clamps are placed across a segment of the ileum, two at each end. The surgeon then divides the ileum in both locations, cutting between the sets of clamps with the ESU. The proximal end of the ileum is closed with a double layer of absorbable suture. The surgeon identifies the ureters and may place a small Penrose drain around them for retraction. The ureters are divided from the bladder, and an end-to-side anastomosis is made between the ureters and the isolated segment of the ileum. The anastomosis is performed with 4-0 interrupted sutures of absorbable material.

Stoma Formation
To perform the ileostomy, the surgeon first incises the skin over the area of the proposed stoma, excising a small disc of tissue from the abdominal wall. Dissection is taken down to the rectus muscle. A Kelly clamp is passed bluntly through the rectus muscle. The open end of the ileal segment is then brought through the hole and everted. The edge of the stoma is sutured to the abdominal wall with 3-0 interrupted absorbable sutures. The wound is then irrigated, and a suction drain is placed in the abdomen. Closure is routine, as described for a laparotomy. The approach used for the ileal conduit is illustrated in Figure 26-24.

URINARY INCONTINENCE

Many procedures to correct urinary incontinence have been developed in recent years. There is public demand for rapid, relatively noninvasive procedures. Special devices and equipment have been quickly developed and marketed to meet the technical requirements of these procedures. Some have shown promise, whereas others have been discarded because of failure or technical difficulty and a steep learning curve for the surgeon.

No longitudinal studies have been performed to analyze the long-term success of these newer procedures, which are all based on the classic Marshall-Marchetti-Krantz and Burch procedures. In all cases, the bladder neck and urethra are suspended from and anchored to the pubic symphysis or pubourethral ligaments with various devices, such as sutures, screws, needles, tape, mesh, or biological material. Laparoscopic and vaginal procedures are preferred over open

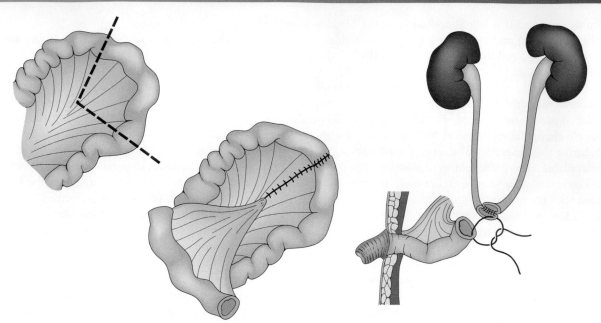

Figure 26-24   **Ileal conduit.** *(From Garden O, Bradbury A, Forsythe J, Parks R: Principles and practice of surgery, ed 5, Edinburgh, 2007, Churchill Livingstone.)*

retropubic techniques. Other procedures, such as implantable electronic devices that control the symptoms of incontinence and a synthetic sphincter, also have been approved in the United States.

The procedures in this section are limited to standard surgeries. The surgical technologist will be able to adapt these to implantation of devices and newer procedures that may or may not have technological longevity.

VESICOURETHRAL SUSPENSION (MARSHALL-MARCHETTI-KRANTZ PROCEDURE)

Surgical Goal

Vesicourethral suspension (Marshall-Marchetti-Krantz procedure) is a suspension of the bladder neck and urethra to the cartilage of the pubic symphysis to treat urinary stress incontinence in the female.

Pathology

Urinary incontinence is involuntary loss of urine. The condition has many causes, including multiple childbirths, prolonged or obstructed labor in childbirth, diabetes, neurological injury, and age. Stress incontinence occurs during exertion of the pelvic muscles, or "bearing down." Functional incontinence can be classified as a bladder or a urethral disorder. In most cases, loss of urethral support at the ureterovesical junction or proximal urethra is seen. Overflow incontinence is caused by an "overactive" detrusor muscle with a normal urethra.

Urinary incontinence is both a hygienic and a psychosocial problem. The number of new cases has increased as the population of aging adults has grown.

TECHNIQUE

1   A lower midline or Pfannenstiel incision is made, and the space of Retzius is entered.
2   The bladder is retracted upward.
3   Several sutures are inserted into the bladder neck and attached to the back side of the symphysis pubis.
4   The wound is closed.

Discussion

The patient is placed in the low lithotomy position and prepped and draped for a combined suprapubic and perineal procedure. A vaginal prep is performed, and a Foley catheter is inserted.

The surgical technologist should have long instruments available, including long needle holders and long Allis clamps.

A suprapubic incision is made and carried through the space of Retzius. A wide Deaver or bladder blade retractor is placed over the bladder to retract it upward, exposing the urethra; this is managed by the assistant.

The surgeon grasps the bladder neck with several long Allis clamps. Several 2-0 interrupted sutures of Dexon or Dacron, mounted on a small, stout, tapered needle, are then placed through the bladder neck and cartilage of the symphysis pubis. Several of these sutures are placed in succession. The sutures are left long.

The assistant lifts the urethra by applying transvaginal pressure on the urethra; this releases tension on the sutures to allow the sutures to be tied. After this maneuver, the scrub must reglove the assistant. This completes the procedure. A large Penrose drain is placed in the space of Retzius, and the wound is closed in routine fashion.

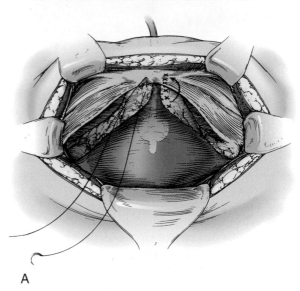

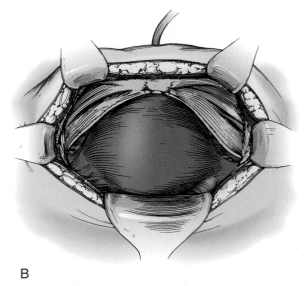

A

B

Figure 26-25 Marshall-Marchetti-Krantz procedure (vesicourethral suspension). **A,** Sutures are secured through the bladder neck. **B,** The vaginal wall is sutured to the symphysis. *(Modified from Walsh PC, Retik AN, Vaughan ED, et al: Campbell's urology, ed 8, Philadelphia, 2002, WB Saunders.)*

The Marshall-Marchetti-Krantz procedure is illustrated in Figure 26-25.

PUBOVAGINAL SLING

Surgical Goal

The bladder neck is held in suspension with a biosynthetic strip or fascia graft that is attached to the abdominal wall.

TECHNIQUE

1 A low transverse incision is made to expose the rectus muscle.
2 The anterior vaginal mucosa is incised, and the incision is carried to the urethra and bladder neck.
3 An anterior vaginal wall flap is created, and dissection is carried to the pubic bone.
4 The graft is measured and positioned.
5 Cystoscopy is performed to assess tension on the graft.
6 The graft is secured.
7 A suprapubic catheter is inserted.
8 The wounds are closed.

Discussion

Material for the sling is taken from the rectus fascia, abdominal fascia, or fascia lata (requiring a separate small incision in the thigh). Biosynthetic materials include polypropylene mesh, Mersilene, Silastic, or Gore-Tex, which are marketed under various proprietary names. Commercially prepared sling systems may include accessory attachments and instruments for securing the sling.

The graft of the fascia lata may be an allograft or an autograft. An autograft is fascia lata that has been removed from the patient's own fascia in one of two ways. In the abdominal approach, the rectus fascia is removed laterally from one iliac crest to the other through a Pfannenstiel incision. The fascia also may be removed in the lateral thigh through two vertical incisions midthigh and above the knee. The graft is dissected out through a tunnel created between the two incision sites.

An allograft may be freeze-dried or fresh-frozen fascia lata obtained from a cadaver. Fresh-frozen fascia lata is the preferred material for repair, because it produces a stronger repair with minimal dissection and a faster recovery time than an autograft or synthetic material. If an allograft is used, the patient may have the procedure performed on an outpatient basis. If an autograft is used, the patient may need to be hospitalized for up to 3 days for postoperative pain management.

In the pubovaginal sling procedure, the graft is attached to the pubic bone. Therefore, in addition to the normal instrumentation required for cystoscopic and bladder suspension procedures, the scrub must have a drill and an anchoring system available.

The patient is anesthetized and placed in the lithotomy position with Allen stirrups. A lower abdominal and vaginal prep is performed. If a fascia lata autograft is to be obtained from the thigh, a separate setup for prepping, draping, and instrumentation is needed for the operative leg. The patient is draped with lithotomy drapes. Cystoscopy is performed, and a Foley catheter is inserted.

The labia majora may be sutured laterally for retraction. An Auvard weighted vaginal speculum is inserted, and a local anesthetic with epinephrine is injected into the lower abdominal incision site and the vaginal mucosa to maintain hemostasis.

A lower transverse incision is made just above the symphysis pubis. The tissue is spread by blunt dissection to expose the anterior rectus muscle. The incision is packed with sponges moistened with an antibiotic solution.

The vaginal portion of the procedure is then performed. The surgeon inserts a Foley catheter into the urethra and measures the length of the urethral meatus by placing the Foley catheter and inflating the balloon at the internal vesicle neck. The catheter is marked, deflated, and removed. The balloon on the catheter is then reinflated, measured, and again deflated. The catheter is reinserted into the patient.

To create space for the sling, the surgeon incises the anterior vaginal mucosa, raises the vaginal mucosal flap, and continues dissection to expose the pubic bone. The surgeon perforates the endopelvic fascia and enters the retropubic space. The power drill is used to create small holes in the pubic bone for anchoring the sutures.

The sutures are then anchored to the pubic bone.

A Stamey needle is passed through one of the vaginal incisions to the pubic bone. The free end of the suturing system is passed parallel to the posterior symphysis pubis. The needle is guided through the fascia and periurethral tissues along the bladder neck. The Foley catheter is again removed, and a cystoscope is used to check the position of the needle. The same process is followed at the other vaginal incision site.

The free end of the suture then is placed through the graft. The Stamey needle is used to pass the graft to the pubic site. The graft is sutured to the pubic bone or paraurethral fascia. The free end of the graft is passed between the urethra and vaginal mucosa. The surgeon places the free end of the graft into the opposite vaginal wound. The excess graft is excised, and the process is repeated for the other side.

The tension of the graft (ability to stop the urinary flow) is tested before the sling is sutured in place. The surgeon performs this step with the cystoscope and by inflating the bladder with fluid. The surgeon may directly visualize the flow of urine, and as the assistant applies tension and pulls the suture upward, the flow of urine should stop. The surgeon then sutures the graft in place. Testing is repeated on the opposite side of the graft before it is secured.

A suprapubic catheter is inserted while the bladder is still full of fluid. The abdominal incision is closed with an absorbable suture. The vaginal mucosa is closed with an absorbable suture, and a packing coated with sulfa cream is inserted into the vagina.

The pubovaginal sling procedure is illustrated in Figure 26-26.

Related Procedures
- Tension-free vaginal tape
- Needle urethropexy
- Inter-Stim implantation
- Artificial urethral sphincter

PROSTATE PROCEDURES

Prostatectomy traditionally has been performed by cystoscopic resection or open surgery using various perineal and suprapubic techniques. Modern prostatectomy is performed laparoscopically, robotically, or through an open approach (perineal or suprapubic) and by cystoscopic resection. Brachytherapy, which involves the implantation of radon seeds, and cryosurgery also are done to treat prostate cancer.

BRACHYTHERAPY

Brachytherapy is the implantation of radioactive seeds into tissue for the treatment of cancer. Brachytherapy of the prostate is generally performed as an outpatient procedure under regional or general anesthetic. The procedure requires a team including a urologist, radiation oncologist, dosimetrist, radiation safety personnel, anesthetist, and scrub personnel. The implantation takes place under transrectal ultrasound and fluoroscopic guidance using iodine-125 or palladium. In order to place the seeds accurately in the most advantageous positions, a coordinating grid attached to the probe receives needles with the preloaded seeds.

The prostate volume is scanned in real time with transrectal ultrasound, and a dosimetrist calculates the exact dose based on special software. Following the procedure, the patient may undergo cystoscopy to further verify position of the seeds. The procedure may be repeated over several days or a week.

PERINEAL PROSTATECTOMY

Surgical Goal

Perineal prostatectomy is the removal of a prostatic adenoma through a perineal approach. In the past, prostatectomy often resulted in impotence and incontinence. Nerve-sparing procedures now are practiced to prevent these complications.

Pathology

Cancer of the prostate is a slow-growing cancer. There are about 230,000 cases and 40,000 deaths per year in the United States. A prostate-specific antigen (PSA) blood test and digital rectal examination are the initial tests. A percutaneous biopsy is performed if the results of these tests are abnormal. Surgical intervention is discussed with the patient, and all treatment options are provided in counseling.

TECHNIQUE

1. The patient is placed in the high lithotomy position.
2. An inverted **U**-incision is made in the perineum and carried through the muscle and fascia.
3. The central tendon is isolated and divided.
4. The rectourethral muscles are divided and retracted.
5. Frozen section biopsies are removed from the prostate.
6. The urethra is clamped and divided.
7. The prostatic capsule is incised, and the prostate is removed.
8. The capsule is closed.
9. A Foley catheter is inserted.
10. The urethra is anastomosed for continuity.
11. The wound is closed in layers.

Discussion

A perineal approach to prostatectomy may include laparoscopic removal of lymph nodes during a combined or a separate procedure. Lymph node analysis is performed for cancer staging.

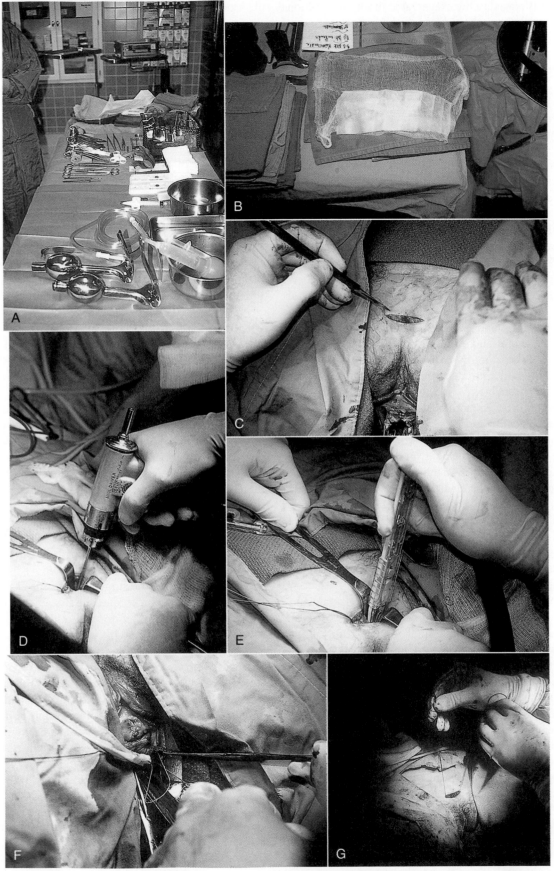

Figure 26-26   Pubovaginal sling. A, Back table setup. **B,** Fresh-frozen fascia lata graft. **C,** Pubic incision. **D,** A power drill is used to create holes for the sutures. **E, F,** The free end of the graft is passed between the urethra and vaginal mucosa and sutured in place. **G,** Wound closure. *(From Nagle GM: Genitourinary surgery: perioperative nursing series, St Louis, 1997, Mosby.)*

The patient is placed in the exaggerated lithotomy position with the legs well above the pelvis and the buttocks brought to the edge of the operating table break. To further lift the sacrum and pelvis, a gel pad is placed under the sacrum. This is an extreme position that puts strain on the lower back, hips, and sacrum. Positioning must be performed by trained personnel with attention to risk factors.

The patient is prepped for a perineal incision extending to the abdomen, midthigh, anus, and lower sacrum. A Foley catheter is placed in the bladder. Draping exposes the perineum. An adherent barrier drape with anal pouch is used for the procedure. The pouch provides an inlet through which the surgeon can digitally support the roof of the rectum during dissection.

To start the procedure, the surgeon passes a Lowsley traction device through the urethra and into the bladder. This pushes the bladder down toward the perineum. A U-shaped incision is made in the perineum with the skin knife. Bleeders are controlled with the ESU. The surgeon then places several Allis clamps on the incision edges for retraction. The incision is extended to muscle and fascia with the ESU.

The central tendon and rectourethral muscle are isolated and divided. The levator muscle is retracted to expose the prostatic capsule and prostate gland. The surgeon may use digital support through the anus to assist dissection. Small sponge dissectors, Metzenbaum scissors, and the ESU are used to extend the dissection and isolate the prostate.

Important points or planes of dissection are those between the prostate and urethra, bladder neck, anterior bladder, seminal vesicles, and rectum. Right-angle clamps are needed to isolate the neurovascular pedicles and to divide and ligate with suture, LigaSure, or ligation clips. Dissection of the vascular system is carefully extended on both sides of the prostate. In nerve-sparing procedures, no electrosurgical coagulation is used to separate the prostate from the surrounding tissue, which contains the nerves and blood vessels that innervate the penis for erectile function.

The urethra is isolated from the base of the prostate and bladder neck. It is then double-clamped and divided, preserving the bladder neck. This leaves a small urethral stump at the bladder neck. The wound is irrigated, and bleeders are controlled with the ESU and fine suture ligatures.

With dissection completed, the prostate can be enucleated from the capsule. The urethral stumps are then anastomosed to bypass the prostate. Before the anastomosis is completed, a Foley catheter is inserted. The anastomosis is done with fine nylon or some other synthetic monofilament suture. The closure is tested by instilling saline into the bladder.

When bleeding has been controlled, the wound is irrigated with warm saline. Drains are placed in the wound and brought out through the incision or a separate stab incision. Closure is completed in layers with 2-0 and 3-0 absorbable synthetic sutures. The skin is closed with 3-0 or 4-0 subcuticular or interrupted sutures. The wound is dressed with gauze fluff squares and an absorbent pad to absorb drainage.

NOTE: *Lymph node dissection is performed before or after the perineal portion of the surgery.*

A perineal prostatectomy is shown in Figure 26-27.

An indwelling Foley catheter is left in place for 1 to 2 weeks after the procedure. This allows the urethral anastomosis to heal. Recovery from an open procedure takes considerably longer than from laparoscopic or robotic-assisted surgery.

Complications include postoperative bleeding, retrograde ejaculation, failure to ejaculate, and urinary retention.

SUPRAPUBIC PROSTATECTOMY

Surgical Goal
In a suprapubic prostatectomy, the prostate is removed through a suprapubic incision.

Pathology
Prostatectomy is performed to treat benign prostatic hypertrophy and for cancer of the prostate. If the patient has been diagnosed with cancer, the lymph nodes are removed to stage the disease.

Discussion
The patient is placed in the supine position. Padded shoulder braces may be required for the Trendelenburg position. However, these are used only if absolutely necessary because of the increased risk to the brachial plexus, discussed in Chapter 19. A Foley catheter is inserted before the prep. The patient is prepped and draped for a suprapubic incision.

The surgeon makes a transverse or longitudinal suprapubic incision into the space of Retzius. A self-retaining retractor is placed in the wound. Two traction sutures or Allis clamps are placed in the bladder wall, and an incision is made between them. The bladder edges are then grasped with Allis clamps and retracted upward. The scrub should have suction available to drain the bladder. A Judd or Deaver retractor is placed in the bladder, and the prostatic mucosa is incised with the ESU. The bladder retractors are then removed.

Using the fingers, the surgeon performs an *enucleation* of the prostate. In this technique, the tissue is removed en bloc without trauma to the fossa or bed of the tissue. The bladder retractors are replaced, and the wound is checked for bleeding. The fossa may be packed with sponges to secure hemostasis. Large bleeding vessels are ligated with size 0 or 2-0 absorbable suture ligatures. Capillary bleeding is controlled with hemostatic agents (e.g., Surgicel, Avitene, or Gelfoam). A Malecot or Pezzer catheter is placed in the wound and brought out through a small stab incision near the wound edge. The bladder is then closed in two layers with absorbable sutures. The wound is irrigated, and a wound drain is placed in the cavity. The incision then is closed in layers.

Related Procedures
RETROPUBIC PROSTATECTOMY In a retropubic prostatectomy (Figure 26-28), the surgery is approached from a lower midline incision. The prostate is dissected from the anatomical attachments discussed previously and enucleated. The prostatic capsule is closed with sutures, and the urethra is anastomosed to the bladder neck. In this approach, the margins of the prostate are sent for frozen section, and lymph node removal

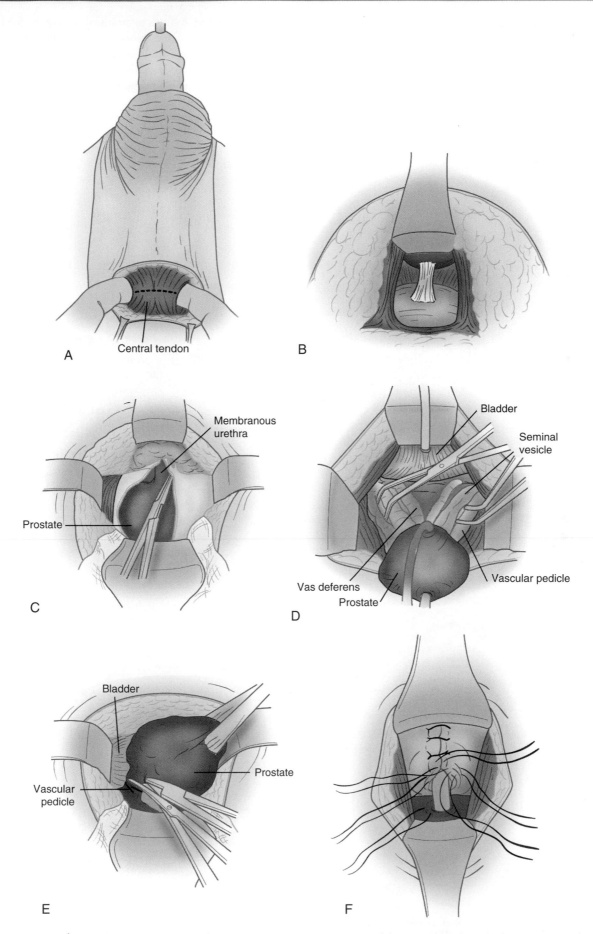

A, Central tendon

B

C, Membranous urethra — Prostate

D, Bladder — Seminal vesicle — Vas deferens — Prostate — Vascular pedicle

E, Bladder — Vascular pedicle — Prostate

F

Figure 26-27   Perineal prostatectomy. **A,** Incision through the perineum. **B,** Exposure of the central tendon. **C,** The preprostatic fascia (gray) has been incised to expose the prostatic capsule. **D,** Mobilization of the vascular pedicle. **E,** The vascular bundle is severed. **F,** Closure of the bladder neck. *(From Rothrock J: Alexander's care of the patient in surgery, ed 17, St Louis, 2007, Mosby.)*

is performed at the time of prostate surgery. The results of the frozen section determine the need for wider pelvic excision.

LAPAROSCOPIC PROSTATECTOMY Laparoscopic prostatectomy is performed with the patient in the low lithotomy position. Three or four trocar ports are used, including an umbilical site for the camera port. After a pneumoperitoneum has been established, the camera port is placed and the remaining trocars are inserted under direct vision.

The procedure follows anatomical dissection for the open prostate technique. The prostate is systematically dissected from the bladder, seminal vesicles, urethra, rectum, and vascular bundles. The ESU or LigaSure system is used to coagulate and to cut away the margins of the prostate, which contain the neurovascular supply necessary for erectile function. Endoscopic clips are used to ligate the two vascular bundles on either side of the prostate.

Once the dissection planes have been established and the prostate can be enucleated from the capsule, the urethra is

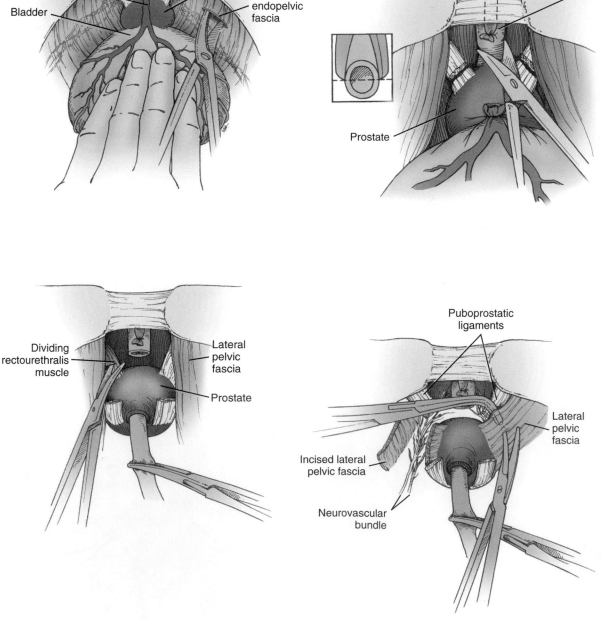

Figure 26-28 **Radical retropubic prostatectomy.** *(From Droller MJ: Surgical management of urologic disease, St Louis, 1992, Mosby.)*

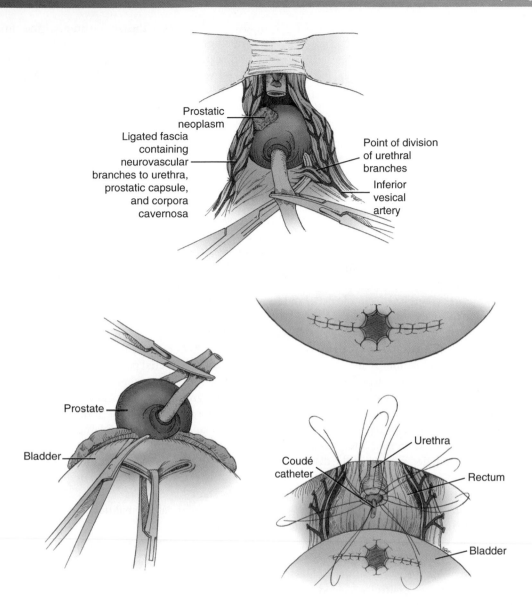

Figure 26-28, cont'd

divided as in an open procedure. The prostate is removed through an endoscopic collection sac.

Continuity of the urethra is reestablished after insertion of a Foley catheter. Anastomosis of the urethra to the bladder is performed in two layers using continuous fine monofilament sutures. The Foley catheter remains in place.

Bleeding is controlled, and the wound is irrigated with warm saline. The ports are withdrawn, and the incisions are closed with one or two layers of absorbable synthetic suture and Steri-Strips.

Following laparoscopic or robotic-assisted surgery, the patient can be discharged from the hospital within 1 or 2 days. The urethral catheter remains in place to allow the urethral anastomosis to heal. Patients experience some level of incontinence in the recovery period. Nerve-sparing procedures provide a greater level of continence and erectile function.

ROBOTIC-ASSISTED PROSTATECTOMY

Robotic-assisted laparoscopic prostatectomy follows the surgical techniques used in the routine laparoscopic procedure, with some technical differences. The robotic arms are used to guide the instruments, and the monitor view is three-dimensional and magnified by 10.

Discussion

The preparation of the patient is the same as for laparoscopy. The patient is placed in the lithotomy position, and the robotic arms enter from the side. The surgical technologist and the surgeon's assistant operate at the bedside. A Foley catheter is inserted and manipulated during the surgery to elevate and identify the urethra intraoperatively.

The surgeon initially scrubs in with the sterile team in order to site and place the cannulas that receive the camera and

TECHNIQUE

1 The patient is prepped and draped for an abdominal laparoscopic procedure in the lithotomy position.
2 A pneumoperitoneum is established using a Veress needle.
3 An optical trocar is inserted through a small periumbilical incision, and the robotic camera is placed.
4 The remaining trocars are sited and placed.
5 The robot is docked and arms locked into the cannulas.
6 The prostate is dissected from the surrounding structures.
7 The major prostatic vessels are identified and ligated.
8 Dissection is completed.
9 The urethra is reattached to the bladder neck.

robotic instruments. She or he then shifts to the robotic console to perform the surgery.

At the start of surgery, the surgical technologist should have instruments available for insertion of cannulas. The anatomical and surgical steps of the procedure are the same as those described for laparoscopy. After placement of the optical trocar, the remaining trocars and cannulas are inserted. The surgeon may use a ruler to measure the distance between the camera and other cannula sites. Once the trocars are in place, the surgical technologist removes instruments used in the trocar placement from the Mayo and replaces these with robotic instruments. A 0-degree camera is most commonly used during the procedure. A major portion of the dissection is performed using a bipolar fenestrated grasper, ESU hook probe, and dissection scissors. A Hem-o-Lok applier and clips should be available for bleeders. One of the advantages of the robotic procedure is the reduction of intraoperative bleeding owing to the pneumoperitoneum, which acts as a tamponade on the large veins that normally bleed profusely during open prostatectomy. Also, robotic surgery allows a much finer dissection and greater control of blood vessels because the robotic instruments are able to enter into much smaller spaces than is possible with open or even MIS surgery alone.

As the dissection continues, the Foley catheter is manipulated by the surgeon's assistant or the surgical technologist as directed by the surgeon to verify the course of the urethra through the prostate. The prostate is dissected from the bladder, urethra, rectum, seminal vesicles, and vascular bundles. The dorsal vein is ligated using size 0 Vicryl or Monocryl. Once the urethra has been dissected from the prostate tissue, it is anastomosed to the bladder neck using 2-0 Monocryl on a double-arm suture. The bladder is irrigated at this point with a catheter tip syringe to check for any gaps in the anastomosis. Gelfoam and Surgicel topical hemostats may be used for hemostasis at the anastomosis.

The prostate is removed through one of the trocars using a specimen retrieval bag (see Specimen Retrieval in Chapter 24). Before removing the trocars, a small drain may be inserted and attached to the skin during closure. A final count is performed and the robotic instruments withdrawn.

The incisions are closed using size 1 PDS or 0 Vicryl for the fascia and 4-0 Monocryl for the skin. Dermabond is also applied over the skin sutures, and finally Band-Aid dressings.

The patient retains a Foley catheter in the immediate postoperative period up to 1 week or more. Most patients are able to be discharged after robotic prostatectomy after 1 to 3 days. The patient will return for follow-up testing and further treatment as required.

SURGERY OF THE URETER AND KIDNEY

URETERAL DIVERSION

Surgical Goal

Injury, disease, or a congenital anomaly of the ureter may result in a distended, obstructed, or nonfunctional ureter. Ureteral diversion surgery is performed to restore continuity between the kidney and the bladder.

Pathology

Diseases that constrict the ureter result in reflux or a buildup of filtrate in the renal pelvis. This is referred to as *hydronephrosis*. Over time, the ureter or its proximal junction at the kidney becomes grossly distended and damaged. The term *vesicourethral reflux* refers to conditions of backward flow from the bladder and the ureter. Examples of common obstructive pathological conditions include the following:

- Calculi that can constrict the ureters and cause injury
- Ureteral scarring related to ureteral scarring
- Prostatic hyperplasia
- Congenital abnormalities that result in stricture or malfunction
- Retroperitoneal or abdominal tumor that impinges on the ureters
- Disease or a congenital defect that arises at the ureterovesical junction in the bladder

Discussion

Ureteral diversion surgeries vary according to the severity of disease in the ureter. The goal of surgery is to reimplant the ureter in a new location and provide continuity of urine flow.

The site of implantation determines the technique and approach to surgery. Ureteral procedures, both open and laparoscopic techniques, use an approach from the flank or abdomen. Patient positioning, instruments, and equipment correspond to these approaches. General surgical instruments, including delicate dissection scissors, clamps, and forceps, are required. Vascular forceps often are used to prevent injury to the ureter.

The ureter itself is extremely small, and in all cases a ureteral stent is required at some point in the surgical and postoperative period. The ureter is anastomosed with 4-0 to 7-0 absorbable sutures. Traction sutures and Silastic vessel loops are used in all cases. A Penrose drain often is used for ureteral retraction. The muscles and fascia surrounding the ureters are dissected with standard instruments and small sponge dissectors.

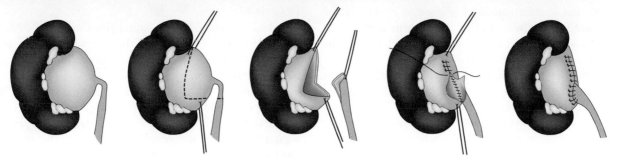

Figure 26-29 **Pyeloplasty.** *(From Garden O, Bradbury A, Forsythe J, Parks R: Principles and practice of surgery, ed 5, Edinburgh, 2007, Churchill Livingstone.)*

The following are some of the terms used to describe ureteral surgery:

- *Pyeloplasty* (Figure 26-29): *Pyelo* (renal pelvis) and *plasty* (reconstruction). Pyeloplasty is the reconstruction of the ureter at the level of the renal pelvis.
- *Uretero:* Indicates a procedure of the ureter. (Do not confuse *uretero* with *urethro*, which pertains to the urethra.)
- *Ureteroplasty:* Reconstruction of the ureter.
- *Ureterostomy:* Anastomosis of the ureter with another hollow structure to provide continuity.
- *Transureteroureterostomy: Trans* (across or joining), *uretero* (pertaining to the ureter), *ostomy* (joining two hollow or tubular structures). Transureteroureterostomy is the crossing of one ureter to another to create an anastomosis between the two ureters. This technique may also be called a *ureteroureterostomy*.
- *Vesicoureterostomy: Vesico* (bladder), ureterostomy (anastomosis of the ureter). Vesicoureterostomy is the reimplantation of the ureter in the bladder.

PERCUTANEOUS NEPHROLITHOTOMY

Surgical Goal

In percutaneous nephrolithotomy, large stones in the kidney or upper ureter are removed percutaneously through the nephroscope.

Pathology

Percutaneous nephrostomy, which involves the insertion of a tube into the renal pelvis for drainage, is indicated for selected patients with calculi lodged in the renal pelvis or upper ureter. It is performed under the following circumstances:

- The stone (or stones) are extremely large (larger than 2.5 cm), such as a **staghorn stone**.
- Conservative treatment, such as oral medication to dissolve the stones, has failed.
- The patient exceeds the weight limit (300 pounds [135 kg]) for extracorporeal shock wave therapy.
- The stone cannot be reached through the endoscopic ureteroscope.
- The stone is infected (the percutaneous method allows evacuation of infectious material at the time of the procedure).

TECHNIQUE

1 The patient is placed in the prone position, and the flank and back are prepped and draped.
2 A hollow needle is inserted near the renal pelvis under ultrasound or fluoroscopy.
3 The first needle is replaced by a second needle with a stylet, which is inserted into the renal pelvis.
4 A guidewire is passed into the renal pelvis.
5 A catheter is placed over the guidewire and inflated to expand the space.
6 Contrast medium is infused into the renal pelvis.
7 The nephroscope is inserted into the tunnel.
8 Stones are fragmented and removed through the nephroscope.
9 A ureteral catheter is positioned in the renal pelvis.
10 The scope is withdrawn.

Discussion

The procedure is performed under fluoroscopic guidance. Staff members must don lead aprons before the procedure. Intraoperative CT or ultrasound scanning also may be used.

A local anesthetic with monitored intravenous anesthesia is used. The patient is placed in the prone position, prepped, and draped for a midback procedure.

A rigid or flexible nephroscope may be used. The standard rigid scopes are available in sizes 19.5 to 26 Fr. Accessories include a working channel that accepts stone crushing and grasping instruments, a holmium:YAG laser fiber, and an ultrasonic lithotripter. A flexible nephroscope has a deflectable tip that is used to reach inside the calyx from its position in the renal pelvis. Warm isotonic irrigation fluid (0.9% saline) is used to flush the operative site during nephroscopy. Precautions for preventing extravasation are same as those used in cystoscopic procedures. The surgical technologist and circulator must keep track of the amount of irrigation fluid used and the outflow to determine the amount absorbed.

To start the procedure, the surgeon uses a small-bore needle to puncture the skin near (but not into) the renal pelvis. The puncture site is located, under fluoroscopic or ultrasound guidance, between the 12th rib and the ilium. The small needle then is replaced with a larger needle with a stylet. The stylet is removed, and contrast medium is injected into the renal pelvis to identify the diseased calyx. The C-arm is rotated to provide optimal views. A guidewire is then passed through the needle sheath and positioned in the renal pelvis.

To pass the nephroscope, the surgeon must make a tract through the tissue. This is done by inserting balloon dilators over the guidewire, which is continually observed on the fluoroscope. When the tract is large enough to admit the nephroscope, the dilator is removed, and the scope is inserted into the tract.

Stone-crushing forceps, stone baskets, and crushers are used to fragment the stone, which is flushed from the tract through the endoscope's working channels. Rigid and flexible endoscopes may be used during the same procedure. The surgical technologist should have accessories and equipment available for both sets. Large stones are fragmented and flushed through the working channel of the nephroscope. These must be retained as specimens. Staghorn stones are particularly sharp, and the fragments may require extraction with a grasping forceps.

When all stone fragments have been removed and the operative site has been irrigated, a nephrostomy tube is inserted into the tract. Foley or Malecot catheters are commonly used for this purpose. A Foley catheter provides continuous tamponade (pressure) within the operative site to control postoperative bleeding. A staged lithotomy may be required for several days after the surgery. In this case, a Malecot catheter is used. Occasionally a ureteral stent is implanted at the close of surgery.

Patients are monitored closely for postoperative bleeding and loss of kidney function. A chest radiograph may be taken in the postanesthesia care unit to make sure the lung was not punctured during insertion of the guidewire. Complications include recurrent stones, urinary fistula, and ureteral obstruction.

SIMPLE NEPHRECTOMY (FLANK INCISION)

Surgical Goal

Simple nephrectomy is the surgical removal of one kidney.

Pathology

A nephrectomy is performed most often for severe hydronephrosis, obstruction, localized tumor, stones with infection, and trauma to the kidney. A kidney also may be removed from a live donor for transplantation.

TECHNIQUE

1 A flank incision is made and carried through the oblique and transverse muscles.
2 A rib resection may be performed.
3 The ureter is cross-clamped, divided, and ligated.
4 The kidney pedicle is divided.
5 The kidney is removed.
6 The wound is closed.

Discussion

The patient is placed in the lateral position with the flank over the table break or kidney lift. The individual is then prepped for a subcostal flank incision. A Foley catheter is inserted before the start of surgery.

The surgeon makes the flank incision along the 12th rib, extending to the border of the rectus muscle. If a rib must be resected, the 11th or 12th rib is first stripped of periosteum with a Doyen elevator or with osteotomes. This is necessary to allow the rib cutter to cut through the bone effectively. The surgeon grasps the rib with an Ochsner or Kocher clamp and then uses a Bethune shears or rib cutter to cut the rib. The scrub should have bone putty available to be placed over the cut portions, which also may require some trimming to remove sharp edges.

The incision is carried through the subcutaneous and oblique muscles with the ESU. A self-retaining retractor is placed in the wound after the surgeon protects the edges of the wound with laparotomy sponges.

The Gerota capsule (perirenal fascia) is identified, and perirenal fat is removed. The scrub must preserve all perirenal fat in a small basin because it may be used to help control bleeding later in the surgery.

The ureter is identified, double-clamped with Mayo clamps, divided, and ligated with size 0 or 2-0 absorbable sutures. The surgeon mobilizes the kidney pedicle, including the renal vessels, by sharp and blunt dissection. To ensure that the renal artery is occluded securely, the surgeon triple-clamps the vessels, and suture ligatures are placed through each vessel. An endovascular stapler can be used to ligate the vessels. This pedicle is then divided. The ligatures are not cut but are left long and tagged with a small hemostat.

The surgeon then removes the kidney from the wound. All bleeding is controlled with the ESU. The pedicle ligatures are cut, and the wound is irrigated with warm saline.

Before closure, the operating table is returned to a flat position to release tension on the flank tissues.

A Penrose drain is placed in the kidney fossa and brought out through a separate stab wound. If a rib was removed, the periosteum may be closed separately. The incision is then closed in layers. The fascia and muscle layers are closed with interrupted absorbable sutures. The skin is closed with staples.

LAPAROSCOPIC RADICAL NEPHRECTOMY

Surgical Goal

In a laparoscopic radical nephrectomy, the kidney and lymph nodes are removed to treat cancer.

Pathology

A primary tumor of the kidney arises from the renal cortex (the most common site) or the renal pelvis. The incidence is higher in men than in women. Risk factors include smoking, obesity, and exposure to industrial chemicals (e.g., petroleum products) and heavy metals.

TECHNIQUE

1 Pneumoperitoneum is established, and trocar ports are placed.
2 The kidney and ureter are mobilized from the bowel, mesentery, muscle, and fascia attachments.
3 The renal artery and vein are isolated and divided.
4 The adrenal vessels are isolated, divided, and ligated with surgical clips.
5 The ureter is divided and ligated with surgical clips.
6 A specimen sac is introduced through a 12-mm cannula, and the kidney is placed inside.
7 The cannula is withdrawn, and the opening is exposed. (The kidney may be withdrawn through an extended incision in the abdomen.)
8 A morcellator is introduced inside the specimen sac, and the kidney is fragmented.
9 The specimen is removed with suction, and the sac is withdrawn.
10 The pneumoperitoneum is released, and the wounds are closed.

Discussion

General laparoscopic instruments, a vessel-sealing system, an ultrasonic scalpel, and vessel clips are needed for the procedure. The surgical technologist must also be ready to convert to an open procedure. A separate setup with laparotomy, kidney, and vascular instruments should be immediately available for conversion to an open case.

The patient is placed in the modified lateral position with the flank positioned over the table break. A soft, padded lift may be used to expand the flank, or the table may be flexed to achieve the same effect. Wide tape is placed over the ilium and secured to the table frame to maintain the patient in the lateral position. A combined flank and abdominal prep is performed, and a Foley catheter is inserted.

The initial trocar ports are inserted with the table rolled for access to the abdomen. After pneumoperitoneum has been established, the table is rolled back and the remaining ports are placed. A 10- or 12-mm port and one or two 5-mm ports are used.

With pneumoperitoneum established, the 10-mm trocar is inserted near the umbilicus. The table then is tilted, and the remaining ports are inserted. Sutures may be used to secure the ports.

After examining the peritoneal cavity, the surgeon begins the dissection by using scissors, a Harmonic scalpel, and an ESU hook to separate the colorenal ligaments and mesentery from the kidney. This frees the bowel and provides access to the kidney and ureter.

The ureter is identified, and dissection continues along the lower pole of the kidney. The dissection may be completed using only the Harmonic scalpel, probe, and ESU hook, although dissecting scissors and forceps also may be used. The renal vein and artery are ligated with surgical staples before they are divided from the hilum. The adrenal vessels are ligated, and smaller vessels are coagulated with the vessel-sealing system or clips.

To divide the ureter, the surgeon places two sets of surgical clips across the structure and incises the section between the clips. The kidney is moved to the abdomen by gentle manipulation.

The specimen can be removed by morcellation, or it can be brought out of the abdomen intact. Intact removal is performed through the 12-mm port using a specimen removal sac. The patient is rolled to expose the abdomen. The sac is inserted through the port and opened in the abdominal cavity. The specimen is pulled into the sac, which is pulled into the trocar. The trocar is withdrawn with the neck of the sac exposed. The incision is extended to accommodate the sac and specimen.

If the morcellation technique is used, the neck of the sac is brought out through the 12-mm trocar incision. The morcellator is inserted into the sac, and the specimen is fragmented. The fragments are removed from the sac with a suction tube, and the sac is withdrawn. The incision is closed.

The wound is then irrigated and checked for hemorrhage. All trocars are removed, and the incisions are closed with 2-0 and 3-0 absorbable sutures. The skin is approximated with interrupted monofilament sutures or skin staples.

KIDNEY TRANSPLANTATION

Surgical Goal
Kidney transplantation involves removing a kidney from a living or deceased donor and implanting it into the patient.

Pathology
Kidney transplantation is performed for acute or chronic end-stage renal disease.

Discussion
Kidney transplantation is performed by a transplant team, and the routines are well established. In this procedure, surgeons operate on the living donor and recipient simultaneously. However, the kidney can be perfused to preserve the tissues. This discussion is limited to essential points in the procedure.

Before the transplantation process begins, the patient's name, date of birth, side of the kidney, and ABO blood compatibility should be confirmed with the team and transplant coordinator.

The operating rooms should connect to minimize contamination if the kidney is removed from a living donor.

The donor kidney is removed as described in the section Simple Nephrectomy (Flank Incision), with several major differences. The renal pedicle, which contains the vascular supply, is isolated and ligated before the kidney is removed. The Gerota fascia may be left intact on the donor kidney.

After removal, the donor kidney is preserved in a cold solution and perfused with the surgeon's choice of electrolyte solution. When the recipient team is ready to receive the kidney, the surgeon transports it in a covered container, maintaining the correct temperature. The donor wound is closed as previously described.

The recipient patient is prepped and draped for a right iliac incision. An incision is made in the right lower quadrant and carried to the retroperitoneum. A self-retaining retractor is placed in the wound. The surgeon dissects through the rectus muscle and preserves the epigastric vessels for anastomosis later in the procedure. In a male, the spermatic cord is identified and retracted; in a female, the round ligament is identified and ligated. Vascular forceps and fine dissecting scissors are used to mobilize the hypogastric artery to the level of the bifurcation of the aorta.

The donor kidney then is brought to the field, and the vessels are trimmed as needed to accommodate the recipient structures. The kidney is returned to the cold solution until the surgeon is ready for implantation.

The internal iliac artery is divided after it has been cross-clamped with a curved or an angled vascular clamp. The proximal side of the artery remains clamped. All the remaining venous tributaries must be ligated with 2-0 or 3-0 silk with the double-clamp and tie method. To prepare the iliac vein for the end-to-side renal anastomosis, the surgeon places Fogarty clamps proximal and distal. The iliac vein is flushed with heparinized saline, and six vascular sutures are put in place to secure the anastomosis later.

The kidney is secured in a slush "sling," and the anastomosis of the iliac vein and renal artery is sutured with 5-0 or 6-0 vascular sutures. The renal artery then is anastomosed to the proximal arm of the iliac artery. The iliac artery clamps are removed, and the anastomosis is observed.

To begin ureteral implantation, the surgeon incises the anterior bladder. The donor ureter is then placed through the bladder wall, and the edges are anastomosed to the inner bladder lining with fine absorbable sutures. A catheter stent is placed into the ureter through the anastomosis. It is advanced into the renal pelvis superiorly and brought out through the urethra. The surgeon then closes the bladder incision in two layers, using 4-0 or 5-0 absorbable sutures for the bladder lining and 2-0 sutures for the muscle layer. The bladder is irrigated to check for leakage.

The fascia is closed with size 0 running absorbable suture. The subcutaneous tissue is closed with a 2-0 or 3-0 interrupted stitch, and the skin is closed with fine nylon. One or two suction drains may be placed in the wound during closure. The wound is dressed with gauze fluffs and tape.

Patients are monitored closely for acute organ rejection, hemorrhage, and infection in the immediate postoperative period. Immunosuppression therapy leaves patients who have undergone transplantation at increased risk of infection and cancer.

ADRENALECTOMY

Adrenalectomy is the removal of one or both adrenal glands. Adrenalectomy usually is performed by conventional (open) surgery, or a minimally invasive approach may be used in selected patients.

Adrenalectomy is indicated for pheochromocytoma, Cushing syndrome, adrenocortical carcinoma, renal carcinoma, and hyperaldosteronism. Hypersecretion of adrenocorticotropic hormone (ACTH) may cause neuroblastoma and affect the growth of other tumors that depend on adrenal secretions. Adrenal diseases are often life-threatening, and the procedure has many potential postoperative metabolic complications.

A number of techniques may be used for adrenalectomy, including open surgery through an abdominal or thoracoabdominal, back (posterior), retroperitoneal incision or laparoscopic surgery. However, the choice of approach depends on many factors, such as the size and location of the tumor, associated structures, the length of the procedure, and the patient's condition.

KEY CONCEPTS

- Knowledge of key anatomical structures of the genitourinary system contributes to the surgical technologist's ability to anticipate the need for instruments, sutures, and other equipment during a surgical procedure.
- Familiarity with diagnostic procedures of the genitourinary system contributes to an understanding of the pathology and may also involve a surgical procedure.
- Many procedures of the genitourinary system are performed using endoscopic techniques that require specific instruments and cystoscopic techniques. The surgical technologist must be familiar with these techniques in order to anticipate the need for instruments and also to assist the urologist during cystoscopic procedures.
- Common pathology of the genitourinary system is important to patient care and understanding of the surgical objectives.
- Familiarity with common surgical procedures of the genitourinary system is necessary for case planning and to perform in the scrub role during surgery.

REVIEW QUESTIONS

1. Explain the purpose of continuous irrigation during transurethral surgery.
2. Explain how a urethral catheter is used as a tamponade.
3. What is a French (Fr) size? What is the most common catheter size for an adult?
4. Explain why testicular torsion is an emergency.
5. The lateral position is used for many procedures of the genitourinary tract. List at least five critical safety considerations for this position. Include specific anatomical locations and risk factors.
6. What surgical approaches are used to enter the retroperitoneal cavity?
7. What specific psychological considerations are important for the male patient undergoing surgery of the external genitalia?
8. Many patients undergoing transurethral surgery are older. List four methods you would use to communicate with these patients.

9. Testicular cancer is the most common cancer among young men. How would you approach a 26-year-old patient undergoing surgery for testicular cancer? Be specific. Define the patient's emotional needs at the time of surgery as part of your response.

BIBLIOGRAPHY

Arthur D: *Smith's textbook of endourology*, ed 2, London, 2007, BC Decker.

Graham SD: *Glenn's urologic surgery*, ed 6, Philadelphia, 2004, Lippincott Williams & Wilkins.

Greenberg R, Surgical management of carcinoma of the penis, *Urologic Clinics of North America* 37:3, 2010.

Pietrow P, Karellas M: Medical management of common urinary calculi, *American Family Physician* 74:86, 2006.

Tanagho EA: *Smith's general urology*, ed 17, New York, 2008, McGraw Hill.

Walters MD: *Urogynecology and reconstructive pelvic surgery*, ed 3, Philadelphia, 2007, Mosby.

27

Ophthalmic Surgery

CHAPTER OUTLINE

Introduction
Surgical Anatomy
Refraction

Diagnostic Testing
Case Planning

Surgical Techniques in Eye
Surgery

Role of the Scrubbed Surgical
Technologist
Surgical Procedures

LEARNING OBJECTIVES

After studying this chapter the reader will be able to:
1. Identify key anatomical structures of the eye
2. Discuss common diagnostic procedures of the eye
3. Describe ocular diseases and disorders

4. Discuss specific elements of case planning for eye surgery
5. Discuss surgical techniques used in eye surgery, including use of the operating microscope
6. List and describe common surgical procedures of the eye

TERMINOLOGY

Accommodation: A process in which the lens continually changes shape to maintain the focus of an image on the retina.

Bridle suture: In ophthalmic surgery, a temporary traction suture placed through the sclera used to pull the globe laterally for exposure of the posterolateral surface. It is called a *bridle suture* because of its resemblance to the reins of a horse's bridle.

Cataract: Clouding of vision caused by a disease in which the crystalline lens of the eye, its capsule, or both become opaque. This prevents light from focusing on the retina, resulting in visual distortion. Cataracts may develop as a result of disease or injury.

Cryotherapy: A technique in which a cold probe is used to freeze tissue, such as the sclera, ciliary body (for glaucoma), or retinal layers, after detachment.

Diathermy: Low-power cautery used to mark the sclera over an area of retinal detachment.

Enucleation: Surgical removal of the globe and accessory attachments.

Evisceration: Surgical removal of the contents of the eyeball, with the sclera left intact.

Exenteration: Removal of the entire contents of the orbit.

Focal point: The point where light rays converge after passing through a lens.

Glaucoma: A group of diseases characterized by elevation of the intraocular pressure. Sustained pressure on the optic nerve and other structures may result in ischemia and blindness.

Keratoplasty: Surgery of the cornea. The term *penetrating keratoplasty* refers to corneal transplantation.

Muscle recession: Surgery in which the eye muscle is repositioned to release the globe.

Muscle resection: Surgical shortening of an eye muscle to pull the globe into correct position.

Phacoemulsification: A process whereby high-frequency sound waves are used to emulsify tissue, such as a cataract.

Pterygium: A triangular membrane that arises from the medial canthus; the tissue may extend over the cornea, causing blindness.

Refraction: A phenomenon of physics in which light rays are bent as they pass through a transparent medium that is denser than air. In the eye, refraction occurs as light enters the front of the eye and passes through the cornea, lens, aqueous humor, and vitreous.

Spatula needle: A flat-tipped suture needle commonly used in ophthalmic surgery.

Strabismus: Inability to coordinate the extraocular muscles, which prevents binocular vision.

INTRODUCTION

The goal of ophthalmic surgery is to restore vision lost as a result of disease, injury, or congenital defect. Procedures include those performed on the external and internal structures of the eye.

Eye procedures are particularly delicate and precise. Teamwork and attention to detail are critical in ophthalmic

surgery, because the surgeon's attention is focused on the focal area of the microscope, and it cannot be easily diverted from the operative site. Ophthalmic surgery is performed in a variety of health care settings, including the hospital and outpatient center. Regardless of the setting, preparations and procedures for the patient's safety are fully implemented in

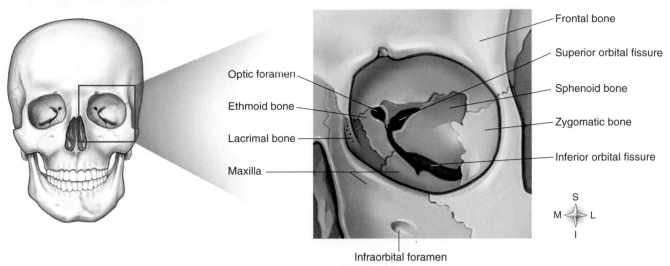

Figure 27-1 The orbital cavity (bony orbit) showing the composite bones. *(From Thibodeau G, Patton K: Anatomy and physiology, ed 6, St Louis, 2007, Mosby.)*

the perioperative period. Of particular concern are verifying that the operative site and the implants are correct, positioning precautions, and drug and environmental safety.

SURGICAL ANATOMY

ORBITAL CAVITY

The basic structure of the eyeball, the globe, is contained within the orbital cavity (also called the *bony orbit*). Seven separate bones come together to form the orbit: the frontal, lacrimal, sphenoid, ethmoid, maxillary, zygomatic, and palatine bones. The paired palatine bones form a part of the orbital floor. These can be seen in Chapter 29, Figure 29-3. The cavity is lined with connective tissue to cushion the eye. Although most of the orbit is composed of thin bone, the rim is particularly thick and therefore more protective. The optic nerve enters the posterior orbital cavity through the optic foramen (Figure 27-1).

EYELIDS

The eyelids are composed of fibrous connective tissue (referred to as the *tarsal plate*) covered with skin. The lids protect the eye from injury and light. The term *palpebral* refers to the eyelids. The space or interval between the upper and lower lids is called the *palpebral fissure*. Each juncture of the eyelids is called a *canthus*. Sebaceous glands located along the lid margin and in the lacrimal caruncle secrete waxy oil that seals the eyelids when they are closed. The eyelashes, which extend along the tarsus, protect the eye from airborne particles (Figure 27-2).

GLOBE

The globe has separate cavities, each of which contains functional structures. The posterior cavity lies at the back of the

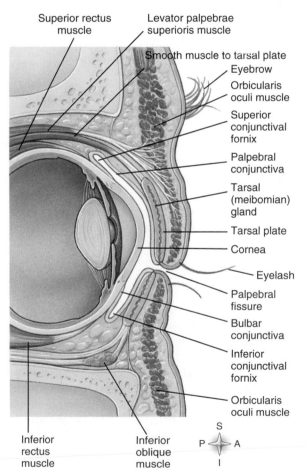

Figure 27-2 The external structures of the eye. *(From Thibodeau G, Patton K: Anatomy and physiology, ed 6, St Louis, 2007, Mosby.)*

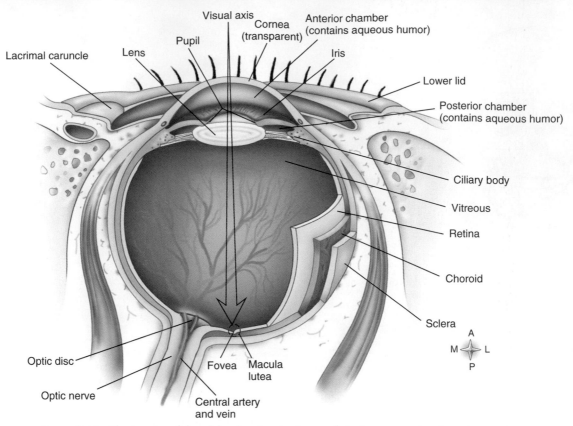

Figure 27-3   The interior of the globe showing the layers of the inner eye, chambers, lens, retina, and optic nerve. *(From Thibodeau G, Patton K: Anatomy and physiology, ed 6, St Louis, 2007, Mosby.)*

eyeball and contains a gel called vitreous. The anterior cavity is divided into two spaces, the anterior chamber and the posterior chamber.

The globe is enclosed by separate tissue layers, each very distinctive in structure and function (Figure 27-3).

EYE MUSCLES

Six muscles attach the sclera to the bony orbit and move the eyeball around various axes. This allows both eyes to focus on a single point. Each eye has four rectus muscles: the superior, inferior, lateral, and medial rectus muscles. Each eye also has two oblique muscles, the superior and inferior oblique muscles. The visual field is the area we see when the eyes are focused on a single point. Vision normally is binocular; that is, each eye has a nearly separate visual field, and the two are brought together as one image in the brain. The visible area consists of central and peripheral vision (Figure 27-4).

CONJUNCTIVA

The palpebral conjunctiva is a thin, transparent mucous membrane that lines each eyelid and reflects onto the globe, where it is called the bulbar conjunctiva. It moves anteriorly encompassing the globe up to the anatomic junction of the cornea and sclera at the *limbus* sclera junction. The bulbar conjunctiva appears white, because the sclera lies directly beneath it.

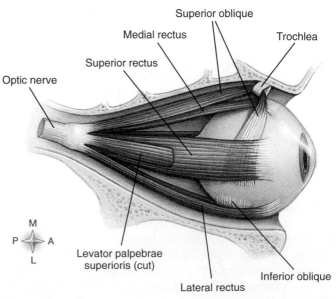

Figure 27-4   The extrinsic muscles of the eye. *(From Thibodeau G, Patton K: Anatomy and physiology, ed 6, St Louis, 2007, Mosby.)*

CORNEA

The cornea is a clear tissue layer overlying the front of the eyeball. Light enters the eye through the cornea and is refracted (bent); this allows images to be focused on the retina. The cornea has no blood vessels. It is composed of three tissue layers: the epithelium (superficial layer), the stroma, and the endothelium. The circular boundary of the cornea extends to the sclera. The two tissues come together at the limbus. During cataract surgery, the initial incision is made in the limbus.

SCLERA

The sclera is a thick, white, fibrous tissue that encloses about three fourths of the eyeball. It is the external supporting layer of the eyeball. The sclera is contiguous with the cornea at the front of the eye. The sclera communicates with the optic nerve sheath.

CHOROID AND CILIARY BODY

The highly vascular pigmented choroid layer lies directly beneath the sclera. The primary function of the choroid is to prevent the reflection of light within the eyeball. An extension of the choroid layer, the ciliary body, is located at the periphery of the anterior choroid. It is composed of smooth muscle tissue to which suspensory ligaments are attached.

IRIS

The iris is a pigmented membrane composed mainly of muscle tissue that surrounds the pupil. The actions of the muscle fibers cause the pupil to close or open, to exclude light, or to admit light into the inner eye. The pupil may appear dilated or constricted, depending on the action of the iris.

RETINA

The innermost layer of the posterior globe is called the *retina.* The retina is the photoreceptive layer of the eye; it receives and transmits images to the brain via the optic nerve. Light energy projected onto the retina from the front of the eye is converted into nerve impulses that are transmitted to the brain, creating sight. The two types of photoreceptive cells are those that transmit black and white and those that enable color perception. The macula is a distinct area of acute vision that lies near the optic nerve. The center of this structure is called the *fovea centralis.* The optic nerve exits the globe in an area of dense neurons called the *optic disc.* The optic disc has no photoreceptors.

LENS

The lens lies directly behind the iris in the anterior chamber. It is a clear biconvex disc contained in a transparent capsule. The lens is held in place by suspensory ligaments called *zonules,* which are attached to the capsule and ciliary body. The suspensory ligaments change the shape of the lens to bend light that passes through the lens. This focuses the images that are projected onto the retina.

ANTERIOR AND POSTERIOR CHAMBERS

The anterior cavity of the eye is divided into two chambers—the anterior and posterior chambers. The pupil is the only passageway between the two chambers. The anterior chamber lies in front of the iris whereas the posterior chamber lies behind the iris but in front of (anterior to) the lens. A clear fluid produced by the ciliary epithelium, called *aqueous humor,* fills the anterior chamber. The pupil allows aqueous humor to pass between the two chambers through a space between the lens and the iris. From there it passes into the canal of Schlemm and is shunted directly into the venous system.

LACRIMAL APPARATUS

The lacrimal apparatus produces tears. This group of structures includes the lacrimal gland, caruncle, tear ducts, lacrimal sac, and nasolacrimal duct (Figure 27-5). Tears are produced by the lacrimal gland located laterally in the orbit. Each gland has numerous ducts that drain into the conjunctiva. The lacrimal ducts extend from the inner canthus to the lacrimal sac. The opening of each duct is called the *lacrimal punctum.* The lacrimal sac is an enlarged portion of the nasolacrimal duct, which is a passageway that connects the punctum and the nasal sinus.

Tears are composed of many chemicals, including proteins, mucus, sodium chloride, glucose, and enzymes capable of breaking down the cell membrane of bacteria. Tears continually bathe the eye and protect it from dehydration and infection. Tearing is stimulated by chemical and physical irritants and strong emotion. Tears produced as a result of emotion have a different composition than those arising from irritation and pain.

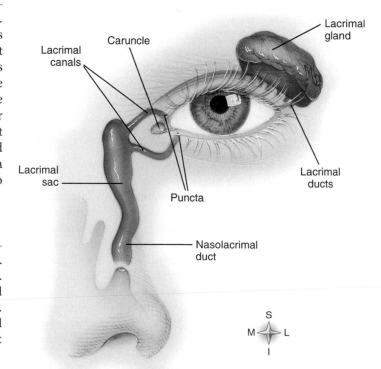

Figure 27-5 **The lacrimal apparatus, including the lacrimal gland and ducts, lacrimal canals and sac, and nasolacrimal duct.** *(From Abrahams P, Marks S, Hutchings R: McMinn's colour atlas of human anatomy, ed 5, Oxford, 2003, Mosby.)*

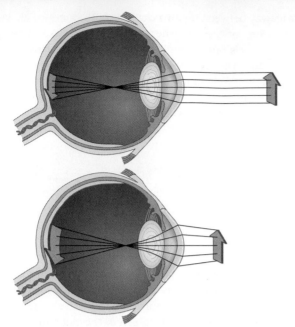

Figure 27-6 Light rays are refracted as they enter the eye and are bent through the lens. Images are focused on the retina and transmitted as nerve signals to the brain. *(From Thibodeau G, Patton K:* Anatomy and physiology, *ed 6, St Louis, 2007, Mosby.)*

REFRACTION

Refraction is the bending of light rays through a transparent medium. Refraction occurs as light enters the front of the eye and passes through the lens. The light rays are refracted as they pass through the cornea, aqueous humor, lens, and vitreous, and the rays converge at the **focal point.** The image produced by the light rays is brought into focus by **accommodation.** This is a complex process in which the lens continually changes shape to keep the image focused on the fovea. This enables us to view objects at various distances and keep them in focus (Figure 27-6).

DIAGNOSTIC TESTING

Refraction is a test for visual acuity, performed with a *photo-opter.* This device has a range of corrective lenses that allow the patient to compare different combinations while viewing an eye chart. The term *refraction,* described earlier as the bending of light rays through a transparent medium, is also used to describe this test. Both uses of the term describe a phenomenon of physics. A *slit lamp* is used to examine the anterior chamber of the eye. Details of the lid margins, conjunctiva, tear film, cornea, and iris can be studied. The pupil can be dilated and the lens and anterior vitreous examined. Fluorescein is used to stain the cornea and highlight irregularities of the epithelial surface. A tonometer is used to measure the intraocular pressure (IOP).

Direct examination of the eyes is performed with an *ophthalmoscope.* This is a handheld instrument that magnifies the focal point, allowing the examiner to evaluate the fundus and other internal eye structures. An indirect binocular ophthalmoscope is used to examine the retina and other structures within a wider focal point.

Fluorescein angiography is used extensively in the diagnosis and evaluation of retinal and choroid diseases. It delineates areas of abnormality and is essential for planning laser treatment of retinal vascular disease. In this test, fluorescein dye is injected intravenously. When the dye reaches the retina and choroid, the vessels and epithelium are clearly delineated and images are recorded.

Ophthalmic ultrasonography is used to measure the density of eye tissues and detect abnormalities. Two types of ultrasound can be used, A-scan ultrasound or B-scan ultrasound. B-scan ultrasound produces an image of the target tissue that shows a series of spots, the brightness of which corresponds to tissue density. As tissue density increases, the image appears darker. For example, vitreous appears very dark or black on ultrasound. The A-scan ultrasound depicts tissue density as amplitude on two axes. The output is represented in waveform, resembling an electrocardiogram. High-density tissue produces an amplified wave.

Magnetic resonance imaging and computed tomography are used in the evaluation of the orbital and intracranial structures. Computed tomography may have some disadvantages in ophthalmology, because it is unable to differentiate between structures of similar density and those that are very small.

CASE PLANNING

PSYCHOLOGICAL CONSIDERATIONS IN EYE SURGERY

Ophthalmic surgery can be frightening to patients. Although many look forward to correcting medical problems to improve or restore their eyesight, they often have unspoken fears that a poor outcome will result in blindness. In most ophthalmic surgeries, the patient receives a regional anesthetic, and monitored sedation is used. The patient therefore is awake and able to hear sounds in the surgical environment. In addition, the patient can see the objects and instruments that are placed in the eye. This can increase preoperative anxiety.

A reassuring environment is always important to the patient's psychological and physical well-being; however, it is particularly important in ophthalmic surgery, because anxiety can result in increased hemorrhage and IOP. The surgical technologist can help the patient by maintaining a calm, supportive atmosphere. Patients find it reassuring to be given simple explanations of what they will feel or sense as the procedure starts. During the procedure, the surgeon usually warns the patient of any steps that involve pressure or pain, such as the initial sting of an anesthetic or loss of sensation.

VERIFICATION OF THE OPERATIVE SITE

The Universal Protocol for verification of operative site and side and other critical information was introduced in Chapter 21. In ophthalmic surgery, particular concerns arise because marks around the eye may be covered by drapes before the verification process is started. This means that the team must be especially vigilant during the TIMEOUT. Verification of implants has historically been a problem in ophthalmic surgery. The consequences of implanting the wrong lens implant during cataract surgery are extremely serious. Intraocular implants *must be verified before insertion*. Lens implants are treated in much the same way as a drug distributed to the field. To prevent insertion of the wrong implant, the American Association of Ophthalmologists (AAO) has developed a sample protocol. The surgical technologist participates in this protocol:

1. Before surgery, the surgeon selects the intraocular lens (IOL) based on the patient's records available *in the operating room*.
2. The circulating nurse shows the surgeon the box and verbally verifies the IOL model number and lens power. The surgeon acknowledges this communication.
3. The circulating nurse *repeats this procedure with the surgical technologist*.
4. The scrubbed surgical technologist *verbally states the model number and lens power* as the IOL is passed to the surgeon.

Documentation of implants is discussed more fully later in this chapter.

POSITIONING THE PATIENT FOR OPHTHALMIC SURGERY

Ophthalmic surgery is performed with the patient in the supine position with the head stabilized on a circular headrest (sometimes called a *doughnut*). The top of the head may be level with the end of the table, or the patient may be positioned several inches lower (toward the feet), depending on the surgeon's operating needs. A wrist rest is attached to the head of the table to aid the surgeon in steadying the hands during the procedure (Figure 27-7).

Many health care facilities use a combination stretcher–operating table for transporting the patient and performing surgery. Shifting the patient immediately after surgery may result in increased IOP and eye injury.

If a standard gurney is used, the patient must be transferred cautiously and slowly. The older patient may have difficulty moving across the gurney onto the operating table. The patient

should be warned of the narrow table, and the safety strap should be secured as soon as possible. The circulator then can stabilize the patient into a comfortable position with gel or foam supports as needed. The patient should be covered with warm blankets to prevent hypothermia and for comfort.

As mentioned, most eye procedures involve a regional block and monitored sedation. The position of the patient for eye surgery must be safe and comfortable. An uncomfortable patient may become restless during surgery, and this can result in injury to the eye. It is critical that patients remain still. Some patients may benefit from lumbar support and a cushion for the popliteal region. The arms may be tucked at the sides, but without contacting any part of the metal frame or attachments.

PREPPING AND DRAPING

The skin prep commonly is performed after the patient has been anesthetized. Because regional anesthesia often is used, the circulator should have all prepping supplies ready before anesthesia is induced to prevent delay. The standard approved eye prep antiseptic is dilute povidone-iodine (5% or as directed by the surgeon). Supplies needed for the sterile prep setup include the following:

- Small basins for the solutions
- Surgical towels
- Plastic towel drapes
- Lint-free gauze sponges
- Cotton balls
- Cellulose eye sponges
- Balanced salt solution (BSS)

The prep area includes the eyelid and margins, inner and outer canthus, brows, and face, ending usually at the chin. Before starting the prep, the circulator secures an adhesive towel drape at the hairline. Surgical towels are placed to absorb any solution runoff. However, runoff is prevented by squeezing excess solution from each sponge. A small piece of cotton may be placed in the operative side ear and the head turned toward the operative side. Irrigation of the eye may be required before the skin prep. BSS or a mild antiseptic of the surgeon's choice is used. The prep is performed starting at the

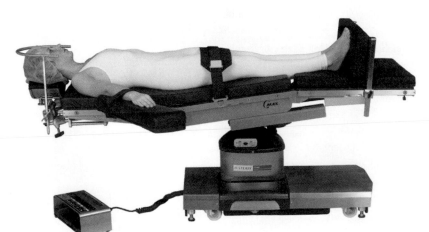

Figure 27-7 Positioning of the patient, showing a wrist rest at the head of the bed. (© 2008 by STERIS Corporation. All rights reserved.)

eyelid and extending outward. The eyelid margins are cleansed using cotton-tipped applicators. The canthus is considered a contaminated area, and any sponge that touches this area is discarded. Skin prep of the eye may include instillation of drugs to prepare the eye for surgery.

A number of techniques are used to drape the eye. It is important to isolate the hairline and nonoperative side of the face. Some surgeons use a head drape. This usually is followed by a fenestrated drape to expose the operative eye. A body sheet is used to maintain a wide sterile field, or the procedure drape may be large enough to extend over the sides of the operating table.

ANESTHESIA

Most ophthalmic surgery is performed using a regional anesthetic with monitored sedation. A topical anesthetic, local infiltration, peribulbar nerve block, or a combination of these is most often used. A retrobulbar block may be used in selected patients. However, this approach is associated with a number of serious risks and has more limited uses. Pediatric patients receive a general anesthetic.

For local anesthesia, a dedicated setup is prepared according to the surgeon's preferences. Anesthetic, syringes, infiltration needles (25 to 27 gauge), transfer needles, and sponges are needed. Lidocaine with epinephrine may be used to maintain vasoconstriction at the operative site. A topical anesthetic is applied over the cornea before injection. Patients generally tolerate the local anesthetic procedure well. The circulator is present at the patient's side to assist and to reassure the patient.

OPHTHALMIC DRUGS

Ophthalmic surgery requires the use of many types of drugs, which are administered preoperatively, during surgery, and in the postoperative period. Many of these drugs have potent effects, and a medication error could irreparably damage the eye. Chapter 13 discusses the appropriate protocol for receiving drugs on the sterile field. Important highlights are:

- *All drugs on the sterile field must be labeled as soon as they are received; this is critical.*
- Every drug passed to the surgeon must be identified and acknowledged by the surgeon—no exceptions.
- Preoperative topical drugs may be administered by the surgeon or the circulating registered nurse.
- The amounts of all drugs used must be recorded on the intraoperative report.

Table 27-1 presents a list of ophthalmic drugs and their uses.

Adverse reactions to medications used during eye surgery are a serious consideration. Many different drugs are used in combination, and the circulator must be vigilant in observing for signs and symptoms that might indicate allergy or sensitivity. The scrub should notify the circulator and surgeon of any symptoms reported by the patient. The technologist does not assess the patient medically but should immediately report any observed changes in the patient's appearance or behavior.

Table **27-1** Medications Used During Ophthalmic Surgery	
Drug (Brand Name)	Description/Uses
Mydriatics (Drugs that dilate the pupil but permit focusing)	
Phenylephrine (Neo-Synephrine, Mydfrin), 2.5%, 10%	Objective examination of the retina, testing of refraction, and easier removal of lenses; mydriatics may be used alone or with a cycloplegic drug.
Cycloplegics (Drugs that paralyze accommodation and inhibit focusing)	
Tropicamide (Mydriacyl), 1%	Anticholinergic, dilation of the pupil, examination of the fundus, and refraction.
Atropine, 1%	Dilates the pupil, inhibits focusing; anticholinergic, potent, and has a long duration of action (7 to 14 days).
Cyclopentolate (Cyclogyl), 1%, 2%	Anticholinergic; dilates the pupil, inhibits focusing
Scopolamine hydrobromide (Isopto Hyoscine), 0.25%	Anticholinergic; dilates the pupil, inhibits focusing
Homatropine hydrobromide (Isopto Homatropine), 2%, 5%	Anticholinergic; dilates the pupil, inhibits focusing
Epinephrine (1:1,000) preservative free (PF)	Dilates the pupil; added to bottles of balanced salt solution (BSS) for irrigation to maintain pupil dilation during cataract surgery or vitrectomy.
Miotics	
Carbachol (Miostat), 0.01%	Potent cholinergic; constricts the pupil, used intraocularly during anterior segment surgery.
Carbachol (Isopto Carbachol), 0.75%, 1.5%, 2.25%, 3%	Potent cholinergic; constricts the pupil, used topically to reduce intraocular pressure (IOP) in glaucoma.
Acetylcholine chloride (Miochol-E), 1%	Cholinergic; rapidly constricts the pupil, used intraocularly during anterior segment surgery; reconstitute immediately before using.
Pilocarpine hydrochloride, 1%, 4%	Cholinergic; constricts the pupil, used topically to lower IOP in glaucoma.

Table **27-1**	**Medications Used During Ophthalmic Surgery—cont'd**
Drug (Brand Name)	**Description/Uses**
Topical Anesthetics	
Tetracaine hydrochloride (Pontocaine), 0.05%	*Onset:* 5-20 sec *Duration of action:* 10-20 min
Proparacaine hydrochloride (Ophthaine), 0.05%	*Onset:* 5-20 sec *Duration of action:* 10-20 min
Injectable Anesthetics	
Lidocaine (Xylocaine), 1%, 2%, 4%	*Onset:* 4-6 min *Duration of action:* 40-60 min, 120 min with epinephrine
Methylparaben free (MPF)	Preservative free; adjunct to topical anesthetic.
Bupivacaine (Marcaine, Sensorcaine), 0.25%, 0.50%, 0.75%	*Onset:* 5-11 min *Duration of action:* 8-12 hr with epinephrine; often used in 0.75% strength in combination with lidocaine for blocks
Mepivacaine (Carbocaine), 1%, 2%	*Onset:* 3-5 min *Duration of action:* 2 hr (longer with epinephrine)
Etidocaine (Duranest), 1%	*Onset:* 3 min *Duration of action:* 5-10 hr
Additives to Local Anesthetics	
Epinephrine, 1:50,000 to 1:200,000	Combined with injectable local anesthetics to prolong anesthesia and reduce bleeding.
Hyaluronidase	Enzyme mixed with anesthetics (75 units per 10 mL) to increase diffusion of anesthetic through tissue, improving the effectiveness of the block; contraindicated if skin inflammation or malignancy is present.
Viscoelastics	
Sodium hyaluronate (Healon, Amvisc, Provisc, Vitrax) in a sterile syringe assembly with blunt-tip cannula	Lubricant and support; maintains separation between tissues to protect the endothelium and maintain the anterior chamber intraocularly; removed from anterior chamber to prevent postoperative increase in pressure; should be refrigerated (except Vitrax); allow 30 min to warm to room temperature.
Sodium chondroitin–sodium hyaluronate (Viscoat) in a sterile syringe assembly with blunt-tip cannula	Maintains deep chamber for anterior segment procedures, protects epithelium of cornea, and improves visualization; may be used to coat intraocular lens before implantation; should be refrigerated.
Duovisc	Packages of separate syringes of Provisc and Viscoat in the same box.
Viscoadherents	
Hydroxypropyl methylcellulose 2% (Occucoat) in a sterile syringe assembly with blunt-tip cannula	Maintains a deep chamber for anterior segment procedures, protects epithelium of cornea, and may be used to coat intraocular lens before implantation; removed from anterior chamber at end of procedure; stored at room temperature.
Hydroxyethylcellulose (Gonioscopic Prism Solution)	Bonds gonioscopic prisms to the eye; stored at room temperature.
Hydroxypropyl methylcellulose 2.5% (Goniosol)	Bonds gonioscopic prisms to the eye; stored at room temperature.
Irrigants	
Balanced salt solution (BSS, Endosol)	Used to keep the cornea moist during surgery; also used as an internal irrigant in the anterior or posterior segment.
BSS enriched with bicarbonate, dextrose, and glutathione (BSS Plus, Endosol Extra)	Used as an internal irrigant in the anterior or posterior segment; must be reconstituted immediately before use by adding part I to part II with the transfer device.
Hyperosmotic Agents	
Mannitol (Osmitrol)	Intravenous (IV) osmotic diuretic; increases the osmolarity of the plasma, causing the osmotic pressure gradient to pull free fluid from the eye into the plasma, thereby reducing the IOP.
Glycerin (Osmoglyn, Glyrol)	Oral osmotic diuretic given in chilled juice or cola; increases the osmolarity of the plasma, causing the osmotic pressure gradient to pull free fluid from the eye into the plasma, thereby reducing the IOP.

Continued

Table 27-1 Medications Used During Ophthalmic Surgery—cont'd

Drug (Brand Name)	Description/Uses
Antiinflammatory Agents	
Betamethasone sodium phosphate and betamethasone acetate suspension (Celestone)	Glucocorticoid; injected subconjunctivally after surgery for prophylaxis; also used to treat severe allergic and inflammatory conditions.
Dexamethasone (Decadron)	Adrenocorticosteroid; injected subconjunctivally after surgery for prophylaxis; also used to treat severe allergic and inflammatory conditions and intraocularly for endophthalmitis.
Methylprednisolone acetate suspension (Depo-Medrol)	Glucocorticoid; injected subconjunctivally after surgery for prophylaxis; also used to treat severe allergic and inflammatory conditions.
Antiinfective Drugs	
Polymyxin B/bacitracin (Polysporin ointment)	Topical treatment of superficial ocular infections of the conjunctiva or cornea; also used prophylactically after surgery.
Polymyxin B/neomycin/bacitracin (Neosporin ointment)	Topical treatment of superficial infections of the external eye; used prophylactically after surgery; hypersensitivity to neomycin is possible.
Neomycin and polymyxin B sulfates and dexamethasone (Maxitrol ointment or suspension)	Topical treatment of steroid-responsive inflammatory ocular conditions or bacterial infections of the external eye; hypersensitivity to neomycin is possible.
Tobramycin/dexamethasone (TobraDex)	Topical treatment or prevention of superficial infections of the external part of the eye; also has antiinflammatory properties.
Cefazolin (Ancef, Kefzol)	Injected subconjunctivally for prophylaxis after eye procedures; also used topically, intraocularly, and systemically for endophthalmitis.
Gentamicin sulfate (Garamycin)	Injected subconjunctivally for prophylaxis after eye procedures; also used topically, subconjunctivally, and intraocularly for endophthalmitis.
Ceftazidime (Fortaz, Tazicef, Tazidime)	Injected subconjunctivally and intraocularly for the treatment of endophthalmitis.
Other Drugs	
Cocaine, 1% to 4%	Used topically only, never injected; used on cornea to loosen epithelium before debridement and on nasal packing to reduce congestion of mucosa.
5-Fluorouracil (5-FU)	Antimetabolite used topically to inhibit scar formation in glaucoma-filtering procedures; handle and discard in compliance with the regulations of the Occupational Safety and Health Administration (OSHA) and health care facility's policies for safe use of antineoplastics.
Mitomycin (Mutamycin)	Antimetabolite used topically to inhibit scar formation in glaucoma-filtering procedures and pterygium excision; handle and discard in compliance with OSHA's and health facility's policies for safe use of antineoplastics.
Tissue plasminogen activator (TPA) (Activase)	Thrombolytic agent; used for the treatment of fibrin formation in patients who have had vitrectomy and for the lysis of clots on the retina.
Fluorescein	*IV diagnostic aid:* Used in fluorescein angiography to diagnose retinal disorders. *Topical stain:* Fluorescein strip temporarily stains the cornea yellow-green in areas of denuded corneal epithelium.
Timolol maleate (Timoptic)	Beta-adrenergic receptor blocking agent; used in the treatment of elevated IOP in ocular hypertension or open angle glaucoma.
Acetazolamide sodium (Diamox)	Carbonic anhydrase inhibitor; given IV to reduce the secretion of aqueous humor, resulting in a drop in IOP; also has a diuretic effect.
Dextrose, 50%	Added to BSS, Endosol, BSS Plus, or Endosol Extra for diabetic patients during intraocular procedures.

From Rothrock JC: *Alexander's care of the patient in surgery,* ed 13, St Louis, 2007, Mosby.

INSTRUMENTS

Ophthalmic instruments (Figures 27-8 to 27-11) are delicate and expensive. All surgical personnel must take special care to ensure that the edges and tips of microsurgical eye instruments are not dulled or damaged by careless handling. Before the procedure begins, the scrub should check all instruments. Sharp items must be smooth, and scissor blades must align properly. Needle holders are particularly susceptible to injury. The scrub should make sure that catches and spring mechanisms are working properly. Suction tips should be checked

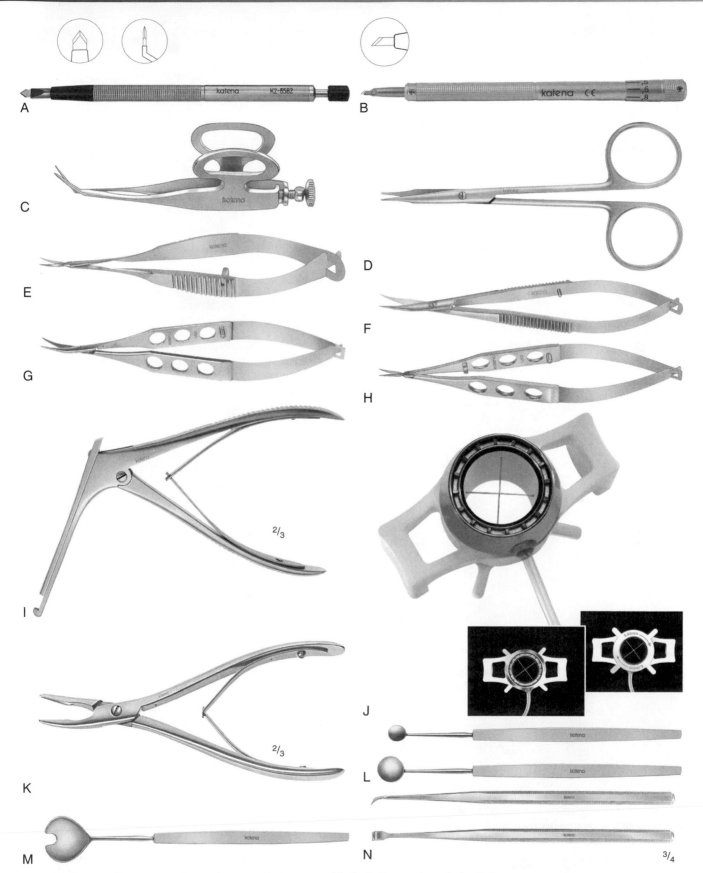

Figure 27-8 **Cutting instruments.** **A,** Diamond knife. **B,** Diamond step knife. **C,** Barraquer iris scissors. **D,** Stevens scissors. **E,** Vannas scissors. **F,** Westcott stitch scissors. **G,** Westcott tenotomy scissors. **H,** Katena-Vannas scissors. **I,** Kerrison rongeur. **J,** Barron vacuum trephine. **K,** Beyer rongeur. **L,** Enucleation spoon. **M,** Wells enucleation spoon. **N,** Freer lacrimal chisel. *(Courtesy Katena Eye Instruments, Denville, NJ.)*

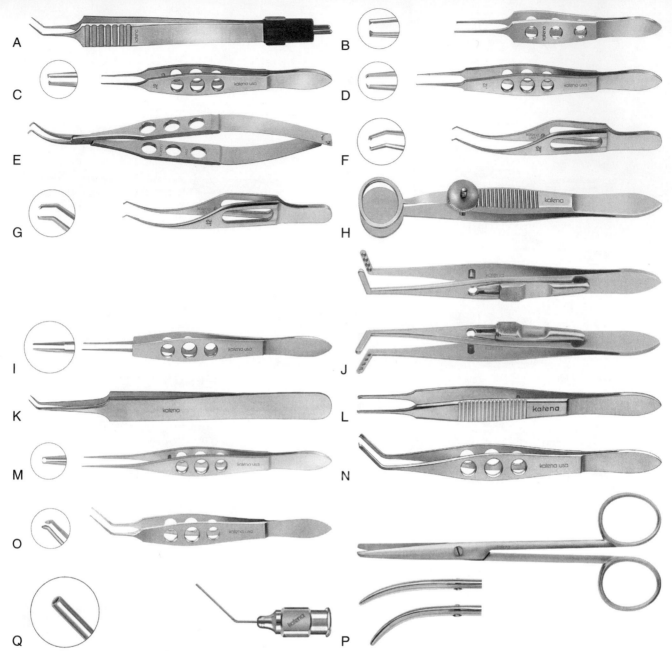

Figure 27-9 **Forceps, calipers, and needle holders. A,** Bipolar forceps. **B,** Bishop-Harmon forceps. **C,** Bonn forceps. **D,** Castroviejo needle holder. **E,** Clayman lens-holding forceps. **F,** Colibri forceps. **G,** Harms-Colibri forceps. **H,** Hunt chalazion forceps. **I,** Jaffe tying forceps. **J,** Jameson muscle forceps. **K,** Jeweler forceps. **L,** Lester fixation forceps. **M,** Pierce corneal forceps. **N,** Troutman rectus forceps. **O,** Utrata capsulorrhexis forceps. **P,** Enucleation forceps. **Q,** Castroviejo caliper. *(Courtesy Katena Eye Instruments, Denville, NJ.)*

for patency. All instruments must be kept in order on the Mayo stand. Surgery often is performed with the overhead lights dimmed. A neat instrument table is essential.

EQUIPMENT AND SUPPLIES

Electrosurgical Unit

Two types of electrosurgical systems are commonly used in eye surgery, the single-use, battery-powered cautery and the bipolar unit. The handheld battery unit has a very small

filament tip that becomes hot when the unit is activated. Unlike monopolar or bipolar electrosurgical units (ESUs), this unit is a true cautery instrument. The filament is used to coagulate very small vessels of the eye; however, it does not have cutting capability. The bipolar or radiofrequency ESU is used for procedures in which fine cutting and coagulation are required. The bipolar unit is used in conjunction with bipolar instruments, which are connected to the unit by a thin cable. (A complete discussion of these technologies and safety precautions can be found in Chapter 18.)

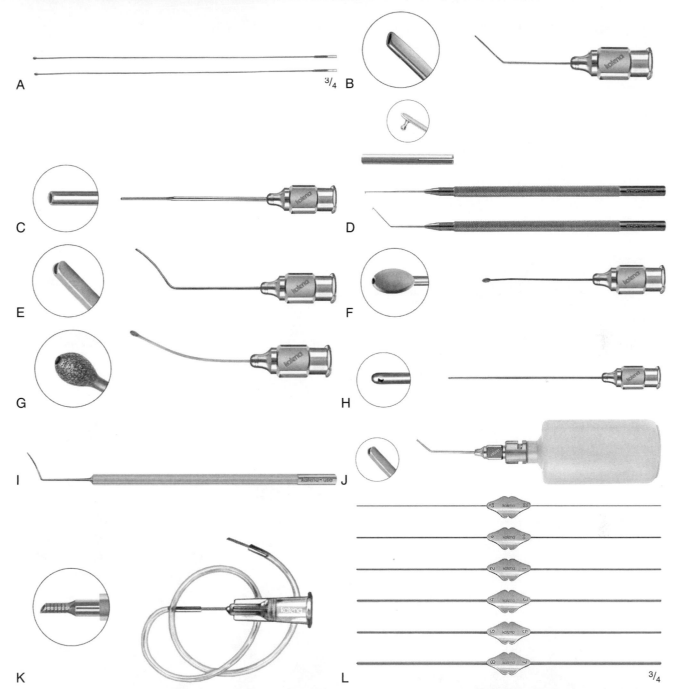

Figure 27-10 **Cannulas, irrigators, and probes. A,** Crawford lacrimal intubation. **B,** Hydrodissection cannula. **C,** Lacrimal cannula (23 gauge). **D,** Lester intraocular lens (IOL) manipulator. **E,** Randolph cyclodialysis cannula. **F,** Welsh olive-tip cannula. **G,** Jensen polisher. **H,** Air injection cannula. **I,** Barraquer iris spatula. **J,** Bishop-Harmon A/C irrigator. **K,** Chamber maintainer. **L,** Bowman lacrimal probe set. *(Courtesy Katena Eye Instruments, Denville, NJ.)*

Eye Sponges

Eye sponges are made of lint-free cellulose or similar material. These are supplied commercially attached to a short plastic rod (Figure 27-12). Sponges must be separated from supplies that might discharge lint particles. During surgery, the scrubbed surgical technologist may be required to blot blood or fluid from the surgical site. The sponge is never used on the cornea. The sponge absorbs fluid by wicking. This is done by holding the tip of the sponge in contact with the fluid and allowing the sponge to absorb it. Fresh sponges must always be available to maintain a clean operative site.

Sutures

Eye sutures are supplied in a wide range of materials in sizes 4-0 to 12-0. These must be handled gently and carefully. Sutures should be handled as little as possible, and the points of the needles should be protected from damage. Double-arm sutures frequently are used in eye surgery to close circumferential

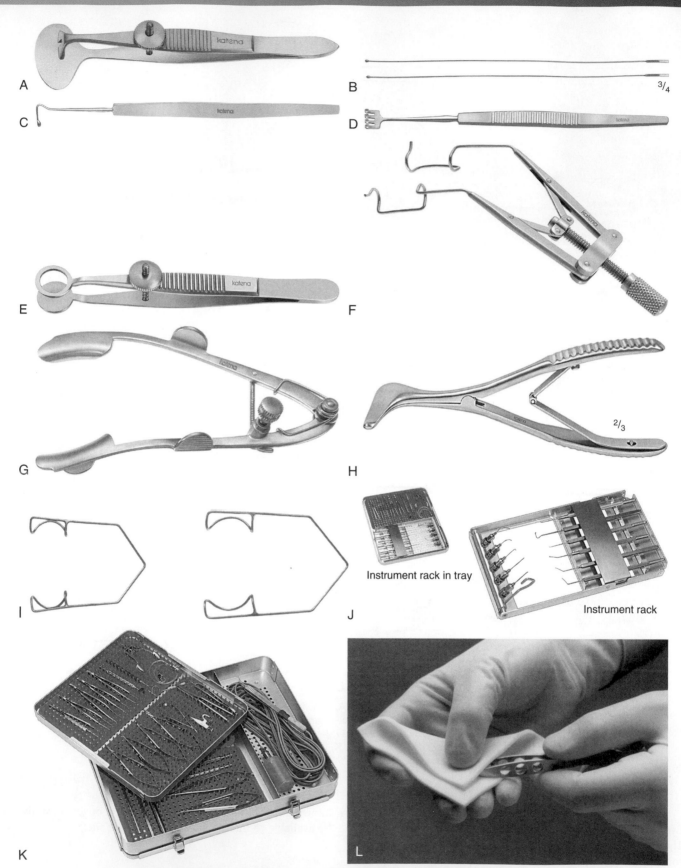

Figure 27-11   **Retractors and speculums. A,** Erhardt lid forceps. **B,** Graefe muscle hook. **C,** Jameson muscle hook. **D,** Knapp retractor. **E,** Lambert chalazion forceps. **F,** Lieberman speculum. **G,** Lester-Burch eye speculum. **H,** Nasal speculum, adult. **I,** Barraquer wire speculum. *Instrument care:* **J,** Instrument rack. Eye instruments must be maintained in racks to prevent damage. **K,** Sterilization case for eye instruments. **L,** Lint-free instrument wipe. *(Courtesy Katena Eye Instruments, Denville, NJ.)*

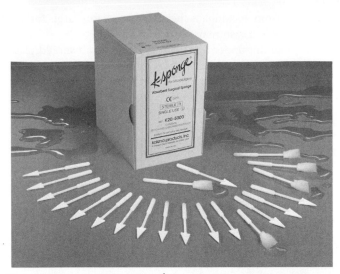

Figure 27-12   Eye sponges and K-sponge spears. *(Courtesy Katena Eye Instruments, Denville, NJ.)*

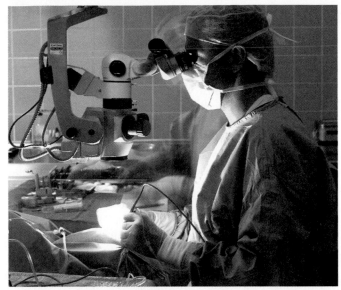

Figure 27-13   The surgeon at the microscope. *(Courtesy Carl Zeiss, Dublin, Calif.)*

incisions. Ophthalmic needles may be as small as 4 mm at the widest part. A magnetic needle pad is necessary for tracking needles during surgery. Sutures should not be allowed to contact cloth towels, which can transfer lint to the needle and suture material.

Ophthalmic Dressings

A soft dressing or hard shield may be used to protect the eye after surgery. Soft, lint-free gauze eye patches are supplied for a simple dressing that absorbs fluid and prevents debris from entering the eye. A rigid eye shield is taped over the eye to provide protection from bumping or abrasion, which may cause dehiscence of an incision.

SURGICAL TECHNIQUES IN EYE SURGERY

MICROSURGERY

Microsurgery presents challenges to the scrub for several reasons:

- The surgeon's field of vision is magnified, but the scope (i.e., the area of vision) is very limited. Special technique is required for passing instruments, because the surgeon must not look away from the field to receive them.
- When required to look away from the field, the surgeon loses concentration and the rhythm of the surgery. To prevent such interruptions, the scrub should prepare for each step of the procedure. Using the proper method to pass instruments reduces the risk of patient injury.
- The patient and surgical field must be completely still. The scrub must prevent even slight movement of the microscope. When passing instruments or preparing items near the field, the scrub must have a steady hand and create as little movement as possible. Remember that if the patient raises his or her head or if any instruments are jarred while touching the eye, the patient can be injured.

Box 27-1   Microscope Terminology

Assistant binoculars: A separate optical body with a nonmotorized, hand-controlled zoom.

Beam splitter: A device that transmits an image from the primary ocular to an observer tube, producing an identical picture.

Broad-field viewing lens: A low-power magnifying glass attached to the front of the oculars that produces an overview of the field.

Coaxial illuminator: A light source (usually fiberoptic) transmitted through the lens or body of the microscope. It illuminates the area in the field of view of the objective lens.

Compound microscope: A microscope that uses two or more lenses in a single unit.

Illumination system: The lighting system of the microscope.

Magnifying power: The ability to enlarge an image.

Objective lens: The lens that establishes the working distance and produces the greatest magnification.

Ocular or eyepiece: The component of the microscope that magnifies the field of view.

Paraxial illuminators: One or more light tubes that contain incandescent bulbs and focusing lenses. Light is focused to coincide with the working distance of the scope.

X-Y attachment: A mechanism that allows the scope to move precisely along a horizontal plane.

Zoom lens: A lens that increases or decreases magnification and is operated by the foot pedal.

Operating Microscope

The operating microscope is a heavy piece of equipment, but it also has delicate components (Figure 27-13). The technologist should become familiar with all components to prevent injury to the patient and to protect the microscope from damage. Box 27-1 lists common microscope terminology.

HANDLING THE MICROSCOPE The following guidelines should be observed when the microscope is handled:

1. Before moving the microscope, secure the arms. This prevents them from swinging out and striking the wall or other equipment.
2. The microscope must be balanced before use. This is necessary to ensure that the head of the microscope does not drift up or down. Always consult the manufacturer's instructions for balancing.
3. The microscope must be adjusted to accommodate the surgeon's and assistant's eyesight. Always test the microscope before moving it to the surgical field.
4. Check the brake and other controls to ensure that they are tight before using the microscope.
5. Take special care to ensure that the microscope head control knob is secure before surgery.
6. Check all cords for fraying or loose wires. Light bulbs also should be tested before surgery, and an extra bulb should be kept in the surgical suite.
7. Some microscopes are equipped with an X-Y axis carrier; this must be centered before the microscope is positioned at the field.
8. When moving the microscope, handle it with *both hands* on the vertical column. Moving the microscope by the head can cause it to tip over.
9. Make all adjustments to the vertical oculars before surgery.

CARE OF THE MICROSCOPE

1. The microscope should be damp-dusted before use. Follow the manufacturer's recommendations for use of a disinfectant. Never use detergent or disinfectant on the lenses. They should be cleaned with a lens cleaner or water and wiped with lens paper. Do not use cloth, which leaves lint on the lens.
2. Do not touch the lenses.
3. The scope and all its openings and attachments should be covered at the end of the day to prevent the accumulation of dust.

ROLE OF THE SCRUBBED SURGICAL TECHNOLOGIST

Assisting in eye surgery is a specialty that requires particular skills and techniques. The scrubbed technologist must learn to focus on minute detail, develop steadiness, and communicate clearly with the surgeon.

- When preparing microsurgical instruments, the scrub should check for burrs (rough or jagged spots on sharp instruments). This is done by inspecting the instruments visually under microscope magnification or by running a lint-free microsurgical wipe gently along the edges of the instrument to feel for any sharp edges.
- Instruments are kept clean during each procedure. Only lint-free microsurgical wipes are used on instruments.
- Practice is required to handle and load sutures properly. When a locking needle holder is used, gentle pressure is applied on the shaft. Too much pressure prevents the needle

holder from locking. A needle that is too large for the needle holder also may prevent locking.

- To cut suture under a microscope, the scrub should place the scissors within the scope's field of vision. Only then should the scissors' tip be positioned at the suture. The scissors are then gently lowered for cutting.
- To cut sutures, the forefinger is placed over the center point on the shank of the scissors. This steadies the instrument and the hand. The point of the scissors is lowered over the suture to cut the ends.
- The scrub must keep all instruments in a specific order on the Mayo stand. When returning instruments to the Mayo stand, the scrub should place them in their original position and not rearrange them.
- Microsurgery requires dexterity and a steady hand. What appears as a small tremor to the naked eye can be severe under magnification.
- Experienced scrubs do not remove their eyes from the microscope to orient an instrument to the surgeon's hand (Figure 27-14).
- The eye normally produces lubricating fluid that nourishes and protects it from infection and drying. The scrub is required to irrigate the eye periodically during surgery to prevent drying. BSS (commercially supplied in a small squeeze vial) is used for this purpose. During irrigation, the tip of the vial is held over the tissue *but never touches the tissue.*

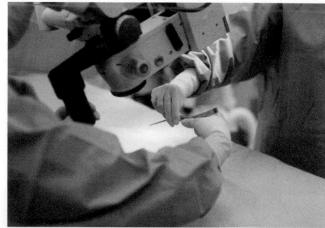

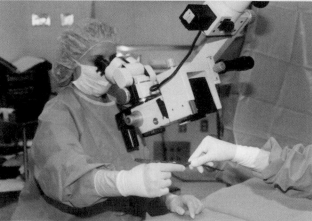

Figure 27-14 Passing instruments under the microscope.

SURGICAL PROCEDURES

EXCISION OF A CHALAZION

Surgical Goal

In excision of a chalazion, nodal tissue arising from a sebaceous gland is excised from the tarsal plate.

Pathology

A chalazion is an inflammatory benign growth that originates in a sebaceous gland of the eyelid. As in other areas of the body, a sebaceous gland may become impacted, causing inflammation. A chalazion is not infectious, but a granuloma (semisolid tissue) develops, which can enlarge and rupture. Surgery is indicated when conservative treatment fails.

TECHNIQUE

1 The lid is injected with a local anesthetic.
2 A chalazion clamp is applied to the lid.
3 A vertical incision is made into the tarsal plate.
4 The contents of the chalazion are removed with a curette.

Discussion

The patient is placed in the supine position, prepped, and draped for an eye procedure. The eyelid is instilled with a local anesthetic. The surgeon clamps the lid with a chalazion clamp. The lid is everted, and a vertical incision is made through the tarsal plate with a no. 11 blade. A curette is used to remove the contents of the chalazion. Bleeding on the edges of the tarsal plate is controlled with the bipolar ESU or eye cautery. A pressure dressing is applied, because suturing is not necessary.

REPAIR OF AN ENTROPION

Surgical Goal

Entropion is an abnormal inversion of the lower eyelid. The goal of surgery is to restore the eyelid to correct anatomical position by resection.

Pathology

An entropion is an inwardly turned eyelid, which causes the eyelashes to rub on the cornea. The condition occurs primarily in older individuals and is caused by weakness and imbalance of eyelid muscles. The condition almost always affects the lower, rather than the upper, eyelids.

TECHNIQUE

1 The lid is retracted.
2 A triangular incision is made into the lid.
3 The lid is sutured.

Discussion

In preparation for an entropion repair, the scrub should have chalazion clamps, a dye marking pen, calipers, and a metal ruler available. A basic eye soft tissue set is used, and the procedure is performed using local anesthesia.

The patient is placed in the supine position with the head stabilized on a doughnut headrest. Before the procedure begins, the circulator instills tetracaine ophthalmic drops into the operative eye. The eye then is prepped and draped. The incision is outlined before or after the skin prep.

The most common approach to an entropion is a triangular excision into the tarsal plate. The surgeon retracts the lid with a chalazion clamp. The incision is made with a #15 Bard-Parker blade mounted on a #3 handle. Straight iris scissors may be used to free the tissue excised by the scalpel. Small bleeders are controlled with the bipolar ESU or eye cautery unit. During the procedure, the scrub irrigates the incision and blots away excess fluid as necessary.

After the triangle has been excised, the scrub should prepare 5-0 or 6-0 absorbable sutures swaged to a **spatula needle**. The surgeon places the sutures and leaves the suture ends untied until all sutures have been placed. Tying forceps are used to secure the knots, which are cut short to prevent them from touching the cornea.

When hemostasis has been achieved, the surgeon releases the chalazion clamp and instills an antibiotic ointment into the eye. The eye is dressed with a cotton eye patch, which is taped in place. Repair of an entropion is illustrated in Figure 27-15.

REPAIR OF AN ECTROPION

Surgical Goal

Ectropion is drooping of the lower eyelid. This creates an overflow of tears and exposes the conjunctiva, which becomes dry and irritated. The goal of surgical treatment is to restore the eyelid to its normal position. Many approaches to ectropion repair can be used. In the lateral canthotomy and tarsal strip procedure, a wedge of tissue is removed from the lower tarsal plate, and the canthal tendon is secured to the periosteum of the orbital rim.

Pathology

An ectropion is an outwardly turned eyelid. The condition most often is associated with age, although it may also occur congenitally, as a result of scarring, or secondary to facial nerve paralysis (Bell palsy). Aging may cause the orbicularis muscle to relax. If it is not repaired, the condition may lead to thickening of the mucosal surface on the inside of the eyelid (conjunctiva) and inflammation of the eye itself.

TECHNIQUE

1 The lateral canthus is incised in the lower lid.
2 The canthal tendon is exposed and sutured to the periosteum.
3 The wound is closed.

Discussion

A basic soft tissue eye setup, cotton-tipped applicators, a metal ruler, and calipers are needed for the ectropion repair procedure.

The patient is prepped and draped for a single or bilateral eye procedure. The incision may be outlined before or after the skin prep. A corneal shield is placed in the eye. The incision is made with fine-toothed forceps and a no. 15 knife blade or straight tenotomy scissors. The surgeon extends the

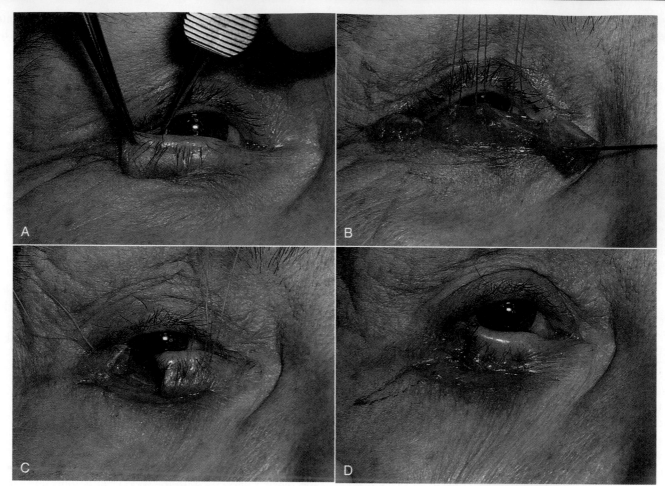

Figure 27-15   Entropion surgery. A, A marginal strip of lid is overlapped to estimate the amount of lid shortening. **B,** A tarsal incision is made and 4-0 traction sutures are placed in the conjunctiva and lower lid. The redundant tissue is removed. **C,** Double-arm sutures are passed anterior to the tarsal plate and through the skin inferior to the lashes. **D,** The lid margin is closed. *(From Tyers AG, Collin JRO: Colour atlas of ophthalmic plastic surgery, ed 2, Oxford, 2001, Butterworth-Heinemann.)*

incision using the bipolar ESU for coagulation. The scrub irrigates the cornea and blots any excess blood or irrigation fluid as necessary.

To perform the repair, the surgeon places one or more sutures of 4-0 absorbable suture swaged to a spatula needle through the tarsal plate and canthal ligament. This prevents the ectropion from recurring. The surgeon then closes the deep tissue layers with several 4-0 or 5-0 absorbable sutures. After the deeper layers have been closed, the technologist should pass several interrupted sutures of 5-0 or 6-0 silk swaged to cutting needles for skin closure. Fine-toothed tissue forceps are used in skin closure. Antibiotic ophthalmic ointment may be instilled into the eye and a soft dressing applied. Repair of an ectropion is illustrated in Figure 27-16.

Related Procedure
Blepharoplasty: Please refer to Chapter 30.

EXCISION OF A PTERYGIUM

Surgical Goal
In excision of a pterygium, the pterygium membrane is surgically removed to prevent loss of vision.

Pathology
A **pterygium** is a patch of degenerative elastic tissue that proliferates from the conjunctiva in response to chronic irritation. It appears as a white or yellowish vascular mass. The lesion begins at the medial canthus and develops laterally. Bilateral pterygium occurs in individuals with a history of extensive exposure to ultraviolet light and dust or sand. If a person is asymptomatic and vision is not impaired, treatment consists of artificial tears and vasoconstrictors. Because a pterygium usually is progressive, surgery is indicated when documented growth has occurred, the lesion is close to the visual axis, or vision is impaired.

TECHNIQUE

1   A topical or regional anesthetic is administered.
2   The pterygium is excised from the cornea.
3   The lesion is dissected and excised from adjacent structures.
4   Mitomycin or the excimer laser may be used to prevent recurrence.
5   The conjunctiva is closed.

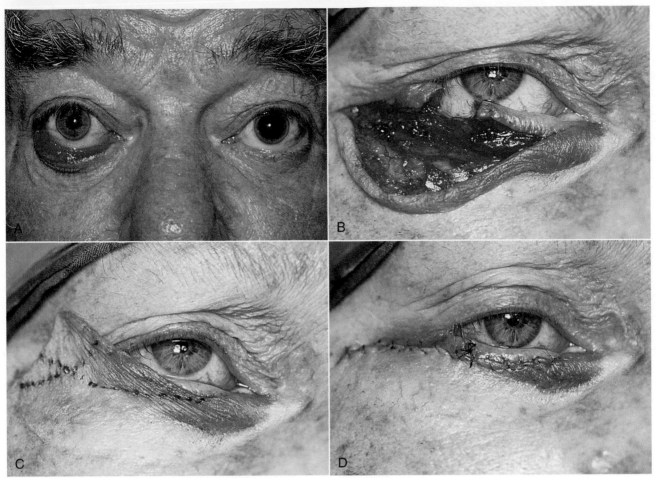

Figure 27-16 **Ectropion surgery. A,** Before surgery. **B,** A skin flap is raised and redundant tarsal tissue is removed. **C,** The area of resection is measured. **D,** Completed closure. *(From Tyers AG, Collin JRO: Colour atlas of ophthalmic plastic surgery, ed 2, Oxford, 2001, Butterworth-Heinemann.)*

Discussion

The patient is placed in the supine position, prepped, and draped for bilateral surgery. The surgeon inserts an eye speculum and instills a local anesthetic into the conjunctival tissue. The technologist should have a ½-inch (1.25-cm), 27-gauge needle available for injection.

An eye scalpel or a #15 surgical blade is used to incise the neck of the pterygium. Using Westcott scissors and toothed forceps, the surgeon incises the conjunctiva on both sides of the pterygium, including any scar tissue. The incision is extended from the limbus. The tissue is then removed and retained as a specimen.

NOTE: If recurrence is likely, mitomycin or the excimer laser may be used.

The conjunctiva is approximated with 5-0 or 6-0 nonabsorbable suture. The speculum is removed, and antibiotic ointment is instilled into the eye.

DACRYOCYSTORHINOSTOMY

Surgical Goal

Dacryocystorhinostomy is the creation of a permanent opening in the tear duct for the drainage of tears.

Pathology

Dacryocystitis is an inflammation of the lacrimal sac, causing pain, redness, and swelling at the site of the medial canthus. This condition appears as a red mass in the septo-orbital area. Pus or a mucoid material may be seen in the punctum. This condition arises from an obstruction or stricture of the nasolacrimal duct.

Lacrimal sac inflammation and infection usually are seen in two groups of patients, adults older than 40 and infants. Dacryocystorhinostomy surgery reestablishes drainage into the lacrimal duct system by enlarging the opening into the nasal sinus. A tube may be inserted to eliminate the obstruction. In infants, the lacrimal duct usually is probed and the duct irrigated.

TECHNIQUE

1 An incision is made over the lacrimal sac.
2 The muscle is dissected to the level of the periosteum.
3 The periosteum is incised.
4 A probe is inserted through the punctum.
5 The anterior lacrimal crest is perforated with a drill.
6 The lacrimal sac and nasal mucosa are incised.
7 The anterior flaps are closed.
8 The incision is closed.

Discussion

The patient is positioned supine and the head is placed on a head ring or headrest for stability. A local anesthetic (usually 2% xylocaine with epinephrine) may be infiltrated into the operative site to promote hemostasis. The nasal sinus may be packed with gauze impregnated with a topical anesthetic. The skin prep starts at the medial canthus and includes the nose, orbital rim, and cheek.

To begin the procedure, the surgeon makes an incision along the medial canthus of the nose with a # 15 blade. Small bleeding vessels are cauterized. A 4-0 suture is placed in the flap for traction. Stevens tenotomy scissors are then used to dissect the muscle until the bone is exposed. A self-retaining retractor is placed into the wound if a traction suture was not placed. The surgeon incises the periosteum and uses a Freer or periosteal elevator to elevate the periosteum, which can be retracted back with a small malleable retractor. This exposes the lacrimal sac.

The nasal packing is removed at this time for better visualization of the nasal mucosa. The sac is then separated from the fossa. A Bowman probe is inserted into the punctum to identify the location.

The technologist should prepare a power drill with a 4- to 5-mm ball burr. This is used to excise the bony lacrimal crest. During drilling, the scrub irrigates the drill site. Suction is used simultaneously to remove bits of bone. The bone excision can be enlarged with a small Kerrison rongeur.

A vertical incision perpendicular to the previous incision is made into the lacrimal sac, forming an H. The surgeon approximates the flaps of the lacrimal sac to the nasal mucosa with 4-0 or 6-0 chromic sutures. The anterior limb of the medial canthal tendon is attached to the edge of the periosteum with 6-0 chromic gut and the incision is closed with 6-0 nylon. A dacryocystorhinostomy is illustrated in Figure 27-17.

Alternative Technique

The lacrimal duct may be stented with silicone tubing. A small number of infants are born with a dacryocystocele and obstruction, causing dacryocystitis. In these cases, the punctum is dilated with a probe and fluorescein dye is used to determine patency. The probe and tube are passed down the nasolacrimal duct and retrieved via the inferior turbinate.

LACRIMAL DUCT PROBING

Surgical Goal

In lacrimal duct probing, the lacrimal duct is opened and an obstruction is removed.

Pathology

During the development of the lacrimal system, three anomalies may occur: (1) the passage may not develop fully; (2) the punctum of the lower eyelid may be absent; or (3) a congenital dacryocystocele or mucocele may occur, causing an obstruction. The most common sign of abnormality of the lacrimal system is constant tearing.

TECHNIQUE

1 A chalazion clamp is applied over the punctum.
2 A 2-mL syringe filled with saline is inserted into the canthus.
3 A Bowman probe is passed through the punctum.
4 Silicone tubing may be implanted.

Discussion

Lacrimal instruments and a soft tissue setup are used for the procedure. The patient is placed in the supine position, prepped, and draped for a unilateral eye procedure. Regional anesthesia with monitored sedation is commonly used. Pressure is applied over the upper canthus, or a chalazion clamp is applied over the punctum. The punctum is checked for patency with a 2-mL syringe and cannula. The superior punctum is dilated with Bowman probes. The probe is advanced until the obstruction is met, and then gentle pressure is exerted. The surgeon will feel a slight pop and the probe is advanced to the naris. The probe is removed, and fluorescein solution is instilled. A yellow-green solution should be suctioned through the naris via a suction cannula, indicating patency.

A silicone tube may be implanted if probing does not relieve the obstruction. The scrub may be required to thread the silicone tube over the Bowman probe, which is inserted as previously described. The probe is advanced through the naris. The tubing is removed from the probe and secured with fine suture.

MUSCLE RESECTION AND RECESSION

Surgical Goal

Muscle resection and **muscle recession** are performed to correct deviation of the eye caused by strabismus. In this procedure, the affected muscles are detached and reattached to the proper location.

Pathology

Strabismus is a condition in which the eyes are unable to focus on point because the muscles lack coordination. One eye (the fixing eye) looks directly at the object of attention, but the other eye (the deviating eye) does not.

Two surgical procedures are commonly used to treat strabismus. In lateral rectus resection, a portion of the muscle is excised and the severed end is reattached at the original site of insertion. This limits the drift of the eye. In medial rectus recession, the muscle is detached from its insertion, moved posteriorly, and reattached. This releases the eye and allows it to move farther in a lateral position.

NOTE: In some textbooks the procedure may be referred to as squint surgery.

TECHNIQUE

1 The conjunctiva is incised.
2 The muscle is measured with calipers.
3 A portion of the lateral rectus muscle is excised.
4 The medial rectus muscle is detached.
5 The muscle is moved posteriorly and reattached.
6 The conjunctiva is closed.

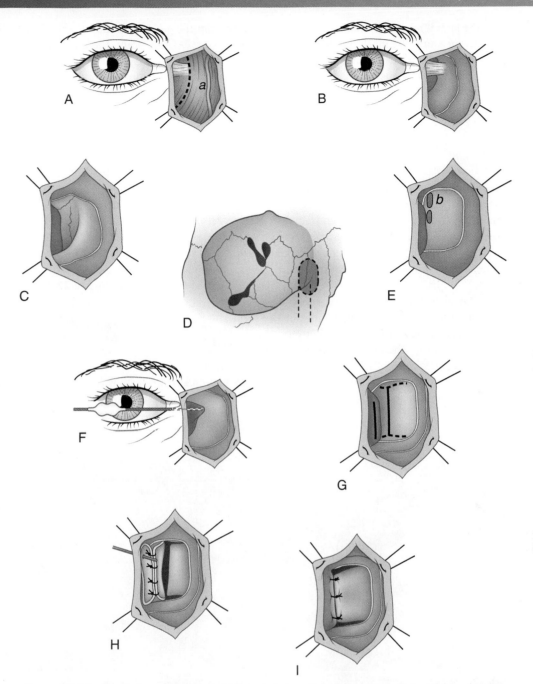

Figure 27-17 Dacryocystorhinostomy. A, The medial canthal tendon is exposed and the orbicularis muscle is separated at the point of insertion. *a.* Medical canthal tendon. Dotted line represents incision. **B,** The periosteum is incised and reflected back. **C,** The canthal tendon and lacrimal sac are retracted to expose the lacrimal fossa. **D,** Bone is removed. **E,** The bony osteum is formed. *b.* Opening (ostomy) drilled into the bony lacrimal crest. **F,** A probe is passed into the lacrimal sac. **G,** The sac and nasal mucosal incisions are drawn. **H,** The posterior mucosal flaps are sutured with the probe or catheter in place. **I,** The anterior mucosal flaps are sutured. *(Modified from McNab A: Manual of orbital and lacrimal surgery, ed 2, Oxford, 1998, Butterworth-Heinemann.)*

Discussion

The procedure requires an eye muscle setup and minor soft tissue instruments. General anesthesia is used for pediatric patients. Routine eye prep and draping are performed. A retrobulbar block may be used in addition to the general anesthetic.

During the procedure, traction on the muscles can cause a vagal response, which can result in bradycardia. If this occurs, the surgeon temporarily releases traction on the muscles.

Resection of the Lateral Muscle

To begin a lateral rectus resection, the surgeon inserts an open-ended eyelid retractor and grasps the limbus with Castroviejo forceps. With tenotomy or Westcott scissors, the surgeon then makes a buttonhole incision in the conjunctiva at the limbus. Bleeding is controlled with cautery. A muscle hook is used to separate the attachments between the Tenon capsule and the muscle sheath. An incision is made with the scissors to expose the tip of the muscle hook. Two Stevens hooks are guided down the lateral rectus muscle, exposing the sclera. A caliper is used to measure and mark the muscle.

The muscle is clamped and cut with tenotomy scissors, and a piece of the muscle is retained as a specimen. The muscle then is reattached to its original site with 6-0 double-arm, nonabsorbable synthetic suture. The conjunctiva can be closed with absorbable suture or left open, depending on the surgeon's preference.

Recession of the Medial Muscle

The procedure for medial rectus recession is identical to that for lateral rectus resection to the point of the conjunctival incision. The surgeon uses tenotomy scissors to undermine the conjunctiva. Using a previously adjusted caliper, the surgeon then measures the distance from the original insertion point to its new one. The new insertion point is indicated with a marking pen.

Two sutures of 5-0 or 6-0 absorbable material are placed at the end of the muscle but are not tied. A straight mosquito clamp or muscle clamp is placed across the muscle between the sutures and the insertion point. The clamp is allowed to remain on the muscle for up to 3 minutes to provide hemostasis. After the clamp is removed, the technologist passes a muscle hook, which is placed under the muscle to elevate it

away from the globe. The muscle then is incised with straight iris scissors. At this point, the ESU may be needed to control bleeding.

The technologist now passes an empty needle holder and smooth tissue forceps and the surgeon moves the muscle back to the scribe mark and secures it with the previously placed sutures. The conjunctival incision is closed with 5-0 or 6-0 absorbable sutures swaged to a spatula needle. Antibiotic ophthalmic ointment is instilled, and the eye is dressed with a cotton eye pad and rigid shield.

Postoperative Considerations

Patients, especially children, who undergo muscle procedures often experience postoperative nausea and vomiting, which are caused by the vagal reflex during surgery. These are treated with antiemetics and are self-limiting. Muscle resection and recession are illustrated in Figure 27-18.

PENETRATING KERATOPLASTY (CORNEAL TRANSPLANTATION)

Surgical Goal

Penetrating **keratoplasty** is full-thickness transplantation of a donor cornea to restore vision.

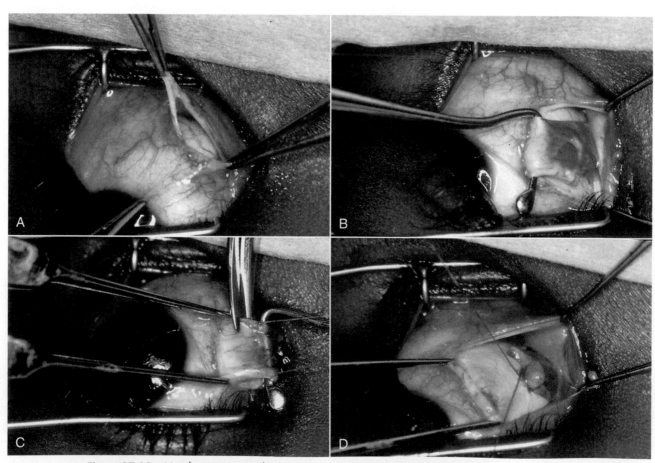

Figure 27-18   **Muscle resection and recession. A,** The sclera is incised. **B,** A muscle hook is inserted to expose the insertion of the muscle. **C,** With the muscle hook in place, the attachment is divided with Westcott scissors. **D,** Sutures are placed across the muscle attachment in its new location. *(From Jaffe N: Atlas of ophthalmic surgery, ed 2, St Louis, 1995, Mosby.)*

Pathology

The cornea may become opaque as a result of disease or injury. Chemical and thermal burns, infection, and degenerative disease are the most common causes of corneal opacification.

TECHNIQUE

1 The donor cornea is prepared.
2 A scleral support ring may be sutured for additional support of the trephine.
3 Partial penetration is performed with the sharp trephine.
4 The anterior chamber is entered and the diseased cornea is excised.
5 The cornea is lifted off and replaced with the donor cornea.
6 The corneal graft is secured with a running or interrupted suture.
7 The anterior chamber is filled.

Discussion

Two types of corneal transplantation are commonly performed: the lamellar (or partial penetrating) keratoplasty and the penetrating (or full-thickness) keratoplasty. In the partial penetrating technique, the anterior chamber is not entered, and one half to two thirds of the cornea is transplanted. In the penetrating technique, the anterior chamber is entered, and a full-thickness corneal graft is transplanted.

In full-thickness keratoplasty, a separate instrument table and Mayo setup are required to prepare and transplant the donor tissue. The two setups are isolated from each other, and instruments are not shared to prevent cross-contamination. The donor cornea is supplied through a routine community tissue bank procedure or by the health care facility's bank. Banked corneal tissue is tested for human immunodeficiency virus and hepatitis B.

The patient is placed in the supine position with the head stabilized. Before beginning the patient prep, the circulator or scrub positions the microscope above the patient and the surgeon adjusts it to his or her needs. The microscope then is locked into position and rotated out of the field.

The eye is prepped in a routine manner. If a regional block anesthetic is to be used, the postauricular area also is prepped. The patient then is draped for an eye procedure.

The donor cornea is prepared for transplantation. After determining the size of cornea required, the surgeon places the donor tissue on a silicone block and uses a disposable circular trephine to incise the cornea. The donor trephine is larger than the recipient's cornea. The donor tissue is placed in saline or the surgeon's choice of preservative and protected from contamination or injury.

The surgeon inserts a lid speculum in the patient's operative eye and positions the microscope. A scleral support ring is sutured to the cornea with 6-0 silk sutures. A calibrated marker can then be used to indicate the location of suture sites for closure. The surgeon excises the superficial corneal layer with a trephine.

A small stab incision is made into the anterior chamber with the diamond knife and extended with corneal scissors.

The surgeon gently lifts off the full-thickness cornea and passes it to the technologist as a specimen.

At this point in the procedure, the eye is extremely vulnerable to environmental contamination; this phase often is referred to as "open sky." The donor tissue is lifted out of its container with a 0.12-mm forceps and manipulated onto the recipient's eye. The surgeon uses 10-0 nonabsorbable interrupted or running sutures to close the cornea. If needed, sodium hyaluronate can be injected into the anterior chamber to replace lost fluid. The scleral ring support is removed, and antibiotic and steroid injections are given. Antibiotic ointment is applied and an eye patch with shield is secured with tape.

Full visual recovery after surgery may take up to 1 year. Most patients with successful corneal transplants enjoy good vision for many years. In some cases the body rejects the transplanted tissue, but this is a rare occurrence. Other risks of corneal transplantation include bleeding, infection of the eye, glaucoma, and swelling of the front of the eye. Corneal transplantation is illustrated in Figure 27-19.

LASIK (LASER-ASSISTED IN SITU KERATOMILEUSIS)

Surgical Goal

LASIK surgery is performed to shape the curvature of the cornea and correct a refractory problem. This procedure is performed with the excimer laser. The laser is focused on the cornea, and the stromal tissue is removed (for nearsightedness), or the cornea is reshaped.

Pathology

The shape of the optic globe and cornea determine the eye's visual acuity (see Refraction). The shape can change through development, or an incorrectly shaped globe may occur at birth. This results in an incorrect focal distance and loss of image clarity. If the anterior-posterior distance of the globe is too short, images that are close are blurred because the focal point is behind the retina; this condition is called *hyperopia*, or farsightedness. If the anterior-posterior distance is too long (i.e., an elongated globe), the focal point lies in front of the retina, resulting in blurred vision of distant objects; this condition is called *myopia*, or nearsightedness. A third condition, *astigmatism*, results from an uneven curvature of the refractive medium caused by defects of the cornea, lens, or retina.

TECHNIQUE

1 The surgeon tests the microkeratome before use.
2 An eyelid speculum is inserted.
3 Corneal alignment is marked.
4 The microkeratome is inserted and the corneal flap is created.
5 The excimer laser is used to ablate the stromal bed.
6 The corneal flap is refloated into the correct position.
7 The flap is sealed after 2 to 3 minutes.
8 Antibiotic-steroid ointment is instilled and the flap alignment is rechecked in 20 to 30 minutes.

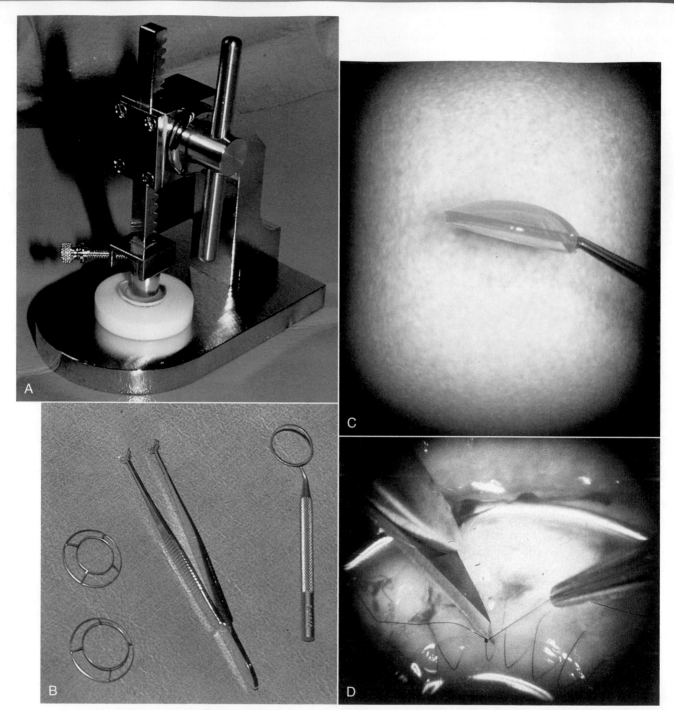

Figure 27-19 Corneal transplantation. **A,** Bourne punch, a mechanical punch that uses disposable trephines on the donor tissue. **B,** Stabilization instruments. *Left to right,* Flieringa rings, Flieringa-LeGrand fixation forceps, Thornton fixation ring. **D,** Excision of the host button by suction trephine. **E,** A running suture is placed to secure the transplant. *(From Jaffe N: Atlas of ophthalmic surgery, ed, 2, St Louis, 1995, Mosby.)*

Discussion

The patient is positioned under the laser and prepped in routine manner. The head is realigned on a head ring under the laser, and a topical anesthetic is instilled into the eye. All instrumentation is tested, and particular attention is paid to the microkeratome to prevent errors.

The surgeon inserts the speculum into the eye, making sure the eyelashes are out of the operative view. The lid and lashes may be taped to the drape. Corneal alignment marks are placed on the cornea. A tonometer is used to verify the IOP of the eye, and a suction ring is placed on the eye to keep it immobilized. The eye is irrigated with BSS.

The microkeratome is inserted through the suction ring and activated. The corneal flap is incised and retracted with a spatula, and the patient is instructed to fix her or his gaze on a pilot light. The surgeon verifies the laser alignment for the last time and then proceeds to ablate the stroma. The stroma is dried at completion, and the flap is folded back over the stroma with an irrigation cannula. The flap is irrigated to remove debris and realigned. Antibiotic drops are instilled and the flap is left to seal for 2 to 3 minutes. An additional assessment is made after 20 to 30 minutes. The eye then is dressed with a protective shield.

Patients must avoid activities that require bending or kneeling for the first week after surgery. Surgical complications occur in 3% to 6% of patients. Complications include visual effects, such as halos, double vision (ghosting), loss of contrast, persistent pain, and glare.

EXTRACAPSULAR CATARACT EXTRACTION (PHACOEMULSIFICATION)

Surgical Goal

Phacoemulsification is the fragmentation of tissue by ultrasonic vibration. This technique is the most common form of cataract removal. The goal of cataract extraction is to remove an opaque lens (cataract) and replace it with an IOL implant to restore vision.

Pathology

A **cataract** is opacity of the lens. The disease has many causes, including genetic defect, injury, overexposure to ultraviolet light, metabolic disease (e.g., diabetes), and age. Certain drugs, such as corticosteroids and busulfan, are known to cause cataracts. Age-related cataracts are the most common type, because the composition of the lens changes with age and as metabolic changes occur. This leads to progressive loss of transparency and visual distortion, glare, and myopia.

TECHNIQUE

1 A traction suture is placed in the superior rectus.
2 A conjunctival incision is made at the limbus.
3 The anterior chamber is inflated with Healon.
4 A capsulorrhexis is performed.
5 Balanced salt solution (BSS) is used to irrigate the eye to free the lens.
6 The phacoemulsification probe is introduced, and the lens is emulsified.
7 Residual fragments of lens are removed.
8 Healon is used to inflate the chamber.
9 An intraocular lens is implanted.
10 The incision may be sutured or left open to heal.

Discussion

Cataract extraction most often is performed using the extracapsular cataract extraction technique. This is removal of the lens only, leaving the lens capsule intact. Historically, intracapsular cataract extraction has been performed with a cryoprobe to remove both the lens and the capsule. This procedure requires enzymatic destruction of the zonules that attach the lens. The intracapsular method has been largely replaced by the extracapsular technique. Current technology allows the phacoemulsifier to be tuned to a frequency that destroys only the target tissue. After the tissue is fragmented and liquefied, it can be safely aspirated.

The patient is placed in the supine position with a headrest or phacovacuum pillow to immobilize the head. During the prep, several drops of povidone-iodine, diluted according to the surgeon's orders, are instilled into the eye for antibacterial effect. The patient is draped for an eye procedure with a head drape and adhesive eye drape. The patient receives conscious sedation or a combination of topical and regional anesthetics.

To begin the procedure, the surgeon places a **bridle suture** of 3-0 or 4-0 silk in the superior rectus muscle and creates a conjunctival flap with Westcott scissors and toothed forceps. A diamond knife or keratome is then used to make a stab incision at the limbus into the cornea. This creates a triangular cut. A second incision is made into the anterior chamber, and a viscoelastic substance such as sodium hyaluronate (Healon) is injected. A *capsulotomy* (incision into the capsule) is performed with a cystotome or capsulorrhexis forceps. The surgeon mobilizes the lens by instilling BSS into the eye with a 27-gauge needle.

The phacoemulsification probe is then introduced. Many surgeons groove the nucleus of the cataract and separate it into four quadrants before proceeding. The phacoemulsification probe fragments and emulsifies most of the lens. However, some small pieces may remain. The surgeon manipulates the probe toward the edges to aspirate the remaining pieces. This is called "polishing the posterior capsule." If the probe is placed in the center, the vitreous may be brought forward from the posterior capsule. This is a complication of the surgery and may necessitate an anterior vitrectomy.

The scleral incision is enlarged, and an IOL is manipulated into the posterior chamber of the capsule. Healon is injected into the chamber and onto the lens. The incision either is closed with 6-0 or 7-0 suture or is left open to heal. Many styles of IOLs are available, but the design primarily consists of a central biconvex optic and two tabs to maintain the lens in position. The newest posterior chamber lenses are made of flexible materials, such as silicone and acrylic polymers. This allows the lenses to be folded, and the size of the incision to be reduced. Multifocal optics are available; the goal of this design is to provide the patient with good near and distance vision without the need for glasses. Cataract extraction is illustrated in Figure 27-20.

ANTERIOR VITRECTOMY

Surgical Goal

An anterior vitrectomy is performed to remove the vitreous from the anterior chamber.

Pathology

An anterior vitrectomy may be performed for a variety of conditions, such as opacity of the anterior segment of the vitreous and loss of vitreous during cataract extraction. This is a complication in which rupture of the posterior capsule allows vitreous to prolapse into the anterior chamber. The phacoemulsification equipment can quickly be adapted to

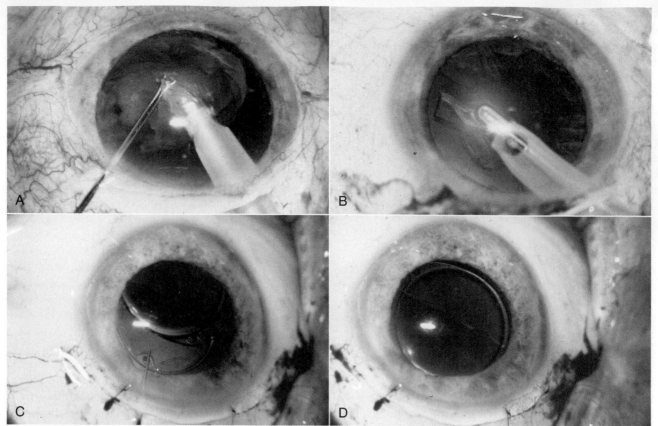

Figure 27-20 **Extracapsular cataract extraction. A,** The nucleus is displaced toward the 6 o'clock position with a bent-tip needle; this is done inside the capsular bag. **B,** Irrigation-aspiration of the residual cortex is performed inside the capsular bag, and the posterior capsule is polished. **C,** The loop is passed under the superior capsular flap. **D,** The lens now is completely within the capsular bag. The opening in the anterior capsule is shown. *(From Jaffe N: Atlas of ophthalmic surgery, ed 2, St Louis, 1995, Mosby.)*

vitrectomy mode. Surgery for removal of vitreous in the anterior chamber is described here.

TECHNIQUE

1 A vitrector, infusion line, and suction line are attached to the phacoemulsification machine.
2 The vitrectomy is performed.
3 A spatula is placed in the anterior chamber to check for vitreous strands.
4 An anterior chamber lens is placed in the eye.
5 The conjunctiva is closed.

Discussion

Once the posterior chamber rupture is assessed, the phacoemulsification instrument is stopped and only the irrigation cannula is used. The primary corneal incision may be closed to prevent loss of vitreous. Usually a stab incision is made at the limbus to allow entry of the vitreous cutter. The irrigation cannula is maintained above the vitreous cutter. A cyclodialysis spatula is used to sweep the vitreous strands posteriorly. The vitreous can also be teased through the incision using a Wek-Cell sponge and detached with Wescott scissors. This

process is called *manual vitrectomy.* The anterior chamber is reformed with viscoelastic solution. The original incision can then be opened and the IOL inserted. Finally the conjunctiva is closed using 10-0 nylon suture.

After the surgery, patients use eye drops for several weeks or longer to allow the surface of the eye to heal. Heavy lifting is avoided for several weeks. Along with the usual complications of surgery, such as infection, vitrectomy can result in retinal detachment. More common complications are high IOP, bleeding in the eye, and recurrent cataracts.

SCLERAL BUCKLING PROCEDURE FOR DETACHED RETINA

Surgical Goal

Scleral buckling surgery is performed when the sensory layer of the retina becomes separated from the pigment epithelial layer. The surgical goal is to restore the layers to their normal positions and prevent blindness.

Pathology

The vitreous normally adheres to the retina in several locations. A tear in the retina causes sudden painless loss of vision, or "shadowing," which appears as a curtain that descends over

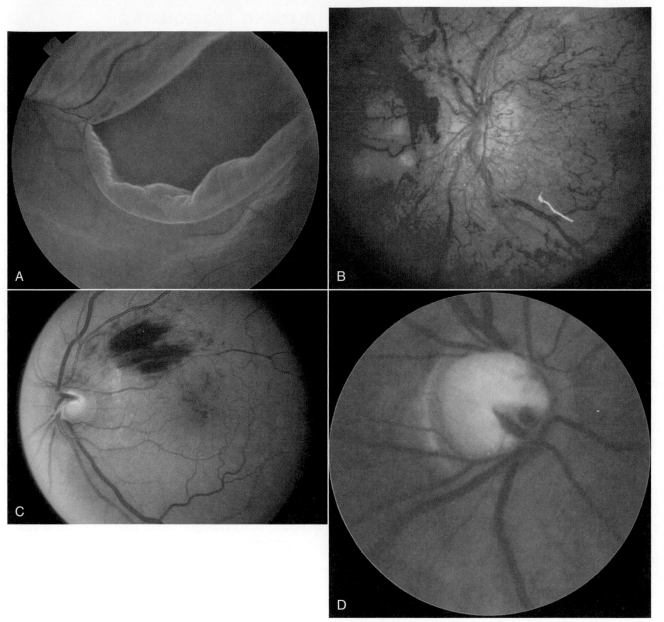

Figure 27-21 **Pathological conditions of the retina. A,** Retinal tear and detachment. **B,** Diabetic retinopathy, showing hemorrhages. **C,** Hypertensive retinopathy, showing the "flame hemorrhages" characteristic of the condition. **D,** Glaucoma (note the cupping of the optic disc caused by intraocular pressure). *(From Thibodeau G, Patton K: Anatomy and physiology, ed 6, St Louis, 2007, Mosby.)*

the patient's field of vision. Light flashes and "floaters" often accompany the vision loss.

A tear in the retina (called a *rhegmatogenous detachment*) creates a passage for the vitreous to seep between the pigment epithelium and the neural layer of the retina. This seepage separates the layers and may extend the tear. A vitreous tear usually is caused by aging, because the vitreous begins to shrink, exerting traction on the retina. Detachment also may be caused by trauma or diabetes mellitus. Retinal tears and other pathological conditions of the retina are shown in Figure 27-21.

TECHNIQUE

1 The Tenon capsule is separated from the sclera with blunt dissection.
2 Diathermy is applied to the area of detachment or tear.
3 Sutures are placed in the sclera.
4 The buckling components are implanted.
5 The site is examined under the indirect headlight for the position of the retinal detachment and break.
6 Intravitreous gas may be injected.
7 The Tenon capsule and the conjunctiva are closed.

Discussion

Retinal detachment requires immediate repair. Several techniques are used to repair detached tissue. A common technique is to produce adhesions between the layers using **cryotherapy** (freezing of the tissue) or **diathermy** (mild heat created by a diathermy unit or laser). Neither treatment damages the eye, and both create points of scar tissue. This is followed by immediate scleral buckling, in which a Silastic or foam band is attached to the sclera. Several synthetic "buckles" are placed over the band, causing it to indent. This technique puts the tissue in close contact with the retina during healing.

Another common technique is to perform a vitrectomy in conjunction with scleral buckling. In this procedure, the vitreous gel is replaced with Healon or gas through a small puncture wound. This method is used to eliminate traction and tearing on the retina. Two puncture sites are made in the sclera to accommodate the microinstruments used to perform cryotherapy or diathermy. The eye remains pressurized throughout the microsurgical procedure. The procedure described here is for scleral buckling and cryotherapy.

The patient is placed in the supine position, prepped, and draped for an eye procedure. Conscious sedation is used for the surgery unless the procedure is expected to last longer than 2 hours. A retrobulbar block also may be used.

An open-ended retractor is placed in the eye. Toothed forceps and Westcott scissors are used to make two incisions in the Tenon capsule, one under each rectus muscle. Some surgeons place two 4-0 bridle sutures under the rectus muscles for traction. The bridle suture is left long and used to retract the globe for access to the posterolateral surface.

Using the diathermy unit, the surgeon makes many small burn marks or "spot welds" over the area of detachment. The diathermy electrode produces a high-frequency electrical current that causes mild burning. If the cryosurgical probe is used, the detached area is treated in the same manner.

The assistant steadies the eye by holding the bridle sutures while the surgeon compresses the globe with cotton-tipped applicators. The sclera then is approximated with fine suture of 4-0 Prolene. A double-arm suture of Dacron or other synthetic material is placed in the sclera and secured over Silastic sponges. This compresses the eye inward at the area of detachment. A Silastic band may be placed 360 degrees around the eye and a scleral buckle sutured into place under the muscles. Sutures are secured to the buckle so that it remains in place.

Intravitreous Gas Injection

Intravitreous gas injection is the injection of intraocular gas through a handheld syringe. The gas infusion exerts pressure on the retina while subretinal fluid is reabsorbed and scarification takes place. The gases include sulfur hexafluoride (SF_6) and perfluoropropane (C_3F_8).

The scleral buckling procedure is illustrated in Figure 27-22.

FILTERING PROCEDURES AND TRABECULECTOMY

Surgical Goal

A **trabeculectomy** is performed to create a channel from which the aqueous humor may drain from the anterior chamber. This procedure is performed for the treatment of glaucoma.

Pathology

Glaucoma is a group of diseases characterized by optic nerve damage and visual field loss. In the past, glaucoma was defined by an IOP above the normal range in association with nerve damage. However, more recent definitions include cases in which IOP is normal. In most types, IOP is elevated and the unrelieved pressure can result in ischemia of the optic nerve, which leads to progressive blindness. The IOP is normally maintained by the aqueous humor, which is secreted by the ciliary epithelium (posterior chamber) and drained between the lens and iris, through the pupil into the anterior chamber. Fluid exits through the trabecular network and the canal of Schlemm. The balance in pressure is maintained by the rate of secretion and drainage. A number of pathological conditions can disturb this balance. In nearly all cases of glaucoma, the problem is with drainage rather than overproduction of aqueous humor (Figure 27-23).

There are many different types of glaucoma. The most common are described below[1]:

- *Primary angle closure glaucoma*: This type of glaucoma accounts for 30% of all cases. The incidence is higher in women. A sudden rise in IOP is caused by total blockage or obstruction of the aqueous humor at the root of the iris (the limbal drainage system). This is considered a medical emergency, because blindness may result if the blockage is not relieved.
- *Primary open angle glaucoma*: This is a chronic disease occurring in both eyes. It develops in the middle years or later. In this condition, the outflow of aqueous humor is obstructed in the trabecular meshwork, which can be caused by different factors.
- *Normal tension glaucoma*: This is a subtype of open angle glaucoma in which IOP is normal. There is retinal damage and visual field loss with migraine and optic disc hemorrhage.
- *Congenital glaucoma*: In congenital glaucoma, the fluid drainage system is abnormal at birth. The infant's eye distends, and corneal haziness occurs. Symptoms include light sensitivity and excessive tearing. Surgery is indicated to prevent blindness.

TECHNIQUE

1. The limbus is incised.
2. A scleral flap is created.
3. A small portion of the trabecular meshwork is excised and removed.
4. An iridectomy may be performed.
5. The conjunctiva is closed.
6. The anterior chamber is reinflated as needed.

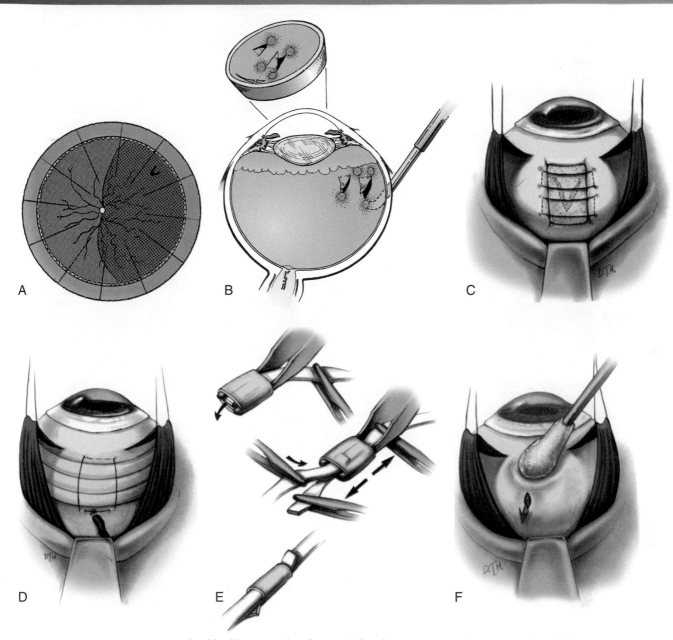

Figure 27-22 Scleral buckling procedure for retinal detachment. **A,** A retinal tear at equator of globe at the 1:30 o'clock position. **B,** The surgeon visualizes the field and places the electrode beneath the retinal tear; a burn mark is made on the sclera at the site of the retinal tear with the diathermy electrode. **C,** A sponge is sutured in place over the treated site of the retinal tear. **D,** A band and tire are used to encircle the eye. **E,** A Watzke silicone sleeve is placed to secure the encircling band. **F,** An incision is made in the sclera and a fine incision is made in the choroids to allow subretinal fluid to drain. *(From Ryan S, Ogden TE, editors: Retina, ed 2, St Louis, 1994, Mosby.)*

Discussion

The patient is prepped and draped in a routine manner. To begin the procedure, the surgeon inserts a lid speculum. Size 4-0 bridle sutures may be placed in the superior rectus muscle. The conjunctiva is incised at the limbus with toothed forceps and the knife. The Tenon capsule is separated from the sclera with Westcott scissors in the direction of the limbus. This creates a conjunctival flap.

The limbal area is gently scraped with a Beaver blade to remove any blood clots. This technique prevents accidental puncture of the conjunctiva. The sclera then is cauterized in

the shape of the flap. The surgeon uses the Beaver blade to make an incision in the sclera, following the outlines of the cautery. Dissection of the scleral flap starts at the apex and extends upward toward the iris.

A stab wound is made through the cornea to drain the aqueous humor. This incision is self-sealing and can be used later to reinflate the anterior chamber. If necessary, the scleral flap is retracted, and Vannas scissors are used to excise a portion of the trabecular meshwork.

A complication of the procedure may occur at this point; that is, the iris may spontaneously prolapse into the wound.

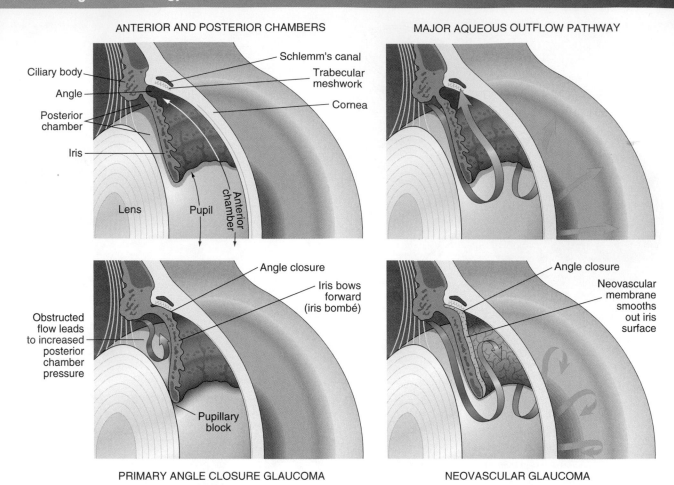

ANTERIOR AND POSTERIOR CHAMBERS

MAJOR AQUEOUS OUTFLOW PATHWAY

Ciliary body

Angle

Posterior chamber

Iris

Lens

Pupil

Anterior chamber

Schlemm's canal

Trabecular meshwork

Cornea

Obstructed flow leads to increased posterior chamber pressure

Angle closure

Iris bows forward (iris bombé)

Pupillary block

PRIMARY ANGLE CLOSURE GLAUCOMA

Angle closure

Neovascular membrane smooths out iris surface

NEOVASCULAR GLAUCOMA

Figure 27-23 **Pathology of glaucoma.** *Upper left,* A normal eye, showing the drainage pathway of the aqueous humor. *Lower left,* Primary closure glaucoma, in which the iris is in close contact with the lens. Increased pressure obstructs the trabecular meshwork. *Lower right,* Contraction of the myofibroblasts in the vascular membrane causes the iris to obstruct drainage. *(From Kumar V, Abbas A, Fausto N: Robbins and Cotran pathologic basis of disease, ed 7, Philadelphia, 2004, WB Saunders.)*

In such cases, an iridectomy is performed. The surgeon grasps the iris with forceps and removes a portion, taking care not to damage the ciliary body.

In an uncomplicated procedure, BSS is instilled into the anterior chamber to reinflate it. The scleral flap is closed with 10-0 nylon sutures. The conjunctiva and Tenon capsule are approximated with 8-0 absorbable suture. BSS then is instilled into the anterior chamber. An eye sponge is placed over the incision site to check for leakage. Subconjunctival antibiotics and steroids are injected, and antibacterial ointments are instilled into the eye.

Adjunctive Chemotherapy

If the filtering procedure is at risk of failure or if a low IOP is indicated, the surgeon may use a chemotherapeutic agent, such as 5-fluorouracil (5-FU), and mitomycin. If this is the case, a sponge soaked with the agent is placed at the surgical site for approximately 1 minute. After removal of the sponge, the entire field is irrigated with BSS, and the instruments that were exposed to mitomycin are removed from the field. Because of the potential toxicity of the drugs, protocols for their disposal and for instrument decontamination are required in most health care facilities.

The trabeculectomy will fail if a flat bleb does not form in the first postoperative days. If a bleb leak develops, a bandage contact lens may be inserted and repair may be necessary. Cataract formation may occur as a result of the trabeculectomy, and additional surgery may be required.

The trabeculectomy procedure is illustrated in Figure 27-24.

ARGON LASER TRABECULOPLASTY

Surgical Goal

In argon laser trabeculoplasty, the argon laser is used to shrink collagen and stretch the canal of Schlemm, thereby expanding the canal, increasing drainage, and reducing IOP.

Pathology

Glaucoma is classified as open angle or closed angle and then further categorized as primary or secondary. Argon laser trabeculoplasty is indicated for primary and secondary open angle glaucoma. Primary open angle glaucoma has a genetic component and is more common in individuals with diabetes and African Americans. Secondary open angle glaucoma is differentiated by the obstruction of the outflow of aqueous

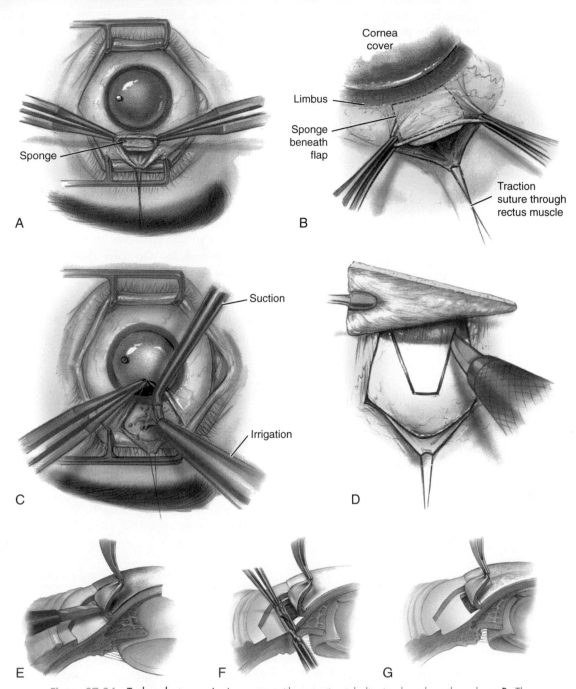

Figure 27-24 **Trabeculectomy.** **A,** A sponge with an antimetabolite is placed on the sclera. **B,** The sclera is drawn over the sponge. **C,** Irrigation. **D,** Scleral flaps are created. **E,** An incision is made into the anterior chamber. **F, G,** A fistula is created by the removal of a flap from the limbus. *(From Rothrock JC: Alexander's care of the patient in surgery, ed 17, St Louis, 2007, Mosby.)*

humor, which causes an increase in IOP (see earlier, Filtering Procedures and Trabeculectomy).

Discussion

The surgeon makes a superior conjunctival incision and dissects the conjunctiva up to the level of the limbus. The sclera is incised, and a flap is dissected. An incision is made into the anterior chamber, and the trabecular meshwork is exposed.

Laser burns are placed at 180 to 360 degrees on the trabecular meshwork. An indirect gonioscopy lens with an antireflective laser coating is used for the procedure. The laser

TECHNIQUE

1 A conjunctival incision is made, and then another incision is made into the anterior chamber.
2 The trabecular meshwork is exposed.
3 An indirect gonioscopy lens with an antireflective laser coating is used for the procedure.
4 Laser burns are placed at 180 to 360 degrees on the trabecular meshwork.
5 The surgeon places 20 to 25 laser burns in each quadrant.

burns are evenly spaced and applied to the anterior portion of the trabecular meshwork. The surgeon places 20 to 25 laser burns in each quadrant.

A laser spot is a burn of 50 mm applied for 0.1 second. Laser energy of 800 to 1200 mV with an argon blue-green laser is recommended. After the procedure, a drop of epinephrine is instilled into the eye. Steroid therapy is started postoperatively.

Complications of laser trabeculoplasty are rare. The most common complication of laser surgery for glaucoma is an increase in the pressure in the eyes. This complication can be prevented by the use of apraclonidine or brimonidine before or after laser surgery, especially in people with a high IOP before laser surgery.

ORBITAL DECOMPRESSION

Surgical Goal

In orbital decompression, one or more bony sections of the orbital cavity are removed to reduce pressure on the optic nerve. This decompresses the globe and allows the eyelids to approximate normally.

Pathology

Orbital decompression most often is performed to treat hyperthyroidism (Graves disease). In this disease, the globe is displaced and protrudes anteriorly, preventing the eyelids from closing. Another indication for orbital decompression is pressure on the optic nerve caused by tumor or swelling.

TECHNIQUE

1 The lower lid is incised.
2 The orbital rim is exposed and the periosteum is incised.
3 The orbital floor is exposed.
4 The infraorbital nerve is located, and bone is removed with rongeurs or chisels.
5 The incision is closed.

Discussion

The patient is placed in the supine position, prepped, and draped. A general anesthetic is administered. The lower lid and anterior orbit are injected with xylocaine with epinephrine to maintain hemostasis.

The most common approach to orbital decompression is through the lower lid. A horizontal incision is made approximately 2 mm under the eyelashes, extending from the punctum to the medial canthus.

The orbital rim is exposed and the incision line is drawn with a marker. The lower lid is incised with tenotomy or Westcott scissors to the bony rim. A malleable retractor is used to displace the globe. This exposes the orbital floor and nerve bundle. An osteotome or power drill is used to incise through the orbital floor. When the drill is in use, the technologist must provide irrigation over the drilling site. The bone is removed in small pieces with a Kerrison or other small-tipped rongeur. This exposes the nerve and vessels across the antrum.

Incisions are made on each side of the inferior rectus muscle with Stevens tenotomy scissors. The periosteum is closed with 4-0 chromic gut. The wound is closed in two layers. The muscle is approximated with 5-0 chromic gut and the skin is closed with 6-0 nylon.

Complications of traditional methods of orbital decompression vary with the approach. They include diplopia, leakage of cerebrospinal fluid, oral-antral fistula, nasolacrimal duct obstruction, and scarring.

ENUCLEATION

Surgical Goal

Enucleation is complete removal of the eyeball (globe). **Evisceration** is a similar procedure in which the contents of the eye are removed, but the outer shell of the sclera and the muscle attachments are left intact.

Pathology

Enucleation is performed to treat intraocular malignancy (e.g., retinoblastoma, melanoma), a penetrating ocular wound, a painful blind eye, or an eye that is blind and painless but disfigured. An artificial prosthesis may be inserted to replace the globe.

A similar procedure is used for a severely traumatized eye.

TECHNIQUE

1 The conjunctiva is incised.
2 The four rectus muscles are identified, clamped, and severed.
3 The rectus and inferior oblique muscles are anastomosed.
4 The optic nerve is severed.
5 A sphere is introduced into the socket.
6 The conjunctiva and Tenon capsule are sutured over the sphere.
7 A tarsorrhaphy is performed (the eyelids are sutured together).

Discussion

Enucleation usually is a psychologically traumatic experience for the patient. Many hospitals now perform this surgery in an outpatient setting. This increases the anxiety and grief experienced by the patient and family, because little professional support is available after the surgery. Great care is taken to provide a comforting environment in the operating room. All team members must be sensitive to the psychosocial and emotional effects of losing an eye. General anesthesia is preferred, for obvious psychological reasons. However, hospital protocol may require a regional anesthetic with monitored sedation.

After enucleation, an implant is inserted to shape the orbital cavity. This implant is called a *sphere*. A *conformer* is placed over the sphere and covers its surface. The conformer and sphere are replaced by an artificial eye after the wound has healed. Orbital implants are designed to allow blood vessels to infiltrate the implant material. Porous polyethylene and hydroxyapatite are the most common implant materials.

The patient is placed in the supine position and prepared for routine eye surgery, as previously discussed. A closed eye retractor is placed in the eye. A circular incision is made as close to the limbus as possible. This conserves as much conjunctiva as possible for closure later in the procedure. The incision is made with a #15 blade or with iris scissors. The surgeon undermines the conjunctiva and Tenon capsule and prepares to sever the rectus and oblique muscles from the globe.

Because the rectus muscles will be sutured to the inferior oblique muscles, both muscles are tagged with sutures of silk or 4-0 or 5-0 absorbable synthetic material. The superior oblique muscle is severed and allowed to retract. The surgeon then severs the previously tagged inferior oblique muscle, secures it to the lateral rectus muscle with 4-0 sutures, and pulls the globe anteriorly (forward).

The technologist should have a muscle hook available at this time. The surgeon passes the hook around the globe to ensure that all connections except the optic nerve have been severed. A Mayo clamp is placed across the optic nerve for 30 to 60 seconds. The clamp is then removed, and curved enucleation scissors are used to sever the optic nerve across the area crushed by the Mayo clamp. This frees the globe, which is passed to the technologist as a specimen. If any intraocular contents have been extruded into the socket, they must be cleaned out with irrigation solution and a 4×4 gauze sponge. Hemostasis is secured with pressure and the ESU.

The optic nerve is cut beyond the implant. The technologist should have several sizes of implant spheres available from which the surgeon can choose the correct size. Adult sizes usually range from 14 to 18 mm.

The surgeon selects the implant and conformer, and the sphere is introduced into the orbit. A sphere introducer may be used to place the implant. The rectus muscles are sutured to the sphere with 4-0 or 5-0 absorbable sutures. Next, the Tenon capsule is pulled over the sphere and sutured into place with scleral biting forceps and 4-0 absorbable synthetic suture. A purse-string suture may be used for this step. The conjunctiva is closed with 5-0 sutures.

The conformer may be placed over the sphere. The silk retraction sutures are removed, and antibiotic ointment is instilled into the eye. The eyelids are then sutured together. The eye is dressed with a soft pad secured with tape. The patient will return for additional surgery to replace the damaged eye with an orbital implant—usually in about 6 weeks, when healing is complete.

ORBITAL EXENTERATION

Surgical Goal

Orbital **exenteration** is the removal of the entire eye and orbital contents, including the eyelids, ocular muscles, and orbital fat. This procedure is performed for the treatment of cancer.

Pathology

Orbital exenteration generally is performed to treat cancers and infections or to treat severe orbital pain and deformities. Because this is a radical procedure and because of the relatively poor reconstruction alternatives, orbital exenteration is performed only after all other therapies have failed.

The number of orbital exenteration procedures performed has declined over the years. In the past, squamous cell cancers and melanomas were treated with exenteration, but the preferred treatment for these cancers has become local resection without exenteration, as long as the tumor remains superficial.

Orbital exenteration may also be required for radical treatment of fungal infection involving the paranasal sinuses and extending into the orbit.

TECHNIQUE

1 The skin, orbital fat, and periosteum are removed with a knife or ESU.
2 Soft tissue is separated from the circumference of the bony orbit.
3 Reconstruction is performed.

Discussion

General anesthesia is used for exenteration. The patient is prepped and draped for an eye procedure. To begin the procedure, the surgeon sews the eyelids closed, and the sutures are left long for retraction. The bony orbit then is marked with a skin scribe.

The knife or ESU is used to remove the skin, orbital fat, and periosteum down to the bony orbit. Depending on the extent of the tumor, some skin and muscle may be saved for reconstruction. Otherwise, dissection of the tumor is continued until the frozen section margins are clear of disease.

A ribbon retractor and periosteal elevator are used to separate soft tissue from the circumference of the bony orbit. Careful dissection at the superior area of the orbit is completed.

The nasolacrimal duct and drainage system and part of the nose may be removed at this stage of the procedure. The enucleation scissors are used to separate the orbital contents from the bony orbital rim. The specimen is removed, and the orbital cavity is packed with moist gauze to achieve hemostasis. After 5 to 10 minutes, the packs are removed and any bleeding vessels are controlled with the ESU. Any additional excision needed for tumor removal is performed at this time, until the margins are free of tumor.

A number of techniques can be used for reconstruction:
- A split-thickness skin graft may be used for closure.
- A dermal graft can be substituted for skin grafts.
- Regional flaps and composite grafts may be used for reconstruction.

KEY CONCEPTS

- Knowledge of key anatomical structures of the eye is necessary to understand a surgical procedure.
- Familiarity with diagnostic procedures of the eye contributes to an understanding of the pathology involved and appropriate patient care.
- Most surgical procedures of the eye are performed using the operating microscope, which requires distinct techniques for handling and passing microinstruments.

- Familiarity with common surgical procedures of the eye is necessary for safe handling of instruments and equipment, and for assisting in eye surgery.

REVIEW QUESTIONS

1. Ophthalmic surgery requires that the patient be very still during the procedure. What steps and precautions are used to ensure this?
2. What is the rationale for documenting lens implants in the patient's medical record?
3. List the categories of drugs commonly used in ophthalmic surgery. Give an example of each.
4. Why do children experience nausea following strabismus surgery?
5. What methods might the surgical technologist use to keep ophthalmic needles from becoming caught in instruments and drapes?
6. What procedure is used for verification of the correct site and side in ophthalmic surgery? Describe or list the steps of the procedure.
7. Explain the anatomical locations of the anterior and posterior chambers.
8. List the ophthalmic procedures discussed in this chapter that might be performed as emergencies. Explain briefly *why* each example might be an emergency.
9. One of the responsibilities of the surgical technologist during ophthalmic surgery is to frequently irrigate the operative site. Describe the typical appearance of dehydrated eye tissues (e.g., cornea, sclera, conjunctiva). How should the tissues appear when irrigated frequently?
10. Define *trabeculectomy*.

REFERENCE

1. Yanoff M, Duker J, Augsburger J, et al: *Ophthalmology*, ed 2, St Louis, 2004, Mosby.

BIBLIOGRAPHY

Foster CS, Azar DT, Claes HD, editors: *Smolin and Thoft's the cornea: scientific foundations and clinical practice*, ed 4, Philadelphia, 2005, Lippincott Williams & Wilkins.

Riordan-Eva P, Whitcher J: *Vaughan and Asbury's general ophthalmology*, ed 17, New York, 2008, McGraw-Hill.

Tyers AG, Collin JRO: *Colour atlas of ophthalmic plastic surgery*, ed 2, Oxford, 2001, Butterworth-Heinemann.

Yanoff M, Duker J, Augsburger J, et al: *Ophthalmology*, ed 2, St Louis, 2004, Mosby.

Surgery of the Ear, Nose, Pharynx, and Larynx

28

CHAPTER OUTLINE

LEARNING OBJECTIVES

After studying this chapter the reader will be able to:
1. Identify the key anatomical structures of the ear
2. Discuss diagnostic procedures of the ear
3. Discuss key aspects of case planning, including instrumentation, for ear procedures
4. Describe common procedures of the ear
5. Identify the key anatomical structures of the nose
6. Discuss diagnostic procedures of the nose

7. Discuss key aspects of case planning, including instrumentation, for nasal procedures
8. Describe common procedures of the nose
9. Identify the key anatomical structures of the neck
11. Discuss key aspects of case planning, including instrumentation, for neck procedures
12. Describe common procedures of the neck

TERMINOLOGY

Cerumen: A substance produced by the cerumen glands of the ear (i.e., ear wax).

Cholesteatoma: A benign tumor of the middle ear caused by shedding of keratin in chronic otitis media.

Effusion: Fluid in the middle ear.

Epistaxis: Bleeding arising from the nasal cavity.

Evert: To turn outward or inside out.

Hypertrophy: Enlargement of an organ or tissue.

Nasolaryngoscope: A flexible endoscope that is passed through the nose to visualize the larynx.

Ossicles: The bones of the middle ear that conduct sound (i.e., the malleus, incus, and stapes).

Ototoxic: A substance that can injure the ear.

Packing: A method of applying a dressing to a body cavity. In nasal procedures, ¼- or ½-inch (0.63- or 1.25-cm) gauze strips are inserted into the nasal cavity to absorb drainage, control bleeding, or expose the mucosa to topical medication. "Packing" a wound may refer to any dressing that is introduced into an anatomical space or cavity.

Papilloma: A benign epithelial tumor characterized by a branching or lobular tumor (also called a *papillary tumor*).

Paranasal sinuses: Air cells surrounding or on the periphery of the nasal cavities. These are the maxillary, ethmoid, sphenoid, and frontal sinuses.

Paresis: Paralysis of a structure (e.g., vocal cord paresis).

Perforation: A defect in the tympanic membrane caused by trauma or infection.

Phonation: Vibration of the vocal cords during speaking or vocalization.

Polyp: Excessive proliferation of the mucosal epithelium.

Sensorineural hearing loss: Hearing impairment arising from the cochlea, auditory nerve, or central nervous system.

TM: The tympanic membrane.

Transsphenoidal: Literally, "across or through the sphenoid bone." Surgery of the pituitary gland may be performed by approaching it through the sphenoid bone.

Tympanostomy tube: A tube that is placed in a myringotomy to produce aeration of the middle ear.

SECTION I: THE EAR

INTRODUCTION

Otorhinolaryngology is the medical specialty concerned with the ear, nose, and throat. Surgery of the ear includes procedures of the outer, middle, and inner ear. Procedures are performed under microscopy.

Many patients undergoing ear surgery have a hearing deficit. The perioperative team should adjust their communication methods to accommodate the patient's needs. The patient may state which method is best for communication and which ear has the deficit, and whether written communication is needed.

Some patients with a hearing deficit develop a sense of isolation. The hearing world often is impatient when individuals are unable to communicate quickly and easily. Equality in patient care sometimes requires extra effort for patients with sensorial loss. One of the primary goals of the perioperative protocol is to provide comfort and healing whenever possible. This begins with compassionate patient communication.

SURGICAL ANATOMY

The anatomy of the ear is divided into three regions: the *external ear*, the *middle ear*, and the *inner ear*.

EXTERNAL EAR

The structures of the external ear include the outer surface of the *tympanic membrane* (**TM**) and all structures lateral to it (Figure 28-1). This includes the *auricle* or *pinna*, the *external auditory meatus*, and the *external auditory canal*. The auricle is a cartilaginous structure covered by skin. Its function is to gather sound waves. The center of the auricle contains the external auditory meatus, which leads to the external auditory canal. The lateral third of the external auditory canal is surrounded with cartilage and is lined with glands that secret a waxy substance called **cerumen.** The external auditory canal measures approximately 1 inch (2.5 cm) and terminates at the TM. The TM also serves as a barrier between the external and middle ears.

MIDDLE EAR

The middle ear extends from the TM to the medial wall of the middle ear cleft. It includes the TM, the **ossicles** (i.e., the *malleus, stapes,* and *incus*), the opening to the eustachian tube, the opening of the mastoid cavity, and the intratympanic portion of the facial nerve.

The TM, which is elliptical and conical in shape, aids in the process of hearing by transmitting sound waves to the ossicles, which are just posterior to it. The three ossicles together can fit on a dime. The malleus (hammer bone), the most lateral of the ossicles, is partly embedded in the TM. The incus (anvil) connects the stapes to the malleus. The stapes (stirrup) transmits the vibrations of the TM and the other ossicles to the inner ear via the oval window.

The proximal *eustachian tube* is composed of connective tissue and lined with mucous membrane. It extends into the nasopharynx at its distal end and assists in equalizing pressure between the external environment and the middle ear. It also is a pathway for bacteria to spread from the nasopharynx to the inner ear, causing *otitis media* (middle ear infection).

INNER EAR

The inner ear contains receptors for hearing and balance and is composed of a series of hollow tunnels called *labyrinths*. The inner ear has two separate labyrinth systems. The *bony labyrinth* is formed by the temporal bone and is filled with *perilymph fluid*. Within the bony labyrinth is the *membranous labyrinth*. This structure has three parts: the cochlea, the semicircular canals, and the vestibule.

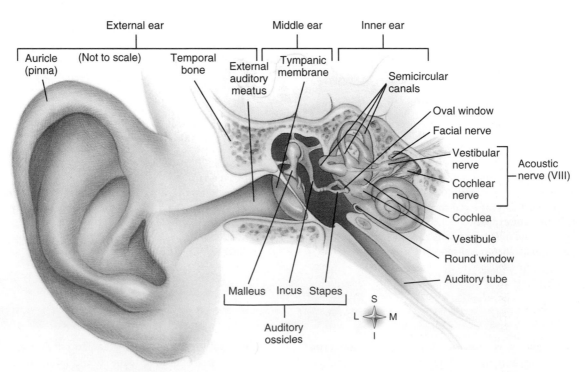

Figure 28-1   Structures of the ear. *(From Thibodeau G, Patton K: Anatomy and physiology, ed 6, St Louis, 2007, Mosby.)*

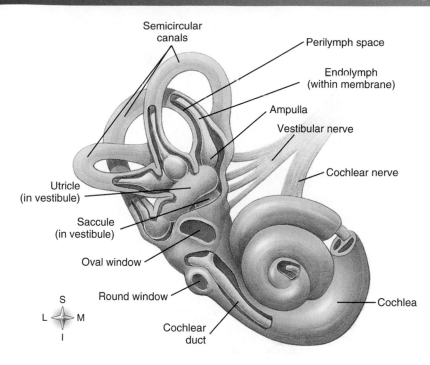

Semicircular
canals

Perilymph space

Endolymph
(within membrane)

Ampulla

Vestibular nerve

Cochlear nerve

Utricle
(in vestibule)

Saccule
(in vestibule)

Oval window

Round window

S

L ◆ M

I

Cochlear
duct

Cochlea

Figure 28-2 Structures of the inner ear. *(From Thibodeau G, Patton K:* Anatomy and physiology, *ed 6, St Louis, 2007, Mosby.)*

The spiral-shaped *cochlea* contains the cochlear duct and the organ of hearing, the *organ of Corti*. This organ extends along the length of the membranous labyrinth in the cochlea. The organ of Corti is lined with cilia, which project into the endolymph and receive the sound waves transmitted by the middle ear.

The *semicircular canals* communicate with the middle ear via the oval and round windows. These are located within the temporal bone and contain endolymph. Each of the semicircular canals contains an enlarged space called the *ampulla*. The *crista ampullaris*, located within the ampulla, is responsible for equilibrium of the body in motion (called *dynamic equilibrium*). Figure 28-2 illustrates the structures of the inner ear.

SOUND TRANSMISSION IN THE EAR

Hearing is the neural interpretation of sound transmission. Sound waves in the air enter the ear and are transmitted to the TM. The membrane vibrates against the malleus, which is attached on the posterior side. This causes vibration in the incus and in the stapes, which is connected to the oval window. From there, sound is transmitted into the perilymph of the cochlea, through the vestibular membrane, to the basilar membrane of the organ of Corti. Nerve transmission occurs from the basilar membrane to the cochlear nerve. This pathway is illustrated in Figure 28-3. Some common pathological conditions are shown in Figure 28-4.

DIAGNOSTIC PROCEDURES

CLINICAL EXAMINATION OF THE EAR

- The external auditory canal, auricle, mastoid, and surrounding tissues are examined for signs of infection, inflammation, neoplasm, scars, and lesions.

- An *otoscope* is used for the initial examination of the TM. If necessary, any cerumen is removed to allow complete visualization of the TM.
- If further examination of the TM is warranted, microscopic examination may be performed with a 250-mm lens and an ear speculum.
- Nasal and oropharyngeal examinations are performed with a tongue blade and a penlight (or the light from an otoscope) to detect any blockage of the eustachian tube by infection, inflammation, or tumor.
- Computed tomography or magnetic resonance imaging scans may be ordered if any abnormalities are noted, such as asymmetrical hearing loss, mass in the nasopharynx, oropharynx, or ear, or if cholesteatoma or infection are suspected.

CASE PLANNING

As mentioned previously, many patients undergoing ear surgery have a hearing deficit. Sensitivity to the patient's needs is extremely important because the environment can be frightening, and communication can be difficult. A dry erase board, hand signals, and other methods of communication should be used if necessary.

The results of diagnostic tests should be made available in the operating room during surgery. These include imaging studies and sensory evaluations made in the preoperative period. Table 28-1 lists common diagnostic tests of the ear.

POSITIONING

Surgical procedures of the ear generally are performed with the patient in the supine position with the head turned. A doughnut headrest is used to stabilize the head and prevent pressure on the opposite ear. It is important that the patient

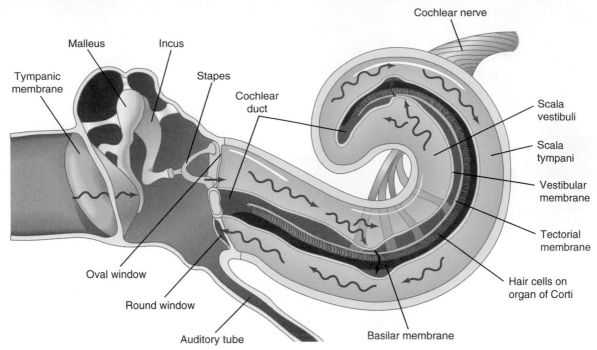

Figure 28-3   **Transmission of sound waves.** *(From Thibodeau G, Patton K: Anatomy and physiology, ed 6, St Louis, 2007, Mosby.)*

remain perfectly still during surgery. The slightest movement while under the microscope can cause injury. Special positioning accommodations may be required for a patient with a previous neck injury or other skeletal problems that might cause discomfort during surgery.

PREPPING AND DRAPING

Prepping and draping for ear procedures focus on the ear and postauricular area. A secondary site is prepped for a skin graft. Selected procedures may require clipping a small amount of hair in the preauricular region.

Before prepping begins, the circulator verifies that the correct prepping solution is being used, because some prepping solutions are **ototoxic** and may damage the ear if allowed to drain into the middle ear through the incision or a puncture in the TM. A sterile cotton ball is placed in the ear canal to prevent prep solution from entering the canal. The circulator then preps the surgical site, extending to the cheek medially, the occiput laterally, the temporal bone superiorly, and the upper neck inferiorly.

The ear is draped with four towels, which are covered with a fenestrated transparent drape. The drape may be stapled in place. Next, a split sheet is draped over the patient and around the ear.

IRRIGATION

Irrigation is used frequently during surgery to remove blood and tissue debris from the operative field. Because the site is extremely small, even small particles of tissue or blood can obscure the entire field. A suction irrigator provides a fine stream of saline or lactated Ringer solution and removes fluid from the field. The suction irrigator also is used to remove

bone fragments and to irrigate the drill tip during bone drilling. The suction irrigator is a combination Frazier suction tip and a smaller irrigator.

INSTRUMENTS

The primary instruments used in ear surgery include a small number of plastic surgery instruments: hook retractors, mosquito forceps, # 15 knife, and delicate skin forceps. Ear instruments are designed with a short fulcrum and long shanks, which are extremely delicate and easily damaged. The working tips are short (2 to 5 mm). These include grasping forceps, cup forceps, scissors, picks, elevators, and knives with different-shaped cutting surfaces. Several types of small spring retractors are also used. Various sizes of ear speculums are included in the set. These are designed to fit into the outer ear canal without external support. Ear instruments are maintained in a rack on the instrument table or Mayo stand. They must be arranged so that the tips are easily visible.

Microinstruments are considerably smaller than regular ear instruments. A dedicated light source should be directed over the Mayo stand so that the instruments can be identified. Like all microinstruments, ear instruments must be handled gently and protected from damage. Ear instruments are shown in Figure 28-5.

Speculum Holder

The speculum holder provides external structural support to the ear speculum; this allows the surgeon to use both hands to operate in the external auditory canal. Several styles of speculum holders are available. They include a bed (table) bracket, a blade that connects to the bed bracket, a flexible arm, and the speculum holder itself, which attaches to the flexible arm.

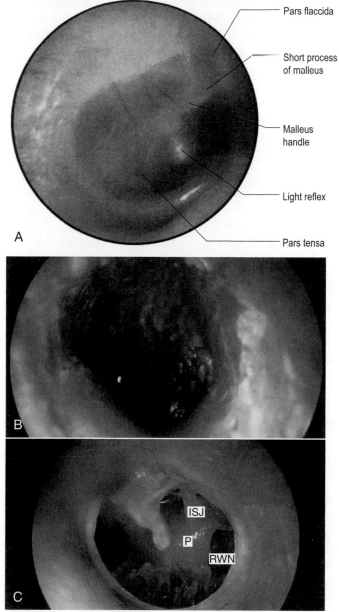

Figure 28-4 **Pathology of the ear. A,** Normal tympanic membrane. **B,** Otitis media. **C,** Subtotal perforation of the tympanic membrane. *ISJ,* Incudoostapedial joint; *P,* promontory; *RWN,* round window. *(From Dhillon RS, East CA: Ear, nose, and throat and head and neck surgery, ed 3, Edinburgh, 2006, Churchill Livingstone.)*

Table **28-1**	**Diagnostic Tests of the Ear**
Test	**Description**
Tuning fork test (Rhine and Weber tests)	Test bone conduction and sensorineural hearing function of cochlea.
Audiological testing (hearing test)	Usually conducted by an audiologist; can include air conduction, bone conduction, and speech recognition tests.
Electronystagmography (ENG) testing	Tests for **nystagmus.**
Head positioning tests	Test for benign paroxysmal positional **vertigo** (BPPV).
Balance testing	Tests stance, gait, and balance for signs of vertigo.
Caloric testing	Tests for vertigo and nystagmus; warm or cool water is instilled into the external ear canal to determine whether those conditions are elicited.
Auditory brainstem response (ABR)	Usually conducted by an audiologist or neurologist; measures the response of the brainstem to electrical stimulus as it relates to the ear.

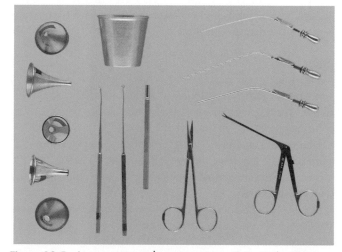

Figure 28-5 **Instruments used in ear surgery.** *(From Tighe SM: Instrumentation for the operating room, ed 7, St Louis, 2007, Mosby.)*

Otology Endoscope

The otology endoscope is used occasionally during surgery. The size of an endoscopes can be 2.7 mm or 4 mm and are 4.4 inches (11 cm) long. The endoscope is used with a standard fiberoptic light source and digital imaging equipment.

EQUIPMENT AND SUPPLIES

Power Drill

A power drill is needed in all ear surgery that involves bone. For example, a drill is used to open the mastoid bone, to enlarge the bony portion of the ear canal, and to drill through the small stapes footplate.

All drills are used with small cutting or diamond burrs, which vary in size from 0.5 to 7 mm. The scrub must irrigate the tip of the drill during operation to prevent tissue heating. A suction irrigator or a 3- to 5-mL syringe fitted with an 18-gauge angiography catheter is used for irrigation. If an angiography catheter is used, it is important that only the tip of the Angiocath be visible in the operating field so that the surgeon's vision under the microscope is not obscured.

Operating Microscope

The operating microscope is used in all procedures of the middle or inner ear. The standard operating lens for ear surgery has a focal length of 250 mm. However, some surgeons prefer a 200- or 300-mm lens. For simple procedures, such as a myringotomy, a small operating microscope on a floor stand may be used. Complex procedures, such as a tympanoplasty or mastoidectomy, require a larger, more mobile operating microscope on a floor stand or ceiling mount. Gross adjustments are made before surgery, and the microscope is draped within an hour of use. (Chapter 27 presents a complete discussion of the use and care of the operating microscope.)

Sponges

Cotton pledgets, such as those used during neurosurgery, are commonly used in ear procedures. Square 4 × 4 sponges should also be available. Even though the operative site may be small, sponge and sharps counts are routinely performed for all ear surgeries.

Dressings

Two types of dressings are used in ear procedures, the mastoid dressing and the Glasscock dressing. The mastoid dressing is applied after complex procedures of the ear, especially those that require drilling of the mastoid. The dressing consists of several fluffed gauze sponges to cover the ear and incision, as well as rolled gauze (Kling or Kerlix), which is wrapped around the patient's head to hold the dressing in place. The Glasscock dressing is used after minor procedures of the ear, such as a stapedectomy or tympanoplasty. This dressing, which comes prepackaged, is composed of gauze sponges with Velcro straps to secure the dressing in place.

Medications

Medications used during ear surgery include anesthetics, hemostatic agents, antibiotic solutions, and irrigation solutions. Lidocaine with epinephrine is used in most ear surgeries to control bleeding by vasoconstriction.

Hemostatic agents are used to control active bleeding. The primary hemostatic agents are Gelfoam and Helistat. Pledgets of Gelfoam may be soaked in epinephrine and applied directly to bleeding tissue.

Antibiotic solution often is instilled into the ear. Gelfoam soaked in a solution composed of an antibiotic and a corticosteroid may be used at the end of a procedure to control postoperative inflammation.

SURGICAL PROCEDURES

MYRINGOTOMY

Surgical Goal

A myringotomy is a surgical opening made in the TM to release fluid from the middle ear.

Pathology

Fluid in the middle ear is referred to as an **effusion.** This can be caused by inflammation of the mucosa. It also can be caused by eustachian tube dysfunction, in which airflow between the nasopharynx and the middle ear is inadequate; the result is negative pressure in the middle ear and retraction

of the TM. Eustachian tube dysfunction can be caused by a congenital anomaly, inflammation of the nasal mucosa, or enlarged adenoids. If left untreated, the effusion may lead to infection, mastoiditis, hearing loss, or perforation.

TECHNIQUE

1 A speculum is placed in the ear canal and the microscope is used to visualize the tympanic membrane (TM).
2 Excess cerumen is removed from the ear canal.
3 A small incision is made in the TM.
4 Fluid is suctioned.
5 A tympanostomy tube is placed if necessary.

Discussion

A middle ear effusion can be treated by making a small incision in the TM (myringotomy). This allows trapped fluid to drain. To maintain open drainage, a **tympanostomy tube** often is placed in the incision. A myringotomy allows equalization of the pressure between the middle ear and the outside barometric pressure. Tubes usually are not removed, but are left in place until they fall out (Figure 28-6). The procedure most often is performed on children.

The patient is placed in the supine position with the head supported on a doughnut headrest. Skin prep and draping usually are omitted. General anesthesia is administered by mask, because the procedure is brief. The surgeon sits while operating and uses a microscope with a 250-mm lens. The microscope is brought into position as soon as the surgeon is seated.

To begin the procedure, the surgeon inserts a Farrior speculum into the external ear canal. The speculum size is determined by the diameter and depth of the ear canal. With the speculum in place, the surgeon removes any wax or debris from the external auditory canal with a cerumen curette. Then, a 2- to 3-mm incision is made in the TM with a myringotomy knife. Fluid behind the TM is suctioned with a small Frazier microsuction (no. 3 or no. 5). If a tympanostomy tube is to be implanted, the scrub uses alligator forceps to grasp the

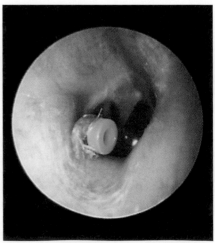

Figure 28-6   **Myringotomy tube in place.** *(From Thibodeau G, Patton K: Anatomy and physiology, ed 6, St Louis, 2007, Mosby.)*

tube. The surgeon inserts the tube into the myringotomy incision. Next, a Rosen needle is used to seat the tube in the incision. Combinations of antibiotic and steroid drops or antibiotic drops alone are then instilled into the external canal, and the speculum is removed. The external canal is packed with cotton.

MYRINGOPLASTY

Surgical Goal

A myringoplasty is performed to close a small nonhealing hole in the TM. The procedure is performed without entering the middle ear.

Pathology

Causes of **perforation** of the TM may include a persistent opening after removal of a tympanostomy tube, a blast injury, or a penetrating foreign body in the ear.

TECHNIQUE

1 A speculum is placed in the external canal for microscopic examination.
2 Debris is removed from the ear canal.
3 The edges of the tympanic membrane are everted and roughened.
4 A fat graft is removed if necessary.
5 A small patch (or fat graft) is placed over the perforation.

Discussion

The patient is placed in the supine position with the head positioned on a doughnut headrest. General anesthesia is administered by mask. Endotracheal intubation seldom is required, because the anesthesia time is short. The patient is prepped and draped for an ear procedure. Because the TM is open during the prep, special care is taken to prevent any prep solution from entering the ear canal.

The operating microscope is fitted with a 250-mm lens. The microscope usually is not draped for the procedure. To begin the procedure, the surgeon places a Farrior speculum into the external auditory canal. The external canal is cleaned with a cerumen curette and Frazier suction. The surgeon then can **evert** (turn back) the edges of the perforated TM and score them with either a fine Rosen needle or a fine right angle pick. Several types of patches can be used to close the defect (e.g., Gelfoam, Gelfilm, Steri-Strip, fat graft).

Fat Graft

The surgeon makes a small incision (approximately 5 to 8 mm) on the posterior side of the ear lobe with a # 15 blade. Single skin hooks are used to expose the subcutaneous tissue. A small piece of the tissue is excised with a # 15 blade and a hemostat or toothed Adson forceps. The graft is placed in a small amount of saline to keep it moist until the surgeon is ready to implant it. The donor site is closed with 4-0 Vicryl suture.

The graft is positioned over the defect in the TM. The external auditory canal is packed with gelatin sponges soaked

in a steroid-antibiotic solution, and a Glasscock-style dressing is applied.

TYMPANOPLASTY

Surgical Goal

A tympanoplasty is the surgical removal of a **cholesteatoma** and mastoid bone, with or without reconstruction.

Pathology

A tympanoplasty is performed to treat a number of disorders affecting the TM. These conditions include a nonhealing perforation of the TM, a dysfunction of the eustachian tube that causes retraction of the TM, and a cholesteatoma. In dysfunction of the eustachian tube, inadequate airflow between the nasopharynx and the middle ear causes negative pressure in the middle ear and retraction of the TM. This causes the TM to vibrate improperly and can lead to a perforation or cholesteatoma. A cholesteatoma may cause infection, otorrhea, bone destruction, hearing loss, and paralysis of the facial nerve.

TECHNIQUE

1 An incision is made posterior to the ear.
2 A fascia graft is removed.
3 The native tympanic membrane (TM) is removed or prepared for grafting.
4 The ear canal is enlarged with a drill (canalplasty).
5 The TM is reconstructed.
6 The incision is closed, and the ear canal is packed.

Discussion

Two methods are commonly used to perform a tympanoplasty. The approach depends on the condition of the TM, the size and position of the perforation, and the surgeon's preference.

In the underlay technique, the TM is lifted away and the middle ear is filled with Gelfoam to support a graft on the undersurface of the TM perforation. This is used for a small visible perforation with minimal signs of infection.

The overlay technique is used for a large perforation, for a severely damaged TM, or for extensive infection. In this procedure, the TM remnants and bony canal skin are removed. The bony canal is enlarged with a drill, and the TM is recreated with a fascia and skin graft (usually from the abdomen, upper arm, or pinna).

The patient is placed in the supine position with the head supported on a doughnut headrest. The arm on the operative side is tucked at the patient's side. General anesthesia is used.

If a skin graft from the arm or abdomen is planned, it may be removed before the skin prep and draping. The arm is prepped and draped with towels. The surgeon removes the graft with a sharp, double-edged razor blade (e.g., a Gillette or a Watson) or a Weck skin graft knife. The graft is placed in a small basin and protected from damage or contamination. A small amount of saline is used to keep the graft moist. The donor site is covered or may be dressed. The patient is prepped and draped for the ear procedure.

The surgeon makes a postauricular (behind the ear) incision and carries it through the temporalis fascia to the mastoid tip. A temporalis fascia graft is harvested with Brown Adson forceps and a # 15 blade. A *fascia press* is used to flatten and shape the graft. A separate sterile table may be set up for this, or the surgeon may use an area of the back table to prepare the graft. The fascia press with the graft on it should be left in the open position unless the surgeon requests otherwise. This allows the graft to dry so that it can be trimmed and placed in the ear later in the procedure.

The microscope is fitted with a 250-mm lens and moved into position. The TM is exposed with a gimmick or House knife and removed with Bellucci scissors or knife. If a **canalplasty** (reconstruction of the canal) is to be performed, the ear canal is enlarged with a small cutting drill and a small 4 × 5 suction irrigator. This permits better visualization of the middle ear and a larger space in which to work.

The middle ear is then prepared to receive the graft. The surgeon trims the fascia to the appropriate size using the fascia press and a # 15 blade. The graft is grasped with a smooth alligator forceps and removed from the fascia press. The surgeon reconstructs the middle ear by placing the fascia graft in position with the alligator forceps and a fine Rosen needle. The skin grafts, if taken, are then laid over the fascia graft with alligator forceps and Rosen needle. The ear is packed with small pledgets of Gelfoam or Helistat to hold the graft in position. The wound is closed in layers with 3-0 absorbable sutures and the skin is closed with 4-0 absorbable sutures. The ear is dressed with a mastoid dressing.

MASTOIDECTOMY/ TYMPANOMASTOIDECTOMY

Surgical Goal

A mastoidectomy or tympanomastoidectomy is the removal of diseased bone, the mastoid air cells, and the soft tissue lining the air cells of the mastoid.

Pathology

The mastoid is composed of many air cells similar to the nasal sinuses. Inadequate flow of air through the sinuses can lead to infection and erosion of the surrounding bone. Cholesteatoma, eustachian tube dysfunction, neoplasm, or congenital malformation of the middle ear may block airflow to the mastoid and cause chronic mastoiditis. An advanced cholesteatoma may spread into the mastoid. In this case, mastoidectomy with tympanoplasty is performed.

TECHNIQUE

1 A postauricular incision is made.
2 The skin flaps are elevated.
3 Temporalis fascia is harvested.
4 Diseased mastoid is removed with a drill.
5 The ossicles are removed if diseased.
6 The cholesteatoma is removed.
7 The mastoid cavity and middle ear are packed.
8 The incisions are closed and dressings are applied.

Discussion

The patient is placed in the supine position, and the arm on the operative side is tucked at the patient's side. General anesthesia is used. A skin graft is taken before the ear prep, as described previously. A 28-gauge needle is used to inject the ear incision site with lidocaine with epinephrine. The patient is then prepped and draped for an ear procedure.

The surgeon makes a postauricular incision. The temporalis fascia graft is removed, smoothed onto the fascia press, and allowed to dry. The incision is carried to the bone, and the diseased mastoid tissue is excised with a power drill with a large cutting burr. The surgeon may use a variety of burrs to remove the bone. A Rosen needle, gimmick, or picks are used to assess the patency of the mastoid and determine the need for continued drilling. The surgeon removes the cholesteatoma with a gimmick or Rosen needle.

With the cholesteatoma removed, the surgeon places the fascia graft over the remaining ossicles; this is done as described for a tympanoplasty. The skin graft is placed in position over the fascia. The surgeon then uses a serrated alligator forceps and a gimmick to pack the mastoid cavity and middle ear with Gelfoam sponges that have been soaked in saline solution or a combination steroid-antibiotic. The incisions are closed in layers with 3-0 absorbable sutures. The skin is closed with 4-0 absorbable sutures. The external auditory canal is also packed with Gelfoam, as for the mastoid cavity. A mastoid dressing is applied.

STAPEDECTOMY/OSSICULAR RECONSTRUCTION

Surgical Goal

A stapedectomy is the reconstruction of the ossicles to restore conduction to the oval window.

Pathology

A stapedectomy, or ossicular reconstruction, is performed to treat profound hearing loss related to sclerosis of the stapes. Sound normally is received at the TM, which transmits vibrations through the ossicles and the oval window, which amplifies the sound. If the bony chain is immobile or discontinuous, not only is amplification lost, but sound perception can be severely dampened. The most common cause of ossicle immobility is *otosclerosis* of the stapes. This is abnormal bone growth that locks the stapes into place and prevents it from vibrating and carrying the stimulus (Figure 28-7). Otosclerosis generally begins at age 30 and progresses with age. After surgery, 90% of patients have a permanent hearing gain, and 1% have a permanent hearing loss.

The most common cause of a break in the ossicle chain is a cholesteatoma, which erodes the ossicles. The shape and articulation of the ossicles provides minimal sound amplification (1.7:1). The size ratio between the TM and the oval window provides most of the amplification (17:1). This is important, because a mobile connection between the TM and the oval window can improve hearing.

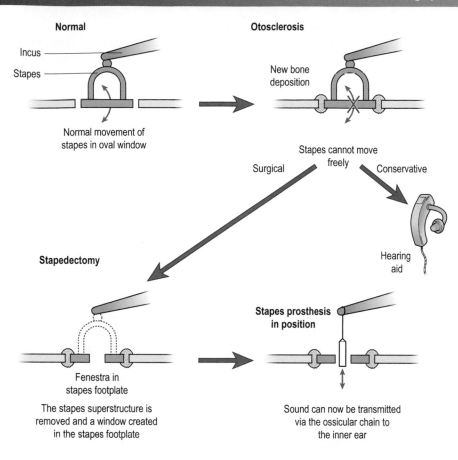

Figure 28-7 Stapedectomy for the treatment of otosclerosis. *(From Dhillon RS, East CA: Ear, nose, and throat and head and neck surgery, ed 3, Edinburgh, 2006, Churchill Livingstone.)*

TECHNIQUE

1 The auditory canal is injected with lidocaine and epinephrine.
2 A speculum is placed in the external auditory canal.
3 The tympanic membrane (TM) is elevated.
4 The affected ossicles are freed or removed.
5 A hole is drilled in the stapes footplate.
6 The prosthesis is implanted and secured.
7 The TM is replaced.
8 The external canal is packed and a dressing is applied.

Discussion

The patient is placed in the supine position, and the arm on the operative side is tucked at the patient's side. General anesthesia is used. The external ear canal is injected with a local anesthetic before prepping. The patient is prepped and draped for an ear procedure.

The operative microscope with a 250-mm lens is used to examine the middle ear. The external ear canal is irrigated and cleaned with a 7-Fr Frazier suction tip. In this procedure, a speculum holder is used. The surgeon places the speculum in the external canal and attaches it to a universal speculum holder for stabilization. This allows the surgeon to operate with both hands while the speculum is held in the external canal. The surgeon then changes to a 5-Fr Frazier suction tip to clear any fluid from the ear.

The TM is elevated and the posterior bony ledge is removed with a House knife. With the TM elevated, the surgeon can visualize the ossicular chain. The incudostapedial joint is cut with a joint knife and the stapedial tendon is severed with Bellucci scissors. The stapes superstructure is then fractured with a fine Rosen needle and micro cup forceps.

The surgeon then drills a hole in the stapes footplate with a Skeeter drill or similar micro drill using a 1-mm cutting burr. The prosthesis, which has been previously loaded onto a serrated alligator forceps or hook, is implanted in the hole in the footplate. The surgeon secures the prosthesis in place by *packing* the ear with gelatin sponges soaked in normal saline or steroid antibiotic ointment. A gimmick and a fine Rosen needle are used to replace the TM. The external auditory canal is packed with gelatin sponges soaked in saline or an antibiotic-steroid solution. A Glasscock or mastoid dressing is applied.

COCHLEAR IMPLANT

Surgical Goal

A cochlear implant is used to transmit external sound directly to the eighth cranial nerve. It is used in the treatment of sensorineural deafness (Figure 28-8).

Pathology

Sensorineural deafness can be congenital or acquired. It has many different causes including:

- Viral or bacterial infection causing damage to the cilia
- Acoustic trauma (caused by loud noise), which results in permanent injury to the cilia
- Tumor of the ocular nerve

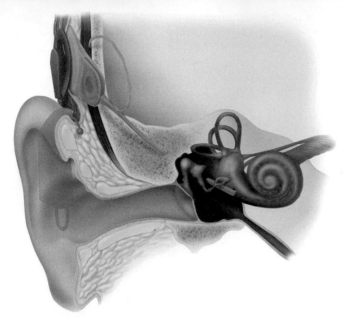

Figure 28-8 Cochlear implant. *(Courtesy Cochlear Ltd, Macquarie University NSW, Australia, 2009.)*

- Drugs such as certain antibiotics that cause permanent hearing loss
- Autoimmune disease, stroke, or brain tumor

A cochlear implant provides the perception of sound. However, significant postoperative rehabilitation is required for the patient to turn this into cognitive information. Congenital deafness in the child can be treated with a cochlear implant, but surgery is delayed until age 2.

TECHNIQUE

1 A postauricular incision is made and extended superiorly.
2 The cranium is exposed.
3 A recessed space for the internal receiver is created in the bone.
4 The facial nerve is identified.
5 The medial wall of the middle ear is identified.
6 The internal electrodes of the implant are placed into the cochlea via the round window.
7 The internal receiver is implanted and secured.
8 The incision is closed.

Discussion

Patients with **sensorineural hearing loss** have functional outer and middle ear structures. However, the cilia, which receive and transmit sound to the ocular nerve and brain, are damaged or absent. The cochlear implant is a device that receives sounds and transmits them as electrical impulses to the brain.

The cochlear implant has two primary components. An electronic processor, which is implanted outside the ear over the temporal bone, captures sound and sends it in digital form to an internal transmitter. The transmitter conveys signals to electrodes, which are implanted in the cochlea. The transmitter takes over the functions of the cochlear cilia. Instead of moving the cilia to transmit sound, the signals are interpreted directly by the acoustic nerve. The patient must learn to interpret the sounds and make sense of their meaning. This requires extensive postoperative rehabilitation and psychological support.

A facial nerve monitor is used to protect the nerve during surgical dissection and implantation of the implants. The monitoring electrodes are placed before the prep and draping.

The patient is placed in the supine position. The surgeon may clip the hair in the temporal region and outlines the incision with a skin scribe. The site is injected with 1% lidocaine with epinephrine 1:100,000. The surgeon implants the electrodes for facial nerve monitoring and connects them to the monitor. The patient then is prepped and draped for an ear procedure.

The surgeon makes a postauricular incision and extends it superiorly using a # 15 blade. A skin flap is elevated with a needle-tip electrosurgical unit (ESU) and retracted with double-prong skin hooks or wire rakes. The flap is extended deeper to include the muscle. With the flaps elevated, the surgeon places a Beckman-Adson retractor or similar self-retaining retractor under the flaps to expose the cranium. The receiver template is placed in position and outlined with a skin scribe or the ESU. The surgeon then drills out the circumscribed area of the temporal bone using a medium cutting burr with irrigation. The template periodically is positioned in the drilled space to ensure a correct fit. A medium diamond burr is used to finish the edges of the temporal bone. Suture tunnel holes are placed, two on each side of the recess. These are used to secure the processor.

Next, a mastoidectomy is performed. The surgeon drills the mastoid with a large cutting burr and suction irrigator, preserving the bony ear canal and the opening of the facial recess. The medial wall of the middle ear is identified.

The implant is opened onto the sterile field. Implants are packaged individually and must be opened in a manner that limits or prevents the discharge of static electricity created during opening, because a static charge can interfere with the function of the implant electrodes. The circulator opens the outer package slowly onto the instrument table. The inner (sterile) package may then be submerged in a basin of normal saline and opened below the surface.

The surgeon places the internal processor into the drilled recess of the temporal bone. The active electrode is passed through the facial recess and round window into the cochlea. This is done using the electrode positioner provided in the implant kit. The active electrode is secured in the round window with a gimmick or Rosen needle.

The surgeon secures the internal processor by placing 2-0 or larger Prolene suture through the suture holes and tying the knots diagonally across the holes. Bleeding is controlled with the bipolar ESU (monopolar ESU is not used, because it could cause current to be passed through the receiver). With the implant secured, the fascia overlying the cranium is closed with 2-0 absorbable suture. A 3-0 absorbable suture is used to close the subcutaneous tissue. The skin then is closed with a nonabsorbable suture. A mastoid dressing is placed over the wound.

To allow wound healing, the implant is activated several weeks after surgery. It is activated slowly so that the patient can adjust to the hearing world.

SECTION II: THE NASAL CAVITY, OROPHARYNX, AND LARYNX

INTRODUCTION

Surgery of the nose, oropharynx, and larynx is performed by an otorhinolaryngologist. Most of the structures in these anatomical regions are related to respiration and vocalization, although some share functions with the digestive system. Surgery of lymph and secretory glands in the oropharynx are included in this specialty.

Procedures for pharyngeal and laryngeal tumors may extend into the neck, which contains large blood vessels and nerves that must be protected. Head and neck surgery requires meticulous dissection to avoid injury to these vital structures.

SURGICAL ANATOMY

EXTERNAL NOSE

The external nose is formed by two U-shaped, cartilaginous structures called the *lower lateral cartilages,* two rectangular structures called the *upper lateral cartilages,* and two nasal bones. The nares are the flared portions of the lower nose (nostrils). These are lined with skin. Fine hairs in this area filter the air as it enters the nasal cavity. The right and left nostrils are divided by the nasal septum, which is composed of cartilage.

NASAL CAVITY

The nasal cavity is located over the palatine bone, which is the "floor" of the nose; the "roof" of the nose is formed from the cribriform plate in the ethmoid bone. This is a significant structure, because it separates the nasal cavity from the cranial cavity. Infection or disease arising from the nose may enter the cranial cavity and spread to brain tissue. The nasal cavity has **paranasal sinuses,** or spaces. These are formed by extensions of the ethmoid bone and the frontal, maxillary, and sphenoid bones. The extensions are referred to as the *turbinates* or *nasal conchae.* The sinuses are lined with a highly vascular mucosa. As air passes through the sinuses, it is warmed, humidified, and filtered.

The nasal cavities drain into the superior, inferior, and middle meatus. The nasolacrimal duct drains into the inferior meatus. The posterior aspect of the nasal cavities is the choana, which separates them from the nasopharynx. This is an important structure because of the congenital anomaly known as choanal atresia. In this condition, infants are born with one or both choanae obstructed, requiring emergency surgery to restore airflow (see Chapter 35).

PARANASAL SINUSES

The paired *maxillary sinuses* are the large sinuses below the ocular orbits. The apices of the tooth roots are found in the floor of these sinuses. The paired frontal sinuses lie behind the lower forehead. The ethmoid sinuses consist of many small air cells in the lateral wall of the nasal cavity between the lateral nasal wall and the turbinates. The sphenoids lie at the posterosuperior extent of the nasal cavity. The optic nerves and carotid arteries are within the lateral wall of these sinuses, and the pituitary gland lies behind and above them. Surgery of the pituitary gland may be performed through a **transsphenoidal** approach. The anatomy of the sinuses is shown in Figure 28-9.

NASOPHARYNX

The *nasopharynx* is situated behind the nasal cavity and above the oral cavity. It communicates with the nasal sinuses and the oropharynx below it.

ORAL CAVITY

The oral cavity is divided into two sections, the vestibule and the oral cavity proper. The *vestibule* lies between the inner surface of the lips, the buccal mucosa (cheeks), and the lateral aspects of the mandible and maxilla. The oral cavity proper lies within the medial surface of the maxillary and mandibular teeth. The roof of the oral cavity proper consists of the hard and soft palates, which separate it from the nasal cavity (Figure 28-10). The soft palate meets in the middle to form the uvula.

The floor of the mouth contains the ducts for the paired submandibular and lingual salivary glands. The tongue is attached in the midline to the floor of the mouth by a membranous structure called the *frenulum.* The tongue is a muscular structure covered by mucous membrane. The surface of the tongue is covered by papillae, or projections that contain taste buds. These are divided by type and regions of the tongue. Various types of papillae and taste buds are capable of separate sensations of taste. The undersurface of the tongue is highly vascular and has large blood vessels. The *sublingual* salivary gland ducts open into each side of the sublingual area.

PHARYNX

The *pharynx* is a tubular structure extending from the nose to the esophagus. It is separated into three areas: the *nasopharynx, oropharynx,* and *hypopharynx* (Figure 28-11). The nasopharynx extends from the posterior *choanae* of the nose to the palate. The adenoids lie in the posterosuperior aspect of the nasopharynx, and the eustachian tubes open on each side of the adenoids. The oropharynx extends from the palate to the hyoid bone. The soft palate, tonsils, and posterior third of the tongue (the base of the tongue) lie in the anterior portion of the oropharynx. The *hypopharynx* extends from the hyoid bone to the esophagus.

LARYNX

The larynx is composed of nine segments of cartilage, three paired sets and three unpaired segments. The unpaired cartilages are the cricoid, thyroid, and epiglottis segments; the paired sets are the arytenoids, corniculate, and cuneiform segments.

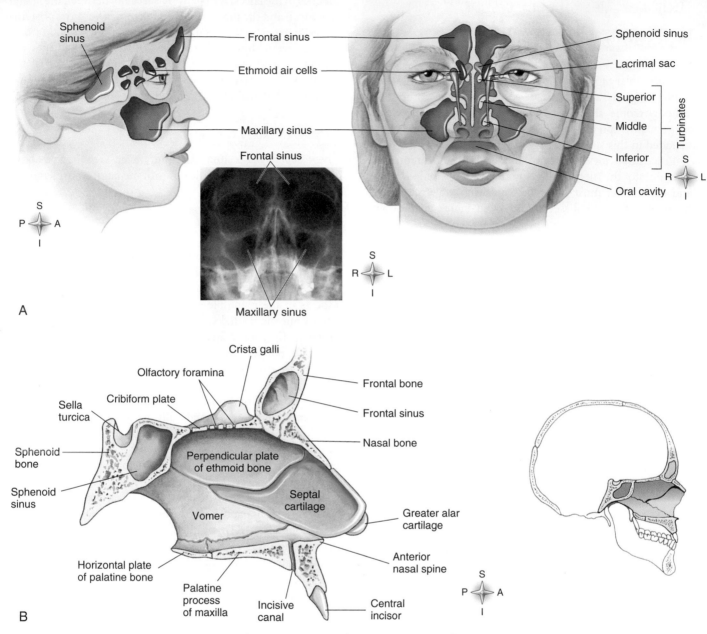

Figure 28-9   **A**, Paranasal sinuses. **B**, Bones of the nasal cavity. (**A** *from Abrahams PH, Marks SC, Hutchings RT:* McKinn's color atlas of human anatomy, *ed 5, St Louis, 2002, Mosby;* **B** *from Thibodeau G, Patton K:* Anatomy and physiology, *ed 6, St Louis, 2007, Mosby.)*

The larynx is separated into three spaces (Figure 28-12). The *supraglottis* lies above the true vocal cords and contains the vestibule, false vocal cords, and *epiglottis*, which is composed of cartilage. The *glottis* extends from the true vocal cords to about ½ inch (1 cm) below the free edge of the true vocal cords. The subglottis extends below this position to the inferior edge of the cricoid cartilage. The arytenoid cartilages lie in the posterior larynx and have processes that extend anteriorly (the vocal processes) and that lie within the true vocal cords. The area between the arytenoids is called the *posterior commissure*.

The true vocal cords meet anteriorly at the anterior commissure and connect to the thyroid cartilage. The free edge of the true vocal cords has a loosely covered membrane that vibrates to produce the voice.

The trachea extends from the cricoid to the carina. It is composed of approximately 20 incomplete cartilaginous rings. The cricoid is the only closed ring of the upper airway. The posterior aspect of the trachea is membranous and has no cartilaginous structures.

DIAGNOSTIC TESTS

Diagnostic endoscopy procedures of the upper respiratory tract (larynx and pharynx) are commonly performed for direct visualization of the anatomy. Procedures include

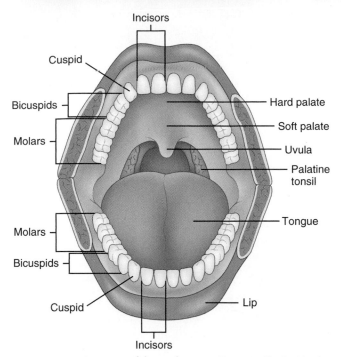

Figure 28-10 **Anatomy of the oral cavity.** *(From Herlihy B, Maebius NK: The human body in health and illness, ed 2, Philadelphia, 2003, WB Saunders.)*

Labels on Figure 28-10:
- Incisors
- Cuspid
- Bicuspids
- Molars
- Molars
- Bicuspids
- Cuspid
- Incisors
- Hard palate
- Soft palate
- Uvula
- Palatine tonsil
- Tongue
- Lip

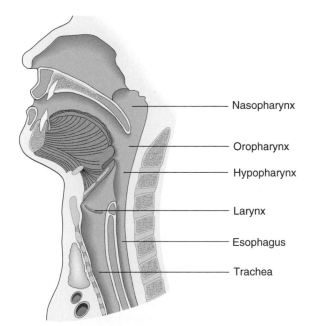

Figure 28-11 **The pharynx.** *(From Garden O, Bradbury A, Forsythe J, Parks R: Principles and practice of surgery, ed 5, Edinburgh, 2007, Churchill Livingstone.)*

Labels on Figure 28-11:
- Nasopharynx
- Oropharynx
- Hypopharynx
- Larynx
- Esophagus
- Trachea

sinusoscopy, laryngoscopy, and bronchoscopy. Selected operative procedures such as biopsy and removal of small lesions may also be performed using endoscopic techniques. Pathology specimens are obtained by removing tissue or by cell washing, in which the mucosa is irrigated with saline and cells are collected with a biopsy brush. Fine-needle aspiration and biopsy are also performed before surgical excision.

Imaging studies such as magnetic resonance imaging, computed tomography, and ultrasonography are commonly used to confirm or rule out of disease or structural abnormalities.

CASE PLANNING

PREPPING AND DRAPING

Patients undergoing nasal procedures generally are prepped from the forehead to the upper neck, including the entire face. Patients having intranasal and endoscopic procedures may not be prepped, because these are considered clean rather than sterile cases. For nasal procedures, the patient is draped with a head drape. A three-quarter sheet is placed under the patient's head. The face then is draped with four towels secured with towel clips, and a split sheet is placed over the patient's body and around the face.

Procedures of the pharynx and larynx are approached transorally, and little or no prep is necessary because these are clean procedures. Often these patients are draped with a three-quarter sheet over the chest. A head drape may be applied and the eyes protected.

EQUIPMENT AND SUPPLIES

Microscope

The operating microscope is used frequently in surgery of the upper airway. The microscope is not draped for procedures of the mouth and throat. While the microscope is in use, the scrub must insert and guide the microinstruments into the laryngoscope, because the surgeon does not turn away from the microscope to receive instruments. (Chapter 27 presents a complete discussion of the use and care of the operating microscope.)

Sponges

Flat cottonoid sponges (patties), cotton pledgets, and round gauze sponges are commonly used in procedures of the nasal cavities, mouth, and throat. All sponges have strings sewn into them for identification and retrieval to prevent loss and aspiration, which can result in injury or death. All sponges are counted according to routine policy.

Dressings

No dressings are applied to the mouth and throat after the procedure. A variety of nasal dressings may be used, depending on the procedure. The interior nasal passages may be "splinted" or packed with a continuous ¼- or ½-inch gauze strip (Figure 28-13). Packing material may be impregnated with a bacteriostatic agent before insertion. **Packing** is the process of placing long strips of fine gauze material inside the nose to provide support and absorb fluid.

Nasal packing also helps control bleeding or drainage after septoplasty or rhinoplasty. Exterior nasal splints are used to maintain the shape of the nose in the immediate postoperative period. Several types of external splints are available, including metal, foam, and fiberglass splints.

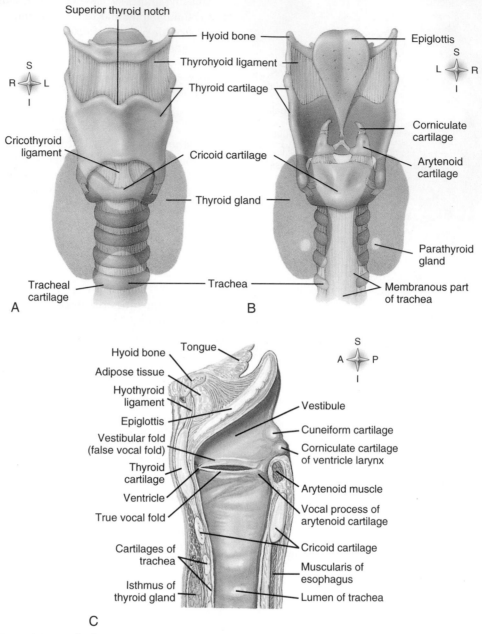

Figure 28-12   **The larynx. A,** Anterior view. **B,** Posterior view. **C,** Sagittal view. *(From Thibodeau G, Patton K: Anatomy and physiology, ed 6, St Louis, 2007, Mosby.)*

Medications

Medications used for procedures of the nose, mouth, and throat include regional anesthetics, vasoconstrictive agents, and decongestants. A local anesthetic with epinephrine is injected into the nasal mucosa and turbinates for most nasal procedures. Cocaine in solution may be used as a vasoconstrictive agent in the nose or larynx for topical use only. Solutions are administered by infiltration (injection) or may be applied topically with flat cottonoid sponges.

NASAL INSTRUMENTS

Specialty nasal instruments are designed for use on soft tissue and bone. Soft tissue instruments are needed for skin, submucosa, and soft connective tissue; bone and cartilage require heavier instruments. In many cases, the complex structure of the nasal cavity requires the surgeon to alternate frequently between these two types of instruments during a surgical procedure. All nasal instruments must be designed to reach deep into the nasal cavities from the outside. Instruments are balanced so that the hinge or fulcrum is much farther from the finger rings than in general surgery instruments. Instrument tips are available in an angled configuration for optimum access. Figure 28-14 shows commonly used nasal instruments.

Retractors

A nasal speculum is used for viewing tissue just inside the nares. Fine skin hooks or rakes are used to retract skin tissue in this area. Common retractors include the following:

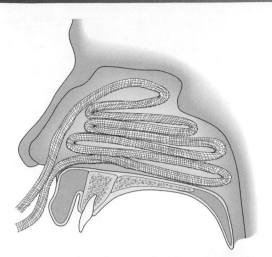

Figure 28-13 Nasal packing is placed in the nasal cavity for tamponade. Packing material is available in 1/4- and 1/2-inch (0.63- and 1.25-cm) long gauze and often is identified by its brand name, Adaptic. *(From Garden O, Bradbury A, Forsythe J, Parks R: Principles and practice of surgery, ed 5, Edinburgh, 2007, Churchill Livingstone.)*

- Alar retractor
- Fomon retractor
- Aufricht retractor
- Cottle retractor

Knives

Knives must have a delicate tip so that they can be manipulated in the small space of the nasal cavity. A # 15 scalpel blade (knife) mounted on a # 7 knife handle often is used for skin and submucosal incisions in the naris. The following are used for deeper dissection:

- Joseph knife
- Ballenger swivel knife
- Button knife

Elevator or Dissector

Elevators are used to lift the periosteum or submucosa from the surface of bone or cartilage. They are available in a wide variety of designs to conform to the complex structure of the nasal cavity. The edge of the elevator is beveled but not sharp. Commonly used elevators include the following:

- Cottle knife or elevator
- Lempert elevator
- Freer elevator
- Penfield dissector

Forceps

Forceps are used for grasping and modeling tissue. The tips of the forceps may be cupped or beveled for cutting, or flat and serrated. An example of the cutting type of forceps is the Takahashi ethmoid forceps, which has small cupped tips. The term *alligator forceps* refers both to a design and to an instrument. Alligator forceps have a long shank, short "working" tips, and two hinges, one at the base of the movable tips and one at the fulcrum that opens the tips. The distinction is made clear by the individual surgeon during the procedure.

Dressing forceps are bayonet-shaped and used to handle nasal packing.

Commonly used tissue forceps include the following:
- Takahashi ethmoid forceps
- Noyes alligator forceps
- Blakesley-Wilde forceps
- Walsham septum straightening forceps
- Knight septum forceps

Rongeur

The rongeur is used specifically to cut bone. To provide enough leverage to cut through bone, many rongeurs have two hinges; these are identified as *double-action* rongeurs. A common double-action rongeur is the Jansen-Middleton rongeur.

Rongeurs with long shanks are used to reach deep into small spaces, such as the nasal sinus. Some of the rongeurs used in nasal surgery also are used in other specialties, such as neurosurgery. An example is the Kerrison rongeur. Commonly used rongeurs include the following:

- Kerrison rongeur
- Hartman rongeur
- Wilde rongeur
- Jansen-Middleton septum-cutting forceps

Gouge, Chisel, and Osteotome

The gouge, chisel, and osteotome are used with a small mallet to model nasal bone. Those used in nasal surgery are smaller and finer than those used in orthopedics. The sharp end of the instrument is angled against the bone and lightly struck with the mallet. This cuts the tissue by increments, producing bone shavings, which are removed with a forceps. The gouge is V-shaped, although the chisel and osteotome are straight. The chisel tip is beveled on both sides, but the osteotome has only one bevel.

Rasp and Saw

A nasal rasp is used to shave bone tissue. The handheld rasp usually is bayonet shaped. Note that the endoscopic shaver or micro debrider is used for the same purpose (discussed later). The bayonet saw is angled (right and left) and used to reduce small defects in bone.

TONSIL AND ADENOID INSTRUMENTS

Tonsil and adenoid instruments include the Crowe-Davis mouth gag, tonsil snares, adenoid curettes, elevators, clamps, and scissors. The Crowe-Davis mouth gag is placed in the patient's mouth and attached to the edge of the Mayo stand during surgery. Tonsil snares are loaded with short strands of stainless steel wire. The snare is looped around the tonsil and retracted to transect the tonsillar fossa and release the tissue. Basic tonsil and adenoid instruments are shown in Figure 28-15.

Shaver and Drills

The micro debrider is used to excise tissue during nasal and laryngeal surgery. It is a small powered handpiece with rotating blades (Figure 28-16). The micro debrider removes small

Figure 28-14 Basic nasal instruments. **A,** *Top,* Five Ludwig wire applicators. *Bottom, left to right,* 1 Bard-Parker knife handle, # 3; 1 Bard-Parker knife handle, # 7; 1 Cottle columella forceps; Brown-Adson tissue forceps with teeth (7 × 7); 1 Beasley-Babcock tissue forceps; 1 Jansen thumb forceps, bayonet shaft, serrated tips; 1 Joseph button-end knife, curved; 1 Freer septum knife; 1 Cottle nasal knife; 1 McKenty elevator; 1 Cottle septum elevator; 1 Freer elevator; 2 Joseph skin hooks; 1 Cottle knife guide and retractor. **B,** *Left to right,* 1 Bauer rocking chisel; 1 Lewis rasp; 1 Maltz rasp; 1 Aufricht rasp, large; 1 Aufricht rasp, small; 1 Wiener antrum rasp; 2 Ballenger swivel knives; 1 Ballenger chisel, 4 mm; 2 Converse guarded osteotomes; 1 Cottle osteotome, round corners, curved, 6 mm; 4 Cottle osteotomes, straight (4, 7, 9, and 12 mm); 1 mallet, lead-filled head. **C,** *Top, left to right,* 1 Ferris-Smith fragment forceps; 1 mastoid articulated retractor; 1 Cottle bone crusher, closed; 1 Aufricht retractor. *Bottom, left to right,* 1 Kerrison rongeur, upbite; Killian nasal speculum, 2 inches (5 cm), front view; Killian nasal speculum, 3 inches (7.5 cm), side view; 1 Vienna nasal speculum, 1⅜ inches, front view; 1 Vienna nasal speculum, 1⅜ inches, side view; Asch septum forceps; 2 Army-Navy retractors, side view and front view. *(From Tighe SM: Instrumentation for the operating room, ed 6, St Louis, 2003, Mosby.)*

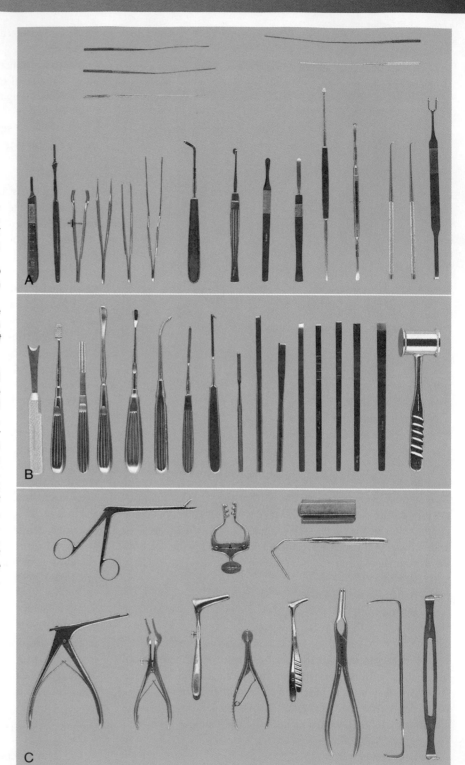

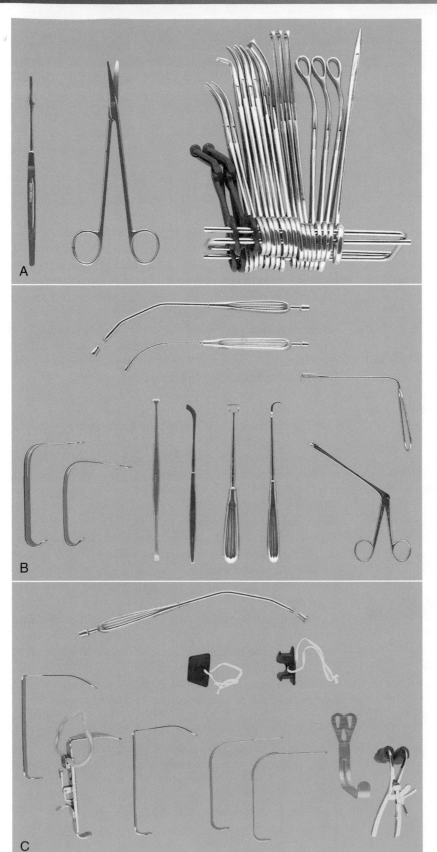

Figure 28-15 **Basic tonsil and adenoid instruments. A,** *Left to right,* 1 Bard-Parker knife handle, # 7; 1 Metzenbaum scissors, 7 inches (17.5 cm); drape clips; 3 Crile hemostatic forceps, 6 ½ inches; 1 Westphal hemostatic forceps; 4 tonsil hemostatic forceps; 1 Allis tissue forceps, long, curved; 1 Allis tissue forceps, long; 3 Ballenger sponge forceps, curved; 1 Crile-Wood needle holder, 8 inches (20 cm). **B,** *Top to bottom,* 1 Andrews-Pynchon suction tube with tip; 1 adenoid suction tube, tip connected. *Bottom, left to right,* 2 Weider tongue depressors; 1 Hurd tonsil dissector and pillar retractor; 1 Fisher tonsil knife and dissector; 1 LaForce adenotome, small, front view; 1 LaForce adenotome, large, side view. *Right, top to bottom,* 1 Lothrop uvula retractor; 1 Meltzer adenoid punch, round, with basket. **C,** *Top to bottom,* 1 Andrews-Pynchon suction tube with tip; 2 bite blocks: child and adult. *Left to right,* 1 McIvor mouth gag frame with blade and two additional blades; 3 Weider tongue depressors, two side views and one front view; side mouth gag. *(From Tighe SM: Instrumentation for the operating room, ed 6, St Louis, 2003, Mosby.)*

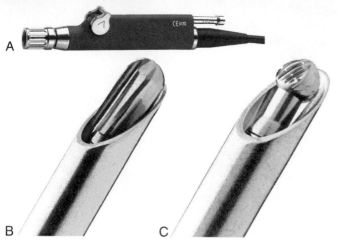

Figure 28-16 A, Tissue shaver for use on cartilage and other soft connective tissue. **B,** Shielded shaver blade. **C,** Shielded spherical blade. *(Courtesy Conmed, Utica, NY.)*

segments of tissue and suctions them, removing blood and debris from the surgical field. Blades are available in a variety of lengths and as straight blades or blades with a 15- or 30-degree bend. A high-speed drill is used to drill bone in the ear and in nasal surgery.

Sinus Scope

The sinus endoscope (sinus scope) is used to visualize the sinus passages of the nose and face. The endoscope is available in focal angles of 0, 30, and 70 degrees. The 0-degree scope is used for sinus exploration and evaluation in all procedures. The 30-degree scope is used for maxillary, sphenoid, and ethmoid sinus procedures. The 70-degree scope is used for procedures of the frontal sinus.

NASAL PROCEDURES

ENDOSCOPIC SINUS SURGERY

Surgical Goal

Endoscopic sinus surgery is performed to treat disease of the paranasal sinuses, nasal cavity, and skull base and to improve nasal airflow. Endoscopic techniques are used in the following procedures:

- Polypectomy
- Maxillary antrostomy
- Ethmoidectomy
- Turbinectomy
- Sphenoidectomy

Pathology

Most endoscopic procedures of the nose are done to treat inflammatory or infectious diseases. A **polyp** is redundant mucosal tissue that prevents airflow and drainage of the paranasal sinus. In rare cases, intranasal neoplasms, **epistaxis** (nasal bleeding), and cerebrospinal fluid leakage may be treated endoscopically.

TECHNIQUE

1 The nasal mucosa is injected with a local anesthetic.
2 The nasal cavities are treated with decongestant compresses.
3 The endoscope is inserted into the nasal cavity.
4 Diseased tissue is removed.
5 Bleeding is controlled.
6 Nasal packing is inserted if needed.

Discussion

The patient is placed in the supine position with the head stabilized on a doughnut headrest and the arms tucked at the sides. General anesthesia is used. A local anesthetic (usually 1% lidocaine with epinephrine 1:100,000) is injected into the nasal mucosa to provide hemostasis. The surgeon uses a nasal speculum and bayonet forceps to pack the nose with small cottonoids soaked in topical anesthetic or a vasoconstrictor (e.g., cocaine solution, topical adrenaline 1:1,000 or Afrin). The patient is prepped and draped for a nasal procedure. The 0-degree sinus endoscope is inserted.

Polypectomy

Under direct visualization with the nasal endoscopes, the surgeon uses either a Wilde forceps or micro debrider to remove the nasal polyps. A # 12 Frazier suction device is used to remove the morcellated tissue.

Maxillary Antrostomy

Under direct visualization with the 0-degree endoscope, the surgeon displaces the middle turbinate with a Freer elevator. The uncinate process is then removed with the sickle knife and Cottle elevator. An alternative technique is to displace the mucosa with a Lusk osteum-seeking probe and then use the micro debrider.

A ball-tip suction probe is used to identify the maxillary antrum. The surgeon may change to a 30-degree endoscope at this point to view the maxillary sinus. The antrum is enlarged with a micro debrider or a reverse biting forceps. Redundant mucosa and polyps are removed from the maxillary sinus with a micro debrider, Wilde forceps, or Takahashi forceps.

Ethmoidectomy

Under direct visualization with a 0-degree endoscope, the surgeon removes (medializes) the middle turbinate up to the midline and removes the uncinate, as in the maxillary antrostomy. This allows visualization of the middle meatus. The ethmoids are removed with either a micro debrider or a Wilde forceps.

Turbinectomy

Under direct visualization with a 0-degree endoscope, the middle turbinate is displaced and the uncinate is removed, as in the maxillary antrostomy. This allows visualization of the middle meatus. The surgeon changes to a 30- or 70-degree endoscope. Any bony obstruction at the frontal sinus osteum is excised with a Wilde forceps or with a micro debrider with a curved blade.

Sphenoidectomy

The posterior ethmoids are removed with a micro debrider or Wilde forceps. A 30-degree endoscope is used to view the sphenoid sinus. The osteum is opened with the micro debrider or Wilde forceps. Diseased tissue is removed with the Wilde forceps or Takahashi forceps.

Bleeding is controlled with nasal packing saturated with a vasoconstrictive agent. The packing is removed after several minutes, and if necessary, fresh packing saturated with antibiotic ointment is inserted.

CALDWELL-LUC PROCEDURE

Surgical Goal

A Caldwell-Luc procedure is a technique used to enter the maxillary sinus in which an incision is made in the gingival-buccal sulcus (the junction of the gum and upper lip). The procedure is commonly performed for drainage of an abscess in the maxillary sinus and surgical removal of granulation tissue that has accumulated as a result of chronic sinus infection.

Pathology

Access to the maxillary sinus and orbital floor is required for treatment of neoplasms and infectious diseases of the orbital cavity.

TECHNIQUE

1　An incision is made in the gingival-buccal sulcus.
2　The periosteum over the canine fossa is elevated.
3　The infraorbital nerve is identified.
4　The anterior wall of the antrum is opened.
5　Cysts and tumors are removed.
6　The gingival-buccal incision is closed.

Discussion

The patient is placed in the supine position with the head on a doughnut headrest and the arms tucked at the sides. General anesthesia is used. Skin prep is omitted for procedures in which an oral approach is used. The patient is draped as for a nasal procedure.

The lip is retracted upward with a gauze sponge, and the gingival-buccal sulcus (gum line) is incised with the ESU. The incision is extended from the lateral incisor to the second molar and carried to the periosteum. The mucous membrane is retracted superiorly to expose the periosteum overlying the canine fossa. The periosteum is elevated with a periosteal elevator to the level of the infraorbital nerve. The nerve is identified and preserved.

Once the periosteum has been removed, the surgeon uses a drill and small cutting burr to enter the maxillary sinus. The opening is enlarged with Kerrison bone-cutting forceps; this exposes the diseased tissue. Cysts and tumors are removed with small cutting instruments, such as a Wilde or Takahashi forceps. Small bone curettes may also be used. The

sinus is irrigated, and small fragments are removed with suction. The gingival-buccal incision is closed with 3-0 absorbable sutures. The Caldwell-Luc procedure is illustrated in Figure 28-17.

TURBINECTOMY/TURBINATE REDUCTION

Surgical Goal

Turbinectomy is removal of the bony turbinate to increase airflow through the nose.

Pathology

Nasal airflow may be impaired by chronic engorgement of the inferior turbinate or congenital malformation of the middle turbinate, called *concha bullosa*. Turbinectomy generally is performed at the same time as septoplasty.

TECHNIQUE

1　A local anesthetic is injected and a vasoconstrictive agent is applied to the nasal mucosa.
2　A nasal speculum is inserted into the nose to expose the affected turbinate.
3　The affected turbinate is removed or reduced.
4　The nasal cavity is packed if necessary.

Discussion

The patient is placed in the supine position with the head on a doughnut headrest and the arms tucked at the sides. General or local anesthesia may be used. The patient is prepped and draped for a nasal procedure. The surgeon begins by infiltrating the turbinate with a local anesthetic with epinephrine. The nose may be temporarily packed with gauze packing (gauze strips) impregnated with a vasoconstrictive agent such as lidocaine with epinephrine. The surgeon then places a nasal speculum in the nose to retract the nostril and expose the turbinates.

If a turbinectomy is to be performed, a # 15 blade is used to make an incision into the mucosa at the anterior border of the inferior turbinate. The mucosa is elevated from the underlying bone with a Freer or Cottle elevator. A portion of the bone is removed with a Wilde forceps. The mucosa may be closed with 3-0 chromic suture.

If a turbinate reduction is planned, a sharp, two-prong bipolar electrode (ESU), sometimes called a *turbinate bipolar*, is inserted into the turbinate and activated for several seconds, causing desiccation of the tissue. The surgeon also may use coblation or somnus cauterization, which uses radiofrequency energy to desiccate the turbinate. This will result in physical shrinkage of the turbinates, allowing greater flow of air. The nasal cavity is packed as necessary to absorb drainage.

SEPTOPLASTY

Surgical Goal

A septoplasty is surgical manipulation of the septum to return it to the correct anatomical position or to gain access to the sphenoid sinus for removal of a pituitary tumor.

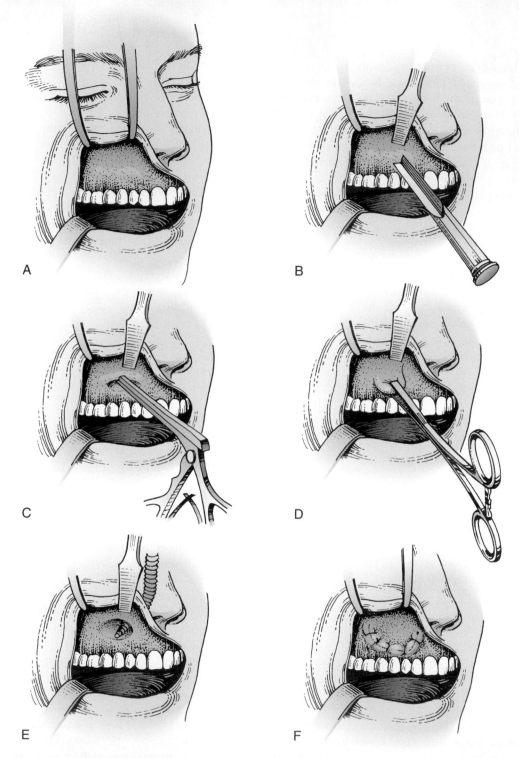

A

B

C

D

E

F

Figure 28-17 **Caldwell-Luc procedure. A,** An incision is made under the upper lip, creating a flap. **B,** The flap is retracted and a perforation is made in the canine fossa. **C,** The perforation is enlarged with a Kerrison rongeur. **D,** The diseased antral membrane is removed. **E,** An antral window is created with a rasp. **F,** The incision is closed. *(Modified from Rothrock JC: Alexander's care of the patient in surgery, ed 12, St Louis, 2003, Mosby.)*

Pathology

Septal deformity may be caused by trauma, infection, neoplasm, or birth trauma, and it may contribute to nasal obstruction, disrupted sleep patterns, headaches, and cosmetic deformities. Septoplasty may be performed with other procedures, such as rhinoplasty or sinus surgery.

TECHNIQUE

1 Local anesthetic is injected into the nasal mucosa.
2 An incision is made ahead of the obstruction on one side.
3 The nasal septum is freed.
4 The deviated bone is removed.
5 The incision is closed.
6 Internal nasal splints are placed.

Discussion

The patient is placed in the supine position with the head on a doughnut headrest and the arms tucked at the sides. General anesthesia often is used, but local anesthesia with monitored intravenous (IV) sedation also may be employed. Before prepping and draping, the surgeon instills the nose and turbinates with a local anesthetic (1% lidocaine with epinephrine 1:100,000) and then packs the nose with $\frac{1}{2}$-inch × 6-inch (0.63-cm × 15-cm) cotton strips soaked in a vasoconstrictive agent (e.g., adrenaline 1:1,000, cocaine, Afrin, or a local anesthetic with epinephrine). The patient is then prepped and draped for a nasal procedure.

The surgeon removes the nasal packs and inserts a nasal speculum. An incision is made in the nasal septum below the obstruction with a # 15 blade. Small tenotomy scissors are used to gently dissect the membranous nasal septum and expose the cartilaginous portion of the septum. The septum is raised from the underlying tissue with a Freer or Cottle elevator. With the nasal septum free, the surgeon removes the deviated bone with a 4-mm chisel and a small mallet. The fractured portions of the septum are grasped with a Takahashi forceps and removed. The incision is closed with 4-0 chromic suture, and internal nasal splints are positioned bilaterally to stabilize the septum. These are sutured to the membranous septum with 3-0 nonabsorbable suture.

RHINOPLASTY

Surgical Goal

Rhinoplasty is performed to reshape the external nose for aesthetic or functional purposes.

Pathology

Deformity of the external nose is caused by injury, congenital defect, or disease. These conditions may lead to functional obstruction, including narrowing and collapse of the cartilage on inspiration. Aesthetic surgery is performed to provide a smooth slope to the nose or to change the width. Rhinoplasty often is performed in conjunction with septoplasty, especially if cartilage is needed for support of external nasal structures.

TECHNIQUE

1 Local anesthetic is injected into the nasal mucosa.
2 An incision is made in the nasal skin and carried to the periosteum.
3 The periosteum and perichondrium are elevated.
4 The nasal bone is remodeled.
5 Septoplasty is performed if necessary.
6 Soft tissue correction and grafting are performed if necessary.
7 The incisions are closed.
8 Internal splints are placed.
9 An external nasal splint is applied.

Discussion

Each rhinoplasty is approached differently, depending on the specific pathological condition. This section provides an overview of the techniques.

The patient is placed in the supine position with the head on a doughnut headrest and the arms tucked at the sides. General anesthesia is used. Before prepping and draping, the surgeon instills a local anesthetic (1% lidocaine with epinephrine 1:100,000) into the nose and turbinates and then packs the nose with $\frac{1}{2}$-inch × 6-inch (0.63-cm × 15-cm) cotton strips soaked in a vasoconstrictive solution (e.g., adrenaline 1:1,000, cocaine, Afrin, or local anesthetic with epinephrine). The patient then is prepped and draped for a nasal procedure, including a head drape.

After removing the nasal packs, the surgeon makes an incision in the nasolabial angle with a # 11 or # 15 blade, and double-prong hooks are inserted to retract the edges of the incision. Frazier suction is used on the incision margins. The *perichondrium* and the *periosteum* are elevated with a Freer elevator and tenotomy scissors. Bony overgrowth is removed with either a rasp or chisel and a small mallet.

Next, the surgeon performs a septoplasty, if necessary. Any cartilage or bone removed from the septum should be placed in normal saline and protected on the back table, because it may be used for grafting later in the procedure. The surgeon then reconstructs the nasal tip, if necessary, by inserting cartilage or bone grafts to provide support or shape.

Finally, lateral osteotomies (bone removal) may be performed with a 3- or 4-mm chisel and small mallet. This is done to straighten a curved nose or to make it narrower. The mucosa then is closed with 3-0 and 4-0 chromic sutures. After the wounds have been closed, internal and external nasal splints are placed. These splints may be made of metal, fiberglass, or tape.

TONSILLECTOMY

Surgical Goal

Tonsillectomy is performed to eradicate infection, improve the airway, or remove a cancer.

Pathology

Tonsillectomy is indicated for a number of different diseases. Among the most common are chronic infection, **hypertrophy** (enlargement), and suspected cancer. Recurrent tonsillitis, chronic tonsillitis, or peritonsillar abscess can lead to hypertrophy, causing disturbed sleep. Hypertrophy also may interfere with swallowing. The tonsil is a common site of cancer in adults, especially smokers.

TECHNIQUE

1 The Crow-Davis mouth gag, including tongue blade, is inserted into the mouth and attached to the Mayo stand.
2 The tonsil is retracted medially with an Allis clamp.
3 The tonsil is separated from the underlying musculature.
4 Bleeding is controlled.

Discussion

The patient is placed in the supine position with a doughnut headrest and a shoulder roll, and the arms are tucked at the side. General anesthesia is administered so that the airway can be supported by endotracheal intubation. The patient is rotated 90 degrees to give the surgeon full access to the head. Draping includes a head drape and a body sheet (usually a three-quarter sheet). Prepping is not necessary, because this procedure takes place in the mouth, which cannot be prepped to reduce bacteria. The surgeon uses a headlight to illuminate the surgical site.

A Crow-Davis retractor is inserted into the oral cavity and secured to the edge of the Mayo stand. This is mechanical retraction, not under direct control of the assistant, surgeon, or scrub. After the retractor has been positioned in the mouth and attached to the Mayo stand, the stand is slowly elevated. This holds the jaw open and provides access to the throat. When the retractor has been secured, the Mayo stand must not be moved or jarred, because this can cause injury. During a tonsillectomy, suction must be available at all times. It is important to protect the lip from burns when a suction ESU is used.

The surgeon grasps the tonsil with a straight or curved Allis clamp and retracts it toward the midline. A peritonsillar incision is made with the ESU or a # 12 blade. The initial incision exposes the tonsillar capsule. The tonsil is separated from the underlying muscle and tonsillar fossa (tonsil bed) with Metzenbaum scissors, a Fisher knife, or a Hurd dissector. Schnidt clamps are used to clamp large bleeding vessels. A tonsil snare may be used to sever the pillar from the tonsil bed. The snare is prepared by inserting fine precut lengths of stainless steel through the tip. This forms a loop, which is used to encircle the tonsil and sever it. Throughout the procedure, the assistant uses suction to remove smoke from the oral cavity and to remove blood and oral secretions. The tonsils are kept as separate specimens and identified as right and left.

Bleeding from the fossa usually is brisk after tonsillectomy. Large vessels are clamped with Schnidt clamps and ligated with 3-0 absorbable suture, or suture ligatures may be used. Tonsil sponges are placed in the tonsil fossa to control bleeding. The oral cavity is irrigated with warm saline, and a final assessment of the operative site is made. The tension of the retractor is then released.

Bleeding is a primary concern after a tonsillectomy. Instruments must remain available for immediate use until the patient has been extubated and transported to the postanesthesia care unit, where immediate surgical care is available in case of postoperative bleeding after extubation.

ADENOIDECTOMY

Surgical Goal

An adenoidectomy is the surgical removal of the adenoids.

Pathology

The primary reasons for an adenoidectomy are chronic infection and obstruction caused by hypertrophy of the tissue. This often leads to obstruction of the eustachian tube and chronic otitis media. Enlarged adenoids may also contribute to upper airway obstruction, resulting in snoring and sleep apnea. Children are affected more often than adults, because the tissue naturally atrophies during adolescence. Adenoidectomy often is performed during tympanostomy and insertion of myringotomy tubes or tonsillectomy.

TECHNIQUE

1 The Crow-Davis mouth gag is inserted.
2 Retraction is applied to the soft palate.
3 The adenoid tissue is removed, and bleeding is controlled.

Discussion

The patient is placed in the supine position, and a doughnut headrest and shoulder roll are used. The arms are tucked at the sides. General anesthesia is administered so that the airway can be supported by endotracheal intubation. The patient is prepped and draped as for a tonsillectomy.

The surgeon stands at the head of the bed and uses a headlight to light the field. A Crow-Davis retractor is inserted into the oral cavity and secured on the edge of the Mayo stand, as described previously. All precautions regarding the Crow-Davis retractor are observed.

The surgeon retracts the palate using a straight (Robinson) catheter (12 or 14 Fr) inserted through the nose and brought out of the mouth. The ends of the catheter are secured with a clamp. Next, the surgeon uses a dental mirror to inspect the adenoids. Dipping the mirror in antifog or Hibiclens solution helps prevent fogging.

If the adenoid tissue is substantial, the surgeon uses an adenoid curette to remove it. The size of the curette depends on the size of the nasopharynx. Adenoid tissue may also be treated with suction ESU (Figure 28-18). After the tissue has been removed, the oral cavity and nasopharynx are irrigated with an Asepto syringe. The surgeon again uses the mirror to ensure that bleeding has stopped and that all of the adenoid tissue has been removed. Tension is carefully released from the Crow-Davis mouth gag, and the catheter and mouth gag are removed.

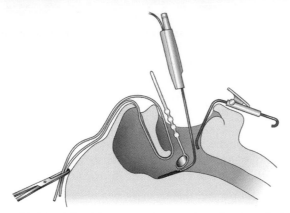

Figure 28-18 Adenoidectomy using suction electrosurgical unit. *(From Dhillon RS, East CA: Ear, nose, and throat and head and neck surgery, ed 3, Edinburgh, 2006, Churchill Livingstone.)*

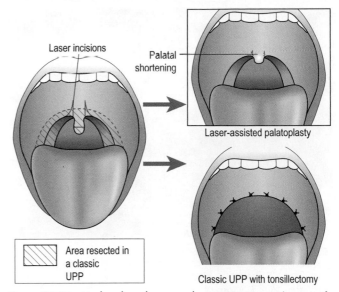

Figure 28-19 Uvulopalatopharyngoplasty (UPP). Surgical options for shortening the palate in the treatment of upper airway obstruction. *(From Dhillon RS, East CA: Ear, nose, and throat and head and neck surgery, ed 3, Edinburgh, 2006, Churchill Livingstone.)*

UVULOPALATOPHARYNGOPLASTY

Surgical Goal

Reconstruction of the uvula and oropharynx, or *uvulopalatopharyngoplasty*, is performed to reduce and tighten oropharyngeal tissue.

Pathology

Enlarged or redundant oropharyngeal mucosa may collapse on inspiration during the deep stages of sleep as muscles lose tone (Figure 28-19). This leads to high intrathoracic pressure as air is pulled through the obstruction, causing sleep apnea or interruption of deep sleep. Obstructive sleep apnea can cause a variety of sleep disorders, ranging from sleep deprivation to dangerous pulmonary and cardiovascular complications, including hypertension, cardiac arrhythmias, and neurological dysfunction.

TECHNIQUE

1 The Crow-Davis mouth gag with tongue blade is inserted.
2 A tonsillectomy is performed.
3 The uvula and soft palate are retracted posteriorly with an Allis clamp.
4 The uvula and a portion of the soft palate are excised.
5 Bleeding is controlled.
6 The soft palate is closed.

Discussion

The patient is positioned as for a tonsillectomy. General anesthesia is used to protect the airway. A tracheotomy setup should be available in case of difficult intubation. The patient then is draped as for a tonsillectomy. Prepping is unnecessary.

A Crow-Davis retractor is inserted and secured to the Mayo stand. The tonsils are removed as necessary, as described previously. After the tonsillectomy, the uvula is grasped with an Allis clamp and retracted posteriorly. The surgeon excises the redundant soft palate and uvula with the ESU. The incision is approximated with 2-0 absorbable sutures. The oropharynx

is irrigated, and any residual bleeding is controlled with the ESU. The tension on the retractor then is released. The tonsils and uvula are preserved as separate specimens and labeled appropriately.

Instruments are kept for immediate use until the patient has been transported to the postanesthesia care unit because of the risk of bleeding after extubation. Selected patients remain in the hospital overnight to ensure that no airway complications arise.

LARYNGOSCOPY

Surgical Goal

Laryngoscopy is endoscopic assessment of the larynx. Tissue specimens may be removed for pathological examination. Instruments for direct laryngoscopy are shown in Figure 28-20.

Pathology

Laryngeal lesions include neoplasms, foreign bodies, papillomas, laryngeal polyps, leukoplakia, and laryngeal web (Figure 28-21). A **papilloma** is a benign proliferative overgrowth of epithelium. Leukoplakia is a benign lesion of the laryngeal epithelium.

TECHNIQUE

Indirect Laryngoscopy
1 A mirror is inserted into the oral cavity.
2 The tongue is retracted manually.
3 The patient is asked to phonate.
4 The vocal cords are visualized.

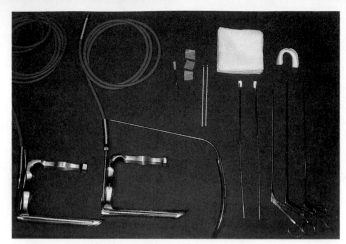

Figure 28-20   **Direct laryngoscopy instruments.** *Left to right,* Rigid laryngoscopes, suction tips, sponge carriers, and forceps for biopsy. *(From Shah JP, Patel SG: Head and neck surgery and oncology, ed 3, London, 2003, Mosby.)*

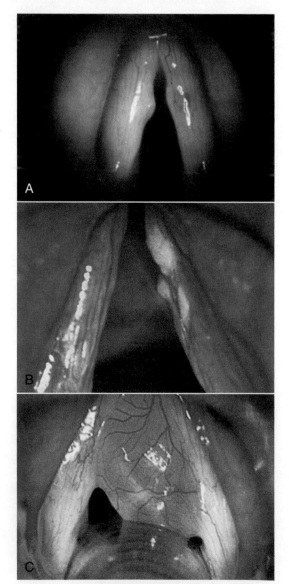

Figure 28-21   **Lesions of the vocal cords. A,** Vocal cord nodules. **B,** Hyperplastic leukoplasia. **C,** Polyp of the right vocal cord. *(From Dhillon RS, East CA: Ear, nose, and throat and head and neck surgery, ed 3, Edinburgh, 2006, Churchill Livingstone.)*

Discussion

The patient is placed either in the sitting position or supine with a doughnut headrest. If the patient can cooperate throughout the procedure, no anesthetic is necessary. However, sedation or general anesthesia may be needed. After examining the mouth, the surgeon retracts the patient's tongue manually with a gauze sponge. The surgeon then positions an examination mirror against the uvula to inspect the larynx, base of the tongue, and pharyngeal wall. The patient may be asked to speak (**phonation**) if possible, so that the surgeon can observe the larynx in motion. The mirror then is removed.

TECHNIQUE

Direct Laryngoscopy
1   A tooth guard is positioned in the mouth.
2   The laryngoscope is introduced into the mouth.
3   The laryngoscope is advanced through the vocal cords.
4   Biopsies are performed.
5   The laryngoscope is removed.

Discussion

The patient is positioned supine with the neck hyperextended, using a shoulder roll as described in Chapter 19. The head is stabilized on a doughnut headrest. General anesthesia is used. The operating table is tilted into reverse Trendelenburg to allow full access to the operative area.

The surgeon introduces a tooth guard to protect the teeth from injury during the procedure. The rigid laryngoscope is introduced on the right side of the mouth and advanced into the upper airway.

Oral secretions are suctioned with an open-tip or a velvet-tip laryngeal suction device. The scrub assists by guiding the instruments into the working channel of the laryngoscope and advancing them a short distance into the scope. The surgeon then continues to advance the scope to the level of the larynx and vocal cords. The surgeon also examines the subglottic region and the upper portion of the trachea. Any suspicious tissue is biopsied with a long, cupped biopsy forceps. The scrub receives biopsy tissue and ensures that all specimens are kept separate and identified by the exact location and side. *It is extremely important that all tissue be collected from the tips of the biopsy instrument and carefully labeled.*

Bleeding is controlled by applying flat pledgets soaked in a vasoconstrictive agent (e.g., adrenaline, Afrin, or cocaine). The scope is gently withdrawn after all specimens have been removed and bleeding has been controlled.

TRACHEOTOMY/TRACHEOSTOMY

Surgical Goal

A tracheotomy or tracheostomy is performed to provide a patent airway.

Pathology

Tracheostomy is indicated for patients who require emergency or elective airway management for prolonged ventilator dependence or acute or chronic upper airway obstruction.

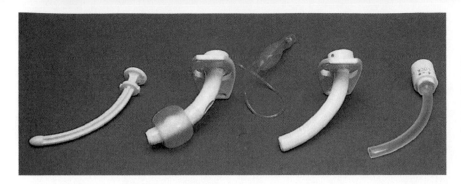

Figure 28-22 Tracheostomy tubes. *Left to right,* Introducer, cuffed fenestrated outer tube, uncuffed nonfenestrated outer tube, inner tube. *(From Dhillon RS, East CA: Ear, nose, and throat and head and neck surgery, ed 3, Edinburgh, 2006, Churchill Livingstone.)*

Upper airway obstruction may be the result of mechanical obstruction, redundant pharyngeal mucosa (causing sleep apnea), a tumor, foreign body, infection, or secretions. Obstruction also may be caused by congenital, neurological, or traumatic conditions. Such obstructions can include a foreign body in the larynx or hypopharynx, acute laryngotracheal bronchitis in children, laryngeal edema, or some other condition that obstructs the airway.

TECHNIQUE

1 An incision is made over the anterior tracheal wall.
2 The tracheal wall is visualized.
3 A tracheal incision is made, usually between the third and fourth tracheal rings.
4 The endotracheal (ET) tube is partly removed to the point superior to the tracheal incision.
5 The tracheotomy tube is inserted.
6 Bleeding is controlled.
7 The tracheotomy tube is secured.
8 Dressings are applied.
9 The obturator from the ET tube is sent with the patient.

Discussion

The patient is placed in the supine position with the head on a doughnut headrest and the arms tucked at the sides with the neck hyperextended. General anesthesia is used. The patient is prepped and draped for a neck procedure.

Using a # 15 blade, the surgeon makes an incision to the midline of the neck; the incision may be vertical or horizontal. The skin flaps are elevated with double-prong skin hooks and a # 15 blade. With the flaps elevated, the strap muscles are separated in the vertical midline, at the median raphe, with a hemostat or the ESU. The isthmus of the thyroid also may be divided to allow visualization of the anterior tracheal wall. A tracheal hook then is placed into the cricoid cartilage to elevate the trachea.

An incision is made into the trachea between the second and third or third and fourth tracheal rings with a # 15 blade. In adults, the tracheal incision is vertical and may include removal of an anterior square of tracheal cartilage. In infants, the tracheal incision is made vertically, and no tracheal cartilage is removed.

After the tracheal incision is made, the anesthesia provider withdraws the endotracheal (ET) tube to the level just above the tracheal incision. A tracheostomy tube then is placed into the tracheal incision with the obturator in place.

When patient ventilation through the tracheostomy tube has been established, the ET tube is completely removed. Bleeding is controlled with the ESU. The tracheostomy tube may be sutured to the skin with 2-0 nonabsorbable suture (e.g., Prolene or silk). Drain sponges and tracheostomy ties are then applied. The obturator must be sent along with the patient after surgery. Figure 28-22 shows an assortment of tracheostomy tubes and a tracheostomy is illustrated in Figure 28-23.

The obturator of the tracheostomy tube is kept with the patient as long as the tracheal tube is in place. If the tube becomes dislodged or is traumatically removed, the obturator is needed to replace the tube.

SECTION III: THE NECK

INTRODUCTION

Surgery of the neck most often is performed to remove or debulk tumors arising from the mouth or upper respiratory system and for surgery of the salivary and thyroid glands.

SURGICAL ANATOMY

NERVES, VASCULAR SUPPLY, AND MUSCLES OF THE NECK

The neck is anatomically organized into triangles for identification. These triangles are called anterior and posterior triangles. Each side of the neck is divided into two large triangles separated by the sternocleidomastoid muscle (SCM), which attaches at the superior end to the mastoid process below the ear and inferiorly to the sternum and clavicle. Below the SCM is the carotid sheath, which contains the carotid artery and its bifurcation, the internal jugular vein, and the vagus nerve (Figure 28-24).

The spinal accessory nerve (cranial nerve XI) crosses the posterior triangle of the neck behind the SCM. The anterior cervical triangle is located anterior to the SCM. The digastric muscle crosses this triangle. Finally, the submandibular triangle occurs above the digastric muscle. This section contains the submandibular gland and the hypoglossal nerve (cranial nerve XII).

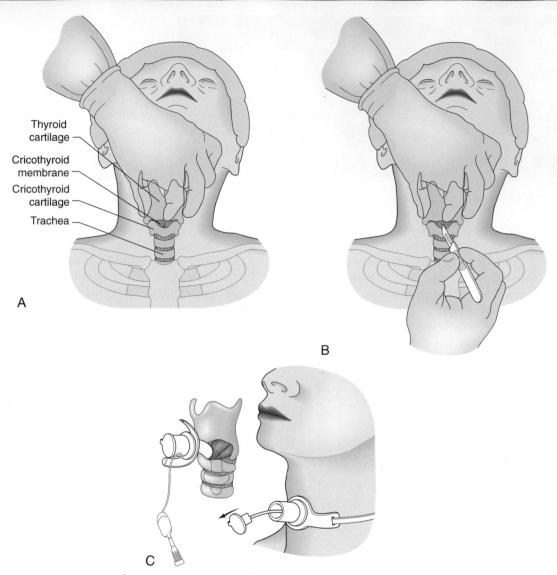

Thyroid cartilage
Cricothyroid membrane
Cricothyroid cartilage
Trachea

A

B

C

Figure 28-23   Tracheostomy. **A,** Palpation of the thyroid cartilage. **B,** An incision is made through the cricoid cartilage. **C,** Insertion of the tracheostomy tube. *(From Garden O, Bradbury A, Forsythe J, Parks R:* Principles and practice of surgery, *ed 5, Edinburgh, 2007, Churchill Livingstone.)*

The space below the digastric muscle contains an important structure, the carotid sheath. The larynx, pharynx, thyroid gland, and parathyroid glands lie on the medial side of the carotid sheath.

Cervical lymph nodes are located throughout the anterior neck. The thoracic duct, which connects the body's entire lymphatic system to the vascular system, is located in the left lower neck behind the carotid sheath, where it inserts at the junction of the left internal jugular vein and subclavian vein.

SALIVARY GLANDS

There are three pairs of salivary glands: the parotid, submandibular, and sublingual salivary glands. Many minor salivary glands are found throughout the oral cavity and pharynx. The largest of the glands, the parotid gland, is situated over the mandible, anterior to the ear. It extends anteriorly to the masseter muscle. The tail of the parotid gland extends below the mandible into the upper neck. The parotid duct drains into the mouth and the cheek opposite the upper second molar. The facial nerve passes through the gland, where it branches and then exits from the anterior aspect (Figure 28-25, *A*).

The submandibular gland is the second largest salivary gland. It is C-shaped and wraps around the lower (inferior) border of the mandible (see Figure 28-25, *B*). The submandibular duct, or Wharton duct, emerges from the deep anterior portion of the gland and drains into the anterior floor of the mouth. A branch of the facial nerve lies within the superficial fascia of the gland. The hypoglossal nerve (cranial nerve XII) and the lingual nerve lie beneath the gland.

The smallest of the salivary glands, the sublingual glands, lie in the floor of the mouth just beneath the mucosa and empty into the oral cavity via multiple small ducts (ducts of Rivinus).

The salivary glands produce saliva, which irrigates the oral cavity and contains enzymes for breaking down simple carbohydrates. Buffers in saliva reduce acidity in the mouth and protect against pathogenic bacteria and demineralization of the teeth.

THYROID GLAND

The thyroid gland is located in the midneck and overlies the trachea below the larynx. It has two lobes, which are connected by a central band of thyroid tissue called the *isthmus*. A thin strip of thyroid tissue also projects from the superior edge of the isthmus (Figure 28-26). The thyroid secretes the hormones thyroxine (T_4) and triiodothyronine (T_3). These thyroid hormones (THs) are necessary for regulating cell metabolism and growth. Calcitonin, which also is secreted by the thyroid, is necessary for calcium regulation. The parathyroid glands are situated within the lobes of the thyroid. These small glands produce parathyroid hormone (PTH), which influences calcium and phosphate levels in the blood.

The thyroid gland is highly vascular and is composed of follicles that synthesize the thyroid hormones.

CASE PLANNING

POSITIONING THE PATIENT FOR NECK SURGERY

Procedures of the neck are performed with the patient in the supine position with the head stabilized on a doughnut headrest. The arms are secured on arm boards at an angle of less than 90 degrees for venous access during general anesthesia. The neck may be hyperextended for better access; this is achieved by placing a padded roll at the shoulders. The roll must be carefully positioned to prevent compression of the cervical nerve.

DRAPING

Patients undergoing procedures of the neck are draped to exclude the face and to maintain a sterile field. The surgical site is draped with towels, which are secured with towel clips or skin staples. A clear incise drape commonly is used to cover

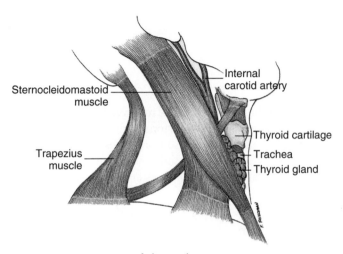

Figure 28-24 **Anatomy of the neck.** *(From Potter PA, Perry AG: Fundamentals of nursing, ed 5, St Louis, 2001, Mosby.)*

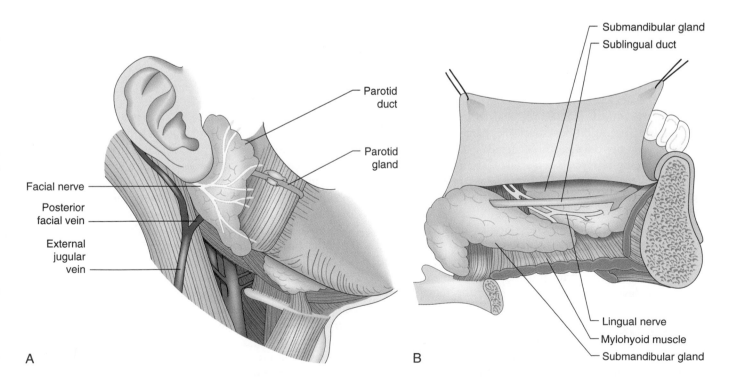

Figure 28-25 **The salivary glands. A,** Anatomy of the parotid gland. **B,** The submandibular gland. *(From Garden O, Bradbury A, Forsythe J, Parks R: Principles and practice of surgery, ed 5, Edinburgh, 2007, Churchill Livingstone.)*

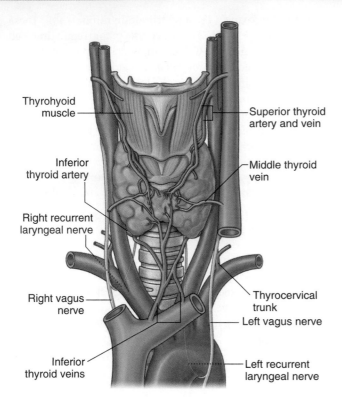

Thyrohyoid muscle

Inferior thyroid artery

Right recurrent laryngeal nerve

Right vagus nerve

Inferior thyroid veins

Superior thyroid artery and vein

Middle thyroid vein

Thyrocervical trunk

Left vagus nerve

Left recurrent laryngeal nerve

Figure 28-26   Relationship of the thyroid to the trachea and larynx. *(From Drake R, Vogl W, Mitchell A: Gray's anatomy for students, Edinburgh, 2004, Churchill Livingstone.)*

the towels and operative site. The patient then is draped with a split sheet that surrounds the head. It may be helpful to cover the patient's chest with a towel and place a magnetic drape on top of the towel to prevent instruments from dropping to the floor during surgery.

INSTRUMENTS

General surgical instruments are required for procedures of the head and neck. Additional special instruments are included in tracheal and thyroid sets. These include neck retractors and thyroid grasping clamps. Vascular clamps may be added for radical neck procedures. Numerous vital nerves and large blood vessels in the neck require soft retraction with a Penrose drain or surgical vessel loops made of Silastic or cotton. Numerous right angle clamps are needed during extensive neck dissection.

Neck dissection involves a significant risk of injury to peripheral nerves. A peripheral nerve stimulator or nerve monitoring device often is used to prevent this injury.

DRESSINGS

Neck dressings vary according to the procedure. Tracheotomy incisions generally are dressed with drain sponges (4 × 4 gauze that has been split to include the tracheotomy tube) and tracheal ties. Other procedures of the neck may be dressed with Telfa and Tegaderm or 4 × 4 sponges and tape. After radical

neck procedures, a suction drain may be placed in the wound before closure.

MEDICATIONS

The medications most often used in head and neck surgery are local anesthetics and hemostatic agents. Hemostatic agents such as Gelfoam and thrombin should be available for extensive neck dissection.

SURGICAL PROCEDURES

EXCISION OF THE SUBMANDIBULAR GLAND

Surgical Goal
The submandibular gland is removed.

Pathology
The submandibular gland may be removed because of chronic infection (bacterial or viral), stone formation, or neoplasm (benign or malignant). These conditions are much more common in adults than in children. In children, however, about 60% of salivary gland masses are malignant.

TECHNIQUE

1 A skin incision is made 0.8 inch (2 cm) below the mandible.
2 The submandibular gland is exposed.
3 The facial artery and vein are ligated.
4 The gland is separated from the mandible.
5 The submandibular duct and nerve are ligated.
6 The gland is removed.
7 Bleeding is controlled.
8 The incision is closed.

Discussion
The patient is positioned for neck surgery. General anesthesia is used. The patient is prepped and draped for a neck procedure, which includes inferior mandibular access.

The surgeon makes an incision with a # 10 or # 15 blade just below the inferior border of the mandible within a naturally occurring tissue fold. The incision is carried through the platysma muscle with the knife or Metzenbaum scissors. The skin-muscle flaps are retracted with double-prong skin hooks or small rake retractors. The surgeon does this carefully to avoid injuring the marginal mandibular branch of the facial nerve.

The knife or Metzenbaum scissors is used to make an incision in the inferior border of the gland. The facial artery and vein are identified, clamped, and ligated with 2-0 or 3-0 silk ties.

The tissue and vessels overlying the gland are retracted superiorly with a dull Senn retractor or three-prong dull rake. The gland then is retracted with an Allis clamp or manually with a surgical sponge. Metzenbaum scissors and bipolar ESU are used to separate the gland from the inferior border of the mandible. The submandibular branch of the lingual nerve is identified, clamped, and ligated with 2-0 or 3-0 silk ties.

Next, an Army-Navy retractor is inserted to retract the myohyoid muscle anteriorly. This exposes the hypoglossal nerve. The submandibular duct is identified and ligated. The remaining soft tissue attachments are excised with a monopolar ESU. Bleeding is controlled with the ESU. The wound is irrigated and a drain is put in place as necessary. The incision is closed in layers with 3-0 absorbable sutures. The skin may be closed with absorbable or nonabsorbable sutures.

PAROTIDECTOMY

Surgical Goal
A parotidectomy is the surgical removal of the parotid gland.

Pathology
A parotidectomy most often is performed for the treatment of a neoplasm. The facial nerve splits the parotid gland into superficial and deep lobes. Disease most often occurs in the superficial lobe and rarely involves the deep lobe. Involvement of the deep lobe usually indicates malignancy. However, most neoplasms of the parotid are benign.

TECHNIQUE

1 A skin incision is made anterior to the ear.
2 The parotid gland is exposed.
3 The gland is mobilized and the sternocleidomastoid muscle is retracted.
4 The gland is separated from the cartilaginous portion of the external auditory canal.
5 The facial nerve is identified.
6 The superficial portion of the parotid gland is removed.
7 The deep portion of the parotid gland is excised if necessary.
8 Bleeding is controlled.
9 The wound is closed.

Discussion
The patient is positioned and draped for a neck procedure. General anesthesia is required. However, neuromuscular blocking agents are not used to allow stimulation of the facial nerve for identification.

The skin incision begins just anterior to the helix of the ear and extends downward to the tragus. If necessary, the incision can be extended for greater access.

The surgeon creates skin flaps by dissecting the subcutaneous layer with Metzenbaum scissors. The skin flaps are retracted with skin hooks or dull rakes. The gland is separated from the SCM and the cartilaginous portion of the external auditory canal with Metzenbaum scissors. The facial nerve trunk then is identified. A nerve stimulator or monitoring device may be required to identify the nerve.

Dissection is continued along the facial nerve branches, either superiorly or inferiorly, with a mosquito clamp and bipolar ESU or McCabe dissector until the superficial portion of the gland is removed. If the deep lobe of the parotid must be excised, the facial nerve is elevated and retracted with vessel loops. With the facial nerve retracted, the facial nerve branches are elevated off the underlying deep lobe of the parotid gland with a hemostat and bipolar ESU.

Dissection continues using the same technique to separate the gland from the underlying masseter muscle. Allis clamps are used to grasp the gland and provide countertraction as it is elevated. After the gland is removed, the wound is irrigated and a drain is placed. The wound then is closed in layers with absorbable sutures. The skin may be closed with either absorbable or nonabsorbable sutures. A parotidectomy is illustrated in Figure 28-27.

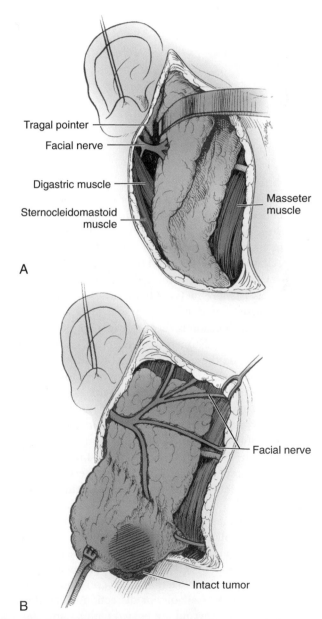

Tragal pointer
Facial nerve
Digastric muscle
Sternocleidomastoid muscle
Masseter muscle

A

Facial nerve

Intact tumor

B

Figure 28-27 **Parotidectomy. A,** Blunt dissection of the parotid gland, exposing the facial nerve. **B,** Removal of tissue with the facial nerve intact. *(From Cummings CW, Haughey BH, Thomas JR, et al: Otolaryngology: head and neck surgery, ed 3, St Louis, 1998, Mosby.)*

THYROIDECTOMY

Surgical Goal

A thyroidectomy is the surgical removal of one or more lobes of the thyroid gland.

Pathology

A thyroidectomy is performed to treat known or suspected malignancy or for the treatment of hyperthyroidism in selected cases. Benign enlargement of the thyroid (*goiter*) may compress the airway or esophagus. Removal of all or one lobe of the thyroid relieves the obstruction. In hyperthyroid disorders, such as Graves disease, the patient may select partial removal of the hyperfunctioning gland or treatment with radioactive iodine.

TECHNIQUE

1 The neck is incised.
2 The platysma muscle is divided.
3 The thyroid is mobilized.
4 The recurrent laryngeal nerve is identified and preserved.
5 The parathyroids are identified and preserved.
6 The thyroid is removed.
7 Bleeding is controlled.
8 The wound is closed.

Discussion

The patient is positioned for a neck procedure with the neck hyperextended. General anesthesia is administered. Before beginning the procedure, the surgeon may mark the proposed incision in a naturally occurring tissue fold over the thyroid.

The neck is incised with a # 10 or # 15 blade. The subcutaneous tissue is incised with the ESU, exposing the platysma muscle. The assistant retracts the tissue layers with rake retractors. The surgeon then divides the muscle layer with the deep knife or ESU. The incision is carried deeper with the ESU and Metzenbaum scissors. Numerous bleeders are encountered in the deep tissue, and these are controlled with the ESU.

As the dissection continues, deeper retractors are used, such as a Green retractor designed for thyroid surgery. When the thyroid gland is exposed, two Lahey spring retractors, or a Mahorner thyroid retractor, are placed in the wound. The surgeon then grasps the gland with one or two Lahey tenacula. As the surgeon dissects the gland from the surrounding tissues, the parathyroid glands, the superior laryngeal nerves, and the recurrent laryngeal nerve are identified and preserved.

The thyroid gland is an extremely vascular structure. Therefore, to mobilize it, the surgeon successively double-clamps small sections of tissue, divides the tissue between the clamps, and ligates each section. Most surgeons use Kelly or mosquito clamps for mobilization. The scrub should have at least 12 to 15 clamps available for dissection of the thyroid. Large arteries of the thyroid are ligated with suture ligatures of 2-0 or 3-0 silk mounted on a fine needle. When mobilization and excision are complete, the gland is passed to the scrub. A frozen section may be required for determination of malignancy.

The wound is irrigated, and a Penrose drain is placed in the wound if necessary. The tissue layers of the neck are closed individually. The skin is closed with staples or fine nonabsorbable suture. The incision is dressed with flat gauze. Fluff gauze may be used if a drain has been inserted.

TECHNIQUE

1 The skin is incised and the skin flaps are elevated using sharp dissection.
2 The platysma muscle is divided.
3 The thyroid sheath is dissected.
4 Bleeders are serially clamped and ligated.
5 The upper and lower poles of the thyroid are explored bilaterally for parathyroid glands.
6 Affected glands are dissected and removed.
7 The wound is closed.

Injury of the recurrent laryngeal nerve can alter airway function. The surgeon may want a flexible laryngoscope available to examine the vocal cords in the recovery room when the patient is sufficiently awake to follow commands. A tracheotomy set should be available in the event of a bilateral cord paralysis. A thyroidectomy is illustrated in Figure 28-28.

THYROPLASTY

Surgical Goal

A thyroplasty involves moving the vocal cord to one side and stabilizing it with a Silastic or Gore-Tex implant.

Pathology

Unilateral vocal cord paralysis, or **paresis,** is the primary reason for performing a thyroplasty. Paralysis may be caused by a variety of conditions, including surgical trauma to the laryngeal nerves or prolonged intubation. Cord paralysis may prevent the vocal cords from meeting at the midline during speaking. Open, closed, or unilateral paralysis can cause difficulty with speech, such as hoarseness and aspiration. The most common type of thyroplasty is medialization, in which the paralyzed cord is fixed in the midline so that the moving cord may push against the fixed cord to close the glottis. This improves speech volume and stamina and reduces aspiration. A paralyzed cord may also obstruct the airway and require lateral fixation.

TECHNIQUE

1 An incision is made over the larynx.
2 The incision is carried to the thyroid cartilage.
3 A "window" is cut into the thyroid cartilage to expose the paraglottic space.
4 A nasolaryngoscope is inserted to view the vocal cords.
5 The true vocal cord is medialized.
6 The patient is asked to speak to assess the position of the vocal cord.
7 An implant is positioned in the paraglottic space.
8 The incision is closed.

Discussion

The patient is positioned for a neck procedure as described previously. The patient is awake for most of the procedure; therefore, it is important that the person be comfortable. IV sedation is given, and a local anesthetic (1% lidocaine with epinephrine 1:100,000) is infiltrated into the surgical site.

The surgeon makes a 0.8- to 1.2-inch (2- to 3-cm) incision in the neck at the midline with a # 15 blade. The skin edges are retracted with double-prong skin hooks. The skin and subcutaneous tissue are dissected from the underlying tissue and elevated. This exposes the platysma, which is divided with a # 15 blade and toothed Adson forceps. A small Weitlaner retractor is placed to expose the strap muscles, which are retracted laterally to expose the thyroid muscle.

A Freer elevator is used to release the thyroid muscle from the thyroid cartilage. With the thyroid cartilage exposed, the surgeon marks the cartilage for the window (Figure 28-29, A to E). This can be done with a caliper or freehand.

When the window has been marked, a small sagittal saw is used to cut a window measuring 5 × 10 mm. The assistant keeps the cartilage moist with sterile saline to prevent the cartilage from being burned during dissection with the sagittal saw. The surgeon then dissects the incised tissue with a single-prong skin hook and a Freer elevator (see Figure 28-29, F and G).

Medialization of the cord is performed by pushing the thyroarytenoid cartilage to the midline. The anesthesiologist passes a flexible **nasolaryngoscope** to visualize the medialization.

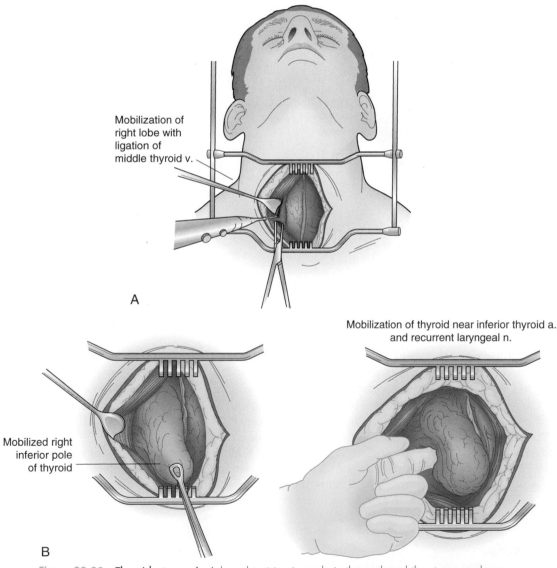

Figure 28-28 **Thyroidectomy. A,** A lateral incision is made in the neck and the strap muscles are retracted with a Green retractor. The thyroid vein is exposed and ligated. **B,** Traction is placed on the thyroid for continued mobilization.

Continued

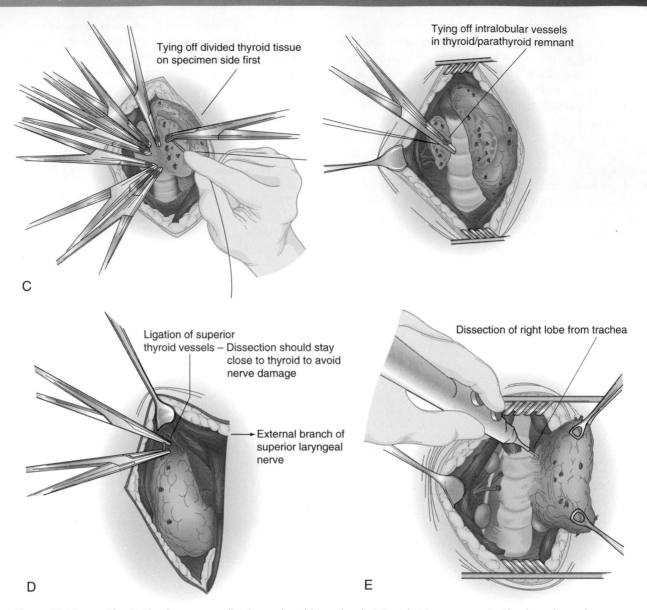

Tying off divided thyroid tissue on specimen side first

Tying off intralobular vessels in thyroid/parathyroid remnant

C

Ligation of superior thyroid vessels – Dissection should stay close to thyroid to avoid nerve damage

External branch of superior laryngeal nerve

D

Dissection of right lobe from trachea

E

Figure 28-28, cont'd   C, Bleeders are serially clamped and ligated with 3-0 and 4-0 suture ties. **D,** The thyroid vessels are carefully dissected free and ligated. **E,** The lobe is dissected from the trachea with the electrosurgical unit. *(From Sabiston DC Jr, Gordon RG, editors:* Atlas of general surgery, *Philadelphia, 1994, WB Saunders.)*

The surgeon asks the patient to speak while the nasolaryngoscope is in place. This step is taken to confirm that the paralyzed cord has been medialized. On confirmation of medialization, the surgeon places an implant. Medialization can be achieved with a portion of a Silastic block that has been carved by the surgeon; a Gore-Tex patch, mesh, or implant; or a prefabricated implant.

The surgeon approximates the strap muscles with 3-0 or 4-0 absorbable suture. A small drain may be placed below the platysmal layer. The platysma is closed with absorbable suture. The skin then is closed and dressed.

NECK DISSECTION

Surgical Goal

Neck dissection is performed to remove a tumor and affected lymph nodes.

Pathology

Many head and neck cancers, including malignant tumors of the oral and pharyngeal cavities, cutaneous malignant melanoma, and skin cancer, metastasize to the cervical lymph nodes.

Three types of neck dissections may be performed, depending on tumor staging. *Radical neck dissection* is the removal of all cervical lymph nodes and surrounding structures, including the spinal accessory nerve, the internal jugular vein, and the SCM. *Modified radical neck dissection* is the excision of all lymph nodes with the preservation of one or more of the nonlymphatic structures (e.g., spinal accessory nerve, internal jugular vein, or SCM). *Selective neck dissection* is the removal of the upper two thirds of the cervical lymph nodes and structures with preservation of the neurovascular and musculoskeletal structures.

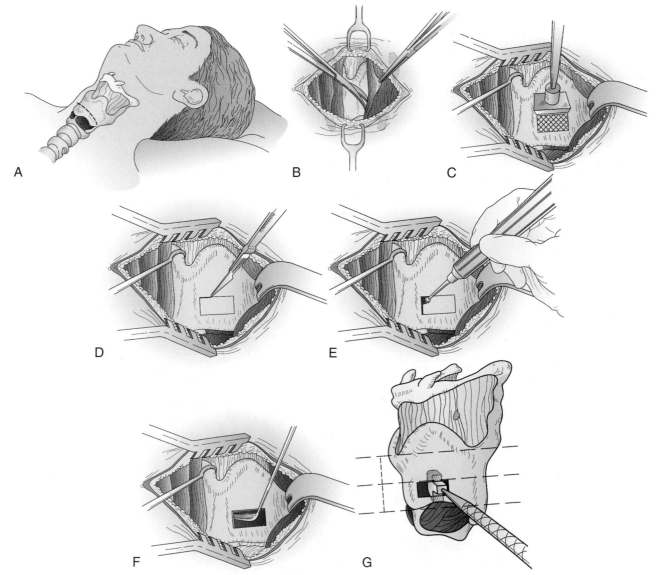

Figure 28-29 **Thyroplasty (vocal cord medialization).** **A,** An incision is made in the midline in the neck. **B,** Skin flaps are created to expose the platysma. **C,** The template for the window is positioned. **D,** The cartilage is marked. **E,** The window is removed. **F,** The window is elevated. **G,** The vocal cord is shifted medially and the implant is positioned. *(Modified from Cummings CW, Haughey BH, Thomas JR, et al: Otolaryngology: head and neck surgery, ed 3, St Louis, 1998, Mosby.)*

TECHNIQUE

1 A skin incision is made.
2 The structures of the neck are exposed.
3 The affected structures are removed.
4 Bleeding is controlled.
5 A tracheotomy is performed if necessary.
6 A drain is placed and the wound is closed.

Discussion

The patient is placed in the supine position on a doughnut or Mayfield headrest with the affected side of the neck upward. The arms are tucked at the patient's sides, and a shoulder roll is placed to hyperextend the neck slightly. General anesthesia is used. The patient is prepped, including the face, neck, and chest, and draped for a head and neck procedure.

The skin incision is made with a # 15 blade. The incision is extended through the platysma, and the ESU and double-prong skin hooks are used for retraction. Bleeding vessels may be ligated with 2-0 or 3-0 silk ties.

The surgeon mobilizes the SCM using blunt dissection and then retracts it laterally with an Army-Navy retractor. If the SCM is to be sacrificed, it is cut with the ESU. This allows the surgeon to visualize the neurovascular sheath. Dissection continues along the neurovascular sheath to expose the anterior portion of the specimen. This dissection is performed bluntly with hemostats.

With the neurovascular sheath exposed, the surgeon identifies the carotid artery, internal jugular vein, and vagus nerve. The neurovascular sheath is retracted with a Cushing vein retractor. If the internal jugular vein is to be sacrificed, it is double-clamped, transected, and ligated with multiple 2-0 silk ties and 2-0 stick ties. The surgeon then retracts the SCM anteriorly, exposing the lateral cervical triangle. The subcutaneous tissue is removed with blunt dissection or Metzenbaum scissors. Bleeders are clamped with hemostats and 2-0 silk ties or the ESU. A tracheotomy is performed if necessary. The wound is then irrigated with normal saline. A drain is placed in the wound, and the wound is closed in layers with absorbable suture. A radical neck dissection is illustrated in Figure 28-30.

GLOSSECTOMY

Surgical Goal

A glossectomy is the removal of the tongue for the treatment of cancer. A partial glossectomy is removal of less than half of the tongue *(hemiglossectomy)*. Simple excision includes primary closure or application of a split-thickness skin graft (STSG) to the anterior tongue. A secondary goal is to ensure that closure of the floor of the mouth prevents a fistula or leakage of saliva from the oral cavity into the neck tissues.

Pathology

The entire neurovascular supply of one side of the tongue passes through the base of the tongue; therefore, if one side of

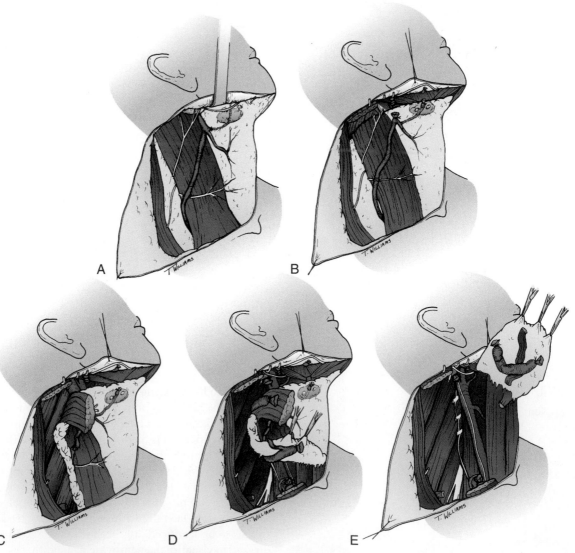

Figure 28-30 **Radical neck dissection. A,** Elevation of the skin flaps. **B,** Dissection and ligation of the facial vessels and dissection of the submandibular fascia. **C,** Sacrifice of the sternocleidomastoid muscle (SCM) superiorly. **D,** Sacrifice of the SCM inferiorly and ligation of the internal jugular. **E,** Removal of the specimen. *(Modified from Cummings CW, Haughey BH, Thomas JR, et al: Otolaryngology: head and neck surgery, ed 3, St Louis, 1998, Mosby.)*

the base of the tongue requires excision, that entire side must be removed. A total glossectomy is the excision of tissue in the anterior two thirds of the tongue. A pectoralis major myocutaneous (PMC [also called PMMC]) flap or a free flap is constructed to produce a watertight seal. A total glossectomy is almost always combined with a total laryngectomy to treat laryngeal metastasis or problems with aspiration. A PMC or free flap is required to provide a watertight seal.

TECHNIQUE

Partial Glossectomy

1 The tongue is grasped with a towel clip, or heavy silk sutures are placed through the tongue.
2 The affected portion of the tongue is excised with the electrosurgical unit.
3 The defect is closed or a split-thickness skin graft is placed.

Discussion: Partial Glossectomy—Primary Closure or STSG Closure

Radical procedures of the neck require instruments used in general surgery and vascular surgery, as well as fine orthopedic instruments, including a drill.

The patient is placed in the supine position on a doughnut or Mayfield headrest with the arms tucked at the sides. General anesthesia is used. The patient is prepped and draped for a head and neck procedure.

The surgeon grasps the tongue either by using large towel clips at the midline or by suturing the midline with a size 0 silk suture and grasping the ends of the suture with a hemostat. The tongue is pulled anteriorly to expose the affected tissue. The surgeon excises the tumor and a wide margin with the ESU blade or needle tip. The tongue is then closed. If primary closure is possible, the tongue is closed with 3-0 absorbable sutures. If primary closure is not possible, the defect is closed with an STSG. The graft is sutured into place with 3-0 absorbable suture.

TECHNIQUE

Hemiglossectomy

1 An incision is made at the midline of the lip and extended to the submental region.
2 The soft tissue is retracted to expose the anterior surface of the mandible.
3 A titanium plate is placed over the proposed site of division and then removed.
4 The mandible is divided at the midline.
5 The tongue is divided at the midline for hemiglossectomy.
6 An incision is made in the floor of mouth between the tongue and the mandible.
7 The tumor is excised.
8 The mandible is approximated and internally fixated.
9 The incision is closed.

Discussion: Glossectomy with Mandibulotomy and PMC Flap

The patient is placed in the supine position on a doughnut or Mayfield headrest with the arms tucked at the sides. General anesthesia is used. Often, a tracheotomy has been performed or will be performed before the glossectomy. The patient is prepped and draped for a head and neck procedure, including the chest in case a PMC flap is needed.

A # 15 blade is used to make an incision through the midline lip; the incision is extended to the submental border. Skin flaps are elevated with the ESU. Senn rakes are used for retraction.

When the mandibular surface is exposed, a titanium plate is positioned in the region of the planned division. The screw holes are drilled with a small power drill. The plate is secured to the mandible with screws. The surgeon removes the plate after placement and splits the mandible at the midline, using a small power saw with a medium saw blade. If a mandibulectomy is to be performed, segmental resection of the bone may be performed at this stage of the procedure. The top of the mandible may have to be sacrificed and further resection is performed after verification of tumor margins.

The surgeon then grasps the mandible with atraumatic rake retractors or a self-retaining retractor (e.g., a Weitlaner retractor). In a hemiglossectomy, the anterior part of the oral floor and the body of the tongue are divided at the midline with the ESU. The incision is extended to the tongue base. The affected side of the tongue is then excised with the ESU.

The incision is closed primarily or with a skin graft. The mandible is approximated and internally fixed with the plate. The incision is closed in layers with absorbable suture. For a total glossectomy, the incision is made between the floor of the mouth and the mandible and extended to the base of tongue with the ESU. The tongue is excised from the epiglottis with the ESU. A neck dissection is performed on one or both sides of the neck (see neck dissection).

If the incision cannot be closed primarily or with an STSG, a PMC flap is harvested (see later, Pectoralis Major Myocutaneous and Deltopectoral Flaps). The flap is sutured into the defect with the skin taking the place of the tongue. The skin is sutured to the remaining mucosa of the floor of the mouth (and to the epiglottic or pharyngeal mucosa if a total laryngectomy was performed concomitantly). Size 3-0 absorbable suture is used for closure. The mandible is reapproximated and internally fixed with the titanium plate.

The lip incision, oral mucosa, and deep portions of the skin incisions are closed with 3-0 absorbable sutures. The skin is closed with fine nonabsorbable suture. A nasal feeding tube is placed and secured with 2-0 silk suture through the nasal septum. The skin incisions are then coated in antibiotic ointment.

The patient is transferred to the intensive care unit for airway monitoring. A gastrostomy tube may be inserted to provide nutrition.

LARYNGECTOMY

Surgical Goal

A laryngectomy is the removal of the larynx, usually with wide excision and tissue grafting.

Pathology

A laryngectomy may be performed for four reasons:

- Cancer of the larynx
- Diversion for total separation of the respiratory and digestive tracts
- Chondroradionecrosis
- Major trauma that precludes open reduction and internal fixation

TECHNIQUE

1 A skin incision is made.
2 The larynx and neck contents are exposed.
3 A neck dissection is performed if necessary.
4 A tracheotomy is performed.
5 The larynx is removed.
6 The pharynx is closed
7 Bleeding is controlled.
8 Drains are placed.
9 The wound is closed.

Discussion

The patient is placed in the supine position on a doughnut or Mayfield headrest with the arms tucked at the sides. A shoulder roll may be placed to hyperextend the neck. General anesthesia is used. The patient is prepped from the level of the nose to the level of the umbilicus and draped for a head and neck procedure, including the face, neck, and chest.

Using a # 15 blade, the surgeon begins by making an apron incision, either from mastoid to mastoid (for laryngectomy with neck dissection) or from midsternocleidomastoid muscle to midsternocleidomastoid muscle (for laryngectomy alone). The flaps are elevated about ½ to 1 inch (1 to 2 cm) above the sternal notch from below and ½ to 1 inch (1 to 2 cm) below the hyoid bone. The flaps generally are secured back with fishhook retractors or suture.

The surgeon detaches the strap muscles from the sternum using the ESU or Mayo scissors and retracts them laterally with Army-Navy retractors. This exposes the carotid sheath, the thyroid, and a portion of the trachea. The carotid sheath is dissected laterally and retracted with a Cushing vein retractor. The thyroid veins may be ligated with hemostat clamps and 2-0 silk ties. The surgeon removes the thyroid lobe on the affected side by dividing the isthmus of the thyroid down the middle with the ESU or scissors.

The thyroid lobe then is dissected free. Scissors are used to remove the fat and lymph tissue from the gland. The inferior thyroid artery is ligated and transected, and the recurrent laryngeal nerve is transected. The dissection of the thyroid continues with blunt dissection to the level of the trachea. The remaining portion of the gland is grasped with a Kocher clamp and divided from the trachea with the ESU.

A cricoid hook is placed in the right side larynx to allow rotation of the larynx and exposure of the constrictor muscles on the thyroid cartilage. These muscles are detached from the cartilage with the ESU.

A periosteal elevator then is used to remove the soft tissue from the underside of the thyroid cartilage. The larynx is rotated to the left with a cricoid hook to free the larynx from the remaining muscle and soft tissue of the thyroid. The surgeon then uses Metzenbaum scissors or a hemostat clamp to dissect the thyroid cartilage from the hyoid bone. Any vessels and nerves that are exposed at this point in the dissection are ligated. All muscular attachments between the tongue base and hyoid bone are separated with the ESU.

With the hyoid bone exposed and free, the surgeon uses heavy Mayo scissors to sever the attachments of the hyoid bone. The tracheotomy is performed at this point because the surgeon is ready to enter the airway. The surgeon sews the anterior tracheal wall to the posterior skin flap to secure it in place. The ET tube then is removed and the anesthesia circuit is switched to the tracheotomy tube.

The surgeon then uses scissors or the ESU to make an incision into the hypopharynx in the midline over the hyoid bone. The hypopharynx is opened with a hemostat, and the epiglottis is grasped with an Allis clamp and rotated out of the larynx. The lateral pharyngeal walls are incised with heavy Mayo scissors, with as much mucosa as possible spared. The larynx then is opened out. The tracheal tube is removed and the posterior membranous trachea is incised with a # 15 blade. The trachea is dissected from the anterior esophageal wall with Metzenbaum scissors. The surgeon also transects any fibrous attachments to the larynx at this point. The larynx is removed, and the tracheal tube is replaced.

With the larynx removed, the pharyngeal mucosa is closed with or without a PMC flap (discussed later) in two layers. The first layer is closed with a long 3-0 absorbable suture on a tapered needle, and the second layer is closed with 3-0 absorbable horizontal mattress sutures. With the pharynx closed, the surgeon creates a stoma by closing the anterior tracheal wall to the inferior skin flap and the posterior tracheal wall to the superior skin flap, using either absorbable or nonabsorbable sutures, depending on the surgeon's preference. The wound is irrigated with normal saline. Drains are placed, and the skin is closed in layers with absorbable suture.

The patient is transferred to the intensive care unit. Chemotherapy and radiation are initiated as soon the wound is sufficiently healed to tolerate them. Laryngectomy is illustrated in Figure 28-31.

Related Procedure

Partial cricoidectomy is subtotal and submucosal resection of the cricoid performed in the treatment or control of chronic aspiration after radical pharyngeal surgery, including removal of the tongue. In this procedure the pharyngeal inlet is enlarged and the laryngeal inlet reduced so that the voice is preserved and aspiration is controlled.

PECTORALIS MAJOR MYOCUTANEOUS AND DELTOPECTORAL FLAPS

Surgical Goal

PMC (or PMMC) and deltopectoral (DP) tissue flaps are created to provide coverage for a soft tissue defect.

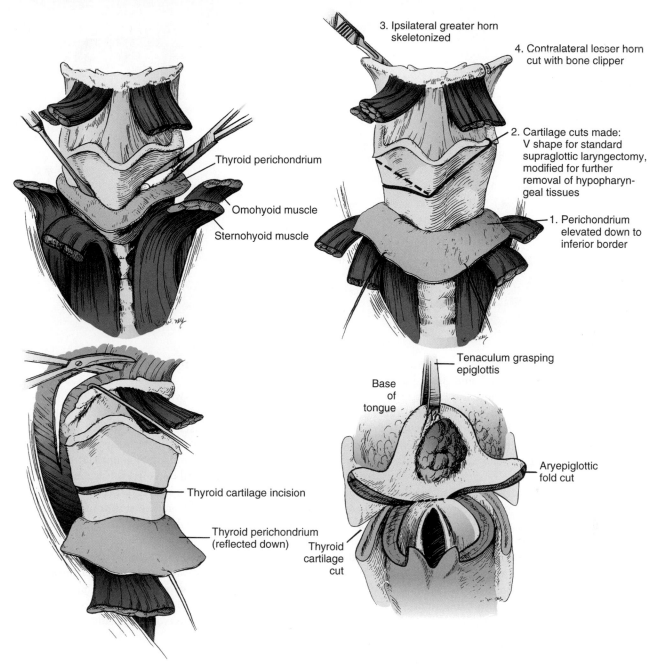

Figure 28-31 **Laryngectomy.** *(Modified from Cummings CW, Haughey BH, Thomas JR, et al: Oto-laryngology: head and neck surgery, ed 3, St Louis, 1998, Mosby.)*

Pathology

PMC and DP flaps replace soft tissue, usually after surgical excision of cancer in the head and neck region. A DP flap usually is used to close postirradiation fistulas and to resurface large cutaneous defects in the neck. A PMC flap may be used in the reconstruction of the pharynx, tongue, face, or neck. It is especially useful for covering the carotid artery when it may be at risk because of previous irradiation.

TECHNIQUE

Deltopectoral (DP) Flap

1 The DP flap incision is made.
2 The flap is elevated.
3 The flap is rotated.
4 The flap is inset.
5 The donor site is closed with a skin graft.

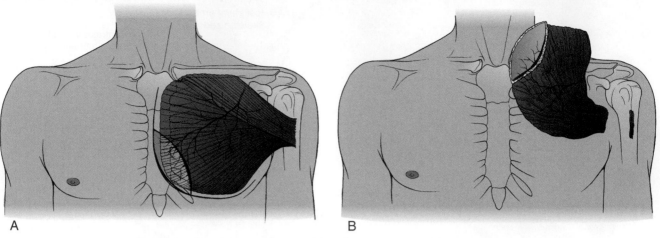

Figure 28-32   Pectoralis major myocutaneous (PMC) flap. **A,** Location of skin flap outlined and incised down to the underlying fascia. **B,** The skin flap is elevated and the lower border of the pectoralis major is identified. *(Modified from Silver CE, Rubin JS: Atlas of head and neck surgery, ed 2, Philadelphia, 1999, Churchill Livingstone.)*

Discussion: Deltopectoral Flap

The patient is positioned, prepped, and draped as for a neck dissection or laryngectomy, because the DP flap often is performed in conjunction with either of these procedures. The surgeon begins by outlining the proposed incision with a skin scribe. The incision typically goes from the acromion process to the sternum, extending to the space between the third and fourth ribs.

The incision is made with a # 10 blade, and the flap (skin, vascular supply, subcutaneous tissue, and fascia) is elevated from the underlying pectoralis major muscle in a lateral to medial fashion. This is done with the ESU or a scalpel. Bleeders are controlled with the ESU. The flap is left attached at the medial border (because this is where its vascular supply enters) and is rotated to cover the defect of the neck). The flap then is sutured into place with 3-0 absorbable sutures. The donor site then is covered with a skin graft, which is secured with 3-0 absorbable sutures or skin staples.

TECHNIQUE

Pectoralis Major Myocutaneous (PMC) Flap
1 An incision is made and the tissue flap is elevated.
2 The flap is "tunneled."
3 The flap is inset into the defect.
4 The donor site is closed.

Discussion: Pectoralis Major Myocutaneous Flap

The patient is positioned, prepped, and draped as for a neck dissection or laryngectomy, because the PMC flap often is performed with one of these procedures. The surgeon begins by measuring from the inferior border of the defect to the midclavicle with a lap sponge. This distance marks the superior portion of the skin paddle, which is drawn as a rectangle with rounded edges between the nipple and the sternum inferiorly to the inferior border of the pectoralis major muscle.

A line is then drawn from the superolateral portion of the rectangle to the axilla.

The incision is made with a no. 10 blade. The skin, subcutaneous tissue, and fascia superior to the incision are elevated off the underlying muscle over the clavicle, making a tunnel into the neck. The flap (skin, vascular supply, subcutaneous tissue, fascia, and pectoralis major muscle) is elevated from the underlying chest wall in an inferior superior fashion. This may be done with either a scalpel or the ESU. The ESU is used to separate the muscle from the sternum and humerus. The muscular portion of the flap should be slightly larger than the skin paddle.

When the flap has been elevated to the level of the clavicle, it is rotated 180 degrees and tunneled under the skin and over the clavicle to reach the defect (Figure 28-32). The flap then is sutured in place with 3-0 absorbable sutures. Two drains are placed in the donor site, which usually is closed with 3-0 absorbable suture.

KEY CONCEPTS

- Knowledge of key anatomical structures of the ear is necessary to understand surgical procedures.
- Familiarity with diagnostic procedures of the ear contributes to an understanding of the pathology involved and appropriate patient care.
- Surgery of the ear requires case planning to include specialty instruments, including microinstruments for the ear, and special materials and drugs designated for use in the ear.
- Familiarity with common surgical procedures of the ear is necessary for safe patient care and for assisting in the role as scrub.
- Knowledge of key anatomical structures of the nose and facial sinuses is necessary to understand surgical procedures.

- Familiarity with diagnostic procedures of the upper respiratory system contributes to an understanding of the pathology involved and appropriate patient care.
- Surgery of the nose and facial sinuses requires case planning to include specialty instruments, materials, and drugs designated for use in the nasal cavities.
- Familiarity with common surgical procedures of the nasal cavities is necessary for safe patient care and for assisting in the role as scrub.
- Knowledge of key anatomical structures of the throat and neck is necessary to understand surgical procedures.
- Familiarity with diagnostic procedures of the throat contributes to an understanding of the pathology involved and appropriate patient care.
- Surgery of neck ear requires case planning to include specialty equipment, including endoscopic instruments and instruments used in soft tissue dissection.
- Familiarity with common surgical procedures of the throat and neck is necessary for safe patient care and for assisting in the role as scrub.

REVIEW QUESTIONS

1. Why is a myringotomy performed?
2. When is a cochlear implant procedure performed on a child?
3. Why is it important to submerge the cochlear implant in normal saline after it is opened onto the sterile field?
4. Explain the difference between indirect laryngoscopy and direct laryngoscopy.
5. List three causes of upper airway obstruction that result in the need for placement of a tracheostomy.
6. Why is the obturator of a tracheotomy tube kept with the patient in the recovery period?
7. Which nerve is identified and preserved in thyroidectomy?
8. Why is a thyroplasty performed?

BIBLIOGRAPHY

Bailey BJ, editor: *Head and neck surgery: otolaryngology*, vols 1 and 2, ed 2, Philadelphia, 1998, Lippincott-Raven.

Boston Medical Products: *Montgomery thyroplasty system: surgeon's implant guide*, Westborough, Mass, 1998, Boston Medical Products.

Brackmann D, Shelton C, Arriaga MA: *Otologic surgery*, ed 2, Philadelphia, 2001, WB Saunders.

Coker NJ, Jenkins HA: *Atlas of otologic surgery*, Philadelphia, 2001, WB Saunders.

Cummings CW, Haughey BH, Thomas JR: *Otolaryngology: head and neck surgery*, ed 3, St Louis, 1998, Mosby.

Dhillon RS, East CA: *Ear, nose, and throat and head and neck surgery*, ed 3, Edinburgh, 2006, Churchill Livingstone.

Herman C: Medialization thyroplasty for unilateral vocal cord paralysis, *AORN Journal* 75:511, 2002.

Marks SC: *Nasal and sinus surgery*, Philadelphia, 2000, WB Saunders.

Montgomery WW: *Surgery of the upper respiratory system*, ed 3, Baltimore, 1996, Williams & Wilkins.

Seiden AM, Tami AM, Pensak ML, et al, editors: *Otolaryngology: the essentials*, New York, 2002, Thieme.

Silver CE, Rubin JS: *Atlas of head and neck surgery*, ed 2, Philadelphia, 1999, Churchill Livingstone.

Weerda H: *Reconstructive facial plastic surgery: a problem-solving manual*, New York, 2001, Thieme.

Oral and Maxillofacial Surgery

LEARNING OBJECTIVES

After studying this chapter the reader will be able to:

1. Identify key anatomical structures of the face and oral cavity
2. Discuss diagnostic procedures used in the maxillofacial specialty

3. Discuss specific elements of case planning for oral and maxillofacial surgery
4. Discuss pathology of the facial bones and oral cavity
5. List and describe common oral and maxillofacial surgical procedures

TERMINOLOGY

Arch bars: Metal plates wired to the teeth to occlude the jaw during maxillofacial surgery or during healing. Arch bars maintain the patient's normal bite (occlusion).

Bicoronal incision: An incision made between the frontal and the parietal bones bilaterally.

Bicortical screws: Screws that penetrate both cortical layers and the intervening spongy layer of the bone.

Blowout fracture: A severe fracture of the orbital cavity in which a portion of the globe may extrude outside the cavity.

Dentition: The number, type, and pattern of the teeth.

Le Fort I fracture: A horizontal fracture of the maxilla that causes the hard palate and alveolar process to become separated from the rest of the maxilla. The fracture extends into the lower nasal septum, lateral maxillary sinus, and palatine bones.

Le Fort II fracture: A fracture that extends from the nasal bone to the frontal processes of the maxilla, lacrimal bones, and inferior orbital floor. It may extend into the orbital foramen.

Inferiorly, it extends into the anterior maxillary sinus and the pterygoid plates.

Le Fort III fracture: This fracture involves separation of all the facial bones from their cranial base. It includes fracture of the zygoma, maxilla, and nasal bones.

Mastication: Chewing.

Maxillomandibular fixation (MMF): See arch bars.

Occlusion: In maxillofacial surgery, this refers to the patient's bite pattern when the jaw is closed.

Odontectomy: Tooth extraction.

Oromaxillofacial surgery: Surgery involving the bones of the face, primarily for repair of fractures and reconstruction of congenital anomalies.

Subciliary incision: Skin incision made approximately 2 mm inferior to the lower eyelashes.

Transconjunctival incision: Incision made through the conjunctiva.

Transosteal implants: Bone plates with retaining posts used in the procedure for dental implants.

INTRODUCTION

Surgery for facial trauma may involve the many bones of the face and frontal sinus. The face is vulnerable to injury in motor vehicle and industrial accidents, high-speed sports, and intentional violence. Maxillofacial injuries can be quite complex, involving skin, muscle, nerves, and blood vessels. The long-term physiological effects of injury or congenital anomalies can affect speech, **mastication** (chewing), and development of the teeth. The psychological effects are equally important, because disfigurement often results in social and emotional isolation. Maxillofacial procedures are performed primarily by surgeons specializing in oromaxillofacial, plastic, or otorhinolaryngology surgery. Specific techniques needed for orthorpedic repair, such as the use of power drills, screw, and plate fixation, are discussed in Chapter 31.

SURGICAL ANATOMY

BONES OF THE FACE

The bones of the face are divided into three regions: the upper face, the midface, and the lower face.

Upper Face

The upper face is composed of:

- The frontal bone

The frontal bone is part of the cranium. It forms the forehead and contains portions of the nasal sinuses (see Chapter 28 for more detail on ear, nose, and throat surgery). The superior margin of the bony orbit is formed by the frontal bone. This area generally is injured in a blow to the forehead. Injury to the dura (one of the protective layers of the brain) also may be sustained in trauma to this area.

Midface

The midface is composed of:

- The ethmoid
- The nasal bone
- The zygoma
- The maxillary bones

The ethmoid bone is a complex structure that contributes to the floor of the cranium and also contains a number of sinus cavities.

The nasal bone forms the bridge of the nose and articulates with the ethmoid and the maxilla. Fractures of the nasal ethmoid area may injure the lacrimal apparatus, including the ducts and lacrimal gland. The dura also is vulnerable and may require neurological surgery.

The zygoma forms the lateral walls and floor of the bony orbit, which houses the eyeball. The zygomatic arch is the cheekbone. Fractures in this area are important because of their association with injury to the eye, especially in displaced fractures. The most common causes of injury are assault, motor vehicle accidents, and sports injuries. The bony orbit is formed by the frontal bone, but it also contains portions of other bones of the face, including the zygoma, maxilla, lacrimal, ethmoid, sphenoid, and palatine bones. The orbital floor is formed by the maxillary sinus.

The bilateral maxillae come together to form the upper jaw, the anterior hard palate, and a portion of the orbital cavities.

Lower Face

The lower face is composed of:

- The mandible

The mandible is the only movable bone of the face. It is a U-shaped bone suspended from the temporal bone. The condyles insert into the glenoid fossa of the temporal bones to form the temporomandibular joints. The ramus extends inferiorly from the condyle to the angle, where it joins the body of the mandible and extends anteriorly and medially to join the other half of the mandible. The teeth are embedded in the alveoli of the body of the mandible. Fractures of the alveoli frequently require dental surgery. Figure 29-1 shows the bones of the face and cranium. Figure 29-2 illustrates the skull as viewed from below, and Figure 29-3 illustrates the mandible.

DIAGNOSTIC PROCEDURES

Facial fractures and structural deformities are most commonly assessed by imaging studies. Plain radiographs are taken for a baseline assessment or for simple fractures. However, extensive tissue swelling may obscure complex anatomical features and injuries. Computed tomography scanning therefore is used for complex facial fractures and reconstruction procedures.

CASE PLANNING

EQUIPMENT AND INSTRUMENTS

Oromaxillofacial surgery focuses on reconstruction and repair of the facial bones and may include structures of the oral cavity. The instrumentation used for these procedures, therefore, includes fine orthopedic instruments, implants, and grafting materials. (Chapter 31 presents a complete discussion of the biomechanical and surgical techniques used in bone trauma and reconstruction, including power drills and techniques for their use.) Nasal instruments may be required for surgery of the midface (see Chapter 28). Facial facture instruments are shown in Figure 29-4.

Power Drill

For procedures involving facial fractures, a small power drill is required to prepare bone for plates and screws and to remodel bone. The drill bits for the screws are included as components of the plate system used. (Chapter 31 presents a complete discussion of drills and techniques.)

Plates and Screws

Plates and screws are the primary means of repairing facial fractures. Miniplate systems are small, malleable mesh plates that can be molded to fit over the contours of facial bone. Small cortical screws or **bicortical screws** are used to implant the titanium or stainless steel mesh plates, which provide stability during healing. Many systems are available, including Synthes, Leibinger, W Lorenz, Osteomed, and KLS. Each of these systems includes implants and the instrumentation required for the repair, including the following:

- Plates with screws
- Plate benders
- Plate cutters
- Holding forceps
- Screwdriver handles and blades
- Depth gauge

For mandibular fractures, the plates and screws most often are at least 2 mm in size. For midface, orbital, and frontal sinus fractures, the plates and screws are 1 to 2 mm. The scrub must keep track of all plates and screws used during surgery for documentation in the patient's record.

PREPPING AND DRAPING

Facial fractures are prepped with dilute povidone-iodine scrub and paint because it has been shown to be the safest and most effective antiseptic for use on the face. Note that hexachlorophene and chlorhexidine are not used on the face because they are ototoxic. The entire face is prepped, from the hairline to the sternal notch, as described in Chapter 20. An endotracheal tube usually is part of the surgical field and therefore must be

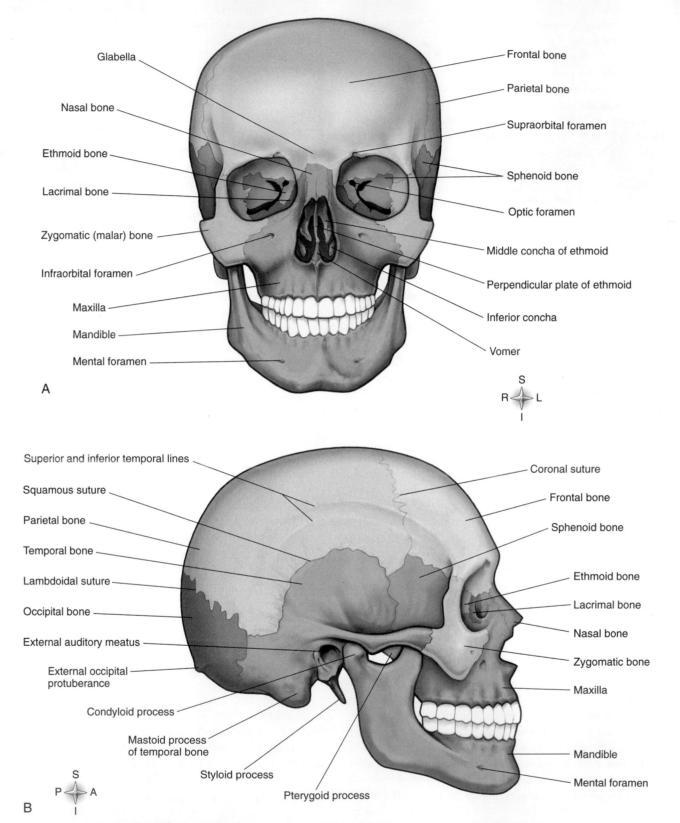

Glabella

Nasal bone

Ethmoid bone

Lacrimal bone

Zygomatic (malar) bone

Infraorbital foramen

Maxilla

Mandible

Mental foramen

Frontal bone

Parietal bone

Supraorbital foramen

Sphenoid bone

Optic foramen

Middle concha of ethmoid

Perpendicular plate of ethmoid

Inferior concha

Vomer

A

Superior and inferior temporal lines

Squamous suture

Parietal bone

Temporal bone

Lambdoidal suture

Occipital bone

External auditory meatus

External occipital protuberance

Condyloid process

Mastoid process of temporal bone

Styloid process

Pterygoid process

Coronal suture

Frontal bone

Sphenoid bone

Ethmoid bone

Lacrimal bone

Nasal bone

Zygomatic bone

Maxilla

Mandible

Mental foramen

B

Figure 29-1   The cranium. A, Anterior view. **B,** Side view. *(From Thibodeau GA, Patt KT: Anthony's textbook of anatomy and physiology, ed 17, St Louis, 2003, Mosby.)*

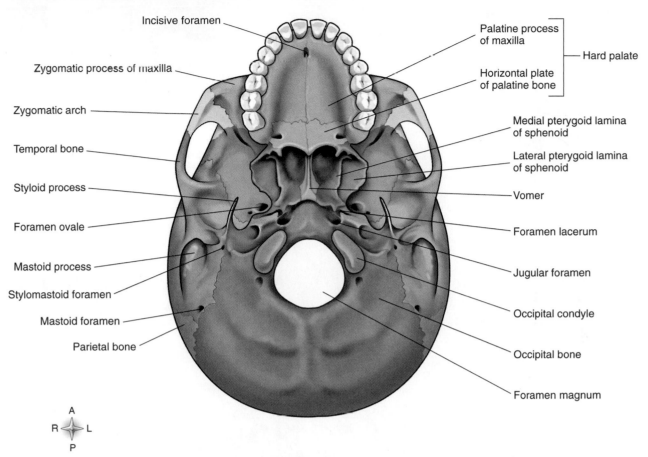

Figure 29-2 **The skull (viewed from below).** *(From Thibodeau GA, Patt KT: Anthony's textbook of anatomy and physiology, ed 17, St Louis, 2003, Mosby.)*

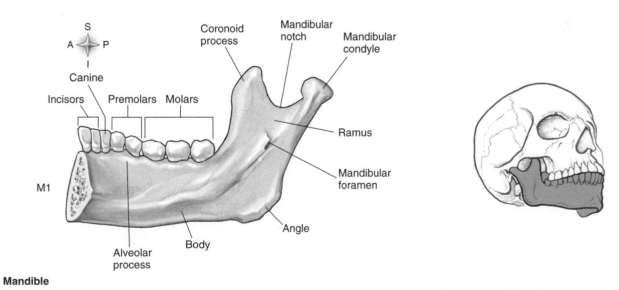

Figure 29-3 **The mandible.** *(From Thibodeau GA, Patt KT: Anthony's textbook of anatomy and physiology, ed 17, St Louis, 2003, Mosby.)*

included in the prep. If a bicoronal incision (behind the hairline) is planned, the patient's head may be shaved, and the prep may be carried from the posterior head to the sternal notch. After the patient has been draped, the mouth may be irrigated with diluted povidone-iodine paint and the teeth gently cleaned as part of the presurgical medical assessment to assist the surgeon in identifying bone fragments and foreign bodies.

The patient is draped with four towels secured with towel clips to expose the surgical site. A split sheet then is draped

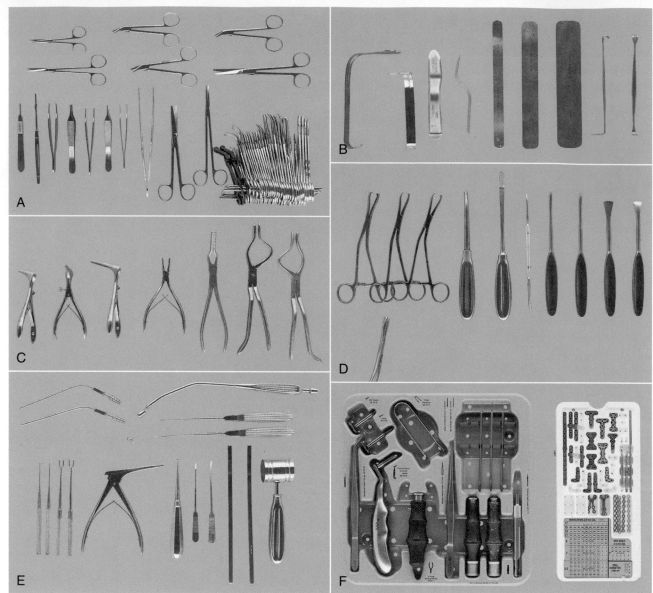

Figure 29-4 Instruments used in the repair of facial fractures. **A,** *Top, left to right,* 1 Stevens tenotomy scissors, curved; 1 plastic scissors, straight, sharp; 3 wire-cutting scissors; 1 Mayo dissecting scissors, straight. *Bottom, left to right,* 1 Bard-Parker knife handle, # 3; 1 Bard-Parker knife handle, # 7; 2 Adson tissue forceps with teeth (1 × 2), front view and side view; 2 Adson tissue forceps without teeth, front view and side view; 1 Brown-Adson tissue forceps with teeth (9 × 9), front view; 1 bayonet dressing forceps, 7½ inches (18.75 cm); 1 Mayo dissecting scissors, curved; 1 Metzenbaum scissors; 2 paper drape clips; 2 Backhaus towel forceps, small; 2 Backhaus towel forceps; 6 Halsted mosquito hemostatic forceps, curved; 2 Halsted mosquito hemostatic forceps, straight; 2 Providence hemostatic forceps, curved; 2 Halsted hemostatic forceps, straight; 4 Crile hemostatic forceps, curved; 2 Allis tissue forceps; 2 Webster needle holders, 4 inch; 2 Crile-Wood needle holders, 6 inch; 2 Johnson needle holders, 6 inch. **B,** *Left to right,* 1 Weider tongue retractor, large, side view; 1 Weider tongue retractor, small, front view; 2 University of Minnesota cheek retractors, front view and side view; 3 ribbon retractors, assorted sizes; 2 Senn-Kanavel retractors, side view and front view. **C,** *Left to right,* 1 Cottle nasal speculum, # 1, side view; 1 Cottle nasal speculum, # 2, front view; 1 Cottle nasal speculum, # 3, side view; 1 Friedman rongeur, single action; 1 Asch forceps; 2 Rowe disimpaction forceps, left and right. **D,** *Top, left to right,* 3 Dingman bone-holding forceps; 1 Dingman zygoma elevator; 1 Gilles malar elevator; 1 Freer elevator; 2 Langenbeck elevators; 1 Langenbeck periosteal elevator, straight; 1 Langenbeck periosteal elevator, angled. *Bottom left,* Tip of Dingman bone-holding forceps. **E,** *Top, left to right,* 2 Frazier suction tubes with stylets; 1 Yankauer suction tube with tip; 2 zygomatic arch awls. *Bottom, left to right,* 2 Joseph skin hooks, single; 2 Joseph skin hooks, double; 1 Kerrison rongeur, 90-degree upbite; 1 Lucas curette, # 0, short; 2 mandibular awls; 1 Cottle osteotome, curved; 1 Cottle osteotome, straight; 1 metal mallet. **F,** Titanium 2-mm microfixation system instrumentation, trays 1 and 2 of 3 (labeled); facial fracture set.

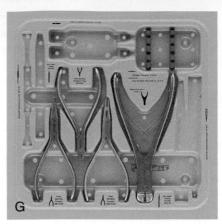

Figure 29-4, cont'd **G,** Titanium 2-mm microfixation system instrumentation, tray 3 of 3 (labeled). *(From Tighe SM: Instrumentation of the operating room, ed 6, St Louis, 2003, Mosby.)*

over the patient and around the face, with the mouth, nose, and eyes included in the surgical field.

NOTE: *During procedures in which oral and orthopedic (facial bone) techniques are required, the instruments used within the oral cavity (a nonsterile area) must be isolated from the orthopedic setup and procedure, which is sterile.*

SPONGES AND DRESSINGS

Sponges

Both 4 × 4 sponges and cottonoids may be used. As with all surgical procedures, all sponges and sharps are counted before, during, and at the end of the procedure.

Dressings

Dressings are used to protect the wound and to absorb exudate. Antibiotic ointment may be applied to the incision, and Telfa or other nonadherent dressing may be placed directly over the site. Flat gauze or gauze fluffs may be placed on top of the dressing. Kerlix (rolled) wrap can be used to secure dressings on the head or face. Kerlix is soft and expandable and conforms to the contours of the skull and facial bones.

SURGICAL PROCEDURES OF THE FACE

MAXILLOMANDIBULAR FIXATION (APPLICATION OF ARCH BARS)

Surgical Goal

Arch bars are applied to realign the teeth or to maintain the patient's normal bite position. A fundamental goal of any maxillomandibular procedure is to preserve the patient's unique bite pattern or normal **occlusion** between the mandible (lower jaw), the maxilla (upper jaw), and the midface bones. Therefore, in many maxillofacial procedures, the teeth are aligned and fixated in a closed (occluded) position. This is called **maxillomandibular fixation (MMF).** In this procedure, a thin metal strap called an **arch bar** is wired to each row of teeth.

The bars are then wired together with stainless steel sutures to occlude the jaw. MMF preserves the patient's normal bite position during repair and healing. MMF may be removed at the end of surgery if the fractures are stable and do not need the support of the arch bars during the healing process. If the fracture is still unstable, the bars may be left in place for several weeks.

NOTE: *If the arch bars remain in place postoperatively, wire cutters must be sent with the patient to the postanesthesia care unit so that the mouth can be opened in the event of an airway emergency.*

TECHNIQUE

1 Arch bars are wired to the teeth with 24- or 26-gauge wire sutures.
2 The arch bars are wired together.

Discussion

Application of arch bars requires a basic facial fracture instrument setup, which includes wire and plate cutters, stainless steel sutures, and arch bar material. Stainless steel suture ends are counted as sharps and isolated to prevent glove puncture or loss in the surgical wound. Wires are always cut with wire cutters rather than suture scissors.

Steel wire is passed to the surgeon mounted on a needle holder. The ends of the suture must be controlled to prevent contamination or injury. A designated clamp may be fixed to the end of the suture for this purpose.

The surgeon shapes an arch bar to fit over the patient's upper teeth and gums. With the cheek and tongue retracted by a cheek retractor, intraoral sweetheart or cloverleaf retractor, the bar is wired into place with 24- or 26-gauge stainless steel suture wires, which are cut into thirds. A wire is clamped with a Rubio needle holder, threaded between the teeth, wrapped around the bar, and twisted to tighten. The suture ends are cut with a wire cutter. Three wires are placed on each side of the mouth if there is sufficient space to accommodate them. The procedure is repeated for the lower teeth.

When the arch bars have been applied to both the upper and lower teeth, the jaw is closed in normal position, and the top and bottom arch bars are approximated with precut lengths of steel suture. Size 24- or 26-gauge stainless steel suture is twisted into a clockwise loop and wrapped around the upper and lower bars with the needle holder. The wire is twisted clockwise until tight against the arch bars and then is cut with a wire cutter. To prevent the suture ends from injuring the soft tissues, a "rosebud" is made in the suture ends by grasping the wire with a hemostat and crimping it inward. The end may be buried in the patient's gingiva.

Standard protocol dictates that wires be tightened in a clockwise fashion so that any other surgeon knows to remove them in a counterclockwise direction.

Wire cutters are kept with the patient at all times during the postoperative period to allow immediate access to the mouth in the event of an airway emergency. Figure 29-5 shows the application of arch bars.

OPEN REDUCTION/INTERNAL FIXATION: MIDFACE FRACTURE

Surgical Goal

In open reduction and internal fixation (ORIF) of midface fractures, fractures of the midface are reduced and fixed in place. The buttressing structures (those under force during dental occlusion) are also reinforced.

Pathology

Fractures of the midface historically have been classified for treatment and identification. These classifications do not reflect the realities of high-impact facial fractures, which often exceed the boundaries defined. However, they are still used by some surgeons.

- **Le Fort I fracture:** This is a horizontal fracture of the maxilla that causes the hard palate and alveolar process to become separated from the rest of the maxilla. The fracture extends into the lower nasal septum, lateral maxillary sinus, and palatine bones.

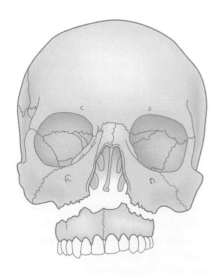

Figure 29-5 Application of arch bars. (From Dingman RO, Natvig P: Surgery of facial fractures, Philadelphia, 1964, WB Saunders.)

- **Le Fort II fracture:** This type of fracture is pyramidal in shape. It extends from the nasal bone to the frontal processes of the maxilla, lacrimal bones, and inferior orbital floor, and it may extend into the orbital foramen. Inferiorly, it extends into the anterior maxillary sinus and the pterygoid plates. This type of fracture also is associated with leakage of cerebrospinal fluid (CSF) into the nasal sinuses.
- **Le Fort III fracture:** This fracture involves separation of all the facial bones from their cranial base. It includes fracture of the zygoma, maxilla, and nasal bones. The fracture line extends through the ethmoid bone and bony orbit, with severe facial flattening and swelling.

Figures 29-6 and 29-7 show Le Fort fractures.

TECHNIQUE

1. Arch bars are applied as required.
2. An incision is made transorally or externally.
3. The fracture is exposed and reduced.
4. The fracture is fixated internally with miniplates and screws.
5. The incisions are closed.
6. The arch bars may be removed.

Discussion

The patient is placed in the supine position on a doughnut or Mayfield headrest with the arms tucked at the sides. General anesthesia is administered through a nasotracheal tube. For extensive trauma, a tracheotomy may be performed first.

The patient is prepped and draped for a facial procedure. If other fractures are present, the patient may be placed in MMF. The surgeon makes the incision in the upper gingival mucosa on the affected side with a # 15 blade. The incision is extended through the mucosa to the level of the maxilla. The surgeon then elevates the periosteum with a Freer or periosteal elevator. The zygoma is reduced with Hohmann retractors or a bone hook, or both.

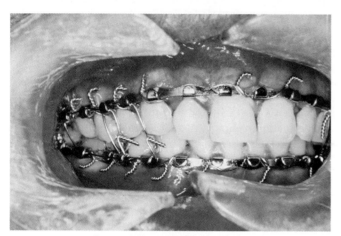
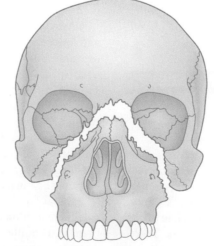
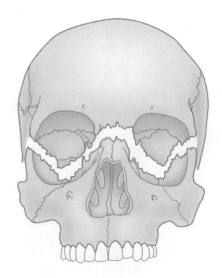

Le Fort type I   Le Fort type II   Le Fort type III

Figure 29-6 Overview of Le Fort fractures. (From Townsend CM, Beauchamp DR, Evers MB, Mattox KL: Sabiston textbook of surgery, ed 18, Philadelphia, 2008, WB Saunders.)

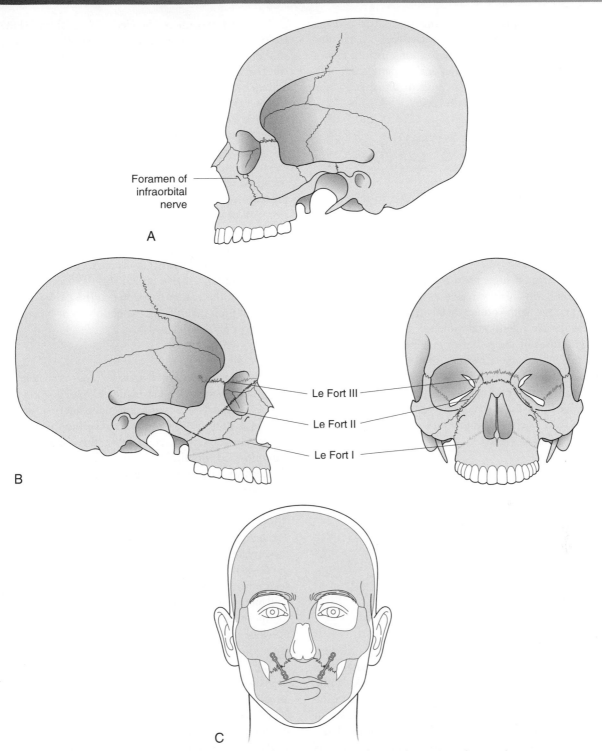

Figure 29-7 **Detail of Le Fort fractures. A,** Malar fracture. **B,** Side and front views of Le Fort factures. **C,** Maxillary fracture with manipulation used for fixation. *(From Dhillon RS, East CA: Ear, nose, and throat and head and neck surgery,* ed 3, Edinburgh, 2006, Churchill Livingstone.)

The surgeon then chooses the size and type of plate to be used. The plates usually are 1.7 or 2 mm. Cortical screws are used to secure the plate to the bone. The plate is held in place with a plate-holding forceps or hemostat. The appropriate drill bit (according to the size of the screw) is loaded onto a small power drill and the screw holes are drilled. The surgeon then chooses the screw length or a depth gauge may be used to determine the depth of the screw holes. The

correct screw is loaded onto the screwdriver and is screwed into place. This process is repeated until all of the screws have been placed and the plate has been secured to the bone. The incision then is closed with 3-0 absorbable sutures. The wound is dressed with flat and fluffed gauze. A Kerlix wrap is used to secure the dressing. If the patient is to remain in MMF, a wire cutter must accompany the patient to the recovery room.

Patients are closely observed for hemorrhage, CSF leakage, and a patent airway in the postoperative period. Healing usually requires 4 to 8 weeks. Complications include dehiscence of oral lesions, especially when oral hygiene is suboptimal. Nerve injury may occur as a result of tissue retraction during the surgery or from the injury itself.

OPEN REDUCTION AND INTERNAL FIXATION: FRONTAL SINUS FRACTURE

Surgical Goal

ORIF of a frontal sinus fracture is performed to repair CSF leakage, prevent obstruction of the frontal sinus ducts, and restore an aesthetic contour to the forehead.

Pathology

Fractures of the frontal sinus are a result of direct trauma to the frontal bone, which may result in bone impaction and fragmentation. As with other facial fractures, the most common causes are intentional violence and motor vehicle accidents. Fractures of the posterior wall of the frontal sinus may result in CSF leakage or herniation of brain tissue. These fractures present a real risk of life-threatening complications, including brain abscess and meningitis. Other complications include damage to the ducts that interferes with normal drainage. This can lead to chronic infection or a mucocele (a cyst arising from a mucous gland).

TECHNIQUE

1 A bicoronal incision is made.
2 The periosteum is separated from the skull.
3 The fractures are exposed.
4 A fat graft is implanted in the sinus and the fractures are repaired.
5 The incision is closed.

Discussion

Before frontal sinus fractures are repaired, the sinus mucosa must be removed and the duct occluded. The sinus then is often filled with a fat graft. In rare cases, a small leak can be patched and the anterior walled plated. Severe fracture of the posterior sinus wall may require *cranialization* of the sinus. In this procedure, the posterior wall of the sinus is removed, the sinus ducts are occluded, and the frontal sinus mucosa is removed. The brain is allowed to move into the previous frontal sinus space, and the fractures are repaired. A neurosurgeon usually is present to participate in the surgery.

The patient is placed in the supine position with the head on a Mayfield or similar headrest and the arms tucked at the sides. General anesthesia is administered. The incisions are made based on accessibility through the existing wounds or the need for entry through an alternative site. If the existing wounds are not used, a **bicoronal incision** may be made (i.e., following a line starting at the junction of the coronal and frontal sutures on one side of the head and extending to the other side, behind the hairline).

Using a #10 blade or the electrosurgical unit (ESU) with a Colorado needle tip, the surgeon makes the incision from the root of the helix of one ear to the root of the helix of the other ear. If a knife is used, Raney clips are applied to the scalp with a Raney clip applier to aid hemostasis (see illustrations in Chapter 36). The incision is carried deep to the periosteum, which is elevated to the level of the superior orbital rims and anterior wall of the frontal sinus.

The surgeon examines the anterior and posterior walls of the frontal sinus. If the posterior wall of the frontal sinus is fractured, the frontal sinus will be obliterated. This is done to prevent the possibility of recurring infection. Both the posterior wall of the sinus and mucosal lining of the frontal sinus are removed using hemostats and a cutting or diamond burr loaded onto a small power drill. The mucosa of the frontal osteum is removed with a small acorn burr. The frontal osteum is packed with muscle or fascia. This separates the frontal sinus cavity from the rest of the sinuses. The cavity then is packed with a fat graft taken from the abdomen or bone cement may be used to fill the space.

Fat Graft

The surgeon makes a small incision (approximately 2 to 3 mm) in the abdomen with a #15 blade. A small portion of fat tissue is excised using a #15 blade and hemostat or a toothed Adson forceps is used to tease out and grasping the tissue. Double-prong skin hooks are used to retract the wound edges. Bleeders are controlled with the ESU. The graft is placed in normal saline to keep it moist until the surgeon is ready to place it in the frontal sinus. The graft site is closed with 4-0 absorbable sutures.

Repair

The anterior wall of the frontal wall is repaired with micromesh plates. Commonly used sizes are 1 or 1.3 mm. The free portions of the bone are secured to the mesh before it is secured to the stable portions of the bone. The appropriate drill bit is loaded onto a small power drill, and holes are drilled for the mesh plate. Screws are inserted as described in the previous procedure. These steps are repeated until the mesh is secured in place and the fracture has been reduced.

The incision is closed in layers. The periosteum is replaced over the cranium, and the subcutaneous tissue is closed with 3-0 absorbable sutures. The skin is closed with skin staples or a locking silk stitch. The wound is covered with antibiotic ointment or with a Telfa and gauze dressing.

Patients are monitored carefully for symptoms of infection and CSF leakage in the postoperative period. Bone fragments remaining in the sinuses can cause injury in the postoperative period. Patients are followed with computed tomography scans for at least 1 year after surgery.

OPEN REDUCTION AND INTERNAL FIXATION: ORBITAL FLOOR FRACTURE

Surgical Goal

ORIF of an orbital floor fracture is performed to reduce a fracture of the orbital floor, to prevent entrapment of the extraocular muscles, and to support the orbital contents.

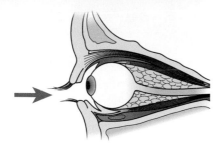

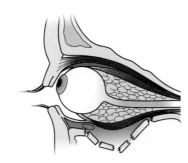

Figure 29-8 **Orbital blowout fracture.** *(From Dhillon RS, East CA: Ear, nose, and throat and head and neck surgery, ed 3, Edinburgh, 2006, Churchill Livingstone.)*

Pathology

Orbital floor fractures, or **blowout fractures**, are caused by high-speed blunt force to the globe (Figure 29-8). Fractures of the orbital floor usually result from the increased orbital pressure caused by the impact on the globe. A portion of the globe may extrude into the nasal sinus (enophthalmus), or the globe can be displaced posteriorly. Entrapment of the eye muscles can result in diplopia (double vision). The most common causes of the injury are assault and being struck by a high-velocity object.

TECHNIQUE

1 A subciliary or a transconjunctival incision is made.
2 The orbit is exposed.
3 The fractures are reduced and repaired.
4 The incision is closed.

Discussion

The patient is positioned and prepped as for a facial fracture. General anesthesia is administered. Ophthalmic ointment may be placed in the eyes before the skin prep. The prep is performed carefully to prevent solution from draining into the eyes and ears.

The surgeon begins by placing corneal protectors in the operative eye. Ophthalmic balanced salt solution is instilled into the eye to provide moisture at this stage and as needed throughout the case.

With the cornea protected, the surgeon makes the incision. Either of two incisions can be used, a subciliary incision or a transconjunctival incision. A **subciliary incision** is made

2 mm under the eyelashes with a #15 blade. A **transconjunctival incision** is made in the conjunctiva of the inferior eyelid. The surgeon exposes the orbit by placing small, malleable retractors or brain spatula retractors into the wound and retracting superiorly and inferiorly. The wound is exposed to the level of the orbital rim, and the periosteum is elevated with a Freer elevator. The surgeon then elevates and retracts the orbital contents superiorly with a small malleable retractor.

After assessment, the surgeon may reconstruct the floor of the orbit using nylon sheeting, mesh, Gelfilm, Silastic sheeting, or an orbital floor plate. Typically, a 1-, 1.3-, or 1.5-mm plate or mesh is selected for orbital fractures. The surgeon cuts the selected material to size with plate cutters or scissors (depending on the material) and positions it between the orbital floor and the orbital contents. An orbital floor plate is secured in place with screws in the infraorbital rim. This technique is performed as previously described (see Prepping and Draping).

With the orbital contents supported, the retractors are removed and the wound is closed. Subciliary incisions are closed with 5-0 absorbable sutures. Transconjunctival incisions are not closed. The surgeon removes the corneal protector after the incisions have been closed. Antibiotic ophthalmic ointment may be placed in the eye and on the incision. A small dressing may be applied.

OPEN REDUCTION AND INTERNAL FIXATION: MANDIBULAR FRACTURE

Surgical Goal

In ORIF of a mandibular fracture, the mandibular fracture is repaired and occlusion is restored.

Pathology

ORIF of the mandible is performed to treat facial trauma involving the mandible. Assault is the most common cause of a mandibular fracture.

TECHNIQUE

1 Arch bars are applied.
2 A transoral or external incision is made.
3 The fracture is exposed and reduced.
4 Miniplates and screws are used to fix the fracture.
5 The incisions are closed.
6 The arch bars may be removed.

Discussion

The patient is placed in the supine position with the head stabilized on a doughnut headrest and the arms tucked at the sides. General anesthesia is administered through a nasotracheal tube. Extensive trauma of the face results in massive swelling and may result in airway occlusion. Therefore, a tracheotomy may be performed before the ORIF. The patient is prepped and draped for a facial procedure.

After administration of anesthesia, the surgeon assesses the fractures. If necessary, arch bars may be applied before fracture reduction and fixation. An incision is made in the gingival-buccal mucosa with the ESU or in the skin over the fracture site with a #10 or #15 blade. The site of the skin incision depends on the location and extent of the fracture. After the skin incision is made, Senn retractors are used to retract the skin and subcutaneous tissue. This exposes the mandible and periosteum, which can be elevated with a Freer or other type of periosteal elevator. The surgeon then reduces the fracture with a small bone clamp. Radiographs or fluoroscopy may be used to evaluate the reduction.

The surgeon selects the plates needed for fixation. The 2-, 2.4-, and 2.7-mm plates are commonly used. Most mandibular fractures require two plates per fracture: a large plate is used on the inferior side, and a miniplate or tension band device is used on the superior aspect. A small drill bit is fitted to a high-speed drill. The plate is stabilized against the mandible with a plate-holding forceps, and the screw holes are drilled. A drill guide may be used to stabilize the drill bit. If a drill guide is used, a depth gauge is used to measure the required screw length. The appropriate screw is loaded into a screwdriver and inserted. When all of the fractures have been reduced and fixed, the incisions are closed. Transbuccal incisions are closed with 3-0 absorbable sutures, external incisions are closed in layers with 3-0 absorbable sutures, and the skin is closed with 4-0 absorbable sutures. The arch bars may be removed or left in placed as needed.

ORAL SURGERY PROCEDURES

Procedures involving the teeth are performed primarily by an oromaxillofacial surgeon.

DENTAL IMPLANTS

Surgical Goal

Dental implants are used to replace lost teeth.

Pathology

An implant may replace a single tooth or multiple teeth. Three types of dental implants are commonly used: endosteal implants, subperiosteal implants, and transosteal implants.

Discussion

An endosteal implant is a threaded screw, cylinder, or flat blade that is implanted in the alveolus of the maxilla or mandible and then covered with soft tissue. After several months (3 months for the mandible and 6 months for the maxilla), a post is connected to the implanted fixture. This post extends slightly above the gingiva, allowing the artificial tooth to be attached.

Subperiosteal implants are placed beneath the periosteum directly on the alveolar bone. This type of implant is used primarily when bone is insufficient to support an endosteal implant.

Transosteal implants are bone plates with retaining posts; they resemble a staple. This type of implant is used only when the patient has severe loss of bone in the mandibular alveolar ridge.

TOOTH EXTRACTION

Surgical Goal

Extraction is the surgical removal of one or more teeth.

Pathology

Odontectomy, or tooth extraction, may be performed for a variety of reasons, including damaged or decayed teeth or impaction, which often affects the third molars (wisdom teeth).

TECHNIQUE

1 An incision is made in the gingiva of the affected tooth.
2 The tissue surrounding the tooth is elevated to the level of the bone.
3 The tooth is elevated out of the alveolus, making it mobile.
4 The tooth is extracted with a dental extractor.
5 The incision is closed if necessary.

Discussion

The patient is placed in the supine position with the arms tucked at the sides. A prep is unnecessary, because the procedure is performed inside the mouth. Povidone-iodine may be needed for irrigation. The patient is draped to allow adequate access to the mouth. The surgeon reviews radiographs to ensure that the correct teeth are extracted. A #15 blade is used to make a gingival incision to the level of the bone. A Molt elevator is used to elevate the tissue, including the periosteum, surrounding the tooth.

The surgeon then elevates the tooth out of the alveolus with an elevator; this breaks the attachment of the ligament holding the tooth in place, allowing the tooth to become mobile. The tooth is extracted with the appropriately sized dental extractor. The size of the extractor varies, depending on the tooth being extracted and the patient's age. If necessary, the incision is closed with absorbable 3-0 sutures (this is usually required with impactions). Dental packs may be placed to prevent postoperative bleeding.

ORTHOGNATHIC PROCEDURES

MANDIBULAR ADVANCEMENT

Surgical Goal

Mandibular advancement is performed to correct a bony deformity of the mandible.

Pathology

Mandibular defects may be acquired or congenital and usually are represented by a recessed mandible. Surgical correction of the defects may help the patient for medical and psychological reasons. Surgery generally is delayed until the patient has developed sufficiently and has most of the permanent teeth.

TECHNIQUE

1 Arch bars are applied.
2 Intraoral incisions are made.
3 The maxilla is cut at a predetermined location.
4 The bone is advanced.
5 Grafts are placed, if necessary, and the bones are wired in place.
6 The intraoral incisions are closed.

Discussion

The patient is placed in the supine position with the arms tucked at the sides. A general anesthetic is used. The patient is prepped and draped to allow full exposure of the lower third of the face.

The surgeon begins by placing arch bars. This aligns the teeth and provides postoperative immobilization. Then, intraoral incisions are made to expose the mandible. This may be done with the knife or ESU. The incisions are carried to the periosteum. The periosteum is elevated with a periosteal elevator to expose the bony surface of the mandible. An oscillating saw is used to make cuts through the mandible at predetermined locations. After the mandible has been split, it can be advanced to the proper position. Bone grafts or biosynthetic material may be used to fill any space between the advanced mandible and the fixed mandible.

The grafts and mandible are fixed in place with wire or a mandibular plating system. The incisions are closed with 3-0 absorbable sutures. The patient remains in MMF for several weeks.

Wire cutters are kept with the patient at all times in the postoperative period in case of an airway emergency.

MIDFACE (MAXILLARY) ADVANCEMENT

Surgical Goal

Midface advancement is performed to correct a bony deformity of the maxilla.

Pathology

Maxillary defects may be acquired or congenital. A recessed maxilla can result in misalignment of the teeth and social isolation. Surgery generally is delayed until the permanent teeth have developed.

TECHNIQUE

1 Arch bars are applied.
2 Intraoral incisions are made.
3 The maxilla is incised.
4 The bone is advanced.
5 Grafts are placed, if necessary, and the bones are wired in place.
6 The intraoral incisions are closed.

Discussion

The patient is placed in the supine position with the arms tucked at the sides. The patient is prepped and draped to allow full exposure of the lower third of the face. Arch bars are placed at the start of surgery. This allows alignment and stabilization of the **dentition** and provides postoperative immobilization.

The surgeon makes intraoral incisions to expose the maxilla. This may be done with the scalpel or ESU. The incisions are carried to the periosteum. A small area of the periosteum is removed with a periosteal elevator. The surgeon then uses an oscillating saw to make cuts through the maxilla at predetermined locations. After the maxilla has been split, it can be advanced to the proper position. Bone graft or biosynthetic material is used to fill any space between the advanced maxilla and the fixed maxilla.

The grafts and maxilla are fixed in place with wire or a mandibular plating system. The incisions are closed with 3-0 absorbable sutures. The patient remains in arch bars for several weeks. Postoperative considerations are the same as for previously described procedures in which arch bars are placed.

TEMPOROMANDIBULAR JOINT ARTHROPLASTY

Surgical Goal

Temporomandibular joint (TMJ) arthroplasty is performed to reduce pain and increase mobility of the joint.

Pathology

Temporomandibular joint disease is characterized by persistent pain and dysfunction of the TMJ. It usually is associated with stress-related muscle tension and grinding of the teeth (bruxism), malocclusion, trauma, or arthritis.

TECHNIQUE

1 A preauricular or postauricular incision is made.
2 The temporalis fascia is exposed.
3 The joint capsule is incised and opened.
4 The disc is replaced or repositioned.
5 Drains are placed.
6 The wound is closed.

Discussion

The patient is placed in the supine position with the arms tucked at the sides. General anesthesia is administered. The patient then is prepped and draped to expose the TMJ, including a head drape.

The surgeon begins by making a preauricular or postauricular incision with a #15 blade. The skin flaps are elevated with either the ESU or scissors to expose the temporalis fascia with small retractors in place and a # 9 Molt elevator is used to dissect the underlying periosteum to the level of the arch. Next, blunt dissection is performed with a hemostat.

A horizontal incision is made into the joint capsule, and a flap is created to expose the condyle. The condyle is distracted inferiorly. Any adhesions are split with the ESU or mobilized with a scalpel. If any perforations are noted in the disc of the joint, the joint usually is removed and an artificial joint is placed. If the disc has rotated, it is repositioned and sutured in place with 2-0 nonabsorbable sutures. A drain then is placed if necessary, and the wound is closed.

NOTE: Endoscopic surgery for this procedure is now available in some dental and oromaxillofacial clinics.

KEY CONCEPTS

- Oral and maxillofacial surgery requires knowledge of the surgical anatomy of the bony structures of the face and oral cavity.
- Imaging studies are performed to diagnose oral and maxillofacial pathology.
- Careful case planning is required for oral and maxillofacial surgery to include specialty instruments, power equipment, draping, and fine reconstruction devices for use on bone.
- An understanding of the pathology involved in oral and maxillofacial disease and deformity is necessary for patient care.
- Knowledge of specific techniques and procedures in oral and maxillofacial surgery is necessary for patient care and for assisting in the role as a scrubbed surgical technologist.

REVIEW QUESTIONS

1. Why are wire cutters sent with the patient after maxillomandibular fixation?

2. Why are arch bars used during open reduction and internal fixation of facial fractures?
3. How should stainless steel sutures be handled? (Review Chapter 22 if necessary.) Expand your answer to include care of sharp ends, and preparation.
4. Describe the three regions of Le Fort fractures.
5. What type of facial fracture might result in leakage of cerebrospinal fluid?
6. Give two reasons for performing tooth extraction.

BIBLIOGRAPHY

Flint PW, Haughey BH, Lund VJ, Niparko JK: *Cummings otolaryngology: head and neck surgery*, ed 5, Philadelphia, 2010, Mosby.

Fortunato N, McCullough SM: *Plastic and reconstructive surgery: perioperative nursing series*, St Louis, 1998, Mosby.

Marks SC: *Nasal and sinus surgery*, Philadelphia, 2000, WB Saunders.

Moody FG: *Atlas of ambulatory surgery*, St Louis, 1999, Mosby.

Porth C: *Pathophysiology: concepts of altered health states*, ed 6, Philadelphia, 2002, Lippincott Williams & Wilkins.

Silver CE, Rubin JS: *Atlas of head and neck surgery*, ed 2, Philadelphia, 1999, Churchill Livingstone.

Thibodeau GA, Patt KT: *Anthony's textbook of anatomy and physiology*, ed 17, St Louis, 2003, Mosby.

Thumfart WF, Platzer W, Gunkel AR, et al: *Surgical approaches in otorhinolaryngology*, New York, 1998, Thieme.

Weerda H: *Reconstructive facial plastic surgery: a problem-solving manual*, New York, 2001, Thieme.

Plastic and Reconstructive Surgery

30

CHAPTER OUTLINE

Introduction
Surgical Anatomy
Case Planning

Techniques in Plastic and
 Reconstructive Surgery
Surgical Procedures

LEARNING OBJECTIVES

After studying this chapter the reader will be able to:

1. Identify key anatomical features of the integumentary system and face
2. Discuss specific elements of case planning for plastic and reconstructive surgery
3. Discuss techniques used in plastic and reconstructive surgery
4. List and describe common plastic and reconstructive surgical procedures

TERMINOLOGY

Aesthetic surgery: Surgery that is performed to improve appearance but not necessarily function; also called *cosmetic surgery.*

Allograft: A tissue graft in which the donor and recipient are of the same species.

Autograft: The surgical transplantation of tissue from one part of the body to another in the same individual.

Biological grafts: Grafts derived from live tissue, whether human or animal.

Biosynthetic: A type of graft or implant material made of synthetic absorbable material.

Composite graft: A biological graft composed of different types of tissues such as skin and muscle.

Debridement: The surgical removal of dead skin, debris, and infectious material from a wound.

Dermatome: A medical device used for removing single thickness skin grafts.

Eschar: Tissue that has been burned (second- and third-degree burns) but remains adherent to the wound. Eschar is nonelastic and may constrict underlying structures, impairing vital functions.

Escharotomy: Excision of eschar to release stricture in surrounding tissues.

Fasciotomy: Longitudinal incisions made in the fascia to release severe swelling or stricture which can result in necrosis.

Full-thickness skin graft (FTSG): A skin graft composed of the epidermis and dermis.

Hydrodressing: A dressing impregnated with a water-based gel. This type of dressing prevents the wound from drying.

Hypertrophic scar: A raised scar characterized by excess collagen.

Implant: A synthetic, natural, or biosynthetic substance used to fill in or replace an anatomical structure.

Keloid: A hypertrophic scar occurring in dark-skinned individuals. The scar may become bulbous and usually does not reduce over time.

Mohs surgery: A procedure in which a malignant tissue mass is removed and cut into quadrants before frozen section. These quadrants are used to map the tumor and determine the exact location of malignant margins.

Photodamage: Damage to the skin caused by ultraviolet light.

Plication: Folding of tissue and securing it in place surgically.

Porcine: Derived from pig tissue.

Ptosis: Drooping or sagging of any anatomical structure.

Split-thickness (or partial-thickness) skin graft (STSG): A skin graft that consists of the epidermis and a portion of the papillary dermis.

Synthetic grafts: Grafts derived from synthetic material compatible with body tissue. Synthetic grafts may be soft, semisolid, or liquid.

Undermine: A surgical technique in which a plane of tissue is created or an existing tissue plane is lifted, such as skin from the fascia.

Xenograft: A graft made up of tissue taken from one species and grafted into another species (e.g., a porcine graft implanted in human tissue).

INTRODUCTION

Plastic and reconstructive surgery involves the treatment of congenital defects and anatomical abnormalities caused by disease and injury. Restoration of form and function is the primary goal of treatment. Plastic and reconstructive surgery crosses nearly all subspecialties and varies from simple procedures to extremely complex and technically demanding operations.

Aesthetic surgery, also called *cosmetic surgery,* is performed to improve the appearance but does not always address function.

An individual's goals are deeply connected with social and cultural standards of acceptable appearance. In Western culture, body image is highly influenced by pressure to appear youthful (i.e., smooth, wrinkle-free skin; a slim body; and high definition of secondary sexual characteristics). Many plastic and reconstructive procedures are specifically intended to provide these changes. The basis of surgery is to fulfill a fundamental need for social acceptability. Individuals who have been disfigured by trauma, a congenital defect, or disease may experience a level of self-consciousness that prevents them from achieving a fulfilling life. For these patients, plastic surgery offers the hope of integration and acceptance into their social culture.

Whether the patient arrives in surgery for an elective or a nonelective procedure, special psychological needs must be met. Patients usually benefit from an honest, straightforward manner and should receive emotional support throughout the perioperative period.

SURGICAL ANATOMY

INTEGUMENTARY SYSTEM (SKIN)

The skin, or integumentary system (Figure 30-1), performs a number of vital functions:
1. It protects underlying tissues and organs.
2. It excretes organic waste and stores nutrients.
3. It excretes water and dissipates heat as a means of thermoregulation.
4. Its sensory organs transmit touch, pressure, pain, and temperature, which alert the body to possible injury.

Epidermis
The epidermis is the outer layer of the skin. The primary tissue cells of the epidermis are the keratinocytes. Five distinct epidermal layers represent various developmental stages of the keratinocyte:
• The *stratum corneum* is the most superficial layer. It is relatively transparent and composed of dead keratinocytes that are filled with a protein called *keratin*. The stratum corneum is thicker on areas of the body that are weight bearing or exposed to friction, such as the hands and feet.

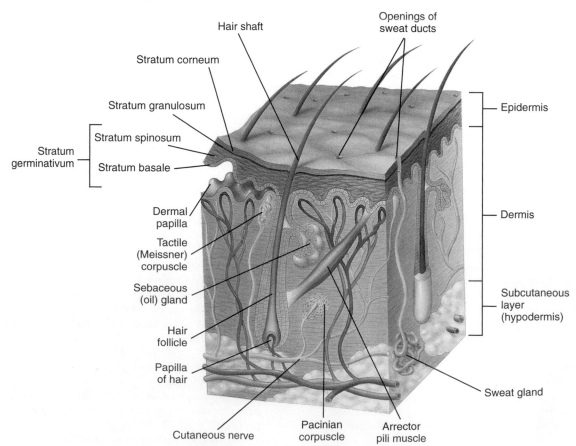

Figure 30-1 The skin, including the dermis and epidermis. *(From Thibodeau GA, Patton KT: Anthony's textbook of anatomy and physiology, ed 17, St Louis, 2003, Mosby.)*

- The *stratum lucidum* is composed of dead or dying cells that are flattened and densely packed. This layer is extremely thin (approximately five cells thick). It may not be found on regions of the body with thin skin.
- The *stratum granulosum* is several cells thick and produces keratin.
- The *stratum spinosum* contains undifferentiated cells that become specialized as they migrate to the skin surface.
- The *stratum germinativum,* also called the *stratum basale,* is the deepest layer of the epidermis attached to the dermis. The cells in this layer undergo mitosis, producing daughter keratinocytes that migrate through the layers of the epidermis. The melanocytes also are found in this layer; these cells are responsible for the production of melanin, a substance that gives rise to skin pigmentation.

Dermis

The dermis lies between the epidermis and the subcutaneous fatty layer. It provides nourishment and innervation to the epidermis. The blood vessels of the dermis are responsible for oxygenation of the tissue and thermoregulation. A large portion of the vascular plexus in the dermis bypasses the capillaries through an arteriovenous network in which small arteries flow directly into venules. This allows the vessels to dilate and constrict as the environmental temperature rises and falls. The dermis has numerous sensory receptors (i.e., for pain, touch, heat, cold, and pressure), which inform the brain about environmental change or danger.

Skin Appendages

Skin contains several specialized structures called *appendages,* such as hair, sweat, and oil glands, which have protective functions.

Hair is a protective structure that covers most areas of the body, except the palms and the soles of the feet. Each hair is surrounded by a follicle located in the dermis. The follicle consists of the hair itself, a sebaceous gland, muscle, and sometimes an apocrine (sweat) gland. The hair shaft, the visible portion of the hair, varies in size, shape, and color. The *sebaceous glands* discharge a waxy, oily secretion called *sebum* into the hair follicles. Sebum acts as a lubricant. The hair muscle (arrector pili muscle) aids thermoregulation of the body by contracting in a cold environment; this reduces the surface area of the skin and prevent heat loss.

Two types of *sweat glands* are found in the human body. The *apocrine sweat glands* arise from the dermis and are located mainly in the axilla and groin. They open out into the hair follicle. The oily secretion has no odor unless it comes in contact with bacteria. The *eccrine glands* secrete sweat over the surface of the body through small tubules. Sweat helps regulate the body temperature by cooling it through evaporation.

As mentioned, sebaceous glands produce sebum, a combination of wax, lipids, cholesterol, and triglycerides. These glands are distributed over the entire body, except on the palms and the soles of the feet. Their functions are to lubricate the skin and hair and to prevent evaporation in a cold environment. The sebaceous glands are responsive to hormonal influence, and their size is proportional to the amount of sebum produced.

ANATOMY OF THE FACE

The soft tissues of the face include skin, fat, muscle, fascia, and ligaments (Figure 30-2). The subcutaneous fatty tissue is separated into deep and superficial layers by a tissue plane called the *superficial musculoaponeurotic system* (commonly called the SMAS). The fat of the superficial layer is composed of lobes, which are deposited unevenly over the surface of the face and integrated within the fibrous tissue of the SMAS. The fat is the most dense in the cheek and neck region. The deep fat layer, under the SMAS, is thinner and divided by fibrous bands. The ligaments of the face support the soft tissue and attach it to the bone.

CASE PLANNING

PREPPING AND DRAPING

Povidone-iodine is used to prep the skin for procedures other than the face. The face and graft sites are prepped with nonstaining solutions. Regardless of the prep solution used, care must be taken not to allow the prep solution to drain into the eyes or ears.

Draping routines in plastic and reconstructive surgery follow the general techniques described in Chapter 20. Extra draping towels, plain sheets, and adhesive drapes should be available for complex draping routines. For procedures involving the face, most surgeons use a head drape. This prevents the hair from falling into the field and allows the surgeon to visualize the entire face during the procedure. If a head drape is used, the front edge of the drape may be placed behind the hairline. Fenestrated or split sheets are used for draping a limb. Whenever large amounts of solution are required, such as during debridement, an impervious pocket drape should be used to collect and isolate runoff. Multiple draping sites are commonly required during plastic and reconstructive surgery.

INSTRUMENTS

Plastic surgery instruments (commonly called *plastic instruments*) include a variety of devices for cutting, retracting, and grasping tissue. Most cosmetic surgery involves only the skin; therefore the instruments are short and have fine tips.

Sharp dissection is performed with tenotomy or fine Metzenbaum scissors and toothed tissue forceps. Many other delicate scissors are available, and most plastic surgeons have one or two favorites, which the scrub should have available.

The skin is retracted with skin hooks or small rakes. These are available in a wide variety of widths and lengths. Instruments used for slightly deeper retraction, such as those needed for combined skin and subcutaneous tissue, are less delicate and may be blunt-tipped to prevent puncturing of blood vessels. Senn retractors commonly are used for skin and subcutaneous retraction. A vein retractor may also be required for procedures in which tendons or large nerves are exposed.

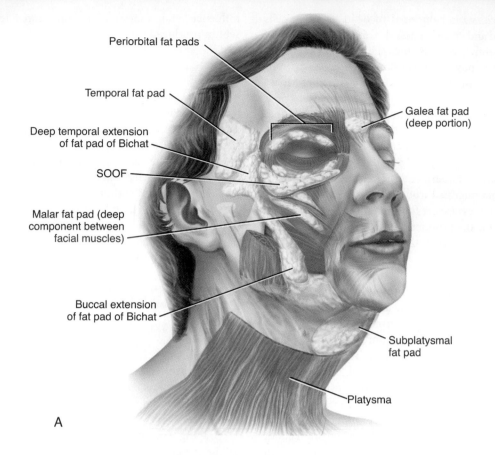

Periorbital fat pads

Temporal fat pad

Deep temporal extension
of fat pad of Bichat

SOOF

Malar fat pad (deep
component between
facial muscles)

Buccal extension
of fat pad of Bichat

Galea fat pad
(deep portion)

Subplatysmal
fat pad

Platysma

A

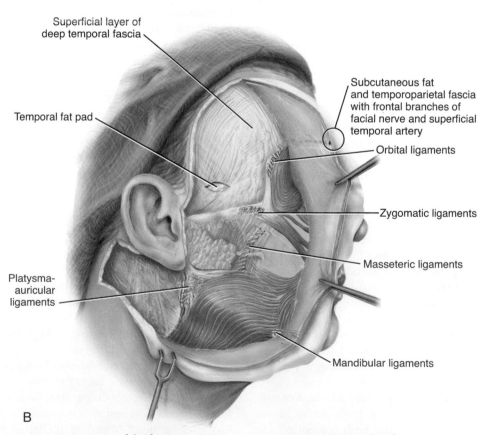

Superficial layer of
deep temporal fascia

Temporal fat pad

Subcutaneous fat
and temporoparietal fascia
with frontal branches of
facial nerve and superficial
temporal artery

Orbital ligaments

Zygomatic ligaments

Masseteric ligaments

Platysma-
auricular
ligaments

Mandibular ligaments

B

Figure 30-2   **Anatomy of the face. A,** Fat deposits deep to the superficial musculoaponeurotic system
(SMAS). **B,** The sub-SMAS anatomy, showing muscles and ligaments. *SOOF,* Suborbicularis oculi
fat. (*A from Fortunato N, McCullough SM: Plastic and reconstructive surgery, St Louis, 1998, Mosby;
B from LaTrenta G: Atlas of aesthetic face and neck surgery, Philadelphia, 2004, WB Saunders.)*

Skin forceps are toothed to prevent the skin from slipping out of the instrument. Adson or fine single-toothed forceps are used for procedures that do not require magnification. Hemostats are not used on the skin but are required for superficial blood vessels or for tagging suture. Fine mosquito forceps are commonly used.

Reconstruction procedures may require fine orthopedic instruments, including small bone clamps, toothed tissue forceps, and small Kocher clamps. Rasps, small osteotomes, and fine curettes also should be available during procedures involving bone tissue. Curved and straight Mayo scissors are needed for trimming cartilage and soft implants.

EQUIPMENT

Dermatome

Skin grafting is a common technique in plastic and reconstructive surgery. Grafts taken from the patient's own body are used to extend the edges of a wound or to cover an area in which skin has been lost in trauma or disease. A large split-thickness graft is removed with a **dermatome**.

MECHANICAL DERMATOME A mechanical dermatome has a flat, oscillating blade housed within an adjustable head. The instrument head is placed over the lubricated graft site and advanced forward. The blade dips just below the epidermis, removing a uniform layer of epidermis.

The dermatome set includes blade guards, a screwdriver, and a disposable blade (Figure 30-3, *A*). The surgeon sets the cutting depth before use. However, the scrub must make sure the blade knife and guards are properly assembled and the correct blades for that instrument are mounted. This is a critical process, because if incorrectly installed, the blade guard and knife can work loose and damage the graft site or tear the graft.

This type of mechanical dermatome may be powered by compressed air or electricity. The most commonly used models are the *Brown* (most common), *Padgett*, and *Zimmer* dermatomes. A handheld, battery-operated dermatome can be used for very small grafts.

DRUM DERMATOME A drum dermatome (*Reese* and *Padgett* dermatomes) is used less often than other types. This type of dermatome requires a skin adhesive, which is painted on the donor site in the shape and size of the graft required. The edge of the donor site is fixed to the drum, which elevates the skin while an oscillating blade separates the skin from the underlying tissue.

Graft Knife

A graft knife is used to remove a full-thickness skin graft. This is a hand instrument that has a handle and an adjustable operating end for the blade (see Figure 30-3, *B*).

Graft Mesher

A split-thickness skin graft is usually modified before implantation in the recipient site. The graft is "aerated" by transforming it from a solid sheet of skin to a mesh configuration.

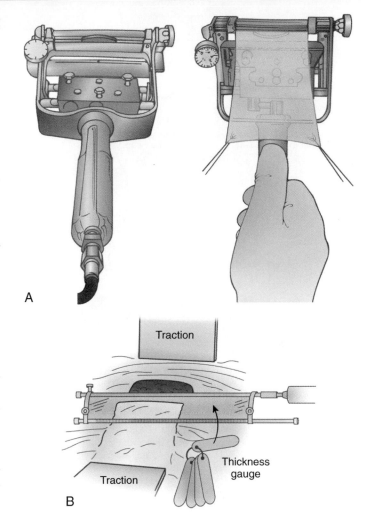

Figure 30-3 **A,** A Brown dermatome is used to remove a split-thickness skin graft. Note the skin emerging from the back of the blade as the dermatome is advanced over the tissue. **B,** A graft knife is used to obtain a full-thickness skin graft by hand. (*From Fortunato N, McCullough SM: Plastic and reconstructive surgery, St Louis, 1998, Mosby.*)

This is done with a graft mesher (Figure 30-4). The graft is placed on a flexible carrier plate and carefully fed into the mesher, which cuts small, diamond-shaped holes in the skin.

The purpose of aeration is to prevent blood and serum from accumulating under the graft during healing. The meshing process also allows the graft to stretch, increasing its surface area and providing a more precise fit over the donor site.

Power Drill

A pneumatic power drill is used in plastic and reconstructive surgery for the following techniques:

- To model bone tissue with a rotating burr or cutter
- To create anchor holes for wire or screws
- To cut through bone with an oscillating saw blade

Power drills are available in a wide variety of sizes and designs. The scrub is responsible for proper assembly and safe management of the drill on the sterile field. Techniques for handling power instruments are presented in Chapters 8 and 31.

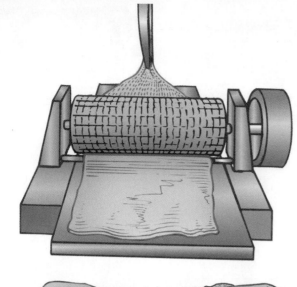

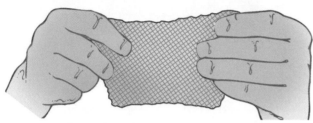

Figure 30-4 **Skin graft mesher.** The skin graft is placed on a carrier plate, which is fed into the mesher. The blades of the mesher create a uniform pattern of diamond-shaped holes, which allow the graft to be expanded and fitted over the defect. *(From Rothrock J: Alexander's care of the patient in surgery, ed 13, Philadelphia, 2007, Mosby.)*

Endobrow Instruments

Endobrow instruments include a 4- or 5-mm endoscope in 0- and 30-degree angles, cannulas, and a variety of periosteal elevators and instruments for blunt and sharp dissection. These instruments usually are included in a self-contained set.

Carbon Dioxide Laser

The carbon dioxide (CO_2) laser is used for facial resurfacing procedures. The principles of laser safety are detailed in Chapter 18.

DRESSINGS

Dressings in plastic and reconstructive surgery provide wound protection and physical support to remodeled structures. Surgery involving only the dermis and epidermis requires a simple protective dressing, such as gauze squares, collodion spray, Steri-Strips, or Tegaderm.

Complex reconstructive procedures require a variety of materials and techniques. Dressing routines in these procedures are exact and are considered a critical step of the procedure. Remodeling procedures require a dressing that provides anatomical support and protection to the affected part. An exact shape and position of the remodeled structure must be maintained throughout the initial healing period to ensure a successful outcome. A support or elastic dressing protects the operative wound but must allow sufficient circulation. Limb surgery requires roller dressings such as Kling, Kerlix, or Ace bandages. Rolled or molded cotton is used to provide barrier protection and support after reconstruction.

Stenting is a specific dressing technique used in skin grafting. The objective of stenting is to apply pressure over the graft site to prevent the accumulation of serum or blood between the graft and the recipient site. Continuous contact also ensures that the graft becomes integrated with the recipient site during healing. (The procedure for stenting is described under Grafting.) A more recent technology is to use Dermabond or some other tissue adhesive to maintain contact between the skin and graft site.

TECHNIQUES IN PLASTIC AND RECONSTRUCTIVE SURGERY

The surgical objectives of plastic and reconstructive surgery are:

- To restore function lost because of trauma, disease, or a congenital anomaly
- To produce a physical outcome that is acceptable to the patient within the individual's cultural and social environment

GRAFTING

Grafting is the surgical implantation of biological or manufactured material into an area of the body. A graft can replace tissue that has been lost, or it can *augment* (build up) tissue for aesthetic and functional purposes. The scrub must be familiar with the type of graft planned for a particular surgery. This information determines the preoperative preparation; the instruments, equipment, and supplies used; and the procedural steps of the surgery.

The two fundamental types of grafts are **biological grafts** (those derived from living tissue) and **synthetic grafts** (those derived from manufactured materials). **Biosynthetic** grafting material is absorbed by the body or enhances healing but is not derived from biological tissue.

Biological Grafts

The scrub should become familiar with terms used to describe implants and grafting techniques in these categories:

- **Allograft:** A graft transferred from one individual (human) to another. Allografts, also called *homografts*, are harvested from donors and preserved by the tissue bank until needed. Skin, bone, and cartilage are commonly used allografts. Allografts are subject to partial reabsorption over time.
- **Autograft:** A biological graft taken from one area of the body and transplanted to another area in the same patient. Commonly used tissues are skin, bone, cartilage, and fat.
- **Composite graft:** A biological graft consisting of more than one tissue type (e.g., skin and subcutaneous tissue). Several types of composite grafts are available and they are classified according to the method of transplantation (described with the surgical procedures later in the chapter).

- **Split-thickness (or partial-thickness) skin graft (STSG):** A graft that contains epidermis and papillary dermis, which is a highly bioactive portion of the dermis.
- **Full-thickness skin graft (FTSG):** A graft that contains the complete dermis and epidermis.
- **Xenograft:** A graft made up of tissue taken from one species that is grafted into another species (e.g., **porcine** [pig] skin grafted into a patient).

IMPLANTS

An **implant** is a synthetic, natural, or biosynthetic substance used to fill in or replace an anatomical structure. Breast tissue can be replaced with a soft implant made of silicone. In chin augmentation, a silicone chin implant is surgically inserted to replace bone tissue. Stainless steel orthopedic implants often are used to replace a joint. A number of different synthetic materials can be used to replace or augment tissue.

Silicone

Silicone has been used as an implant material since the 1950s. It has proven to be both safe and effective. The harder the silicone, the more stable it is. These implants are easily sculpted. Silicone can be used for a variety of purposes, including chin and cheek implants. The silicone implant must have sufficient soft tissue coverage to prevent chronic inflammation.

Polyethylene

Polyethylene (Medpor) implants are porous, cause little inflammatory reaction, and remain stable in the body. These characteristics make it a desirable implant material. However, it is difficult to sculpt, and when it is removed, it can damage surrounding soft tissue.

Gore-Tex

Gore-Tex implants have been used in cardiovascular procedures for many years. Gore-Tex implants are now frequently used in facial augmentation. Gore-Tex is quite inert, and tissue infiltration into the implant is minimal. This allows the implant to be removed at a later date, if necessary.

DEBRIDEMENT

For diseased or traumatized tissue to heal, all devitalized or infected areas must be removed. Damaged or dead cells prevent the formation of fibrin, collagen, and other matrix tissue that binds the healing tissues. The process of removing the diseased, damaged, or infected tissue is called *debridement*.

Debridement often is performed outside the operating room unless prolonged deep anesthesia is required. Burn patients require frequent debridement during the healing process. Grafting cannot take place until debridement is complete.

Several methods of debridement can be used. Procedures vary according to the extent and depth of the affected tissue:

- *Chemical debridement:* Enzymes are used to dissolve tissue. These are impregnated into wound dressings or may be applied at the time of debridement.

- *Surgical debridement:* Tissue is removed using sharp dissection with surgical instruments. Note that all debrided tissue must be removed from the field, isolated, and confined. Debridement is considered a contaminated procedure.
- *Pressurized saline:* Debridement is performed using a fine jet spray of saline. This technique is used commonly in burn and trauma patients.

TISSUE REMODELING

Many plastic and reconstructive procedures require tissue remodeling. The techniques for remodeling are sculpting or augmentation of tissue. Soft tissue is sculpted by sharp and blunt dissection or with the laser. Dense connective tissue is sculpted with a variety of drills and bone cutters. Augmentation procedures require synthetic or biological grafts and implants.

SURGICAL PROCEDURES

EXCISION OF SUPERFICIAL LESIONS

Surgical Goal

Skin lesions are removed for diagnostic purposes and to prevent or treat malignancy.

Pathology

Malignant lesions usually result from excessive exposure to ultraviolet light (sun or artificial) in combination with genetic susceptibility. The most common types of lesions are basal cell carcinoma, squamous cell carcinoma, and malignant melanoma. Of these, malignant melanoma is the lesion of most concern. Many benign lesions are excised for cosmetic purposes, to prevent recurrent infections, and for diagnosis.

TECHNIQUE

1. The lines of excision are drawn on the skin.
2. The surgeon excises the lesion.
3. Frozen sections may be performed and further tissue removed.
4. The wound is closed.

Discussion

The patient is positioned to allow the surgeon access to the surgical site:

- Prone for lesions of the back and buttocks
- Lateral for lesions of the hip and shoulder
- Supine for facial or limb procedures

A local anesthetic is used if the surgical wound can be closed by primary intention. If the procedure will be more extensive or if frozen section with wide excision is planned, general anesthesia may be more appropriate.

During **Mohs surgery,** a malignant skin lesion is removed and divided into quadrants before frozen section. These quadrants are used to map the tumor and determine the exact location of malignant margins (Figure 30-5). Further excision is performed until the specimen is clear of all malignancy.

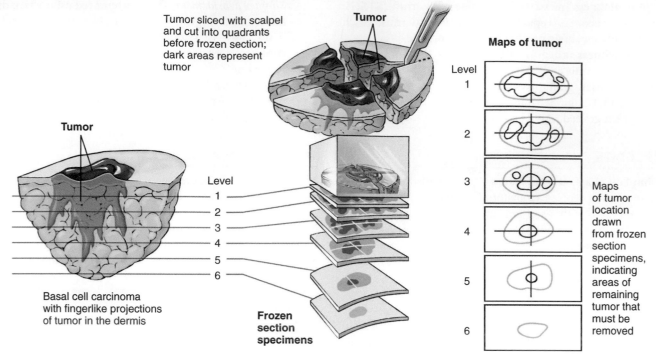

Tumor sliced with scalpel and cut into quadrants before frozen section; dark areas represent tumor

Tumor

Maps of tumor

Level 1

Tumor

Level 1
2
3
4
5
6

Basal cell carcinoma with fingerlike projections of tumor in the dermis

Frozen section specimens

Level 2

3

Maps of tumor location drawn from frozen section specimens, indicating areas of remaining tumor that must be removed

4

5

6

Figure 30-5   **Mohs surgery.** A frozen section is quartered and sliced into multiple layers to obtain a clear view of tumor margins. This technique preserves as much tissue as possible while excising any containing cancer cells. *(From Thibodeau G, Patton K: Anatomy and physiology, ed 6, St Louis, 2007, Mosby.)*

The surgeon marks the incision and possible skin flaps before the prep. Planning includes the possibility of total excision with adequate margins.

The patient is prepped and draped to allow access to the lesion. Using a #15 blade, the surgeon makes a skin incision that is carried to the subcutaneous layer. Any subcutaneous extension of the lesion is dissected away with tenotomy scissors, a hemostat, or the scalpel. The assistant may use double-prong or single-prong skin hooks to retract the skin flaps. Small bleeders are controlled with the electrosurgical unit (ESU), unless obliteration of malignant margins that must be identified by frozen section is a concern.

After the lesion has been removed and delivered from the wound, the surgeon may place orientation sutures in the specimen. The lesion is sent to the pathology department for frozen section or review. The wound is irrigated and closed with subcutaneous and dermal absorbable sutures. The wound is dressed with a simple gauze dressing.

SCAR REVISION

Surgical Goal

Scar revision is performed to remodel a previous scar or to remove a keloid.

Pathology

Scar formation is a normal phase of healing. Clean surgical wounds usually heal with minimal scarring, especially when little or no tension is put on the wounds. However, infection, excess pressure, or tension on a wound may result in a scar

that appears ragged, misshapen, or undulating. Scars resulting from traumatic injury are particularly prone to uneven scar formation. A **hypertrophic scar** is one that develops excess tissue and may be red or raised. This type of scar generally heals after 6 months and may resolve over a period of years. However, **keloid** scars, which often develop in dark-skinned individuals, continue to form at the wound site and may become bulbous and unsightly. Keloids also can invade nearby tissue. This type of scar is difficult to treat and usually does not resolve naturally.

Discussion

The surgeon begins by marking the planned revision. The scar is incised with a #15 blade and Adson toothed forceps. Allis clamps may be used to provide traction on the scar during excision. The surgeon's next step is to **undermine** the surrounding tissue with Metzenbaum scissors to release the scar. The wound edges are closed with 4-0 or 5-0 absorbable synthetic suture.

DEBRIDEMENT OF BURNS

Surgical Goal

Debridement is the removal of nonviable tissue from a nonhealing or traumatic wound. Burn wounds require repeated debridement to remove dying and dead tissue so that healing can continue.

Pathology

Burns are caused by flame, scalding (liquid), electrical current, radiation, or chemicals. The current system for classifying burns established by the American Burn Association, http://www.ameriburn.org, describes the depth of tissue injury.

- *Superficial partial-thickness first-degree:* Only the outer layer of the epidermis is injured. The skin is red or pink, dry, and painful to touch.
- *Partial-thickness second-degree:* The epidermis and various degrees of the dermis are injured. The skin is blistered, red, and moist. The burn is very sensitive to environmental exposure and touch.
- *Full-thickness second-degree:* The epidermis and full dermis are injured. These burns are characterized by a white, smooth, shiny surface with dry blisters and edema.
- *Full-thickness third-degree:* The skin, subcutaneous tissue, muscle, and bone are burned. The third-degree burn is centered in an area of second-degree injury. The skin may be white, brown, or black and appears waxy. There is no pain because nerves have been destroyed.

Third-degree burns develop **eschar**, which is devitalized nonelastic tissue that adheres to the wound site. Eschar is removed during debridement to allow healing and to reduce constriction.

Extensive second- and third-degree burns can result in fluid and electrolyte imbalance, infection, inadequate nutrition, respiratory deficit, and vascular damage. Circumferential eschar has a tourniquet effect on the affected body part and thus can extensively damage underlying muscle, bone, and vascular tissue. In this case, an **escharotomy** (eschar removal) or **fasciotomy** (multiple incisions through the fascia) is performed to release the stricture.

TECHNIQUE

1. Nonviable tissue is removed.
2. Bleeding is controlled.
3. The debrided area may be covered with a graft.
4. Dressings are applied.

Discussion

Preparation of the burn patient requires extensive thermoregulation and physiological monitoring. The temperature in the operating room is raised to reduce the risk of hypothermia.

The patient is positioned to allow for adequate exposure of the burns. General anesthesia is used. The patient is prepped with povidone-iodine spray and draped with towels and three-quarter sheets. A pneumatic tourniquet may be used for burns of the extremities.

The surgeon begins by removing all nonviable skin with a Braithwaite blade or USF debrider. The tissue is removed until only a viable layer remains. Lap sponges soaked in a solution of sterile saline and topical epinephrine (1:1,000) are applied to control bleeding. The concentration most often used is 1,000 mL of normal saline, with 4 mL of topical epinephrine (1:1,000) added according to the surgeon's orders.

When hemostasis has been achieved, an allograft may be applied. The graft is stapled over the debrided burns to create a layer of protection until autografting can be performed (usually several days after the initial debridement).

Nonadherent dressings (e.g., Xeroform) and fluffs are applied. The extremities are wrapped with Ace bandages.

Patients may recover in the *burn intensive care unit*. Multiple debridement surgeries and multiple skin grafts may be required before the rehabilitation process can begin. After the healing process, burn patients undergo extensive physical and occupational therapy to regain full use of the burned areas.

SPLIT-THICKNESS SKIN GRAFT

Surgical Goal

Skin grafting is performed to replace skin that has been lost as a result of trauma, disease, or infection.

Pathology

Skin is necessary for protection and nourishment of underlying tissues. Minor injuries or defects can regenerate sufficient skin to create a scar. Large defects require a skin graft to protect underlying tissues from infection, *desiccation* (drying), and injury.

TECHNIQUE

1. The donor site is pulled taut.
2. The donor site is covered with lubricant.
3. The graft is removed with a dermatome.
4. The donor site is dressed.
5. The graft is applied to the prepared recipient site.
6. The recipient site is dressed.

Discussion

The patient is positioned to allow exposure of the donor site (i.e., supine position for the lower extremities and trunk; prone position for the buttocks and back). The donor and recipient sites are prepped and draped separately.

The surgeon removes the skin graft with either a free-hand skin graft knife (full-thickness graft) or a dermatome (split-thickness graft).

DERMATOME The scrub must prepare the dermatome, inserting the appropriate blade and guard. (In some facilities, the surgeon prepares the equipment.) The dermatome should always be handed to the field with the depth gauge set at 0. This allows the surgeon to select the depth setting for the blade, usually 0.012 to 0.015.

Mineral oil is applied to the graft site to reduce friction as the blade glides over the skin. To assist the surgeon in taking the graft, the assistant pulls the donor skin taut using either 4 × 4 gauze sponges or tongue blades. The surgeon positions the dermatome at the donor site and advances forward to remove the top layer of skin (Figure 30-6). The graft emerges from the back of the instrument as the dermatome is advanced across the skin. The assistant grasps and elevates the graft with forceps as it is produced (the surgical technologist may be asked to perform this task).

When sufficient skin has been removed, the dermatome is angled upward; this severs the graft. If it is not released, the graft can be separated from the donor bed with fine scissors.

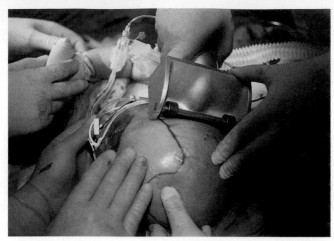

Figure 30-6 Removal of a split-thickness graft with a dermatome. *(From Barret JP, Herndon DN: Color atlas of burn care, Philadelphia, 2001, WB Saunders.)*

The scrub accepts the graft in a basin to protect it from contamination and injury. Alternatively, the surgeon may transfer the graft immediately to a carrier plate for meshing (see next section). The graft should be kept moist but not wet and covered with gauze, according to facility protocol.

The donor site is covered with a sponge soaked in saline or a solution of saline and topical epinephrine (1:1,000) to aid hemostasis. Xeroform gauze also is used to cover the wound.

GRAFT PREPARATION Most split-thickness grafts require meshing before implantation. In this process, the graft is fed into a blade and roller mechanism that perforates the graft. The surgeon places the skin on a plastic carrier plate, spreading it evenly over the surface with the exterior side facing upward. The plate is inserted into the mesher, which is hand-operated.

PLACING THE GRAFT The recipient site may require debridement before grafting. When the site is ready, the carrier plate is held near the recipient site, and the skin is gently teased onto the prepared tissue bed. The surgeon spreads the graft over the defect and trims any excess with curved iris scissors. The graft is attached to the skin surrounding the defect with staples or absorbable suture. If the graft is implanted on an exposed area of the body, such as the hands or face, it is sutured in place. On areas that are not exposed, such as the abdomen or back, the graft may be stapled.

The donor site is dressed with an OpSite transparent dressing or a nonadherent dressing covered with Kerlix gauze roll.

A stent dressing may be placed over the graft (see Chapter 22).

STENT DRESSING A *stent* is a type of pressure dressing that is placed over the graft site to prevent the accumulation of serum or blood under the graft. To prepare a stent, four or more opposing sutures are placed at the periphery of the graft site. The ends are not cut but left long. Petroleum gauze is cut to fit over the entire graft. Saline-moistened gauze is molded to fit over the petrolatum. The gauze is tied in place with the long

suture ends. The site is dressed with gauze fluffs. A soft splint made of cotton and gauze may be applied to prevent displacement of the graft in the immediate postoperative period.

PEDICLE GRAFT

Surgical Goal
Pedicle grafts provide coverage and vascularization to a soft tissue defect.

Pathology
A pedicle graft (also called a *flap graft*) is raised from the donor site but not immediately severed free. The donor site tissue is partly severed, and the flap is brought in contact with the recipient site. The graft is sutured in place to cover the defect. During the healing process, the graft tissue infiltrates and develops over the recipient wound. When healing is complete, the flap is released and the donor site defect is closed primarily with sutures. This type of graft is used when the recipient site requires skin and deep tissue to fill a large tissue defect resulting from radical surgery or trauma.

Types of Pedicle Graft
Pedicle grafts are classified as near or distant. A near graft is created in adjacent tissue (e.g., from the palm for use on the finger). Distant grafts are created from the trunk or other areas for use on a limb.

An advancement flap (see the following section) is raised from the tissues in the immediate area of the defect. Rotational flaps are semicircular and require some degree of turning to reach and cover the recipient tissue defect.

Pedicle flaps have large blood vessels that infiltrate the recipient site during healing. A pedicle graft to the finger is shown in Figure 30-7. A rotational flap is shown in Figure 30-8.

TECHNIQUE

1. The defect is measured.
2. The incision lines of the flap are measured and drawn on the skin.
3. The flap is elevated.
4. The flap is positioned over the defect.
5. The flap is sutured into place.
6. The donor site is closed.

Discussion
ADVANCEMENT FLAP The patient is placed in a position that allows access to both the defect and the donor site. Depending on the size of the defect, general or local anesthesia may be used. The surgeon begins by measuring the defect and the proposed flap to ensure complete coverage. The incision lines are drawn with a skin scribe. Both surgical sites are prepped. The surgeon cleans any rough, uneven edges of the defect with a # 15 blade.

Next, the donor site is incised. The flap is elevated with the knife or tenotomy scissors. Retraction is applied with double-prong skin hooks. When the flap has been raised sufficiently, it is advanced into position over the donor site. The surgeon

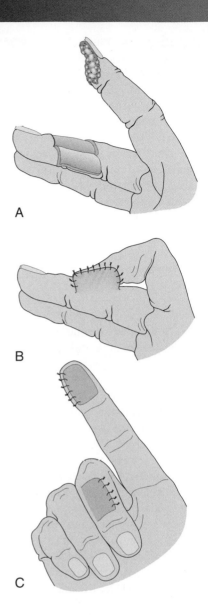

Figure 30-7 Pedicle graft of the finger. **A,** The flap is raised on the middle finger. **B,** The injured first digit is placed in contact with the flap and sutured in place. **C,** The flaps are closed after healing. (*From Garden O, Bradbury A, Forsythe J, Parks R: Principles and practice of surgery, ed 5, Edinburgh, 2007, Churchill Livingstone/Elsevier.*)

does this by simply approximating the edges of the skin flap to cover the defect; 3-0 or 4-0 absorbable sutures are used for deep tissue, and 5-0 or 6-0 nonabsorbable sutures are used for the skin.

BLEPHAROPLASTY

Surgical Goal

Blepharoplasty resection of the eyelid is done to improve vision of the upper visual fields.

Pathology

With advancing age, the eyelids lose elasticity and tone and may obscure vision. The procedure also may be performed for cosmetic purposes.

TECHNIQUE

1. The lids are injected with a local anesthetic.
2. The skin and subcutaneous tissue are incised.
3. The excess skin is removed from the eyelid.
4. The incision is closed.

Discussion

The patient is placed in the supine position with the head on a doughnut headrest and the arms tucked at the sides. General or local anesthesia may be used. A local anesthetic is instilled into the lid. The patient is prepped and draped with a head drape and split sheet.

UPPER LID BLEPHAROPLASTY The surgeon determines the exact location of the incisions and marks the sites with a skin scribe. The incision is made with a #15 blade. Dull rakes are used to retract the skin and expose the subcutaneous tissue. Depending on the amount, the fatty tissue may be excised with tenotomy scissors. A needlepoint bipolar ESU is used to control bleeding in the fatty tissue. If excess muscle also is present, it is removed with curved iris scissors. The incision is closed with nonabsorbable subcuticular suture and several interrupted sutures to reinforce the primary suture line. The ends of this suture are left long for easy removal. Upper lid blepharoplasty is illustrated in Figure 30-9.

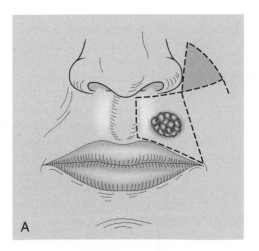

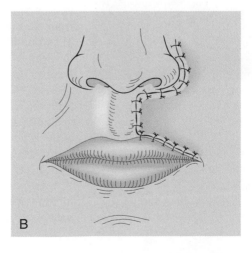

Figure 30-8 Rotational flap from the face. **A,** The lesion is removed, and a flap is raised from the perialar area. **B,** The flap is rotated to fit over the defect, and the graft site skin is closed after healing. (*From Garden O, Bradbury A, Forsythe J, Parks R: Principles and practice of surgery, ed 5, Edinburgh, 2007, Churchill Livingstone/Elsevier.*)

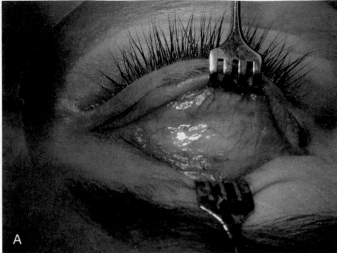

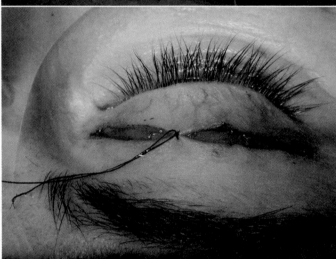

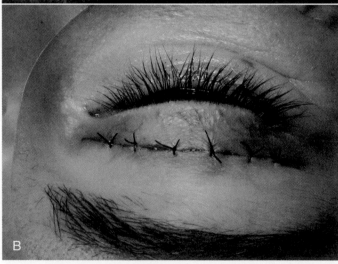

Figure 30-9 **Upper lid blepharoplasty. A,** The skin incision is retracted with dull rakes. Small bleeders have been coagulated with the bipolar ESU. The fat pad is exposed and may be removed with Westcott scissors. **B,** Closure with 6-0 Vicryl sutures. *(From Chen W, Khan J, McCord C: Color atlas of cosmetic oculofacial surgery, Edinburgh, 2004, Butterworth-Heinemann.)*

LOWER LID BLEPHAROPLASTY: SUBCILIARY APPROACH Using a #15 blade, the surgeon makes the incision in the subciliary region, 2 to 3 mm below the lower lash line. The lower lid skin is elevated upward and outward to determine the amount to be removed. The skin is excised with a #15 blade. To gain access to the infraorbital fat pads, the surgeon makes an incision into the orbicularis muscle. Double-prong skin hooks are used to retract the skin. The excess fat is removed with iris scissors. The orbicularis oculi muscle is reattached to the periosteum at the lateral orbital rim with clear, nonabsorbable sutures. This prevents the lower lid from drooping after blepharoplasty. The incisions are closed as described previously. Lower lid blepharoplasty is illustrated in Figure 30-10.

BROW LIFT (OPEN AND ENDOSCOPIC TECHNIQUES)

Surgical Goal
Brow lift procedures are done to lift the supportive structures of the brow and alleviate drooping of skin, muscle, and fascia.

Pathology
The soft tissues of the brow may droop with age and deepen the furrows over the eyes. This may also lead to eyebrow **ptosis** and upper lid "hooding" of the eye.

Discussion
OPEN TECHNIQUE The patient is placed in the supine position with the head of the table raised. The arms are tucked at the sides. The surgeon pulls the hair back and secures it with rubber bands. The face is prepped and draped using a head drape and split sheet.

A number of approaches can be used for a brow lift (Figure 30-11). These include the coronal approach (behind the hairline), the pretrichial approach (at the hair line), or the direct approach (at the level of the brow itself). The selected incisions are drawn carefully with a skin scribe. The incisions are made with a #15 blade. A periosteal elevator is used to lift the periosteum from the cranium to the level of the superior orbital rims. The periosteum is incised at the level of the orbital rim with the elevator. This allows for mobility of the brows. The muscles at the bridge of the nose are incised with scissors, ESU, or the elevator. The excess skin of the inferior flaps is excised with the #15 blade. The inferior flap is suspended from the superior periosteum with a nonabsorbable suture. The wound is closed in layers. Absorbable sutures are used for the deep layers. Absorbable or nonabsorbable sutures are used for the skin, or staples may be used in a coronal approach.

ENDOSCOPIC TECHNIQUE The patient is placed in the supine position with the head of the bed raised. The arms are tucked at the sides. The hair is pulled back and secured with rubber bands. The face is prepped and draped with a head drape and split sheet.

Using a #10 blade, the surgeon makes three central scalp incisions behind the hairline, one in the midline and two just medial to the superior temporal line. The incisions are

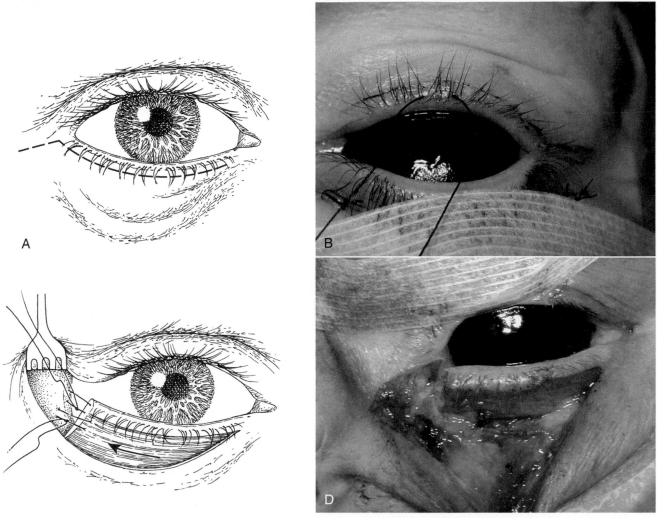

Figure 30-10 **Lower lid blepharoplasty. A,** Infraciliary incision. **B,** Upside-down view of the lower lid margin. **C,** Canthotomy and resection. **D,** The lid after resection. *(From Chen W, Khan J, McCord C: Color atlas of cosmetic oculofacial surgery, Edinburgh, 2004, Butterworth-Heinemann.)*

extended, and a periosteal elevator is used to dissect the forehead flap from bone. The 30-degree 4- or 5-mm endoscope is passed through the rim of one of the incisions. Undermining is continued to a point approximately 0.8 inch (2 cm) above the supraorbital rim.

Next, a straight periosteal elevator is used to elevate the temporal fascia with the endoscope in place. The two temporal dissections are connected with a straight periosteal elevator and the 30-degree endoscope. The surgeon elevates the frontal fascia to the level of the supraorbital rim.

When the periosteum has been mobilized, the surgeon elevates and fixes the lateral brow. (The medial brow usually is not fixed, because if it is elevated too much, the brow looks unnatural.)

The tissue may be fixed by drilling into the bone and passing absorbable sutures through the holes and soft tissue. The incision is closed with staples. A head dressing consisting of Kerlix fluffs and rolled gauze is applied. An endoscopic brow lift is shown in Figure 30-12.

RHYTIDECTOMY

Surgical Goal

Redundant and sagging supportive tissue of the face is reduced or modified to provide a more aesthetic appearance.

Pathology

The aging process and gravity affect the skin and the structures that lie beneath it. This results in hollow infraorbital regions, nasolabial folds, jowls, and excess skin below the chin. Certain environmental factors contribute to laxity and wrinkling of the skin. Wrinkles are a normal product of aging. However, **photodamage** occurs with extended, excessive exposure to ultraviolet light. Smoking also causes extreme wrinkling of the skin.

Discussion

The patient is placed in the supine position with the head stabilized on a doughnut or Mayfield headrest and the head of the bed raised. The surgeon marks the skin with a skin scribe before the prep is performed. The patient is prepped and draped for a face procedure.

The surgeon may inject the excisional areas injected with local anesthetic containing epinephrine as a vasoconstrictor to provide hemostasis. The scrub should verify the type and exact strength ordered by the surgeon. A fine-gauge spinal needle and 10-mL syringe are used for the injection. This area includes the cheek to the submentum (under the chin) and posteriorly over the mastoid and into the neck. Skin incisions are made with a #15 blade, and double-prong skin hooks are used for retraction. The surgeon may staple a sponge to the posterior aspect of the incision to reduce the amount of blood that collects in the hair.

The dissection continues with rhytidectomy scissors. The bipolar ESU is used to control small bleeders. The surgeon may use a fiberoptic retractor to aid exposure during dissection. At this point, the surgeon may overlap the underlying fascial attachment with 2-0 or 3-0 absorbable suture. A surgical option is to excise a strip of fascia in the preauricular area with Metzenbaum scissors. This tissue should be saved on the back table in saline in case it is needed for further augmentation procedures.

If the surgeon is performing a deep plane rhytidectomy, the fascia is elevated from the parotid gland and surrounding area in the neck. This dissection is performed with the rhytidectomy or Metzenbaum scissors. The two ends of the fascia are then folded over and secured with 2-0 or 3-0 absorbable suture.

Excess skin is excised with Metzenbaum scissors, and the subdermal layer is closed with 3-0, 4-0, and 5-0 absorbable sutures. A small Penrose drain may be placed during closure.

The skin is closed with a combination of staples and 5-0 absorbable or nonabsorbable sutures. A head dressing is placed to support the incisions. Gauze sponges with an Ace wrap or a fascioplasty splint are commonly used to dress the wound. Figure 30-13 shows rhytidectomy techniques.

LASER SKIN RESURFACING

Surgical Goal

Laser skin resurfacing removes the epidermis and a portion of the dermis to reduce facial lines and wrinkles.

Pathology
See Rhytidectomy.

> **TECHNIQUE**
>
> 1. The patient is anesthetized.
> 2. The operative area is draped with moist towels.
> 3. The skin is resurfaced with either the carbon dioxide or the erbium-YAG laser.
> 4. The wounds are dressed.

Discussion

All laser precautions must be followed before the start of surgery. This includes safety attire for the operating team (correct goggles for the type of laser), safety signs, and strict attention to sources of combustion on the operative field. (Chapter 18 presents a complete discussion of laser use.)

The patient is placed in the supine position with the arms tucked at the sides. The head of the operating table is elevated according to the technical requirements of the procedure. The

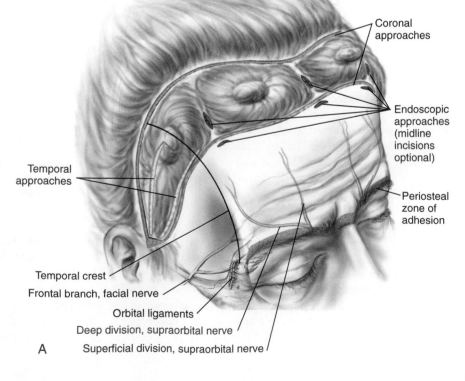

Figure 30-11   Open brow lift. A, Incisions for a brow lift.

Coronal approaches

Endoscopic approaches (midline incisions optional)

Periosteal zone of adhesion

Temporal approaches

Temporal crest

Frontal branch, facial nerve

Orbital ligaments

Deep division, supraorbital nerve

Superficial division, supraorbital nerve

A

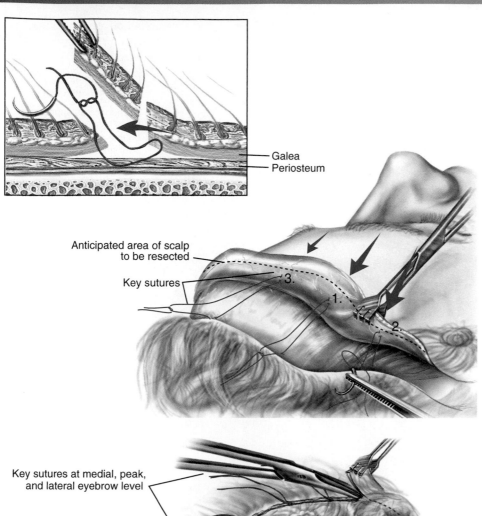

Galea
Periosteum

Anticipated area of scalp
to be resected

Key sutures

Figure 30-11, cont'd **B,** Closure and removal of redundant scalp tissue. *(From LaTrenta G:* Atlas of aesthetic face and neck surgery, *Philadelphia, 2004, WB Saunders.)*

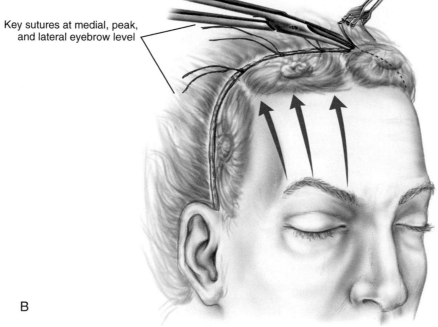

Key sutures at medial, peak, and lateral eyebrow level

B

type of anesthesia depends on the extent and length of the procedure. Short cases are done using local anesthesia, whereas more extensive surgery requires general anesthesia. If general anesthesia is used, a laser endotracheal tube must be used to prevent an airway fire.

The face is prepped with a nonalcohol prepping agent and draped with a head drape and split sheet. Moist towels are placed around the surgical site to reduce the risk of peripheral

thermal damage and fire. The patient's eyes must be protected from injury with laser safety goggles.

The surgeon adjusts the laser settings before resurfacing. The handpiece is passed over the skin using the computer guidance system of the unit. Each pass removes a layer of the epidermis, reducing the appearance of wrinkles. When the entire face has been resurfaced, a **hydrodressing** is applied.

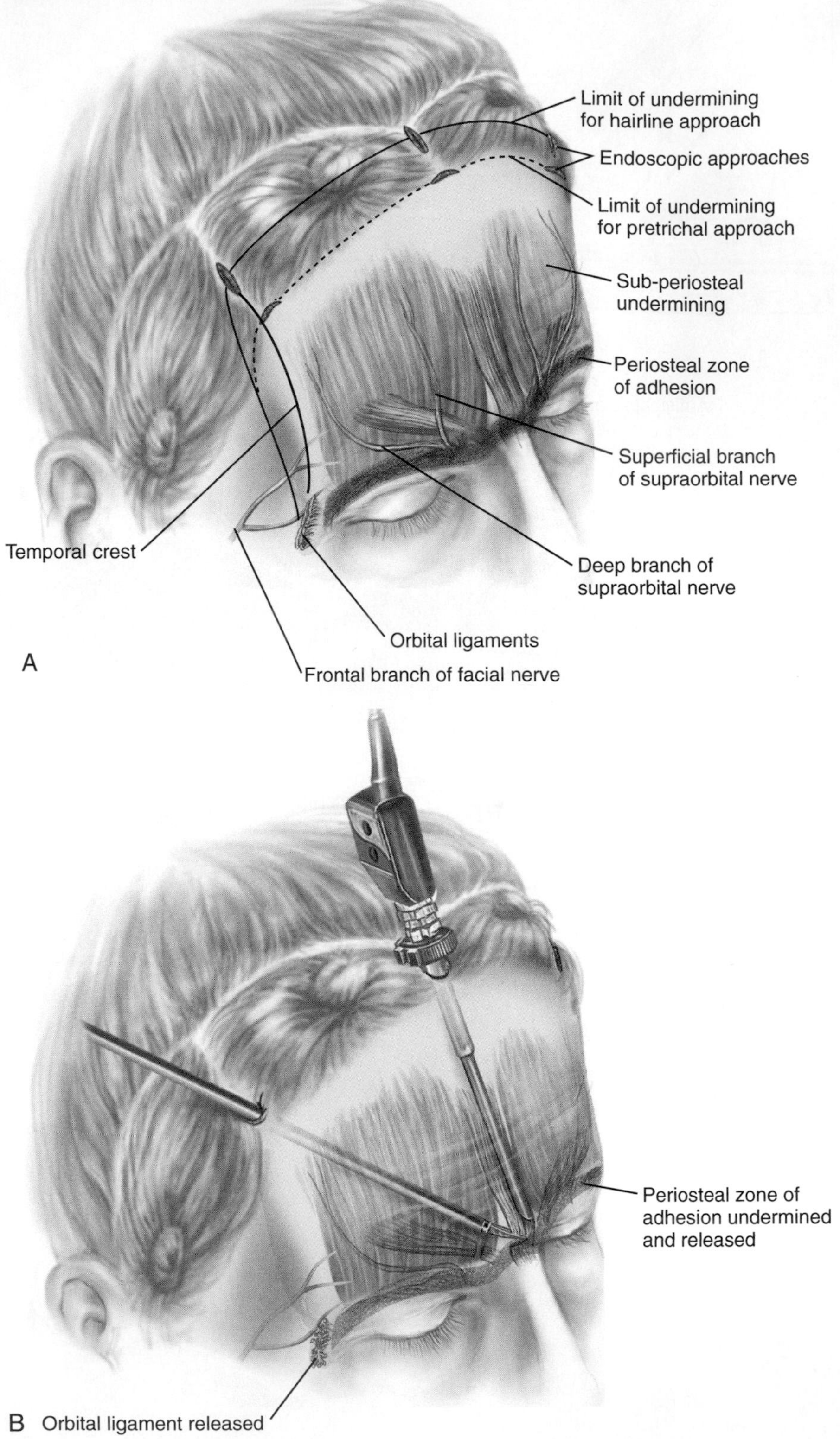

Figure 30-12 **Endoscopic brow lift. A,** Incisions for endoscopic lift. **B,** Subperiosteal dissection. *(From LaTrenta G: Atlas of aesthetic face and neck surgery, Philadelphia, 2004, WB Saunders.)*

Labels on figure A:
- Limit of undermining for hairline approach
- Endoscopic approaches
- Limit of undermining for pretrichal approach
- Sub-periosteal undermining
- Periosteal zone of adhesion
- Superficial branch of supraorbital nerve
- Deep branch of supraorbital nerve
- Orbital ligaments
- Frontal branch of facial nerve
- Temporal crest

A

Labels on figure B:
- Periosteal zone of adhesion undermined and released
- Orbital ligament released

B

FACIAL IMPLANT

Surgical Goal

Facial augmentation is performed to give normal contours to the chin or cheek. This is achieved by inserting a molded implant in the affected area. Many different materials are used as implants, including silicone, acrylic polymers, polyethylene, Gore-Tex, and mesh. Several types of subdermal and subcutaneous injectable filler materials are available. These include Dermalogen, Alloderm, Restylane, collagen,

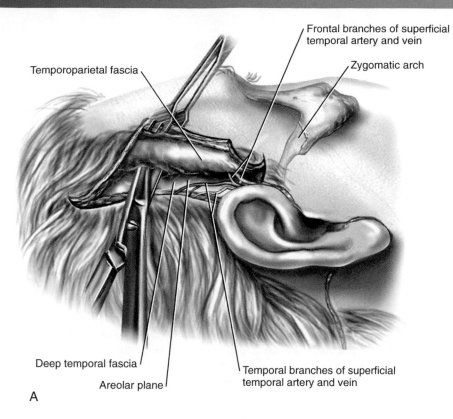

Temporoparietal fascia

Frontal branches of superficial temporal artery and vein

Zygomatic arch

Deep temporal fascia

Areolar plane

Temporal branches of superficial temporal artery and vein

A

SKIN TENSION VECTORS AND CLOSURE SEQUENCING
1 → 2 → 3

3. Set the upper face last

2. Set the midface next

1. Set the neck first

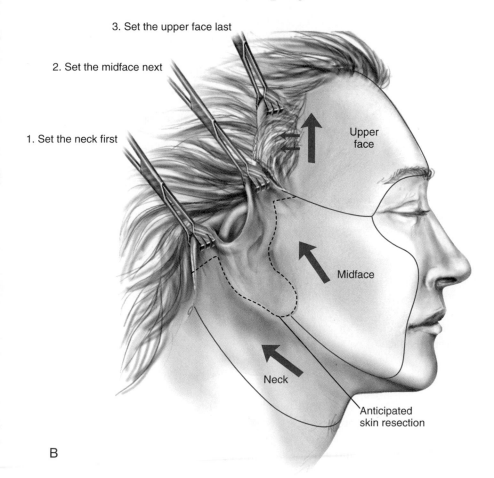

Upper face

Midface

Neck

Anticipated skin resection

B

Figure 30-13 Rhytidectomy techniques. A, Undermining in the temporal area. **B,** Closure of skin flaps and areas of resection. *(From LaTrenta G: Atlas of aesthetic face and neck surgery, Philadelphia, 2004, WB Saunders.)*

and liquid silicone. An autograft (fat, bone, or cartilage) may also be used. The type of implant chosen depends on the surgeon's preference and the type of defect to be filled.

Pathology

Facial augmentation corrects malformation or loss of facial tissue caused by congenital anomaly, trauma, or radical surgery in which bone and other connective tissue was removed. Patients may also seek augmentation for aesthetic reasons in the absence of deformity.

TECHNIQUE

1. The incision is planned and the skin is marked.
2. The skin is incised.
3. The skin is undermined.
4. The superficial SMAS is imbricated, incised, and plicated.
5. The skin is closed.
6. Dressings are applied.

Description

MENTOPLASTY (CHIN AUGMENTATION) The patient is placed on the operating table in the beach chair position with the arms tucked at the sides. General anesthesia may be used or local anesthetic is instilled into the region of the mental nerve, the incision line, and the surrounding soft tissue. Draping fully exposes the face to allow the surgeon to assess the projection given by the implant. A head drape and a split sheet are commonly used.

A 10- to 15-mm incision is made vertically in the midline on the chin with a #15 blade. The incision extends through the subcutaneous fat and muscle to the layer of the periosteum. The assistant retracts the skin flaps with double-prong skin hooks. The periosteum is incised with a #15 blade.

Next, the surgeon elevates the periosteum with a periosteal elevator (e.g., Joseph elevator). The implant is eased into position; the periosteum is elevated with a Senn retractor during implantation. Absorbable sutures may be placed in the distal end of the implant and periosteum to prevent the implant from shifting.

The wound is closed in two layers. The periosteum is closed with interrupted 3-0 absorbable sutures and the skin is closed with 6-0 nonabsorbable suture or a 5-0 fast-absorbing suture. Gauze dressings are applied.

MALAR AUGMENTATION (CHEEK AUGMENTATION) The patient is prepped and draped as described previously. An intraoral incision is made below the parotid duct with a #15 blade and extended to the periosteum. The periosteum then is incised and elevated superiorly and laterally over the malar and zygoma. The implant is positioned, and the wound is closed in layers with 3-0 absorbable sutures. No dressing is applied, because the incision is intraoral.

TECHNIQUE

1. The incision is made.
2. The periosteum is elevated.
3. The implant is inserted.
4. The wound is closed.

OTOPLASTY

Surgical Goal

Otoplasty is surgical creation of the external ear.

Pathology

Otoplasty is performed to correct a congenital malformation of the external ear or to re-create an ear destroyed by trauma.

TECHNIQUE

1. Incisions are made in the periauricular skin.
2. Keith needles are inserted.
3. Sutures are placed.
4. The incisions are closed.

Discussion

Procedures for otoplasty often involve multiple surgeries. These procedures are somewhat complex, and many approaches can be used, depending on the pathological condition and the patient's needs.

The patient is placed in the supine position with the head of the table raised. A doughnut headrest is used to stabilize the head and allow access to the posterior ear. If the procedure is a bilateral one, the patient is prepped and draped to allow access to both ears.

An incision is made in the postauricular skin with a #15 blade to expose the cartilage. The soft tissue is dissected from the perichondrium. Keith needles are then used to recreate the antihelix on the anterior surface of the ear. The Keith needles are used as guides on the posterior surface to help the surgeon "break" the spring of the cartilage so that the antihelix can be recreated. This can be done by incising strips of skin with the #15 blade. Wedges of tissue are then released with a triangular Farrior knife. A diamond-tip drill may be used to thin the strips. Once the spring has been broken, the cartilage is fixed in position with nonabsorbable sutures. If necessary, a strip of cartilage is removed from the lateral portion of the conchal bowl and the cartilage is reapproximated with nonabsorbable sutures. Techniques for pinning the ear usually involve suturing the posterior portion of the conchal bowl to the mastoid periosteum with nonabsorbable suture. The skin then is closed with absorbable suture.

The reconstructed ear is reinforced with ointment-impregnated cotton balls and a mastoid dressing.

AUGMENTATION MAMMOPLASTY

Surgical Goal

Augmentation mammoplasty is performed to increase the size and improve the shape of the breast. Mastopexy (reduction of excess skin over the breast resulting in ptosis or dropping of the breast tissue) may also be performed during the procedure.

Breast implants are constructed with a silicone outer layer and a saline or silicone inner space. Implants may be round or anatomical in shape. Round implants are used for an elective procedure on an intact breast, whereas anatomical implants are used after mastectomy or if the breast is very small.

Mammoplasty can be performed using open surgery or endoscopic instruments (used in patients who are small in stature).

Discussion

POSTMASTECTOMY RECONSTRUCTION The patient is placed in the supine position, prepped, and draped for a breast procedure, including the sternal notch and xiphoid process. This allows the surgeon to use midline anatomical marks that have not been altered by previous surgeries.

The surgeon excises the mastectomy scar with Allis clamps and the skin knife. Hemostasis is maintained with the ESU. The scar is referred for pathological evaluation to ensure that no abnormal cells are present.

TECHNIQUE

1. The mastectomy scar is excised.
2. A pocket is created under the pectoralis major muscle.
3. A tissue expander is implanted in the pocket with the saline port in the subcutaneous tissue of the midaxillary line (allowing easy access for expansion over the following weeks).
4. The saline reservoir is filled (the initial amount is 150 to 300 mL of saline solution).
5. The wound is closed.

The surgeon creates a pocket in the musculofascial tissue of the pectoralis major. This is done with a blunt hemostat or with gentle digital separation of the tissue. A tissue expander with a saline reservoir is inserted into the pocket. The reservoir is filled to 150 to 300 mL. The injection port is placed in the subcutaneous tissue at the midaxillary line of the affected side. The incision then is closed with 3-0 and 4-0 absorbable suture (e.g., Vicryl). The skin is closed with a running subcuticular suture of 4-0 synthetic absorbable material.

The surgeon uses the saline-filled tissue expander to slowly stretch the skin and underlying tissue by gradually filling the saline reservoir. When the tissue has stretched sufficiently, the tissue expander is removed and replaced with a permanent implant.

For insertion of the permanent implant, the patient is placed in the supine position, prepped, and draped as previously described.

A #15 blade is used to make an incision in the axillary region, around the lower half of the areola and nipple, or in the inframammary fold. Hemostasis is maintained with the ESU.

The surgeon creates a pocket under the pectoralis major. A tissue expander is inserted into the pocket and filled in 60-mL increments. The scrub must record the amount of fluid used in the expander, because the same amount will be used in the implant.

The surgeon may assess the symmetry and position of the breast by placing the patient in the sitting position. In this case, the patient's arms and head must be fully supported with the assistance of the anesthesia care provider. The permanent implant is inserted and filled with the appropriate amount of saline. The incision is closed with 3-0 and 4-0 absorbable suture. The skin is closed with a subcuticular suture.

TECHNIQUE

Augmentation

1. The incision is made according to the selected approach.
2. A pocket is created under the pectoralis major muscle.
3. A temporary sizer is placed and filled with the appropriate amount of saline.
4. The sizer is removed and the permanent implant is placed.
5. The wound is closed.

The procedure is repeated for the other breast. At the conclusion of the procedure, the scrub must document the amount of saline used in each implant.

REDUCTION MAMMOPLASTY

Surgical Goal

In a reduction mammoplasty, excess breast tissue is removed and the breast is reconstructed to provide an anesthetic appearance.

Pathology

Reduction mammoplasty may be performed for cosmetic or medical reasons. Macromastia (excessively large breasts) is related to the weight and size of the breast. The increased forward weight can cause cervical and thoracic pain. Patients also may suffer socially and psychologically. Macromastia in males is referred to as *gynecomastia*.

TECHNIQUE

1. The incision lines are marked (this may be done before surgery admission).
2. An incision is made around the areola and extended in a wide triangle to the inframammary line.
3. The skin tissue is undermined.
4. The breast tissue is removed through the inframammary incision.
5. The inframammary and triangular incisions are closed.
6. A circular incision is made at the apex of the breast; the nipple is brought up and sutured in place.
7. The wound is closed and dressed with gauze fluff and a pressure dressing.

Discussion

Many different techniques are used to perform reduction mammoplasty. Preoperative preparation of the patient takes place in the surgeon's clinic. The procedure is planned using computer modeling and calibration. The incisions are clearly marked with an indelible skin scribe.

For the surgery, the patient is positioned in the supine or semi-Fowler position, prepped, and draped for a breast procedure as previously described.

The surgeon begins by making a circular incision around the areola with the breast held in extension. Next, the surgeon makes a triangular or anchor-shaped incision with the apex at the nipple margin and the base along the inframammary fold. The skin is undermined with a #15 blade, Adson toothed forceps, or Metzenbaum scissors. The breast then is manually retracted superiorly, and the glandular and fatty tissue are excised. This step is performed with sharp dissection. Any tissue removed is passed off the field to be weighed. This is done to ensure that approximately the same amount of tissue is removed from each breast.

The surgeon then approximates the breast tissue at the midline by bringing the sides of the triangle together and suturing them with absorbable 3-0 suture on a curved needle. Any excess skin at the inframammary incision is trimmed with Metzenbaum scissors or a # 15 blade. The incision is closed with 3-0 absorbable suture. Both skin incisions then are closed with 4-0 subcuticular suture.

The surgeon uses a nipple marker to make a circular incision at the apex of the triangular incision. The tissue is excised with a #15 blade. This creates a new position for the areola and nipple, which are pulled through the incision line and sutured in place with nonabsorbable subcuticular suture. Raising the position of the breast is referred to as mastopexy. Gauze fluffs and supportive dressings are then applied.

TRANSVERSE RECTUS ABDOMINIS MYOCUTANEOUS FLAP

Surgical Goal

A transverse rectus abdominis myocutaneous (TRAM) flap procedure is performed to reconstruct the breast without the use of implants.

Pathology

A TRAM flap can be used in a variety of plastic and reconstructive procedures, including breast reconstruction after

TECHNIQUE

1. The mastectomy scar is excised.
2. An elliptical incision is made in the transverse plane in the lower abdomen, at the level of the umbilicus, to include the umbilicus and the area above the symphysis pubis.
3. The incision is extended along the border, with attention paid to avoiding the large vessels of the rectus muscle.
4. The skin superior to the incision site is undermined at the level of the fascia.
5. The rectus sheath is incised.
6. The inferior epigastric artery and vein are ligated.
7. The flap is dissected up the costal margin, leaving the central edge of the rectus sheath attached to the rectus muscle.
8. The flap is delivered through the subcutaneous tunnel that has been created.
9. The transverse rectus abdominis myocutaneous (TRAM) flap is inserted into the area created by the elevated skin flaps of the mastectomy site.
10. The flap is trimmed to fit the defect and a new breast is constructed.
11. Excess portions of the flap may be defatted and used to create a breast mound.
12. The flap is sutured in place.
13. The abdominal wound is closed and a new umbilicus is created.

mastectomy. In this procedure, a tissue flap containing skin, subcutaneous tissue, and muscle is raised from the lower abdomen and transferred to the mastectomy site. The flap continues to receive its blood supply from the pedicle (the portion of the flap that remains attached to the point of origin). This allows reconstruction of the breast without the use of implants.

Discussion

The patient is placed in the supine position and prepped from the neck to the pubis. Draping exposes the abdomen and the breasts.

The surgeon grasps the mastectomy scar with Adson toothed forceps or Allis clamps and excises it with a #15 blade. The transverse abdominal incision extends from one iliac crest to the other. The upper margin includes the umbilicus. The surgeon then creates a subcutaneous tunnel that connects the mastectomy site with the abdominal incision, usually along the costal margin. This step is performed with large clamps and Metzenbaum scissors. The flap is elevated, and the upper border of the elliptical incision is carried into the abdominal wall. A small amount of subcutaneous tissue is left intact over the rectus sheath to preserve the vascular supply to the area.

The lower incision is carried to the level of the anterior fascia. The lateral margins, or "tails," of the incision are then mobilized. The rectus sheath and muscle are incised, and the inferior epigastric artery (found on the posterior surface of the rectus muscle) is ligated with a 2-0 silk tie. Sharp dissection is used to mobilize the rectus muscle, including the sheath, to the level of the costal margin.

The flap is brought through the subcutaneous tunnel in the direction of the mastectomy site. When the flap is in place over the mastectomy incision, it is trimmed. Excess skin is excised with scissors or a knife, and the flap edges are aligned with the skin flaps of the mastectomy incision.

The surgeon shapes the breast, trimming excess skin and subcutaneous tissue as needed with Metzenbaum scissors or the scalpel. The scrub must save all trimmed portions of the flap, because the subcutaneous tissue can be used to fill in the axillary region and to add more tissue to the breast mound itself.

A suction drain is placed in the wound before closure. Absorbable synthetic sutures (e.g., Vicryl) are used to secure the flap to the chest wall. Next, the skin flaps are closed with 4-0 nonabsorbable suture (e.g., Monocryl). Nipple reconstruction may be done at a later date if the patient desires. Additional surgeries also may be needed to contour the breast mound.

The surgeon closes the abdomen in layers. The rectus sheath is approximated with 2-0 absorbable synthetic suture. The skin is closed with staples or an absorbable subcuticular suture. Synthetic mesh may be used to reinforce the closure. (This process is described in Chapter 23.)

Nipple Reconstruction

After a TRAM flap reconstruction, some women may want the nipple and areola reconstructed to create a more natural appearance. The areola is constructed from a full-thickness graft taken from the medial thigh crease or postauricular region. The nipple is created with a full-thickness skin graft taken from the labia.

The nipple may be tattooed to provide color contrast at the time of reconstruction or at a later date. Figure 30-14 illustrates the process of TRAM flap breast reconstruction.

LIPOSUCTION

Surgical Goal

Liposuction is performed to remove excess deep fat.

TECHNIQUE

1. The incisions are marked before surgery with a skin scribe.
2. Tissue to be removed is injected with a local anesthetic mixed with lactated Ringer solution.
3. The incisions are made.
4. The fat is aspirated.
5. The incisions are closed.
6. Dressings are applied if needed.

Pathology

No physical pathological condition requires the use of liposuction.

Discussion

LIPOSUCTION INSTRUMENTS Liposuction is performed with high-vacuum suction, a rigid cannula, and a large-bore suction tube (at least $\frac{3}{8}$ inch [0.9 cm] in diameter). Large-bore tubing is required because adipose tissue is dense and would clog normal suction tubing. A high-vacuum apparatus is required to pull the tissue through the tubing.

The patient is placed in the supine position with the arms at a 90-degree angle to the body. Depending on the extent of the procedure, either general anesthesia or local anesthesia with intravenous sedation is used. The patient is prepped and draped with towels and three-quarter sheets to allow exposure of all the sites to be treated.

The surgeon begins by injecting an anesthetic into the soft tissue. A large volume of lidocaine and epinephrine diluted in lactated Ringer solution is injected into the targeted tissue until it is taut. The injection provides local anesthesia and hemostasis and expands the operative area, making it easier to insert the liposuction cannula.

Multiple incisions are made into each target area. This is done to allow easier access to the target tissue and to prevent depressions around the access sites. The liposuction cannula is connected to the large-bore suction tubing and high-vacuum suction. Superficial aspiration is performed with a 2- or 3-mm cannula. Deep aspiration requires a 4- or 5-mm cannula.

Aspiration is continued until the desired volume of fat has been removed or the desired shape has been achieved. The cannula is removed, and the incisions are closed with 3-0 absorbable suture. If the extremities have been treated, a compression stocking is applied to provide support and reduce postoperative swelling.

PANNICULECTOMY (ABDOMINOPLASTY)

Surgical Goal

Panniculectomy is performed to remove excess skin and adipose tissue from the abdominal wall.

Pathology

Abdominoplasty usually is performed as a cosmetic procedure, but it also can be performed for medical reasons. After significant weight loss, the skin of the abdomen hangs flaccid and can interfere with normal body movement. In some cases, the redundant skin can hang to the level of the knees. This "apron" makes movement and activities of daily living very difficult. In these cases, a panniculectomy is considered a medically necessary procedure.

TECHNIQUE

1. With the patient in the standing position, the incision line is marked in the natural skin fold of the lower abdomen.
2. A low transverse incision is made, extending to both inguinal areas.
3. The skin or subcutaneous tissue flap is elevated away from the anterior abdominal wall.
4. **Plication** (folding) of the rectus abdominis may be performed from the level of the xiphoid process to the mons pubis.
5. The skin and subcutaneous tissue flaps are pulled inferiorly, and the excess tissue is excised.
6. A small midline incision is made through which the umbilicus may be delivered.
7. The umbilicus is sutured in place.
8. The abdominal incision is closed in two layers with drains in place.
9. Postoperatively the patient is placed in high Fowler position to reduce tension on the abdomen.

Discussion

The patient is placed under general anesthesia and placed in semi-Fowler position to reduce tension on the abdominal tissue. The individual is prepped from the nipples to the thighs and draped for an abdominal procedure. A transverse, U-shaped incision is made in the lower pelvis and extended to the fascia. Skin flaps are elevated with the ESU and Metzenbaum scissors. The umbilicus is excised and left in its natural position. The skin flap is further elevated to the level of the xiphoid process and the inferior sternal borders.

The abdominal wall may be folded (plicated) from the xiphoid process to the mons pubis. This is done with 2-0 nonabsorbable suture (e.g., Prolene). The skin flap then is pulled inferiorly, and the excess skin is excised with the ESU. A small midline incision is made in the skin flap with a #15 blade to allow for delivery of the umbilicus into its natural position. The umbilicus is sutured into place with 3-0 absorbable suture. The abdominal wound is closed in two layers with absorbable suture. Dressings are applied, and the patient is maintained in semi-Fowler position to prevent tension on the suture line.

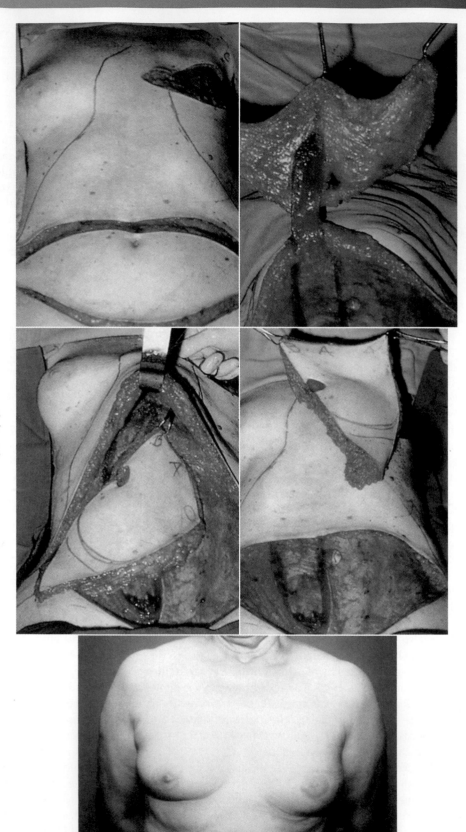

Figure 30-14 Transverse rectus abdominis myocutaneous (TRAM) flap for postmastectomy breast reconstruction. *(From Fortunato N, McCullough SM: Plastic and reconstructive surgery, St Louis, 1998, Mosby.)*

KEY CONCEPTS

- *Plastic and reconstructive surgery* involves the treatment of congenital defects and anatomical abnormalities caused by disease and injury. Restoration of form and function is the primary goal of treatment.

- *Aesthetic surgery,* also called *cosmetic surgery,* is performed to improve the appearance but does not necessarily address function.

- Most cosmetic surgery involves only the skin; therefore, the instruments are short and have fine tips.

- Reconstruction procedures may require fine orthopedic instruments, including small bone clamps, toothed tissue forceps, and small Kocher clamps. Rasps, small osteotomes, and fine curettes also should be available during procedures involving bone tissue.

- The dermatome is used to remove split-thickness skin grafts. The Brown-type dermatome is the most commonly used.

- Dressings in plastic and reconstructive surgery provide wound protection and physical support to remodeled structures. Complex reconstructive procedures require a variety of materials and techniques. Dressing routines in these procedures are exact and are considered a critical step of the procedure.

- Grafting is the surgical implantation of biological or manufactured material into an area of the body.

- A split-thickness skin graft (STSG) contains only the dermis, whereas a full-thickness skin graft (FTSG) contains both dermis and epidermis. A composite graft is one that contains two or more types of tissue.

- An implant is a synthetic, natural, or biosynthetic substance used to fill in or replace an anatomical structure.

- For diseased or traumatized tissue to heal, all devitalized or infected areas must be removed. The process of removing the disease, damaged, or infected tissue is called debridement.

- During *Mohs surgery,* a malignant skin lesion is removed and cut into quadrants before frozen section. These quadrants are used to map the tumor and determine the exact location of malignant margins (see Figure 30-6). Further excision is performed until the specimen is clear of all malignancy.

- Burns are classified according to the depth of tissue injury.

- In a superficial partial-thickness, first-degree burn, only the outer layer of the epidermis is injured. The skin is red or pink, dry, and painful to touch.

- A partial-thickness, second-degree burn is one in which the epidermis and various degrees of the dermis are injured. The skin is blistered, red, and moist. The burn is very sensitive to environmental exposure and touch.

- In a full-thickness, second-degree burn, the epidermis and full dermis are injured. These burns are characterized by a white, smooth, shiny surface with dry blisters and edema.

- Proper assembly of the dermatome blade and head is critical to prevent skin tissue from tearing during the procedure.

- The skin graft mesher is used to perforate a skin graft. This increases its surface area and prevents serum from accumulating under the graft once it is in place.

- In a full thickness, third-degree burn, the subcutaneous tissue, muscle, and bone are burned. The third-degree burn is centered in an area of second-degree injury. The skin may be white, brown, or black and appears waxy. There is no pain because nerves have been destroyed.

- Third-degree burns develop *eschar,* which is devitalized, nonelastic tissue that adheres to the wound site.

- Mineral oil is applied to the donor skin graft site to reduce the friction between the skin and dermatome blade.

- A stent is a special dressing applied over a skin graft. The dressing provides continuous pressure on the site to keep the graft in contact with the wound during healing.

- A pedicle graft is a composite graft in which a flap of tissue is partially released from one area of the body and attached to the wound site. When healing is complete, the flap is released and the donor site defect is closed primarily with sutures.

- Blepharoplasty resection of the eyelid is done to improve vision of the upper visual fields.

- Brow lift procedures are done to lift the supportive structures of the brow and alleviate drooping of skin, muscle, and fascia.

- The normal aging process and certain environmental factors such as smoking and exposure to excessive ultraviolet light contribute to sagging and wrinkling of the skin. Rhytidectomy is performed to remodel the skin and underlying tissue.

- Facial augmentation is performed to give normal contours to the chin or cheek. This is achieved by inserting a molded implant in the affected area.

- Otoplasty is performed to correct a congenital malformation of the external ear or to re-create an ear destroyed by trauma. Procedures for otoplasty often involve multiple surgeries. These procedures are somewhat complex and many approaches can be used, depending on the pathological condition and the patient's needs.

- Augmentation mammoplasty is performed to increase the size and improve the shape of the breast. The procedure is performed in postmastectomy patients and those desiring larger breasts for aesthetic reasons.

- Reduction mammoplasty may be performed for cosmetic or medical reasons. Macromastia (excessively large breasts) is related to the weight and size of the breast. The increased forward weight can cause cervical and thoracic pain.

- A transverse rectus abdominis myocutaneous (TRAM) flap procedure is performed to augment the breast without the use of implants. In this procedure a flap is raised from the abdomen and transferred to the chest wall as a pedicle graft.

- Panniculectomy (abdominoplasty) is performed for cosmetic reduction of abdominal fat. An "apron" of tissue is removed in severe cases to improve the patient's quality of life.

REVIEW QUESTIONS

1. What are the three classifications of burns? Describe them.
2. When is debridement necessary for the treatment of burns?
3. What is compartment syndrome?
4. Differentiate full-thickness and split-thickness skin grafts.
5. Explain the purpose of a flap graft.
6. What is a biosynthetic material?

BIBLIOGRAPHY

Aston SJ, Beasely RW, Thorne CHM: *Grabb and Smith's plastic surgery*, ed 5, Philadelphia, 1997, Lippincott-Raven.

Cummings C, Flint P, Haughey B, et al: *Cummings otolaryngology—head and neck surgery*, Philadelphia, 2005, Mosby.

Marks MW, Marks C: *Fundamentals of plastic surgery*, Philadelphia, 1997, WB Saunders.

Phillips N: *Berry and Kohn's operating room technique*, ed 11, St Louis, 2007, Mosby.

Rothrock JC: *Alexander's care of the patient in surgery*, ed 13, St Louis, 2007, Mosby.

Sandberg DJ, McGee WP, Denk MJ: Neonatal cleft lip and cleft palate repair, *AORN Journal* 75:490, 2002.

Tyers AG, Collin JRO: *Colour atlas of ophthalmic plastic surgery*, ed 2, Oxford, 2001, Butterworth-Heinemann.

Weerda H: *Reconstructive facial plastic surgery: a problem-solving manual*, New York, 2001, Thieme.

Orthopedic Surgery

CHAPTER OUTLINE

LEARNING OBJECTIVES

After studying this chapter the reader will be able to:

1. Identify anatomy of the skeletal system and connective tissues
2. Discuss diagnostic procedures of the skeletal system
3. Discuss specific elements of case planning in orthopedic surgery
4. Discuss skeletal system pathology
5. Describe surgical techniques and technology used in orthopedic surgery
6. Discuss common surgical approaches and procedures in orthopedic surgery

TERMINOLOGY

Alloys: Substances that are mixtures of pure metals.

Aponeurosis: A tendinous sheet that separates muscles or attaches a muscle to bone.

Arthrodesis: Surgical fusion of a joint.

Bioactive implant: An orthopedic implant that releases calcium to enhance healing.

Biocompatibility: A term that describes a material that is compatible with tissue (i.e., causes no toxic or inflammatory effect).

Biomechanics: The relationship between movement and biological or anatomical structures.

Broaches: Fin-shaped rasps used to enlarge the medullary canal for insertion of an implant. The broach is the same shape as the implant.

Cannulated: A device having a hollow core; for example, an instrument with a central channel that can be fitted over a guidewire or pin.

Casting: A method of immobilizing a limb by the application of rigid or semirigid material along the length of the limb. A cast can be fully or partially circumferential.

Closed reduction: Alignment of bone fragments into anatomical position by manipulation or traction.

Comminuted: A fracture in which there are multiple bone fragments.

Compartment syndrome: Extreme tissue swelling within a closed compartment of the body or closed external device such as a cast. Edematous tissue can exceed the capacity of the space it is held in, causing sufficient pressure to cause tissue necrosis.

Compression: Mechanical force in which a structure is compacted or pressed together. Compression is used to repair tissue. A compression injury (e.g., compression fracture) results when bone or other tissue is compacted.

Cruciate: Cross-shaped.

Dislocation: Displacement of a joint from its normal position.

Distraction: A mechanical process in which a structure is elongated. Distraction can be used to suspend a limb (and thereby stretch the soft tissue and bones) during surgery. A distraction injury is caused by the pulling apart or stretching of tissue (the opposite of a compression injury).

Examination under anesthesia (EUA): Fracture and dislocation may be fully assessed when general anesthesia is used.

External fixation: A method of stabilizing bone fragments in anatomical position from outside the body. A cast is an example of an external fixation device.

Internal fixation: A method of surgically repairing a fracture by implanting a device that holds the bone fragments in place. Metal plates, rods, pins, and screws are examples of internal fixation devices.

Open reduction: Surgical access (through an incision) to bring bone fragments into anatomical alignment.

Orthopedic system: A specific (usually patented) set of instruments and implants used for an orthopedic technique. For example, arthroplasty implants are marketed as systems that include the joint components and instruments that are designed for use with that implant.

Press-fit: To impact or press a joint implant into position. Press-fitted implants do not require bone cement.

Ream: To enlarge a preexisting hole, depression, or channel, such as the medullary canal.

Replantation: Surgical attachment of the hand, thumb, or fingers after traumatic amputation.

TERMINOLOGY (cont.)

Reduction: The process of manipulating a bone structure to restore anatomical position.

Skeletal traction: Traction device in which bone fragments are connected by pins or rods that are surgically inserted into the bone.

Traction: A mechanical method of applying pulling force to fractured bone in order to bring the fragments into alignment.

INTRODUCTION

Orthopedic surgery is a specialization of the body's connective tissues. These tissues are the framework of the body in a supporting and binding function. Surgery is performed to treat or to correct injuries, congenital anomalies, and disease of the bone, joints, ligaments, tendons, or muscle. Most orthopedic procedures focus on restoring bone and joint function that has been lost or diminished because of traumatic injury or disease. Alleviating pain is also a primary goal of surgical intervention. This chapter is presented according to the anatomical location of the pathology and surgery and encompasses bone and soft tissue repair.

Proficiency in orthopedic techniques relies heavily on a thorough understanding of the instrumentation and implants used for repair and reconstruction. Orthopedic techniques and **biomechanics** share many of the principles and language used in carpentry and engineering. Many procedures rely on the use of an **orthopedic system**, which is a set of instruments and a technique specific for one surgical approach. For example, a fracture can be repaired with a plate, screws, wire, or rod placed through the medullary canal for stability during healing. A typical system for any of these repairs might include the hardware (plate, screws, or rod) and specialty instruments designed for use with that particular company's hardware. Most manufacturers' system components are not interchangeable with those of another manufacturer, although some generic hardware does exist.

Although a daunting number of systems are available and in development, the biomechanical principles of orthopedics remain constant. Surgical approaches (systems, procedural technique, technology) to orthopedic injury and disease may seem complex but they follow a basic pattern based on the mechanical and physiological aspects of bone structure. This chapter explains the basic techniques and mechanics and introduces common approaches while pointing out the possibility for variation. The key to developing advanced skills is to learn basic principles and apply them to complex systems.

SURGICAL ANATOMY

SKELETON

The skeleton (Figure 31-1) provides structural support for the soft tissues of the body. For classification purposes, the *skeleton* is divided into two parts: the *axial* skeleton, which includes the skull, face, ear bones, hyoid, sternum, and ribs; and the *appendicular skeleton*, which includes the bones of the legs, feet, hands, trunk, and spine. Individual bones usually articulate or join other bones at a joint.

Axial Skeleton

The axial skeleton is composed of the skull and facial bones, vertebral column, sternum, and ribs. The skull, or *cranium*, has eight main bones that are connected by tough connective tissue called *sutures*. The brain is encased within the cranium, which includes the floor of the skull, and the sphenoid bone. At birth, the cranial bones are loosely fused. In the prenatal period, the sutures are wide and soft, which allows the head to mold as it passes through the mother's pelvis during birth. The *fontanels* are areas where the joint space is particularly wide. These occur in the posterior skull at the junction of the parietal and occipital bones and in the anterior skull between the parietal and frontal bones. The posterior fontanel usually closes by 8 weeks of age and the anterior fontanel at 3 to 18 months of age.

The fetal cranium is shaped to allow rapid growth of the brain, which occurs in the first several years of life. In infants, the head accounts for 25% of the total height of the body and is much wider from front to back than the adult skull.

The *facial bones* are more complex and form the structure of the nasal sinus, orbit of the eye, and jaw. Only the *mandible* (lower jaw) is freely moveable. The *zygoma* and *orbital rim* are common sites of fracture in sports and motor vehicle accidents. These bones usually are repaired with small mesh plates. Reconstructive surgery of the face and cranium is a surgical specialty known as *oromaxillofacial surgery*. This type of surgery is performed to treat congenital malformations, as well as injuries or disease that result in disfigurement and loss of function.

The *vertebral column* consists of 24 individual vertebrae: 7 *cervical,* 12 *thoracic,* and 5 *lumbar.* In adults, the sacrum is composed of five vertebrae that are fused. The coccyx is formed by the fusion of four or five vertebrae.

The sternum forms the anterior chest wall and is composed of three sections: the *manubrium,* the *body,* and the *xiphoid process.*

Twelve pairs of ribs connect to their corresponding vertebrae. Ribs 1 through 8 attach to the sternum and are connected by costal cartilage. Ribs 11 and 12 are "floating" ribs (i.e., they are not attached anteriorly).

Appendicular Skeleton

The appendicular skeleton is composed of the upper extremities, the lower extremities, and the pelvis.

Upper Extremities

The shoulder includes the *scapula* and *clavicle.* The long bone of the upper arm is the *humerus.* It articulates proximally with the *glenoid fossa.* The *ulna* and *radius* form the forearm, and the *carpal* and *metacarpal* bones form the hand and wrist.

Lower Extremities

The pelvis consists of the *ilium,* the *ischium,* and the *pubis.* The *femur,* or thigh bone, is the longest bone of the body. The *patella* is a sesamoid bone located between the femur and the lower leg. The lower leg bones are the *tibia* and the *fibula.* The foot is made up of the *calcaneus,* the *cuboid* and *navicular* bones, and the five *tarsals* and *metatarsals* (toes).

BONE TISSUE

Two types of bone tissue are found in the body: *cortical* bone and *cancellous* bone. Cortical bone (also called *compact bone*) is found on the surface of bones and is organized in tubular units called *osteons.* Osteons resemble the rings of a tree. Each tubular unit has a central canal (the *haversian*

canal), which provides nutrition and carries away cellular waste products. Blood vessels are located in the central canals. The concentric layers (lamina) of each osteon are composed of calcified tissue.

The ends of bones and the inner layer are composed of softer, less dense cancellous bone (also called *spongy bone*). Cancellous bone is less dense than cortical bone and has no geometric structure. Instead, the structure resembles a sponge, and the spaces are filled with red or yellow marrow, a soft connective tissue. Red marrow, which produces blood cells, is found in the center of certain long bones, in the vertebrae, and in pelvic bones. Important components of the immune system originate as precursor cells in marrow. These include lymphocytes, monocytes, and macrophages. The structure of bone tissue is illustrated in Figure 31-2.

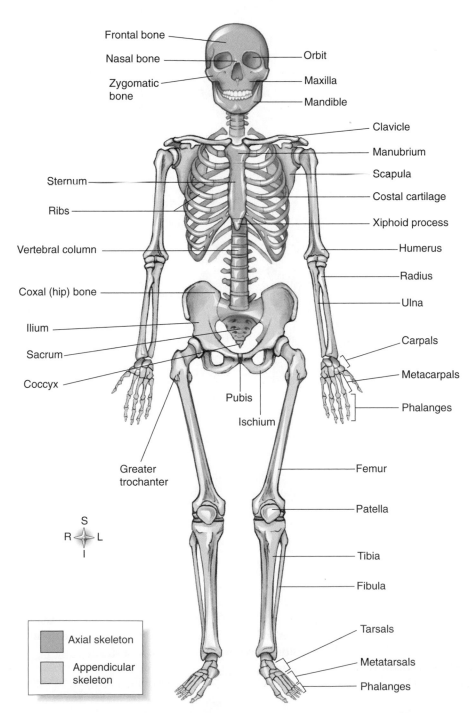

Frontal bone
Nasal bone
Zygomatic bone
Orbit
Maxilla
Mandible
Sternum
Ribs
Vertebral column
Coxal (hip) bone
Ilium
Sacrum
Coccyx
Greater trochanter
Pubis
Ischium
Clavicle
Manubrium
Scapula
Costal cartilage
Xiphoid process
Humerus
Radius
Ulna
Carpals
Metacarpals
Phalanges
Femur
Patella
Tibia
Fibula
Tarsals
Metatarsals
Phalanges

Axial skeleton
Appendicular skeleton

Figure 31-1 **Axial and appendicular skeleton.** *(From Thibodeau G, Patton K: Anatomy and physiology, ed 6, St Louis, 2007, Mosby.)*

Continued

Figure 31-1, cont'd

BONE MEMBRANES

Bones are covered with a tough bilayered membrane called *periosteum*. The function of the periosteum is to protect the bone surface and provide attachment for tendons. It also contains osteoblasts. These are the bone's growth cells; they provide a source of development and repair in the same way that tree bark functions.

NOTE: *The periosteum is an important tissue in orthopedic surgery. It must be scraped away from the bone before cutting or remodeling. This is done with a periosteal elevator.*

The *endosteum* lines the inner channels of long bones. It also fills the *interstitial spaces* (i.e., the spaces between cells) of cancellous bone, as well as the haversian canals. The endosteum initiates bone growth and provides nutritional substances to bone.

BONE STRUCTURE AND SHAPE

The long bones are characterized by a middle shaft, called the *diaphysis,* and the two ends, called the *epiphyses* (sing., epiphysis). Bones with these features include the bones of the legs, arms, and digits (i.e., the fingers and toes). The shaft is composed mostly of compact bone and has a hollow center. The transition between the diaphysis and epiphysis is not readily apparent except during development, when the region is filled with cartilage. This developmental tissue is called the *epiphyseal plate* or *metaphysis*. It is significant in fracture pathology, because a break in this area may delay growth of the bone in a child. The hollow cavity inside a mature long bone is called the *medullary canal*. The epiphyses are wider and have bony outcroppings and protrusions where the ligaments are attached. The epiphyses, which are composed of cancellous bone, form the joints, which are covered with cartilage, a resilient connective tissue that increases the strength of the joint and reduces friction between the bones.

Figure 31-3 illustrates the parts of a long bone and its membranes.

Bones can be classified by their shape. The *short* bones are those of the wrist and ankle. *Irregular* bones include the vertebrae, spine, and face. A few irregularly shaped bones occur singly; these are referred to as *sesamoid bones*. The patella is an example of a sesamoid bone.

Flat bones usually are thin compared to other types of bones. In adults, the inner cancellous layer of the flat bones

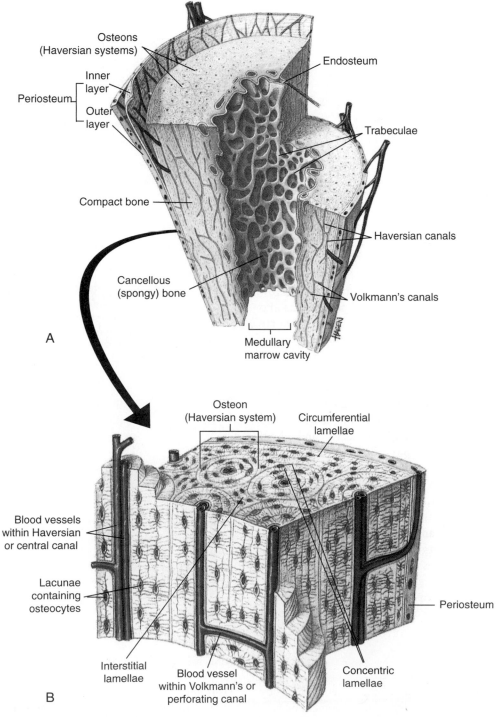

Figure 31-2 **Structure of bone tissue.** A, Longitudinal section of a long bone. B, Compact bone.

Continued

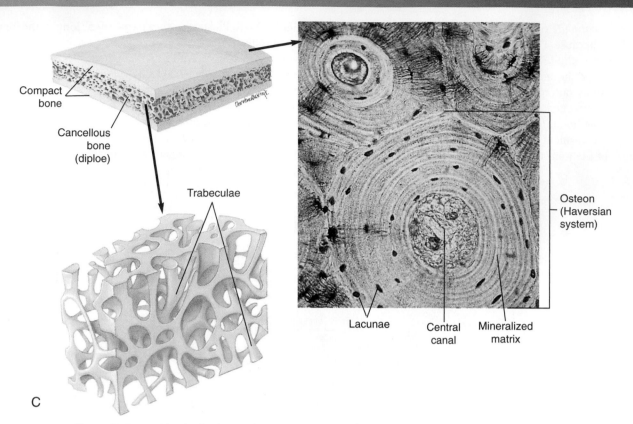

Compact bone

Cancellous bone (diploe)

Trabeculae

Osteon (Haversian system)

Lacunae

Central canal

Mineralized matrix

C

Figure 31-2, cont'd   C, Flat bone, showing compact and cancellous layers, haversian system, and trabeculae. *(From Thibodeau G, Patton K:* Anatomy and physiology, *ed 6, St Louis, 2007, Mosby.)*

contains red marrow. (In other types of bones, red marrow converts to yellow marrow during childhood and persists into adulthood.) The ribs, cranial bones, scapula, and sternum are examples of flat bones.

LANDMARKS

Bones have many different irregularities, called *landmarks*. These function as areas of attachment for tendons and ligaments or provide a passageway for nerves and blood vessels. They appear as raised projections, bumps, ridges, channels, and tunnels. Some common types of landmarks are listed in Box 31-1. The body has many hundreds of bone landmarks. Differentiating the different types of landmarks is less important than recognizing them as identifiers of significant or common anatomical sites. Specific landmarks are referred to in surgical procedures to clarify the technique. For example, "an osteotomy was performed in the femoral neck." This means that the neck of the femur was incised, or cut. Another example of an important landmark is the *iliac crest*, which is a common site for harvesting a bone graft.

JOINTS

The articular system (joints) includes the areas of the body where two bones meet and some degree of movement occurs. The movement may be small, as in the ossicles of the ear, or large, as in the hip joint.

Box **31-1**	**Common Landmarks of Bone**
Condyle	A knuckle-shaped portion of bone generally found in association with a joint.
Crest	A ridge of bone (e.g., iliac crest).
Foramen	A rounded orifice in a bone (e.g., olfactory foramen); usually a passageway for blood vessels or nerves.
Fossa	A depression in a bone (e.g., iliac fossa).
Neck	A narrow bridge of bone between two other structures (e.g., neck of the femur, neck of the humerus).
Process	A projection of bone (e.g., coracoid process).
Sinus	A cavity within a bone (e.g., nasal sinus).
Spine	A sharp, narrow projection (e.g., spinous process).
Sulcus	A groove in a bone.
Tubercle	A small rounded projection (e.g., deltoid tubercle).
Tuberosity	A large rounded projection (e.g., ischial tuberosity).

Classification

Joints are classified according to the degree of movement they allow and also by the shape of the articulating surfaces (Figure 31-4). Joint classifications are as follows:

- *Synarthrosis (suture joint):* A joint with limited movement or fixed articular surfaces, such as between the skull bones.

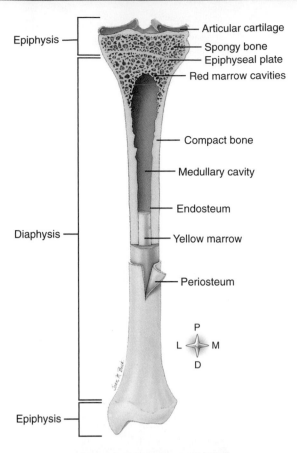

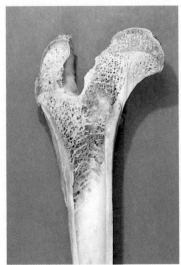

Figure 31-3 **Parts of a long bone.** *(From Thibodeau G, Patton K: Anatomy and physiology, ed 6, St Louis, 2007, Mosby.)*

- *Amphiarthrosis (cartilaginous joint):* A joint in which the bones are connected by cartilage and only slightly moveable. The symphysis joints are included in this category (e.g., symphysis pubis).
- *Diarthrosis (synovial joint):* A joint that is freely moveable, such as the hip or the shoulder. Most joints of the body are diarthroses. They are also called *synovial joints* because the joint capsule contains a fluid called *synovial fluid.* The synovial joint is the most important type for the study of surgical technology.

SYNOVIAL JOINTS A synovial joint is composed of articulating bone ends and the connective tissues that surround them (Figure 31-5). The joint capsule surrounds the joint and contains nerves and blood vessels. The capsule is lined with a synovial membrane, which produces a viscous fluid that lubricates and nourishes the joint. The synovial fluid flows out of the joint capsule when it is injured or incised. The articular surfaces of the bones in the joint are covered with cartilage, which aids smooth gliding of one bone surface over the other. The space inside the joint capsule is called the *joint cavity.* During endoscopic joint surgery *(arthroscopy),* the telescope and instruments are inserted into the joint cavity through the capsule.

NONSYNOVIAL JOINTS Nonsynovial joints are separated by immoveable cartilaginous or fibrous tissue. These joints are said to have a *fixed* articulation, and there is no joint cavity. Nonsynovial joints include the *sutures, synchondroses, symphyses,* and *syndesmoses.*

Joint Movement

The flexibility of the joints is the basis of body movement. When a joint becomes diseased or is injured, movement becomes difficult or impossible because of mechanical restrictions or pain.

Joint movement is carefully described in medicine. In surgery, movement terminology often is used during assessment of a joint. Terms are also used to direct patient positioning. In both cases, the surgeon may ask other team members to move a limb in a certain direction or in a spatial orientation. For example, the surgeon may request "more internal rotation" or "increased abduction." Specific terminology is used because less precise terms may cause confusion, resulting in injury to the patient.

Anatomically, a joint moves within its normal range of motion. Each moveable joint of the body is classified according to specific anatomical movements (Figure 31-6). These are described in mechanical terms. The important point is that joints must be manipulated *only within their normal range of motion* to prevent injury. (Chapter 19 reviews terms and presents illustrations related to joint movement.) The types of moveable joints are as follows:

- *Hinge joint:* A joint that has rocker and cradle components, which allow extension and flexion only (e.g., the elbow).
- *Saddle joint:* A joint in which the two components have a complementary convex-concave shape, and the bones slide over each other. The body has only one saddle joint, which is in the thumb. This joint allows flexion, extension, *abduction,* and *adduction.*
- *Gliding joint:* A joint in which relatively flat surfaces of bone slide over each other (e.g., the vertebrae, movement of which allows the spine to flex).
- *Ball-and-socket joint:* A joint with a spherical component and a concave component. Movement occurs in several planes, making this joint the most freely

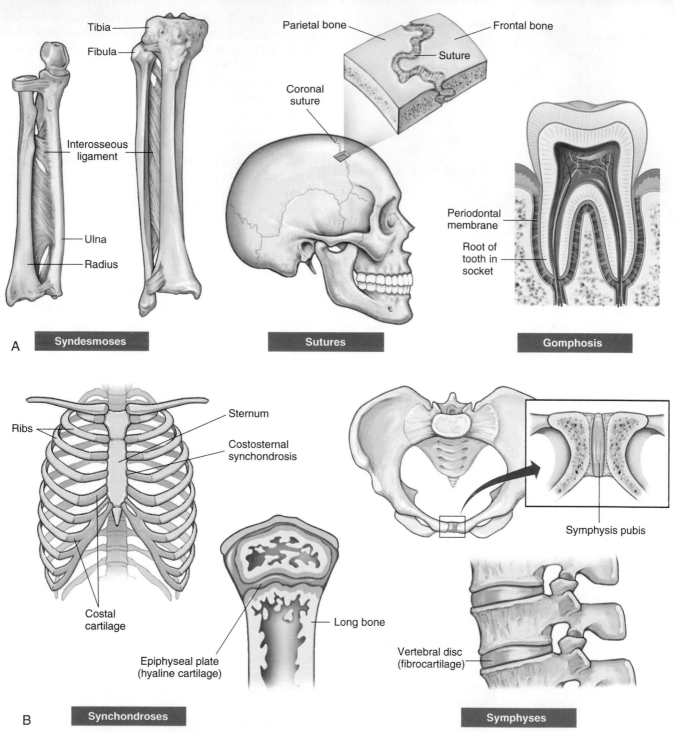

Figure 31-4 Classification of joints. A, Fibrous joints. **B,** Cartilaginous joints. *(From Thibodeau G, Patton K:* Anatomy and physiology, *ed 6, St Louis, 2007, Mosby.)*

moveable type (e.g., the hip and the humerus). Ball-and-socket joints allow flexion, extension, abduction, adduction, rotation, and circumduction.

- *Pivot joint:* A joint composed of a bony protuberance and an open collar component (e.g., the first and second vertebrae of the neck). This type of joint allows rotation.
- *Condyloid joint:* A joint in which a small protrusion (condyle) slides within a slightly elliptical component (e.g., the carpal bones of the wrist). Condyloid joints allow flexion, extension, abduction, and adduction.

SOFT CONNECTIVE TISSUES

Tendons and Ligaments

Muscles and bones are attached by tendons and ligaments:
- Tendons attach muscle to bone.
- Ligaments attach bone to bone.

The fibers of tendons and ligaments can withstand very high levels of stress and tension along the fiber axis. Tendons move within a protective sheath filled with a type of synovial fluid. Their movement to move the muscles often resembles a pulley system. Tendons can take the form of a fibrous cord or

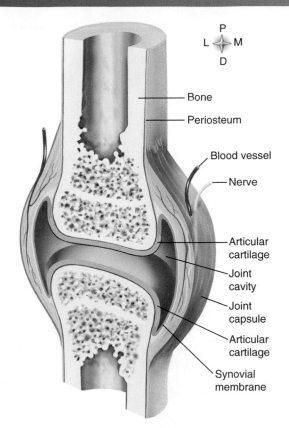

Figure 31-5 **Synovial joint structure.** *(From Vidic B, Suarez FR: Photographic atlas of the human body, St Louis, 1984, Mosby.)*

a sheet of connective tissue called an **aponeurosis**. Ligaments attach bones to each other, providing flexibility and strength to the skeletal structure. When attached to the cartilage, they stabilize the joint and limit movements that might injure it. Neither tendons nor ligaments have a significant blood supply.

Muscle

The three major muscle types in the human body are striated muscle, smooth muscle, and cardiac muscle.

STRIATED MUSCLE *Striated muscle,* also commonly called *skeletal muscle,* is composed of fibers that are bound together by sheaths of fascia. Each group of fibers and its associated sheath are bound together to form one muscle. Striated muscle is under voluntary control and makes up most of the body's muscle tissue (Figure 31-7). The primary functions of muscle are to provide skeletal movement, support the body's posture, and to maintain body heat through anaerobic metabolism. Muscle groups are attached to bone by tendons at two fixed points in order to allow skeletal movement. These points are called the origin and insertion of the muscle. When a muscle contracts, it moves the bone in a specific directions which are determined by the type of joint.

SMOOTH MUSCLE Smooth muscle is also called *involuntary muscle* because it is not under conscious control. These muscles are found principally in the internal organs, especially the digestive tract, respiratory passages, urinary and genital ducts,

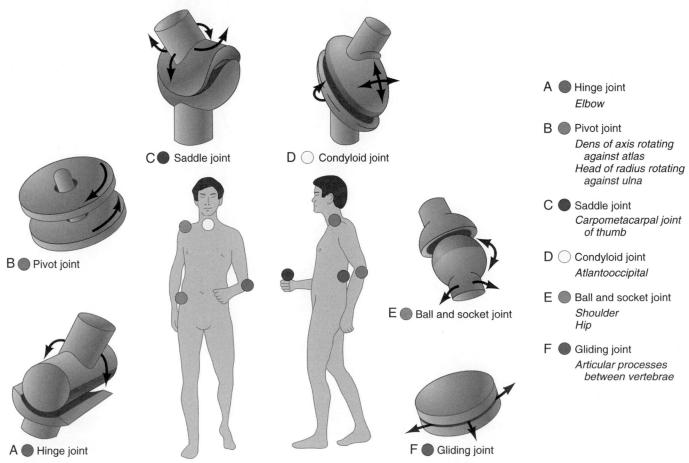

Figure 31-6 **Types of moveable joints.** *(From Thibodeau G, Patton K: Anatomy and physiology, ed 6, St Louis, 2007, Mosby.)*

urinary bladder, and gallbladder, and in the walls of blood vessels. In structures such as the bladder and intestine, smooth muscle has two layers, an outer longitudinal layer and an inner circular layer. When the smooth muscles such as those in the intestine contract and relax, the contents are moved along the length of the intestine. This is referred to as *peristalsis*. Peristalsis occurs in many other tubular structures of the body such as the esophagus, ureters, and fallopian tubes, which also contain smooth muscle.

CARDIAC MUSCLE As the name implies, cardiac muscle is the muscle of the heart. Like voluntary muscle, cardiac muscle is striated, but these muscles are involuntary. Cardiac muscle is responsible for the sustained contractions of the heart and for movement of blood into and out of the heart. This mechanism, as well as the rate of contraction, is driven by a complex series of impulses from the autonomic nervous system.

DIAGNOSTIC PROCEDURES

A variety of imaging procedures are used to diagnose orthopedic trauma and disease, including the following:

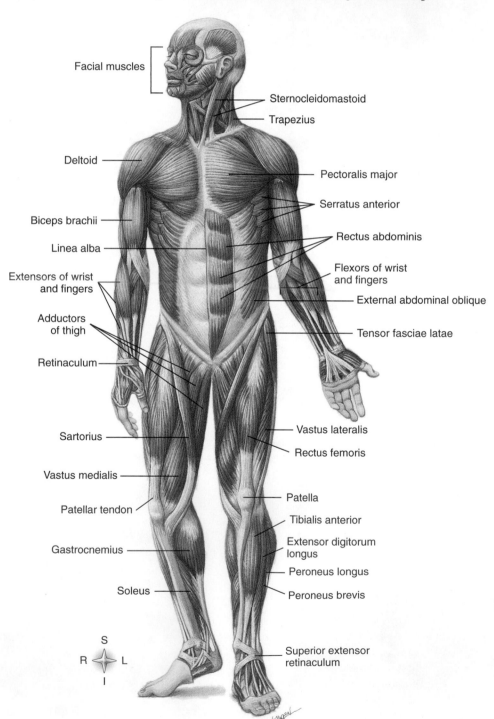

Figure 31-7   Striated muscles of the body. *(From Thibodeau G, Patton K: Anthony's textbook of anatomy and physiology, ed 17, St Louis, 2003, Mosby.)*

Facial muscles
Sternocleidomastoid
Trapezius
Deltoid
Pectoralis major
Serratus anterior
Biceps brachii
Rectus abdominis
Linea alba
Flexors of wrist and fingers
Extensors of wrist and fingers
External abdominal oblique
Adductors of thigh
Tensor fasciae latae
Retinaculum
Sartorius
Vastus lateralis
Rectus femoris
Vastus medialis
Patella
Patellar tendon
Tibialis anterior
Extensor digitorum longus
Gastrocnemius
Peroneus longus
Soleus
Peroneus brevis
Superior extensor retinaculum

S
R ◆ L
I

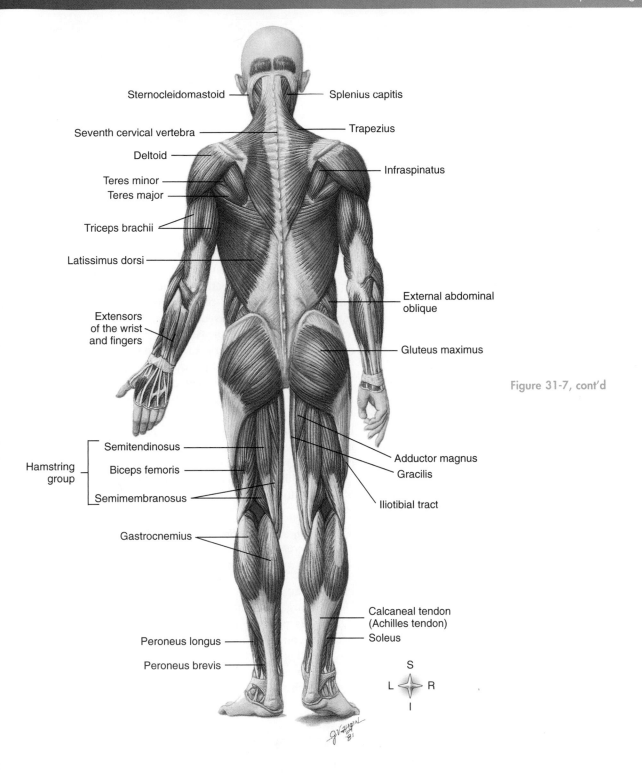

Sternocleidomastoid

Splenius capitis

Seventh cervical vertebra

Trapezius

Deltoid

Teres minor

Teres major

Infraspinatus

Triceps brachii

Latissimus dorsi

External abdominal oblique

Extensors of the wrist and fingers

Gluteus maximus

Semitendinosus

Adductor magnus

Hamstring group

Biceps femoris

Gracilis

Semimembranosus

Iliotibial tract

Gastrocnemius

Calcaneal tendon (Achilles tendon)

Peroneus longus

Soleus

Peroneus brevis

S
L — R
I

Figure 31-7, cont'd

- *Radiography:* Radiographs are the first-level assessment in most cases of orthopedic trauma.
- *Magnetic resonance imaging (MRI):* MRI scans generally are not used for routine diagnosis of fractures, but they commonly are performed for spinal cord injuries and for tumors of the musculoskeletal system.
- *Computed tomography (CT):* CT scans are used for complex fractures, joint disease, and trauma. The scans produce cross-sectional images that are valuable in the diagnosis of tumors and internal injury caused by trauma.

- *CT-angiography:* In orthopedics, angiograms are used to diagnose vascular injury caused by trauma.
- *Ultrasonography:* Ultrasound scans routinely are done in cases involving complex traumatic injuries.

SPECIAL STUDIES

Selected trauma cases require assessment for soft tissue damage associated with injury and disease. Refer to Chapter 37 for a discussion of trauma injury.

CASE PLANNING

PATIENT TRANSPORT AND TRANSFER

Patients undergoing an orthopedic procedure arrive for surgery either shortly after a traumatic injury or as "well" patients who are having reconstructive or joint replacement surgery. Trauma patients and those with a chronic skeletal injury require special handling during transport and transfer to the operating table.

Trauma patients may arrive in traction (explained later) or external splinting device. The transfer may be completed after administration of an anesthetic to reduce the patient's discomfort. It is important to maintain anatomical alignment of the body at all times during the transfer. This may require extra personnel to complete the transfer safely. Traction equipment must be monitored carefully to ensure that weights and pulleys are not dislodged. Teamwork is essential in transferring a trauma patient.

POSITIONING

Patients are positioned for orthopedic surgery on the standard operating table or on a specialty table. (Chapter 19 presents a complete description of important safety precautions for preventing patient injury during positioning.)

The modern orthopedic table (also called a *fracture table*) is used mainly for surgery of the femur and lower leg. This table supports the operative leg while providing open access to the femur. The open design of the table also allows safe and rapid positioning of the C-arm fluoroscope. Features of the orthopedic table include:

- Jointed (articulated) components to hold the leg in traction
- Open design of the lower portion to allow positioning of the C-arm
- Translucent support surfaces

Many standard operating tables can be converted to allow femoral or lower extremity surgery by removing the foot section and replacing it with adjustable leg suspension devices. The Fowler position can be created for shoulder surgery by adjusting the articulated sections of the table and replacing the normal headboard with an open-design head stabilizer. It is important to allow adequate time to make these modifications before the patient arrives in surgery. Table accessories can be quite heavy; therefore, adequate personnel should be available for assembly.

Positions associated with a specific surgical exposure are described in Table 31-1 and shown in Figures 31-8 through 31-12.

HEMOSTASIS

Bone tissue bleeds briskly when cut; the bleeding arises from capillaries that cannot be ligated. Hip arthroplasty and open reduction of a hip fracture have been associated with a high risk of significant blood loss. However, refined instrumentation and improved surgical techniques have reduced this risk.

Total blood loss is determined by weighing surgical sponges and measuring the volume of blood in the suction canister (and by subtracting the amount of irrigation fluid used at the operative site). Emergency trauma patients are evaluated before surgery, and blood products are administered as needed.

Pneumatic Tourniquet

The pneumatic tourniquet is used in most extremity procedures. The components of the tourniquet are the cuff, the regulator, and the tubing. An appropriately sized cuff must be selected according to the patient's size. The tourniquet cuff is placed proximal to the surgical site before the patient is prepped. Webril bandaging material is wrapped over the tourniquet site carefully to reduce any folds or pinching in the skin. The cuff then is secured over the bandaging. The regulator is adjusted for the patient's blood pressure but not activated. After the surgical prep and draping, a latex bandage (Esmarch bandage) is used to exsanguinate the limb. The bandage is applied in a proximal direction, causing blood to flow out of the limb. The tourniquet then is inflated, providing a nearly bloodless surgical field.

Pneumatic tourniquets have been associated with skin, nerve, and vessel damage and embolus when used improperly. Numerous safety protocols guide their application and use. Before and after application, the skin must be assessed for injury or potential damage. Tourniquet times depend on the patient's overall medical condition and tissue status. (Chapter 22 presents illustrations and a more detailed discussion of the pneumatic tourniquet.)

> A website covering all clinical aspects of tourniquet use, including current guidelines from the Association of periOperative Registered Nurses (AORN), can be found at http://www.tourniquets.org/aorn.html.

Hemostatic Agents

During surgery, a moldable preparation called *bone putty* (Ostene) is pressed into bleeding areas to control oozing. Beeswax combinations (bone wax) traditionally have been used for this purpose, but these have been largely replaced with more effective and safer materials. Other hemostatic agents, such as topical thrombin, are used in peripheral tissues during microsurgery of the hand.

INFECTION CONTROL

Orthopedic surgery is performed with particular attention to the risk of airborne contaminants and droplet contamination. Postoperative infection after joint replacement (arthroplasty) can result in destruction of the joint, with no recourse for further treatment. Osteomyelitis after any orthopedic surgery can result in long-term disability.

Orthopedic procedures are commonly performed in operating suites with laminar airflow or "superclean" air capability. In laminar airflow, air moves in linear patterns, entering at one wall and exiting at another. Superclean air is created with fresh air exchanges that occur at a rate of more than 300 changes per minute. Laminar airflow and systems used to create

Table 31-1	Positions for Surgical Exposure in Orthopedic Surgery	
Anatomical Area	**Position**	**Special Features***
Shoulder and humerus	Beach chair (modified Fowler position)	Head is stabilized with a Mayfield headrest or similar attachment.
		Upper body is flexed 45 to 60 degrees.
		Operative shoulder is slightly over the table edge.
		Nonoperative shoulder is padded at the scapula.
		Vertical foot board may be required.
Forearm and elbow	Supine with hand table extension	Operative arm is extended on a hand table at no greater than 90 degrees of abduction.
	Supine or semilateral using "over chest" extension	Operative arm is abducted and elevated over the thorax with the elbow flexed.
		Stabilizers are used to maintain the semilateral position (table supports, foam wedges).
Wrist and hand	Supine with hand table extension	Operative arm is extended on a hand table at no greater than 90 degrees of abduction.
		Pad or "bump" is placed under the wrist for stabilization.
	Supine with hand suspended in sterile distractor	Separate sterile accessories are required for the distractor.
Pelvis	Supine	Precautions are taken to protect nerves and blood vessels.
	Prone	Lower extremities may be held in traction.
		Precautions are taken for respiratory clearance.
		Lower table section may be removed.
Hip and femur	Supine using standard operating table	No special accessories are required.
	Supine using fracture table	Operative leg is in traction or distraction.
		Nonoperative leg rests on a perpendicular crutch or is extended in a boot accessory.
		Perineal stop (post) requires substantial padding.
		Allows complete clearance above and below lower extremities.
	Lateral	Stabilizers are used to maintain the lateral position (table supports or padded wedges).
Knee and lower leg	Supine	Operative knee is supported in variable flexed position with foot or knee crutch support.
		Operative leg may be suspended over the table edge for intraoperative manipulation.
Ankle and foot	Supine	Supine or prone position is used with the operative leg in free position or elevated on padding.

*Normal precautions to protect nerves, vessels, and respiratory clearance are observed for all positions.

superclean air significantly reduce the number of airborne organisms.

Other methods of reducing airborne contaminants include ultraviolet light and the use of vented operating attire, or "space suits," which consist of a vented head bubble and body suit.

DRESSINGS

Surgical dressings are used to protect the incision from contamination and injury. The orthopedic dressing frequently provides support as well as protection. Casting is one example of external support. However, many other types of soft or semirigid support systems are used on the limbs. Orthopedic appliances such as combined Velcro and hard plastic splints, foot boots, and other postoperative support systems are usually fitted to the patient by a trained physiotherapist shortly after the operative procedure. However, the surgical *dressing* is applied in the operating room at the close of surgery. The surgical technologist becomes familiar with dressing combinations used at her or his facility. Some of the most common materials are:

- *Gauze "fluffs,"* which are made with Kerlix or plain gauze squares that are pulled apart from the center to make them fluffy rather than flat. These are used to provide cushioning in small areas such as between the fingers or toes.

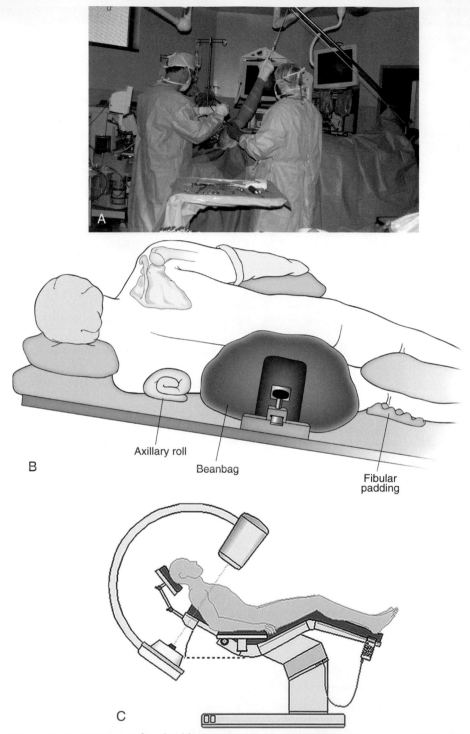

Figure 31-8 **Positioning for shoulder surgery.** **A,** Supine position with the arm suspended in an overhead distractor to allow manipulation. **B,** Lateral position using an arm board for a posterior approach to the shoulder. **C,** Semi-Fowler (beach chair) position with the C-arm in place. (*A from Canale S, Beaty J: Campbell's operative orthopaedics, ed 11, St Louis, 2007, Mosby; **B** from Miller MD, Chhabra AB, Hurwitz SK, Mihalko WM: Orthopaedic surgical approaches, St Louis, 2008, WB Saunders.*)

- *Thick cotton wrap* is used to provide support to a limb.
- *Ace type stretchable fabric bandages* are used to wrap a limb, usually on top of cotton wrap to provide extra support and some compression.
- A *Coban-type dressing* is a common roller bandage with superior stretching and self-sticking capability. This type of

material does not offer as much support as the Ace type of fabric bandage but conforms more easily to the shape of the limb.

- *Stockinet* is commonly used under splits and casts. It is a stretchable tube-shaped fabric that is fitted over the limb and folded over at the top to form a smooth padded edge.

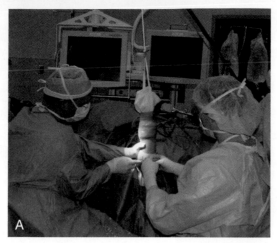

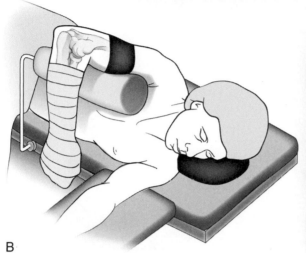

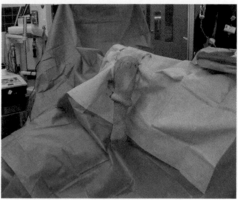

Figure 31-9 **A,** Positioning for elbow surgery using an overhead distractor. The arm can also be left in a free position. **B,** Lateral position using an arm holder for arthroscopy. (**A** from Canale S, Beaty J: Campbell's operative orthopaedics, ed 11, St Louis, 2007, Mosby; **B** from Miller MD, Chhabra AB, Hurwitz SK, Mihalko WM: Orthopaedic surgical approaches, St Louis, 2008, WB Saunders.)

FRACTURE PATHOLOGY

Fractures occur as a result of trauma or disease and represent the majority of pathology requiring orthopedic surgery. Traumatic bone injury may be complicated by soft tissue injury, with critical damage to nerves and blood vessels. Except in cases of pathological fracture, fractures are the result of forceful blunt or sharp impact on bone. Motor vehicle accidents, passenger versus vehicle, sports injuries, and interpersonal violence are the primary causes of fractures. Cases therefore often present as emergencies.

CLASSIFICATION OF FRACTURES

Fractures are medically classified for reporting and treatment purposes. Several classification systems are used. Classification is important to the surgical technologist, because it provides information needed for preparation of the appropriate instrumentation, for positioning, and for the surgical approach. Systems of classification vary by the type of criteria they use:

- *Name of the bone and location:* The distinguishing features are the name of the bone (e.g., tibia, femur, third phalanx)

and the anatomical area (distal or proximal). For example, a fracture might be located in the distal tibia or the proximal humerus.
- *Pattern of fracture:* Fractures may be described by the pattern of the break (explained later). This helps identify the forces involved and the methods required for repair.
- *Level of comminution:* This is the extent of fragmentation. For example, a severely **comminuted** fracture is one that has many fragments. Mild comminution describes a fracture with few fragments. A highly comminuted fracture requires a longer surgical time and complex instrumentation.
- *Displacement:* This factor describes whether the bone fragments are in anatomical alignment. A nondisplaced fracture is one in which the bone fragments are in alignment.
- *Pathological origin:* A pathological fracture can occur with normal load. It is caused by any disease that weakens the structure and composition of bone.

FRACTURE PATTERNS

Fracture patterns can be associated with the impact and environment that caused them (Figure 31-13). Common fracture patterns include the following:

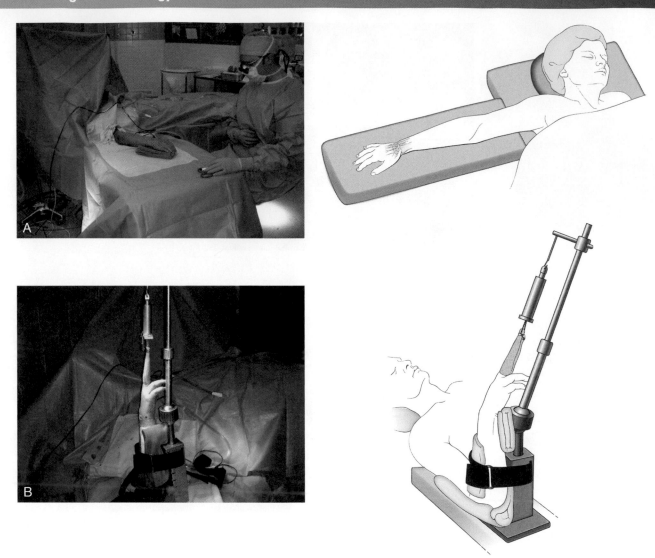

Figure 31-10 **Positioning for hand surgery. A,** The patient is in the supine position with the hand in the prone or supine position. **B,** The hand is stabilized with a sterile distractor. *(From Miller MD, Chhabra AB, Hurwitz SK, Mihalko WM: Orthopaedic surgical approaches, St Louis, 2008, WB Saunders.)*

- *Transverse:* The fracture line is perpendicular to the long axis of the bone.
- *Oblique:* A type of transverse fracture that occurs at an angle.
- *Spiral:* A fracture of the long bone that occurs in a spiral pattern as the result of twisting or torsion on the bone.
- *Impacted:* A fracture in which bone fragments are driven into each other or into another bone.
- *Comminuted:* A fracture with two or more pieces.
- *Open:* A fracture in which the fractured end penetrates the skin.
- *Greenstick:* A fracture of immature bone that is soft and less brittle than mature bone. The fracture is incomplete or the impact results in severe bending and bruising.
- *Depressed:* Refers to cranial fracture in which the fragments are displaced inwardly.

BIOMECHANICAL FORCES ON BONE

Different types of stress or impact and the type of bone determine the pattern of a fracture (Figure 31-14). The following terms are used in biomechanics. They are relevant to fractures and also to methods of repairing bone.

- *Torque or torsion (twisting force):* Torque is the type of force applied to a screwdriver to implant a screw. Torsion injury results when tissue is twisted on itself.
- *Shear force (bending):* The force of an object acting perpendicular or at an angle to another surface. Shear force can apply to any surface or structure acting on tissues, such as skin. For example, shear injuries occur when a patient is dragged across a bed sheet (rather than being rolled or lifted). The friction of the sheet can cause tissue injury that

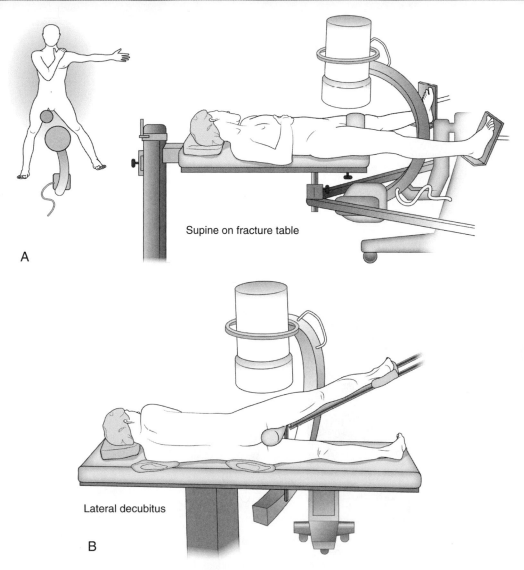

Figure 31-11 **A,** Orthopedic table used for procedures of the hip and femur. The open configuration use allows positioning of the C-arm fluoroscope. The hips may be distracted by adjusting the leg extensions. **B,** Patient in the lateral position. *(From Miller MD, Chhabra AB, Hurwitz SK, Mihalko WM: Orthopaedic surgical approaches,* St Louis, 2008, WB Saunders.)

may not be immediately visible, because the injury can occur in the deeper tissues.

- *Axial or* **compression** *force:* This force or load occurs parallel to the long bone. For example, the weight of the upper body exerts axial force on the long bones of the legs. A compression force may result in the compaction of one bone into another.

FRACTURE REPAIR

Common surgical goals for all types of fractures are:
1. Alignment of the bones (reduction)
2. Stabilization of the bone until healing is complete (fixation)

Reduction

Reduction is the process of bringing the bone fragments into anatomical alignment. Mechanical or manual reduction of the bone fragments is performed with the patient under anesthesia. Reduction is a physical (kinetic) process and may require the mechanical advantage of a traction device that pulls the injured bones into alignment. After injury, severe tissue swelling can make reduction more difficult, requiring mechanical aids. If the fracture is minor, manual reduction may be adequate. The two types of reduction are open and closed:

- **Open reduction** takes place through an incision as part of the surgery.
- **Closed reduction** is performed by manipulation of the bone or with an external traction device that pulls the bone fragments into position. No incision is made in the skin.

The patient may arrive in surgery with a traction device in place, or reduction may be performed internally as part of the surgery. **Distraction** and traction are not quite the same. A *distractor* is used to elongate a limb or structure during surgery. This is done to aid positioning or to increase the "compartment" space that the bones occupy in the tissue.

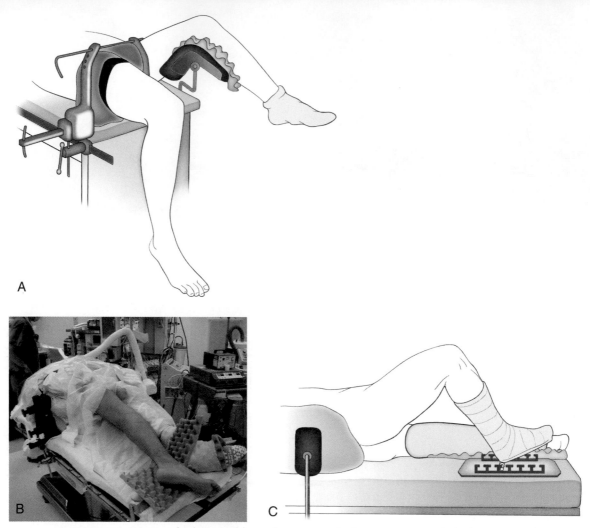

Figure 31-12   **Positions for knee and lower leg surgery. A,** Supine position with the leg positioned in a knee crutch suitable for arthroscopy. **B,** The leg may be draped in a free position resting on the operating table for ease of manipulation during the procedure. **C,** Posterolateral position using a foot stabilizer. *(From Miller MD, Chabra AB, Hurwitz SK, Mihalko WM: Orthopedic surgical approaches, St Louis, 2008, WB Saunders.)*

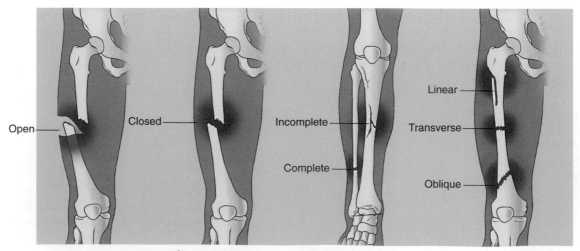

Figure 31-13   Common fracture patterns. *(From Thibodeau G, Patton K: Anthony's textbook of anatomy and physiology, ed 17, St Louis, 2003, Mosby.)*

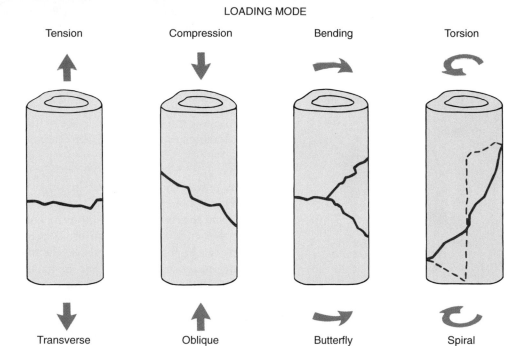

LOADING MODE

Tension   Compression   Bending   Torsion

Transverse   Oblique   Butterfly   Spiral

FRACTURE TYPE

Figure 31-14 **Fracture loading.** *(From Browner B, Jupiter J, Levine A, Trafton P: Skeletal trauma: basic science, management, and reconstruction, ed 3, Philadelphia, 2003, WB Saunders.)*

Fixation

Fixation is the mechanical or structural method used to hold bone fragments in anatomical position during healing. Much of orthopedic surgery focuses on various methods of fixation. The two main types of fixation are:

- **Internal fixation,** which requires surgery to insert or implant a device that holds the bone fragments in place. Metal plates, rods, pins, and screws are examples of internal fixation devices.
- **External fixation,** a means of stabilizing bone fragments in anatomical position from outside the body. A cast is an example of an external fixation device. Other devices, including external frames and cages, are also used. Pins or wires may be inserted through the skin and into the bone to support the external fixation device.

Orthopedic procedures are specifically described according to the type of reduction and repair. The surgical options are:

- *Open reduction and internal fixation:* This procedure involves open surgery to expose the bone and reduce the fracture (i.e., replace the bones in anatomical position). Internal orthopedic implants are used to achieve fixation.
- *Open reduction and external fixation:* In this procedure, reduction requires an incision to align the bones. However, an external device (e.g., a frame or cast) is used to stabilize and hold the bone fragments during healing.
- *Closed reduction and external fixation:* The fracture is reduced manually or with a traction device. Except for casting and other types of noninvasive splinting, an external fixation device requires the insertion of wires,

pins, or other devices to support the external structure. Some devices can be inserted transcutaneously. A very small incision is made in the skin, and the pin or wire is drilled into the deeper tissue and bone.

THE PHYSIOLOGY OF BONE HEALING

Bone healing takes place through a complex physiological process that resembles soft tissue repair. However, the process is slower. Return of full function may take 6 months or longer, especially in weight-bearing bones. The three phases of bone healing are the inflammatory phase, the reparative phase, and the remodeling phase.

Inflammatory Phase

When bone suffers a traumatic injury, blood arising from the bone itself and from the adjacent soft tissue accumulates at the fracture site. The body's clotting mechanism is triggered and fibrin is released to form the basis of platelet aggregation and hematoma (congealed blood), which eventually is absorbed by the body. Fibroblasts in the region of the injury create a network of granulation tissue, which is a soft, spongy matrix of connective tissue and blood vessels.

Reparative Phase

During the reparative phase, growth cells originating from the periosteum develop into rudimentary bone cells and cartilage. These proliferate and form a callus, which fills in the space between the bone fragments. This normally occurs within a few days of injury. Ossification occurs as the soft callus is replaced by bone minerals and bone cells. During this phase, a capillary vascular system develops within the matrix.

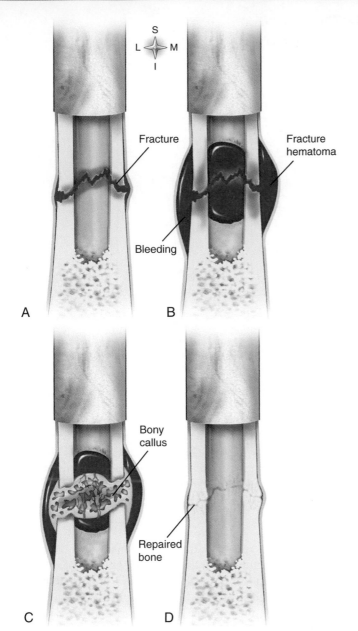

Figure 31-15 **Process of bone healing. A,** Fracture site. **B,** Formation of a hematoma. **C,** Reparative phase with formation of callus. **D,** Remodeling phase. *(From Thibodeau G, Patton K: Anatomy and physiology, ed 6, St Louis, 2007, Mosby.)*

Remodeling

The remodeling stage is characterized by replacement of the initial bone matrix with compact bone cells and absorption of excess callus. This takes place over a period of weeks or months. The process of bone healing is illustrated in Figure 31-15.

ORTHOPEDIC TECHNOLOGY AND INSTRUMENTATION

POWER EQUIPMENT

Power equipment is used in orthopedic surgery to cut, drill, and remodel bone. The surgical technologist should be famil-

iar with the safety and mechanical features of power equipment. The most important points are:

- Safety features of the equipment and power source
- How to connect the power equipment to the power source
- Types of accessories and their function
- How to attach accessories
- Assisting the surgeon during use of the equipment
- Cleaning and reprocessing the equipment

Safety

Most power equipment used in surgery uses compressed nitrogen (pneumatic energy). The force exerted through the hose and instrument is very powerful and can cause serious injury. A complete discussion of gas cylinder and regulator safety can be found in Chapter 8. The following are general safety precautions for use of pneumatic instruments:

1. Inspect the instrument and hose before use. Make sure the instrument is properly assembled.
2. Place the instrument in the safe position (i.e., with the safety catch "on") before attaching accessories or the power hose.
3. Make sure that accessories are attached correctly, using guards where applicable. A drill or saw attachment that is incorrectly seated can be propelled from the handpiece with extreme force and may cause serious injury.
4. Inspect accessories before attaching them. Never attach a bent drill tip or other accessory, because it can wobble and become disengaged from the handpiece. Never use a cracked or chipped cutting accessory.
5. Put the safety catch "on" before passing it to the surgeon.
6. Test the pressure before using the instrument. Make sure the pressure does not exceed the approved level.
7. Always "bleed" the air hose before detaching the handpiece. With the nitrogen tank valve turned off, activate the instrument to remove any remaining gas from the hose.
8. Follow the manufacturer's guidelines for decontamination and sterilization.
9. Power instruments generate heat as a result of friction between the tissue and tip. The temperature can be high enough to destroy tissue in the vicinity of the tip. To prevent tissue injury, make sure to irrigate the tip while the instrument is in use. Irrigation solution is always used with power drills and saws.

Drill

An orthopedic drill is similar to a carpenter's drill. The drill has two main components, the head and the handle. Attachments for the drill are inserted at the drill head. Many different kinds of attachments are available. The surgical technologist must be familiar with the specific functions and handling of surgical drills (Figure 31-16). Drills are used whenever torque is required (torque is rotational energy).

DRILL ATTACHMENTS AND ACCESSORY TOOLS The following are the most commonly used drill attachments and accessories:

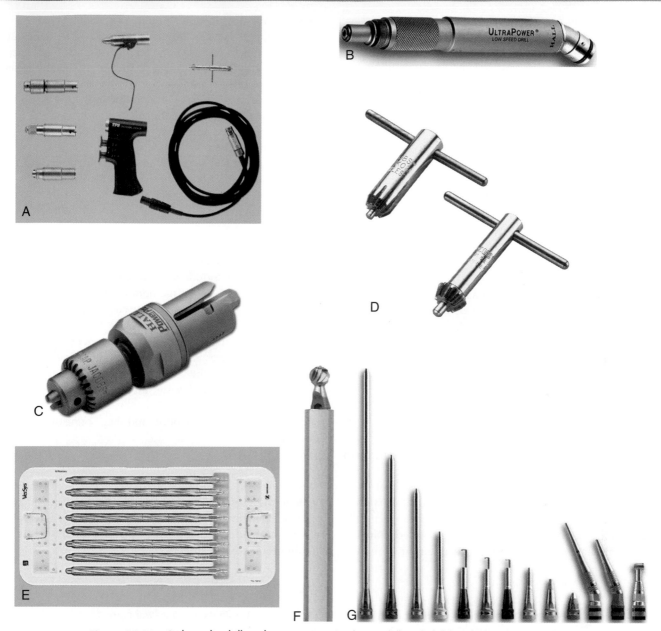

Figure 31-16 **Orthopedic drill and accessories. A,** Electric drill and drill heads. **B,** Pneumatic low-speed drill. **C,** Jacob chuck. **D,** Jacob chuck keys. **E,** Reamers used for canalization of the long bones. **F,** Diamond burr. **G,** Drill tips. *(A and E from Tighe SM: Instrumentation for the operating room, ed 6, St Louis, 2003, Mosby; D, F, and G courtesy Zimmer, Warsaw, Ind.)*

- *Burr:* A round, conical, or tapered tip used for making narrow holes or for smoothing very small areas. Burrs are made from stainless steel, titanium, or diamond.
- *Chuck:* The chuck is attached to the drill head and receives attachments such as reamers, burrs, drill bits, or other rotational cutting tips, which fit into the central hole of the chuck. A chuck key is used to open and close the chuck's jaws, which are shaped like a cloverleaf. Most types of chucks are tightened and loosened manually.
- *Depth gauge:* A small calibrated rod used to measure the depth of a drilled or reamed hole in bone.
- *Drill bit:* A pin with wide cutting threads that is used to make a smooth-sided hole in the bone. Flutes (phalanges) in the drill bit allow cut bone to escape from the thread

channels. Drill bits are supplied singly or in standard sizes in a metal rack.
- *Drill guide (drill sleeve):* An instrument inserted near or at the screw hole to correctly aim the angle of a screw, pin, nail, or wire as it enters the bone. The drill guide may be a single instrument or part of an assembly. Although many designs are available, the function is the same for all types.
- *Reamer:* A rod-shaped or chisel-pointed cutter used to **ream,** or clear, the medullary canal. A rounded or cup-shaped reamer is used for dishing surfaces such as the acetabulum. Reaming is used to prepare the bone for an implant. A reamer may be attached to a power drill or used manually.

- *Shaver:* A type of burr used mainly on cartilage for shaping and removing tissue such as the meniscus.
- *Tap:* An instrument similar to a screw that is used to cut threads in the bone. The tap corresponds to the diameter of the screw, its shape, and the pitch. Pretapping prevents bone from becoming embedded in threads of the screw as it is inserted. However, some screws are self-tapping.

Saws

Power saws are used to cut bone in a precise direction and angle. The saw blades generally are fine-toothed and vibrate or oscillate rapidly. This produces a smooth cut with little bone loss. Orthopedic saws are identified mainly by the movement of the blade. The name of the saw is also the category of blade that the device uses:

- *Reciprocating saw:* The blade moves "in and out" of the handpiece.
- *Sagittal saw:* The blade is fixed at a right angle (90 degrees) to the handpiece and moves along a perpendicular axis.
- *Oscillating saw:* The blade is mounted along the same axis as the handle and moves "back and forth."

Each type of blade is available in many shapes, which are identified by the length of the blade shaft, the type, and the width of the blade edge.

HAND INSTRUMENTS

Many orthopedic instruments have been designed for use with a specific system. These specialized instruments are classified by type (e.g., impactor) and system (e.g., Sirus tibial nail). Generic instruments, which are not associated with a specific system, are classified by type and sometimes more specifically by anatomical region (e.g., hip, knee). Surgical technologists should be familiar with the standard instruments used in their facility.

Retractors and Bone-Holding Clamps

Because bone does not yield to retraction the way soft tissue does, the surgeon most often retracts the surrounding tissue away from the bone or uses a bone-holding clamp or hook to grasp a bone for manipulation. Certain types of bone retractors (e.g., Blount and Bennett retractors) are designed to be used as levers against the bone, to shift its position. Soft tissue retractors are designed for a specific anatomical location, such as the shoulder, and some general surgery retractors (e.g., Army-Navy and Weitlaner retractors) are also used in orthopedic surgery. Figures 31-17 and 31-18 illustrate common bone-holding clamps and retractors.

Rongeurs and Bone Cutters

Rongeurs and bone cutters are used for trimming and modeling bone and cartilage. Double-action instruments have two hinges for increased force at the tips (from increased leverage). Cutting edges may be cupped, anvil tip, or double-bladed. Figure 31-19 shows common rongeurs and cutters. Specialty cutting instruments used in ear, nose, and throat (ENT) surgery, plastic surgery, and neurosurgery are shown in Chapters 28, 30, and 36.

Chisels, Osteotomes, Gouges, and Curettes

Chisels, gouges, and osteotomes are used with a mallet to model bone or to remove bone for a graft. Each has a specific type of cutting tip. Instruments in this group usually are supplied in graduated sizes and secured in a metal rack.

- *Chisel:* Beveled (sloped) on one side only
- *Osteotome:* Beveled on both sides
- *Gouge:* V-shaped chisel

A curette is used without a mallet. It has a cup-shaped cutting edge and is used for scooping out bone and other dense tissue. Figure 31-20 shows instruments in this category.

Elevators and Rasps

A periosteal elevator (or simply, elevator) is used in nearly every open orthopedic procedure. Although it has many uses, its main function is to remove or scrape away the periosteum (the tough outer membrane of the bone) from the bone surface. This is necessary to cut or saw through bone tissue, because the periosteum tends to shred or tear on contact with a rongeur or cutting instruments, preventing a clean cut. Many sizes and types of elevators are available. The most common are the smooth-tip joker elevator and the larger, square-tip Key elevator. Figure 31-21 shows common elevators.

A bone rasp is used to model and shape bone or to roughen the bone surface.

Measuring Devices

Measuring devices commonly used in orthopedic procedures include the protractor, caliper, screw depth gauge, and ordinary ruler (Figure 31-22). Computerized mapping has replaced some but not all of the measuring techniques previously used in joint replacement surgery.

ORTHOPEDIC IMPLANTS

Orthopedic implants or hardware are the devices used to attach or fix bone and other connective tissue (joint replacement implants are discussed separately). Many hundreds of different implants are available for orthopedic repair. However, a relatively simple classification system (i.e., implant type and use) is used for them. The manufacture and use of orthopedic hardware are regulated to protect the public. The U.S. Food and Drug Administration (FDA) requires strict documentation and tracking of implant devices. Infection related to implants is prevented by strict protocols for sterilization.

Hospitals and other health care facilities maintain an inventory or supply of sterile implants for surgical cases routinely performed in that facility. The inventory is organized in a way that protects the implants from contamination and damage while making it easy for staff members to select the correct implant for surgery. A database of all implants is maintained for regulatory purposes and restocking. A surgical technologist (team leader or orthopedic specialist) may be designated to maintain implant inventories and implement the documentation and supply system.

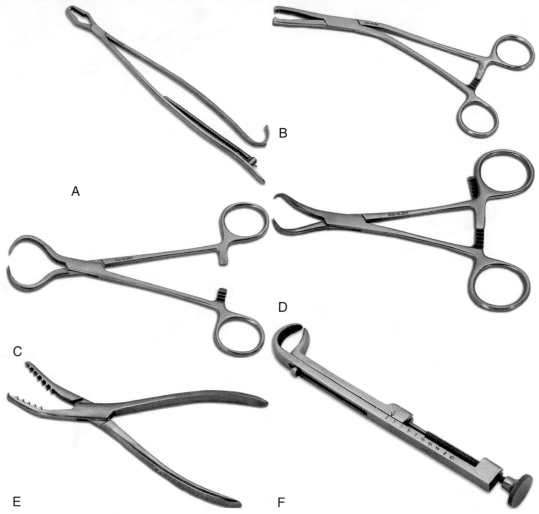

Figure 31-17 **Clamps. A,** Kern. **B,** Dingman. **C,** Lewin clamp. **D,** Bone reduction clamp. **E,** Martin cartilage clamp. **F,** Lowman. *(Courtesy Sklar Instruments, West Chester, Pa.)*

Materials

Metals are commonly used in the manufacture of implants, because metal can withstand the load required of bone. Current research is aimed at creating new metal **alloys** (made from a mixture of different metals) that are highly biocompatible and inert. Stainless steel remains the alloy most commonly used for implants.

Bioactive implants (e.g., absorbable fixation screws that release calcium) are absorbed by the body and stimulate or enhance bone repair. *Bioresistance* is another desirable quality of implant material. Particular materials that make up an implant may make it resistant to infectious agents. **Biocompatibility** means that the implant is compatible with tissue and does not cause injury. This includes a possible allergic reaction or other immune response. A material that is *inert* does not react with other nonorganic or biological substances. This quality is also critical because metals, in particular, can interact at the molecular level, creating ions that are harmful to the body. Reactions also can lead to corrosion or oxidation of the implant, leading to weakness or breakdown. For these reasons, it is important for the surgeon to make sure that devices composed of different metals are not implanted near each other in the body.

Documentation

All implants stored in the operating room must be documented on a database for tracking, retrieving, and stock replacement. When an implant is used, specific information about the implant is recorded in the patient's record. This includes but is not limited to:

- Date and name of the facility
- Type of implant and size (where applicable)
- Location of implant in the body
- Name of the surgeon
- Manufacturer's identification number, including the batch, lot, and serial numbers

IMPLANT LOG The facility keeps information about each implant in a permanent log. This can be an electronic database or a written log. The FDA requires the following information:

- Name and address of the surgical facility
- Manufacturer's identification information
- Implant serial number, lot number, batch number, and any other identifying information (e.g., size, type)
- Patient's identification details

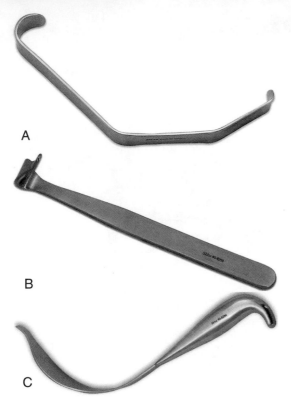

Figure 31-18   Retractors. A, Shoulder retractor. **B,** Blount knee retractor. **C,** Aufranc cobra retractor. *(Courtesy Sklar Instruments, West Chester, Pa.)*

- Surgeon's identification details
- Implant expiration date (if applicable)

Implant Sterilization

Many implants, including joint components, are supplied by the manufacturer individually in sterile packages. Plates, screws, pins, and rods are not wrapped individually but supplied in sterile sets, from which the appropriate size is selected during surgery. Joint and other specialty implants that are sterilized and packaged by the manufacturer are opened onto the sterile field only after the exact size and type have been determined. This reduces environmental exposure during surgery, as well as the need for an excessive implant inventory.

Implants must not be flash-sterilized except in extreme emergency. The Association for the Advancement of Medical Instrumentation (AAMI), which institutes international protocols for patient safety, states that "careful planning, appropriate packaging, and inventory management in cooperation with suppliers can minimize the need to flash-sterilize implants."[1] The Association of periOperative Registered Nurses (AORN) recommends that if an emergency situation makes flash sterilization unavoidable, a biological monitoring device must be used, along with a chemical indicator. The implant must not be used until the biological indicator provides a negative result.[2]

The patient's permanent operative record must reflect the details of the sterilization process and the outcome of the

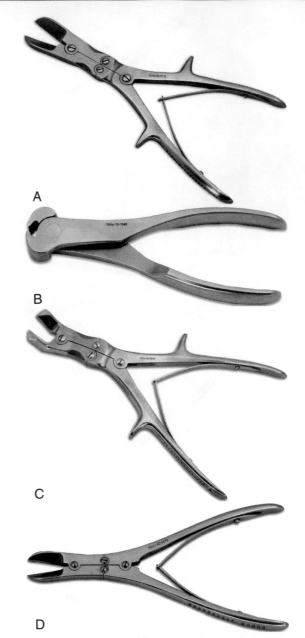

Figure 31-19   Rongeurs and bone cutters. A, Stille-Liston rongeur. **B,** Liston cutting forceps. **C,** Stille-Horsley rongeur. **D,** Ruskin forceps. *(Courtesy Sklar Instruments, West Chester, Pa.)*

biological and chemical indicators. The sterilizer log (computer printout), which includes all sterilization parameters achieved when the implant was flashed, must be included in the patient's chart. The AAMI provides yearly updates of accepted sterilization practices through its *Standards Registry*. Standard *ST79* provides current practices regarding steam sterilization for implants and should be consulted yearly for updated information.

SCREWS

An orthopedic screw is the most commonly used type of orthopedic implant (Figure 31-23). Screws are supplied in different types, sizes, shapes, and designs. They are made of

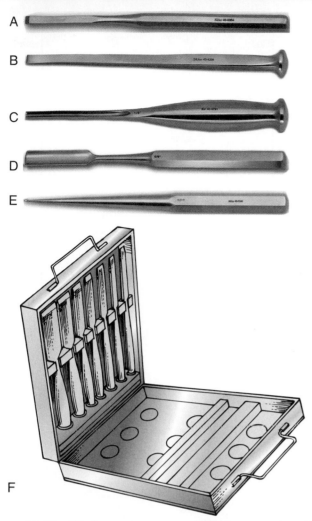

Figure 31-20 **Chisels, osteotomes, gouges, and curettes.** A, Hibbs chisel. B, Hoke chisel. C, Army pattern osteotome. D, Lambotte osteotome (often called simply a "Lambotte"). E, Smith Peterson gouge. F, Instrument rack. *(A-E Courtesy Sklar Instruments, West Chester, Pa. F from Phillips N: Berry and Kohn's operating room technique, ed 11, St Louis, 2007, Mosby.)*

titanium, stainless steel, or bioabsorbable material. To maintain order and allow quick identification of the size needed during surgery, screws are held in screw racks that are color-coded or imprinted with the sizes. The surgical technologist should be able to recognize different types of screws and understand their application. Screws are commonly used to:

- Attach a metal implant to bone
- Attach bone to bone or bone to soft connective tissue

Parts of a Screw

The parts of a screw are as follows:

- *Head:* The flat or conical part of the screw. The recess of the screw may be hexagonal, a straight slot, or cruciform (cross-shaped).
- *Shaft:* The long section of the screw. The outside of the threads (thread diameter) determines the screw's

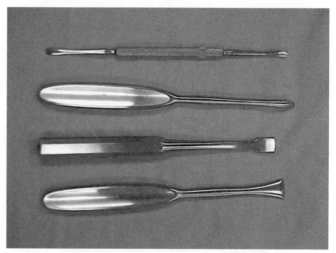

Figure 31-21 **Elevators.** *Top to bottom,* Freer elevator, used mainly in ear, nose, and throat (ENT) and plastic surgery; joker elevator; Key elevator; and Langenbeck elevator. *(Courtesy the College of Southern Idaho, Twin Falls, Idaho.)*

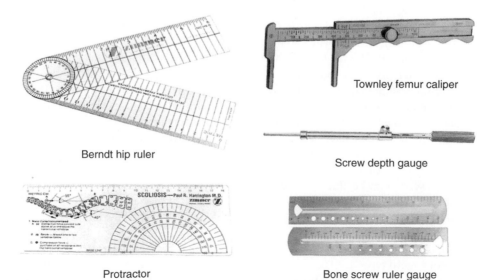

Berndt hip ruler

Townley femur caliper

Screw depth gauge

Protractor

Bone screw ruler gauge

Figure 31-22 **Measuring devices.** *(From Phillips N: Berry and Kohn's operating room technique, ed 11, St Louis, 2007, Mosby.)*

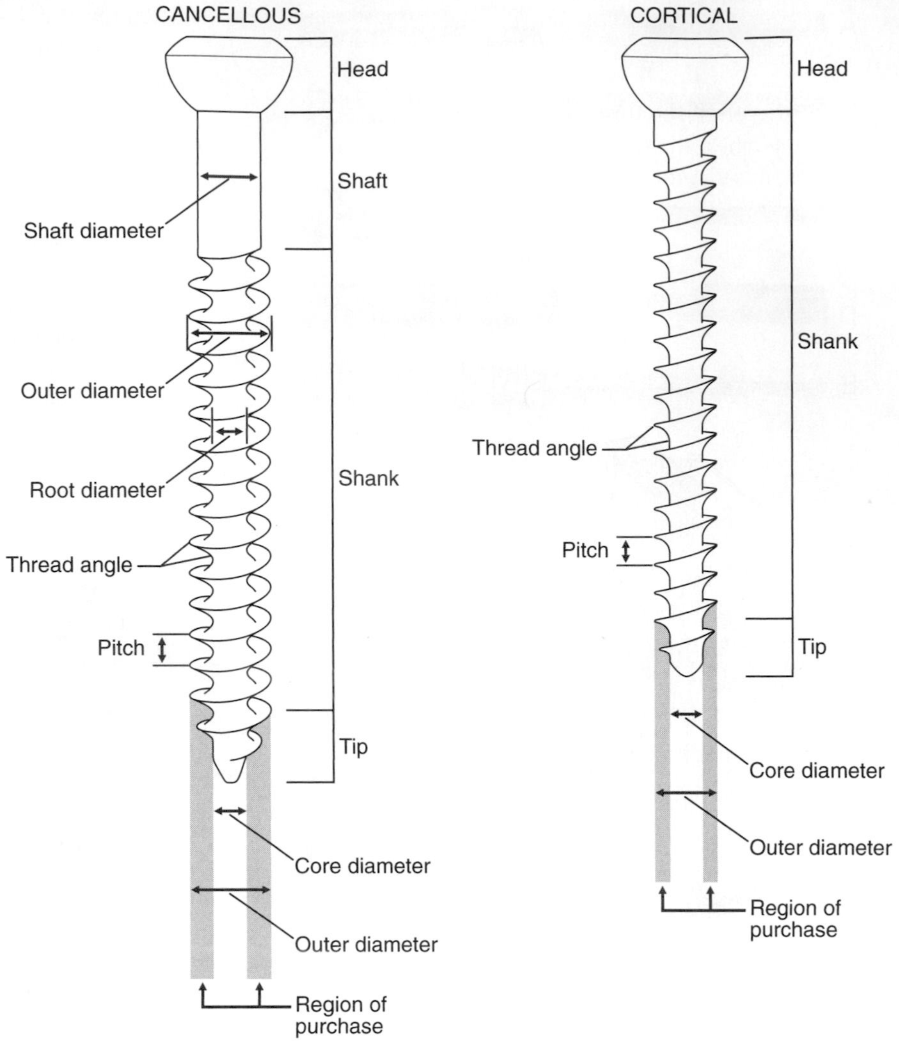

CANCELLOUS

CORTICAL

Figure 31-23　Components of the cancellous and cortical screw. *(From Browner B, Jupiter J, Levine A, Trafton P: Skeletal trauma: basic science, management, and reconstruction, ed 3, Philadelphia, 2003, WB Saunders.)*

numerical diameter. This measurement is important when the surgical technologist selects the correct drill bit size to match the screw size (non–self-tapping screws only) to be used. The main shaft, or root diameter, determines the strength of the screw.

- *Threads:* The spiral-shaped ridges along the screw shaft. The threads on most screws are asymmetrical (i.e., flat on the top and rounded underneath). This provides a wide surface for pulling the screw into the bone. The depth of the thread determines contact with the bone and its "pullout" strength. The number of threads in relation to the length of the shaft determines the pitch. As the pitch increases, so does contact with the bone, giving the screw greater gripping strength. Some screws have no threads near the head. These partly threaded screws have a specific biomechanical function (discussed later).
- *Tip:* The pointed end of the screw may be blunt, corkscrew, or trocar shaped. The shape determines whether the screw is self-tapping or requires a predrilled hole.

Types of Screws
Screws can be classified according to type:
- *Cancellous:* Used mainly in dense (cancellous) bone; large diameter and greater pitch to increase contact with the bone.

- *Cortical:* Small diameter and decreased pitch; used in cortical bone. The bicortical screw is inserted into the cortical bone on one surface and passes through the cancellous portion into the cortical surface on the opposite face of the bone.
- *Lag:* All screws that exert compression on bone fragments, either directly or with a plate.
- *Herbert:* Used for fixation of small bones; a cannulated screw with variable pitch and threads at both ends.
- *Locking:* Used with a special plate that has threaded holes to secure the screw head to the plate.
- **Cannulated**: A screw with a hollow core that is used to join bone fragments. The hollow center allows the screw to be fitted over a prepositioned guidewire to ensure precise placement.
- *Self-tapping:* Has flutes at the tip that cut a passage for the threads as the screw is inserted. Tapping is the process of making a hole in the material to accommodate the screw. A drill bit is used for tapping a hole (Figure 31-24).

The function of a screw is to hold two or more objects together. It can be used to attach a plate that bridges a fracture, and it can be used by itself to join two or more bone fragments or bone and soft connective tissue. When a screw is implanted across two objects, it compresses the materials together by cutting a spiral path in the material. This prevents the screw from backing out. The strength of a screw depends on several factors:

- The depth of the threads
- The pitch of the threads
- The shape of the threads

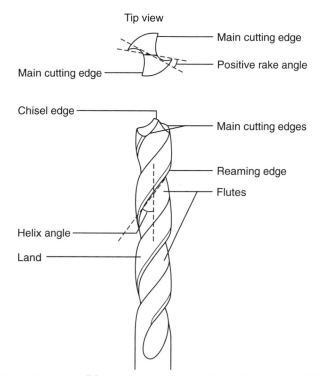

Figure 31-24 **Drill bit.** A bit is fitted to the head of a power drill for tapping (i.e., making a hole to accommodate the screw). *(From Browner B, Jupiter J, Levine A, Trafton P: Skeletal trauma: basic science, management, and reconstruction, ed 3, Philadelphia, 2003, WB Saunders.)*

It is important that surgical technologists understand the lag screw principle. The screw thread applies compression only on the object farthest from the screw head. For example, in the case of two bone fragments, the fragment farthest from the screw head is drawn into the first. This is an important concept for the scrub assisting in orthopedics cases. When tapping is done for this type of screw, the size of the drill tap is slightly larger than the screw diameter. The near side of the hole is drilled out to produce a space for countersinking the screw head. This allows the smooth part of the screw to glide easily through the hole (sometimes called the *glide hole*). When the screw engages in the second fragment, it grabs it and pulls it into position. Figure 31-25 illustrates the application of a lag screw through two bone fragments.

PLATES

Plates span bone and provide stability and support during healing. They are used in simple or comminuted fractures. Plates are made of titanium or stainless steel and are available in a matte or a polished finish. All have screw holes, because screws are used to fix them in place and to aid compression. Plates can be straight, contoured, or beveled to fit smoothly over bone and joint surfaces. The screw holes can be smooth sided, threaded, oblique, or straight.

Different forces are exerted on the fracture, the plate, and the soft tissue, depending on the type of plate used. To be effective at stabilizing, the implant must provide a means of preventing normal movement of the fracture area. This means that twisting, bending, and shearing (force at a right angle to the long axis) must be prevented. Functions of various plating systems are to:

- Protect and neutralize the fracture
- Span the fracture
- Provide compression

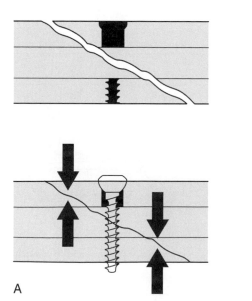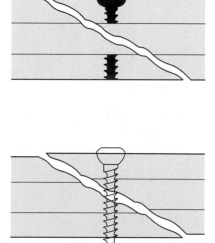

A   B

Figure 31-25 **Application of a lag screw.** The black sections indicate drilling areas. **A,** The cortex is drilled on the near side to produce a glide (countersink hole). **B,** Lack of a countersink results in a gap in the bone. *(From Browner B, Jupiter J, Levine A, Trafton P: Skeletal trauma: basic science, management, and reconstruction, ed 3, Philadelphia, 2003, WB Saunders.)*

- Reduce the fracture (bring the bone fragments together)
- Buttress (support) structures or fragments

Static (Neutralization) Plate

A static, or neutralization, plate spans a two-fragment fracture and is fixed in place with lag screws. This is a simple means of

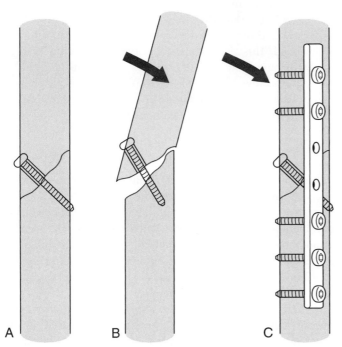

Figure 31-26   Neutralization plate. **A,** Screw fixation without a neutralization plate. **B,** The bone is loaded transversely, showing failure. **C,** The plate is effective at resisting the load as force is distributed across the length of the bone. *(From Browner B, Jupiter J, Levine A, Trafton P: Skeletal trauma: basic science, management, and reconstruction, ed 3, Philadelphia, 2003, WB Saunders.)*

stabilizing (i.e., neutralizing) force acting on the bone fragments with no mechanical action on the fracture line. This type of plate is used when the fragments can be compressed manually and the fracture is stable (Figure 31-26). The plate also is used to reduce a fracture (Figure 31-27).

Reconstruction Plate

A reconstruction plate may be bent to fit the contours of the bone surface. First, an aluminum template is fitted over the bone to duplicate its contour. The template then is taken to the back table and the implant plate is shaped with pliers, a plate press, and other instruments. More delicate reconstruction plates may be shaped and cut to size by hand. This type of plate is used commonly in facial and cranial fractures (Figure 31-28).

Locking Plate

A locking plate has threaded screw holes that lock the screws into the plate. This prevents rocking of the screws, which tends to loosen them or cause them to back out.

Dynamic Compression Plate

A dynamic compression plate has screw holes that are inclined (sloped) and offset. This design feature provides reduction and compression of the fragments. Anchor screws are inserted into one fragment. As the screws are tightened, the plate slides along the bone, drawing the two bone fragments together (Figure 31-29). The term *dynamic* refers to the compression of bone fragments produced by the natural load exerted on the bones by the body itself.

A low-contact dynamic compression plate is designed to reduce contact between the plate and the bone. The plate sits just above the surface of the bone, secured by screws. This prevents direct pressure on the periosteal vascular supply and

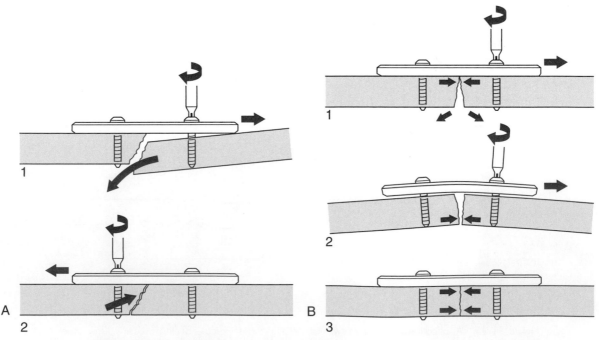

Figure 31-27   **The plate as a means of reducing a fracture. A,** The screws are tightened to produce inward loading and alignment. **B,** The rigid plate draws the displaced fragments into horizontal alignment with the plate. *(From Browner B, Jupiter J, Levine A, Trafton P: Skeletal trauma: basic science, management, and reconstruction, ed 3, Philadelphia, 2003, WB Saunders.)*

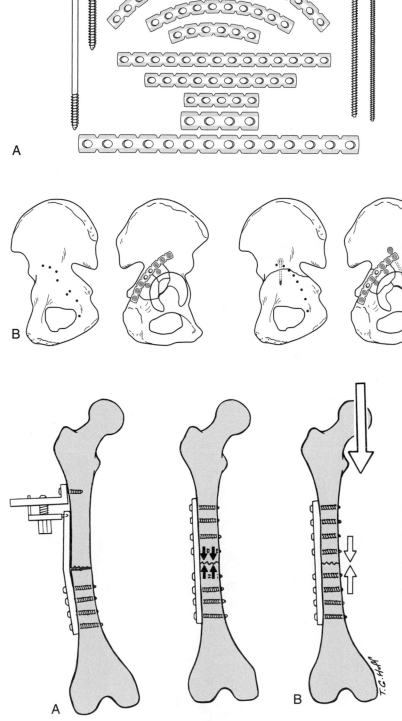

Figure 31-28 **A,** Examples of reconstruction plates. Plates are notched along the sides so that they can be easily bent in all directions to fit the contours of the bone. **B,** Use of plates for fixation of the posterior acetabular wall. *(From Browner B, Jupiter J, Levine A, Trafton P: Skeletal trauma: basic science, management, and reconstruction, ed 3, Philadelphia, 2003, WB Saunders.)*

Figure 31-29 **Compression plate technique.** Both static and dynamic compression are shown. **A,** The plate is applied to the femur to produce static compression. **B,** Normal weight (loading) on the femur further compresses the fragments at the fracture site. *(From Browner B, Jupiter J, Levine A, Trafton P: Skeletal trauma: basic science, management, and reconstruction, ed 3, Philadelphia, 2003, WB Saunders.)*

may enhance healing. Another type of plate is used to reduce contact with the periosteum is the wave plate, which is contoured to intermittently curve away from the bone. This type of plate is used in fractures that have failed to heal by other methods (Figure 31-30).

Tension Band Plate

A tension band plate provides a mechanical advantage in fixation of the long bones. Asymmetrical loading occurs in all long bones; that is, more weight is carried on the concave side

of the long axis of the bone. A partial fracture on the convex side tends to widen under load. The tension band plate is placed on the convex or gap side of the fracture to counteract the load and prevent the gap from widening. The principle of tension banding is also used without plates (Figure 31-31).

Buttress Plate

A buttress is a supporting structure that prevents an adjoining object or structure from collapsing. An example of common buttressing is a lean-to shed. The structure supporting the roof at its highest point is a buttress. The supporting structure is "pushing" on the roof to support it at an angle. In orthopedics, a buttress plate is used to give added strength or to "prop" one structure against another. This technique is commonly applied in fractures of the tibia (Figure 31-32).

Condylar Plate

A condylar plate often is used in conjunction with a compression screw for fixation of fractures of the *condyle* (the rounded

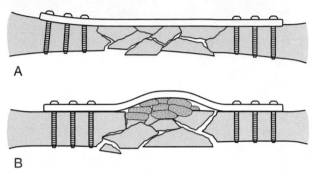

Figure 31-30   Wave or bridge plate. This type of plate is contoured away from an area of severe comminution to preserve blood supply and encourage the growth of new bone cells without external pressure. **A,** Conventional plating. **B,** Wave plate. *(From Browner B, Jupiter J, Levine A, Trafton P: Skeletal trauma: basic science, management, and reconstruction, ed 3, Philadelphia, 2003, WB Saunders.)*

end of a long bone). The end of the plate is contoured to fit over the surface of a condyle, and compression lag screws are inserted through the fracture fragments (Figure 31-33).

Intertrochanteric Nail and Plate Combination

Fractures that occur across the trochanter of the hip often require stabilization from a side plate, which is implanted at the proximal end of the femur. An older prototype of this device is the Jewett nail. Although the Jewett nail is still occasionally used, it has been largely replaced by more efficient systems, such as the dynamic hip screw and the dynamic compression–sliding hip screw. This implant has two primary pieces, a lag screw, which is inserted into the trochanter, and a locking plate, which is inserted over the screw and extends along the proximal femur. During healing, the plate-nail combination shifts the load from the trochanter (normal loading) to the long axis of the femur, removing excess pressure from the trochanter (Figure 31-34).

INTRAMEDULLARY NAIL OR ROD

An intramedullary (IM) nail is a thick rod inserted into the medullary canal of long bones to provide structural support from inside the bone. This device is used for fractures of long bones, such as the femur, tibia, and humerus. IM nails are made of titanium and stainless steel. They are supplied as

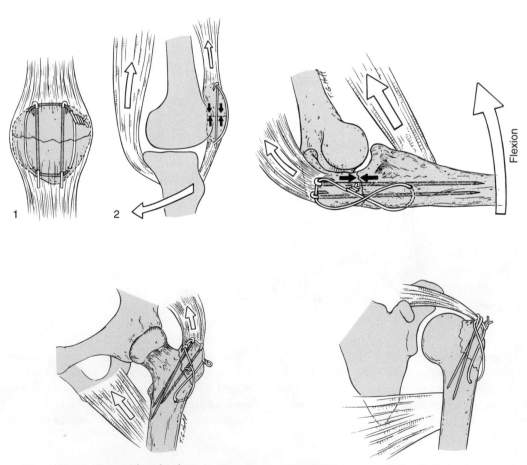

Figure 31-31   Tension band technique. *(From Browner B, Jupiter J, Levine A, Trafton P: Skeletal trauma: basic science, management, and reconstruction, ed 3, Philadelphia, 2003, WB Saunders.)*

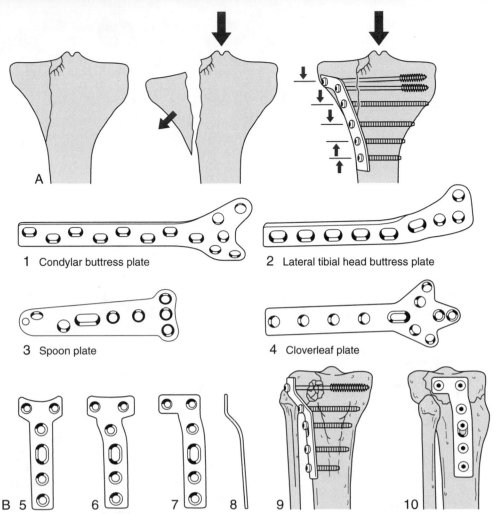

Figure 31-32 **Buttress plating. A,** The plate acts as a retaining wall to support the fractured component. **B,** Views *1 to 10* are types of buttress plates. Views *9* and *10,* Lateral plate used with a cancellous bone graft to buttress a tibial plateau fracture. *(From Browner B, Jupiter J, Levine A, Trafton P: Skeletal trauma: basic science, management, and reconstruction, ed 3, Philadelphia, 2003, WB Saunders.)*

slotted, cannulated (hollow), or solid. Nails are inserted by reaming the intramedullary canal or by impacting the nail through the marrow tissue to seat it. The Ender nail and Rush rod are older style nails that are used in multiples and impacted with a mallet. Modern IM systems include the nail itself plus two or more transverse locking bolts, which increase contact with the bone and provide structural support. Locking bolts are placed at the proximal and distal ends of the nail and prevent it from drifting or backing out of the medullary canal. They also provide rotational support. Figure 31-35 shows a femoral nail with locking bolts.

WIRES AND CABLES

Flexible wire and cable are used in a variety of techniques to approximate bone and soft tissue and for stabilization. Wire most often is used to reduce small bone fragments. This is done by drilling holes in the fragments, inserting a wire through the holes, and drawing the fragments together. The wires are then twisted and the resulting knot is buried in adjacent soft tissue or flattened against the bone. Wire or cable

also is used in cerclage (encircling) reduction to provide added strength to another type of implant, such as an IM nail. Cables are closed at their ends with a cable clamp.

KIRSCHNER WIRES AND STEINMANN PINS

Kirschner wires (K-wires) and Steinmann pins are thick wires that are inserted with a drill. The wires have a sharp, diamond-shaped point that penetrates bone and soft tissue. They are inserted directly into tissue with a drill. They are extremely sharp and can easily puncture gloves and drapes with little impact. They should be handled with caution. After insertion, the surgeon cuts the excess wire with cutters. All pieces are retrieved from the surgical field and placed in a magnetic container to prevent injury or loss in the wound.

The main advantages of K-wires and Steinmann pins are their size and ease of insertion. They cause little trauma to bone and can be easily withdrawn. They commonly are used:

- As a guidewire for cannulated screws and instruments
- To provide temporary or final stabilization for a fracture

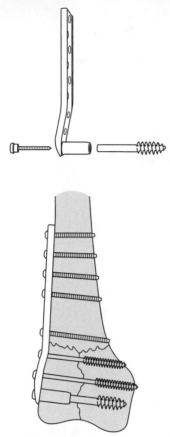

Figure 31-33 Condylar plate and screw. *(From Browner B, Jupiter J, Levine A, Trafton P: Skeletal trauma: basic science, management, and reconstruction, ed 3, Philadelphia, 2003, WB Saunders.)*

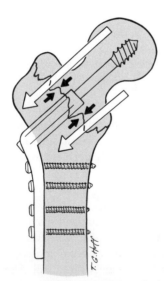

Figure 31-34 Dynamic compression plate with sliding hip screw for fracture of the trochanter. *(From Browner B, Jupiter J, Levine A, Trafton P: Skeletal trauma: basic science, management, and reconstruction, ed 3, Philadelphia, 2003, WB Saunders.)*

- As an intramedullary device to span a fracture in a small bone (e.g., the digits)
- To position multiple fragments of a comminuted fracture
- As a template for cannulated nails
- As a component of traction devices

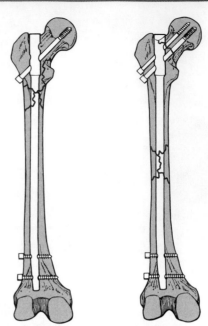

Figure 31-35 Femoral intramedullary nail. This is the second-generation intramedullary nail, which adds locking bolts at each end for added strength and to prevent the nail from backing out or rotating. This type of nail is used for femoral and tibial fractures. *(From Browner B, Jupiter J, Levine A, Trafton P: Skeletal trauma: basic science, management, and reconstruction, ed 3, Philadelphia, 2003, WB Saunders.)*

JOINT REPLACEMENT IMPLANTS

Joint implants are metal or synthetic components used to replace the diseased or injured tissue. The load placed on a joint requires that the implant meet certain criteria. When implant surfaces (called the *bearing surfaces*) rub on each other, minute particles of the implant materials are released into the joint cavity. These particles cause a cellular reaction that leads to the destruction of bone tissue. Different types of implant materials are designed to help overcome this problem through greater resistance to wear. No implant material or design is suitable for all patients. The selection is based on the patient's bone type, age, activity level, and general health.

Materials

METALS Metal alloys are used in the manufacture of joint implants. The metals and alloys most commonly used are:

- Cobalt-chromium-molybdenum
- Titanium-aluminum-vanadium
- Pure titanium
- Tantalum

Metal-on-metal components were the first type to be used in joint replacement. Some researchers have returned to this design, using more advanced metallurgy. However, metal can release ions into the body, causing toxicity. This type of system is not used in patients with kidney disease or in women of childbearing age.

POLYETHYLENE Polyethylene is a highly durable, low-friction plastic in the form of ultrahigh molecular weight, highly cross-linked polyethylene (UHMWPE). This is a modified form of polyethylene made through a process of irradiation. Although very strong, highly cross-linked polyethylene breaks down through wear and delamination (separation of layers). UHMWPE components are commonly used in hybrid joint systems, which use both metal and polyethylene.

CERAMIC Ceramic materials were developed in orthopedic technology to increase resistance to wear. This type of component is mainly limited to hip replacement. Three types of ceramic materials are currently used: alumina, zirconium, and oxidized zirconium. Ceramic materials have been used for the manufacture of femoral heads for several decades. Ceramic-on-polyethylene, ceramic-on-ceramic, and ceramic-on-metal implants are currently available.

The advantages of ceramic are that it is very hard, it can be highly polished, and it remains resistant to scratching. The greatest disadvantage is that the material is brittle and can fracture or shatter.

SURFACE MATERIALS Some implants are roughened and coated to enhance healing and resist wear. Metal fibers or "beads" may be applied to the surface of the implant to create microscopic pores that accept bone cement during implantation. In **press-fit** implants, bone tissue infiltrates the pores during healing. Metal coatings are used or the original surface material may be altered by infusing it with gas or exposing it to nitrogen ions.

Design Structure

The structure and surface of a joint implant are extremely important to the safety and function of the joint postoperatively. Joint stability is achieved by the basic design and surface coating.

Modular and Nonmodular Design

Modular components are now used in many joint replacement systems. These are joint systems that contain several parts. Modular components can be manufactured from different materials or the same material and assembled inside the patient. An inventory of modular components allows surgical facilities to maintain a variety of sizes of components within a single system. Nonmodular systems may provide greater longevity because they have fewer components.

Joint implants may be cemented in place with bone cement or they may be press-fitted by impaction. The choice of cemented or press-fit design depends on the bone quality and the patient's age, health, and desired level of activity.

GRAFTS, BONE CEMENT, AND BIOACTIVE MATERIALS

Grafts

Bone transplantation usually is performed using a segment of the patient's own bone (autograft) or cadaver bone (allograft). Cadaver bone is reprocessed to remove minerals and protein and then is freeze-dried. Bone is stored in the hospital bone bank and supplied in sterile form.

The most common anatomical areas used for autograft donor bone are the iliac crest and tibia. Grafts are usually taken using chisels. The graft site is prepped separately. If it is not closed promptly after the graft is out, the surgical technologist should keep the site covered and protected with sterile towels or a small drape. Bone graft tissue is covered with moist saline sponges and kept on the back table in a basin until needed. Do not soak a bone implant in saline solution unless requested by the surgeon. Never use water to moisten bone implants, as this causes cellular damage.

BONE GRAFT SUBSTITUTES Bone graft substitutes are commonly used to repair and reconstruct bone. A shortage of graft materials and interest in bioactive materials has led to the development of new graft substitutes:
- *Ceramic:* Composites of calcium phosphate, calcium sulfate, and bioactive glass (paste, chips, granules)
- *Polymer:* Cross-linked collagen based or hydroxyapatite coated, resin based

Bone graft substitutes are supplied in the following forms:
- Injectable paste
- Block form
- Granules
- Putty
- Chips

Materials are mixed with intravenous fluids or solutions using a graft preparation device.

Bone Cement

Implants used in arthroplasty (joint replacement) may be cemented in place with polymethylmethacrylate (PMMA). Bone cement is an interface or a grout (rather than glue) between the joint implant and tissue. It is formed by mixing two components, PMMA powder and a liquid monomer of methylmethacrylate. When dry, the cement forms a strong radiopaque filler. Bone cement is supplied plain or with an antibiotic additive that is released into the bone.

Bone cement is prepared during surgery to a doughy consistency. It is instilled into the joint manually or with a cement gun. After mixing, it hardens within 15 minutes. During mixing, the two components create an exothermic (heat-releasing) reaction.

PMMA is a hazardous chemical and must be handled according to regulations established by the National Institute for Occupational and Safety Health (NIOSH) and the hospital's policies and protocols. Exposure to PMMA vapor is an occupational risk and use of the cement is associated with toxic and cardiovascular events in the patient.

OCCUPATIONAL RISKS Vapors released when the dry and liquid components of PMMA are mixed are known to cause serious eye damage and respiratory tract and skin irritation. An allergic reaction may also occur. The effects of vapor inhalation are cumulative and are associated with kidney and liver damage. Inhalation also may cause neurological symptoms and pregnancy complications.

More information on occupational risk is available on the NIOSH website at http://www.cdc.gov/niosh/database.html.

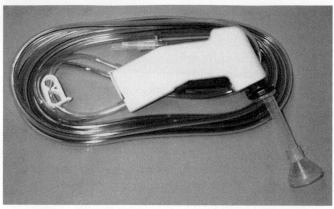

Figure 31-36   Pulse lavage system. Antibiotic solution or saline commonly is used to apply a pulsed stream of pressurized solution to the wound for debridement and irrigation. *(From Townsend CM: Sabiston textbook of surgery, ed 17, Philadelphia, 2001, Saunders.)*

PATIENT RISKS Patient risks associated with PMMA include toxicity and vascular events. Acute toxicity causes sudden cardiovascular complications and possible cardiac arrest. Increased intramedullary pressure may force marrow tissue into the circulation, resulting in embolism. Bone cement implantation syndrome includes life-threatening hypotension, pulmonary edema, and cardiogenic shock. These hazards can be reduced by the use of good surgical technique, such as pulse lavage (Figure 31-36) to clear the medullary canal before the cement and implant are inserted.

SAFETY PRECAUTIONS The cement is supplied to the sterile field in its two components, as a dry powder and a liquid solvent. These are combined and mixed in a closed container specially designed for use with PMMA. The bone cement mixer is fitted with a vacuum tube that shunts vapors away from the surgical field. They then are dissipated through a charcoal filter. The vacuum system also removes air pockets, which destabilize the cement. Surgical technologists can become familiar with the operation and assembly of bone cement mixers used in their facility.

PREPARING BONE CEMENT The manufacturer's instructions for mixing bone cement should always be consulted before the process is started. Cement is injected into a prepared joint with a cement gun. Some mixers have a cartridge that is transferred directly to the cement gun after mixing. General preparation includes the following steps:

1. Assemble the mixing apparatus according to manufacturer's specifications. Attach one end of the vacuum tubing to the mixer. The circulator receives the other end and attaches it to a vacuum pump, which is operated with compressed nitrogen.
2. Pour the powdered and liquid cement components into the mixer.
3. Secure the lid of the mixer. Rotate the lid handle to mix the components.
4. Continue to mix the cement until it reaches a doughy consistency. At this stage, it is removed from the mixer

and molded to shape. When it is no longer sticky, it is ready for use.
5. If a cartridge mixer is used, remove the cartridge from the mixer and transfer it immediately to the cement gun.
6. Change sterile gloves when the cement no longer requires handling.
7. Discard any unused cement according to hospital policy. *Do not handle unused cement.*

CASTING

Casting is a method of external fixation in which a limb is immobilized by applying plaster or synthetic resin. Acute or open fractures are not treated with a cast because of the high risk of complications, such as compartment syndrome and infection. Surgical technologists who are required to learn casting techniques are best trained by the orthopedic surgeons in their facility. The role is usually that of an orthopedic technician, who has completed training in the duties required, including the medical aspects of the role.

Casts differ by location and medical objectives. A cylinder cast is a simple wrap along the length of the limb to immobilize a fracture. A spica cast is used in pediatrics to immobilize hip fractures or deformities. The spica cast covers the trunk and one or both limbs. Casting splints sometimes are applied longitudinally over the arm or wrist to provide rigid support after surgery. The splints do not cover the surgical incision or encase the limb.

Casting materials include plaster and polyurethane resin. Plaster is used less commonly than resins, which are stronger and resistant to breakdown by moisture. Resin casts also are more manageable for the patient because of their light weight. Casting materials are available in 2- to 6-inch (5- to 15-cm) widths.

Before a cast is applied, the limb is wrapped with padding. Two types of padding are commonly used. A stockinet is first applied to the limb. This is followed with felted (batted) cotton Webril. Rolled Webril is applied from the distal to proximal end of the limb. At least two layers of Webril are needed. Extra padding is needed for bony prominences.

Rolls of cast material are immersed in water before use. During application, the limb is lightly supported by the assistant. Plaster hardens within 30 minutes but requires 24 to 48 hours to set completely. Resin casts dry in 15 to 30 minutes. The single largest patient risk associated with casting is **compartment syndrome**. This is edema (swelling) of tissue within a closed compartment of the body (such as the cranium) or inside an external cast. When pressure on the tissues exceed the space in the compartment, the tissue becomes necrotic. In orthopedics this can lead to necrosis of the entire limb and eventual amputation if circulation is not restored. Safeguards to prevent this include using splints rather than cylindrical casting and judicious use of cotton Webril, which can be constricting when improperly applied. Naturally, postoperative swelling must be taken into account when a cast is applied directly after surgery. Careful monitoring of the limb and postoperative instructions to the patient are very important in

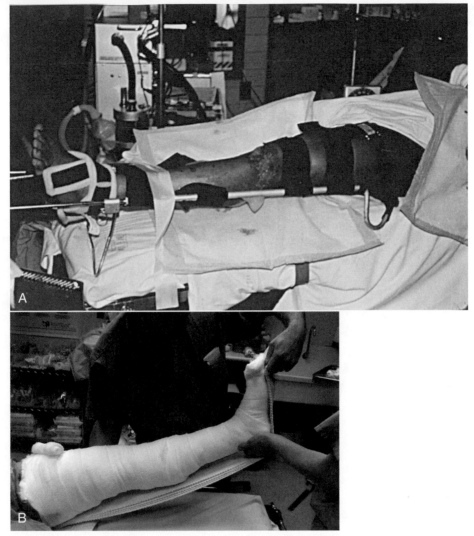

Figure 31-37   Traction. A, Emergency traction using soft straps and rods. **B,** Skeletal traction of the femur after surgery to insert traction pins. (**A** *from Wolinsky PR, Johnson KD: Femoral shaft fractures. In Browner BD, Jupiter TB, Levine AM, Trafteon PG, editors: Skeletal trauma, ed 2, Philadelphia, 1998, WB Saunders; **B** from Townsend CM: Sabiston textbook of surgery, ed 17, Philadelphia, 2001, WB Saunders.)*

the detection of compartment syndrome in the postoperative period.

TRACTION

Traction is a mechanical method of applying pulling force or elongation to fractured bone. Traction is used to:

- Prevent injury to soft tissues, especially blood vessels and nerves near the fracture site
- Align bone after a fracture or **dislocation**
- Prevent movement of a fractured limb
- Reduce pain in acute orthopedic trauma patients before surgical repair
- Reduce muscle spasm in orthopedic injuries

Traction is used much less often in modern orthopedics than it was in the past. Advances in orthopedic implant surgery and techniques have replaced long-term traction as a primary method of treatment except in certain circumstances. The two types of traction are:

- *Skin traction*, which involves taping a traction system to the skin. It generally is used only as a temporary measure (e.g., Buck traction). Skin traction is seldom used in adults. Modern external traction frames provide temporary traction for emergency use (Figure 31-37, *A*).
- **Skeletal traction**, which requires surgical insertion of metal pins or rods through the bone distal to the fracture. The pins are attached to a traction device that applies force or is drawn by a weighted pulley (see Figure 31-37, *B*).

MODULAR ROD AND PIN FIXATION

Modular rod and pin fixation is used mainly for temporary external stabilization of a fracture. The system is very flexible and can be used for fractures of the long bones and pelvis and

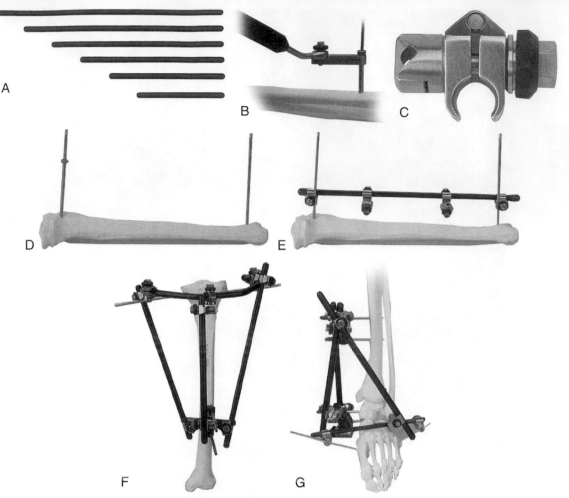

Figure 31-38 **Modular external fixation-distraction device. A,** Modular pins. **B,** Setting the pins. **C,** Clamp. **D,** Building the frame. **E, F,** Building the frame. **G,** Ankle frame in place. *(Courtesy Zimmer, Warsaw, Ind.)*

also for joint-lengthening procedures involving bone loss. This type of system also is used to distract bone in which loss has occurred as a result of trauma or disease. The external framework maintains alignment with expansion of the limb to create space for new bone growth.

The basic design is based on external metal rods, which act as a superstructure to the bone. The rods are held in place with bolts and pins, which are inserted through the bone to support the outer framework. The modular system can be used as a unilateral frame (a single rod attached by internally placed pins) or a modular frame or cage constructed with multiple rods and pins, which are inserted into the bone fragments and connected with clamps (Figure 31-38). Many types of pins do not require predrilling and are inserted with a power drill. This type of traction is commonly used in patients with severe open trauma.

ARTHROSCOPIC SURGERY

Arthroscopic surgery is minimally invasive surgery (MIS) of the joints. This technique is used mainly for diagnostic procedures and for repair and reconstruction of soft tissue. Most

open soft tissue procedures of the joints can be performed arthroscopically.

Before studying the minimally invasive techniques presented in this chapter, the reader should review Chapter 24. The principles are the same; only the instrumentation, patient preparation, and specific operative techniques are different.

Instruments

Many orthopedic MIS instruments resemble those used in open procedures. However, where retraction normally would require an instrument with strong leverage, a hook or probe is used. Because the endoscope penetrates the joint area, mechanical retraction usually is not necessary. Dissection is performed with heavy endoscopic scissors, an electrosurgical unit (ESU) probe, and shears. Power shavers, drills, burrs, and cutters are supplied in endoscopic sets. Graspers contain biting tips for use on cartilage and other fibrous tissues.

A number of sophisticated devices are available for passing sutures through bone and cartilage. The basic principle in all the designs is similar. An eyed, awl-type instrument is used to run the suture through the tissues, or a hole can be made first and the eyed tool, with suture mounted, is passed through it.

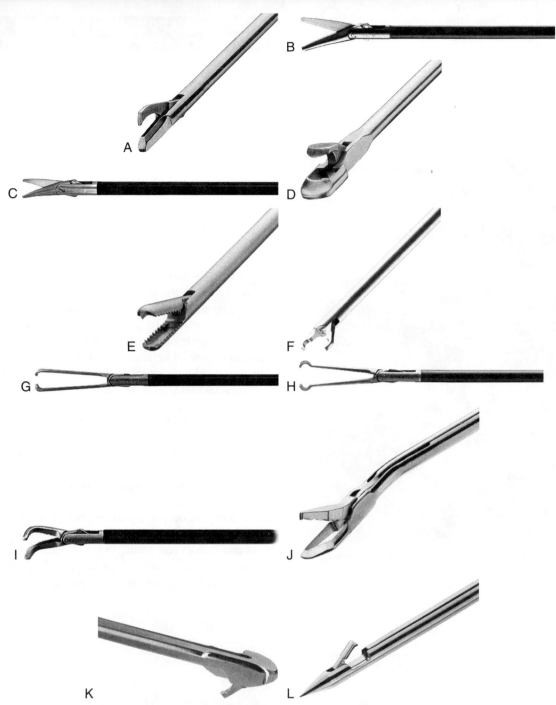

Figure 31-39 **Arthroscopy instruments. A,** Microscissors. **B,** Mayo scissors. **C,** Metzenbaum scissors. **D,** Shovel-nose forceps. **E,** Alligator grasper. **F,** Retrieval forceps. **G,** Allis grasper. **H,** Babcock grasper. **I,** Mixter forceps. **J,** Linear grasper. **K,** Retro punch. **L,** Suture carrier. *(Courtesy Zimmer, Warsaw, Ind.)*

Anchoring devices, which contain a biosynthetic screw with suture attached at the distal end, are easily passed through a large trocar for attachment of the joint capsule to ligaments and muscle. Common arthroscopic instruments are shown in Figure 31-39.

Joint Distention

Joint distention with saline or lactated Ringer solution is necessary for arthroscopy of the shoulder and knee. Fluid is instilled into the joint through one port and exits through another. Inflow tubing and outflow tubing are required to maintain continuous flushing of the joint.

As with other forms of MIS, expansion of the operative field from within allows greater visibility of the structures. Free-flowing solution keeps the operative field free of tissue debris and blood, which can obscure the endoscopic image transmitted to the monitor.

Fluid distention also acts as a tamponade (pressure to control bleeding). This is particularly important in rotator cuff surgery, in which bleeding can be brisk. In knee surgery, the synovial capsule may be inflamed, which can contribute to capillary bleeding. When tamponade is required, the inflow of fluid must be adjusted to keep up with the outflow. The circulator is responsible for making adjustments in the pump system (or gravity system) as necessary. An arthroscopic fluid system is shown in Figure 31-40.

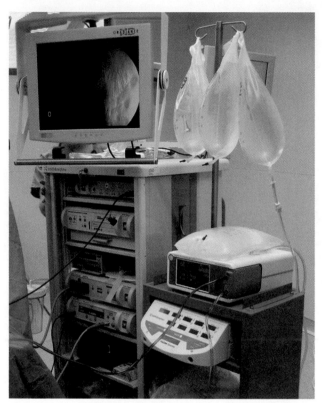

Figure 31-40 Continuous irrigation system used in arthroscopy. Flow pressure is monitored by the control unit. *(From Canale S, Beaty J: Campbell's operative orthopaedics, ed 11, St Louis, 2007, Mosby.)*

SURGICAL APPROACHES TO THE SHOULDER AND ARM

The shoulder is composed of three main bones: the scapula, the clavicle, and the humerus. The head of the humerus fits into the glenoid socket of the scapula; this forms the glenohumeral joint. The socket is surrounded by a rim of cartilage called the *labrum,* which helps stabilize the head of the humerus. The labrum also attaches to several ligaments, which further support the joint.

The clavicle moves in coordination with the humerus and is a primary site of sports injury. Clavicular joints include:

- *Acromioclavicular (AC) joint:* Clavicle to acromion
- *Sternoclavicular (SC) joint:* Clavicle to sternum

The shoulder is a mechanically unstable structure. It is suspended from the skeleton by soft tissue and is mobile in all directions. The head of the humerus technically is a ball-and-socket joint, but the glenoid socket, which holds the head of the humerus, is shallow. As mentioned earlier, the labrum encircles the rim of the glenoid. The labrum is a cartilaginous structure similar to the meniscus in the knee. It increases the amount of contact between the humeral head and the glenoid, but joint stability relies on the ligaments, muscles, and tendons. The muscles that attach the humerus to the glenoid socket are jointly called the *rotator cuff.* These muscles also add to the stability of the joint; however, they can be torn as a result of sports injury or other traumatic stress (Figure 31-41).

The shoulder joint is shown in Figure 31-42. Inside the joint capsule is a layer of connective tissue that is thickened at three points; these are the *glenohumeral ligaments.* When these soft tissues fail because of injury or repetitive stress, shoulder dislocation can occur. Recurrent dislocation requires surgical treatment in most cases. In the past, techniques were used to bind and restrict soft tissues in the shoulder to prevent recurrence of the injury. In modern surgery, the goal is to restore function and range of motion, especially in active patients

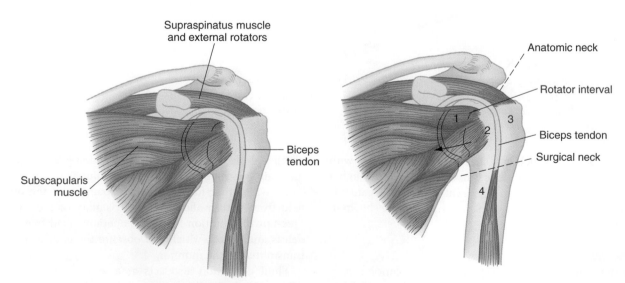

Figure 31-41 Structures of the rotator cuff. *(From Marx J, editor: Rosen's emergency medicine: concepts and clinical practice, ed, 6, Philadelphia, 2006, Mosby.)*

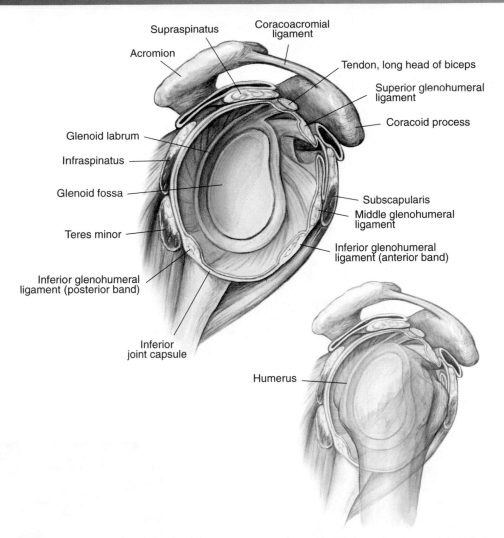

Figure 31-42 Anatomy of the shoulder joint. *(From Miller MD, Chhabra AB, Hurwitz SR, Mihalko WM: Orthopaedic surgical approaches, Philadelphia, 2008, WB Saunders.)*

who want to return to their usual activities. This goal is not always possible; the surgeon discusses surgical alternatives with the patient to determine the best approach to meet the individual's needs.

The *Bankart* and *Putti-Platt* procedures, which involve soft tissue repair and replantation to secure the shoulder, are commonly used for recurrent shoulder dislocation. In the Bankart procedure, the glenoid rim is reattached to the joint capsule; in the Putti-Platt procedure, the subscapularis tendon is severed and attached to the glenoid. Sutures or anchoring devices are used to attach the cartilaginous structures. The Bankart procedure is described in the following section as a representative procedure for recurrent shoulder dislocation. Many variations on the two procedures have been developed, but the principles are similar.

NOTE: *The Bristow procedure, used in the past, has been replaced by safer techniques. In this procedure the coracoid process is severed and transferred as a sling. This technique has largely been abandoned because of intraoperative risk and postoperative complications, including recurrent dislocation.*[3]

During open surgery, an anterior approach is used for many types of shoulder procedures (Figure 31-43, *A*). Another common approach is directly over the deltoid at the acromion (see Figure 31-43, *B*). The posterior approach also is used is some cases.

BANKART PROCEDURE

Surgical Goal

In the Bankart procedure, the glenoid rim is reattached to the joint capsule with a biosynthetic or other anchoring device or with heavy sutures.

Pathology

An important cause of recurrent glenohumeral dislocation is separation of the labrum (the rim of the glenoid capsule) from the joint capsule. This usually is caused by sports trauma in which the humeral head is forced out of the glenoid anteriorly. The condition may affect young healthy individuals.

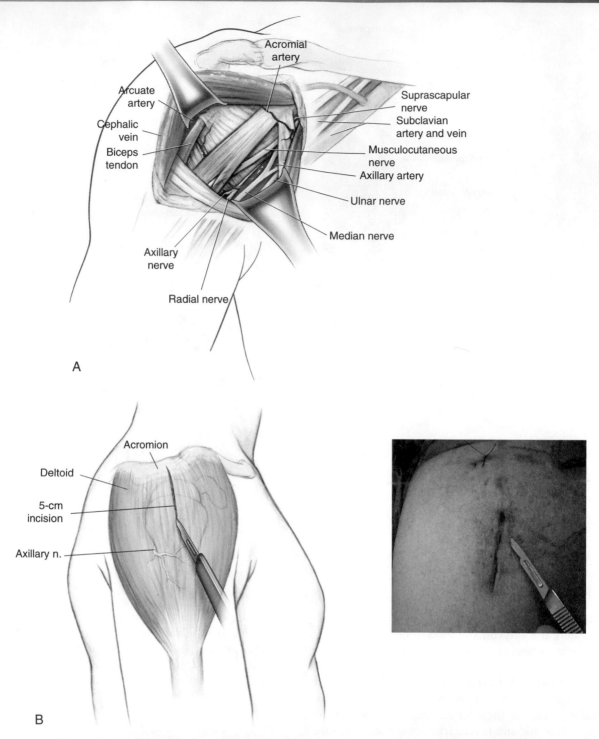

Figure 31-43 Surgical approach to the shoulder. A, Deltopectoral approach. **B,** Deltoid-splitting incision. *(From Miller MD, Chhabra AB, Hurwitz SR, Mihalko WM: Orthopaedic surgical approaches, Philadelphia, 2008, WB Saunders.)*

TECHNIQUE

1. An anterolateral or anterior incision is made and extended to the joint.
2. The conjoined tendon is mobilized and retracted.
3. The joint capsule is incised.
4. The glenoid rim is elevated and trimmed.
5. The capsule is attached to the glenoid with biosynthetic bone anchors, staples, or heavy sutures.
6. The capsule is closed.
7. The wound is closed.

Discussion

The Bankart procedure has been modified since it was developed in the 1920s. It has become less traumatic with the development of absorbable anchoring devices attached to heavy sutures. The device is placed through the joint capsule and the sutures are placed through the glenoid rim to repair the lesion. Heavy sutures may also be used to reattach the glenoid.

The patient is placed in the beach chair position. A pad is placed under the scapula to lift the shoulder and bring the scapula forward. The shoulder and arm are prepped and draped and the arm is left free for intraoperative manipulation.

An anterior or anterolateral incision is made near the axillary crease. The incision is carried into deep tissue using sharp dissection with Metzenbaum scissors and the ESU. Rake retractors are used superficially to expose the muscles. As the incision is extended, deep handheld or self-retaining retractors are used to expose the joint (Figure 31-44).

When the muscles have been exposed, the conjoined tendon is dissected free and retracted. The capsule is divided and the glenoid rim is elevated with a retractor such as a ring retractor. The glenoid is prepared for the anchoring devices. In some cases the tear may require slight remodeling with small rongeurs. An osteotome or rasp is used to score the glenoid rim and produce a raw surface on the bone (to expose the capillary blood supply and initiate bone healing) to which the capsule will be attached.

The capsule is attached with biosynthetic bone anchors, staples, or heavy sutures (Figure 31-45). If anchors are used, the scrub should have several anchors available. For thick bone, a pilot hole may be required. Size 0 or 2-0 Mersilene sutures are used in the traditional method of repair.

After inspecting the repair, the surgeon uses the long suture ends to close the joint capsule. The shoulder then is manipulated into all ranges of motion to test the repair. The wound is irrigated and closed with continuous or running sutures. A simple dressing is applied and the shoulder is placed in a soft immobilizer.

After an open procedure for shoulder instability, dislocation can recur in 30% to 60% of cases. The patient may return to some activity within several months. Physical therapy is required to strengthen the rotator cuff muscles. Healing usually is complete within 6 months.

OPEN ROTATOR CUFF REPAIR

Surgical Goal

The goal of rotator cuff repair is to reattach torn muscles of the rotator cuff to the humerus with sutures or anchor-suturing devices. An open or arthroscopic approach can be used.

Pathology

The rotator cuff is composed of four tendons that attach to the humerus. Each tendon is continuous with a muscle that originates at the scapula. The muscles are the *supraspinatus*, the *subscapularis*, the *infraspinatus*, and the *teres minor*. One or more tendons may be damaged by traumatic injury or as a result of recurrent shoulder dislocation. A rotator cuff tear usually occurs where the supraspinatus tendon inserts into the humerus. The injury can be superficial or can involve the entire tendon. Degenerative conditions, in which the tissue is weakened because of past injury or previous surgery, can also result in tearing.

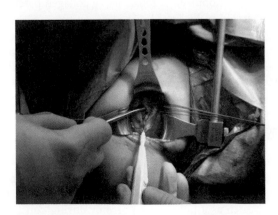

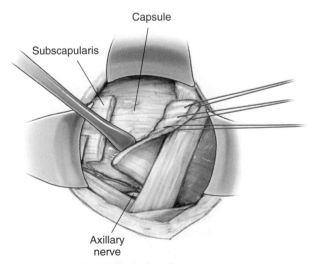

Figure 31-44 Exposure of the shoulder. The subscapularis has been divided and traction sutures have been placed. Note the conjoined tendon at right. *(From Miller MD, Chhabra AB, Hurwitz SR, Mihalko WM: Orthopaedic surgical approaches, Philadelphia, 2008, WB Saunders.)*

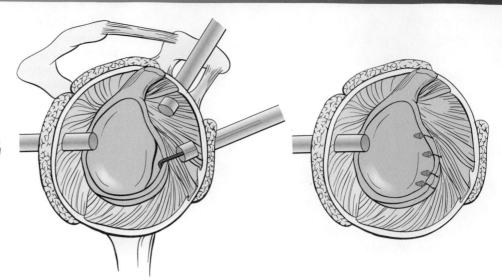

Figure 31-45 Surgical repair for recurrent shoulder dislocation. Multiple sutures are placed in the glenoid rim. *(From Rakel R: Textbook of family medicine, ed 7, Philadelphia, 2007, WB Saunders.)*

TECHNIQUE

1. An anterior or deltopectoral incision is made in the shoulder and carried to the coracoacromial ligament.
2. The ligament is incised and traction sutures are placed through the edge.
3. For suture repair, several suture holes are made in the humerus with a drill or an awl.
4. Sutures are passed through the bone and tendon.
5. Biosynthetic screws or a collagen patch may be used in the repair.
6. The deltoid is attached with heavy synthetic sutures.
7. The wound is closed.

Discussion

The patient is positioned, prepped, and draped for a shoulder procedure with the arm free. In addition to general surgery instruments, the technologist should have a shoulder set, drill, and small drill bits available. The incision is carried to the joint capsule with the ESU and Metzenbaum scissors. A self-retaining retractor (e.g., Gelpi or Beckman retractor) is used to expose the rotator cuff tendons and muscles.

The deltoid muscle may be split with a needle-tip ESU or it may be dissected from the acromion, depending on the exposure needed and the type of repair. The coracoacromial ligament is incised with the ESU. A heavy polyester suture is inserted through the ligament and the long suture ends are tagged with a hemostat. The supraspinatus tendon and bursa are then exposed and the injury is evaluated.

If sutures are used to repair the tear, the acromion must be prepared. If acromioplasty is required after resection of the joint capsule, it may be necessary for the surgeon to perform an osteotomy at the superior acromion and incise the anterior acromion. The cut surfaces are remodeled to remove any spurs or other rough spots on the bone. This technique can also be applied in arthroscopic surgery. Several small holes are made in the surface of the humerus with an awl or drill. Braided polyester sutures are passed through the bone and the tendon; two lines of sutures may be placed. The suture ends are left long and tagged with hemostats. This step is repeated until all sutures are in place. The arm then is raised and the shoulder is adducted to reduce tension on the suture line. The sutures are then tied.

Newer techniques for rotator cuff repair involve the use of biosynthetic or collagen material, which is secured over the repair site to strengthen the tissue. If anchor screws are used for the repair, pilot holes are drilled before insertion of three or more anchors, depending on the size of the tear. The anchor is implanted and the sutures are drawn through the edge of the tendon and then tied. If the deltoid muscle was severed, it is reattached to the acromion with several heavy sutures passed through drill holes. The wound is irrigated with antibiotic solution, and bleeding is controlled with the ESU.

The incision is closed with 2-0 and 3-0 absorbable suture. The subcutaneous tissue is closed with staples or 4-0 absorbable suture and Steri-Strips. The incision is covered with 4 × 4 gauze and a bulky dressing and is immobilized with a sling or shoulder immobilizer. A repair using collagen patch material is illustrated in Figure 31-46.

PLATING OF THE PROXIMAL HUMERUS

Surgical Goal

A fracture of the proximal humerus is repaired using open reduction and internal fixation. A metal plate is secured across the fracture with locking screws.

Pathology

A direct blow to the proximal humerus may result from a fall. This type of injury is common among older people. Other accidents, such as a fall from a horse or during construction work, are also common causes. Only about 20% of proximal humeral fractures require open reduction or pinning. Most heal with immobilization.

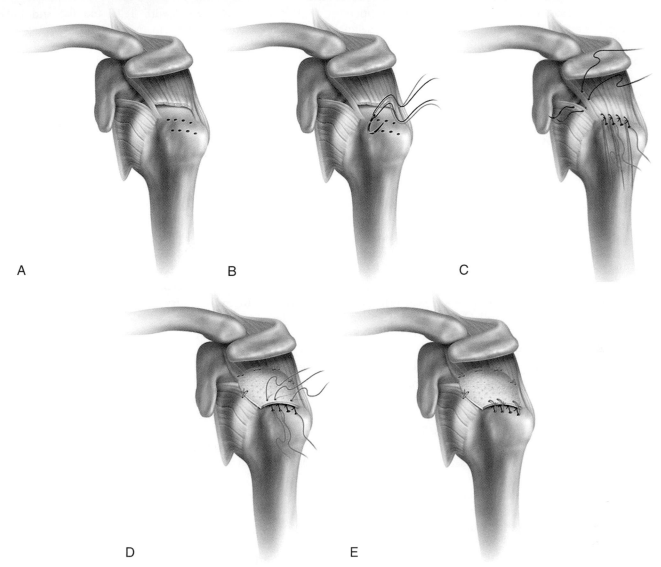

Figure 31-46 **Rotator cuff repair. A,** Preparation of the humerus. Holes are made with a drill or an awl. **B,** Insertion of Mersilene or braided nylon sutures through the bone holes. **C,** The rotator cuff tendon is attached. Additional sutures are placed through the rotator cuff gap *(top)*. **D,** A collagen patch is trimmed and fitted over the repair site. Additional sutures are placed. **E,** Completed repair. *(Courtesy Zimmer, Warsaw, Ind.)*

TECHNIQUE

1. The patient is placed in the beach chair position and prepped for a shoulder procedure.
2. An anterior deltopectoral approach is used.
3. The fracture is reduced and stabilized with K-wires.
4. K-wires are placed in the proximal and distal screw holes with a drill guide.
5. Screw holes are drilled and measured. Screws are inserted and hand-tightened.
6. The K-wires are removed and locking caps are placed on each screw.
7. The wound is irrigated and closed in layers.

Discussion

Humeral plating is a method of restoring continuity after a displaced fracture of the proximal humerus. A number of systems are available. Cannulated screws or a screw-plate combination are commonly used. Plates may be fixed to the lateral side of the humerus, with additional smaller plates on the anterior side.

The instruments required are a basic orthopedic set, power drill, Kirschner wires, and the implant plates and screws, plus any specialty instruments packaged with the plate set (i.e., a drill guide, screwdriver, and bone spacers). C-arm fluoroscopy is needed and the equipment should be adjusted and draped before the start of the case.

The patient is placed in a supine or semi-Fowler position, and a general anesthetic is administered. An anterior (delto-pectoral) approach is used to expose the humerus (see the description of the Bankart procedure). Rake and right angle retractors are placed in the wound.

The fracture is reduced by manipulation and then stabilized with 2-mm K-wires or heavy synthetic sutures. At least two or three wires are used. These are inserted with the power drill. The plate then is fitted over the curve of the proximal humerus and temporarily attached with a K-wire.

A bone spacer may be used, depending on the surgeon's preference. Spacers elevate the plate slightly to prevent direct contact with the periosteum, which can compromise the blood supply to the fracture during healing. Spacers are available in thicknesses of 1 to 3 mm. The position of the plate is assessed fluoroscopically. If the reduction is satisfactory, screws may be inserted.

In preparation for setting the screw holes and fixing the plate, the scrub should have drill bits, a screw rack, drill guide, screwdriver, and depth gauge available. The drill guide and drill bit are needed to drill the screw holes. The drill guide fits over the plate and guides the angle of insertion. The screw holes are drilled under fluoroscopy. A depth gauge is used to measure the depth of the hole and the screw length required. The screws are selected, measured, and implanted; a torque screwdriver is used to hand-tighten the screws. The same technique is used for proximal and distal screws. The K-wires are removed.

The last step in the procedure is to set the locking caps on the screws. This is done with the torque screwdriver. The bone spacers then can be removed and replaced with additional screws. Surgical options include the use of a small bendable side plate that is attached to the main plate with wire and to the bone with small screws. The technique is illustrated in Figure 31-47.

The wound is dressed with Telfa and flat and fluffed gauze for protection. The arm may be put in a sling or an immobilizer.

Physical therapy is required to regain flexibility and strength in the shoulder. Adhesions (scarring) and limited range of motion may result in a stiff arm. Healing normally occurs within about 12 weeks.

SHOULDER ARTHROSCOPY

Surgical Goal

The surgical goals are the same as for open procedures and depend on the nature of the injury.

Pathology

An arthroscopic approach can be used for most types of shoulder injury and disease, except for total joint arthroplasty procedures and when the injury is extensive and wider exposure is needed.

Discussion

The patient is placed in the semi-Fowler or lateral position. The shoulder and arm are prepped and draped free or suspended with a shoulder distractor. A marking pen is used to identify the bony landmarks. The surgeon uses an 18-gauge spinal needle and 60 mL of saline with or without epinephrine to infiltrate and expand the joint space. A small puncture is then made with a #11 blade, and the inflow cannula is inserted.

Irrigation is connected, and the tubing is unclamped. While the joint is being infiltrated, a second incision is made. The scope sleeve and the 30-degree scope are inserted, and the biceps tendon is identified. Figure 31-48 illustrates the placement of the operative scopes and instruments during a routine shoulder arthroscopy.

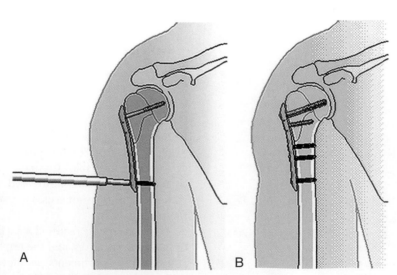

A

B

Figure 31-47 **Proximal plating of the humerus. A,** Bicortical screws are inserted into the proximal and distal ends of the plate. **B,** Completed repair. *(Courtesy Zimmer, Warsaw, Ind.)*

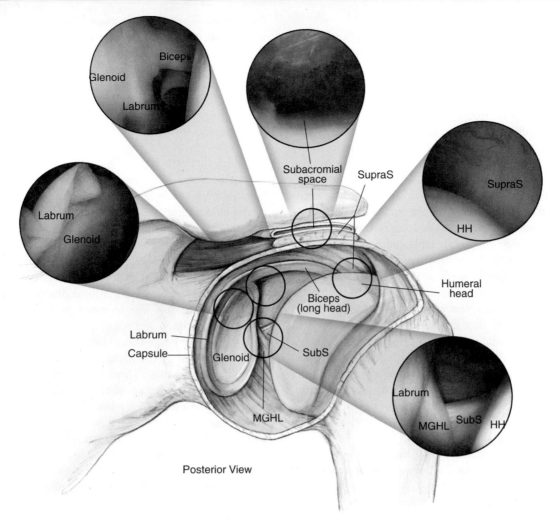

Figure 31-48 **Arthroscopy of the shoulder.** Posterior view for procedures of the glenohumeral joint and subacromial space. *HH,* Humeral head; *MGHL,* medial glenohumeral ligament; *SubS,* subscapularis; *SupraS,* suprascapularis. *(From Miller MD, Chhabra AB, Hurwitz SR, Mihalko WM: Orthopaedic surgical approaches, Philadelphia, 2008, WB Saunders.)*

The patient's arm is rotated and moved as needed to allow the surgeon to visualize the various structures in and around the joint. The shoulder is irrigated, incisions are closed with 4-0 nylon sutures, flat dressings are applied, and either a shoulder immobilizer or an arm sling is applied.

SHOULDER ARTHROPLASTY

Surgical Goal
During total shoulder arthroplasty, the humeral head and glenoid capsule are replaced with artificial components to restore function and relieve pain. In hemiarthroplasty, only the humeral component is replaced.

Pathology
The indications for shoulder arthroplasty are persistent pain that is not relieved by more conservative surgery and inability to perform activities of daily living because of loss of function. Osteoarthritis is the primary cause of these symptoms.

Rheumatoid arthritis, traumatic arthritis, and shoulder instability related to rotator cuff disease are less commonly indicated for joint replacement.

TECHNIQUE
1. An anterolateral incision is made in the shoulder and carried to the glenohumeral joint.
2. The shoulder is dislocated.
3. The humeral head is resected.
4. The humeral shaft is reamed and shaped to receive the implant.
5. The humeral implant is inserted with or without cement.
6. The glenoid fossa is assessed and osteophytes are removed. The rim is lowered as necessary.
7. Holes or a trough is drilled into the fossa as required to receive the glenoid component.
8. The glenoid component is cemented in place.
9. The joint is reduced.
10. The wound is closed.

Discussion

Many shoulder replacement systems are available. The appropriate system for any patient depends on the pathology, the condition of the tissues at the time of surgery, and the patient's age and level of activity. A total joint system includes a humeral component, which is similar to the femoral component used in hip arthroplasty. The stem portion may be press-fit or cemented. The glenoid component is replaced with a pegged cup, usually constructed of polyethylene. Figure 31-49 shows a total shoulder system (the Zimmer Anatomical Shoulder).

In preparation for shoulder arthroplasty, the surgical technologist should have all the components and sizers needed for the selected system. A major orthopedic set and shoulder instruments are added and ample table room should be provided to accommodate the instrument trays. A pneumatic oscillating saw is needed to perform the osteotomy. Reamers are required for medullary canalization of the humerus. **Broaches** (fin-shaped rasps that closely match the contour of the medullary implant) that fit the specific system implant are also needed for canalization. If a cemented prosthesis is planned, provisions should be made for these components (e.g., mixer, tubing). A magnetic instrument pad should be used to prevent instruments placed on the surgical field from falling. ESU and suction are used continuously during the procedure and holsters should be provided for these on the field.

A total arthroplasty procedure has three parts: the approach to the joint, replacement of the humerus, and replacement of

the glenoid. The patient is placed in a semi-Fowler position with the affected side near the edge of the operating table. The shoulder and upper body are prepped as previously described. An anterior (deltopectoral) approach is most commonly used for the procedure. The incision extends to the joint capsule, which is incised to allow the humerus to be lifted from the glenoid fossa. Slotted retractors and a bone hook may be used to release the humerus.

Humeral Component

With the humerus removed from the glenoid fossa, the humeral neck can be severed. A template measuring device is placed either directly over the humerus or over the x-ray to determine the angle of osteotomy (bone cut). The surgeon can mark the cutting line with the ESU. The technologist should have a sagittal saw and irrigation prepared at this point. A retractor may be placed under the humerus to protect the soft tissues during the osteotomy. The sagittal saw then is used to divide the humerus. The removed portion is passed to the scrub as a specimen and may be used during bone grafting.

The medullary canal is prepared for reaming by delivering the humerus out of the incision. A pilot hole is made in the cancellous bone with a small reamer and increasingly larger reamers (8 to 12 mm) are used to enter the medullary canal. An osteotome is used to remove a "fin" of bone to fit the shape of the prosthesis. When the cancellous bone has been penetrated, modular broaches are used to form a space for the humeral stem. When the last modular rasp has been used, it is left in place. Test heads are fitted onto the modular rasp with the attachments specific to the system used. The modular broach then is removed and the actual head component is assembled.

The humeral component now can be inserted. Before insertion, pulse lavage is used to irrigate the medullary canal and clean it of all debris. Antibiotic solution may be used for irrigation.

NOTE: Sutures used to repair the subscapularis may be placed just before the prosthesis is fitted into the canal. Several drill holes are made in the neck of the humerus and Mersilene or other braided suture is passed through the holes. The sutures are tied during closure.

The stem is fitted to the system impactor (driver), and the prosthesis is inserted into the canal with or without bone cement, depending on the type of implant used. Bone or biosynthetic material may be used to fill in any gaps in a press-fit prosthesis. When the prosthesis is fully seated, the impactor is removed and the ball prosthesis is fitted on the stem. If a hemiarthroplasty is planned, the humerus can be replaced in the glenoid cavity by manipulation.

Glenoid Component

When complete arthroplasty is planned, the disarticulated joint is examined before the glenoid side is prepared. The glenoid rim often needs to be trimmed and osteophytes and other bony growths must be removed. The fossa can be lowered (the rim taken down) with rongeurs or by reaming the fossa with a high-speed burr or cup-shaped reamers.

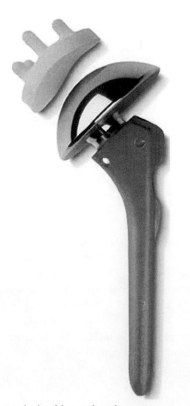

Figure 31-49 Total shoulder arthroplasty components. *(Courtesy Zimmer, Warsaw, Ind.)*

Two types of glenoid prostheses are commonly used, a pegged design or a keeled design. Holes may be drilled to accommodate a pegged component. Pegged systems provide a drill guide for exact placement of the holes. For a keeled component, a trough is drilled with a high-speed drill and round burr. After creation of the holes or trough, the surface is cleaned with pulse lavage. If a cemented prosthesis is used, the cement may be impacted into the peg holes with a sponge and hemostat. The prosthesis is fitted into the holes and held in place manually or with a system tool until the cement has set. Before the humerus is replaced in the glenoid, the joint is irrigated and all bits of cement are removed from the field. The scrub assists by making sure all debris has been removed from the drapes and that fresh sponges are supplied. The joint then is reduced and assessed for mobility and function.

The incision is closed in layers. The subscapularis sutures are secured, and the rotator cuff is closed with synthetic non-absorbable sutures. The superficial layers are closed with absorbable synthetic sutures. A suction drain may be placed before closure. The wound is dressed with Kerlix fluffs and an abdominal pad. A shoulder brace is applied for stability. Shoulder arthroplasty is illustrated in Figure 31-50.

Patients begin passive range-of-motion exercises within 24 hours of surgery. A rigorous physiotherapy routine is begun within the first week and continues for 3 to 6 months.

ELBOW ARTHROPLASTY

Surgical Goal

Elbow arthroplasty is performed to relieve pain and restore function to the elbow (Figure 31-51).

Pathology

Arthroplasty of the elbow most often is performed to treat rheumatoid arthritis or a severe traumatic injury.

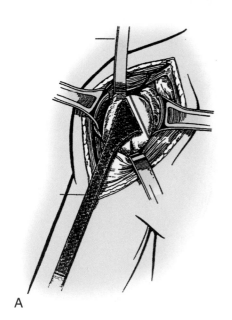

A

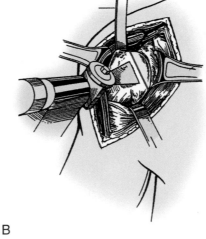

B

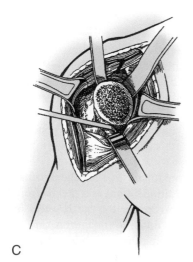

C

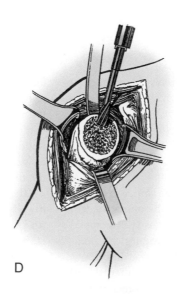

D

Figure 31-50 Shoulder arthroplasty. **A,** The humeral head is measured for an osteotomy with a template. **B,** A sagittal saw is used to perform the osteotomy. **C,** The cut surface of the humerus. **D,** Reamers are used to penetrate the cancellous bone.

Continued

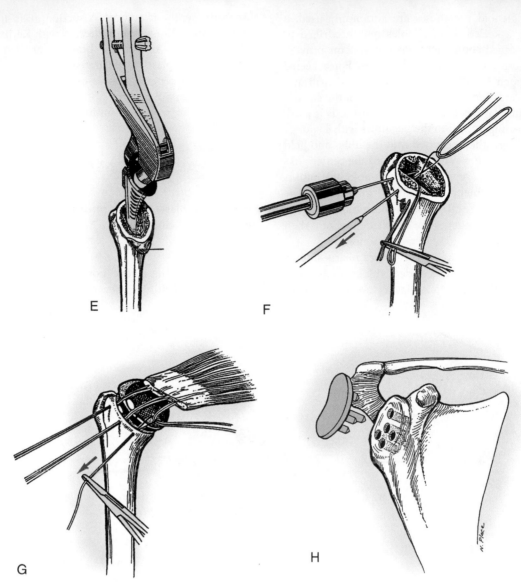

Figure 31-50, cont'd   **E,** Modular broaches are used to form a space for the humeral stem. **F,** Holes are drilled in the humeral neck and sutures are threaded through them. **G,** After the humeral implant is inserted, the sutures are used to secure the subscapular tendon. **H,** Placement of the glenoid component. *(From Matsen FA III, Rockwood CA Jr, Wirth MA, et al: Glenohumeral arthritis and its management. In Rockwood CA Jr, Matsen FA III, Wirth MA, et al, editors: The shoulder, ed 3, Philadelphia, 2004, WB Saunders.)*

Discussion

Elbow arthroplasty is a procedure that currently is in development, and is performed much less often than shoulder or knee reconstruction.

The instruments required for elbow arthroplasty include an orthopedic set, power drill, K-wires, Steinmann pins, pulse lavage, and the selected joint replacement system. A general anesthetic is used.

A pneumatic tourniquet is applied to the upper arm. The patient is placed in the supine position and the operative arm and hand are prepped and draped. The hand is usually wrapped with an occlusive drape to exclude it from the surgical site.

The surgeon makes a posteromedial incision at the elbow. The ulnar nerve is identified and protected. The medial half of the triceps is elevated and the tip of the olecranon is removed. The medial collateral ligament is released to improve exposure. The forearm then is rotated in the lateral position to produce exposure of the distal humerus. An oscillating saw is used to remove a portion of the trochlea. Access to the medullary canal of the humerus is complete. An IM canal finder is inserted and exchanged for an alignment stem with an attached cutting block. An oscillating saw is used to remove the distal humerus.

The surgeon enters the medullary canal of the ulna using a high-speed drill or burr. Additional bone is removed from the tip of the olecranon to make room for the reamers. After reaming, a rasp is impacted into the ulna, with care taken to prevent a proximal ulnar fracture or other complication. The medullary canal is then irrigated to remove all tissue fragments.

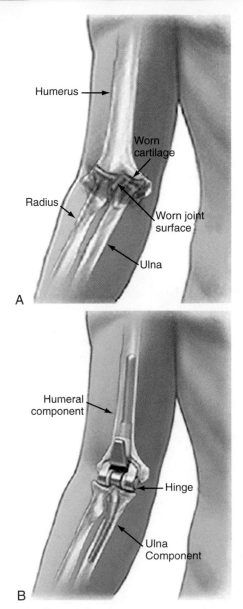

Figure 31-51 Elbow arthroplasty. A, Areas of worn cartilage. **B,** Implant design. *(Courtesy Zimmer, Warsaw, Ind.)*

After the humerus and ulna have been prepared, the surgeon inserts the trials. When the trials are in place, range of motion, including flexion and extension, is tested. The trials are removed and the surgical site is irrigated.

Bone cement is mixed and placed in a cement gun for injection into the humeral and ulnar canals. Bone grafts are placed in any open spaces and behind the humeral implant. The bone graft helps the humerus resist posterior and rotational displacement. The humeral implant is impacted and the ulnar implant is inserted.

When the bone cement has cured, the tourniquet is deflated and hemostasis is obtained with the ESU. The surgical site then is irrigated with an antibiotic irrigant. The incision is closed, a dressing is applied, and the elbow is placed in neutral position with a posterior splint and an arm sling.

SURGICAL APPROACHES TO THE WRIST AND HAND

Wrist and hand surgery is a specialty that combines orthopedics, vascular surgery, and neurosurgery. Technological advances in instrumentation within the past 15 years have greatly improved recovery after complex hand trauma and soft tissue diseases such as fascia contraction and nerve entrapment. Innovative joint replacement procedures are now common for the treatment of joint diseases, such as degenerative and rheumatoid arthritis.

The arm and hand are prepped using standard techniques. The hand may require scrubbing to remove dirt, especially from under the fingernails. Trauma cases involving shards of glass, metal, wood, or other foreign objects that are embedded in soft tissue require more complex **debridement** and lavage. This usually is performed outside the operating room, often in the emergency department. Industrial accidents may result in tissue injection of oil and other chemicals, which also require extensive debridement.

A regional or local anesthetic is used for most hand surgery. A combination of lidocaine and a long-acting local anesthetic (e.g., bupivacaine) is commonly used. Vasoconstrictive agents (e.g., epinephrine) are not used, because they can cause damage to delicate vessels and nerves. A pneumatic tourniquet is used for all hand cases.

Short plastic surgery instruments are used for all hand procedures. Delicate orthopedic instruments are required for joint and trauma surgery involving bone. A small drill and fine Steinmann pins or K-wires are commonly used for internal fixation. Reconstruction procedures require small vascular clamps and short right angle clamps. The bipolar ESU with a fine-needle point and bipolar forceps is used to prevent lateral heating. Silastic vessel loops are used to retract tendons and ligaments. The surgeon may use magnifying loupes or the operating microscope during surgery. Instruments commonly used in hand surgery are shown in Figure 31-52.

Delicate tendons, ligaments, nerves, and blood vessels are critical for precise movement of the hand. These tissues must be kept moist during surgery. The surgical technologist assisting in hand procedures irrigates the surgical wound with saline. A small bulb syringe or standard syringe fitted with an irrigation tip may be used. Low-pressure suction with fine angled suction tips is used to prevent injury to the tissue. Neurosurgical patties and small gauze sponges dipped in saline are also required.

In reconstructive hand surgery, sutures are required for tendon, nerve, and ligament repair. These tissues must heal with as little scar formation as possible to preserve function. Inert suture materials, such as 6-0 and 7-0 polypropylene (Prolene), stainless steel, and polyester (Ti-Cron), are commonly used. A fine ⅜ cutting curve is commonly used. Vascular sutures are required for trauma, reconstruction, and **replantation**, also called *reimplantation* (reattachment of a digit or a portion of the hand). Sutures of 5-0 and 7-0 polyester and polypropylene are commonly used. Double-arm sutures are used for anastomosis of vessels, tendons, and nerves. Figure 31-53 presents an anterior view of the hand.

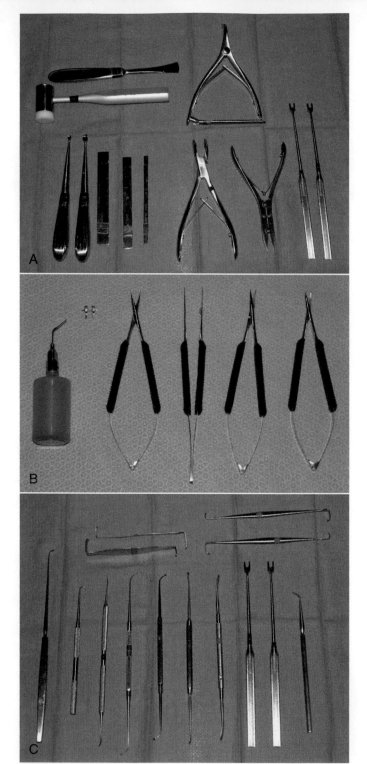

Figure 31-52 **A,** Small bone instruments used in hand surgery. **B,** Selected microinstruments. **C,** Dental and ear, nose, and throat (ENT) instruments useful in hand surgery. *(From Canale S, Beaty J: Campbell's operative orthopaedics, ed 11, St Louis, 2007, Mosby.)*

OPEN REDUCTION AND INTERNAL FIXATION OF THE WRIST

Surgical Goal

Screws or pins are used to repair a fracture of the wrist to stabilize the bone fragments so that healing can occur in the correct anatomical position.

Pathology

The scaphoid is the most common site of a wrist fracture because of its vulnerable location. A common cause of fracture is a fall when the wrists are flexed to break the impact. Simple nondisplaced fractures are treated with casting. Open reduction and internal fixation are required for a displaced fracture.

Discussion

One or more cannulated screws are used for fixation of the scaphoid. The Herbert screw, the Synthes 3.0 cannulated screw, or Steinmann pins are surgical options. C-arm fluoroscopy should be available for the procedure.

The patient is placed in the supine position with the operative arm on a hand table. A tourniquet is applied and the hand and arm are prepped and draped in routine manner. The instruments required for insertion of a cannulated or Herbert screw include a minor orthopedic set, a small drill, K-wires, and a screw system. A compression fracture may require bone grafting.

Exposure

A rolled towel may be placed under the wrist to stabilize it or the hand may be placed in a distractor. A common approach for repair is the volar approach (Figure 31-54). The surgeon makes a small incision over the scaphoid bone and inserts two rake retractors to expose the flexor carpi muscle. This is divided with a curved hemostat and scissors. The tendon sheath is incised and the flexor tendon is isolated and retracted. Depending on the approach, a branch of the radial artery may be encountered. This is divided and ligated with 3-0 or 4-0 nonabsorbable suture. The joint capsule then is incised to expose the scaphoid bone. A small Weitlaner retractor is placed in the wound and Homan small bone elevators used to expose the fractured bone.

Cannulated Screw and Threaded Washer

The cannulated screw and washer set includes instruments required for the procedure described here. The fracture is reduced under fluoroscopy to ensure correct alignment. For placement of a cannulated screw, a threaded guidewire is inserted over the fracture site. A drill sleeve may be used to direct the wire at the correct angle. The screw hole may be predrilled with a small power drill and cannulated drill bit. A space for the threaded washer also is created.

The washer is inserted with the cannulated driver. A measuring device similar to a drill tap is inserted over the guidewire to measure the depth of the predrilled hole and washer. The screw is threaded over the guidewire and tightened with

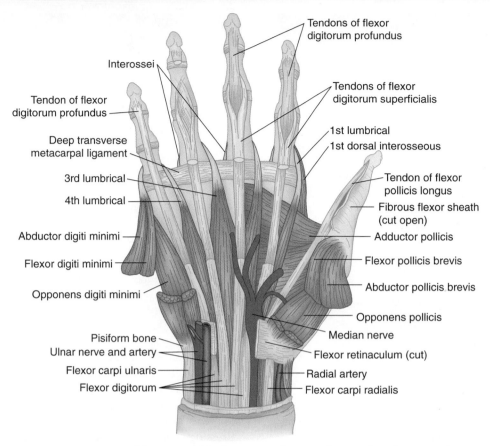

Figure 31-53 **Anatomy of the anterior hand.** *(From Snell RS, Smith MS: Clinical anatomy for emergency medicine, St Louis, 1993, Mosby.)*

a screwdriver. The guidewire is removed by using the power drill in reverse mode.

The wound is irrigated and closed in layers. The capsule is closed with 4-0 synthetic absorbable suture. Skin and subcutaneous tissue are closed with 4-0 nonabsorbable sutures. The wound is dressed with flat gauze. A plaster cast usually is applied over the wrist and arm.

CARPAL TUNNEL RELEASE

Surgical Goal
The goal of surgical carpal tunnel release is to free an entrapped median volar nerve and restore function of the wrist. An open or a minimally invasive technique may be used. Arthroscopic instruments used in carpal tunnel release are shown in Figure 31-55.

Pathology
Carpal tunnel syndrome occurs when the median nerve in the carpal tunnel of the wrist is compressed. A variety of factors may contribute to nerve compression. These include an anatomical decrease in the size of the carpal tunnel, wrist fracture, post-traumatic arthritis, and inflammatory disease, such as rheumatoid arthritis. External conditions, such as vibration, prolonged direct pressure, and repetitive movement, may contribute to or trigger the condition. Carpal tunnel syndrome

occurs most often in adults 30 to 60 years of age and is more common in women than in men. Patients experience numbness and tingling in the fingers and pain in the hand that often radiates up the forearm.

TECHNIQUE

1. A curvilinear or longitudinal incision is made in the palm and extended to the wrist.
2. The carpal ligament is retracted and divided.
3. The tourniquet is deflated and the wound is inspected for bleeding.
4. Hemostasis is maintained.
5. The wound is closed.
6. A compression bandage and splint are applied.

Discussion
The patient is positioned supine on the operating room table with the affected arm resting on a hand table. The procedure is performed using local infiltration, a regional nerve block (Bier block), or general anesthesia. A pneumatic tourniquet is used to create a bloodless field. The open technique is described here.

The surgeon uses a #15 blade to create a longitudinal or curvilinear incision in the skin (Figure 31-56). Blunt dissection with small Metzenbaum scissors exposes the fascia, which

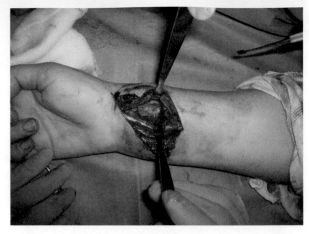

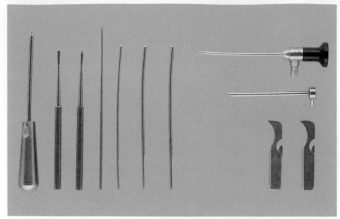

Figure 31-55 Arthroscopic carpal tunnel instruments. *Left to right,* 1 obturator; 2 dissectors; 1 probe; 3 Hegar dilators; small arthroscope and handles for carpal tunnel blades. *(From Tighe SM: Instrumentation for the operating room, ed 6, St Louis, 2003, Mosby.)*

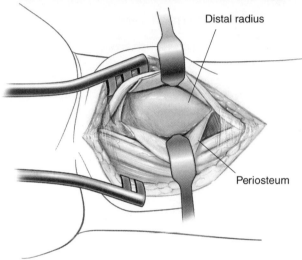

Figure 31-54 Volar approach to the hand. *(From Miller MD, Chhabra AB, Hurwitz SR, Mihalko WM: Orthopaedic surgical approaches, Philadelphia, 2008, WB Saunders.)*

is retracted with small Weitlaner retractors, skin hooks, or sharp Senn retractors. The flexor tendon is exposed and retracted. The surgeon identifies both the flexor tendon and the neurovascular bundle that lies close to the tendon.

The carpal ligament then is well visualized and the midsection is cut either with scissors or with a knife blade to release the carpal ligament and median nerve. The incision is irrigated with sterile saline.

The tourniquet pressure is released and the wound is checked for bleeders, which are controlled with the bipolar ESU. The surgeon may inject the incision with bupivacaine to control postoperative pain. The skin is closed with an absorbable subcuticular suture. A bulky compression dressing using gauze fluffs and a splint is applied.

Arthroscopic Technique

Carpal tunnel release may also be performed as an MIS using Endowrist instruments. The anesthesia considerations, prepping, draping, and tourniquet use are as described for open carpal tunnel release. An advantage of the endoscopic approach is that it uses one or two small incisions over the palm of the

hand instead of the extensive incision described for the open approach. The carpal ligament is directly below the incisions, in the distal area of the palm just below the wrist. The carpal ligament is cut longitudinally. This releases the pressure on the nerve as it passes through the ligament. Wound closure and dressing application are as described for the open technique.

Carpal tunnel release most often is performed in the outpatient setting and the patient is discharged within hours of the procedure. Immediate and long-term postoperative complications are rare.

METACARPOPHALANGEAL JOINT ARTHROPLASTY

Surgical Goal

The surgical goal of metacarpophalangeal (MCP) joint arthroplasty is to eliminate pain and align the joints, producing joint stability.

Pathology

The primary cause of MCP joint disease in adults is advanced rheumatoid arthritis.

Discussion

The patient is placed in the supine position with the affected arm extended on an arm table. A tourniquet is applied. The arm is prepped from the fingertips to the elbow. The arm then is draped with an extremity drape. A small bone set, the implant instruments, and a microburr are needed.

A transverse incision is made over the dorsum of the metacarpals, exposing the tendon. Note that a volar (palm side) approach may be used. Tenotomy scissors and a # 15 blade are used to release the extensor tendon. The joint capsule and collateral ligaments are elevated on both sides of the metacarpal and on the proximal phalanx. A microsaw is used to resect the metacarpal head. Two small (Hohmann) retractors should be placed under the bone to protect the underlying tissue

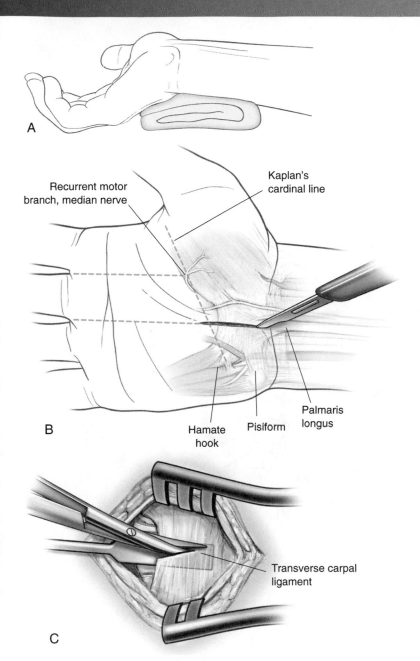

A

Recurrent motor
branch, median nerve

Kaplan's
cardinal line

Hamate
hook

Pisiform

Palmaris
longus

B

Transverse carpal
ligament

C

Figure 31-56 **Open carpal tunnel release. A,** Position on
the hand. **B,** Skin incision and anatomy. **C,** Exposure of the
median nerve with fine dissecting scissors. *(From Miller MD,
Chhabra AB, Hurwitz SR, Mihalko WM: Orthopaedic surgical approaches, Philadelphia, 2008, WB Saunders.)*

when the saw is used. A small diamond rasp is used to smooth
the ends of the bones.

The surgeon uses a microburr to enter the medullary canal.
This burr also widens the canal for the implant. When the
intramedullary canal is open, trials are used to measure the
implant size and the site is irrigated. The implants are inserted,
the joint is again irrigated, and the wound is closed. Dressings
are applied and the hand is placed in a posterior splint with
the finger or fingers held in extension. This procedure is illustrated in Figure 31-57.

DUPUYTREN CONTRACTURE

Surgical Goal
Constricted palmar fascia is incised and released to restore
mobility to the hand and fingers.

Pathology
A Dupuytren contracture is a common condition in which the
fascia of the palm or fingers contracts. The disorder has a
strong familial component, particularly when the onset is in
younger men. The deformity progresses rapidly.

Discussion
The patient is placed in the supine position with the operative
arm on an arm board. A Bier block or general anesthetic may
be used. The hand and lower arm are prepped and draped.

The surgeon uses a #15 blade to make the incision on the
ulnar side of the palmar fascia, as well as the apex of the fascia.
Tenotomy scissors and fine forceps are used to dissect the
tissue and expose the tendons. After the tendons have been
freed and the fingers can be moved without impingement,
the tourniquet is released and the wound is checked for

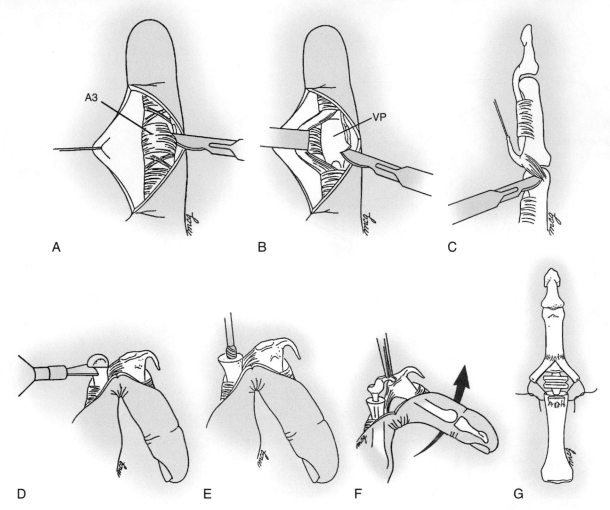

Figure 31-57   Metacarpophalangeal (MCP) joint arthroplasty. A, A V-shaped incision is made to expose the flexor tendon and A3 pulley. **B,** The flexor tendon is retracted to expose the volar plate. **C,** The collateral ligaments are released. **D,** The articular surface is exposed. **E,** The medullary canal is prepared. **F,** Trial implants and the permanent implant are inserted. **G,** The ligaments are reconstructed. *(From Canale S, Beaty J: Campbell's operative orthopaedics, ed 11, St Louis, 2007, Mosby.)*

hemostasis and then irrigated. The skin is closed with interrupted nonabsorbable sutures. A bulky compression dressing using gauze fluffs is applied.

SURGICAL APPROACHES TO THE HIP AND PELVIS

FEMORAL NECK FRACTURES

Surgical Goal

A combination femoral plate and compression lag screw (intertrochanteric component) are inserted to stabilize a fracture of the femoral neck or proximal femur. Fractures that occur above the trochanter also may be repaired with a cannulated screw system using a similar technique.

Pathology

The femoral neck (trochanter) is a common site of injury in a fall. The fracture may occur alone or may be accompanied by

a fracture of the femur itself. Figure 31-58 illustrates common femoral neck fractures.

TECHNIQUE

1. A lateral or posterolateral incision is made over the hip.
2. A guide pin is inserted into the trochanter.
3. The pin is measured for length.
4. A cannulated reamer is fitted over the pin.
5. A lag (compression) screw is inserted through the trochanter.
6. The plate component is fitted over the screw and advanced.
7. The guide pin is removed.
8. Screw holes are drilled and screws are inserted into the side plate.
9. The lag screw is removed.
10. The wound is closed.

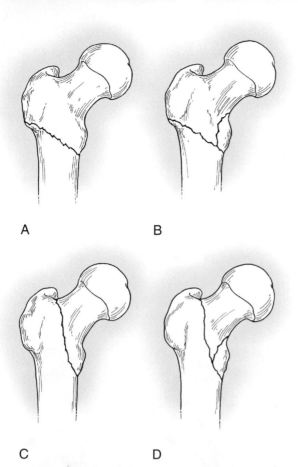

A   B

C   D

Figure 31-58 **Femoral neck fractures. A** does not involve the trochanter. **B** extends below the trochanter. **C** does not involve the lesser trochanter. **D** extends into the lesser trochanter. *(From Canale S, Beaty J: Campbell's operative orthopaedics, ed 11, St Louis, 2007, Mosby.)*

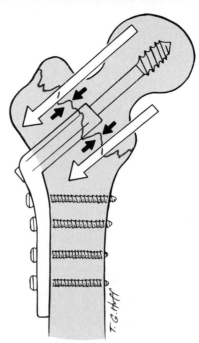

Figure 31-59 **Compression screw-plate system.** A plate-tube assembly is inserted through the trochanter and a compression screw is inserted through the trochanter to pull the fragments together. The screw is then removed. *(From Browner B, Jupiter J, Levine A, Trafton P: Skeletal trauma: basic science, management, and reconstruction, ed 3, Philadelphia, 2003, WB Saunders.)*

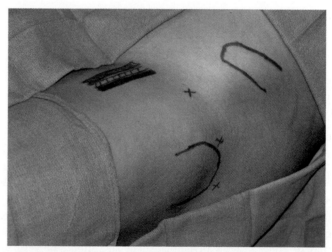

Figure 31-60 **Exposure and alignment of the leg for hip surgery using a fracture table.** *(From Canale S, Beaty J: Campbell's operative orthopaedics, ed 11, St Louis, 2007, Mosby.)*

Discussion

A number of options are available for surgical treatment of a fracture of the femoral neck (located across the trochanter or the neck itself). These include:

- Compression screw and plate system
- Dynamic compression screws alone
- Arthroplasty

A procedure using a compression screw and sliding plate (Figure 31-59) is discussed here. The instruments and supplies needed for the procedure include a major orthopedic set, a drill, K-wires, Steinmann pins, and a screw-plate system. The orthopedic table is used, with the lower extremities in abduction and the affected leg in traction (Figure 31-60). C-arm fluoroscopy and an image intensifier are used intermittently during the procedure.

A general anesthetic is administered and the patient is placed in position for traction. The fracture is reduced using table traction and the position is verified on fluoroscopy. The operative leg is prepped from the lower leg to the chest. The leg is draped with wide exposure.

A lateral or posterolateral incision is used for surgical treatment of a hip fracture (Figure 31-61). Rake retractors are placed in the wound and the ESU is used to divide the subcutaneous tissue and fascia. The muscle then is divided and

retracted. Richardson, Army-Navy, Hibbs, or Deaver retractors may be used for deep retraction.

A guide pin is inserted to establish the correct angle for the trochanter compression screw and plate. A Steinmann (guide) pin and drill are used for this purpose. The guide pin remains in place during most of the procedure, and cannulated instruments are inserted over it. For insertion of the guide pin, a 6.4-mm drill bit is used to make a pilot hole in line with the femoral neck. An angle guide is used to obtain the correct angle of the guide pin. The pin then is drilled following the angle of the guide, viewed under fluoroscopy. Next, the depth

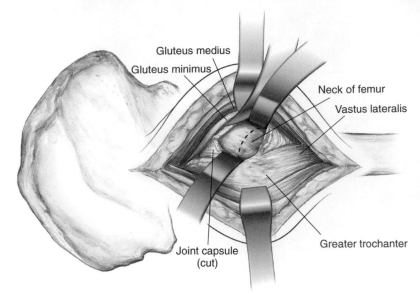

Figure 31-61 Lateral approach to the hip. Tissue layers usually are thin. After the skin incision has been made, the subcutaneous, fascial, and muscle layers are quickly incised with the electrosurgical unit. Note the position of the Hibbs retractor *(top)*. Narrow Deaver or Richardson retractors also are used at this level. *(From Miller MD, Chhabra AB, Hurwitz SR, Mihalko WM: Orthopaedic surgical approaches, Philadelphia, 2008, WB Saunders.)*

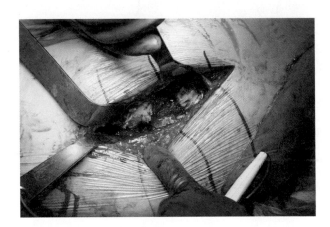

of the guide pin is determined with a cannulated depth gauge. An appropriately sized reamer is used to drill over the guide pin according to the depth gauge measurement. This is the starter channel, or tap. A long reamer designed for lag screw insertion is calibrated for the channel, which then is reamed to the appropriate depth. The reamer is cannulated and fits over the guidewire during this process. The angle of the pin may be checked with a trial plate. The size should be verified with the surgeon before the sterile implant is opened. The scrub may receive the plate from the circulator at this time.

The lag screw is inserted with or without pretapping. A calibrated tap drill (reamer) is used as necessary and the reading is taken from the back of the tap. The surgeon then determines the correct size for the lag screw. The plate component is fitted into the lag screw inserter and the T-handle and lag screw are inserted into the assembly. The assembled unit is placed over the guide pin and into the prepared channel. The surgeon advances the lag screw and plate barrel. The guide pin is removed and the traction is released.

The scrub should prepare a drill, drill guide, and drill bit for attaching the side plate to the femur. The surgeon then drills the holes and measures them with a depth gauge. The scrub selects the correct size of screw and passes it with the screwdriver. When the side screws have been placed, an impactor may be used to secure the plate barrel. A compression screw is inserted into the tube and tightened by hand. This brings the femoral neck fragments into contact. The compression screw then is removed.

The wound is irrigated and checked for bleeders. A suction or gravity drain or may be placed in the wound before closure. The muscle is closed with 2-0 or 3-0 interrupted absorbable synthetic sutures. The fascia is closed with running suture of the same material. Subcutaneous tissue is closed with 3-0 absorbable sutures and the skin is approximated with staples. A compression dressing consisting of flat gauze and an abdominal pad is placed over the incision. The steps of the procedure are illustrated in Figure 31-62. A related procedure is repair using a cannulated screw system (Figure 31-63).

The patient usually is able to begin weight bearing within 24 hours after surgery.

INTRAMEDULLARY FEMORAL NAILING

Surgical Goal

A femoral shaft fracture can be repaired with an intramedullary femoral nail. A femoral nail is a rigid rod that is seated in

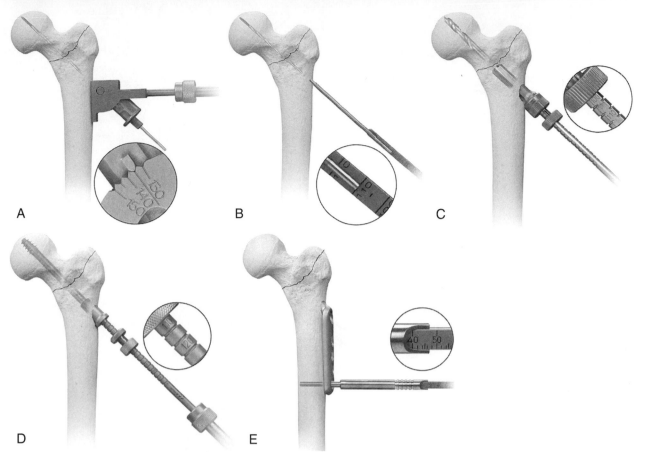

Figure 31-62 Compression screw and plate fixation of a femoral neck fracture. **A**, An angle guide is used to accurately place a Steinmann pin, which is inserted with a drill. **B**, A guide pin depth gauge is used to measure the length of the pin in place. This determines the length of the implant. **C**, A calibrated reamer is used to drill over the guide pin. **D**, Calibrations are shown on the bone tap. **E**, The tube/plate is inserted into the bone, and screw holes are drilled. A depth gauge is used to determine the tap hole depth. *(Courtesy Zimmer, Warsaw, Ind.)*

the medullary canal and held in position with locking screws placed at a 90-degree angle to the nail.

Pathology

The intramedullary technique for repairing a femoral fracture may be used for a comminuted fracture or a proximal and distal fracture.

Discussion

The instruments required for the procedure are an orthopedic set, including hip retractors, a drill, a Steinmann pin set, and a femoral nailing system.

The patient is placed in the supine position on an orthopedic or a standard operating table. A general anesthetic is administered. The operative leg may be placed in traction using the orthopedic table's boot attachment. The position then is assessed fluoroscopically. The prep includes the knee, hip, thigh, buttock, and trunk, including the axilla. Draping is standard, using a large U-drape that extends to the knee. An incision is made over the trochanter and carried through the subcutaneous, fascial, and muscle layers. Richardson or large rake (Israel) retractors are used to expose the trochanter.

An awl is used to form the entry point into the medullary canal. As an alternative, a Steinmann pin can be inserted percutaneously. The awl is rotated to create the entry point. A ball-tip guidewire then is inserted into the canal.

To prepare for medullary reaming, a cannula (metal sleeve) and bushing are placed over the guidewire. The cannula is advanced over the guidewire until it is seated. A cannulated reamer is inserted over the pin to the trochanter. The guidewire then is replaced with a ball-tip wire, which is manipulated into the canal beyond the fracture site. A cannulated nail length gauge is used to measure the depth of the canal. Fluoroscopy is used to assess the position and depth.

Graduated intramedullary reamers are used to increase the space for nail insertion. The technologist should have several reamers of incremental sizes ready for this part of the procedure; sizes 8 to 17 mm in 0.5-mm increments should be available. The first reamer is an 8-mm end-cutting reamer.

When the medullary canal has been prepared, the correct nail is selected and prepared on the back table. An interlocking nail guide is used to align the cross-screw position in the nail. A driver and *slap hammer* attachment are used to drive the nail into the canal while the nail guide maintains correct

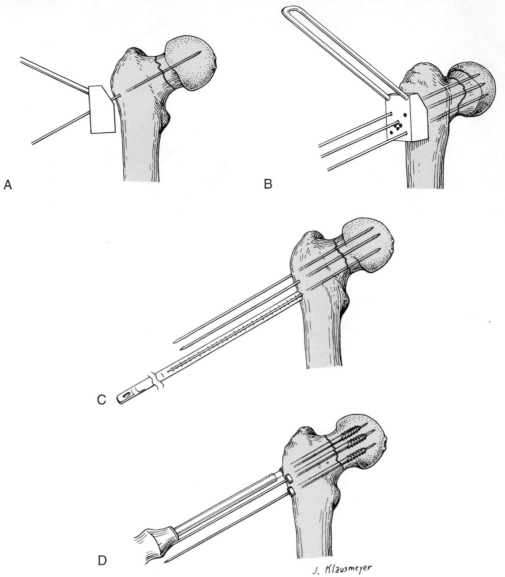

A

B

C

D

J. Klausmeyer

Figure 31-63 Cannulated screw system for a fracture of the trochanter. **A,** The fracture is reduced, and a guidewire (Steinmann pin) is inserted. **B,** Additional guidewires are placed as needed. **C,** A depth gauge is used to determine the length of the pins. **D,** Cannulated screws are placed over the guidewires, which are then removed. *(From Browner B, Jupiter J, Levine A, Trafton P: Skeletal trauma: basic science, management, and reconstruction, ed 3, Philadelphia, 2003, WB Saunders.)*

position. The nail is driven into the medullary canal and the driver is disengaged. Nail caps, if used, are inserted by hand at this time with a nail cap inserter.

A screw guide with protective bushing is inserted into the targeting device and the proximal screw holes are drilled. A depth gauge is used to measure the holes and the appropriately sized screws are placed through the bone and nail by hand. A freehand targeting device is used to locate the distal screw hole with fluoroscopy. The targeting device is positioned over the distal nail hole, and a combination trocar-drill is used to penetrate the bone through the targeting device. The position is confirmed with fluoroscopy. An incision is made over the trocar and the nail hole is located with a hemostat. The trocar is centered in the nail hole and the hole is completed. A depth gauge is used to measure the drill hole and the appropriate-size screw is inserted and hand-tightened.

The scrub and circulator should note the size of the screws and nail used, because these must be documented appropriately. The position of the nail and screws is assessed and the wound is irrigated. All tissue debris is removed from the wound and any potential bleeders are checked with the ESU. The wound is closed with interrupted absorbable synthetic sutures and skin staples. A flat dressing is placed over the incision.

NOTE: *The techniques used in this procedure closely follow those used in tibial nailing, which is discussed later in this chapter.*

Related Procedure: Repair of a Supracondylar Fracture

Distal femoral fractures may be repaired using a lag screw–plate combination. The techniques described previously are used for this procedure. The patient is placed in the supine position with the operative flank raised slightly for better exposure of the distal femur.

HIP ARTHROPLASTY

Surgical Goal

The goal of hip arthroplasty is to replace diseased components of the hip joint, including the acetabulum, trochanter, and ball of the femur, with one or more artificial implants.

Pathology

Hip arthroplasty is performed to treat a number of arthritic conditions:

- *Osteoarthritis:* Results in loss of cartilage and eventual erosion of bone. The disease usually is associated with the aging process.
- *Osteonecrosis:* Death of bone and marrow tissue, usually related to trauma or disease.
- *Acetabular fracture:* Hip trauma, commonly associated with falls and motor vehicle accidents.
- *Femoral neck fracture:* Commonly associated with falls.
- *Avascular necrosis:* Death of bone tissue related to interruption of the blood supply to the hip.

TECHNIQUE

1. An anterior or posterolateral incision is made over the hip.
2. The hip is dislocated.
3. The femoral neck is incised and the ball of the femur is removed.
4. The acetabulum is trimmed and reamed.
5. A trial shell is tested in the acetabulum and the prosthesis is implanted with or without screws.
6. The femoral canal is created with reamers and broaches.
7. The cut end of the femur is trimmed.
8. The trial femoral head is inserted over the broach or femoral implant and tested by reducing the joint.
9. The joint is dislocated and the femoral canal is cleaned.
10. The prosthesis is cemented or press-fitted into place.
11. The wound is irrigated and closed.

Discussion

Many surgical approaches can be used for hip arthroplasty. Aside from variations in the implant design, the main technical differences important to the surgical technologist are:

- One or both components of the hip joint may be replaced.
- The implants may be cemented or press-fitted.
- One or two incisions may be used for the surgical approach.

The surgical options are chosen based on the patient's age and desired level of activity after surgery, the condition of the bone, and the surgeon's specific training.

Hip Components

Modular implant systems for hip arthroplasty include the following components:

- *Femoral component:* Includes the stem, neck, and head. The neck usually is adjustable for angle (called the *offset*) and length. The femoral component may be press-fitted or cemented.

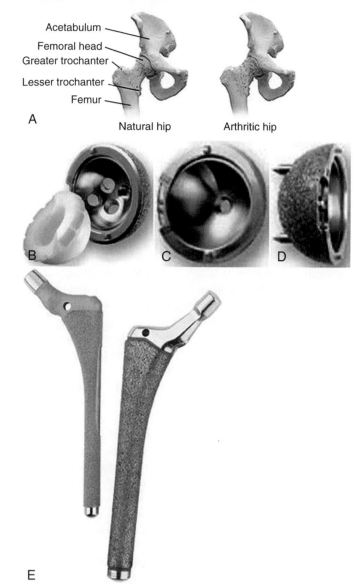

Figure 31-64 **Components of a modular hip arthroplasty.** A, Modular components include the femoral stem, ball, acetabular cup, and polyethylene liner. B, An acetabular cup and liner with screw holes for attachment. C, An acetabular cup with a single screw hole. D, An acetabular cup with pegs. Note the beaded coating. E, Femoral stems. *(Courtesy Zimmer, Warsaw, Ind.)*

- *Acetabular components:* Includes an acetabular liner, which is seated into the prepared acetabulum, and a shell, which fits into the liner. The outside of the shell may be spiked or smooth, or it may have drill holes for screws.

Figure 31-64 shows examples of hip arthroplasty components.

Instruments needed for hip arthroplasty include a standard orthopedic set and hip instruments, including large hip retractors, bone hooks, bone clamps, chisels, and osteotomes. The manufacturer commonly supplies any additional equipment intended for use with a specific type of implant. Special instruments include bone-cutting and measuring devices, an impactor, and screwdrivers. Broaches are used to create a space in the medullary canal for the femoral stem. A power saw and drill are also needed. If a cemented implant is used, components for mixing the cement and an exhaust system are required.

Implants are not opened until the surgeon requests them during surgery. Trial sizers are included in the system setup and are used to test an implant after measurements have been taken and the bone prepared.

The patient is placed in the lateral position and a stabilizing device is used to maintain the position. The skin is prepped from the waist to the foot. Draping exposes the hip and thigh. The foot is not exposed but is wrapped in sterile towels so that the hip and leg can be manipulated during the procedure. The lower leg may be draped with an impervious tube stockinet. An incise drape is used to cover the operative site.

The surgeon makes an anterior or posterolateral incision. An anterior approach is discussed here. After the skin incision has been made, the wound is opened with the ESU. Initially, medium Richardson or similar retractors are placed in the wound edges. The fascia and muscle are then divided, and large rake retractors or right angle retractors can be inserted in the wound. The technologist should have ample lap sponges and suction available during this part of the procedure.

Once the joint capsule has been exposed, the surgeon opens it with the deep knife and the ESU. Hohmann retractors are used to elevate and expose the proximal femur. The hip joint is dislocated using a large bone hook and manual traction. This exposes the acetabular surface. The surgeon trims diseased tissue, including a torn labrum (the rim of connective tissue around the acetabulum). This is done with the knife, ESU, and cup-tipped rongeurs. Pituitary-type rongeurs also may be used for this step of the procedure.

The next step is the osteotomy, in which the femoral head is removed. The technologist should prepare a narrow-width oscillating blade and power saw. A cutting guide or jig is placed over the proximal trochanter and the femoral head is grasped with a sharp bone clamp. The saw then is used to divide the femoral neck. The assistant irrigates the bone during cutting to prevent heating. The scrub receives the femoral head, which is set aside on the back table and preserved with moist saline sponges. The surgeon may need to remove additional bone from the femoral neck after measurements are taken.

To prepare the acetabulum for the implant, the surgeon trims any loose tissue or *osteophytes* (bony spurs) from the rim of the joint. A cup-shaped rongeur (e.g., pituitary rongeur), curette, ESU, and knife are used to remove the tissue. The surgeon then dishes out the surface of the acetabulum using power-operated reamers in graduated sizes. The surgical technologist should clean excess tissue from the reamers and broaches between uses. A basin of sterile water should be available for this.

The trial shell is fitted (but not impacted) into the acetabulum with a positioning instrument. The final component then is impacted by hand with a mallet or with the supplied positioner and slap hammer. If screws are to be inserted through the shell, these can be inserted by hand through predrilled pilot holes. The liner then is fitted into the shell.

To prepare the femoral side of the joint, the surgeon creates an intramedullary space in the femur to accept the femoral stem. The exact depth of the space may be determined before surgery by comparing the radiograph with a transparent template. The surgeon may measure the femur again before reaming. A hand awl or chisel is used to start the opening for the femoral canal. This is followed by broaches. The technologist should have several sizes of intramedullary rasps (broaches). The broach is impacted into the canal with a mallet or slap hammer and guide, which is fitted over the broach. Broaches are used in successively larger sizes. Immersing the rasps in a basin of water is helpful for removing tissue debris from the instruments after each use. When broaching is nearly complete, the handle of the broach is removed and a planer is used to prepare the end surface (calcar) of the femur. This step is optional for some types of femoral implants. The broach may be tested for tightness. Final broaching then is completed and the handle is removed.

In the next phase of the procedure, a trial femoral head is tested for fit. Two surgical options are available: the trial head can be fitted over the broach, or the broach can be removed and a trial stem inserted in its place. The hip is reduced and assessed. The hip is dislocated and the femoral component and neck are implanted. If a broach is still in place, it is removed. A pulse lavage system is used to irrigate the femoral canal, which then is suctioned to remove debris.

NOTE: *If at any time the femur cracks under the broaches, a cabling system should be available to secure the femur and implant.*

Cement is prepared if required for the implant (see the earlier discussion of bone cement). The circulator then opens the appropriate size of implant and distributes it to the scrub. When the cement is ready, it is injected into the femoral space. The implant is impacted into the space by fitting it to a stem inserter. Press-fit components can be inserted by hand and then seated with the mallet and stem inserter. Figure 31-65 illustrates a technique for hip arthroplasty.

Patients are closely monitored for hemorrhage and embolism after arthroplasty. Deep vein thrombosis or a fat

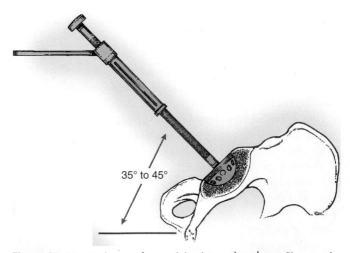

35° to 45°

Figure 31-65 **Technique for modular hip arthroplasty.** Planning for the femoral stem is shown. A template is placed over the radiographic image to determine the depth of intermedullary reaming. (*From Canale S, Beaty J: Campbell's operative orthopaedics, ed 11, St Louis, 2007, Mosby.*)

embolism may occur in the immediate postoperative period or weeks after surgery. Patients are encouraged to begin walking within 24 hours of surgery.

FRACTURE OF THE PELVIS

Surgical Goal

The goal of surgical fixation of the pelvis is to reduce and stabilize a fractured pelvis.

Pathology

Fractures of the pelvis generally are the result of a high-impact injury and often are accompanied by soft tissue injury. An unstable pelvic fracture can be life-threatening as a result of damage to major blood vessels and pelvic organs. Refer to Chapter 37 for a more detailed discussion of severe traumatic pelvic fractures.

Discussion

Open reduction is the preferred method of repair of an unstable fracture. A number of surgical options for fixation are available based on the location of the fracture:

- Fracture of the ilium is fixed internally with lag screws and fragment plates.
- Surgical options for fracture of the pubic rami are percutaneous pins or internally placed screws.
- Sacral fracture is treated with plates, screws, or rods (Figure 31-66).
- External fixation with a rod and pin system may also be used.

The patient is placed in the supine position for access to the pubic symphysis and also for a fracture of the acetabulum. A Pfannenstiel incision is used for access to the pubic rami.

The prone position is used for fractures of the iliac wings, ilium, sacroiliac joint, and some fractures of the acetabulum. When the prone position is used, a chest brace is placed under the thorax with the arms extended on arm boards. Soft padding is placed under the thighs and feet. (Chapter 19 presents a discussion of precautions to use with the prone position and a chest brace.)

Patients with pelvic fractures often have other serious injuries, and simple stabilizing surgery using an external pelvic clamp is the preferred method so that soft tissue injuries such as bladder rupture can be attended to first. More complex procedures are performed after the patient is stabilized. Refer to Chapter 37 for a discussion on stabilizing external fixation of the pelvis. All assessment scans must be available during surgery. These may include CT scans, MRI scans, contrast angiogram, and cystogram. If the patient arrives in traction, weights are attached to the operating table until reduction is secured.

The surgical technologist and circulating nurse are informed about instrumentation for internal or external fixation. However, a decision may be changed during surgery. The scrub should have a major orthopedic set, general surgery instruments, a drill, and the designated implant system available. Extra drapes, towels, and laparotomy sponges are needed for trauma patients. A suprapubic catheter may be inserted during the procedure. Bone-grafting instruments and materials should be readily available but not opened unless requested. Abdominal and pelvic injury may require bowel instruments.

Complications of a pelvic fracture include infection, pulmonary embolism, and urinary problems. Permanent nerve injury also may occur. Recovery from a pelvic fracture can be very long and difficult.

SURGICAL APPROACHES TO THE KNEE AND LOWER LEG

The knee is the most complicated joint of the body. It is vulnerable to a variety of injuries, which are caused mainly by sports and motor vehicle accidents. The knee is the largest joint and it carries a great deal of body weight, especially when in

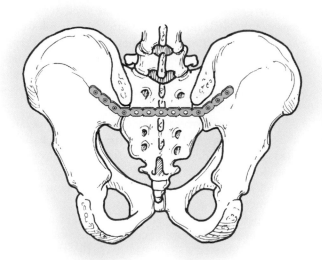
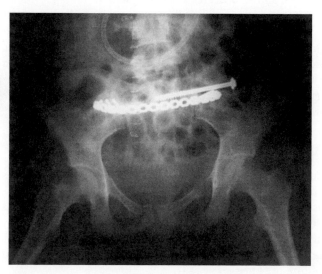

Figure 31-66 **Tension band plate used for a sacral fracture.** *(From Canale S, Beaty J: Campbell's operative orthopaedics, ed 11, St Louis, 2007, Mosby.)*

motion. It also has the longest mechanical levers of the body. Pathogenic conditions in the knee often are very disabling because of the weight-bearing function of the joint. Anterior and posterior views of the knee are shown in Figure 31-67. The joint is divided into separate compartments, which are created by the structures contained within it. However, no separate fibrous capsule binds the joint together. The ligaments and tendons surround the two joints that make up the knee, the tibiofemoral joint and the patellofemoral joint. The patella forms part of the knee joint on the anterior side. The *menisci* separate the femoral and tibial condyles and provide shock absorption.

Many procedures of the knee are approached endoscopically. The open technique most often is used with a parapatellar, medial, lateral, or posterior approach.

KNEE ARTHROSCOPY

Surgical Goal

Knee arthroscopy is a common technique for assessing and correcting problems arising from injury and disease.

Discussion

The patient is placed in the supine position. Spinal or general anesthesia is used. The surgeon examines the knee under anesthesia (**examination under anesthesia [EUA]**), assessing flexion and extension. A tourniquet is applied to the operative leg. The nonoperative leg is placed in a padded leg holder and the operative leg is placed in a stabilizing device that allows countertraction. The leg is prepped from midthigh to the ankle circumferentially and draped in routine manner.

An incision is made lateral to the patella and just above the joint line, allowing an inflow cannula to be inserted into the knee joint without damaging the cartilage.

When the knee has been infiltrated with fluid, a second incision is made medially and a sharp trocar and sheath are inserted into the knee joint. The trocar then is removed and replaced with a blunt trocar. The knee is irrigated, any fluid is removed, and a 30-degree scope is inserted.

An 18-gauge spinal needle is inserted into the knee joint under direct visualization to determine the placement of a third incision. This incision creates an opposite portal for the insertion of the probe and operative instruments. The location of this incision depends on the type of surgery to be performed. Figure 31-68 illustrates visualization of the knee through various ports.

ARTHROSCOPIC MENISCECTOMY

The meniscus is a horseshoe-shaped cartilage that distributes load across the joint and creates stability. A tear in the meniscus is the most common knee injury. The medial meniscus is injured more often than the lateral meniscus. Meniscectomy may be partial or complete. Complete meniscectomy leaves the medial rim of the structure to share load bearing and stabilize the knee.

When the meniscus is in view, the surgeon locates the tear with a probe. The attachment of the meniscus is divided with a hook knife. A motorized shaver is used to remove frayed edges from the cartilage. Complete removal, if required, is performed with meniscus knives and scissors. Figure 31-69 illustrates arthroscopic meniscal surgery.

ARTHROSCOPIC ANTERIOR CRUCIATE LIGAMENT REPAIR

Surgical Goal

The goal of surgery is to repair a torn anterior **cruciate** ligament (ACL) and restore stability to the joint.

Pathology

The ACL stabilizes the knee in the anterior-posterior position, preventing buckling of the knee. It crosses the center of the knee joint, attaching to the femur superiorly and the tibia inferiorly. ACL tears usually occur during a twisting motion of the leg, often during sports or other strenuous activity.

TECHNIQUE

1. The knee is assessed arthroscopically.
2. A tendon graft is harvested from the patella tendon, including bone plugs at each end.
3. The graft is prepared at the back table.
4. The damaged anterior cruciate ligament is removed from the knee joint.
5. Tunnels are drilled in the femur and tibia to receive the graft.
6. The graft is passed through the tunnels and secured with biosynthetic interference screws.
7. The repair is tested by manipulating the knee.
8. The wounds are closed and dressed.

Discussion

Repair of the ACL routinely is performed arthroscopically. A graft is taken from the central portion of the patellar tendon to replace the torn ACL. Surgical options include harvesting a graft from the hamstring or quadriceps tendon or using a cadaver graft. Many options can be used for arthroscopic repair of the ACL; however, the surgical principles are similar. A composite graft of bone and tendon is used to replace the ACL. The graft is secured by passing it through tunnels made in the tibia and femur. The graft is attached with sutures or biosynthetic interference screws, which prevent the graft from being pulled out of the tunnels.

The required instrumentation includes arthroscopy instruments, as well as ACL system instruments, including cannulated burrs, guidewires, and attachment devices. In this procedure, biosynthetic interference screws are used to attach the graft. Power equipment includes drills, a microsagittal saw, and a motorized arthroscopy shaver.

The patient is prepped and draped for a diagnostic arthroscopy. A pneumatic tourniquet is used. The foot of the operating table is lowered slightly. Before starting the procedure, the surgeon manipulates the knee with the patient under anesthesia to assess the injury. An arthroscopic examination is performed before the start of the repair.

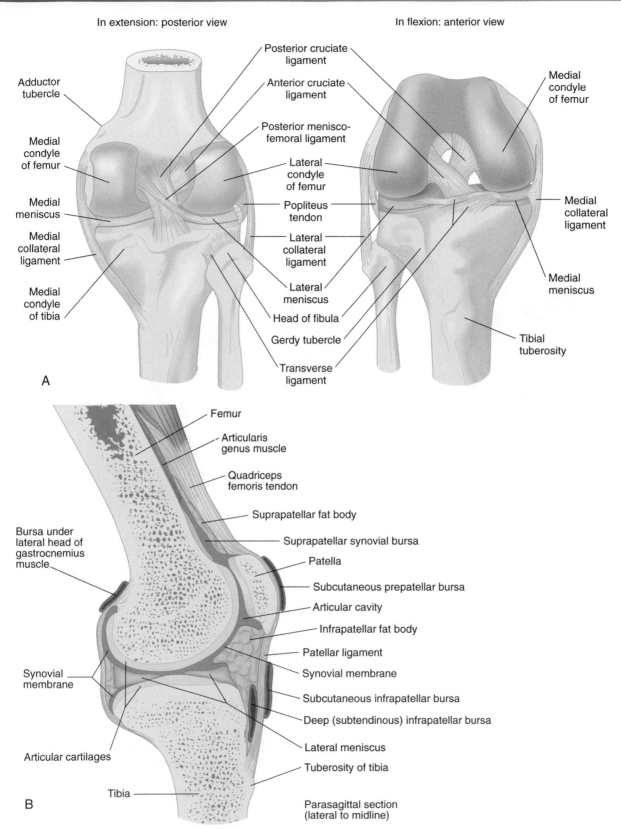

In extension: posterior view

In flexion: anterior view

Adductor tubercle

Medial condyle of femur

Medial meniscus

Medial collateral ligament

Medial condyle of tibia

Posterior cruciate ligament

Anterior cruciate ligament

Posterior menisco-femoral ligament

Lateral condyle of femur

Popliteus tendon

Lateral collateral ligament

Lateral meniscus

Head of fibula

Gerdy tubercle

Transverse ligament

Medial condyle of femur

Medial collateral ligament

Medial meniscus

Tibial tuberosity

A

Femur

Articularis genus muscle

Quadriceps femoris tendon

Suprapatellar fat body

Bursa under lateral head of gastrocnemius muscle

Suprapatellar synovial bursa

Patella

Subcutaneous prepatellar bursa

Articular cavity

Infrapatellar fat body

Patellar ligament

Synovial membrane

Subcutaneous infrapatellar bursa

Synovial membrane

Deep (subtendinous) infrapatellar bursa

Articular cartilages

Lateral meniscus

Tuberosity of tibia

Tibia

Parasagittal section (lateral to midline)

B

Figure 31-67 Anatomy of the knee. A, Anterior and posterior views. B, Sagittal view. (From Marx J, editor: Rosen's emergency medicine: concepts and clinical practice, ed, 6, Philadelphia, 2006, Mosby.)

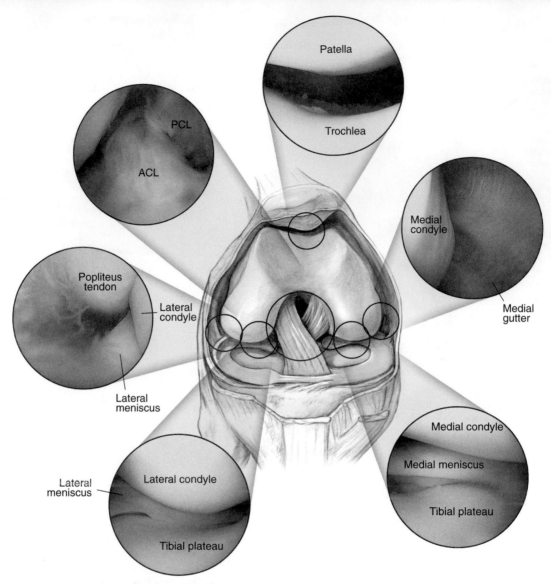

Figure 31-68   Arthroscopy of the knee. *(From Miller MD, Chhabra AB, Hurwitz SR, Mihalko WM: Orthopaedic surgical approaches, Philadelphia, 2008, WB Saunders.)*

Graft Harvesting (Open Surgery)

Although the ACL repair is performed arthroscopically, the graft is removed using open surgical technique. An anterior approach to the patellar tendon is used, which may involve either one or two incisions. After dividing the skin and subcutaneous tissue, the surgeon uses Metzenbaum scissors to separate the paratenon, which lies directly over the tendon. Senn retractors or small rakes are used for retraction. This exposes the patellar tendon. Army-Navy retractors should be available to expose the joint.

The graft is removed from the center patellar tendon. A disposable double-bladed knife or #15 knife blade is used to notch out a section of tendon, which remains attached to the patella at the upper pole and the tibia at the lower pole. An oscillating saw then is used to cut through the bone at each end of the graft. A ¼-inch (0.63-cm) osteotome is used to divide the bone plugs at both ends. This produces a strip of

tendon with small bone plugs attached at each end. The scrub should have a small basin to receive the graft, which is removed to the back table for preparation. The graft should be kept moist with saline.

The bone ends are trimmed with a small, single-action rongeur. The scrub must preserve any bone chips in a basin with a small amount of saline, because they may be replaced in the wound when the graft is placed. The surgeon passes the graft through a 10-mm metal tube to trial the graft to ensure that it fits. The bone plugs are trimmed as necessary. The surgeon then makes a small hole in each bone plug using a small drill and a fine drill bit. Size 0 nonabsorbable sutures are passed through each hole and the ends are left long and tagged with hemostats. The surgeon then uses a surgical pen to mark the graft at the bone-tendon margin. These marks are used to align the graft in the joint during insertion. The graft is ready for insertion. It is preserved in a specimen basin until the surgeon needs it.

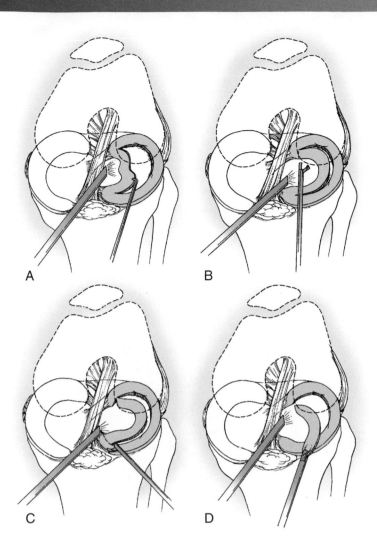

Figure 31-69 **Arthroscopic meniscus repair. A,** A bucket-handle tear is assessed with a probe. **B,** After reduction, the posterior attachment is divided with scissors. **C,** The anterior attachment is divided. **D,** A grasper is used to extract the fragment. *(From Canale S, Beaty J:* Campbell's operative orthopaedics, *ed 11, St Louis, 2007, Mosby.)*

The surgeon irrigates the wound and closes the remaining patellar tendon with 2-0 absorbable suture. Skin closure is delayed until the end of the procedure.

Arthroscopic Insertion of the Graft

To start the arthroscopic portion of the procedure, the surgeon inserts two lateral trocars. The joint is distended with saline or lactated Ringer solution. The surgeon then examines the torn ligament and menisci. A probe is introduced into the joint for the examination.

The motorized shaver is used to remove the damaged ACL. The scrub should have a basin available for periodic outflow drainage. A torn meniscus may be removed at this stage. To prepare the joint for the graft, a drill guide is used to position the tunnel that will receive the graft. A guidewire is drilled into the tibia. A tunnel then is drilled over the guidewire with a cannulated reamer or burr. This step is repeated on the femoral side. A calibrated aiming device may be used to locate the exact angle of the tunnels before drilling.

An eyed pin is drilled through the bone tunnels and brought out through the skin. The scrub should bring the graft to the field when directed by the surgeon. The preplaced sutures are threaded through the eye of the pin and pulled through the tunnel at both ends. Biosynthetic interference screws are placed in the tunnel against the bone plugs to provide a tighter fit. A small guidewire is placed first and the screws are placed over the wire. The screws are seated with a screwdriver. The preplaced sutures are then removed.

The repair is inspected through the arthroscope and the distension fluid is drained. The wounds are closed with synthetic absorbable suture. The wound is dressed with gauze and a leg brace is applied. The technique for ACL repair is illustrated in Figure 31-70.

The patient remains on crutches for 2 to 3 weeks using a leg brace. Physical therapy is initiated within the first week of recovery. The total recovery period is 4 to 6 months. The patient usually is able to return to normal activities after a successful repair.

Related Procedure: Repair of a Torn Lateral Collateral Ligament

A torn lateral collateral ligament can be repaired using the techniques described for repair of the ACL. A patellar tendon graft is used to replace the damaged collateral ligament. With a less severe injury, the ligament may be reattached with biosynthetic screws, staples, or sutures of heavy Dacron.

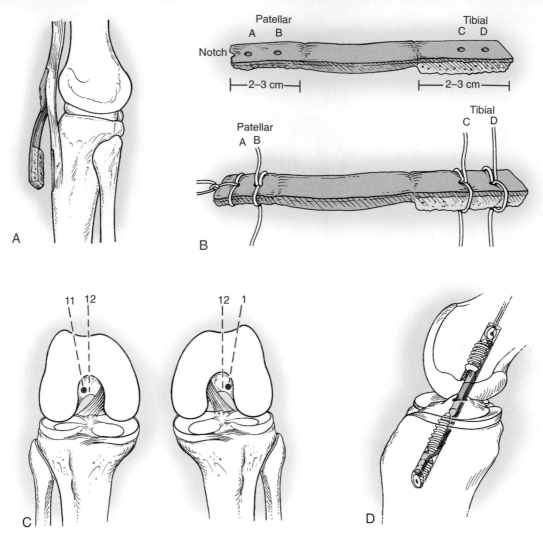

Figure 31-70   Anterior cruciate ligament repair with graft. **A,** Removal of the graft from the tibial tuberosity. **B,** Sutures may be placed at each end of the graft. **C,** The pilot holes are positioned to accommodate the graft. **D,** The graft is secured with biosynthetic screws. *(From Canale S, Beaty J: Campbell's operative orthopaedics, ed 11, St Louis, 2007, Mosby.)*

KNEE ARTHROPLASTY

Surgical Goal

The goal of knee arthroplasty is to relieve pain and allow the patient to resume activity.

Pathology

Three common forms of arthritis affect the knee: osteoarthritis, rheumatoid arthritis, and post-traumatic arthritis. Inflammation and degeneration of the joint surfaces result in pain and loss of function. Osteoarthritis is the most common indication for arthroplasty.

Discussion

The knee has three cartilaginous surfaces: the patella, the tibia, and the femur. Any or all three surfaces may be involved in joint disease. In unicompartmental arthroplasty, the medial or lateral surfaces of the femur and tibia are replaced. In total

knee replacement, all three components are replaced. Unicompartmental replacement often requires total knee replacement later in the patient's life and is suitable for patients with intact supporting structures.

Knee replacement is a complex procedure. Many systems are available and are continually being refined. In particular, the unicompartmental approach has been under intense development. Electronic systems that aid precise alignment of the joint components are now used in some facilities.

As mentioned, during total knee replacement, three components are implanted. (Modular or partial arthroplasty also is performed.) Figure 31-71 shows the knee components:

- A metal femoral component inserted over the distal femur
- A tibial base plate and a metal tray that is placed in the proximal tibia. A polyethylene patellar component is inserted. The components may be implanted with bone cement or they may be press-fitted.

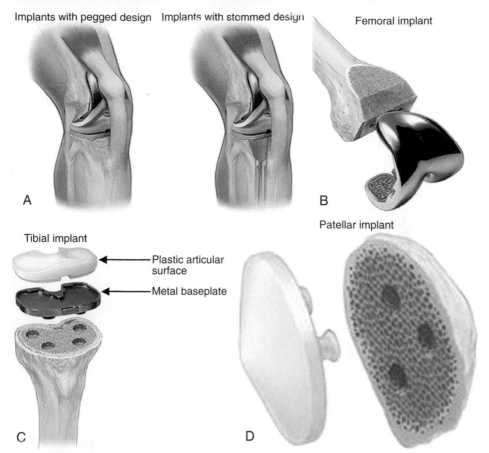

Implants with pegged design   Implants with stemmed design

A

Femoral implant

B

Tibial implant

Plastic articular surface

Metal baseplate

C

Patellar implant

D

Figure 31-71 **Knee arthroplasty. A,** Pegged and stemmed design. **B,** Femoral implant. **C,** Tibial implant. **D,** Patellar implant. *(Courtesy Zimmer, Warsaw, Ind.)*

TOTAL KNEE REPLACEMENT

TECHNIQUE

Femur
1. The knee is opened with an anterior or a midpatellar approach. The patella is retracted.
2. The intramedullary canal is located with a drill.
3. The distal femur cuts are planned with a computer-based system or an alignment system.
4. A distal femoral guide (block) is used to direct the cut.
5. The distal femur is cut with an oscillating saw.
6. Distal femoral holes are drilled to calibrate the femur.
7. The posterior femur is cut.
8. The anterior femur is cut.

TECHNIQUE

Tibia
1. The proximal tibia is cut.
2. The proximal tibia is drilled and sized.
3. The tibia is reamed by hand if a stemmed component will be implanted.

TECHNIQUE

Implantation of Components
1. A press-fit tibial base plate is impacted over the tibial surface.
2. The base plate is stabilized with screws.
3. If a cemented base plate is used, a thin layer of cement is placed over the tibia.
4. The polyethylene insert is fitted over the base plate.
5. The femoral component is implanted with an impactor.

The wound is irrigated frequently during the procedure with pulse lavage to remove all debris, which might contribute to infection.

The incision is closed in layers with 2-0 and 3-0 absorbable synthetic sutures. The skin is closed with staples or 3-0 or 4-0 nonabsorbable sutures. An occlusive dressing is placed over the incision, followed by a support bandage or stocking. Knee arthroplasty is illustrated in Figures 31-72 and 31-73.

The patient is encouraged to ambulate within 24 hours after surgery and is placed on anticoagulant therapy to prevent thrombosis. Continuous passive motion may be used immediately after surgery for a patient who is unable to ambulate. The patient generally is required to remain in the hospital for up to 3 days after surgery and may resume limited activity within 2 to 4 weeks.

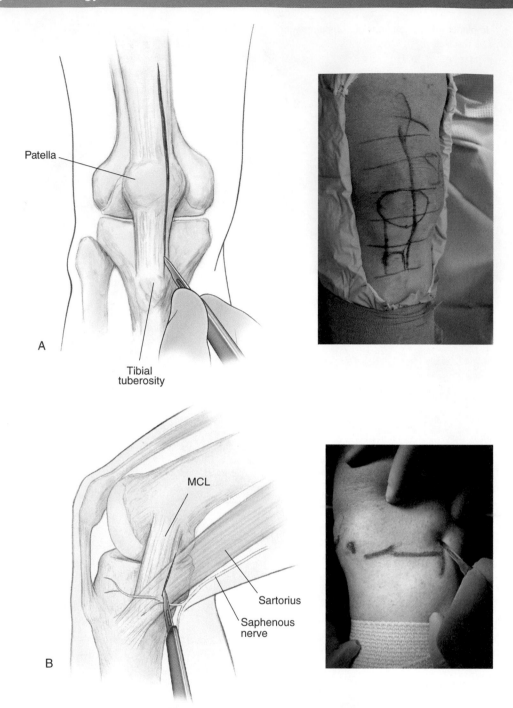

Figure 31-72 Surgical approaches for the knee. A, Parapatellar. **B,** Medial. *MCL, Medial collateral ligament. (From Miller MD, Chhabra AB, Hurwitz SR, Mihalko WM: Orthopaedic surgical approaches, Philadelphia, 2008, WB Saunders.)*

INTRAMEDULLARY NAILING (TIBIA)

Surgical Goal

In intramedullary nailing of the tibia, an intramedullary rod (nail) is inserted into the tibia for fixation and stabilization of a fracture.

Pathology

Fractures of the tibia are commonly the result of a high-velocity impact caused by a motor vehicle accident or sports trauma.

TECHNIQUE

1. The medullary canal is opened.
2. A guidewire is inserted into the canal.
3. The intermedullary canal is reamed.
4. The tibial nail is inserted using a targeting device.
5. The nail is impacted.
6. The guidewire is removed.
7. Locking screws are inserted using a targeting device.

Discussion

The selection of an IM nail for a fracture of the tibia is based on the type and severity of the fracture, the patient's age, and the surgeon's preference. Two types of IM nails are commonly used, the cannulated nail and the solid nail. Although called "nails," these devices are rod implants that are impacted into the intramedullary space along the parallel axis. Stabilizing screws may be placed at the proximal and distal ends to prevent the nail from slipping. The nail may be inserted without preparation of the medullary canal, or the canal may be reamed before insertion of the nail.

The patient is placed in the supine position on a translucent operating table or orthopedic table using distraction. C-arm fluoroscopy is used intraoperatively. The knee will be flexed to 90 degrees during the procedure and appropriate padding and accessories are necessary to maintain safe positioning. A knee

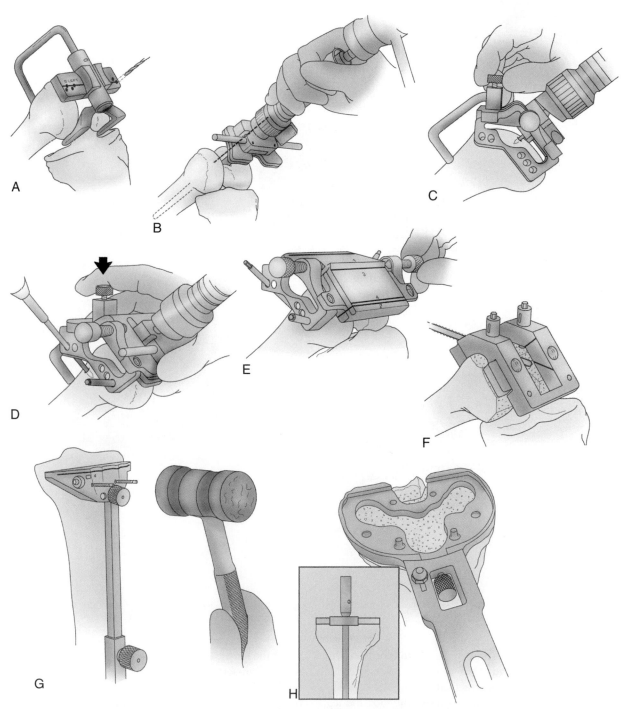

Figure 31-73 **Knee arthroplasty. A,** A femoral sizer is placed over the distal femur. **B,** The femoral canal is reamed and an intramedullary alignment guide is inserted into the medullary canal. **C,** The femoral cutting guide is attached to the alignment guide. **D,** The femoral cutting guide is positioned. **E,** The femur is resected. **F,** The femoral cuts are completed. **G,** A tibial alignment guide is positioned and the tibia incised. **H,** Tibial measurements are taken. (Courtesy Zimmer, Warsaw, Ind.)

Continued

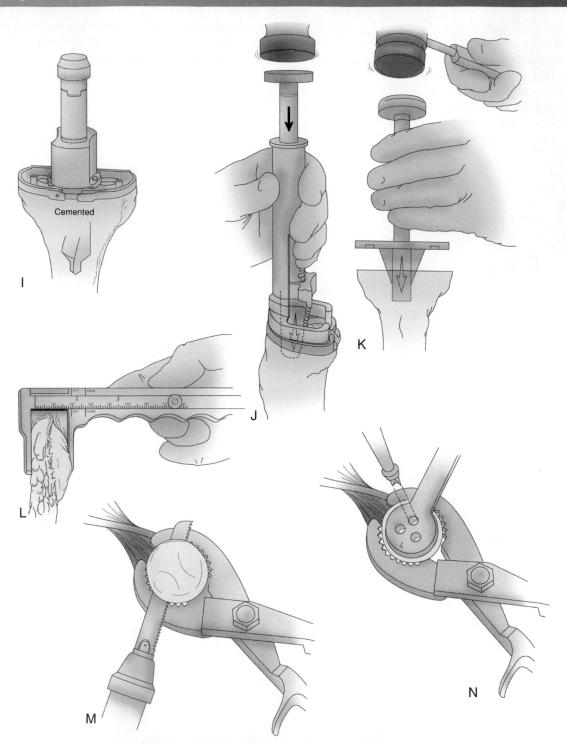

Figure 31-73, cont'd I, The tibia is reamed. J, The tibia is impacted. K, The tibial trial is inserted. L and M, The patella is measured and sized. N, The patella is drilled. *(From Rothrock J: Alexander's care of the patient in surgery, ed 17, Philadelphia, 2007, Mosby.)*

crutch or distraction device may be used to position the affected leg. The C-arm is adjusted before the skin prep to ensure full exposure of the operative site. A pneumatic tourniquet may be used to maintain hemostasis. The foot and leg are prepped up to and including the thigh, because the leg is manipulated during surgery. The foot may be wrapped in an occluding drape before the leg drapes are applied.

Before starting surgery, the surgeon measures the tibia using the image intensifier and a ruler, which is positioned along the long axis of the leg in two places. The skin is marked with a skin scribe. This determines the size of nail required. For complex multiple fractures of the tibia, a distractor may be required to hold the leg in reduction.

The scrub should have a basic orthopedic set available, including knee retractors; general surgery instruments, including superficial retractors; and the instruments, implants, and accessories for the nailing set to be used. A pneumatic drill or hand drill also is required for setting the guide pins. Some types of IM nails are inserted with the drill. The nail may be inserted percutaneously (through the skin) or through an incision and preparation of the medullary canal.

After the prep, draping, and TIMEOUT, the knee is flexed and held in position by the assistant. The surgeon makes an incision over the proximal tibia along the midline of the bone. The scrub should have skin rakes and the ESU immediately available. The patellar tendon then is retracted with a dull rake or a shallow right angle retractor (e.g., Senn retractor). In some procedures, the tendon is split.

To ensure correct positioning of the implant and precise removal of intramedullary tissue, a guide pin or rod and a tissue protection sleeve are positioned in the canal.

A guidewire (threaded Steinmann pin) is inserted into the medullary canal with a power drill or hand drill. A 2.5-mm wire is commonly used. The guidewire is advanced with a drill sleeve, which keeps the pin straight as it is drilled. The position of the pin then is verified fluoroscopically.

A cannulated reaming rod is used to ream the intramedullary canal. Reaming may be by hand or using power instruments. Intramedullary reamers are sized from 8 to 17 mm in 0.5-mm increments. This step may be omitted if reaming is unnecessary. In the nonreamed method, a tissue protection sleeve may be inserted over the guide rod. If reaming is necessary, the cannulated reaming rod is placed over the guidewire and advanced with a hand drill. The turning motion of the reamer creates bits of tissue from the medullary canal. The scrub should be alert to clear these tissue fragments from the field and retain them as specimens. The scrub also must keep the reamer irrigated to reduce tissue heating.

After the canal has been reamed, the hand assembly is removed and the tissue or medullary tube is inserted over the reamer. The reamer then is removed and may be replaced with a guide rod, which is used to guide the IM nail into position.

The selected nail implant then is inserted. At each step, the position of the guidewires is verified and the hollow medullary tubes are used to protect the tissue of the endosteum while drilling takes place. The medullary tube and guidewires are removed only when the IM nail is in place.

Depending on the system and the manufacturer, a number of methods can be used to insert the nail. A hollow nail can be grasped with a targeting device or guide, which keeps the nail straight and angled correctly as it is inserted over the guidewire. The nail is inserted manually with a twisting or oscillating movement. A metal driver may be used to seat the nail.

The position of the implant is verified fluoroscopically and the guidewire is removed. Locking pins are then inserted. These fit into the nail at a right angle through the proximal and distal ends of the nail. To line up the entry point of the locking bolts with the nail, a targeting guide or similar right angle aiming device is used. The IM guidewire is removed and the targeting device is attached. The skin is incised over the site for the locking bolts and the tissue is dissected to bone. The drill holes then are made through the tissue protector. Screw length is determined with a depth gauge. The locking screws are inserted and tightened manually with the screwdriver. Tibial nailing is illustrated in Figure 31-74.

SURGICAL APPROACHES TO THE FOOT

REPAIR OF THE ACHILLES TENDON

Surgical Goal

The goal of repair of the Achilles tendon is to return strength and flexibility to the foot after a traumatic injury.

Pathology

The Achilles tendon may be torn or ruptured in active sports, especially those involving jumping, such as tennis, basketball, gymnastics, and volleyball. A low-level injury may occur in other activities, such as cycling.

Discussion

Surgical treatment for Achilles tendon injuries varies widely. A graft may be used to replace a severely injured tendon. In some cases, the paratenon is stripped to provide a "fresh" wound for more rapid healing.

The patient is placed in the supine position with the affected leg supported by a soft support or gel pad. Spinal or general anesthesia is used, and a pneumatic tourniquet applied. The foot and lower leg are prepped and draped in the routine manner.

A posterolateral approach is used. The incision is made parallel to the tendon on the lateral or median side with a #15 knife. The skin and subcutaneous tissue are retracted with skin rakes or a Weitlaner retractor. This exposes the fascia (paratenon), which is incised to expose the tendon. The tendon is irrigated and trimmed with Metzenbaum scissors. The ends of the torn tendon are approximated with size 0 heavy Mersilene or other synthetic suture. The paratenon is sutured with 2-0 absorbable synthetic sutures. The foot remains flexed while a short leg cast is applied.

TRIPLE ARTHRODESIS

Surgical Goal

Triple **arthrodesis** is the fusion of the talocalcaneal, talonavicular, and calcaneocuboid joints. This is performed by removing the cartilage from each joint and allowing them to heal in approximation. The surgical goal is to prevent movement of these joints and thereby prevent pain and joint instability.

Pathology

Triple arthrodesis is performed to treat a number of painful, chronic joint diseases that are not helped by conservative therapy. These include rheumatoid arthritis, post-traumatic arthritis, and neuromuscular disease.

Discussion

The instruments required for triple arthrodesis include a foot and ankle orthopedic set, including a lamina spreader, bone saw, drill, K-wires, and burrs. Medium-size osteotomes and curettes also should be available, along with a cannulated screw system. A bone graft may be harvested from the iliac crest, or biosynthetic grafting material can be used.

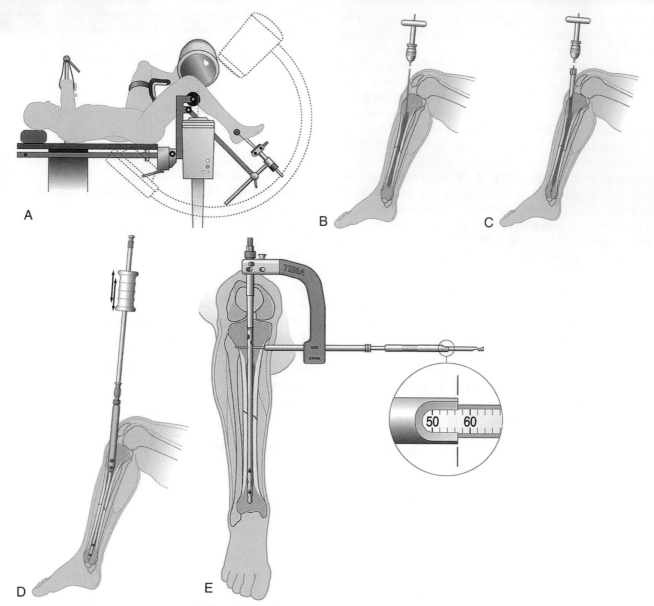

Figure 31-74 **Intermedullary tibial nailing. A,** Patient position using a fracture table. **B,** A guide rod is inserted into the medullary canal. **C,** A ball tip is inserted under image intensification. **D,** The canal has been reamed and a nail has been inserted. A slap hammer is used to impact the nail. **E,** A targeting device is used to locate the screw holes. The screw length is measured (shown), and the locking screws are inserted. *(Courtesy Zimmer, Warsaw, Ind.)*

The patient is placed in the supine position. General or spinal anesthesia is used. The foot and leg are prepped to the knee. The foot is draped in routine manner.

An anterior or anterolateral incision is made. This approach prevents injury to the superficial peroneal nerves. The cartilage and soft tissue are dissected and removed from the joints with single- and double-action rongeurs, a #15 blade, and tissue forceps. The capsules of the talonavicular, calcaneocuboid, and subtalar joints are incised circumferentially to obtain as much mobility as possible. The articular surfaces of the calcaneocuboid joint, the subtalar joint, and the talonavicular joint are removed with an osteotome, a power saw, or a rasp. Any bone removed is preserved on the back table for possible use in grafting.

When all articular surfaces have been cleaned, the foot is placed in correct anatomical position. Bone or biosynthetic grafting material may be used to fill gaps in the bone-to-bone surfaces. K-wires are inserted for temporary fixation. Cannulated screws then are used to bridge the three bones (Figure 31-75). Fluoroscopy is used to check the position of the K-wires and the cannulated screws inserted over them.

Distal locking screws are placed over the cannulated screws. Surgical options include insertion of a cannulated arthrodesis nail, which is inserted from the calcaneus and locked in place with cannulated screws.

A closed drainage system (e.g., Hemovac drain) may be inserted, and the wound is closed in layers. A postoperative nerve block is used to reduce postoperative pain. The ankle is

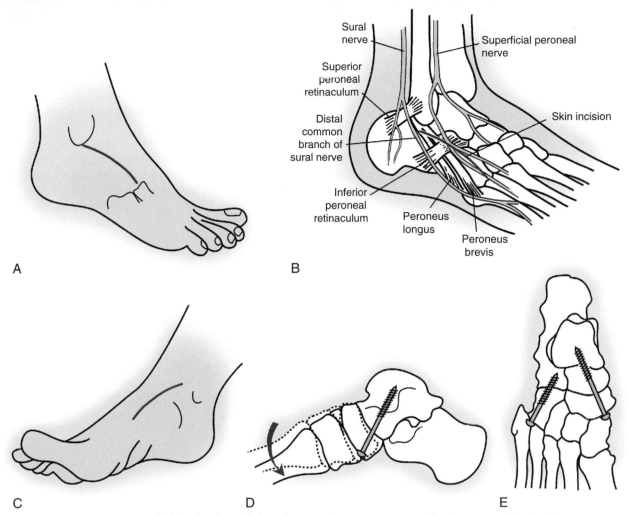

Figure 31-75 **Triple arthrodesis of the ankle. A,** Skin incision. **B,** Superficial anatomy. **C,** Medial incision. **D,** Talonavicular fixation. **E,** Calcaneocuboid and talonavicular screw fixation. *(From Canale S, Beaty J: Campbell's operative orthopaedics, ed 11, St Louis, 2007, Mosby.)*

covered with a compression dressing and a posterior splint is applied.

The patient is weight bearing after 2 weeks. Physical therapy is started as soon as possible to increase range of motion. Complications of triple or hindfoot arthrodesis include failed union, avascular necrosis of the talus, arthritis, and ankle deformity.

FRACTURE OF THE ANKLE

Surgical Goal

Open reduction and internal fixation of the foot is performed to stabilize fractures of the distal tibia, fibula, talus, and calcaneus.

Pathology

Fracture of the ankle is caused by overeversion or overinversion, usually as a result of a sports injury, missed step, or fall. Ankle injury also is common in motor vehicle, motorcycle, and bicycle accidents.

Discussion

Open reduction and internal fixation of the ankle is performed using cannulated screws, pins, wires, and plates. Preoperative assessment, including imaging studies, is performed to determine the best approach. Special instruments are selected based on the approach chosen. Basic instruments and supplies include a basic orthopedic set, soft tissue instruments, a drill, a K-wire set, drill bits, and shallow right-angle retractors. Trauma cases may require a pulse lavage irrigation system. C-arm fluoroscopy is used in most procedures.

The patient is placed in the supine position with the operative leg supported on a padded roll. A tourniquet is positioned around the upper leg. General or spinal anesthesia is used. The foot and leg are prepped to just above the knee.

Surgical options for internal fixation include the following:

- *Insertion of cannulated or lag screws:* K-wires (guidewires) are inserted across the fracture and their position is verified fluoroscopically. Screw holes are made with a cannulated drill and measured with a depth gauge. The cannulated screws are inserted over the guidewires. The position is verified, and the K-wires are removed.

- *Bridge plates with screws:* Small plates (small fragment set) are cut and contoured to fit the fracture site.

BUNIONECTOMY

Surgical Goal

In a bunionectomy, an enlarged metatarsal head (hallux valgus) is reduced or removed. The goal of surgery is to alleviate pain and increase patient mobility.

Pathology

Hallux valgus is a deformity of the first metatarsal head and is associated with various structural anomalies of the entire

toe. Poorly fitting shoes contribute to the pathology. An enlarged metatarsal head is painful and often limits the patient's mobility.

Discussion

The patient is placed in the supine position. Regional anesthesia is administered and a pneumatic tourniquet is applied. The foot is prepped and draped.

An incision is made in the anterior or medial side of the metatarsal shaft and extended through the fascia. Senn retractors are placed in the wound. The joint capsule is incised with the deep knife and tenotomy scissors. Repair is performed by removal of the proximal phalanx with an oscillating power saw. The bony outgrowth of the metatarsal head (bunion) is also removed. To maintain the toe in alignment, one or two fine K-wires are placed through the medullary canal of the

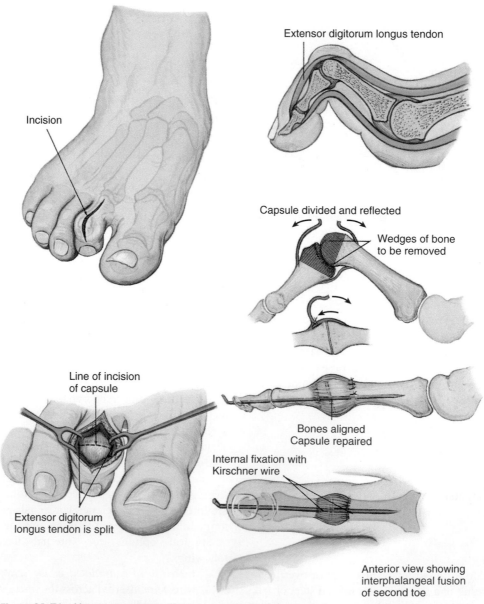

Figure 31-76   Hammertoe repair. *(From Herring JA: Tachdjian's pediatric orthopaedics from the Texas Scottish Rite Hospital for Children, ed 3, Philadelphia, 2002, WB Saunders.)*

phalanx and metatarsal head. Fluoroscopy is used to check the position of the K-wires. The wound is irrigated and closed with absorbable sutures. The foot is dressed with bulky padding and placed in a foot brace.

HAMMERTOE CORRECTION

A hammertoe is a condition in which a toe has contracted at the proximal interphalangeal joint, the middle joint in the toe. Contracture of the ligaments and tendons causes the toes to curl downward. Pain arises from friction between the shoe and the top of the joint. Hammertoe may occur in any toe except the big toe.

To correct a hammertoe deformity, a flexor tenotomy is performed with a #15 knife. Surgical options include resection of the head of the proximal phalanx. A small K-wire is driven through the end of the toe and both joint edges to maintain alignment during healing (Figure 31-76).

KEY CONCEPTS

- Knowledge of the surgical anatomy of the skeletal system, joints, and soft connective tissues is a prerequisite to a complete understanding of the surgical procedures, patient care, and case planning.
- Familiarity with diagnostic and intraoperative imaging procedures is necessary to understanding the pathology of fractures and joint disease and the techniques used in repair and replacement.
- Orthopedic surgery requires complex case planning to include specialty instruments, power devices for use on bone, implant selection and management, special draping techniques, and use of irrigation and hemostatic devices.
- An understanding of fracture and joint pathology is necessary for safe patient care and case planning.
- Orthopedic techniques in surgery involve repair, reconstruction, and replacement specific to bone and joints.

REVIEW QUESTIONS

1. Define these important terms in your own words for surgical technique in orthopedics:
   - Internal fixation;
   - External fixation;
   - Open reduction;
   - Closed reduction.
2. Give an example of a specific orthopedic procedure for each of the four techniques listed in question 1.
3. What techniques and specific instruments must be used to insert simple bone screws that are not self-tapping?

4. Describe the sterilization protocol (rules) for orthopedic implants.
5. What is a lag screw? How does it work?
6. What special equipment is used to mix bone cement? Why is this equipment necessary?
7. Define *torque*.
8. During joint replacement surgery, the limb is often prepped and draped "free." What does this mean and why is it done?
9. What is meant by the term *cannulated* as it applies to orthopedic hardware?
10. What are the most important reasons for immediate stabilization of a fracture?

REFERENCES

1. Association for the Advancement of Medical Instrumentation: *ANSI/AAMI ST79:2006 Comprehensive guide to steam sterilization and sterility assurance in health care facilities*, Arlington, Va, 2006, AAMI.
2. Association of periOperative Registered Nurses (AORN): Recommended practices for sterilization in the perioperative practice setting. In *Standards, recommended practices and guidelines, 2007 edition*, Denver, 2007, AORN.
3. University of Washington Orthopedics and Sports Medicine: *Treatment of recurrent instability in shoulder dislocations*. Accessed January 24, 2007, at www.orthop.washington.edu/uw/tabID_3404Default.aspx.

BIBLIOGRAPHY

Browner B, Jupiter J, Levine A, Trafton P: *Skeletal trauma: basic science, management, and reconstruction*, ed 3, Philadelphia, 2003, WB Saunders.
Canale S, Beaty J: *Campbell's operative orthopaedics*, ed 11, St Louis, 2007, Mosby.
DeLee J, Drez D: *DeLee Drez's orthopedic sports medicine: principles and practice*, Philadelphia, 2003, WB Saunders.
Marx J, editor: *Rosen's emergency medicine: concepts and clinical practice*, ed 6, Philadelphia, 2006, Mosby.
Matsen FA III, Rockwood CA Jr, Wirth MA, et al: Glenohumeral arthritis and its management. In Rockwood CA Jr, Matsen FA III, Wirth MA, et al, editors: *The shoulder*, ed 3, Philadelphia, 2004, WB Saunders.
Miller MD, Chhabra AB, Hurwitz SR, Mihalko WM: *Orthopedic surgical approaches*, Philadelphia, 2008, WB Saunders.
Rothrock J: *Alexander's care of the patient in surgery*, ed 17, Philadelphia, 2007, Mosby.
Thibodeau G, Patton K: *Anatomy and physiology*, ed 6, Philadelphia, 2007, Mosby.
Townsend CM: *Sabiston textbook of surgery*, ed 17, Philadelphia, 2001, WB Saunders.

32

Peripheral Vascular Surgery

CHAPTER OUTLINE

Introduction
Surgical Anatomy

Diagnostic Procedures
Case Planning

Techniques in Vascular
Surgery

Surgical Procedures

LEARNING OBJECTIVES

After studying this chapter the reader will be able to:

1. Identify key anatomical features of the peripheral vascular system
2. Discuss diagnostic procedures of the vascular system

3. Discuss specific elements of case planning in orthopedic vascular surgery
4. Describe surgical techniques used in vascular surgery
5. Discuss vascular pathology
6. List and describe common vascular procedures

TERMINOLOGY

Aneurysm: Ballooning of an artery as a result of weakening of the arterial wall. It may be caused by atherosclerosis, infection, or a hereditary defect in the vascular system.

Angioplasty: Dilation of an artery using endovascular techniques (i.e., an arterial catheter); may include insertion of a supportive stent inside the artery to maintain blood flow.

Arteriosclerosis: A disease characterized by thickening, hardening, and loss of elasticity of the arterial wall.

Arteriotomy: An incision made in an artery, usually to perform an anastomosis with a graft or another artery or to remove plaque or a thrombus.

Atherosclerosis: The most common form of arteriosclerosis, which causes plaque to form on the inner surface of an artery.

Bifurcation: The Y-shape of an artery or graft.

Doppler duplex ultrasonography: A type of ultrasonography that amplifies sounds that pass through tissue and produces a visual image of blood flow.

Embolus: A moving substance in the vascular system. An embolus may consist of air, a blood clot, atherosclerotic plaque, or fat.

Endarterectomy: The surgical removal of plaque from inside an artery.

Hemodialysis: A process in which blood is shunted out of the body and passed through a complex set of filters for the treatment of end-stage renal disease (and in some cases, poisoning); also called *renal replacement therapy*.

Hemodynamic: A term referring to the pressure, flow, and resistance in the cardiovascular system.

Infarction: A blockage in an artery that may lead to ischemia and tissue death.

In situ: A term meaning "in the natural position or normal place, without disturbing or invading surrounding tissues."

Intravascular ultrasound: A diagnostic tool in which a transducer is introduced into an artery and ultrasound is used to translate the physical characteristics of the lumen into a visible image.

Ischemia: The decrease in or absence of blood supply to a localized area, usually related to vascular obstruction.

Lumen: The inside of a hollow structure, such as a blood vessel.

Percutaneous: A term that literally means "through the skin." In a percutaneous approach in surgery, an incision is not made; rather, a catheter or other device is introduced through a puncture site.

Stent: A tubular device placed inside an artery for dilation, support, and prevention of stricture.

Thrombus: Any organic or nonorganic material blocking an artery; generally refers to a blood clot or atherosclerotic plaque but also includes fat or air.

Umbilical tapes: Lengths of cotton mesh tape used to loop around a blood vessel for retraction. See *vessel loop*.

Venous stasis: Pooling of blood in the veins caused by inactivity or disease. Stasis can cause distention of the veins.

Vessel loop: A device used to retract a vessel during surgery. A length of thin Silastic tubing or cotton tape (umbilical tape) is passed around the vessel. The ends can be threaded through a bolster (a ⅛- to ¼-inch [0.3- to 0.6-cm] length of rubber or Silastic tubing) to secure the loop against the blood vessel.

INTRODUCTION

Peripheral vascular surgery is a specialty of the arteries and veins lying outside the immediate area of the heart or brain. Many vascular procedures are performed to treat **arteriosclerosis**, atherosclerosis, or thromboembolic disease. Surgical intervention for vascular disease includes open and minimally invasive procedures. Many conditions that required open surgery in the past may now be performed using an endovascular technique, with far less trauma and a more rapid recovery. Sophisticated diagnostic technology also has contributed to early diagnosis and a decrease in the number of open surgical procedures.

Reconstruction and grafting procedures often require temporary clamping of large vessels or those that contribute the main blood supply to vital organs. Timing is important to minimize the risk of **ischemia** (loss of blood supply) to tissue during selected grafting procedures. An example is clamping the carotid artery during carotid endarterectomy. Even if the blood flow to the brain is decreased because of the disease, complete occlusion presents a risk of ischemia to the brain, which must be managed. The surgical technologist must be attentive to the surgical site at all times, but especially when major vessels are clamped. Complex vascular surgery requires a high level of knowledge and a well-organized instrument table.

SURGICAL ANATOMY

The peripheral vascular system is a complex network of vessels, which carry blood cell components and nutrients (including oxygen) to all parts of the body and remove the waste products of metabolism. The major organs of this system are the arteries, veins, and capillaries.

STRUCTURE OF BLOOD VESSELS

All blood vessels except the capillaries are composed of three layers or walls. From the outside to the inside, they are:
- The *tunica externa* (also called the *adventitia*), which is composed of connective tissue and protects the vessel from injury and provides structural strength.
- The *tunica media*, which is composed of inner layers of smooth muscle bounded by connective tissue. Smooth muscle is under the control of the autonomic nervous system.
- The *tunica intima*, which secretes substances that cause vasodilation or constriction, as well as substances that prevent platelet aggregation in the vessel.

The structure of arteries and veins is shown in Figure 32-1.

ARTERIES

The *arteries* carry oxygenated blood from the heart to the rest of the body. The only exception is the *pulmonary arteries*, which carry deoxygenated blood to the lungs. Arteries and the smaller arterioles have distinct characteristics that enable them to transport a large volume of blood under pressure.

The arteries are thick-walled and highly elastic, and contain mostly smooth muscle. The arteries branch into the arterioles, which transition to the capillaries, where oxygen is released into the tissues. The arterioles provide vascular resistance, regulating the flow of blood into organs and tissues.

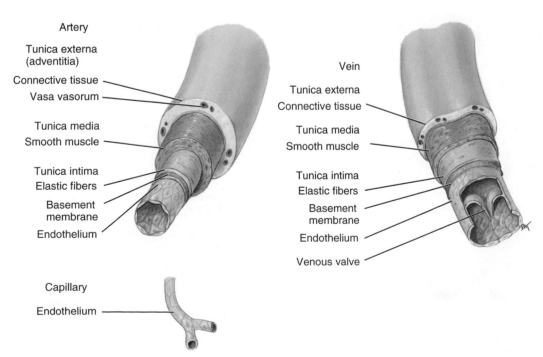

Figure 32-1   **The structure of blood vessels.** *(From Applegate E: The anatomy and physiology learning system, ed 2, St Louis, 2000, WB Saunders.)*

The elastic nature of the arteries allows them to contract during *systole* (ventricular contraction) and relax during *diastole* (the resting phase of the heart) to maintain vascular pressure. The arteries dilate and contract to accommodate the metabolic needs of the body. For example, inflammation causes expansion of the arteries and the release of blood through the arterioles; this increases blood supply to the injured and infected tissue. Vascular dilation lowers the body temperature, because it exposes the blood to surface cooling provided by evaporation of sweat from the skin. Peripheral vasoconstriction occurs during shock and when the body's core temperature is subnormal; this concentrates the greatest volume of blood in the heart and brain and prevents further cooling at the surface of the body.

CAPILLARIES

The *capillaries* are microscopic vessels that function as the transition and exchange mechanism for oxygen and other substances between the vessel walls and the tissue cells. Arterioles transition to the capillaries, which transition to venules and veins. Capillaries are composed of endothelial cells and have no muscle fibers. Precapillary sphincters control the flow of oxygenated blood into the capillary. The walls of the capillary are one cell thick and allow selected substances, including oxygen, to diffuse through the capillary membrane into the tissue. The microcirculation of the capillary system is illustrated in Figure 32-2.

Some tissues, such as the liver and spleen, have a rich supply of capillary networks. Because of this, these tissues bleed easily and profusely when injured. Capillary bleeding sometimes is difficult to control during surgery and topical hemostatic agents are required to maintain hemostasis.

VEINS

The venous system carries blood back to the heart from the peripheral tissues. After passing through the capillary network, blood enters the venules, which transition to increasingly larger branches of veins that run roughly parallel to the arteries on their way to the heart.

Veins are thin-walled, which allows them to expand. They function as vessels for transporting blood and also as storage units for blood. Like arteries, larger veins contain muscle fibers that allow them to constrict. However, unlike arteries, veins have valves that open only one way, preventing blood from backing up.

Blood is not pumped through the veins; rather, it is milked toward the heart by contractions in skeletal muscles in the peripheral system (Figure 32-3) and by intraabdominal and intrathoracic pressure in the trunk of the body. Malfunction of the veins' one-way valves results in **venous stasis** or pooling, which can cause the veins to dilate abnormally (called a *varicosity*). A number of physiological functions prevent blood from clotting in the vessels. Movement is among the most important. Stasis and pooling can cause thrombosis or blood clots in the peripheral or cardiac circulation.

Box 32-1 presents important differences between arteries and veins.

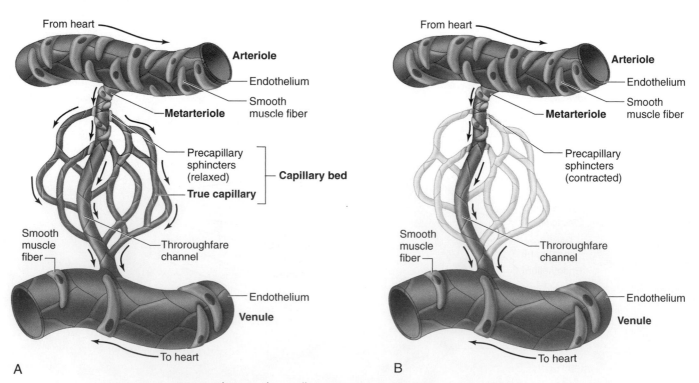

Figure 32-2   Microcirculation in the capillary system. A, Precapillary sphincters relaxed—blood flows through capillary bed. **B,** Precapillary sphincters contracted—blood flows through metarteriole only. *(From Thibodeau G, Patton K: Anatomy and physiology, ed 6, St Louis, 2007, Mosby.)*

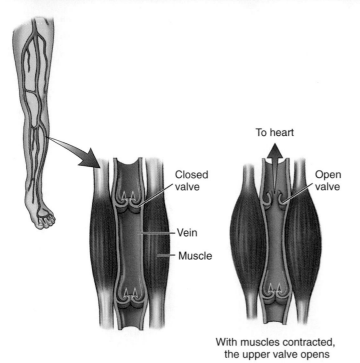

Figure 32-3 Skeletal muscle "pump." One-way valves in the veins prevent blood from backing up. Blood in the extremities is milked toward the heart by skeletal muscle contraction. *(From Herlihy B, Maebius NK: The human body in health and disease, ed 2, Philadelphia, 2003, WB Saunders.)*

| Box **32-1** | **Comparison of Arteries and Veins** |

Arteries
- Thick walls
- Elastic
- Blood moved through arteries by the pumping action of the heart
- No internal valves
- Loss of function can lead to tissue injury or death
- When severed, spurt blood (because of pumping action of the heart)
- Blood loss can be rapid and severe
- Arterial pressure higher than venous pressure

Veins
- Thin walls
- Less elastic than arteries
- Blood moved through veins by contraction of skeletal muscles
- Internal valves prevent backflow
- Loss of function not as medically significant as with arteries
- When severed, tend to bleed slowly
- Tend to be closer to the skin surface than arteries

PULMONARY AND SYSTEMATIC CIRCULATORY SYSTEMS

The circulatory system is divided into two pathways, the pulmonary system and the systemic system. The pulmonary system carries blood from the heart to the lungs for oxygenation (hemoglobin in the red blood cells picks up oxygen

molecules). The oxygenated blood then returns to the heart and is pumped into the systemic circulation, which reaches all tissues of the body.

The systemic and pulmonary systems (Figure 32-4) function simultaneously. The ventricles provide the primary pumping action for the heart. As the ventricles contract, deoxygenated blood flows to the lungs through the pulmonary system while oxygenated blood is pumped into the systemic system. Both systems have arterial, venous, and capillary structures.

- *Systemic circulation:* Oxygenated blood in the left ventricle is pumped through the ascending aorta to the rest of the body. Blood returning from the body passes from the capillaries into the venous system and returns to the left atrium through the vena cavae.
- *Pulmonary circulation:* Deoxygenated blood in the right ventricle is pumped through the *pulmonary arteries* (the only arteries that carry deoxygenated blood) to the lungs. Blood is oxygenated in the capillaries of the alveoli (lungs) and returns to the left ventricle through the *pulmonary veins* (the only veins that carry oxygenated blood).

BLOOD PRESSURE

Blood pressure is the force exerted on the arterial wall by the pumping action of the heart. The *systolic pressure,* the higher pressure, occurs during contraction of the ventricles (systole). The lower pressure, the *diastolic pressure,* occurs during the relaxation phase of the cardiac cycle (diastole).

Regulation of blood pressure is influenced by chemicals released by the autonomic nervous system in response to injury, body position, temperature, pain, and emotion. The complex hormonal regulation of arterial pressure, which is called the *renin-angiotensin-aldosterone system,* is influenced by fluid volume and other factors.

Negative alterations in blood pressure *(hypotension)* can be caused by hypovolemia (a precipitous drop in blood or fluid volume), fluid shifts between the spaces in the body, shock, or infection.

Hypertension, or abnormally high blood pressure, often is caused by cardiovascular disease, such as arteriosclerosis, but it also occurs with chronic renal failure and hypermetabolic conditions (e.g., malignant hyperthermia and hyperaldosteronism).

Normal blood pressure is affected by the following factors:
- *Gender:* Adult females generally have higher blood pressure than males.
- *Age:* A gradual rise in blood pressure occurs from childhood to adulthood.
- *Weight:* Blood pressure is higher in individuals with a high body mass index, regardless of age.
- *Exercise:* Blood pressure rises with strenuous activity but returns to baseline level at rest.
- *Diurnal (daily) fluctuation:* Blood pressure tends to rise during the day and is lowest in the mornings.

Blood pressure also is influenced by specific physiological parameters:

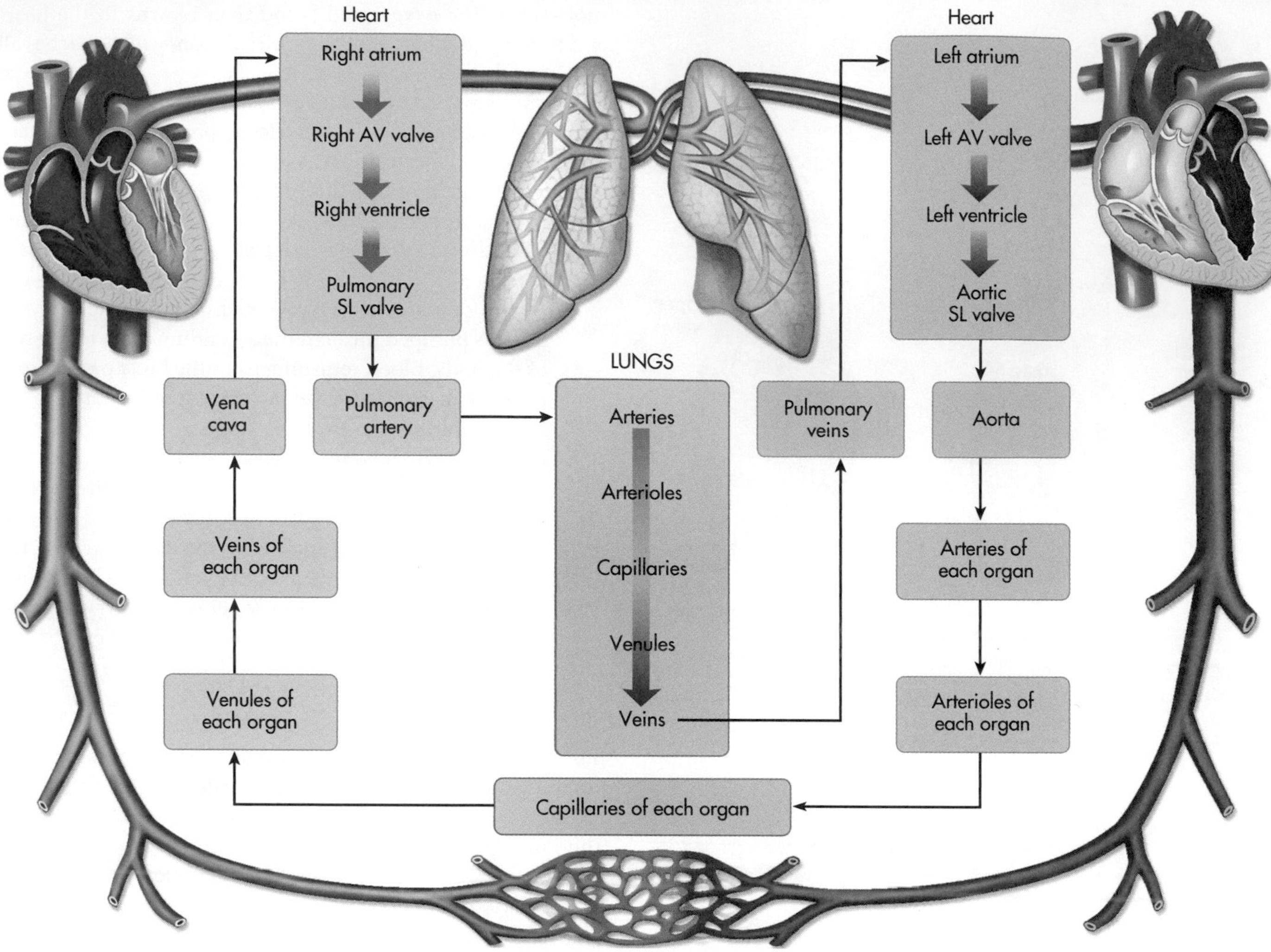

Figure 32-4   The systemic and pulmonary systems. In the pulmonary system, blood leaves the right heart, travels to the lungs, and returns to the heart. In the systemic circulation, oxygenated blood leaves the left ventricle, travels through the ascending aorta, and is transported throughout the body. It passes through the capillary system and returns to the heart via the venous system. (See text for further detail.) *AV,* Atrioventricular; *SL,* semilunar. *(From Thibodeau G, Patton K:* Anatomy and physiology, *ed 6, St Louis, 2007, Mosby.)*

- *Elasticity of the arterial walls:* The ability of the artery to expand and relax affects systemic pressure. Arteries stiffened by atherosclerosis result in hypertension.
- *Total blood volume:* The total amount of circulating blood has a direct effect on blood pressure. The body has mechanisms to constrict peripheral blood vessels when volume is low. However, this protective mechanism cannot overcome large blood loss or fluid shifts.
- *Peripheral vascular resistance:* Vascular resistance occurs when the muscular layer of the artery is unable to relax or arteries are stiff and their diameter is reduced.
- *Blood viscosity:* Viscosity is measured by the amount of fluid in the blood. Lower viscosity or "thicker" blood increases blood pressure.

BLOOD VESSELS OF THE BODY

In many cases, only the major arteries and veins and tributaries of the body are named. Names are often identical among arteries and veins, with a few exceptions.

Major Arteries

The largest artery of the body is the aorta. It emerges from the heart in an arch at the left ventricle and curves downward to descend through the thoracic cavity, passing behind the heart but in front of the spinal column. As it enters the abdomen, it passes through the diaphragm behind the retroperitoneum space. The aorta terminates at the pelvic **bifurcation** (splitting into a Y), which forms iliac arteries.

Thoracic Cavity

The aorta arises from the left ventricle of the heart to form an arch (the *aortic arch*). Three major arteries arise from the top of the arch: the *brachiocephalic* artery, the *left common carotid* artery, and the *left subclavian* artery. Beyond these branches, the aortic arch curves downward and is called the thoracic *descending aorta*. It passes through the diaphragm and leaves the thoracic cavity and enters the abdominal cavity. It is called the *abdominal aorta* at this level. There are many branches of the aorta at all levels.

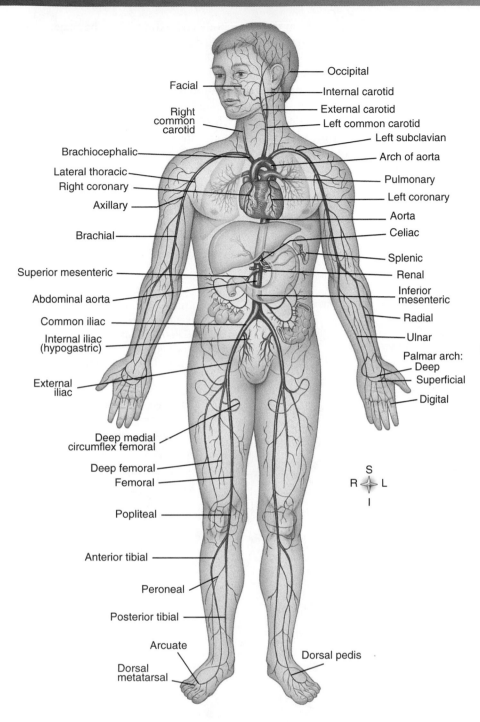

Figure 32-5 Major arteries of the body. *(From Thibodeau G, Patton K: Anatomy and physiology, ed 6, St Louis, 2007, Mosby.)*

Labels on figure:
- Occipital
- Facial
- Internal carotid
- External carotid
- Right common carotid
- Left common carotid
- Left subclavian
- Brachiocephalic
- Arch of aorta
- Lateral thoracic
- Pulmonary
- Right coronary
- Left coronary
- Axillary
- Aorta
- Brachial
- Celiac
- Splenic
- Superior mesenteric
- Renal
- Abdominal aorta
- Inferior mesenteric
- Common iliac
- Radial
- Internal iliac (hypogastric)
- Ulnar
- Palmar arch: Deep, Superficial
- External iliac
- Digital
- Deep medial circumflex femoral
- Deep femoral
- Femoral
- Popliteal
- Anterior tibial
- Peroneal
- Posterior tibial
- Arcuate
- Dorsal pedis
- Dorsal metatarsal

Head

The *brachiocephalic artery* gives rise to the *right common carotid artery*, which branches to the *external carotid artery* and the arteries of the brain. The vertebral artery, which branches from the *brachiocephalic artery*, follows the cervical vertebrae and branches distally to the arteries of the head.

Upper Extremities

The arteries of the upper body begin at the three vessels of the aortic arch discussed earlier. The brachiocephalic artery branches into the right common carotid and the right subclavian arteries. These supply blood to the right side of the head, neck, right shoulder, and upper arm. The left common carotid artery supplies blood to the left side of the neck and head. The left subclavian artery provides blood to the left shoulder and

right arm. The radial and ulnar arteries arise from the brachial artery. Figure 32-5 shows major arteries of the body.

Abdomen

The descending aorta continues through the abdomen and branches to the celiac trunk, a network that gives rise to the gastric, splenic, and hepatic arteries. Other significant arteries in the abdomen include the mesenteric arteries, which provide the blood supply to the intestines, and the renal arteries, which branch directly from the aorta and supply blood to the kidneys.

Lower Limbs

The iliac arteries divide into the internal and external iliac arteries in the pelvis and the external iliac artery converges into the femoral artery in the groin. Traveling distally, the femoral artery communicates with the popliteal artery in the knee area. The popliteal artery branches into the arterial tibial, peroneal, and posterior tibial arteries. The dorsal pedis emerges from the anterior tibial artery and then further divides into smaller arteries of the foot and phalanges.

Major Veins

The largest vein of the body is the vena cava, which is divided into *inferior* and *superior* segments. The venae cavae communicate with the heart through the right atrium. The superior vena cava receives deoxygenated blood from the head, neck, and upper extremities, and the inferior vena cava receives blood from the lower body and extremities. The major veins are illustrated in Figure 32-6.

Portal Circulation

The hepatic portal circulation is unique in structure and function. The superior mesenteric and splenic veins converge to form the portal vein. This large vessel carries nutrients from the digestive system into the liver and also supplies about 60% of that organ's oxygen requirements. The hepatic veins carry blood out of the liver to the vena cava. However, a pressure difference between the hepatic and portal veins allows the liver to store approximately 450 mL of blood. This can be released back into the systemic circulation as needed.

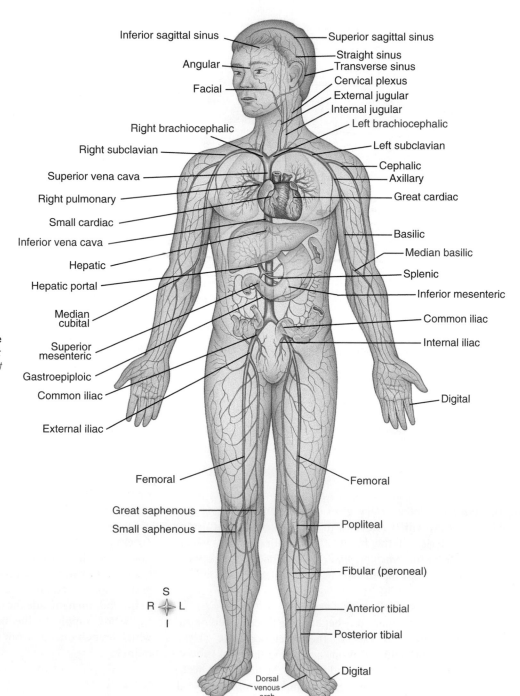

Figure 32-6 Major veins of the body. *(From Thibodeau G, Patton K: Anatomy and physiology, ed 6, St Louis, 2007, Mosby.)*

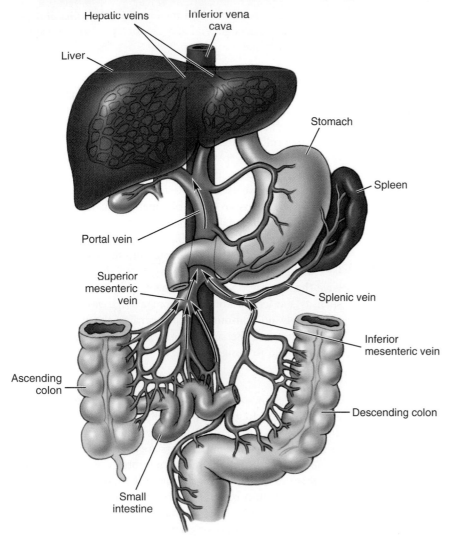

Hepatic veins

Inferior vena cava

Liver

Stomach

Spleen

Portal vein

Superior mesenteric vein

Splenic vein

Inferior mesenteric vein

Ascending colon

Descending colon

Small intestine

Figure 32-7 **The portal circulation.** *(From Herlihy B, Maebius NK: The human body in health and disease, ed 2, Philadelphia, 2003, WB Saunders.)*

Microscopic sinuses (sinusoids) in the liver, which are lined with epithelium, filter and remove bacteria, toxins, and cell remnants from the blood. The blood then is shunted back into the hepatic veins and into the vena cava (Figure 32-7). Because of the structure of the liver and sinusoids, fibrotic diseases of the liver, such as cirrhosis, can prevent the flow of venous blood out of the sinusoids. Blood backs up into the veins of the digestive system, causing varicosities and rupture of the vessels.

LYMPHATIC SYSTEM

The lymphatic system is composed of ducts (vessels), regional lymph nodes, and lymph (fluid). Lymph tissue such as the tonsils, adenoids, and Peyer's patches, in the large intestine, are important surveillance tissues which help to mediate the immune system. Lymph contributes to the formation of plasma, the liquid portion of blood, which is derived from intercellular components. Lymph vessels follow the anatomical pattern of arteries and veins. Like veins, lymph vessels contain valves that prevent reverse flow. The complex lymph system drains into two primary collection ducts. The right lymphatic duct drains lymph from the head, neck, thorax, and right arm. Lymph from the right lymphatic duct enters the

subclavian vein. The second collecting system is the thoracic duct, which receives lymph from other parts of the body and drains into the left subclavian vein. Occlusion of these ducts (e.g., during radical surgery) results in lymphedema or swelling of the lymph vessels. Certain diseases and tumors also cause blockage of the lymph system.

Lymph nodes are located at intervals along the lymph ducts. Nodes are composed of lymphatic tissue that collects and filters fluid from the system. They also produce lymphocytes (white blood cells). Nodes occur in groups or chains in collection areas. For example, the axillary nodes drain lymph from the breasts. Lymph from the pelvic organs drains to nodes in the inguinal area. During lymph node dissection, specific nodes are removed and assessed according to the organ suspected of cancer to determine whether metastasis has occurred.

DIAGNOSTIC PROCEDURES

Diagnosis of peripheral vascular disease is based first on the patient's history and the physical examination findings and on the results of routine blood tests. More specific studies may be performed based on the findings of these tests and the patient's signs and symptoms.

ARTERIAL PLETHYSMOGRAPHY

A pulse volume recorder is used to measure the arterial pulse waveform during systole. For this test, three blood pressure cuffs are placed on the leg and inflated to 65 mm Hg. Each cuff reading produces a waveform, which is compared with the waveforms from the other two cuffs. A reduced wave in one area may indicate reduced blood flow at that point.

DOPPLER SCANNING

Doppler scanning intensifies the sounds made by blood flowing through a vessel. The pitch, rhythm, and quality of the sound reflect pressure, volume, and flow rate. The tip of the Doppler probe is placed over a pulse point or other area that requires evaluation. The high-frequency sound waves generated by the probe are reflected back to a data recorder. Interpretative Doppler scanning is performed with a sterile probe. **Doppler duplex ultrasonography** combines Doppler scanning with ultrasound to produce visual images of the vessel. Blood flow, strictures, thrombi, turbulence (swirling motion of blood characteristic at a stricture), and other abnormalities are displayed on a monitor in real time and can be preserved for permanent documentation.

ARTERIOGRAPHY

Arteriography is radiographic imaging of the artery. This is done as an intraoperative, diagnostic, or interventional procedure to delineate the shape and interior surface of the arteries. A contrast medium is injected into the artery under fluoroscopy or computed tomography. Complex studies that provide three-dimensional images and time flow data are commonly used in diagnosis. Multidetector computed tomography angiography has taken the place of conventional angiography for diagnostic studies of the arterial system. Interventional arteriography is performed in conjunction with the insertion of stents and other devices.

INTRAVASCULAR ULTRASONOGRAPHY

Intravascular ultrasound is used in both peripheral and coronary surgery to map the **lumen** of a vessel. A rotating flexible catheter carrying a transducer is introduced into the vessel. Ultrasonic energy is generated and interpreted by the transducer. The lumen of the vessel can be mapped (including density, accumulation of atherosclerotic plaque, and wall thickness), and a visual image can be produced. Because the catheter is able to rotate, intravascular ultrasound produces a 360-degree image.

CASE PLANNING

INSTRUMENTS

Vascular surgery is performed with general surgical instruments and vascular instruments. Other sets are added according to the regional anatomy. Nearly all vascular procedures require right angle (Mixter type) clamps, tonsil (Schnidt) clamps, and Kelly, Crile, and mosquito forceps. General dissecting scissors and general surgery forceps also are used on nonvascular tissue.

Vascular Clamps

Vascular clamps are specifically designed to prevent trauma to blood vessels. The jaws contain finely serrated inserts that grip the tissue but do not crush or damage the surface of the vessel, even when fully closed. Clamps are available in a wide variety of shapes and sizes to fit around a vessel as it lies in normal anatomical position. Peripheral vascular clamps are much smaller than those used in cardiac surgery. Hundreds of types of vascular clamps are available, many with the same name (e.g., DeBakey clamps). The nature of vascular surgery is such that often little time is available for selection during surgery. It is common practice for the surgeon to specify which vascular clamps are needed before surgery so that the scrub can have them ready on the instrument table. In an emergency, such as sudden hemorrhage from a large vessel, the scrub should rely on common sense regarding the type of clamp needed, because the surgeon may not be able to turn away from the field to designate one.

Scissors

Vascular scissors are extremely sharp and fine. Many are angled so that the tips can be easily inserted into the vessel. The blades must be kept sharp to prevent tissue from buckling or folding between them. Scissors are sharply pointed or have a rounded probe tip. The most commonly used vessel dissection scissors are Potts (angled) and De Martel (straight) scissors. Fine Metzenbaum scissors are also used in vascular dissection. Vascular scissors must never be used to cut any materials such as suture or grafts, because this damages them.

Forceps

Vascular forceps (pickups) have very fine serrations at the tips to allow a secure grip without tearing or slipping. The most common vascular forceps are DeBakey forceps.

Surgeons generally do not ask for a specific type of vascular forceps during surgery. They assume that their personal preference is on record and the scrub has placed these on the instrument table. Vascular forceps are always passed to the surgeon when it is apparent they will be used to grasp a blood vessel or other delicate tissue. Plain general surgical forceps are not suitable for use on vascular tissue, because they do not have the precision or gripping ability of vascular forceps. Toothed forceps are never used on blood vessels, because they can puncture the walls of the vessel.

Retractors

There are few vascular-specific retractors except small vein retractors, which are also used in general surgery. Nonpenetrating shallow retractors are commonly used during superficial vascular surgery. A dull Weitlaner (self-retracting) or spring retractor should be available for skin and subcutaneous retraction in the hand, arm, or superficial leg. Handheld retractors include the Senn retractor, vein retractor, and shallow Richardson retractor. Skin hooks occasionally may be needed.

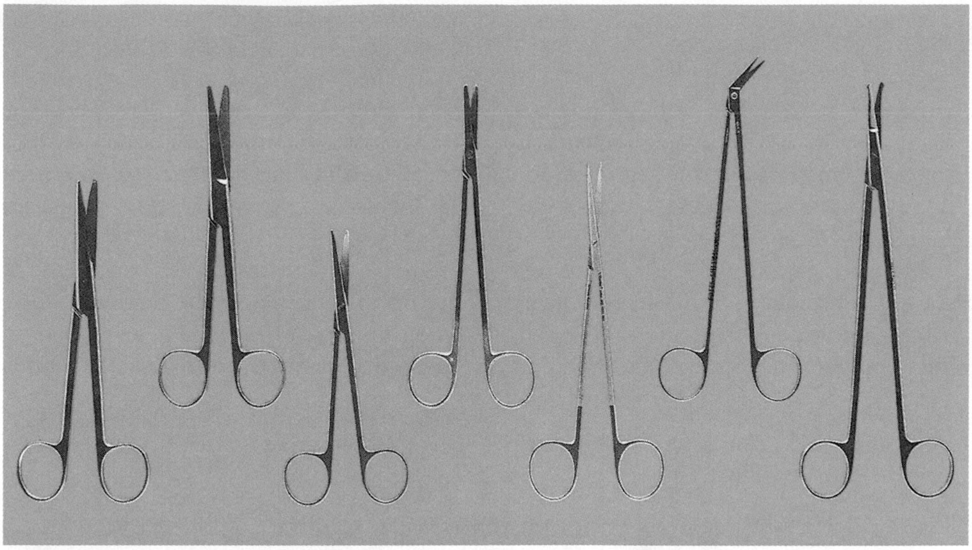

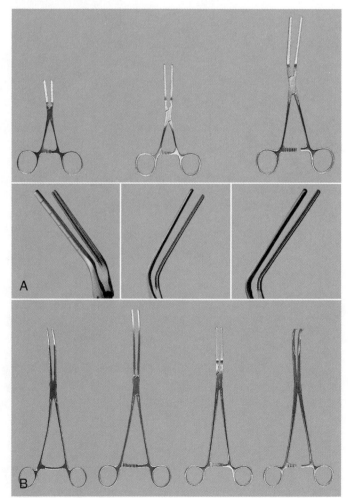

Figure 32-8 **Vascular surgery scissors.** *Left to right,* 1 straight Mayo scissors; 1 curved Mayo scissors; 1 Metzenbaum scissors; 1 Metzenbaum carbide insert scissors; 1 Lincoln scissors; 1 Potts-Smith scissors, 1 Strully scissors. *(From Tighe SM: Instrumentation for the operating room, ed 7, St Louis, 2007, Mosby.)*

For deeper surgery, general surgery retractors are used (e.g., Deaver, Richardson, and Army-Navy retractors). A standard Balfour self-retaining retractor is commonly used for procedures of the abdominal arteries.

Suction Tips

Small suction tips, such as the Frazier tip, are commonly used in most vascular procedures. The suction pressure should be lowered for use on the actual vessels. Frazier suction tips are available in a wide variety of French (Fr) sizes and the size used depends on the tissue. Suction tips must be kept clear of blood and tissue debris by suctioning a small amount of water through the tip. Larger suction tips are used according to the regional anatomy. General surgical tips, such as the Poole (vented) or Yankauer suction tip, are used in abdominal vascular surgery.

A dry surgical site is critical in vascular surgery and suction must be available at all times. Because vascular suction tips (e.g., the smaller Frazier tip) clog easily, the scrub should keep one on the field and another in reserve. This allows the clogged tip to be flushed or cleared with a metal stylet while one remains in use.

Large vessels, such as the abdominal aorta, require larger suction tips. Two suctions may be necessary to maintain a dry field. In general, suction is used more often than sponges to maintain a dry operative field.

Tunneler

A tunneler is used to burrow a channel through connective tissue to make space for a tubular vascular graft. Occasionally during surgery, the graft anastomosis sites are surgically exposed but located some distance apart. The tunneler is inserted into one site and pushed through the subcutaneous tissue to the other wound site. This creates a path for the graft, which can then be pulled through before anastomosis.

Instruments commonly used in vascular surgery are illustrated in Figures 32-8 to 32-10.

Figure 32-9 **Cardiovascular clamps. A,** *Left to right,* College clamp, angled; DeBakey clamp; DeBakey peripheral vascular clamp. **B,** *Left to right,* DeBakey aortic clamp, S-shaped; DeBakey aortic clamp, S-shaped, long; DeBakey multipurpose clamp; Semb ligature-carrying forceps. *(From Tighe SM: Instrumentation for the operating room, ed 7, St Louis, 2007, Mosby.)*

EQUIPMENT AND SUPPLIES

Sutures

Vascular sutures range in size from 3-0 to 11-0. Cutting and taper needles used for anastomosis are ⅜ curved needles. Synthetic monofilament or coated material is preferred over plain braided suture, because it is nonreactive and prevents endovascular clotting and emboli.

Vascular suture materials include polyester (Mersilene), polypropylene (Prolene), polyhexafluoropropylene (Pronova), Gore-Tex, and silk. Suture-needle combinations are very delicate and require careful handling. Only fine-tip needle holders

should be used. Cardiovascular (CV) sutures are available as single needles or double-arm needles.

The CV needle is grasped in the usual position behind the swage and the suture is gently withdrawn from the package. When vascular sutures are removed or passed, care must be taken to avoid snagging the needle on drapes or gloves. Passing of double-arm sutures may be problematic. As the loaded needle holder is passed, the other end may be easily snagged on drapes and instruments. Two needle holders may be used or a small hemostat can be clamped to one of the needles. The whole unit must be passed in a way that prevents tangling. An alternative method is to pass the nonoperative (mounted)

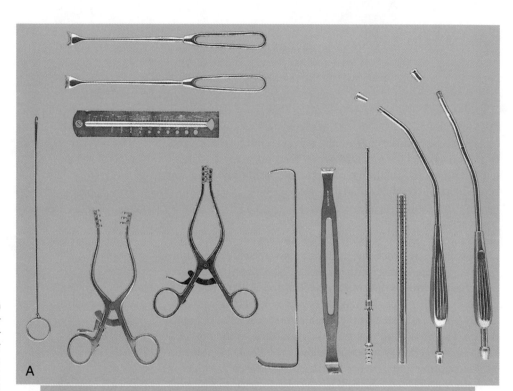

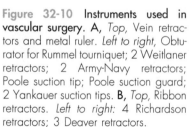

Figure 32-10 Instruments used in vascular surgery. A, *Top,* Vein retractors and metal ruler. *Left to right,* Obturator for Rummel tourniquet; 2 Weitlaner retractors; 2 Army-Navy retractors; Poole suction tip; Poole suction guard; 2 Yankauer suction tips. **B,** *Top,* Ribbon retractors. *Left to right:* 4 Richardson retractors; 3 Deaver retractors.

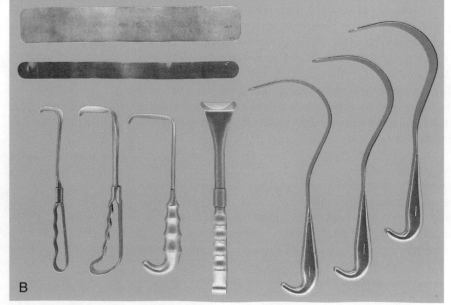

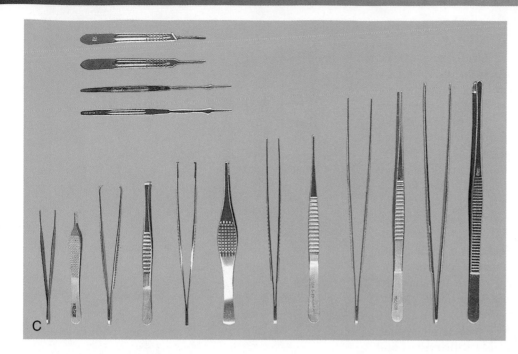

Figure 32-10, cont'd C, *Top,* Knife handles. *Left to right,* 2 Adson forceps; 2 Martin forceps; 2 Ferris Smith vascular forceps; 2 DeBakey vascular forceps, medium; 2 DeBakey forceps, long; 2 Russian forceps. *(From Tighe SM:* Instrumentation for the operating room, *ed 7, St Louis, 2007, Mosby.)*

needle on a folded towel while passing the mounted needle in the usual way. The towel is placed on the field in clear sight of the surgeon and assistant.

NOTE: *During surgery, do not remove a loaded needle holder from the field unless you are certain it is free and clear of the anastomosis. Double-arm sutures are used in tandem and removing one may drag the other out of the tissue.*

Vascular sutures are also supplied with felt pledgets (small squares of felted material) attached to the suture. The pledget prevents the stitch from tearing through the arterial wall.

Vascular Grafts

Vascular grafts are used to replace a blood vessel or to patch a vessel. Synthetic grafts are made of Dacron, polyester, or Gore-Tex. Sources of biological materials are banked human umbilical cord and autograft (usually from the saphenous vein). Grafts may be straight or bifurcated (Y-shaped). The length is measured in centimeters and the diameter reflects the outside diameter.

Synthetic grafts require no preinsertion preparation except trimming. Patch grafts are cut into elliptical sections and sutured in place with a double-arm suture. Bovine grafts were commonly used in the past but are rarely used today. All prepared grafts are intended for use as directed by the manufacturer.

Vascular grafts are extremely expensive. They must not be opened until the surgeon is ready to insert them and has verbally requested the size required. All manufactured grafts are identified by size, lot, and identification number, which must be recorded on the patient's operative record.

Catheters

The most common method of removing thrombi is with a Fogarty-type embolectomy catheter. This is a narrow flexible catheter with a firm tip surrounded by an inflatable balloon.

The length of the catheter varies widely. Balloons are round or elliptical and catheters are available in sizes ranging from 1 to 6 Fr. The balloon is filled with air or saline for testing purposes and with saline for actual use, according to the manufacturer's specification. A tuberculin syringe is used to fill the balloons, which have a volume of 1 mL or less. The balloon must be tested before use and must never be overinflated.

Central Venous Line

The central venous catheter, known commonly as a *central line*, was introduced in Chapter 13 as a method of administering IV drugs, solutions, parenteral nutrients, and for blood draws in patients that require long or medium term therapy. Central line catheters are constructed of polyvinyl choride, Teflon, polyurethan, or silastic (silicone elastomer blend). The main line of the device is a soft tube with an insertion end that remains in the vein and distal end that remains outside the body. The distal end may have two or three extensions (lumens) which are designated for drug, fluid, or blood infusion, or for blood withdrawal. The catheter is inserted into the superior vena cava near the right atrium through a percutaneous (through the skin) entry into the subclavian, internal jugular, or less commonly, the femoral vein. Although a number of companies manufacture and distribute central venous catheters under their own brand name, the generic names remain in use and identify the exact type. The following are common generic types:

Tunnelled catheter: A portion of the catheter is embedded or "tunnelled" in the subcutaneous tissue. There is an insertion site and an exit site. Common tunnelled catheters are the Hickman, Broviac, and Groshong. These are used for long term intravenous therapy and may have single or multiple lumens.

Non-tunnelled catheter: Used for short or medium term intravenous therapy.

Port: This type of catheter has an access port or reservoir which is implanted under the skin.

Central lines, like with other medical devices, have evolved over time and complexity and procedures for insertion have changed. In the past, central lines were place at the patient's bedside and often required repeated sticks with a large bore needle or an incision (called a *cutdown*) to expose the vein directly. This resulted in high infection rates and limited success rates. Modern central line placement is performed using strict aseptic technique, in the interventional radiology department or in the operating room using guided fluoroscopy technique or ultrasound to pinpoint the exact entry site and correct placement of the catheter in the vena cava.

Two techniques are commonly used for central line placement, *tunnelled* and *non-tunnelled* (Seldinger method). Both techniques require wide skin prep using chlorhexidine, draping to expose the sternoclavicular region including the chin, and regional or general anesthesia with routine physiological monitoring by an ACP.

Tunnelling technique: The entry vein (subclavian or inferior jugular) is punctured percutaneously with syringe and *introducer needle* supplied in the catheter insertion kit. With the needle held in position, the syringe is removed and a *guide wire* placed over the needle which is then removed. The guide wire is advanced to the inferior vena cava and the distal end of the catheter threaded over the guide wire. An exit site for the distal end of the catheter is selected a few inches below the insertion site and a plastic *tunneler* inserted near the venotomy site. This is advanced subcutaneously to the exit site where a small stab wound is made with a scalpel over the tip of the tunneler. The catheter is then pulled through the tunnel to emerge through the stab wound. The catheter is flushed, checked for placement, and sutured in place.

Seldinger technique: The entry vein is punctured with an introducer needle. A guide wire is placed over the needle which is then withdrawn, leaving the guide wire in place. The catheter is then threaded over the guide wire for exact placement. The guide wire is removed the catheter is flushed, and sutured in place.

Stents

An endovascular **stent** is a tubular mesh implant that fits against the wall of an artery. The stent thus provides a physical barrier between the atherosclerotic plaque and the vessel lumen. It also holds the vessel open so that blood can flow freely without platelet aggregation. Stents are made of stainless steel, titanium, or a metal alloy called Nitinol.

Stents are implanted permanently. Two common types of stents are the balloon stent and the self-expanding mesh stent. The balloon stent is a fine catheter with a balloon tip. The stent is fixed over the balloon, and when the balloon is expanded, the stent is pushed into position against the vessel wall. The self-expanding stent opens to provide a similar effect.

VESSEL RETRACTION

During vascular surgery, blood vessels are mobilized and positioned for incision and entry. Retraction is performed with a

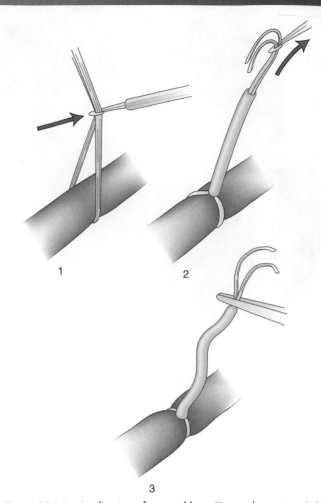

Figure 32-11   Application of a vessel loop (Rummel tourniquet). The two ends of the umbilical tape are grasped and threaded through the tubing. *(From Ouriel K, Rutherford R: Atlas of vascular surgery: operative procedures, Philadelphia, 1998, WB Saunders.)*

vessel loop. Several types of loops are available. The most common is a thin length of Silastic material, which is carried around the vessel with a right-angle clamp. The ends of the vessel loop are clamped together with a hemostat. **Umbilical tapes** (18 inches [45 cm] by ⅛- or ¼-inch [0.3- or 0.6-cm] flat, mesh cotton) are available prepackaged for use as vessel loops. A vessel loop may also be used to occlude a blood vessel by acting as a tourniquet. In this case, the ends of the vessel loop are threaded through a 0.25-mm length of Silastic tubing (called a *bolster*). The ends of the loop are pulled taut through the bolster, which tightens the loop around the blood vessel. When a bolster is used, the scrub threads the loop through the bolster and passes it on a right angle clamp along with a hemostat to secure the ends. A Rummel tourniquet is a longer bolster (Figure 32-11).

DRUGS

Vascular surgery requires a number of important and high-alert intraoperative drugs. Safety protocols for the distribution of drugs and proper labeling must be followed. (These protocols are discussed in detail in Chapter 13.) Specific drugs are used to prevent blood from clotting at the operative site (anticoagulation) or to encourage clotting (coagulation).

Anticoagulation

During vascular surgery, heparinized saline solution is used to prevent coagulation in the area of the operative vessels. This prevents thrombi from forming at the surgical site and reduces the risk of embolus. Systemic heparin may be administered just before arterectomy (incision into the operative artery) begins. Heparinized saline is prepared by the scrubbed surgical technologist. He or she receives both heparin and injectable saline, which are mixed in a ratio according to the surgeon's orders. For use on the field, the solution is drawn up with a 20- or 30-mL syringe fitted with a tapered irrigation tip. Systemic heparin is reversed with protamine sulfate, which is administered by the anesthesia care provider.

Coagulation

Hemostasis is maintained at anastomosis sites with collagen or fibrin products, such as microfibrillar collagen hemostat (Gelfoam, Avitene) or topical thrombin. Topical thrombin is a dry powder that is reconstituted with intravenous saline. Topical hemostatic collagen materials are used on anastomosis sites and capillary beds. Small squares (1 cm) of Gelfoam may be soaked in topical thrombin before use. Surgicel also may be placed on the site of the anastomosis.

NOTE: It is critically important that all medications on the field be clearly marked as soon as they are received. Accidental intravenous (IV) administration of thrombin can cause a fatal embolus.

TECHNIQUES IN VASCULAR SURGERY

ENDARTERECTOMY

Many vascular procedures require removal of atherosclerotic plaque from the inside of the artery (**endarterectomy**). Plaque is a rubbery substance that adheres to the tunica intima, causing stenosis or occlusion. When the surgeon removes plaque, there is a risk it will break apart, causing an embolus when clamps are removed to test blood flow. Endarterectomy requires meticulous technique and fine instruments. Plaque can be removed in one piece (Figure 32-12). The surgeon may use a Penfield or Freer elevator to separate the plaque from the intima while applying gentle traction. An alternative technique is to open the artery at its bifurcation and remove the plaque circumferentially.

VESSEL ANASTOMOSIS

Longitudinal or circumferential incisions in the blood vessel are closed with a double-arm suture. Traction sutures may be placed at one or both ends of the incision. (Figures 32-13 to 32-15).

GRAFT TUNNELING

Vascular grafts often must be tunneled through subcutaneous tissue or other layers to connect one vessel to another. Two techniques are used. The surgeon may use the fingers to separate the tissue digitally or a graft tunneler (discussed previously) can be used. The tunneler is a long metal shaft with blunt tips that is pushed manually through the tissue. As the tunneler is advanced, it leaves a tubular space through which the graft can be threaded. The surgeon usually performs this step by inserting a long clamp (e.g., a Péan clamp) into the tunnel and grasping the graft from the entry site. If the tunnel is short, the surgeon can pass it easily. Longer grafts may require an intermediate incision in the skin and subcutaneous tissue.

SURGICAL PROCEDURES

INTRAOPERATIVE ANGIOGRAPHY

Surgical Goal

Preoperative angiography (arteriography) is the injection of contrast medium into a selected artery and its branches to determine the exact location of strictures, occlusion, or malformation. During surgery, intraoperative angiography is used in conjunction with angioplasty to allow the surgeon to see the position of the stricture and to place the catheter in the correct location.

TECHNIQUE

1 All team members must wear a lead apron during a procedure involving radiography.
2 The circulator distributes the contrast medium to the scrub.
3 The scrub prepares the contrast medium and sterile saline.
4 The operative site is prepared for radiographs or C-arm fluoroscopy.
5 Metal instruments are removed from the field and the operative site is covered with a sterile drape.
6 The surgeon injects the contrast medium into the artery and images are recorded during injection.
7 The contrast medium is flushed from the artery with sterile saline.

Discussion

Intraoperative angiography is performed with intravascular ultrasound and other imaging techniques because it allows the surgeon to see obstructions or emboli distal and proximal to the operative area.

In this procedure, the contrast medium is injected directly into the operative artery and its branches and outline, as well as the interior configuration of the vessel, are observed by radiography or fluoroscopy. The contrast medium is flushed through the vessel with sterile saline at the completion of the procedure. Repeat injections and data recording may be required to clarify an image.

Whenever angiography is planned, all personnel must wear a lead shield over their scrub attire. The equipment needed for intraoperative angiography includes:

- Two or more 30- or 50-mL syringes
- A contrast medium, as specified by the surgeon
- An arterial needle
- One or two vinyl catheters with a stopcock attached
- An IV catheter for injection of the contrast medium
- Sterile IV saline

The circulator distributes the contrast medium to the scrub, who draws it up into two syringes. A solution of 60% Renografin is frequently used. A third syringe of IV saline is prepared to flush the contrast medium from the arteries when radiography has been completed. The scrub attaches one end of the angiography needle to a short length of vinyl tubing and the other end to a syringe of dye. All air bubbles must be removed from the tubing to ensure that air is not introduced into the artery. A Kelly or Mayo hemostat is placed across the tubing to prevent air from backing into it. If a stopcock is used, air bubbles are flushed out and the stopcock is secured in the closed position.

The surgeon may choose one of several techniques to inject the contrast medium:

- If the **arteriotomy** (incision in the artery) has already been sutured closed, an angiography needle is inserted between the sutures.
- A catheter can be inserted into the vessel and secured with a suture tie.

If standard radiographs are to be taken, the scrub uses sterile technique to receive the cassette in a cassette pouch. A deep fold is made in the edge of the cover, making a wide sterile cuff. After the cassette has been dropped inside, the edges of the pouch are turned up and secured. The

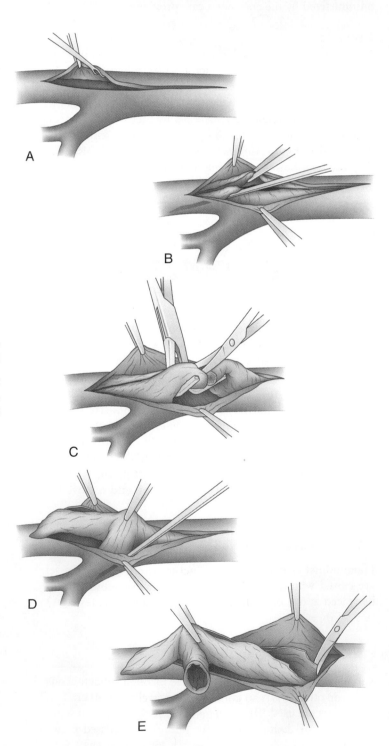

Figure 32-12　Endarterectomy technique. A, An arteriotomy is performed. **B,** A plane is created between the vessel wall and plaque. **C,** The plaque is divided over a right angle clamp. **D,** The plaque is mobilized distally. **E,** The proximal end of the plaque is trimmed. *(From Ouriel K, Rutherford R: Atlas of vascular surgery: operative procedures, Philadelphia, 1998, WB Saunders.)*

cassette is placed under the limb, the radiography machine is positioned, and films are taken. The cassette and cover are removed from the field. If C-arm fluoroscopy is used, the C-arm is draped and images are observed during injection. The artery and branches are immediately flushed with saline.

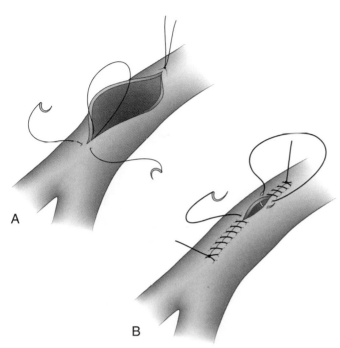

Figure 32-13 Suturing technique for closing a longitudinal arteriotomy. **A,** Double-arm suture is placed at each end. **B,** Continuous sutures are placed to provide a sealed closure. *(From Ouriel K, Rutherford R: Atlas of vascular surgery: basic techniques and exposures, Philadelphia, 1993, WB Saunders.)*

TRANSLUMINAL ANGIOPLASTY

Transluminal **angioplasty** is the insertion of an arterial catheter or stent into an artery to establish patency and normal blood flow.

Pathology

Atherosclerosis is an obstructive arterial disease that causes stiffening and loss of elasticity of the artery wall. In peripheral atherosclerosis, fatty plaque and calcium are deposited on the tunica intima, causing stenosis and loss of circulation. Areas of plaque are most dense near arterial bifurcations. Circulatory obstruction in the lower limbs leads to intermittent *claudication* (severe pain related to obstructed arterial flow) and ischemia. Dry gangrene may develop in untreated severe obstruction.

Discussion

Angioplasty is performed during angiography with C-arm fluoroscopy. The contrast medium is injected to verify correct placement of the stent, embolectomy catheter, or intravascular shaving device. **Percutaneous** angioplasty is performed in interventional radiology.

Balloon Angioplasty

In balloon angioplasty, a stricture in the artery is expanded with a balloon catheter that has been inserted to the level of the plaque. The inflated balloon pushes the plaque against the vessel wall and releases the stricture. Angioplasty balloons are available in graduated lengths and widths.

Before the balloon angioplasty is performed, contrast medium is injected into the artery and the area of stricture is marked on films produced by the data recorder. The balloon catheter is inserted into the artery to the level of the stricture. The catheter is left in place at a specific pressure and for a

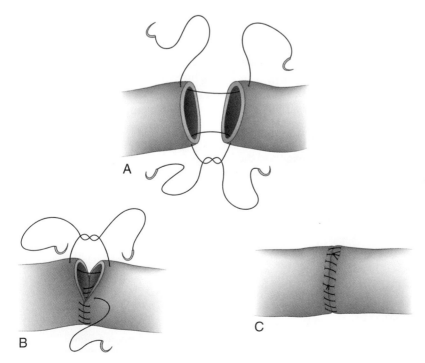

Figure 32-14 End-to-end anastomosis. **A,** Two double-arm sutures are placed in opposite locations. **B,** Continuous sutures are placed circumferentially. **C,** Completed closure. *(From Ouriel K, Rutherford R: Atlas of vascular surgery: basic techniques and exposures, Philadelphia, 1993, WB Saunders.)*

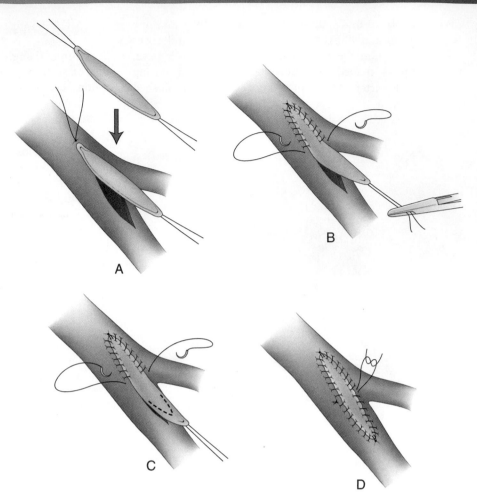

Figure 32-15 Technique for placing a patch graft. **A,** Traction sutures are placed at each end of the graft. **B,** Sutures are applied at both sides of the graft. **C,** The graft may be trimmed as needed *(dotted line).* **D,** Completed graft. *(From Ouriel K, Rutherford R: Atlas of vascular surgery: basic techniques and exposures, Philadelphia, 1993, WB Saunders.)*

specific length of time. The balloon catheter is filled with contrast medium and both the vessel walls and catheter balloon are observed on fluoroscopy. The catheter is withdrawn and final angiography films are taken.

Stent

For implantation of the balloon stent, the patient is placed in the supine position and a large-bore needle is inserted into the vessel distal to the stenting site. A flexible guidewire is passed over the needle, which is withdrawn, and the angioplasty balloon catheter is inserted and filled using a syringe. The stent is discharged and the catheter is removed. A common type of balloon-expandable stent is the Palmaz stent. The self-expanding stent is placed in the same manner except that the stent is preloaded into a delivery system that is passed over the guidewire. When the stent is discharged, it opens and adheres to the lumen wall. The Wallstent is a commonly used self-expanding stent. Figure 32-16 illustrates percutaneous transluminal angioplasty.

INSERTION OF A VENA CAVA FILTER

Surgical Goal

A vena cava filter is a metal, umbrella-shaped filter inserted into the inferior vena cava to prevent emboli from entering the pulmonary system. The filter can be temporary or permanent.

Pathology

Pulmonary emboli occur when one or more thrombi move from the venous system into the pulmonary vascular system. The vena cava filter is a method of capturing and preventing further movement of emboli. Candidates for the surgery include the following:

- Patients who have a venous thrombus but cannot tolerate anticoagulant therapy; these include patients who have had recent surgery or have a history of hemorrhagic stroke.
- Patients who have had a massive pulmonary embolism and survived but for whom a subsequent embolism would be fatal.
- Patients with chronic or venous thromboemboli in spite of anticoagulant therapy.
- Patients at high risk for pulmonary embolism.

TECHNIQUE

1 An incision is made in the groin and a guidewire is inserted.
2 The filter and introducer are inserted over the guidewire under fluoroscopy.
3 The filter is deployed from the introducer and the introducer is withdrawn.
4 The position of the filter is verified.
5 A pressure dressing is applied to the insertion site.

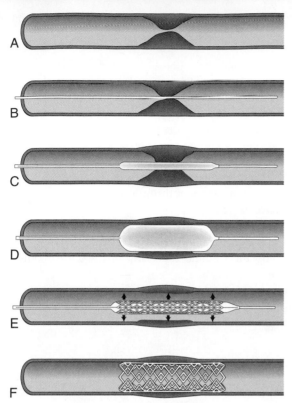

Figure 32-16   Percutaneous transluminal angioplasty. A, Stenosis of the artery. **B,** Insertion of a guidewire. **C,** A balloon catheter is inserted over the guidewire. **D,** The balloon is inflated. **E,** A mesh stent is inserted over the guidewire. **F,** The stent is inflated and the guidewire is removed. *(From Garden O, Bradbury A, Forsythe J, Parks R: Principles and practice of surgery, ed 5, Edinburgh, 2007, Churchill Livingstone/Elsevier.)*

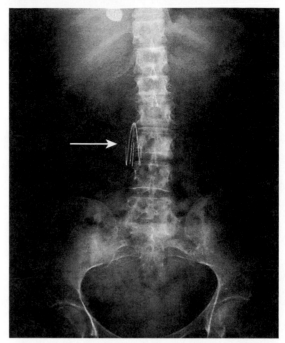

Figure 32-17   Radiograph showing the position of a vena cava filter inserted to prevent emboli. *(From Garden O, Bradbury A, Forsythe J, Parks R: Principles and practice of surgery, ed 5, Edinburgh, 2007, Churchill Livingstone/Elsevier.)*

Discussion

Insertion of a vena cava filter is commonly performed in the interventional radiology department under fluoroscopy. New filter devices can be inserted at the patient's bedside in the intensive care unit (ICU).

The vena cava filter is inserted by percutaneous needle insertion. The procedure requires a guidewire and filter introducer. The guidewire is a fine flexible wire coated with a chemical (e.g., polytetrafluoroethylene [PTFE]), which prevents platelet aggregation and allows the wire to slide easily through the vessel. The filter itself, which resembles an umbrella without fabric, is made of titanium, stainless steel, or Nitinol. When the filter is deployed, it opens out to the edges of the vessel (Figure 32-17).

All personnel working in interventional radiology wear lead aprons over their scrub attire.

The patient is placed in the supine position on the fluoroscopy or radiology table. The groin is prepped with povidone-iodine solution and the area is draped in the usual manner. Local anesthesia with or without sedation is administered.

The surgeon or radiologist begins the procedure by inserting a large-bore needle into the femoral artery. A guidewire is inserted through the needle and the needle is withdrawn. With the aid of fluoroscopy, the introducer is passed over the guidewire and the filter is ejected from the tip. The introducer and guidewire are withdrawn and pressure is applied to the puncture site for 10 to 15 minutes. A pressure dressing is placed over the site. The patient must remain in the flat supine position for at least 4 hours after the procedure to prevent postoperative hemorrhage.

VASCULAR ACCESS FOR RENAL HEMODIALYSIS

Surgical Goal

Patients with severe or end-stage renal disease require frequent hemodialysis. This treatment requires long-term access to the patient's vascular system. An anastomosis between the arterial and venous systems is created surgically to produce this access. Two techniques usually are used to create vascular access: an arteriovenous shunt or an arteriovenous fistula.

Pathology

End-stage and severe renal disease results in severe electrolyte imbalance and uremia (nitrogenous wastes in the blood). When the kidneys' filtering ability drops below 5%, hemodialysis is necessary for survival. During extracorporeal **hemodialysis,** the patient's blood is shunted outside the body through an artery. The blood is pumped through a series of filters to remove the waste products and excess electrolytes that normally would be filtered by the kidneys. The blood then is returned to the body through a vein.

Discussion

ARTERIOVENOUS SHUNT: ARM The patient is placed in the supine position with the arm extended on a large arm board. The arm is prepped and draped free. A local anesthetic usually is administered.

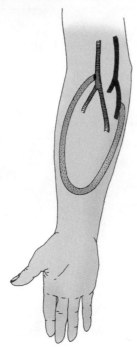

Figure 32-18 **Arteriovenous shunt.** A graft is implanted to form an anastomosis between the arterial and venous circulations. In this technique, the brachiocephalic vein and radial artery have been used. An alternative technique is direct anastomosis between the artery and vein. *(From Wilson SE: Vascular access: principles and practice, ed 3, St Louis, 1996, Mosby.)*

A skin incision is made over the cephalic vein and carried through the fascial layer with a curved hemostat and tenotomy or other plastic surgery scissors. Two small vessel loops are placed around the vein and the ends are clamped with mosquito hemostats. A small bulldog or similar vascular clamp is placed over the proximal end of the vessel. The distal end is divided and ligated with silk or polypropylene suture. This technique is repeated on the artery. A graft tunneler may be used to bring the graft in close approximation to both vessels. The graft is sutured in place with 6-0 or 7-0 polypropylene suture. The incisions are closed in layers and dressed with dry gauze. The completed graft is shown in Figure 32-18.

ARTERIOVENOUS FISTULA An *arteriovenous (AV) fistula* is a direct anastomosis between an artery and a vein. The site is selected for patency and accessibility. After routine prep and draping of the area, an incision is made over the vessels. The vessels are mobilized with sharp dissection and anastomosed as for an arteriovenous shunt. The wound is closed in layers.

Several months may be required for complete recovery of the AV fistula before it can be used for dialysis. Postoperative complications include infection and thrombosis.

THROMBECTOMY (OPEN PROCEDURE)

Surgical Goal
The goal of thrombectomy is to remove a stationary clot in a blood vessel. This restores circulation and prevents emboli.

Thrombectomy is commonly performed with an embolectomy catheter.

Pathology
A **thrombus** is a stationary clot in the arterial or venous system. A thrombus that breaks away from the vessel wall is called an **embolus.** As an embolus travels through increasingly smaller vessels of the vascular system, it may lodge in the heart, brain, kidney, mesentery, or other vital organ. This causes vascular obstruction **(infarction),** leading to tissue death. Thrombectomy therefore can be a life-saving procedure. Common causes of thrombi are:

- Atherosclerosis
- Surgery, especially when large blood vessels are exposed to air and clots form at the surgical site
- Orthopedic trauma, especially of the hip or other large bone
- Pulmonary emboli (those that lodge in the lung) usually originating from the venous system of the lower extremities

TECHNIQUE

1. The surgeon exposes and mobilizes the target vessel.
2. Vessel loops are placed around the artery.
3. The vessel is clamped.
4. An incision is made into the artery (arteriotomy).
5. The embolectomy catheter is threaded into the arteriotomy past the thrombus.
6. The balloon is inflated and the catheter is retracted slowly, pulling the thrombus through the arteriotomy.
7. Intraoperative Doppler duplex ultrasonography may be performed.
8. The arteriotomy is closed.
9. The wound is closed.

Discussion
Patient preparation depends on the location of the thrombus as determined by angiograms, duplex Doppler ultrasonography, and magnetic resonance imaging. Thrombi from the lower extremities often are removed from the groin. Mesenteric thrombi require an abdominal approach (laparotomy). The following discussion presents the techniques of thrombectomy, beginning with isolation of the vessel and use of the embolectomy catheter. Surgical incisions and closures are found in chapters associated with a particular anatomical area.

The patient is placed in the supine position for abdominal, lower extremity, and upper extremity surgery. A general or regional anesthetic is used. The surgical site is prepped in normal fashion.

The scrub should have heparinized saline, vessel irrigation tips, vascular sutures, ties, and hemostatic agents available. A variety of vascular clamps matched to the size of the vessel (or the surgeon's preference) also should be available on the instrument table. Small-bore suction and larger atraumatic suction tips are needed. Vascular forceps are used throughout

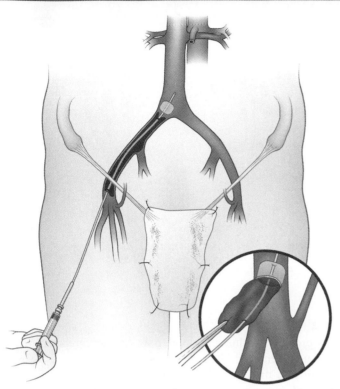

Figure 32-19   A thrombectomy catheter is inserted through a femoral venotomy and advanced past the thrombus. The balloon is inflated and the catheter is carefully withdrawn, pulling the thrombus with it. *(From Ouriel K, Rutherford R: Atlas of vascular surgery: operative procedures, Philadelphia, 1998, WB Saunders.)*

the procedure. Catheters should not be opened until the surgeon requests the size and type needed.

After surgical exposure of the target vessel, the surgeon places several vessel loops around the vessel and its nearby tributaries. This allows manipulation of the vessel and traction as needed.

To perform the embolectomy, the surgeon clamps the vessel distal to the thrombus. A vascular clamp is selected to fit the configuration of the vessel and its position in the wound. An arteriotomy is made with a #11 scalpel blade. Suction is applied at the arteriotomy site.

The prepared embolectomy catheter is carefully threaded into the vessel past the site of the thrombus. The balloon is inflated and the catheter is withdrawn (Figure 32-19). This pulls the thrombus back through the vessel. Angioscopy and angiography may be performed to ensure that the procedure was successful. The removed thrombus should be retained as a specimen.

The arteriotomy is closed with 6-0 or 7-0 nonabsorbable vascular suture. The wound is closed in layers according to the incision site.

CAROTID ENDARTERECTOMY

Surgical Goal

Carotid endarterectomy is the surgical removal of atherosclerotic plaque from the carotid artery. Plaque is removed through an open incision in the artery. This reestablishes the flow of oxygenated blood to the brain.

Pathology

Partial obstruction of the carotid artery forms at the bifurcation of the common carotid artery with the internal and external carotid branches. The obstruction causes restricted arterial blood flow to the brain, which may result in neurological symptoms resulting from transient ischemic stroke and high risk for major stroke. Patients with complete blockage of the carotid artery are generally not considered for carotid endarterectomy.

TECHNIQUE

1 An incision is made along the anterior border of the sternocleidomastoid muscle and carried to deep tissue.
2 The common, external, and internal carotid arteries are mobilized and controlled with vessel loops.
3 The internal, common, and external carotid arteries are clamped.
4 The electroencephalogram is monitored.
5 An arteriotomy is made into the common carotid artery and extended upward.
6 An intraluminal shunt may be put in place to provide continuous cerebral blood flow.
7 Atherosclerotic plaque is dissected from the vessel wall.
8 A graft may be sutured over the arteriotomy or the incision may be closed.
9 The graft is checked for leaks and extra sutures are placed as needed.
10 All bleeders are controlled with the electrosurgical unit (ESU).
11 The wound is closed in layers.

Discussion

During carotid endarterectomy, the surgeon will temporarily occlude the carotid arteries while removing plaque. This is a critical phase in the procedure, because blood flow to the brain is severely compromised. The instruments and Mayo table must be kept neat and organized to ensure maximum efficiency during the procedure. All essential instruments, catheters, and vascular clamps must be prepared and in view. Attention to the surgical wound is important throughout the procedure.

Carotid endarterectomy may be performed using either a general or regional anesthesia. When a regional anesthetic is used, the patient will respond to simple neurological tests, such as hand strength tests or speaking. An *electroencephalogram (EEG)* commonly is used to measure the brain's electrical activity during the procedure. Electrical activity is affected by oxygen supply to the tissue, a critical component of carotid surgery.

The patient is placed in the supine position and the head is turned away from the affected side. A small pad may be placed under the shoulders to hyperextend the neck. If EEG monitoring will be used, electrodes are placed. The skin prep extends from the face to the axillary line. Draping is similar to that for thyroidectomy.

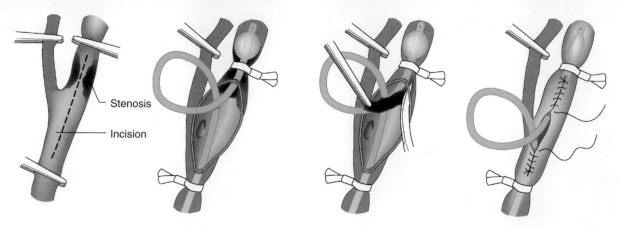

Figure 32-20   Use of the Javid shunt during endarterectomy. The arteriotomy is performed and the shunt is inserted, allowing partial blood flow during the removal of plaque. *(From Garden O, Bradbury A, Forsythe J, Parks R: Principles and practice of surgery, ed 5, Edinburgh, 2007, Churchill Livingstone/Elsevier.)*

The surgeon begins the procedure by incising the neck along the anterior border of the sternocleidomastoid muscle. The incision is carried deeper with the vascular forceps, electrosurgical unit (ESU), Metzenbaum scissors, and sponge dissectors to the level of the common, internal, and external carotid arteries. The scrub should have a variety of retractors available, including two dull Weitlaners, dull rakes, and Army-Navy retractors. The rake retractors should have dull rather than sharp teeth to prevent trauma to the large vessels that lie nearby.

The common, external, and internal carotid arteries are mobilized with fine vascular tissue forceps and Metzenbaum scissors. The bifurcation itself is not mobilized fully. Vessel loops are placed around each of the three arteries. Small hemostats are used to clamps the ends of the loops. Small sections of tubing or Rumel tourniquets also may be placed around the loops for control.

Before the surgeon makes the arterial incision, the anesthesia care provider administers systemic heparin to the patient. This prevents clotting and reduces the risk of emboli. The carotid sinus may be injected with 1% lidocaine to prevent bradycardia and hypotension associated with manipulation with the carotid body.

Before the actual endarterectomy, the scrub should have a number of instruments ready: a #11 scalpel blade, Potts and De Martel scissors, neurosurgical elevators (Penfield or similar), a Freer elevator, and straight hemostats. Wide-tip atraumatic suction also is needed. The surgeon indicates the preferred vascular clamps.

To begin the endarterectomy, the surgeon clamps the internal, common, and external carotid arteries. The surgeon then notifies the anesthesia care provider and circulator that the arteries have been clamped. The length of time the artery is occluded is timed. The EEG is closely monitored until the clamps are released.

The surgeon makes a small incision into the common carotid artery with the #11 scalpel blade. The incision is extended with Potts or De Martel scissors. Arterial plaque is identified as a thick, yellow, rubbery material that adheres to the lumen (intimal layer) of the artery.

Internal Shunt Device

To provide continuous blood flow to the cerebrum while plaque is removed, the surgeon may insert a flexible internal shunt into the internal and common carotid arteries. Many types of shunts are available (e.g., *Javid shunt*). The scrub must flush the shunt with heparinized saline before passing it to the surgeon. Use of a shunt during the procedure is shown in Figure 32-20.

If a shunt is to be used, it is inserted at this point. A shunt ring clamp (called a *Javid clamp*) and vessel tourniquets are used to maneuver and hold the shunt in place. Cross clamps placed on the carotid before the arterectomy. These may be released when the shunt is in place.

The surgeon grasps the edge of the plaque with vascular forceps or a straight hemostat and lifts it gently from the intima. Penfield or Freer elevators are used to create a dissection plane between the plaque and the inner lumen. The arterial plaque and lumen of the artery are flushed with heparinized saline during this part of the procedure.

After dissection, the plaque is passed to the scrub as a specimen. The arterial lumen is flushed with heparinized saline solution.

The arterial incision is closed with 5-0 or 6-0 cardiovascular sutures or a patch graft may be put in place at this time. The patch graft is cut to size from a sheet of PTFE or other grafting material.

Before the arteriotomy is closed, the external, internal, and common carotid artery clamps are opened and closed, in that order. This allows any debris to flow out and restores blood flow. At this point, the arteries are clamped.

NOTE: If a shunt has been placed, it is removed just before the arterial incision is completely closed. The ring clamp holding the shunt is released from the internal carotid artery and the shunt is removed. The arterial clamps are removed sequentially (e.g., external, common, and internal).

When the arteriotomy has been closed, the surgeon removes the clamps from the external, common, and finally the internal carotid arteries.

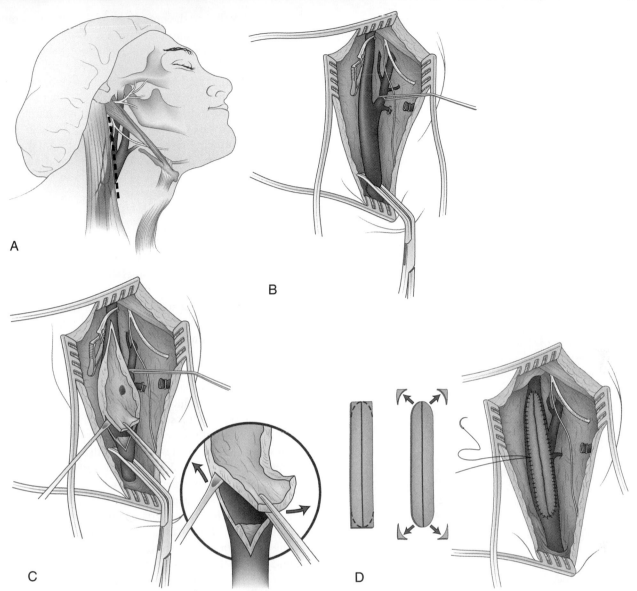

Figure 32-21   Carotid endarterectomy. A, The incision is made parallel to the sternocleidomastoid muscle. **B,** The internal jugular vein is mobilized, and the carotid vessels are exposed. **C,** An arteriotomy is performed and plaque is extracted from the vessel. **D,** Closure with a patch graft. *(From Ouriel K, Rutherford R: Atlas of vascular surgery: operative procedures, Philadelphia, 1998, WB Saunders.)*

The suture line is observed for leaks and blood flow confirmed with Doppler. Any leaks are repaired with additional sutures and controlled with topical hemostatic agents. Protamine sulfate is administered to reverse the effects of systemic heparin.

Angiograms may be taken at this time to check the patency of the vessel superior to the surgical site. Doppler and intravascular ultrasound also may be used. All bleeders are controlled with the ESU and the neck incision is irrigated with warm saline. The deep layers of the arterial incision are closed with 3-0 synthetic absorbable sutures. The skin is closed with 4-0 nylon or other synthetic nonabsorbable material. The wound is covered with a gauze dressing. The procedure for carotid endarterectomy is shown in Figure 32-21.

Patients may be taken to the neurosurgical ICU after the procedure and observed closely for neurological deficit,

hemorrhage, and respiratory complications. Damage to the carotid body, a structure between the external and internal carotid arteries, may result in disruption of the body's hypoxic drive to breathe. Alterations in cerebral perfusion may cause neurological deficit.

ABDOMINAL AORTIC ANEURYSM

Surgical Goal

An abdominal aortic **aneurysm** is a condition in which a section of the abdominal aorta becomes thin and bulges because of atherosclerotic plaque and progressive weakening of the aortic wall. The surgical goal is to implant a graft extending from the aorta to both iliac arteries. This restores circulation to the lower extremities and pelvis.

Pathology

Aortic aneurysms can occur at any location in the artery. However, they usually occur just below the renal arteries and extend to the bifurcation of the common iliac arteries or just above it. If the disease remains undiagnosed, the walls of the aorta become increasingly stretched and finally rupture. A dissecting aneurysm is one in which blood seeps between the layers of the vessel, causing it to tear and split. Atherosclerosis and degeneration of the muscular layer of the vessel are the most common causes of aortic aneurysm. Although the aneurysm may not extend into the iliac arteries, a bifurcated graft often is used in the repair.

TECHNIQUE

1 The surgeon performs a laparotomy through a midline incision extending from the xiphoid to the pubis.
2 The retroperitoneal space is entered.
3 The abdominal aorta is partly dissected.
4 The renal vein may be ligated for access to the perirenal aorta.
5 The aorta is cross-clamped.
6 The aneurysm is incised and opened.
7 Blood clots and plaque are removed from the aneurysm sac.
8 A graft is implanted in the aorta above the proximal end of the aneurysm, extending to the bifurcation of the iliac arteries.
9 Angiograms are taken.
10 The retroperitoneal space is closed.
11 The abdomen is closed as a single layer with polydioxanone surgical (PDS) suture or in multiple tissue layers.

Discussion

Repair of an aortic aneurysm may be scheduled (elective) or an emergency procedure. If the procedure is an emergency, recall that the most important stages of the surgery are exposure of or access to the target tissue, adequate visualization of the trauma site, immediate control of hemorrhage, and rapid repair or restoration of circulation.

The scrub should have long instruments immediately available because the target site is anterior to the posterior body wall or retroperitoneum. Right angle clamps, the surgeon's choice of vascular clamps, abdominal suction tips, and an ESU are needed. A long Penrose drain and vascular loops also should be available for vessel retraction. Because of the depth of the wound, deep handheld retractors (e.g., a Deaver retractor) or a self-retaining retractor (e.g., a Thompson or Bookwalter retractor) with multiple attachments may be required. Grafts should be available but not opened until the surgeon has prepared the vessels. A blood recovery system, such as the Cell Saver or Haemonetics system, usually is used in emergency surgery.

The patient is placed in the supine position, prepped, and draped for a midline incision extending from the xiphoid to the pubis. A Foley catheter is inserted before the skin prep.

The surgeon enters the abdomen through a long midline incision. Many moist laparotomy sponges are used to preserve tissue viability during the procedure. If the intestines must be brought out of the abdominal cavity, a plastic pouch may be used to keep them moist. Long vessel loops should be prepared at this time. Each should be tagged with a hemostat. Right angle clamps are used to pass the loop under the vessels.

Retractors are placed, and the retroperitoneum is incised with a #10 blade mounted on a long scalpel handle. Using blunt and sharp dissection vascular forceps, the surgeon exposes the aorta and places a vessel loop around it.

Occasionally the left renal vein must be clamped and ligated to provide access to the perirenal aorta. (This does not usually have a long-term effect on the kidney, because collateral circulation is sufficient.) Using finger dissection and sponge dissectors, the surgeon frees the upper end of the aorta. There is a risk of damaging the vena cava at this stage. If damage occurs, it is repaired immediately with 4-0 or 5-0 vascular suture. The inferior mesenteric artery is clamped, ligated, and divided.

Dissection continues until the aorta is freed from the vertebral column. If excessive bleeding occurs, pressure is applied with laparotomy sponges. Dissection of the distal aorta is performed to the level of the common iliac arteries for complete exposure. The arteries are mobilized carefully by blunt dissection. The lumbar arteries, which enter the aorta from the posterior side, may be occluded with 4-0 or 5-0 polypropylene or braided polyester sutures. When dissection is complete, the surgeon can decide the type and size of graft needed for the repair. If the iliac arteries are also diseased (aneurysmal), the internal and external arteries are mobilized in order to provide space for cross clamping.

The aneurysm is prepared for opening. If a risk of excessive bleeding exists in spite of cross clamps on the aorta, a Foley catheter with a 30-mL balloon may be prepared for use as an intraluminal tamponade in the aorta. In any event, the scrub should be prepared for excessive bleeding when the aneurysm is opened. Extra aortic clamps, suction, and mounted sutures should be prepared. A basin is used to collect large clots and debris.

Before the aneurysm sac is opened, the patient is heparinized and the common iliac arteries are clamped using DeBakey or similar right angle vascular clamps. The proximal aorta is then cross-clamped using Crafoord coarctation forceps, Satinsky clamp, Potts, or Cooley clamp. Some surgeons place the distal clamps first to prevent the flow of thrombi into the renal arteries. However, this is not a rigid practice and the proximal clamp may also be placed first.

The surgeon uses a #15 blade or the ESU to make a longitudinal incision into the aneurysm sac, leaving the anterior surface of the aorta and aneurysm intact. Any blood clots and debris are scooped out. The plaque is grasped with vascular forceps and gently separated from the wall of the aorta. The scrub should keep the basin on the field to collect the specimens. Any bleeding from the lumbar arteries can be repaired with polypropylene sutures. Bleeding from the inferior mesenteric artery may require clamping or ligation with a vessel loop.

Each artery is opened, and the proximal ends are irrigated with heparinized saline. The bifurcated graft is trimmed and

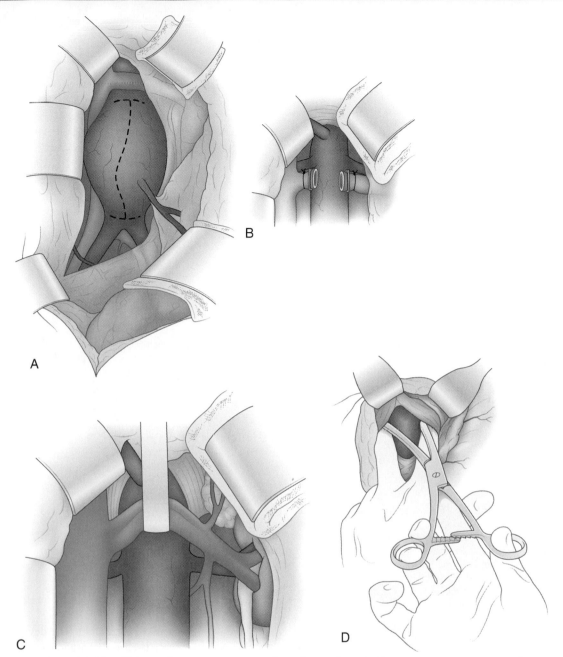

Figure 32-22 Abdominal aortic aneurysm with graft insertion. **A,** The retroperitoneum is incised over the aneurysm. **B,** The left renal vein can be safely divided to gain additional exposure. **C,** Alternatively, a narrow retractor can be used to provide exposure. **D,** The aorta is cross-clamped. *(From Ouriel K, Rutherford R: Atlas of vascular surgery: operative procedures, Philadelphia, 1998, WB Saunders.)*

distal limbs anastomosed with 3-0 or 4-0 polypropylene suture. If only a straight graft is required (e.g., in the case of healthy iliac arteries), the aneurysm sac is approximated over the graft using 3-0 polypropylene vascular suture. The surgeon checks the graft for leaks by slowly releasing the clamps. Additional sutures may be required. Hemostatic agents may be applied to the suture lines until all bleeding has been controlled. Angiograms and ultrasound are used to verify patency of the vessels.

The wound is irrigated with saline solution. The retroperitoneum is closed with 2-0 or 3-0 running absorbable suture. The abdominal contents are replaced, and the abdominal wound is irrigated before closure. A single-layer closure of polydioxanone surgical (PDS) suture may be used or the abdomen can be closed in layers. Figure 32-22 presents the details of this procedure.

Endovascular Approach (Endovascular Abdominal Aneurysm Repair)

In endovascular abdominal aneurysm repair (EVAR), the aortic aneurysm is approached through the femoral artery. A multisectional stent (endograft) is introduced into the aorta through the femoral artery under fluoroscopy. Because the graft is expandable, once it is implanted, the vessel can be

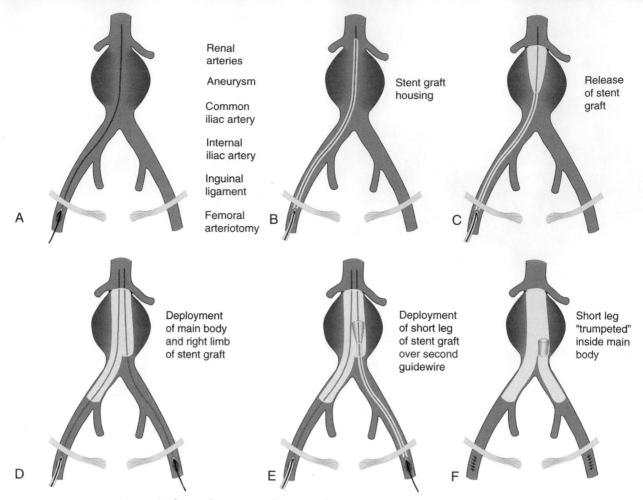

Renal
arteries

Aneurysm

Common
iliac artery

Internal
iliac artery

Inguinal
ligament

Femoral
arteriotomy

Stent graft
housing

Release
of stent
graft

Deployment
of main body
and right limb
of stent graft

Deployment
of short leg
of stent graft
over second
guidewire

Short leg
"trumpeted"
inside main
body

Figure 32-23   **Endovascular stent graft repair of an aortic aneurysm. A,** A guidewire is passed through the aneurysm through the right common femoral artery. **B,** A catheter containing the stent graft is passed over the guidewire and into position in the aneurysm. **C,** The outer cover of the catheter is removed, allowing the proximal end to remain open. **D,** The rest of the graft is removed, allowing deployment of the main body and right limb of the stent graft in the common iliac artery. **E,** A second guidewire is passed through the short limb of the stent graft. **F,** Deployment is complete and the aneurysm sac is excluded from the circulation. *(From Garden O, Bradbury A, Forsythe J, Parks R: Principles and practice of surgery, ed 5, Edinburgh, 2007, Churchill Livingstone/Elsevier.)*

straightened to some degree, reducing the risk of rupture (Figure 32-23). The long-term effectiveness of the EVAR procedure is under statistical review. Short-term results have been favorable.

Discussion

During the procedure, correct placement of the stent graft is verified with a variety of catheters and guidewire systems. The devices used are based on the surgeon's experience and preferences. Each manufacturer of a stent system has a specific design and method of stent deployment. At the time of this writing there are at least four different systems in use. Sectional stents are used in order to accommodate anatomical variations of the aneurysm. Commonly used systems are based on multiple components and three main operative objectives. These are:

• Access to the ileofemoral region.
• Placement (deployment) of the main body of the graft stent.
• Deployment of the stent limbs. The components of the device are deployed separately, and connect by overlapping

"barbs" in the neck of each stent. The devices are made of stainless steel, cobalt-chromium alloy, or Nitinol, whereas the grafts are usually polyester or ePTFE (expanded polytetrafluoroethylene). Components include:

1. The main body of the stent graft, which is bifurcated (Y-shaped)
2. A graft limb (iliac limb)
3. Extensions as needed
4. Cuffs

The patient is positioned on a radiolucent operating table with fluoroscopy available during the procedure. Skin prep and draping are the same as that used for bilateral femoral bypass (see earlier discussion). Both groins are prepped because the stent is inserted through one side while the opposite site is used for angiogram access during stent placement.

A femoral artery on the side of the stent insertion (operative side) introduces the stent guidewire through the femoral artery through direct puncture or mobilization and control of the artery in the standard fashion for arterial cutdown. The angiogram catheter is introduced into the opposite femoral artery. The operative guidewire is advanced under fluoroscopic guidance and advances the stent into the aorta. The stent is then positioned and the graft deployed. The graft barbs attach to the aortic wall and help to stabilize its position. The guidewire is removed.

The angiogram catheter is now removed and the opposite-side iliac limb stent and graft are inserted using a new guidewire under fluoroscopy.

One of the most common complications (and reasons for failure) of EVAR is endoleak, in which blood flows outside the graft and into the aneurysm sac postoperatively. The components of the graft or device can separate at the site of attachment or the sac may enlarge. These complications can be repaired by reentering the wound and placing additional stents or balloon dilation. In more severe cases, coil embolization or ligating the lumbar and inferior mesenteric arteries may be necessary.

Abdominal aortic procedures commonly cause fluid shifts, which require continuous observation and treatment for **hemodynamic** abnormalities. The peripheral pulses are carefully monitored, and chest radiographs and electrocardiograms are routinely obtained in the postoperative period. Complications include hemorrhage, infection, renal failure, and bowel obstruction.

AORTOFEMORAL BYPASS

Surgical Goal

An aortofemoral bypass is performed to treat aortoiliac occlusive disease. A graft is implanted between the aorta and the femoral arteries to bypass the iliac arteries and restore circulation (Figure 32-24).

Pathology

The iliac artery is a common site of atherosclerosis. An aortofemoral bypass is performed instead of an endarterectomy or aortoiliac bypass because it produces increased patency and can be performed in patients with extensive calcification of the arteries.

TECHNIQUE

1 Bilateral groin incisions are made to expose the femoral arteries.
2 A laparotomy is performed through a long midline incision, and the aorta is exposed.
3 The patient is heparinized and the aorta is clamped below or at the renal arteries.
4 The distal portion of the aorta is oversewn with heavy vascular sutures.
5 The proximal end of a bifurcated graft is anastomosed to the distal aorta.
6 Bilateral subcutaneous tunnels are made in the retroperitoneal tissue.
7 The graft is pulled through the tunnels.
8 Bilateral arteriotomies are made in the femoral arteries, and the graft limbs are anastomosed to each artery.
9 Angiography and ultrasound are used to verify patency.
10 The wound is checked for bleeders and closed in the routine manner.

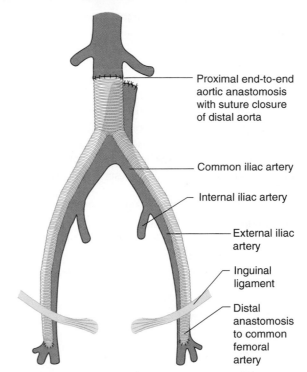

Figure 32-24 **Aortofemoral bypass.** A graft is implanted between the aorta and the femoral arteries to bypass the iliac arteries and restore circulation. *(From Garden O, Bradbury A, Forsythe J, Parks R: Principles and practice of surgery, ed 5, Edinburgh, 2007, Churchill Livingstone/Elsevier.)*

Labels on figure:
- Proximal end-to-end aortic anastomosis with suture closure of distal aorta
- Common iliac artery
- Internal iliac artery
- External iliac artery
- Inguinal ligament
- Distal anastomosis to common femoral artery

Discussion

The patient is placed in the supine position. The prep area extends from the axillary line to the midthighs. Both legs are draped circumferentially and the genitalia are covered with a towel and barrier drape. A Foley catheter is inserted before the skin prep.

The procedure begins with bilateral groin incisions, which are carried deeper to expose the femoral arteries. Dissection is performed with Metzenbaum scissors, sponge dissectors, and the ESU. Weitlaner or Gelpi self-retaining retractors are used superficially and Richardson retractors are used for deeper hand retraction. After the femoral vessels have been exposed, the incisions may be covered with sterile towels during laparotomy.

A midline abdominal incision is made and carried to the aorta, as described in the previous procedure. The proximal portion of the aorta is dissected to the renal veins.

Heparin is administered to the patient and the femoral arteries are clamped with right angle vascular clamps. The inferior mesenteric artery is clamped to prevent an embolus from entering it when the aortic clamp is applied.

The surgeon mobilizes the aorta using blunt dissection and clamps it below the level of the renal arteries. The aorta is divided and the distal end is oversewn with 2-0 or 3-0 polypropylene sutures. The proximal end of a bifurcated graft is trimmed to fit and anastomosed to the distal aorta with 3-0 polypropylene sutures.

Retroperitoneal tunnels are created in the loose connective tissue of the groin to accommodate the graft limbs. The tissue is then separated digitally. The two limbs of the graft are pulled through the tunnels and into the femoral wounds. A vascular clamp may be placed across the graft limb to prevent it from twisting.

Suture scissors are used to trim the ends of the graft to a 45-degree angle, rounding the tips. Each limb of the graft is sutured into the femoral artery through an arteriotomy, commonly with 4-0 double-arm polypropylene sutures.

After completion of the anastomoses, the femoral clamps are slowly released. Angiograms and ultrasound scanning are performed to verify the patency of the grafts. The wound is irrigated and closed as described in the previous procedure.

Patients recover in the ICU or the surgical unit. Doppler testing is performed throughout the first 48 hours of postoperative recovery to ensure that the peripheral circulation remains intact. Complications include infection, renal failure, hemorrhage, fluid shift, and respiratory complications.

AXILLOFEMORAL BYPASS

Surgical Goal

An axillofemoral bypass creates circulation between the femoral arteries and the axillary artery. This restores circulation to the lower extremity or, in an emergency procedure, bypasses an infected aortic graft or aneurysm.

Pathology

Circulation to the lower extremities derives from the descending aorta and the iliac and femoral arteries. Atherosclerotic disease of the aortoiliac region results in obstruction of the lower extremities.

TECHNIQUE

1 A 45-degree incision is made in the subclavicular area on the affected side.
2 The pectoralis major muscle is bluntly divided and the deep fascia is incised.
3 The pectoralis minor muscle tendon is divided.
4 The axillary artery is mobilized and clamped.
5 A synthetic graft is tunneled through the subcutaneous tissue from the axillary incision to the femorofemoral graft.
6 The axillary artery and tributaries are clamped.
7 The axillary artery is incised and the proximal end of the graft is anastomosed to the artery.
8 The groin is entered and the femoral graft is mobilized and controlled.
9 The distal graft is anastomosed to the femorofemoral graft.
10 The incisions are checked for leakage.
11 Angiograms are obtained.
12 The wounds are closed in layers and dressed.

Discussion

An important indication for axillofemoral bypass is an infected aortic graft. Perfusion of the leg (i.e., blood flow and oxygen exchange in the leg tissues) can be restored after excision of the graft. Axillofemoral bypass offers an alternative. It

avoids the risks of major aortic surgery, but long-term patency of the graft is possible only if outflow from the axillary artery is brisk.

The patient is placed in the supine position. The skin prep includes the affected arm, shoulder, clavicular and neck areas, abdomen, and groin. The arm is placed on a wide arm board and draped as for an upper arm procedure (excluding the hand). The groin is occluded with towels and an adhesive drape. Separate drapes are used to expose the operative area, and both legs may be draped with split sheets or U-drapes. A body sheet or procedure drape is placed on top of the drapes.

Two surgeons may work simultaneously, one at the subclavicular incision and the other at the groin. To begin the procedure, the surgeon makes a 45-degree incision in the subclavicular region. The subcutaneous layer is entered with the ESU and rakes or retractors are placed at the incision edges. The pectoralis major muscle is divided manually and the deep fascia is incised. However, the tendon attachment of the pectoralis minor must be severed with the ESU. A deep self-retaining retractor or small Richardson retractor replaces the rakes.

The axillary artery is mobilized and vessel loops are placed around it and nearby tributaries. Small branches are clamped with small bulldog or spring clamps, divided, and ligated.

A graft tunneler may be used to make a tunnel in the subcutaneous incision between the upper incision and the groin. If the patient is very tall, an intermediary incision may be necessary.

The groin is entered as previously described and the femoral artery graft and bifurcation are mobilized. Vessel loops are placed around the graft and controlled with Rummel tourniquets.

The patient is given heparin intravenously and the axillary artery is clamped. The artery is incised with a #11 scalpel blade and the anastomosis is performed with 5-0 or 6-0 polypropylene suture.

The distal end of the graft is brought in contact with the femoral graft. The distal tip of the graft is beveled with scissors and anastomosed with 6-0 Gore-Tex sutures. A double-arm suture is commonly used.

Suture lines are checked for leaks and the heparin is reversed with protamine. An angiogram may be obtained to ensure patency of the graft. Both wounds are irrigated and closed in layers.

FEMOROFEMORAL BYPASS

Surgical Goal

A femorofemoral bypass involves implantation of a prosthetic graft that connects the femoral artery on the affected side to the opposite femoral artery. This is done to bypass unilateral atherosclerotic disease in the iliac artery.

Pathology

A femorofemoral bypass is used only when the iliac system on the donor side is free of disease. Iliac disease usually is bilateral, and in such cases, stenting or balloon angioplasty of the donor iliac system may be necessary.

TECHNIQUE

1 Bilateral groin incisions are made and the common femoral arteries are isolated.
2 A subcutaneous tunnel is created between the groin incisions.
3 A synthetic graft is pulled through the tunnel and anastomosed to each femoral artery.
4 The wounds are closed.

Discussion

The patient is prepped and draped for bilateral groin incisions. A Foley catheter may be inserted and the genitalia are excluded from the prep with towels and an occlusive drape. A general or regional anesthetic may be used.

The procedure begins with groin incisions, which are made with the scalpel and carried to the deeper layers with sponge dissectors, Metzenbaum scissors, and the ESU. Large bleeders may be clamped and ligated with 3-0 silk suture. The scrub should have right angle clamps and two or more self-retaining retractors available for the dissection. Army-Navy retractors and small Richardson retractors also may be needed. The groin incision is carried to the level of the common femoral artery, which is isolated with Silastic loops. The iliac artery also may be looped for manipulation. The procedure is repeated on the opposite side.

The surgeon uses the fingers to create a subcutaneous tunnel in the skin between the two incisions. An aortic clamp is used to puncture the fascia attachments at the midline. The surgeon grasps one end of the graft with the curved aortic clamp and pulls it through the tunnel. The graft must be pulled through the tunnel without kinks or twists.

An end-to-side anastomosis is created between the graft and the profunda femoris on each side. Running sutures of 5-0 or 6-0 polypropylene are commonly used to perform the anastomosis. Air is pushed out of the graft and the vascular clamps are removed. Hemostatic agents are applied to the suture lines. Protamine sulfate may be administered to reverse the effects of systemic heparin. However, this practice is under investigation and current research. When the wound is dry and the suture lines are secured, the wound is closed in layers. A femorofemoral bypass is illustrated in Figure 32-25.

IN SITU SAPHENOUS FEMOROPOPLITEAL BYPASS

Surgical Goal

In situ saphenous vein bypass is a surgical alternative to the use of a synthetic graft to bypass a diseased femoral artery. The saphenous vein is not removed but is left in anatomical position. In the technique described here, a continuous incision is made along the entire saphenous vein. This is the safest method and allows complete ligation of tributaries. The distal

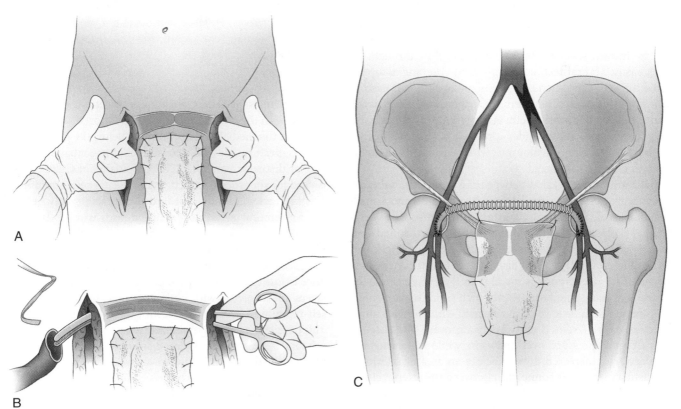

Figure 32-25 **Femorofemoral bypass. A,** A suprapubic tunnel is created digitally. **B,** The midline fascia is pierced with a long clamp, which grasps a Penrose drain or umbilical tape to facilitate delivery of the graft without kinks or twists. **C,** Bilateral end-to-side anastomoses are constructed; each anastomosis is run onto the profunda femoris artery if the superficial femoral arteries are occluded. *(From Ouriel K, Rutherford R: Atlas of vascular surgery: operative procedures, Philadelphia, 1998, WB Saunders.)*

or narrow end of the vein is anastomosed to the popliteal artery and the proximal vein is anastomosed to the large end of the femoral artery. The goal is to produce vascular continuity with an autograft.

TECHNIQUE

1 A single incision or multiple incisions are made on the medial thigh, following the path of the saphenous vein.
2 The branches of the vein are ligated and divided.
3 The proximal and distal ends of the vein are clamped and divided.
4 Internal valves are obliterated with microvascular valve scissors, a valvulotome and angioscope, or a valvulotome alone.
5 The saphenous vein is anastomosed to the femoral and popliteal arteries.

Discussion

The patient is prepped and draped with the operative leg and thigh exposed. The medial aspect of the thigh is incised from above the ankle to the groin, following the saphenous vein. The incision is carried deeper with dissecting scissors and the ESU. This exposes the saphenous vein, which is partly or completely mobilized. Vessel loops are placed along its length for manipulation.

The branches of the vein are clamped with mosquito hemostats or clipped. Each is divided from the vein. Fine silk sutures also may be used to ligate the tributaries. The distal and proximal ends of the saphenous vein are clamped and divided.

Before the anastomoses are performed between the saphenous vein and the femoral and popliteal arteries, the valves must be incised so that arterial blood can flow through the valves easily. Several techniques are used. The angioscope is passed through the lumen of the vein and a system is used to both sever the valves and remove tributaries. This avoids extensive dissection of the vein. An alternative method is to incise the first two valves under direct vision with valve scissors and then to use a valvulotome, with or without the angioscope, to release the others.

Anastomoses are created between the saphenous vein and the femoral artery. The vein is trimmed to a bevel and a small incision is made in the femoral artery with Potts scissors or a #11 scalpel blade. An end-to-side anastomosis is formed with 6-0 or 7-0 nonabsorbable sutures with a double- or single-arm needle. The profunda femoris also can be used for anastomosis. The distal anastomosis is made with the same technique.

Next, the small tributaries that branch from the saphenous vein must be occluded. These are located with Doppler ultrasound unless the vein is completely exposed. The surgeon applies digital pressure over the vein while observing the Doppler wave. Increased flow indicates an area of arteriovenous fistula (a vascular connection between the arterial circulation and the venous flow). These areas are exposed and each individual tributary is clipped or ligated and incised.

Angiography is performed at this time to check for patency. The wounds are irrigated and closed in layers, with absorbable synthetic sutures used for subcutaneous and fascial tissue. The skin is closed with clips or nonabsorbable suture.

The wounds are dressed with a nonadherent dressing and then with gauze squares and roller gauze.

FEMOROPOPLITEAL BYPASS

Surgical Goal

In a femoropopliteal bypass, a synthetic graft or autograft is implanted between the femoral and popliteal arteries. As discussed previously, in situ grafting uses the greater saphenous vein as a shunt.

Pathology

Femoropopliteal bypass is indicated for atherosclerosis of the femoral artery

TECHNIQUE

1 An incision is made on the medial side of the thigh and carried to deep tissues with sharp and blunt dissection.
2 The femoral artery is mobilized and vessel loops are placed around it.
3 The distal incision is made on the medial side of the knee, inferior to the patella.
4 The popliteal artery is located and mobilized.
5 Angiograms are taken.
6 A synthetic graft is tunneled through the subcutaneous tissue, connecting the two wound sites.
7 The femoral artery is clamped and an arteriotomy is performed.
8 The proximal end of the graft is anastomosed to the femoral artery.
9 The popliteal anastomosis is performed.
10 Angiograms are taken and pulses are verified.
11 The wounds are closed after all bleeding has been controlled.

Discussion

The patient is placed in the supine position, prepped, and draped with the affected leg and groin exposed. An incision is made on the medial side of the thigh, below the groin. Dissection is performed with the scalpel, Metzenbaum scissors, sponge dissectors, and the ESU. A Weitlaner or Gelpi retractor is used for superficial retraction. For deeper retraction, Army-Navy retractors or small Richardson retractors may be used.

The femoral artery is mobilized with careful dissection. One or more vessel loops are placed around the artery for retraction and manipulation.

A second vertical incision is made on the medial side of the knee below the patella. The subcutaneous, fascial, and muscle layers are dissected with both sharp and blunt dissection. A self-retaining retractor is used to expose the popliteal space. The popliteal artery is mobilized with sponge dissectors and scissors. A vessel loop is placed around the artery. Angiography may be done at this time to verify that the popliteal artery is patent.

The surgeon chooses the appropriately sized graft. The greater saphenous vein may be used instead of a synthetic graft (see the following section).

A tunnel is made in the subcutaneous tissue and the graft is carried from the upper to the lower wound. The graft is then drawn back into the popliteal space. To perform the anastomosis, the surgeon first places a vascular clamp across the femoral artery. A small incision is made in the artery with a

#11 scalpel blade or vascular scissors. Using running sutures of 5-0 or 6-0 polypropylene, the surgeon creates the anastomosis between the femoral artery and graft.

The popliteal anastomosis is created in the same manner as the femoral anastomosis. During both anastomoses, the scrub should have heparinized saline solution available for irrigation of the arterial sites. Hemostatic agents are used to check bleeding at the anastomosis and additional sutures are placed if needed.

Angiography may be done at this time and the patency of the arterial system is monitored with the Doppler or intravascular ultrasound. The wound is irrigated and closed in layers. The popliteal space is closed with 2-0 or 3-0 interrupted absorbable synthetic sutures. The skin commonly is closed with staples or nylon sutures. The groin incision is closed in layers and dressed with gauze squares.

A femoropopliteal bypass is illustrated in Figure 32-26.

During the immediate postoperative period, the patient's pedal pulses are monitored carefully. Possible complications include blockage of the graft and infection. Patients may experience some numbness of the lower leg. Swelling of the operative leg is common after surgery.

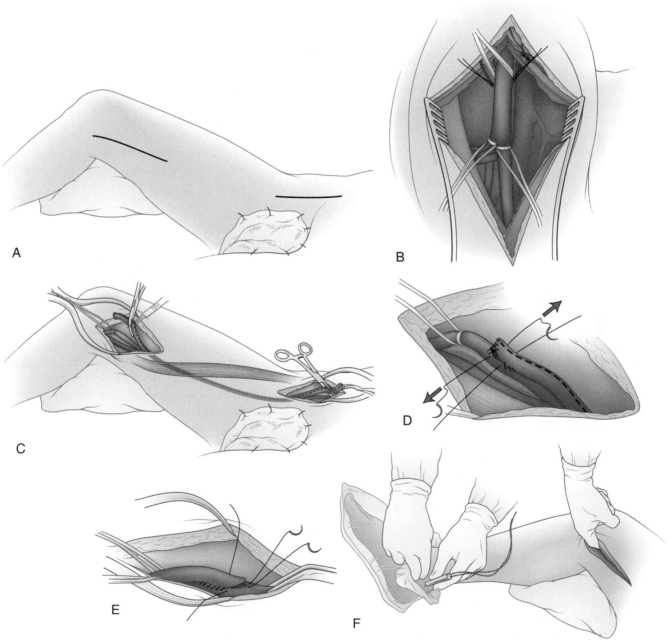

Figure 32-26 **Femoropopliteal bypass. A,** A femoral incision is made at the level of the inguinal ligament. A popliteal incision is made on the medial side of the distal thigh. **B,** The common femoral, superficial femoral, and profunda femoris arteries are exposed in the groin. **C,** A curved hemostat and the knife blade are used to bevel the graft for the anastomoses. **D,** Completion of the popliteal anastomosis. **E,** The proximal anastomosis is completed with a two-suture technique. **F,** Doppler ultrasound is used to assess the hemodynamic result intraoperatively. *(From Ouriel K, Rutherford R: Atlas of vascular surgery: operative procedures, Philadelphia, 1998, WB Saunders.)*

SAPHENOUS VEIN GRAFT

Surgical Goal

For a saphenous vein graft, the greater saphenous vein is removed to provide an autograft for peripheral or coronary artery bypass. The goal is to remove the vein yet retain its structural and physiological soundness.

Pathology

An autograft is an ideal graft for arterial bypass. The greater saphenous vein has been used more successfully than other materials for small-diameter arterial bypass. It is readily accessible and its connective tissue layer thickens with increased pressure. This makes it strong and able to withstand high arterial pressure.

TECHNIQUE

1 The groin and inner aspect of the leg are incised over the saphenous vein.
2 Branches of the vein are clamped, ligated, and divided.
3 The vein is injected with papaverine or lidocaine to prevent spasm.
4 The vein is mobilized and removed.
5 The vein is checked for leaks.
6 Tributaries are clamped and ligated.
7 The leg wound is closed.
8 The graft is preserved in saline.

Discussion

A general anesthetic usually is administered because the procedure is performed in conjunction with peripheral or cardiac bypass surgery. The patient is placed in the supine position and the selected leg is prepped from the groin to the foot. Drapes expose the leg and groin, with the foot occluded.

A common problem during vein harvesting arises from the practice of one surgeon harvesting the vein while the rest of the team prepares the implant site (e.g., during coronary artery bypass). In this case, the two overhead operating lights are dedicated to the top of the surgical field, leaving no direct light for the saphenous vein harvest. A third light or headlight should be available to provide lighting on the leg.

The knee is flexed to gain access to the medial aspect of the leg. To begin the surgery, the surgeon makes a long incision directly over the saphenous vein from the groin to the point of removal, usually below the knee.

The groin incision is made parallel to the upper thigh crease, directly over the saphenous vein. Bleeders are coagulated with the ESU or ligated with 3-0 silk sutures. A dull Weitlaner retractor may be placed in the wound. Branches of the vein are clamped and ligated with silk or clipped and divided. The vein is ligated with heavy silk sutures and divided with scissors.

The surgeon performs the distal excision by first clamping tributaries and ligating them. The vein is carefully dissected along its length to avoid creating wide tissue flaps on each side. The scrub or assistant must keep the vein and incision moist during the surgery. Frequent irrigation with saline solution is necessary. An Asepto syringe can be used for irrigation. Some surgeons inject papaverine or lidocaine into the subcutaneous tissue to prevent vein spasm.

The surgeon places Silastic vessel loops around the vein for retraction rather than using forceps, which can damage the vessel. When all tributaries have been divided, the vein is removed and placed in a basin.

Preparation of the Vein

The scrub attaches a blunt-tipped irrigation needle to a 30-mL syringe. The needle is inserted into the tip of the vein and secured with a heavy silk tie. Saline is used to irrigate the vein during the repair. If ordered, heparinized papaverine may be used. The surgeon injects solution into the vein and occludes the branches with silk ties. The vein must be kept moist at all times.

After preparation, the graft is maintained in a moist saline environment until needed. The vein also may be placed in a basin with heparinized papaverine and normal saline solution. This is called a "vein bath." The vein must be carefully monitored and protected at all times.

The leg incision is closed with interrupted sutures. The skin is closed with staples or monofilament synthetic suture. Harvesting of a saphenous vein is illustrated in Figure 32-27.

MANAGEMENT OF VARICOSE VEINS

Surgical Goal

Surgical treatment of varicose veins involves the removal of dilated and tortuous (varicose) veins and their tributaries to prevent symptoms and to improve cosmetic appearance.

Pathology

Venous blood returns to heart from the extremities aided by the contraction of skeletal muscles. The intraluminal valves of the veins prevent blood from returning by gravity to the extremities. Valve incompetency or chronic inactivity may cause stasis of venous blood and distention in the veins. In primary varicose veins, the superficial saphenous veins are affected. Secondary varicose veins originate from the deep saphenous vein. Surgical treatment includes removal of the deep saphenous vein, superficial saphenous veins, or both. Tributaries of the veins visible through the skin are removed separately.

TECHNIQUE

1 The greater saphenous vein is exposed at the medial malleolus.
2 The vein is ligated and divided.
3 A vein stripper is passed through the vein to the groin.
4 The groin is incised to expose the proximal end of the vein.
5 The proximal end is ligated and all tributaries are divided and ligated.
6 The vein is removed by extracting the vein stripper.
7 Superficial veins are removed by excision.

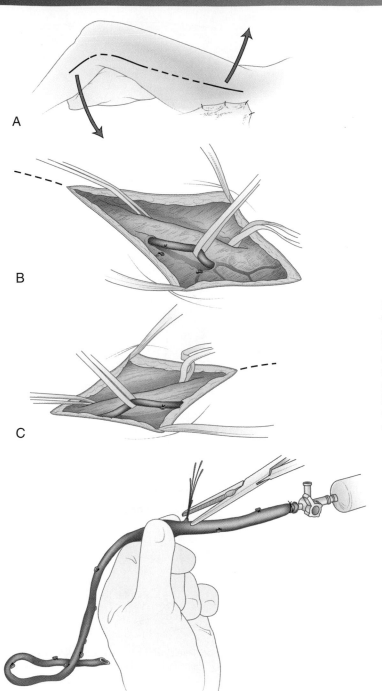

A

B

C

D

Figure 32-27 Harvesting the saphenous vein. The saphenous vein commonly is harvested to replace a diseased coronary artery and for other bypass procedures. **A,** External rotation of the hip exposes the line of incision. **B,** The saphenous vein and artery are exposed. Tributaries are clamped, tied, and divided. **C,** During surgery, the vein is preserved with saline solution (note the Asepto syringe). **D,** The vein has been removed and is tested for leaks, which are clamped and ligated. *(From Ouriel K, Rutherford R: Atlas of vascular surgery: operative procedures, Philadelphia, 1998, WB Saunders.)*

Discussion

Before surgery, the paths of the superficial veins are marked with indelible ink. The patient is placed in the supine position, prepped, and draped with the affected leg and groin exposed. A general or regional anesthetic is administered.

The surgeon makes an incision anterior to the medial malleolus. The incision is carried deeper with a curved hemostat and Metzenbaum scissors. A small Weitlaner retractor or Senn retractors may be placed in the wound.

When the distal saphenous vein is located, it is dissected free. The severed distal end is ligated with 2-0 silk. The surgeon threads a disposable vein stripper through the lumen until resistance is felt. Small tributaries (perforators) that

connect the deep saphenous vein to the superficial vein may impede passage of the stripper. A small incision is made over the tributary, which is clamped, divided, and ligated. The stripper is advanced to the terminal end at the femoral junction.

The groin is incised with the scalpel and bleeders are coagulated with the ESU. A rake or Army-Navy or Weitlaner retractor is placed in the wound. The proximal end of the saphenous vein is isolated with a vessel loop. The branches are double-clamped, divided, and ligated with 3-0 silk suture.

When all branches have been secured, the vein stripper is pulled out at the groin incision while the assistant applies pressure over the calf and thigh using folded towels.

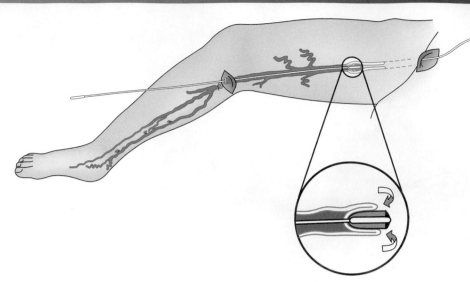

Figure 32-28 Stripping of the saphenous vein. *(From Townsend CM: Sabiston textbook of surgery, ed 17, Philadelphia, 2001, WB Saunders.)*

To remove small superficial tributaries, the surgeon makes an incision directly over them and mobilizes them with a curved hemostat and dissecting scissors. The vessels are double-clamped, divided, and ligated with silk ties.

The leg is dressed with nonadherent gauze strips and rolled gauze and then with an elastic compression bandage. Varicose vein stripping is illustrated in Figure 32-28.

Patients generally have pain, bruising, and swelling after surgery. Serious complications include arterial injury, deep vein thrombosis, and pulmonary embolism.

ABOVE-THE-KNEE-AMPUTATION

Surgical Goal

Above-the-knee amputation involves the surgical removal of the leg.

Pathology

Although amputation may not be considered strictly a vascular procedure, it usually is performed when vascular insufficiency caused by arteriosclerotic or thromboembolic disease results in necrosis of the lower limb. Above-the-knee rather than below-the-knee amputation is chosen when the vascular supply in the lower limb is insufficient for proper healing at the amputation site. The procedures are very similar. Incision sites for all leg amputations are shown in Figure 32-29.

TECHNIQUE

1. The skin and subcutaneous tissue are incised.
2. The incision is carried to the femur.
3. The femur is severed.
4. The popliteal vessels are ligated.
5. The sciatic nerve is ligated.
6. The wound is closed.

Discussion

The patient is placed in the supine position and the affected leg is prepped. Many surgeons prefer to place the gangrenous

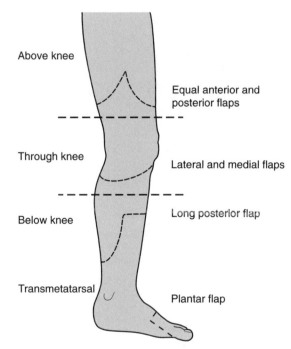

Figure 32-29 Amputation levels with flap designs. *(From Garden O, Bradbury A, Forsythe J, Parks R: Principles and practice of surgery, ed 5, Edinburgh, 2007, Churchill Livingstone/Elsevier.)*

foot in a plastic bag to protect the wound site from possible contamination. The foot is excluded from the scrub prep.

To begin the procedure, the surgeon incises the leg. The incision is carried through the subcutaneous, muscle, and fascial layers with the deep knife, heavy scissors, or electrocautery pencil. Large rake retractors (e.g., Israel rake retractors) often are useful for drawing the wound edges back to expose the femur. The surgeon may sever the femur with a Gigli saw or with an amputation saw (e.g., Satterlee saw).

When the femur has been severed, the surgeon completes the amputation by severing the soft tissues that lie on the posterior side of the femur. The scrub removes the limb from the field and may pass it directly to the circulator. The surgeon ligates the popliteal artery and vein and grasps the sciatic nerve with a Kocher or other heavy clamp. The end of the nerve is crushed with the clamp to prevent the formation of a neuroma (tumor at the end of a nerve). It is ligated with 0 or 2-0 suture ligatures. The end of the nerve is cut with the scalpel or scissors and allowed to retract into the femoral stump.

The stump is closed in layers with 0 or 2-0 Dexon or other absorbable suture. The skin is sutured with the surgeon's choice of material and dressed with bulky gauze and an elastic wrap bandage.

Patients are monitored carefully for hemorrhage and pain in the immediate postoperative period. Complications of surgery include phantom limb pain (pain perceived in an area of the severed limb), limb edema, and damage to the incision area.

KEY CONCEPTS

- Knowledge of the peripheral vascular anatomy is necessary to a complete understanding of surgical procedures.
- Familiarity with diagnostic procedures used in vascular medicine is important to patient care and preparation for intraoperative assessment.
- Case planning for vascular surgery requires knowledge of vascular instruments, surgical techniques, and the materials used in vascular repair, reconstruction, and replacement.
- Techniques in vascular surgery include anastomosis, vessel transplant, repair, and replacement using prostheses.
- An understanding of vascular pathology is required for case planning and for participating in the scrub role.
- A complete understanding of vascular procedures is necessary for participation in surgery that requires advanced surgical skills.

REVIEW QUESTIONS

1. Define *stent*.
2. Why is it important to try and remove sclerotic plaque from an artery in one piece?
3. Why are double-arm needles used for arterial anastomosis?
4. What is the effect of venous stasis on the veins?
5. What are the three layers of the arterial wall?
6. What is the proper method of handling an amputated limb during surgery?
7. A Freer elevator or a Penfield elevator is used to remove atherosclerotic plaque from an artery. In what other surgical specialties are these instruments used?

BIBLIOGRAPHY

Eliason JL, Clouse DW: Current management of infrarenal abdominal aortic aneurysms, *Surgical Clinics of North America* 87:5, 2007.

Garden O, Bradbury A, Forsythe J, Parks R: *Principles and practice of surgery*, ed 5, Edinburgh, 2007, Churchill Livingstone/Elsevier.

Moody F: *Ambulatory surgery*, Philadelphia, 1999, WB Saunders.

Ouriel K, Rutherford R: *Atlas of vascular surgery: operative procedures*, Philadelphia, 1998, WB Saunders.

Porth CM: *Pathophysiology: concepts of altered health states*, ed 7, Philadelphia, 2004, Lippincott Williams & Wilkins.

Rutherford R: *Atlas of vascular surgery: basic techniques and exposures*, Philadelphia, 1997, WB Saunders.

Tinkham MR: The endovascular approach to abdominal aortic aneurysm repair, *AORN Journal* 89:289, 2009.

Thibodeau G, Patton K: *Anatomy and physiology*, ed 6, St Louis, 1997, Mosby.

Townsend CM: *Sabiston textbook of surgery*, ed 17, Philadelphia, 2001, WB Saunders.

33

CHAPTER OUTLINE

LEARNING OBJECTIVES

After studying this chapter the reader will be able to:

1. Identify key anatomical features of the respiratory structures in the thoracic cavity
2. Describe diagnostic procedures of the respiratory system
3. Discuss pathology of the respiratory system
4. Discuss specific elements of the case planning in surgery of the thoracic cavity and respiratory system
5. List and describe common thoracic procedures of the respiratory system

TERMINOLOGY

Arterial blood gases (ABGs): A blood test that determines carbon dioxide and oxygen saturation, pH, and other important parameters of respiration and oxygen perfusion.

Blebs: Areas of overdistention in lung tissue.

Closed chest drainage: A system of removing air or fluid from the thoracic cavity and restoring negative pressure so that the lungs can expand properly after thoracic surgery or penetrating trauma to the chest wall.

Diffusion (oxygen): The molecular passage of oxygen across the alveoli and into the bloodstream.

Dyspnea: Difficulty breathing.

Empyema: A pus-filled area of the lung.

Expiration: The act of breathing out (exhalation).

Hemoptysis: Bloody sputum or bleeding arising from the respiratory tract.

Hemothorax: The presence of blood in the thoracic cavity or between the pleural sac and lungs, usually caused by trauma.

Hypoxia: Lower than normal oxygen perfusion.

Inspiration: The act of taking a breath (inhalation).

Perfusion (oxygen): The distribution of oxygen to tissues.

Pneumothorax: Air in the chest cavity, which prevents the lungs from expanding and may displace the mediastinal structures.

Pulmonary function tests (PFTs): Tests performed to measure the function and strength of the pulmonary system.

Ventilation: The process of inflating and deflating the lungs during breathing.

INTRODUCTION

Thoracic and pulmonary surgery includes procedures of the respiratory system and thoracic cavity, excluding those that involve the heart and cardiac vessels. Thoracic procedures within the specialty involve the lungs, bronchi, and peripheral bronchial system. Surgery involving other organs located within the thoracic cavity, such as the esophagus and thymus, may be performed by a thoracic surgeon or by a general surgeon with assistance of a thoracic specialist. This often depends on whether the surgery involves pulmonary structures.

Surgery of the lungs and other pulmonary structures in the thoracic cavity is frequently preceded by endoscopic assessment of the respiratory structures. Tissue biopsy is performed through the flexible or rigid bronchoscope. Open or video-assisted thoracoscopy may then be used to remove a mass or perform other procedures. Interventional procedures such as foreign body removal, biopsy, and removal of small tumors can be performed through the endoscope, especially the rigid bronchoscope, which has a larger diameter than the flexible scope.

Maintaining lung inflation is an important procedural consideration in thoracic surgery. The thoracic cavity is under *negative pressure*. Under normal circumstances, the lungs expand freely within a vacuum in the chest cavity. An incision, tear, or puncture of the chest wall allows atmospheric air to rush into the thorax. This results in immediate collapse of the lungs. During *thoracotomy* (open chest surgery), the lungs are inflated with the use of a mechanical respirator managed by the anesthesia care provider. In the immediate postsurgical phase and healing phase, the normally negative pressure within the thoracic cavity is maintained with a closed drainage system, which removes air and fluid to allow lung expansion (described later in the chapter).

SURGICAL ANATOMY

The diaphragm is a sealed barrier between the thoracic and abdominal cavities. The function of the respiratory system is to maintain a steady intake of oxygen from the air and eliminate carbon dioxide from the blood. Oxygen is necessary for life, whereas carbon dioxide is a waste product of normal metabolism.

Three processes are involved in respiratory function:

- **Ventilation:** The breathing process; it involves contraction of the diaphragm and accessory muscles and expansion of the ribs to pull air into the lungs.
- **Diffusion (oxygen):** The transfer of oxygen from the alveoli in the lungs to the bloodstream.
- **Perfusion (oxygen):** The movement and absorption of oxygen molecules into body tissues; also called *oxygenation*.

UPPER RESPIRATORY TRACT

The nose is composed of cartilage and bone covered by skin. The external nose flares to form the nares. The internal nose is lined with mucous membrane and is highly vascular. It is divided by the nasal septum, which is composed of cartilage and bone. Nasal hairs in the anterior nasal cavity help filter the air as it enters the upper respiratory tract. Olfactory nerves, which are responsible for the sense of smell, are located in the superior nasal airway and septum.

The nasal sinuses are bilateral structures, each composed of three tiers of bony projections called the *conchae* or *turbinates*. These projections are the superior, medial, and inferior meati (sing., *meatus*). The projections form spaces called the *paranasal sinuses*. Each of these is named after the bone above it (i.e., the maxillary, ethmoid, frontal, and sphenoid bones). The nasal passages are lined with mucous membrane, which warms and humidifies air as it enters the body.

PHARYNX

The pharynx lies behind the oral cavity and communicates with the nasal cavities. It is subdivided into three sections: the oropharynx, nasopharynx, and laryngopharynx or larynx. The oropharynx lies immediately below the mouth. The nasopharynx communicates with the nasal cavities. Two important structures are located in the nasopharynx: the eustachian tube, which drains from the middle ear, and the pharyngeal tonsils (adenoids). The palatine tonsils, the structures commonly referred to as "the tonsils," are located in the oropharynx.

LARYNX

The larynx connects the trachea with the oropharynx. The anatomy of this region is complex and is best understood by studying illustrations of this anatomy. The larynx is a wide, circular cavity formed by cartilage. It contains the vocal cords and prevents food and other foreign bodies from entering the trachea.

The epiglottis is a cartilaginous structure that functions as a flap to close off the entrance to the trachea during swallowing. The epiglottis also is under voluntary control and is closed when a person holds the breath. During defecation, the glottis is voluntarily closed and the intraabdominal muscles are contracted. This is referred to as the *Valsalva maneuver*. This action also causes a momentary decrease in intrathoracic pressure and an increased heart rate. The epiglottis often is confused with the uvula, which is the visible projection of epithelial tissue extending from the soft palate of the mouth.

The larynx is divided into bilateral sections by paired folds of tissue, which are extensions of the epithelial lining of the laryngeal cavity. The upper folds are called the *vestibular folds*. The lower folds form the vocal cords, which produce speech. The space between the folds is the glottis, which is the entrance to the trachea.

Two other important cartilaginous structures in the larynx are the thyroid cartilage and the arytenoid cartilage. The thyroid cartilage is a large "shield" of tissue that forms the anterior wall and protects the larynx from injury. This structure is larger in men than in women. The horn-shaped arytenoids extend superiorly and support the vocal cords. Figure 33-1 illustrates the upper respiratory system.

TRACHEA

The trachea begins at the larynx and branches into two main airways, the right and left primary bronchi and bronchial tree. The trachea is a semirigid tube mainly composed of C-shaped cartilaginous rings. The cricoid cartilage is the only completely closed ring in the structure.

BRONCHI

The trachea branches into the right and left primary bronchi at the carina. Because the right bronchus is straighter than the left, inhaled foreign material is more likely to enter the right lung. As the bronchi enter the lung segments, they branch into smaller and smaller branches, or bronchioles, forming a treelike structure. Cartilaginous rings support the primary bronchi. However, as the branches become smaller, the walls are formed by cartilage plates until the level of the bronchioles, where there is no cartilage. The bronchioles are composed of smooth muscle lined with epithelium.

LUNGS

The lung is divided into anatomical regions. The right lung has three lobes and the left lung has two lobes. Each lung is composed of smaller segments, called *bronchopulmonary segments*, which contain branches of the main bronchi. The hilum (notch) of each lung is located on the medial side. Large blood vessels and primary bronchi enter the lung at the hilum. The apex of the lung is located at the upper portion and extends just above the clavicle.

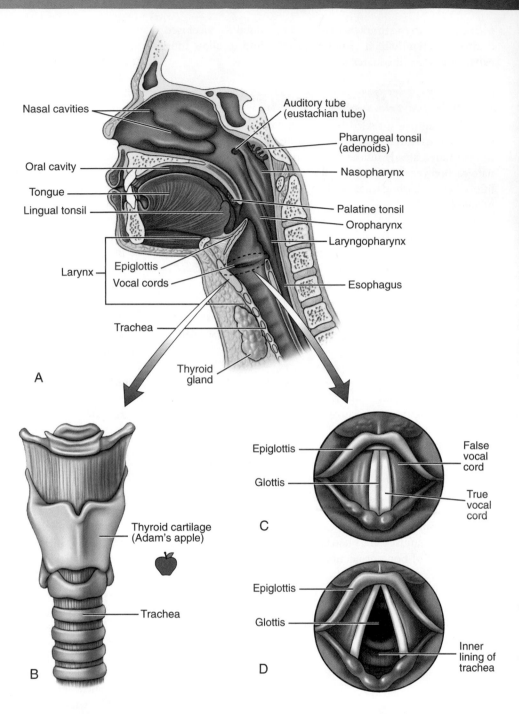

Figure 33-1 A, Upper respiratory system. **B,** Larynx, showing the thyroid cartilage. **C,** Vocal cords and closed glottis. **D,** Open glottis. *(From Herlihy B, Maebius NK: The human body in health and illness, ed 2, Philadelphia, 2003, WB Saunders.)*

The bronchioles terminate in small ducts, alveolar sacs, and individual alveoli. An alveolus exchanges incoming oxygen molecules with carbon dioxide molecules from the blood.

The lungs are separated in the thoracic cavity by the mediastinum. This space contains the heart, large vessels, bronchi, trachea, esophagus, and thymus gland which produces hormones necessary for immune function. Each lung is enclosed in a pleural cavity and covered by a double membrane, the pleural sac. The outer membrane forms the parietal pleura, which lines the thoracic cavity and outer mediastinal walls. The inner, or visceral, pleura covers the lungs. A small amount of pleural fluid is secreted into the pleural space between the two membranes. *Pleuritis* is inflammation of the pleural membranes. An increase in fluid (e.g., serous fluid, pus, or blood) is called a *pleural effusion*. The pleural space is called a

potential space because during respiration, the space increases or decreases as the lungs fill with air. In pleural effusion, the lungs cannot expand fully.

The pleural space normally maintains negative pressure in relation to atmospheric air and the alveoli. If the chest wall and pleural space are opened, such as during trauma or surgery, air rushes in and collapses the lungs in the same way vacuum-packed wrappers fill with air when punctured. Figure 33-2 illustrates the lungs and bronchial tree.

MECHANISM OF BREATHING

Breathing is a complex physiological and mechanical process controlled by the autonomic nervous system but also under voluntary control. The thoracic cavity is a closed space. The

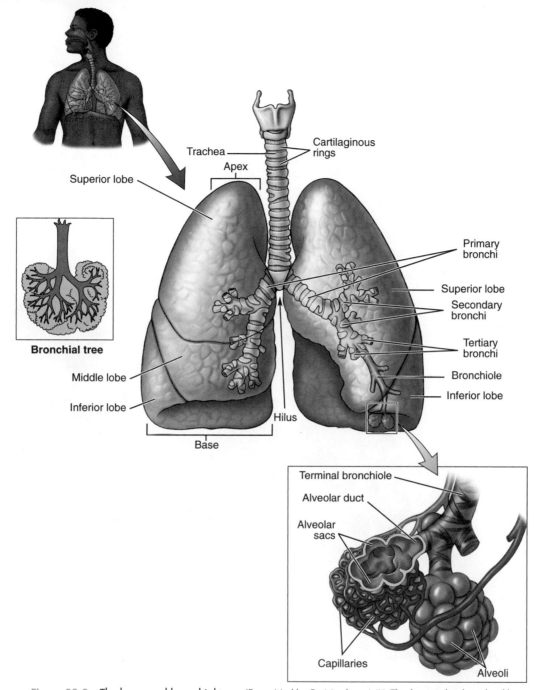

Trachea

Cartilaginous rings

Apex

Superior lobe

Bronchial tree

Middle lobe

Inferior lobe

Hilus

Base

Primary bronchi

Superior lobe

Secondary bronchi

Tertiary bronchi

Bronchiole

Inferior lobe

Terminal bronchiole

Alveolar duct

Alveolar sacs

Capillaries

Alveoli

Figure 33-2 **The lungs and bronchial tree.** *(From Herlihy B, Maebius NK: The human body in health and illness, ed 2, Philadelphia, 2003, WB Saunders.)*

diaphragm is continuous with the parietal pleural membrane. Recall that the pressure between the two pleural membranes is negative, whereas air pressure in the trachea, bronchi, bronchioles, and alveoli is equal to atmospheric pressure outside the body. When the diaphragm contracts during inhalation, the potential space between the two pleural membranes decreases, and air is pulled into the airways and lungs. When the diaphragm relaxes during exhalation, air flows passively out of the lungs (Figure 33-3).

A number of important factors affect breathing:

1. An intact pleural membrane is needed to maintain the negative pressure in the pleural space (keep in mind the analogy to the vacuum-sealed package that is created by removing air from the inside—a hole in the package allows air to rush in).

2. Penetrating trauma to the chest cavity causes air to rush in and collapses the lungs. Air **(pneumothorax),** blood **(hemothorax),** or exudate in the pleural space displaces and compresses the lungs. This prevents their expansion and, if severe enough, may result in full collapse of the lung.

3. The alveoli must have sufficient elasticity to expand and fill with air. Diseases that constrict the alveoli, such as emphysema, cause loss of alveolar elasticity. The result is inability to exchange oxygen with carbon dioxide.

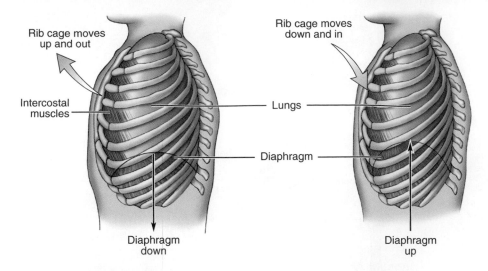

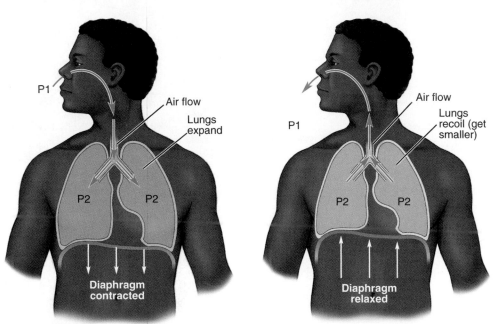

Figure 33-3 **Mechanism of breathing.** *(From Herlihy B, Maebius NK: The human body in health and illness, ed 2, Philadelphia, 2003, WB Saunders.)*

4. An intact central nervous system is required to initiate transmission to the phrenic nerve, which controls the diaphragm. For example, barbiturate drugs can depress the central nervous system to the level at which breathing stops.
5. The chest cavity must be able to expand freely. An example of pathological restriction is eschar from extensive third-degree burns.

DIAGNOSTIC TESTS

Diagnostic tests for the respiratory system assess the function of the lungs, thoracic space, and bronchial system. Terms related to the medical assessment of respiration:

- *Apnea:* Cessation of respiration
- *Dyspnea:* Difficulty or painful respiration
- *Hyperventilation:* Abnormally fast rate of respiration
- *Hyperpnea:* Excessively deep respiration

- *Cyanosis:* Bluish tint to skin seen in patients with poor oxygenation
- *Hyperventilation:* Abnormally rapid rate of respiration

PULMONARY FUNCTION

Pulmonary function tests (PFTs) are a specific group of procedures that measure lung function. These noninvasive tests are performed with a complex breathing machine, which measures the parameters digitally. The following tests are included in this group:

- *Tidal volume:* The amount of air exhaled during normal respiration.
- *Minute volume:* The amount of air exhaled per minute.
- *Vital capacity:* The total volume of air exhaled after maximum **inspiration.**
- *Functional residual capacity:* The volume of air remaining in the lungs after exhalation.

- *Total lung capacity:* The total amount of air in the lungs when fully inflated.
- *Forced vital capacity:* The amount of air expelled in the first, second, and third seconds after exhalation.
- *Peak expiratory flow rate:* The maximum amount of air expelled in forced **expiration.**

LABORATORY TESTS

A complete blood count (CBC), including white blood cell differential, is performed as a basic screening tool for surgical patients. More specific laboratory tests, such as those for tumor markers, are performed according to the suspected pathological condition. Culture and sensitivity tests may be performed on exudate collected from the respiratory tract.

Among the most important blood tests for pulmonary function is determination of arterial blood gas values, commonly called **arterial blood gases (ABGs).** In this test, the arterial blood is assessed for oxygen and carbon dioxide levels and pH (acid-base balance).

IMAGING STUDIES

Imaging studies of the pulmonary and thoracic structures include radiographs, magnetic resonance imaging (MRI), ultrasound scans, and computed tomography (CT). Radiographs are used to screen patients for tuberculosis and other fibrotic diseases. Fluid and air in the pleural space, tumors, and anatomical deformities are also detected on radiographs. MRI and CT scans are used for more definitive analysis of masses.

Pulmonary angiography is performed when CT scans are inconclusive for diagnosis of pulmonary embolism. During angiography, the blood vessels of the lungs are injected with a contrast medium, and fluoroscopy or CT is used to detect any abnormalities (Figure 33-4).

Endoscopic procedures (discussed later in the chapter) are performed to obtain biopsy specimens of cells, fluid, and tissue. Visual examination of the respiratory tract by endoscopy, along with other diagnostic tools, assists in determination of the diagnosis.

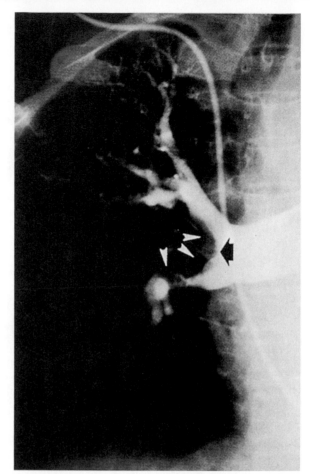

Figure 33-4 Pulmonary arteriogram showing an embolus at the root of the pulmonary artery. *(From Thibodeau G, Patton K:* Anatomy and physiology, *ed 6, St Louis, 2007, Mosby.)*

CASE PLANNING

PREPPING AND DRAPING

The incisions most commonly used in pulmonary surgery are the posterolateral and anterolateral thoracotomy, with the patient in the lateral position (see Chapter 19). The skin prep may extend from the neck to the iliac crest. Minimum draping includes a body sheet, towels for squaring the incision, an incise drape, and a fenestrated thoracotomy drape.

INSTRUMENTS

Open thoracic surgery of the respiratory structures requires the following instruments:

- General surgery instruments, including long instruments (shanks must be at least 9 inches [22.5 cm] for most adult patients).
- Chest wall instruments, including self-retaining chest, rib, and scapula retractors, and rib approximators. Orthopedic rongeurs, periosteal elevators, and rib-stripping instruments also are required for some procedures.
- Lung instruments, including atraumatic tissue-grasping clamps.
- Bronchus clamps, which are large, right angle clamps used to occlude the primary bronchi. The jaws of the clamps are stippled for greater grip on the cartilaginous tissue.
- Surgical stapling instruments, which are commonly used in thoracic surgery (both open and endoscopic procedures). These are used in lung resection and for occlusion of the bronchial stem after resection.
- Vascular clamps are needed for some lung procedures.

With the patient in a lateral position, it is necessary to position a magnetic instrument pad over the top drape to serve as a neutral zone, and also to retain any instruments that are placed on the drape.

Figures 33-5 and 33-6 show thoracic and tracheal instruments.

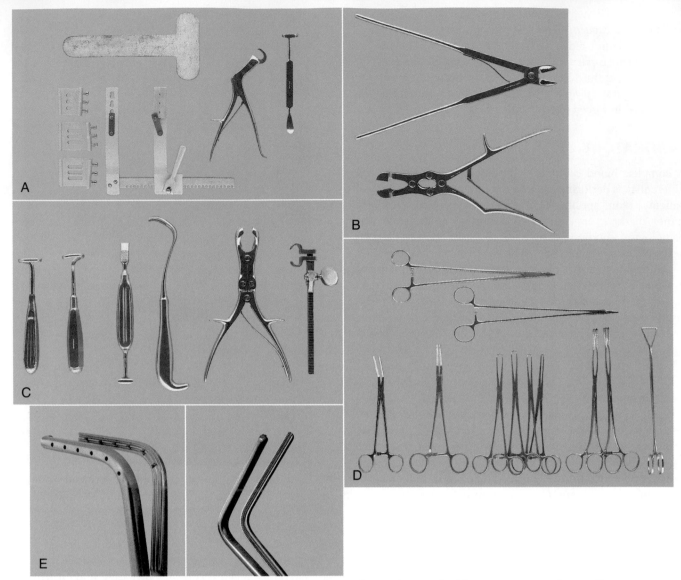

Figure 33-5 **Thoracic instruments.** **A,** Thoracotomy instruments. *Top, left to right,* 1 malleable **T**-retractor, Finochetto self-retaining retractor with blades; 1 Giertz rib rongeur; 1 combination Matson rib stripper and elevator. *Bottom left,* Burford rib spreader with shallow blade attached; 1 shallow blade; 2 deep blades. **B,** Rib rongeurs. *Top,* Bethune rongeur. *Bottom,* Sauerbruch rongeur. **C,** Rib instruments. Left to right, 2 Doyen rib rasps; 1 Alexander rib elevator; 1 Semb lung retractor; 1 Semb rongeur; 1 Bailey rib contractor. **D,** Soft tissue instruments. Top, Crile-Wood long needle holders. Left to right, 1 Sarot bronchus clamp; 1 Lee bronchus clamp; 4 Allis clamps; 3 Duval lung clamps, side and front views. **E,** *Left,* Sarot clamp. *Right,* Lee clamp. *(From Tighe SM: Instrumentation for the operating room, ed 6, St Louis, 2003, Mosby.)*

DRUGS AND SOLUTIONS

Hemostatic agents are commonly used in thoracic surgery to control capillary bleeding from the lung surface and for coagulation at the site of anastomosis of the large vessels. Gelfoam soaked in thrombin and oxidized cellulose or absorbable collagen should be available according to the surgeon's preference. Bone sealant (Ostene) may also be required to seal the cut edges of a rib or sternum. Fibrin sealant is used to prevent the escape of air from a lung or bronchial anastomosis. Refer to Chapter 22 for a review on the pharmacology and preparation of these materials.

CLOSED CHEST DRAINAGE

Negative pressure in the thoracic cavity is lost when the chest wall and pleura are opened or punctured (Figure 33-7). This occurs during trauma, disease, and thoracic surgery. For the lungs to expand, negative pressure must be restored. This is achieved with **closed chest drainage,** also called *closed underwater drainage* (Figure 33-8). One or more chest tubes are inserted through the body wall and into the chest cavity. The distal end of the tubes is connected to a set of connecting chambers. The first container drains blood, fluid, and air from the thoracic cavity. The second container is partly filled with water to prevent air from entering the system from the distal

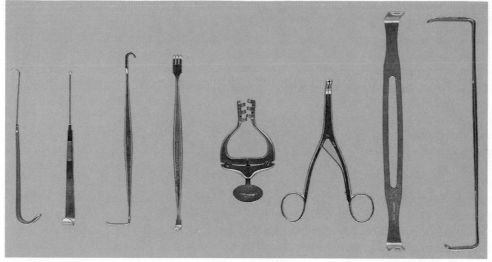

Figure 33-6   **Tracheal instruments.** *Left to right,* 2 tracheal hooks; 2 Senn retractors; 1 mastoid retractor; 1 tracheal dilator; 2 Army-Navy retractors. *(From Tighe SM: Instrumentation for the operating room, ed 6, St Louis, 2003, Mosby.)*

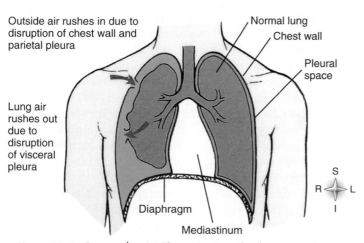

Figure 33-7   **Pneumothorax.** The pressure in the thoracic cavity normally is negative. Air rushes in through an opening in the pleural sac, causing the lung to collapse. *(From Thibodeau G, Patton K: Anatomy and physiology, ed 6, St Louis, 2007, Mosby.)*

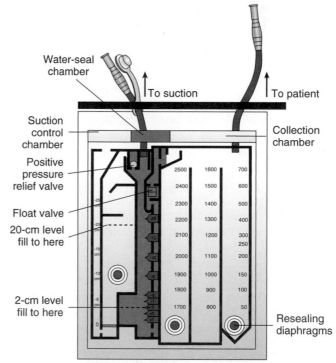

Figure 33-8   A closed chest drainage unit is used to maintain negative pressure in the thoracic cavity after surgery or trauma to the chest cavity. *(From Lewis SM, Heitkemper MM, Dirksen SR: Medical surgical nursing, ed 6, St Louis, 2004, Mosby.)*

end. The system works by gravity or active suction. As long as the sealed chambers remain below the level of the patient's chest, fluid and air drain from the thoracic cavity. However, if the drainage system is raised, fluid flows back into the chest cavity and can collapse the lungs or heart.

NOTE: The prototype for disposable (single-use) closed chest drainage systems was the Pleur-evac (Teleflex Medical, Research Triangle Park, NC), which was introduced in 1967. The term pleur-evac is often used as a generic term for all closed chest drainage systems, although other companies manufacture similar devices.

During closure, a chest tube is placed in one or more locations in the thoracic cavity. If two tubes are required (in one or both pleura), they can be joined with a Y-connector and attached to the drainage system.

A patient with a chest drainage system must be moved carefully to avoid disruption of the chest tubes. If a chest tube becomes dislodged from the thoracic cavity, the proper emergency response is to prevent air from entering the wound. Sterile petroleum gauze is kept with the patient at all times for this purpose. In the event a drainage tube comes out, the gauze is immediately placed over the wound to prevent air from filling the thorax and deflating the lung. The three-chamber unit is always kept upright and never raised to the level of the chest, because this causes fluid to flow back into the chest cavity.

SURGICAL PROCEDURES

INSERTION OF CHEST TUBES

To provide closed chest drainage, chest tubes must be surgically inserted. In the case of a surgical procedure involving thoracotomy, the tubes are inserted just before the chest is closed to establish negative pressure as soon as possible following endotracheal extubation. After a spontaneous or traumatic air leak or a surgical procedure in which the right or left pleural cavity is opened, negative pressure must be restored to allow the lungs to expand. The surgeon achieves this by making an opening into the affected pleural cavity through a small thoracic incision. One or more chest tubes are inserted and connected to a water-seal chest drainage system to remove air, blood, and other fluids from the thoracic or pericardial cavity. Suction is applied.

Chest tubes are made of heavy Silastic or polyvinyl chloride tubing that has numerous perforations at the proximal end. After surgery, the chest tube is inserted through a stab incision away from the surgical incision. Chest tubes may be placed in one or more locations. They are sutured to the chest wall with heavy, nonabsorbable sutures and dressed with petroleum gauze, fluffed, and flat gauze.

BRONCHOSCOPY

Surgical Goal

Bronchoscopy is endoscopic examination trachea and bronchi. The surgical goal is to assess the respiratory structures, remove specimens for biopsy, or perform a minor surgical procedure.

Pathology

The effects of diseases of the bronchi often are visible with the aid of endoscopy. Pathological indications for bronchoscopy include:

- Bleeding arising from the respiratory tract (called **hemoptysis**).
- Suspected tumor
- Infection
- Evaluation of the extent of burn injury from toxic inhalation or smoke inhalation
- Aspirated foreign body (food or objects, usually in pediatric patients)
- Lesions seen during imaging studies

TECHNIQUE

1 A bronchoscope is inserted into the trachea and slowly advanced.

2 The respiratory structures are examined.

3 Interventional procedures, such as removal of tissue or extraction of a foreign body, are performed.

4 Bronchial specimens are removed (washings, cytological biopsy, or sputum samples).

5 The bronchoscope is gently withdrawn.

Two types of bronchoscopy are discussed next—*rigid* and *flexible*. Each has particular advantages and is used according to the patient's requirements:

- Flexible bronchoscopy utilizes a slender fiberoptic endoscope capable of entering the primary and peripheral bronchi. The modern flexible scope may also be used for interventional procedures such as cryosurgery and laser surgery.
- Rigid bronchoscopy is used for interventional procedures, which require a large-bore endoscope and rigid instruments, such as removal of a tissue mass or a foreign body. This is because the lumen of the rigid scope is larger than that of the flexible bronchoscope.

RIGID BRONCHOSCOPY

Discussion

The patient is placed in the supine position with the neck slightly hyperextended. A body drape is applied. The patient's eyes may be protected with pads and a head drape. Before the procedure begins, the scrub should make sure all light cables and fittings are in good working order. An eyepiece adapter should be placed over the scope to protect the surgeon from contamination by the patient's body fluids. A tooth guard is placed in the patient's mouth to protect the teeth.

The surgeon inserts the rigid scope into the trachea. Side channels on the bronchoscope allow for insertion of irrigation and suction devices and other instruments. The scrub should assist by guiding the instruments into the side channels.

If sputum or fluid samples are to be taken, suction tubing adapted with a Lukens trap is attached to the tubing. Cells are washed free from the bronchus and retrieved with the suction cannula attached to a Lukens trap. This small vial collects solutions as they are suctioned. The trap must be held upright to avoid losing the specimen. The surgeon performs bronchial lavage by injecting saline into the side channel.

Biopsy tissue is removed with cup forceps. The scrub is responsible for removing the tissue from the forceps. The sample is placed on a moistened Telfa pad to prevent its loss. The tissue must be handled gently when removed from the forceps so that it is not crushed, because this may distort the pathology.

Foreign bodies are retrieved with a basket similar to that used to remove kidney stones. The basket instrument is threaded into the side channel. Grasping forceps also may be used to retrieve a foreign body.

At the close of the procedure, before the scope is withdrawn, the surgeon suctions the patient free of all secretions. The scope is then withdrawn.

An important complication of rigid bronchoscopy is injury to the tracheobronchial structures if the patient moves during the procedure. The autonomic gag reflex may cause the patient to arch and cough, even during heavy sedation or light general anesthesia. This is called *bucking*. A local anesthetic is sprayed into the trachea before the endoscope is inserted to help prevent bucking during the procedure.

Complications include possible injury to the bronchial tree and lung tissue. Additional complications include laceration of blood vessels near the bronchial tissue and infection. Bronchoscopy is illustrated in Figure 33-9.

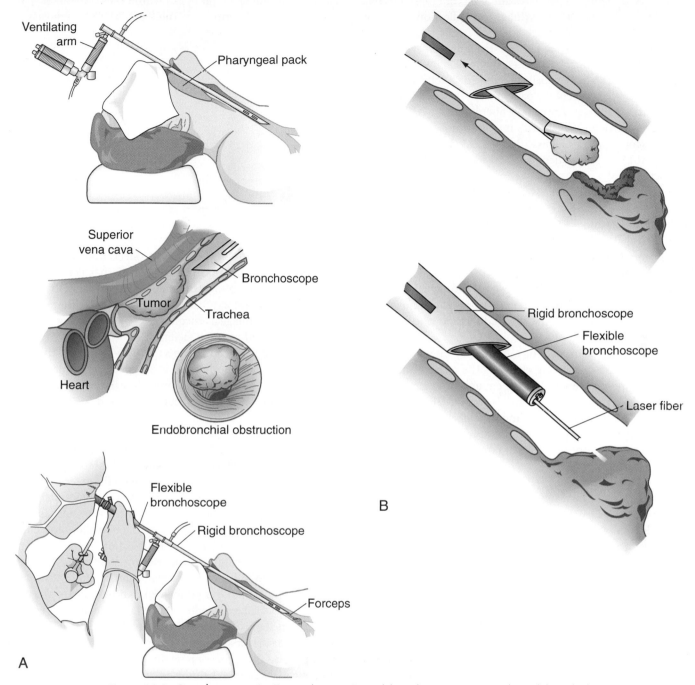

Figure 33-9 Bronchoscopy. A, *Top to bottom,* A rigid bronchoscope is inserted—endobronchial obstruction is encountered. A flexible scope is placed inside the rigid scope for biopsy. **B,** The mass is removed with forceps. Laser removal is performed. *(From Sugarbaker DJ, Strauss G, Fried MP: Laser resection of endobronchial lesions: use of rigid and flexible bronchoscopes, Operative techniques in otolaryngology—head and neck surgery 3:93, 1992.)*

FLEXIBLE BRONCHOSCOPY

TECHNIQUE

1 A fiberoptic tube is inserted through the patient's mouth or nose.
2 The tracheobronchial tree is examined.
3 Cytology or biopsy specimens are taken.
4 The bronchial tree is suctioned.
5 Video data are recorded.
6 The scope is withdrawn.

Discussion

Flexible bronchoscopy is preferred over rigid bronchoscopy for patients in whom hyperextension of the neck or jaw manipulation is difficult or impossible. The flexible bronchoscope can provide a more extensive assessment. Rigid and flexible procedures may be performed sequentially during the same surgery.

Like all endoscopes, the fiberoptic bronchoscope has digital capability, and the images transmitted through the scope are projected onto a monitor. Instruments required include imaging equipment, various sizes and types of biopsy forceps, a cytology brush, a 10-mL syringe, and collection tubes for tissue washings. If cytology specimens are to be taken, microscope slides and fixative are needed. The patient is placed in a semi-Fowler position. A local anesthetic is sprayed into the throat, and the patient usually is sedated. A bite block frequently is used to prevent the patient from biting on the endoscope and damaging it. The flexible fiberoptic tube is lubricated and passed through the patient's mouth or nose. Unlike rigid bronchoscopy, which allows the patient to be ventilated through the tube, the patient must breathe around the flexible endoscope.

The patient is placed in a supine position. There is no prep, although a top drape is used to protect the patient and secure the instruments and leads. The eyes are protected with a towel or head drape. Monitored sedation is often used. The throat may be sprayed with local anesthetic before insertion of the scope to prevent gagging.

The surgeon advances the endoscope through the trachea and bronchial tree. When cancer is suspected or known, the healthy lung is examined first to avoid seeding it with cancer cells.

The surgeon obtains cytology samples by inserting a small brush through the operating channel. The technologist must make sure the instrument is long enough to extend outside the tip of the scope. After the brush is removed, the scrub dips it in a specimen container holding a small amount of saline. This process may be repeated several times. In some cases the tip of the cytology brush may be cut from the wire and placed in the fixative container.

Biopsy forceps may be used to obtain small tissue samples. These forceps must be handled carefully, because they are very small and easily lost. After the forceps is withdrawn from the scope, the sample should be placed immediately in a specimen container or on a Telfa pad. A hypodermic needle is helpful for removing bits of tissue from the biopsy forceps.

A suction cannula is used to remove secretions. These are trapped in the Lukens specimen trap, just as in rigid bronchoscopy.

Innovations in tumor-ablating devices have increased the use of flexible bronchoscopy for tissue debridement. The *microdebrider* used commonly in sinus surgery (see Chapter 28) has been modified for use in flexible bronchoscopy. Cryotherapy and argon laser are also becoming more popular for interventional procedures. These techniques have been discussed in Chapters 18 and 28.

MEDIASTINOSCOPY

Surgical Goal

Mediastinoscopy is endoscopic examination of the mediastinum through an incision. Thymus and lymph node biopsy are performed to establish a diagnosis.

Pathology

Mediastinoscopy is performed for diagnostic or interventional surgery. The thymus gland, which is located in the mediastinal space in children, regresses in adulthood. Biopsy of the thymus

gland and regional lymph nodes within the mediastinal space is performed to determine or rule out a cancer diagnosis.

TECHNIQUE

1 An incision is made in the suprasternal notch.
2 The fascia is incised and a tunnel is created into the mediastinum with digital pressure.
3 The mediastinoscope is inserted into the tissue space.
4 The trachea, bronchial tree, aortic arch, and lymph nodes are examined.
5 Lymph nodes may be removed.
6 The mediastinoscope is withdrawn.
7 The wound is closed.

Discussion

A rigid mediastinoscope is a stainless steel endoscope inserted through a small incision at the suprasternal notch. Video-assisted endoscopy allows the scope's field of vision to be projected on a monitor. Other techniques, including natural orifice (transesophageal) mediastinoscopy, are being assessed and implemented in some facilities.

The patient is placed in the supine position with the neck hyperextended. The individual is prepped and draped for an upper thoracic incision. The procedure is performed using general anesthesia. The surgeon may stand at the patient's head or side.

A small incision is made over the suprasternal notch with a #10 knife blade. The incision is carried through the subcutaneous and muscle layers, commonly with Metzenbaum scissors and tissue forceps. The fascial layer on the anterior surface of the trachea is identified. The surgeon clamps small veins with mosquito hemostats and ligates them with fine silk ties. The electrosurgical unit (ESU) is used for smaller bleeders.

The surgeon uses blunt finger dissection to make a plane between the tissues into the superior mediastinum. The scope is then inserted into this tissue plane and carefully advanced.

Lymph node biopsy is performed routinely during the procedure. A specialized needle attached to a metal stylet is used to pierce the biopsy tissue and aspirate the contents. The technologist attaches a syringe to the stylet before handing it to the surgeon. This procedure is done to verify that the specimen is nodal tissue. When this is confirmed, the surgeon uses cup biopsy forceps to obtain a pathology specimen. The technologist removes the tissue from the forceps and places it in a specimen container or on a Telfa pad moistened with saline.

After specimens have been obtained, the surgeon dries the wound and checks for bleeding. The ESU and hemostatic agents (e.g., absorbable gelatin sponge) may be used to control bleeding. The surgeon then withdraws the scope and closes the incision with synthetic absorbable sutures and skin staples.

THORACOSCOPY (VIDEO-ASSISTED THORACOSCOPIC SURGERY)

Video-assisted thoracoscopic surgery (VATS) is minimally invasive surgery of the thoracic cavity. This technique is similar to other types of minimally invasive procedures in which cannulas are inserted through the body wall and used to receive a rigid scope and telescope instruments. This technique is different from endoscopic (bronchoscopic) surgery in which a flexible or rigid scope is inserted through the airway via the trachea. The term *video-assisted thoracoscopy* or *VATS* was coined at a time when minimally invasive endoscopic surgery was in its early development. At that time, video display from the endoscope to a monitor was a relatively new technology. Thoracoscopy has now been developed to the extent that it has taken the place of most open procedures of the thorax.

CASE PLANNING

Patient Preparation

The patient is placed in the lateral position with the operative side up and a general anesthetic is administered through a double-lumen endotracheal tube. The double lumen allows the operative lung to collapse while the anesthetic and oxygen are administered to the opposite lung.

The patient is prepped from the neck to the iliac crest and from bedside to bedside. The exposed shoulder and arm also may be prepped and the arm placed on an overhead arm board.

Trocar and Cannulas

Endoscopic ports are placed according to the procedure. Three or four ports usually are required. A combination minithoracotomy (small thoracotomy incision) and thoracoscopy may be performed.

Instruments

Thoracoscopy in an adult requires 10-mm lenses in sizes 0 and 30 degrees. The scope, camera, and light source are managed as for all minimally invasive endoscopic procedures (see Chapter 24). Thoracoscopy instruments are shown in Figure 33-10.

THORACOSOPY: LUNG BIOPSY

Surgical Goal

In *thoracoscopic* lung biopsy, a small portion of lung tissue is removed for pathological assessment.

TECHNIQUE

1 The cannulas and telescope are inserted.
2 One or more additional trocar sites are incised for instrumentation.
3 A small section of lung is removed.
4 The edges of the divided lung tissue are assessed for bleeding and air leakage.
5 A chest tube may be inserted through one puncture site.
6 The wounds are closed.

Discussion

The patient is placed in the lateral position and prepped and draped for a thoracostomy. A 2-mm skin incision is made to

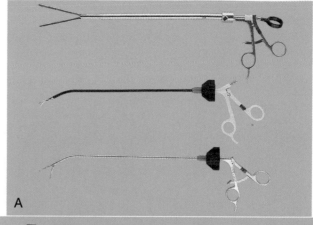

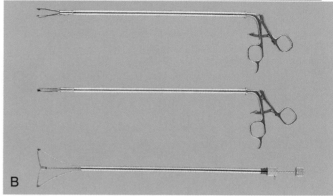

Figure 33-10 Thoracoscopy instruments. **A,** *Top to bottom,* 1 lung grasper; 1 roticulating scissors; 1 roticulating Babcock clamp. **B,** *Top to bottom,* 2 Duval lung clamps; fan retractor. *(From Tighe SM: Instrumentation for the operating room, ed 6, St Louis, 2003, Mosby.)*

accommodate the first cannula. Size 10- or 12-mm trocars are used. A 10-mm thoracic telescope is introduced.

A wedge resection is a large tissue biopsy or the removal of a small peripheral lesion. These are commonly removed with the linear surgical stapler during thoracoscopy.

A small sponge forceps is inserted through one of the instrument ports, and a 30-mm endoscopic linear stapler is introduced through a separate port. The biopsy specimen is removed with the stapling device, which divides the lung and secures the opening. Additional specimens, including lymph node samples, may also be removed.

The surgeon carefully inspects the suture line for air leaks by filling the chest cavity with warm saline solution. The anesthesia care provider then inflates the lung and observes the suture line for bubbles. The surgeon or assistant applies pressure to the site and additional sutures are placed as needed. A wedge biopsy is illustrated in Figure 33-11.

The instruments are withdrawn and a chest tube is inserted into the lower incision. The wounds are sutured with synthetic absorbable suture and skin staples. Steri-Strips may also be used to close the skin.

NOTE: *If a small open incision is necessary for biopsy, the procedure is performed as described with the linear stapler. A chest tube is inserted, and the wound is closed with synthetic absorbable sutures and skin staples.*

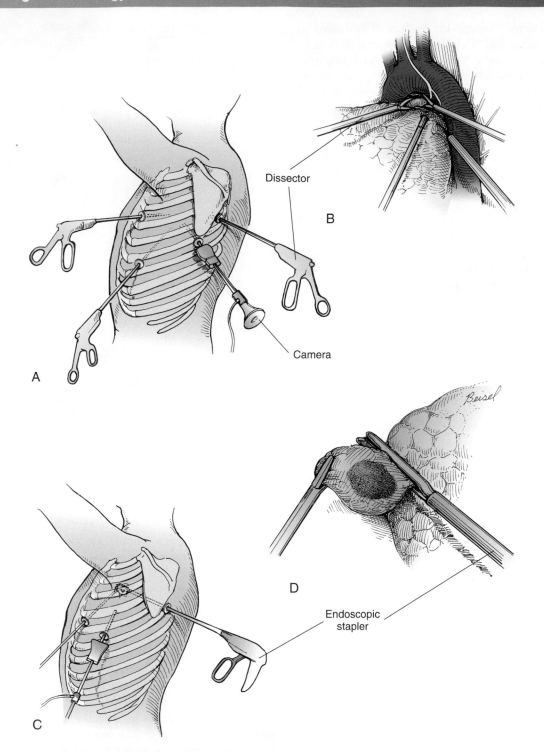

Dissector

B

Camera

A

D

Endoscopic
stapler

C

Figure 33-11   Video-assisted thoracoscopic surgery (VATS). A, The trocar is placed. **B,** The lung tissue is isolated. **C,** The endoscopic stapler is inserted. **D,** The wedge is resected. *(Modified from Waldhausen JA, Pierce WS, Campbell DB: Surgery of the chest, ed 6, St Louis, 1996, Mosby.)*

RELATED PROCEDURE

Pleuroscopy, endoscopic surgery of the thorax, may be performed in place of VATS for diagnostic purposes and some surgical interventions. During this procedure, a flexible fiberoptic endoscopic is inserted through a single incision in the chest wall. Talc poudrage is a procedure commonly performed using the pleuroscope. During this procedure, talc is applied to the pleural space to create adhesions and prevent recurrent spontaneous pneumothorax. The talc is introduced through the endoscopic working channel using an atomizer (Figure 33-12).

LUNG VOLUME REDUCTION SURGERY

Surgical Goal

In lung volume reduction surgery, portions of the lung severely affected by chronic pulmonary emphysema are removed to

The surgeon uses Duval lung forceps or other atraumatic forceps to isolate areas to be resected. The edges of resected lung tissue must be sealed to prevent air from escaping after excision. A leak-proof seal is achieved with a stapling device lined with bovine pericardium, or by placing a polytetrafluoroethylene (PTFE) graft on the edges of the resection. If the bovine implant is used, the scrub receives it from the circulator and rinses it in several baths of normal saline before insertion. PTFE strips do not require special preparation before use.

The selected blebs are transected and removed. The resected sections are examined for leaks. A chest drain is inserted and the thoracoscopy cannulas are removed. Individual incisions are closed in two layers and the chest drains are attached to a sealed chest drainage unit. The patient may be transferred to the postanesthesia care unit or the intensive care unit.

Patients who undergo a VATS technique for resection of blebs may be placed on mechanical ventilation in the immediate postoperative period.

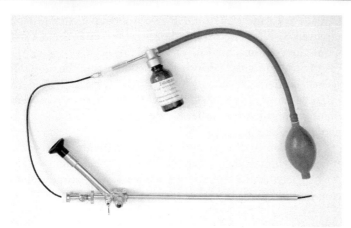

Figure 33-12 **Pleuroscope prepared for poudrage.** An atomizer is used to disperse talc (vial shown) in the pleural space to create adhesions and prevent spontaneous pneumothorax. *(From Mason R et al: Textbook of Respiratory Medicine, ed 5, Philadelphia, 2010, Saunders.)*

improve pulmonary function. Segmental resection is performed by means of a VATS technique using surgical staples.

Pathology

Chronic pulmonary emphysema is marked by loss of elasticity and destruction of lung tissue, usually related to chronic cigarette smoking. The disease is characterized by stiffening of the tissue and inability to empty the alveoli, which results in abnormal enlargement of the lungs. Gas exchange is severely impaired and the result is **dyspnea** (difficulty breathing) and **hypoxia.** Areas of overinflation, or **blebs,** develop in the most severely affected tissue. Segmental removal of diseased lung tissue improves pulmonary function, especially tidal volume.

TECHNIQUE

1 Trocars and cannulas are placed for a video-assisted thoracoscopic surgery (VATS) procedure.
2 Adhesions are dissected.
3 The lungs are deflated to identify areas of trapped air.
4 Lung clamps are used to grasp the portion of the lung to be excised and surgical stapling devices lined with bovine pericardium or polytetrafluoroethylene (PTFE) are applied to each side of the lung tissue to be excised.
5 The lung is inspected to identify residual air leaks; these are closed.
6 Chest tubes are placed in each pleural space.
7 The incisions are closed.

Discussion

The patient is placed in the lateral or supine position and prepped and draped. General anesthesia is administered.

Trocars and cannulas are placed at strategic locations in the chest wall. To inspect the lung, the anesthesia care provider inflates and deflates areas of the pulmonary tissue. This reveals areas of trapped air, indicating severe damage caused by emphysema.

SCALENE NODE BIOPSY

Surgical Goal

Scalene node biopsy is performed on patients with palpable nodes in the area of the scalene fat pads. Biopsy is performed to establish cancer staging or to confirm a diagnosis.

Pathology

Lung cancer spreads through the intrathoracic and mediastinal lymphatics to the supraclavicular nodes. Excision and biopsy of the scalene fat pad are performed before thoracotomy. Scalene node biopsy is performed in conjunction with bronchoscopy and is used to identify patients most likely to benefit from thoracotomy for malignant disease.

TECHNIQUE

1 An incision is made following the clavicle.
2 The incision continues through the platysma muscle.
3 The scalene fat pad is removed, exposing the phrenic nerve and the anterior scalene muscle.
4 The wound is closed.

Discussion

The patient is placed in the supine position with the head turned away from the surgical site. The patient is then prepped and draped for an upper thoracic incision. General anesthesia is used for the procedure. The surgeon makes a transverse incision 2 to 2.8 inches (5 to 7 cm) long, approximately 0.8 inch (2 cm) above the clavicle. Small bleeders are coagulated using the ESU. The incision is carried through the subcutaneous tissue and loose connective tissue. The surgeon places a small self-retaining retractor in the wound or may use a shallow handheld retractor to expose the lymph nodes.

An individual lymph node is dissected from the surrounding connective tissue using Metzenbaum scissors and fine tissue forceps. Fine silk ligatures or the ESU are used to control bleeders. The node is fully dissected free and passed off the field. A frozen section may be ordered.

The wound is closed using fine absorbable synthetic sutures size 3-0 or 4-0. Skin is closed with interrupted sutures of nylon or silk, or fine skin staples may be used. The wound is dressed with a flat gauze dressing.

THORACOTOMY

Surgical Goal

Thoracotomy is the general term for open surgery of the thoracic cavity. The procedure for opening and closing the chest generally is the same for any thoracotomy. Thoracic emergencies involving open or penetrating wounds with severe hemorrhage, may require the thoracotomy to be performed in the emergency department. In these cases, the patient is rushed to the operating room as soon as hemostasis is controlled. Refer to Chapter 37 for a more detailed description of emergency thoracotomy.

Pathology

Thoracotomy may be performed for any condition that requires opening of the chest.

TECHNIQUE

1 The skin is incised.
2 The subcutaneous tissue and muscle layers are divided.
3 A rib may be removed.
4 The intercostal space is entered.
5 The thoracic cavity is entered.

Discussion

Thoracotomy requires a thoracotomy set and long general surgery instruments. Rib instruments usually are included in the thoracotomy set. Once the chest cavity is opened, lung-grasping forceps (Duval type), long tissue forceps, mounted sponges, and Metzenbaum scissors are required. Lung tissue is spongy and delicate and requires smooth rather than toothed instruments (e.g., forceps and other grasping instruments). Various sizes of right angle (Mixter) clamps are needed to reach around vessels for hemostasis and dissection. Deep vascular clamps may be required for some resection procedures. Bronchial clamps (e.g., Sarot clamps) are required for resection. Many surgeons use long vascular forceps for handling tissue.

An extender or long spatula blade is needed for the ESU pencil to reach deeply into the wound. A Finochietto self-retaining retractor commonly is used. Handheld retractors include medium and wide Deaver and malleable ribbon retractors. A scapular retractor should also be available. Silastic vessel loops or a long Penrose drain is used for retraction of large vessels.

The patient is placed in the lateral position, prepped, and draped for a lateral thoracotomy. The incision is made following the curve of the rib. Subcutaneous and muscle layers then are divided with the knife or ESU. Bleeders are coagulated or clamped and ligated with silk ties.

The surgeon inserts a scapular retractor beneath the shoulder muscles and elevates the scapula. An intercostal incision is made with the knife or ESU. Occasionally a rib must be removed. If this is necessary, the surgeon incises the periosteum along its anterior surface. A periosteal elevator or rib rasp is used to strip periosteum from the rib. The surgeon severs the rib from its attachment at the spine and sternum using Bethune or similar rib shears. The entire rib is removed. The surgeon then trims the sharp edges of the remaining rib end using Sauerbruch rib shears.

The edges of the wound are covered with laparotomy sponges to protect them from bruising. A self-retaining retractor is placed in the wound and opened slowly. Surgery then continues as planned.

Closure

After chest tubes have been inserted and instruments have been removed, the surgeon places pericostal sutures (e.g., 1-0 or 2-0 absorbable suture) around the two ribs and tags the suture ends with a hemostat. Four to six sutures usually are required. A rib approximator (e.g., the Bailey approximator) is used to bring the ribs together. The pericostal sutures are tied securely while the approximator is in place.

A size 0 continuous absorbable suture may be used to approximate the periosteum between the two ribs. The surgeon then closes the muscles with a size 0 continuous or interrupted nonabsorbable suture. Subcutaneous tissue is closed with 3-0 nonabsorbable synthetic sutures. The skin is closed with staples or 4-0 nonabsorbable suture. Chest tubes are connected to the sealed drainage system, and the wound is dressed with absorbent pads and tape. A thoracotomy is illustrated in Figure 33-13.

LOBECTOMY

Surgical Goal

In a lobectomy, a lobe of the lung is removed to prevent the spread of cancer or to treat a benign tumor. Lobectomy may be performed as a VATS procedure or as an open procedure. The principles and anatomical divisions are the same for open and closed procedures. If thoracoscopy is planned, instruments for converting to an open procedure must be available.

Pathology

A lobectomy most often is performed to treat tumors, but it may indicate in other conditions, such as cysts, localized infection, or trauma to a portion of the lung.

TECHNIQUE

1 A thoracotomy is performed.
2 The hilum of the lobe is identified and individual arteries and veins are divided.
3 The bronchus is mobilized and separated from the hilum.
4 The lobe is removed.
5 The suture line is tested for leaks and extra sutures are placed as needed.
6 The bronchial stump is covered with pleura.
7 Chest tubes are inserted and the incision or incisions are closed.

Discussion

The patient is placed in the lateral position, prepped, and draped for a thoracotomy incision.

A posterolateral thoracotomy is performed. The surgeon examines the entire lung and mediastinum closely to make certain no evidence of disease exists beyond that previously diagnosed. The lobe then is retracted with lung-grasping forceps, and the pleura incised. The pulmonary artery and vein are dissected free at the hilum. Sponge dissectors are used to help separate the vessels from the connective tissue around the hilum.

Silastic vascular loops may be used to retract the bronchus and large vessels. Smaller vessels are mobilized with scissors and clamped with right angle clamps. Ligation is done with 2-0 silk ties.

The bronchus is occluded with a bronchus clamp. Suction is very important while the bronchus is open to prevent blood or fluid from draining into the opposite lung. The scrub may be needed to manage the suction while the surgeons transect and suture the bronchus. Interrupted sutures of 3-0 silk, 4-0 synthetic absorbable suture, or a linear stapler are used to occlude the proximal bronchus, which is divided with the knife.

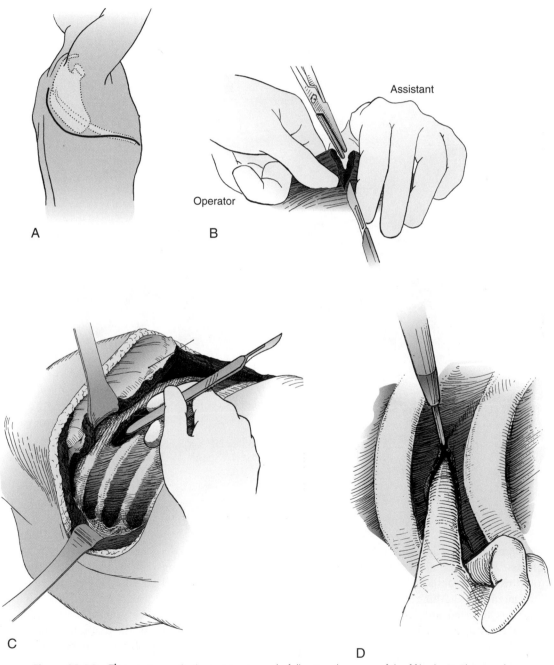

Figure 33-13   **Thoracotomy. A,** An incision is made following the curve of the fifth rib. **B,** The muscles are divided. **C,** A short incision is made in the intercostal muscles. **D,** The incision is extended with the ESU.

Continued

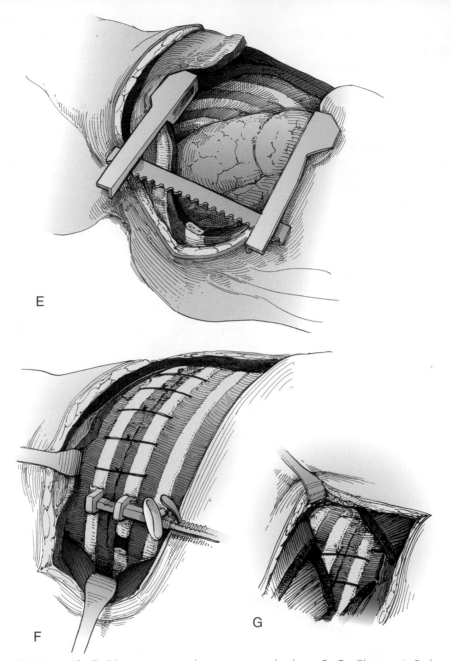

E

F

G

Figure 33-13, cont'd E, Rib retractor in place, exposing the lung. **F, G,** Closure. A Bailey rib approximator is used to close the ribs. *(Modified from Waldhausen JA, Pierce WS, Campbell DB: Surgery of the chest, ed 6, St Louis, 1996, Mosby.)*

When all vessels and the bronchus have been occluded, the lobe can be removed. The bronchial stump is covered with the pleura and sutured with interrupted 3-0 polyethylene sutures. The wound is irrigated and the lung is inflated to check for leaks. A chest tube is inserted and the wound is closed in layers. A lobectomy is illustrated in Figure 33-14.

PNEUMONECTOMY

Surgical Goal
Pneumonectomy is the removal of the entire lung.

Pathology
Removal of a lung reduces the size of a tumor that may be impinging on vital structures. Debulking is also a palliative measure to slow the progression of cancer. Other indications for lobectomy include extensive or chronic abscess or bronchiectasis, which is chronic dilation of the bronchi caused by infection, pulmonary obstruction, or tuberculosis.

Discussion
The patient is placed in the lateral position and a thoracotomy is performed. The entire lung and surrounding tissues are

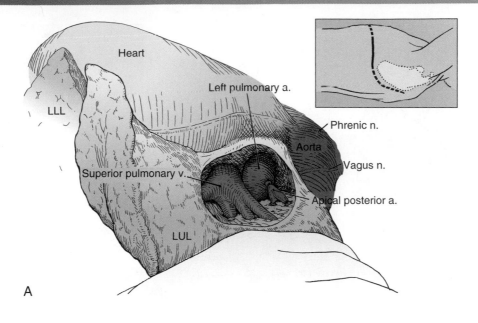

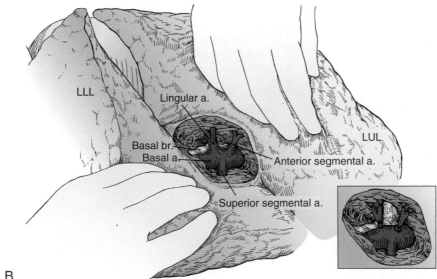

Figure 33-14   **Open lobectomy. A,** The left main pulmonary artery is identified and followed distally to the first upper lobe branch. **B,** The fissure is divided between the upper and lower lobes and opened to allow division of the arteries.

TECHNIQUE

1 A thoracotomy is performed.
2 The mediastinal pleura is incised.
3 The major vessels are divided (i.e., bronchus, pulmonary artery, and superior and inferior pulmonary veins).
4 The vagus, phrenic, and recurrent laryngeal nerves are identified.
5 Regional lymph nodes are dissected.
6 The bronchus is divided and closed.
7 The lung is removed and the wound is closed; chest tubes may be inserted.

examined closely to evaluate the extent of the disease. The lung is retracted with nonmalleable or malleable retractors or Duval lung forceps to expose the mediastinal pleura. The pleura is incised with scissors and smooth tissue forceps. Blunt dissection along the edge of the parietal pleura is performed with sponge dissectors.

Dissection is carried to the hilum. The major structures connected to the lung are isolated, including the bronchus, pulmonary artery, and pulmonary vein. The pulmonary artery and vein are carefully separated, clamped with right angle vascular clamps, and divided. Heavy silk sutures are used to ligate the vessels. The vagus, recurrent laryngeal (left side

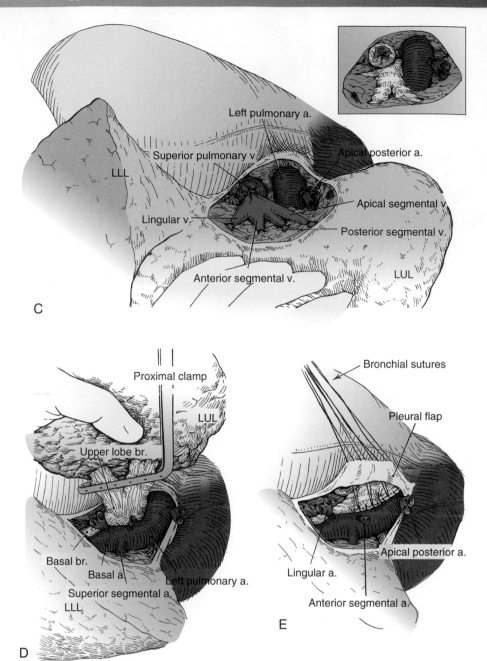

Figure 33-14, cont'd   **C,** Dissection of the superior pulmonary vein. **D,** Proximal clamp in place. **E,** Closure of the upper lobe bronchus. *a.,* Artery; *br.,* bronchus; *LLL,* left lower lobe; *LUL,* left upper lobe; *n.,* nerve; *v.,* vein. *(Modified from Waldhausen JA, Pierce WS, Campbell DB: Surgery of the chest, ed 6, St Louis, 1996, Mosby.)*

only), and phrenic nerves are retracted with vessel loops or moist umbilical tapes.

The pulmonary artery is clamped, divided, and ligated. The surgeon may oversew the cut edges of the artery with fine suture, such as 4-0 or 5-0 silk or polypropylene. The superior and inferior veins are ligated and divided in similar fashion. Ligation clips may be used for smaller vessels.

The bronchus commonly is occluded with a Sarot clamp and divided with the knife. The lung then can be removed from the wound. The open end of the bronchus is closed with interrupted sutures (e.g., 3-0 polypropylene sutures) or the stapler. The bronchus is divided and the lung is removed from the wound.

The wound is irrigated with warm saline and any leaks are identified and repaired with sutures. The pleura is sutured over the bronchus. Chest tubes may be inserted and brought out through stab wounds adjacent to the incision. These are secured with heavy silk sutures. The upper mediastinal pleura is closed with absorbable suture, and the wound is closed in layers.

RIB RESECTION FOR THORACIC OUTLET SYNDROME

Surgical Goal

Thoracic outlet syndrome (TOS) is a rare condition in which the subclavian vessels and the brachial plexus are compressed at the apex of the thorax. The surgical goal is to release the compression of the neurovascular tissue and restore function to the affected upper extremity, neck, or shoulder.

Pathology

The opening of the thoracic outlet is formed by the first ribs, the spine, and the sternum. TOS occurs when the brachial plexus and the subclavian vein or artery are compressed as they pass from the neck into the upper extremity (in the region between the thoracic outlet and the insertion of the pectoralis minor muscle). The obstructing structures may include the first rib, clavicle, or pectoralis tendon. The causes of TOS include trauma, structural anomaly, repetitive motion, and poor posture.

Complete rib resection may help to prevent recurrent symptoms. Soft tissue dissection instruments, as well as rib cutters, elevators, and rongeurs, are needed.

TECHNIQUE

1. An axillary incision is made.
2. Dissection is carried to the cervical or first rib.
3. The rib is resected.
4. A drain is placed and the incision is closed.

Discussion

The patient is placed in the lateral position with the arm abducted up to 90 degrees and suspended by an assistant or mechanical device. The skin prep includes the arm, neck, and upper chest. An incision is made between the pectoralis muscle and the latissimus dorsi muscle on the affected side. The incision is carried to the level of the cervical rib (if present) or the first rib. The ESU is used for this step of the procedure.

A self-retaining retractor is placed in the wound with several lap tapes to protect the edges. The neurovascular bundle is identified and the rib is exposed. The midportion of the rib is dissected using a periosteal elevator.

The midportion of the rib is removed or the entire rib can be extracted using bone shears or double-action rongeurs. A small Penrose drain may be placed in the wound, which is closed using interrupted sutures of absorbable synthetic material.

DECORTICATION OF THE LUNG

Surgical Goal

Decortication of the lung is the surgical removal of a portion of the parietal pleura.

Pathology

Chronic inflammation, infection (**empyema** or tuberculosis), or a lung tumor causes the formation of exudate in the pleural space. Because of the effusion or tumor, fibrin deposits form, and the parietal pleura can adhere to the chest wall, referred to as a *peel*. Removal of the peel or affected pleura aids the treatment of chronic infection and eases restriction of the pleura. Pleurectomy (removal of the pleura) is performed to treat pleural cancer, such as mesothelioma.

TECHNIQUE

1. The patient usually is placed in a posterolateral thoracotomy position.
2. An incision is made in the fifth intercostal space.
3. Blood clots or exudate is removed.
4. Adhesions below the parietal and visceral pleura are sharply divided.
5. When the visceral pleura is reached, the dissection is continued alternately with a gauze pledget or the fingertip until the fibrotic covering is removed sufficiently to allow full expansion of the lung.
6. Drainage tubes are inserted.
7. The incision is closed.

Discussion

A thoracotomy set is required for the lung decortication. Curettes may also be needed for removal of tough fibrous deposits.

After the thoracic incision has been made, the skin, subcutaneous tissue, and muscle are dissected with scissors and ESU. A rib spreader is inserted to expose the affected portion of the lung. A portion of the fifth or sixth rib may be resected with rib shears. Empyema or other fluid is drained and cultured. The anesthesia care provider expands the lung intermittently to demonstrate areas requiring additional decortication. After sufficient dissection and removal of the fibrous membrane, drainage tubes are inserted and the incision is closed.

LUNG TRANSPLANTATION

Surgical Goal

Transplantation of one or both lungs is performed to remove a diseased lung and replace it with a donor lung. Single-lung transplantation increasingly is used as a way to maximize the allocation of donor lungs. If both lungs are diseased, bilateral transplantation is indicated. Living donor transplantation involves removal of the donor's lower lobes only.

Pathology

Single- or double-lung transplantation is indicated for patients with restrictive lung disease, emphysema, pulmonary hypertension, and other noninfectious end-stage pulmonary diseases.

Discussion

The donor patient is placed in the supine position, which allows the best exposure of the various organs to be excised. Procurement of lung tissue (and other organs) is a very precise procedure that requires knowledge of protocols and procedures, as well as problem-solving abilities. Procurement teams are self-sufficient and usually do not require equipment or instruments from the host facility, such as basic thoracic and/or cardiac instruments and supplies (e.g., cold preservative solutions and sterile containers for the organs).

Speed usually is important, because many organs have a limited period of viability. Organ transplantation is a team effort and all members of the staff play a role in a successful transplantation outcome.

TECHNIQUE

Lung Donor

1 The donor is prepped from chin to knees.
2 A median sternotomy is performed
3 A sternal (or rib) retractor is inserted.
4 The pleura is opened longitudinally and the pericardium is divided.
5 Umbilical tapes are placed around the aorta and the superior and inferior venae cavae.
6 Pleural adhesions are divided and the proximal pulmonary arteries are dissected.
7 The superior vena cava is ligated with heavy silk ties.
8 The aortic arch is dissected free and the ligamentum arteriosum (the remnant ductus arteriosus) is divided.
9 The pulmonary artery is encircled with an umbilical tape and separated from the ascending aorta.
10 Cardioplegia solution is infused through the proximal aorta into the heart via the coronary arteries; pulmoplegia solution is infused into the pulmonary organs.
11 Cardiac veins and arteries are separated, and the heart is removed and placed in a cold preservative solution.
12 The pulmonary arteries are separated from the mediastinum.
13 The trachea is dissected free.
14 The lungs are inflated and then stapled and removed.
15 The lungs are placed in a cold preservative solution.

Single-Lung Transplantation (Recipient)

A patient undergoing single-lung transplantation is placed in the lateral position with the affected side up. A double-lumen endotracheal tube is inserted to inflate either lung selectively. Generally, the groin is prepped and exposed in case a femorofemoral bypass is required. Thoracotomy instruments are used in single lung transplantation; cardiopulmonary bypass instruments and supplies should be available in the operating room in case bypass is required. The choice of suture materials depends on the surgeon; the previous description may be different in other institutions.

Techniques used during the procedure include shortening the donor bronchial stump, wrapping the anastomosis with omentum or an intercostal muscle pedicle, and performing an intussuscepting (e.g., telescoping) bronchial anastomosis technique.

TECHNIQUE

Lung Recipient

1 The patient is placed in the lateral position with the operative side up. The individual is prepped from chin to knees.
2 A thoracotomy incision is made and a retractor is inserted.
3 If the recipient's right lung is to be removed, the pulmonary vein, pulmonary artery, and azygos vein are isolated and divided.
4 If the recipient's left lung is to be removed, the ligamentum arteriosum is divided.

5 The lung to be removed is collapsed and the proximal pulmonary artery is occluded. If hemodynamic instability is a factor, a femorofemoral bypass may be performed.
6 The lung is removed.
7 The pulmonary veins are divided and branches of the pulmonary artery are separated.
8 The bronchus is divided and the diseased lung is removed.
9 The bronchus-to-bronchus anastomosis is performed with 3-0 absorbable suture.
10 The pulmonary artery–to–pulmonary artery anastomosis is performed with running 4-0 polypropylene suture.
11 The recipient pulmonary veins are attached to the donor atrial cuff with running 4-0 polypropylene suture.
12 The new lung is inflated and inspected.
13 Chest tubes are inserted and hemostasis is achieved.
14 The chest is closed.
15 Bronchoscopy may be performed to suction secretions and confirm an intact anastomosis.

Bilateral Lung Transplantation (Recipient)

Bilateral lung procedures often require cardiopulmonary support. Bypass may be avoided with the bilateral sequential technique, in which the more diseased native lung is removed first if the other lung is capable of maintaining adequate oxygenation. Femoral cannulation supplies should be readily available.

Complications include rejection and infection. Transplant anastomoses may require repair if persistent bleeding develops. Lung biopsies are done in the postoperative period to detect possible rejection.

TECHNIQUE

Bilateral Lung Recipient

1 The patient is placed in the supine position and prepped from chin to knees. The arms are placed above the head and supported with an ether screen or similar device.
2 A bilateral anterior thoracotomy ("clamshell") incision is made.
3 If bilateral sequential transplantation is to be performed, the most functional lung is inserted first and the process is repeated on the opposite side for the second lung. This often eliminates the need for cardiopulmonary bypass.
4 If a bilateral en bloc procedure is to be performed (both donor lungs are removed and implanted as one unit), cardiopulmonary bypass usually is required.
5 Bronchial pulmonary artery and atrial anastomoses are performed as described for single lung procedures.
6 The procedure is completed as described for single-lung transplant.

KEY CONCEPTS

- Knowledge of the key anatomical structures of the thoracic cavity is necessary for a complete understanding of surgical procedures.

- Familiarity with diagnostic procedures of the respiratory system and thoracic structures is important for patient care and a more complete understanding of pathology.
- An understanding of respiratory system pathology is important for patient care and case planning.
- Case planning in thoracic surgery requires specific understanding of the instruments, hemostatic materials and techniques, drugs, sutures, and patient positioning.
- In order to be effective in the scrub role, the surgical technologist must be knowledgeable about specific surgical procedures and the steps involved in each procedure.

REVIEW QUESTIONS

1. Explain the process of breathing, including the influence of negative pressure in the thoracic cavity.
2. Why must a closed chest drainage unit be kept lower than the patient's body?
3. What are the differences among lobectomy, pneumonectomy, and segmental resection?
4. What is the difference between thoracotomy and thoracostomy?
5. Explain pneumothorax and why it occurs.
6. What is the purpose of debulking a tumor?
7. What instruments are needed to perform a rib resection?
8. What is the Valsalva maneuver? What is the effect of this maneuver on the heart rate?

BIBLIOGRAPHY

Ferri F: *Ferri's clinical advisor 2012*, Philadelphia, 2011, Mosby.

Khatri V, Asensio J: *Operative surgery manual*, Philadelphia, 2003, Saunders.

Lewis SM, Heitkemper MM, Dirksen SR: *Medical surgical nursing*, ed 6, St Louis, 2004, Mosby.

Mason R, et al: *Textbook of Respiratory Medicine*, ed 5, Philadelphia, 2010, Saunders.

Miller RM, Eriksson LI, Fleisher LA, et al: *Miller's Anesthesia*, ed 7, Philadelphia, 2009, Churchill Livingstone.

Roberts J, ed: *Clinical procedures in emergency medicine*, ed 5, Philadelphia, 2009, Saunders.

Townsend C, Beauchamp R, Evers B, Mattox K: *Sabiston textbook of surgery*, ed 19, Philadelphia, 2012, Saunders.

34

Cardiac Surgery

CHAPTER OUTLINE

Introduction
Surgical Anatomy

Diagnostic Procedures
Case Planning

Surgical Procedures
Heart Failure

LEARNING OBJECTIVES

After studying this chapter the reader will be able to:
1. Identify key anatomical features of the heart and great vessels
2. Describe diagnostic procedures commonly used in cardiac medicine

3. Describe specific elements of case planning for cardiac surgery
4. Discuss cardiac pathology
5. List and describe common cardiac procedures

TERMINOLOGY

Aneurysm: A weakness in the arterial wall resulting in ballooning of the artery and possible rupture.

Apex: The lower left tip of the left ventricle of the heart; also, the rounded upper portion of each lung.

Arrhythmia: An abnormal heartbeat (also called *dysrhythmia*).

Arteriosclerosis: Disease of the arteries characterized by loss of elasticity and hardening of the arterial walls.

Atherosclerosis: A disease characterized by the buildup of cholesterol deposits in the arterial lining.

Bradycardia: A slow heart rate (usually a heart rate under 60 beats per minute in an adult).

Cardiac cycle: The pumping action of the heart from one beat to the next.

Cardioplegia: Intentional stopping of the heart during cardiac surgery. This is achieved with a cardioplegic solution, which often contains a mixture of potassium chloride, lidocaine, dextrose, insulin, albumin, tromethamine, and Plasmanate.

Coarctation: A congenital narrowing or stricture in the descending thoracic aorta.

Congenital: A condition present at birth.

Cross-clamp: To place a clamp across a structure to occlude it.

Diastole: That phase of the cardiac cycle when the ventricles contract.

Endovascular repair: Endoscopic surgery of the vascular system.

Fibrillation: Uncoordinated muscular activity in the heart muscle, which results in a "quivering" rather than pumping action.

Fusiform aneurysm: A type of aneurysm that involves the entire circumference of a blood vessel.

Heart-lung machine: Medical device used during cardiac bypass. Systemic blood is shunted out of the body via cannulas, which are implanted in the heart. The device collects the blood, removes excess carbon dioxide, oxygenates it, and returns it to the body through separate cannulas.

Infarction: Necrosis and death of tissue related to obstruction of blood flow.

Ischemia: Reduced blood supply to tissue. Ischemia may be a result of obstruction within the blood vessels or external pressure, which acts as a tourniquet.

Off-pump procedure: A procedure performed without a cardiopulmonary bypass (i.e., "the pump").

Pacemaker: A device that stimulates the heart muscle to contract.

Preclotting: The process of soaking a graft or patch of synthetic graft material in the patient's blood or plasma before insertion. Most grafts no longer need preclotting.

Saccular aneurysm: A type of aneurysm in which a saclike formation with a narrow neck projects from the side of the artery.

Shunt: To bypass a structure or carry fluid from one anatomical location to another.

Stenosis: The narrowing of a hollow structure such as a blood vessel or duct.

Sternotomy: An incision made into the sternum.

Systole: A phase of the cardiac cycle in which the ventricles contract.

Tachycardia: A fast heart rate (usually over 120 beats per minute in the adult).

Thoracotomy: An incision made into the thoracic cavity.

INTRODUCTION

Cardiac surgery includes procedures of the heart and associated great vessels performed to treat acquired or **congenital** disease. Open techniques and minimally invasive endoscopic procedures are used. The techniques used in cardiac surgery build on those used in thoracic, general, and vascular procedures. However, cardiac procedures generally are more complex and require equipment not used in other specialties (e.g., cardiac bypass). The surgical technologist may become a specialist in cardiac surgery after training in general, peripheral vascular and thoracic surgery. This specialty requires a thorough understanding of cardiothoracic anatomy and cardiac function, as well as the ability to work in a complex surgical environment with multiple technologies.

SURGICAL ANATOMY

The thoracic cavity contains the heart and its great vessels, the lungs and their associated respiratory structures, the mediastinum, and a portion of the esophagus.

HEART

The heart is a muscular organ that consists of four hollow spaces, or chambers. The two upper chambers are the right atrium and the left atrium; the two lower chambers are the right ventricle and the left ventricle (Figure 34-1). The heart is contained within a closed cavity called the *mediastinum*,

between the two lungs, posterior to the sternum, and anterior to the vertebrae and esophagus. Most of the heart lies to the left of the midline.

The heart is enclosed by a double-layered membrane called the *pericardium*. Pericardial fluid between the outer parietal and inner visceral pericardium lubricates the layers and prevents friction. The walls of the heart have three layers: the outer epicardium, the middle myocardium, and the inner endocardium. Myocardium is specialized muscle tissue (cardiac muscle) capable of generating electrical impulses, which cause the heart to contract.

The heart's four chambers are divided by a septum (Figure 34-2). The right ventricle receives deoxygenated blood from the right atrium. From the right ventricle, the blood is pumped through the pulmonary artery to the lungs, where it is oxygenated. The left ventricle receives oxygenated blood from the left atrium. From the left ventricle, the blood is pumped into the aorta and the systemic circulation. The valves of the heart maintain one-way flow through the cardiac chambers.

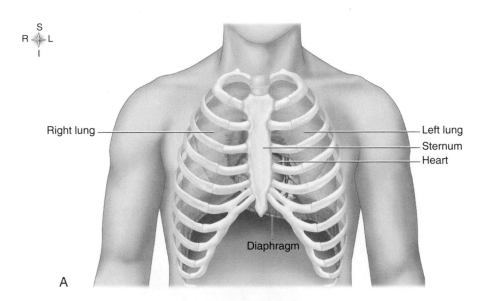

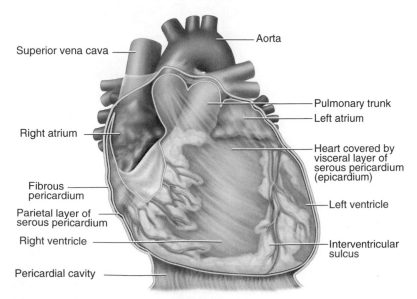

Figure 34-1 **A,** Anterior view showing the heart in relation to the lungs. **B,** Detail of the heart with the pericardial sac open. *(From Thibodeau G, Patton K: Anatomy and physiology, ed 6, St Louis, 2007, Mosby.)*

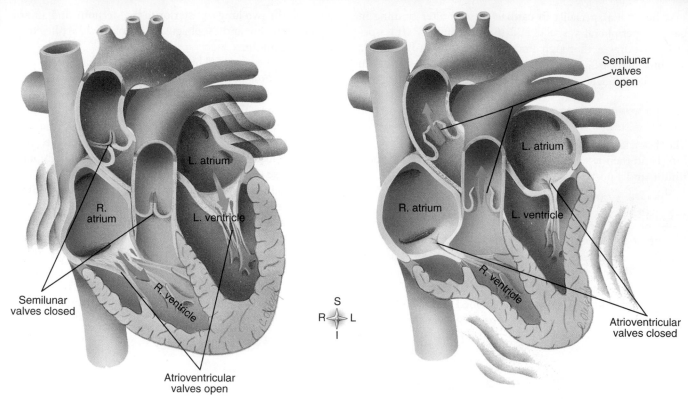

L. atrium

R. atrium

L. ventricle

R. ventricle

Semilunar valves closed

Atrioventricular valves open

Semilunar valves open

L. atrium

R. atrium

L. ventricle

R. ventricle

Atrioventricular valves closed

S
R ✦ L
I

Figure 34-2 Chambers and valves of the heart. *L.,* Left; *R.,* right. *(From Thibodeau G, Patton K: Anatomy and physiology, ed 6, St Louis, 2007, Mosby.)*

Figure 34-3 Coronary arteries, which supply blood to the heart tissue. *(From Thibodeau G, Patton K: Anatomy and physiology, ed 6, St Louis, 2007, Mosby.)*

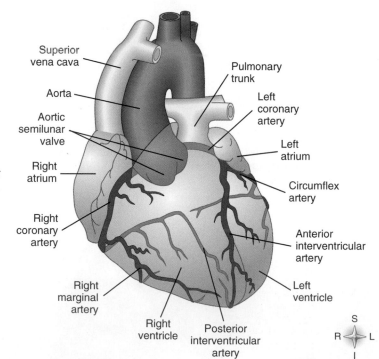

Superior vena cava

Aorta

Aortic semilunar valve

Right atrium

Right coronary artery

Right marginal artery

Right ventricle

Pulmonary trunk

Left coronary artery

Left atrium

Circumflex artery

Anterior interventricular artery

Left ventricle

Posterior interventricular artery

S
R ✦ L
I

The heart's own blood supply is delivered by the coronary artery circulation (Figure 34-3).

HEART VALVES

The valves of the heart maintain unidirectional blood flow. The atria are separated from the ventricles by the atrioventricular (AV) valves. The tricuspid valve lies on the right side and the bicuspid (mitral) valve lies on the left side. The leaflets of the valves open as blood is pumped and close when the pressure on the other side of the valve exceeds the entry pressure. The AV valve leaflets are attached to the papillary muscle of the ventricles by connective tissue called *chordae tendineae*. The large vessels of the heart also have valves. The

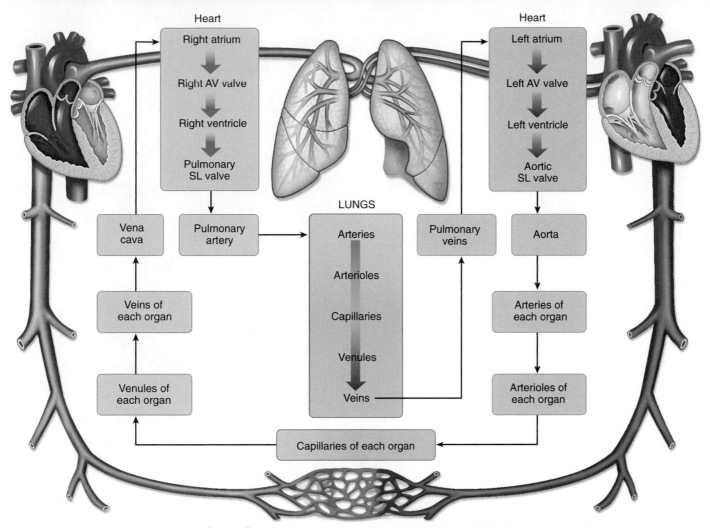

Figure 34-4 **Cardiac cycle**. *AV, Atrioventricular; SL, semilunar. (From Thibodeau G, Patton K: Anatomy and physiology, ed 6, St Louis, 2007, Mosby.)*

semilunar valves connect the ventricles to the large vessels. The pulmonary valve connects the right ventricle with the pulmonary artery. The left aortic valve connects the left ventricle to the aorta.

CARDIAC CYCLE

The pumping action of the heart from one beat to the next is called the **cardiac cycle**. The cycle occurs in two phases, systole and diastole. During **systole**, the ventricles contract; in **diastole**, they relax and fill with blood. The cycle is fully defined by the electrical impulses that occur in specific areas of the heart, the muscular activity, and the flow of blood through the chambers and vessels. The electrical activity of each cycle is demonstrated on an electrocardiogram (ECG). The complete cycle is shown in Figure 34-4.

CONDUCTION SYSTEM

The electrical conduction system contains a network of specialized cells, which generate electrical activity along conduction pathways. These cells, which are found in several areas of

the heart, transmit nerve signals that cause the heart muscle to contract in a coordinated way.

The sinoatrial (SA) node initiates the cardiac cycle and is sometimes called the heart's pacemaker. Impulses travel from the SA node to the AV node in the interatrial septum. From the AV node, they travel to the bundle of His at the AV junction. Conduction continues through the right and left bundle branches, ventricular walls, and Purkinje fibers. Disease or interference in the conduction system results in uncoordinated electrical activity in the cardiac muscle and may cause ineffective contractions. The conduction system is illustrated in Figure 34-5.

DIAGNOSTIC PROCEDURES

Before surgery, the patient undergoes diagnostic studies to identify pathological conditions or anomalies. Many of these studies are performed in the interventional radiology department, and the surgical technologist occasionally may be involved in the procedures. Cardiac function tests may require sophisticated imaging techniques, injection of radionuclide, and physical stress tests.

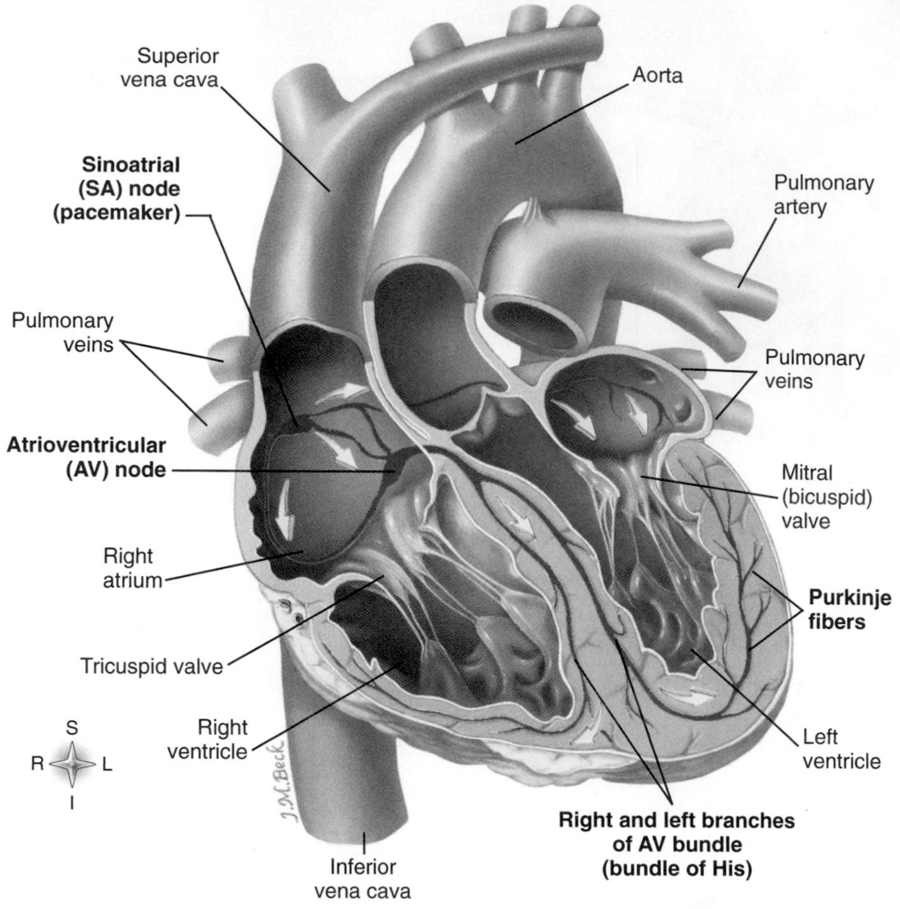

Figure 34-5 Conduction system of the heart. *(From Thibodeau G, Patton K: Anatomy and physiology, ed 6, St Louis, 2007, Mosby.)*

Labels: Superior vena cava; Aorta; Sinoatrial (SA) node (pacemaker); Pulmonary artery; Pulmonary veins; Atrioventricular (AV) node; Pulmonary veins; Mitral (bicuspid) valve; Right atrium; Purkinje fibers; Tricuspid valve; Right ventricle; Left ventricle; Right and left branches of AV bundle (bundle of His); Inferior vena cava

---

Box 34-1 Cardiac Diagnostic Tests

Resting electrocardiogram (ECG)
Exercise ECG (stress test)
Chest radiography
Echocardiogram
Radionucleotide scanning
Computed tomography (CT) scan
Positron emission tomography (PET) scan with or without stress test
Magnetic resonance imaging (MRI) and magnetic resonance angiography (MRA)
Pulmonary function tests
Aortography
Electrophysiology
Cardiac catheterization
Endomyocardial biopsy
Mediastinoscopy

Routine laboratory tests are performed to identify abnormalities of the blood, urine, cardiac enzymes, and waste products, which may indicate myocardial damage. Common tests are listed in Box 34-1.

CARDIAC CATHETERIZATION

Cardiac catheterization is an interventional radiology procedure that involves insertion of a cardiac catheter into the heart chambers and large vessels via a peripheral artery or vein.

Specific tests are then performed inside the heart and vessels, such as intravascular ultrasonography, angiography (including coronary artery imaging), and endocardial biopsy.

Left heart catheterization most often is performed to assess the coronary arteries, systemic vascular resistance, aortic and mitral valve function, and left ventricular pressure. These tests are performed through a percutaneous puncture of the femoral, radial, or brachial artery, with catheterization through these vessels.

Right heart catheterization is performed to assess the right atrium and ventricle and the pulmonary artery. Pulmonary artery occlusion pressure (PAOP) is a significant test that determines cardiac volume and output. Valve function may also be tested through right heart catheterization. In this procedure, a catheter is inserted percutaneously through the femoral, subclavian, or internal jugular vein, advanced into the right atrium, and then advanced farther, into the pulmonary artery, via the tricuspid valve, right ventricle, and pulmonary valve.

Cardiac imaging has become increasingly complex in the past 10 years. In addition to standard angiography, in which a contrast medium is injected to obtain real-time images of the cardiac system, digital subtraction angiography also is used. In this process only the vessels and chambers in which contrast medium is injected are shown on the fluoroscopic image. All other tissues are masked or subtracted. Aortic imaging is performed for the assessment of **coarctation** of the aorta, valve regurgitation, congenital anomalies, and **aneurysm**. Ventricular angiography demonstrates the movement

Table 34-1 | Angiographic Data

Angiographic Data	Findings
Coronary arteries	Anatomy/function of the coronary vascular bed, distal coronary flow, atrioventricular fistula, atherosclerosis, anomalous origin of coronary arteries
Ventriculography	Anatomy/function of ventricles and associated structures, left ventricular aneurysm, congenital abnormalities, valvular stenosis/regurgitation, shunts
Valvular angiography	Intact mitral/tricuspid complex, valvular incompetence/stenosis/regurgitation
Pulmonary angiography	Pulmonary embolism, congenital abnormalities
Aortography	Patency of aortic branches; normal mobility, competence, and anatomy of aortic valve; aneurysms (saccular, fusiform); origin of aortic dissection; shunts or anomalous connections; congenital defects or obstructions

Modified from Pagana KD, Pagana TJ: *Mosby's diagnostic and laboratory test reference*, ed 7, St Louis, 2005, Elsevier/Mosby.

of blood through the valves and can be used to measure the ejection fraction (the amount of blood pumped from the ventricles) and end-systolic and end-diastolic volumes. Cardiac imaging data are shown in Table 34-1.

Intravascular ultrasound is performed with an end catheter transducer, which can be advanced into the lumen of the blood vessel to determine the rate of blood flow.

Oxygen saturation can be measured at various points in the heart and large vessels during catheterization. This information determines whether blood is being shunted (taking an abnormal route).

Cardiac output is measured by calculating the amount of blood ejected through the heart per minute.

Cardiac muscle biopsy is performed to detect tissue rejection after heart transplantation.

CASE PLANNING

POSITIONING

Procedures of the heart and associated structures are performed with the patient in the supine or lateral position with the affected side up. The following are the incisions most commonly used in open cardiac surgery:

- *Median* **sternotomy** *(supine):* A partial or full midline incision is made through the sternum.
- *Paramedian (supine):* The incision is made to the right or left of the sternum. This position is used for minimally invasive procedures and lymph node biopsy.
- *Anterolateral, posterolateral:* This is a modification of the lateral position in which the patient is supine with soft padding under the hip and shoulder of the affected side. This rolls the thorax slightly upward. The shoulder of the

affected side then is abducted and the arm is suspended safely on an overhead table brace.
- *Minithoracotomy (supine):* The 2-inch (5-cm) right or left minithoracotomy is made between the ribs for access during minimally invasive and robotic procedures.

Common thoracic incisions are described in Table 34-2.

INSTRUMENTS AND EQUIPMENT

Cardiac surgery requires a general surgery set augmented with cardiac instruments, general thoracic instruments (including stapling devices), and lung instruments, depending on the procedure. Specific instruments for coronary artery, valve, aneurysm, chest wall, and lung surgery may be added (Figure 34-6). Instrumentation can be quite complex, requiring experience and advanced organizational skills to anticipate the steps of a procedure.

The Rumel tourniquet, commonly used in cardiovascular surgery, is a short length of synthetic tubing either commercially prepared or cut from a straight (Robinson) urinary catheter. The tourniquet is threaded over cannulation sutures to help hold them in place. The Rumel tourniquet also is used when large vessels are occluded or isolated with a vessel loop or umbilical tape (a length of cotton passed under a vessel for retraction). A stylet, such as that from a Rumel tourniquet, is used to snare the strands of suture or tape and bring them through the lumen of the tubing. The tubing is tightened against the cannula or vessel by pulling on the strands, which are held using a hemostat placed at the upper end.

Coronary Artery Instruments

Coronary artery instruments are extremely delicate. They include scissors, forceps, and needle holders, which are similar to routine vascular instruments. Many are angled at the tips.

Minimally invasive coronary procedures require longer instruments with the same precision tips. In off-pump coronary anastomosis, a flexible, suction tip coronary stabilizing device can be positioned on either side of the coronary artery to minimize cardiac movement. Figure 34-7 shows the stabilizer attached to a sternal retractor and an apical suction device to expose the posterolateral heart.

Valve Instruments

Valve instruments include special retractors to expose the valve, suture holders, and accessories for the valve prosthesis. These include sizers and holders.

Aneurysm Instruments

During aneurysm repair, large vessels must be clamped and meticulous dissection performed on the inside of the diseased vessel. This requires dissecting instruments and vascular clamps. Median sternotomy or **thoracotomy** is needed, depending on the approach selected by the surgeon.

Endoscopic Instruments

Endoscopic cardiac instruments are used during video-assisted thoracoscopy (VATS). Robotic instruments used in the da Vinci system are illustrated in Chapter 24, which also describes the care and handling of endoscopic instruments.

Table 34-2 Thoracic Incisions

Incision	Position of Patient	Indications	Special Patient Needs
Median sternotomy: Incision down the center of the sternum	Supine	Most adult cardiac procedures except those on branch pulmonary arteries, distal transverse aortic arch, and descending thoracic aorta; OPCAB	Padding for the hands, elbows, feet, back of head, and dependent bony prominences
Ministernotomy: Partial upper or lower sternal incision starting either from the sternal notch or the xiphoid process and extending to the midportion of the sternum; lower end sternal splitting (LESS)	Supine	MAS, on-CPB or off-CPB procedures	Same as for a median sternotomy
Parasternotomy: Resection of the right or left costal cartilages (from the second to the fifth cartilage, depending on the surgical target)	Supine; a small roll may be placed under the affected side	Left: MAS CABG Right: MAS CABG, valve procedures	Same as for a median sternotomy; risk of postoperative chest wall instability
Anterolateral thoracotomy: Curvilinear incision along the subpectoral groove to the axillary line	Supine with a pad or pillow under the operative site; arm on the affected side is supported in a sling or overarm board; the arm on the unaffected side may be tucked along the side	MAS, MIDCAB, trauma to the anterior pericardium and left ventricle; repeat sternotomy	Padding for extremities; pad or other device to elevate the affected side; arm board or sling for the arm on the affected side
Left anterior small thoracotomy (LAST), right anterior minithoracotomy: Curvilinear incision along the subpectoral groove, right or left side	Supine with a small roll under the affected side	Left: MAS, MIDCAB Right: MAS valve procedures or CABG	Same as anterolateral thoracotomy
Lateral thoracotomy: Curvilinear incision along the costochondral junction anteriorly to the posterior border of the scapula	Placed on the side with the arms extended and the axilla and head supported; the knees and legs are protected	Lung biopsies; first rib resection; lobectomy	Arm board, overarm board, axillary roll, padding for extremities, padding between the legs; sandbags, straps, wide tape, or other devices to support the torso
Posterolateral thoracotomy: Curvilinear incision from the subpectoral crease below the nipple, extended laterally and posteriorly along the ribs almost to the posterior midline below the scapula (the location of the intercostal incision depends on the surgical site); used less often with the availability of VATS techniques	Lateral with the arms extended and the axilla and head supported; the knees and legs are protected	First rib resection; lobectomy	Similar to needs for a lateral thoracotomy
Transsternal bilateral anterior thoracotomy (clamshell): Submammary incision extending from one anterior axillary line to the other across the sternum at the fourth interspace	Supine	Lung transplantation; emergency access to the heart when a sternal saw is not available	Same as median sternotomy; requires transection of left and right IMA
Subxiphoid incision: Vertical midline incision from over the xiphoid process to about 4 inches (10 cm) inferiorly (the lower portion of the sternum may be divided to improve exposure)	Supine	Pericardial drainage, pericardial biopsy, attachment of pacemaker electrodes, MAS	Same as median sternotomy
Thoracoabdominal incision: Low curvilinear incision on the left side, extended to the anterior midline, and continued vertically down the abdomen	Anterior thoracotomy with the chest at a 45-degree angle to the table; abdomen supine	Thoracoabdominal aneurysm	Same as anterolateral thoracotomy

Modified from Rothrock JC: *Alexander's care of the patient in surgery*, ed 13, St Louis, 2007, Mosby; Waldhausen JA, Pierce WS, Campbell DB: *Surgery of the chest*, ed 6, St Louis, 1996, Mosby; and Zipes DP, Libby P, Bonow RO, Braunwald E, editors: *Braunwald's heart disease*, ed 7, Philadelphia, 2005, Elsevier/Saunders.

CABG, Coronary artery bypass grafting; *CPB*, cardiopulmonary bypass; *IMA*, internal mammary artery; *MAS*, minimal access surgery; *MIDCAB*, minimal access direct coronary artery bypass; *OPCAB*, off-pump coronary artery bypass; *VATS*, video-assisted thoracoscopic surgery.

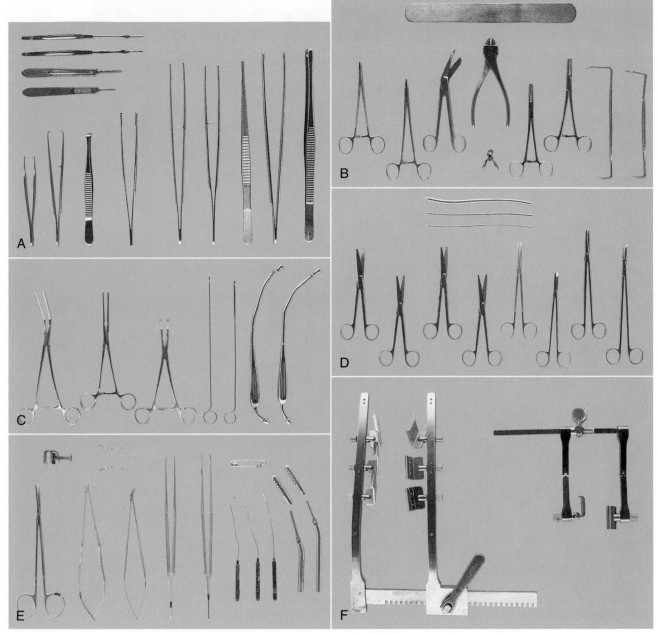

Figure 34-6 **Cardiac instruments. A,** *Top left,* 2 Bard-Parker knife handles, #7; 1 Bard-Parker knife handle, #4; 1 Bard-Parker knife handle, #3. *Bottom, left to right,* 1 Adson tissue forceps with teeth (1 × 2); 2 Hayes Martin tissue forceps, front view and side view; 1 Ferris-Smith tissue forceps; 3 DeBakey vascular Atraugrip tissue forceps with post, long, 2 front views and 1 side view; 2 Russian tissue forceps, long, front view and side view. **B,** *Top,* 1 Ochsner malleable retractor, medium. *Bottom, left to right,* 1 Jarit sternal needle holder, 7-inch; 1 Jarit sternal needle holder, 8 inch; 1 bandage scissors, heavy; 1 wire cutter, heavy; 1 bed cord–holding clip; 2 Jarit (Vorse) tubing occluding clamps; 2 Army-Navy retractors. **C,** *Left to right,* 1 DeBakey multipurpose vascular clamp, obtuse angle, 60 degrees, jaw length 4 cm, overall length 9 inches; 1 Glover patent ductus clamp, straight; 1 Beck aorta clamp; 2 eyed obturators (stylets) for Rumel tourniquet; 2 Yankauer suction tubes with tips. **D,** *Top,* 3 Hegar dilators: 7 and 8, 5 and 6, 3 and 4. *Bottom, left to right,* 1 Mayo dissecting scissors, curved; 3 Mayo dissecting scissors, straight; 2 Metzenbaum scissors, 7-inch; 1 Metzenbaum scissors, 8-inch; 1 Strully scissors with probe tip. **E,** *Top, left to right,* 1 tubing clamp; 1 Parsonnet epicardial (self-retaining spring) retractor, sharp, 3 × 3 prongs; 1 safety pin with rings. *Bottom, left to right,* 1 Snowden-Pencer scissors, straight; 1 Yasargil scissors, bayonet handle, 125-degree angle; 1 You-Potts scissors, fine, thin 10-mm blades, 45-degree angle; 2 Snowden-Pencer dressing forceps, 8-inch; 3 Garrett dilators: 2-, 1- and 1.5-mm; 2 metal coronary suction tubes with tips. **F,** *Left to right,* 1 Ankeney sternal retractor; 1 Himmelstein sternal retractor.

Continued

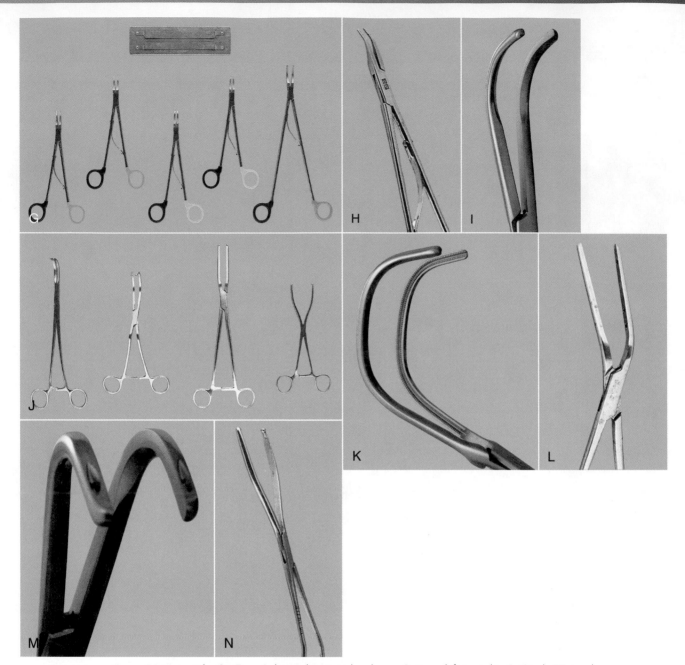

Figure 34-6, cont'd   **G,** *Top,* 1 hemoclip cartridge base. *Bottom, left to right,* 5 Weck EZ Load hemoclip appliers: 2 medium, 7.75-inch; 2 small, 7.75-inch; 1 large, 10.75-inch and tip. **H,** Close-up of Weck hemoclip applier. **I,** Semb ligature-carrying forceps, 9-inch; **J,** *Left to right,* 1 Semb ligature-carrying forceps, 9-inch; 1 Lambert-Kay aorta clamp; 1 Fogarty clamp-applying forceps, angled; 1 bulldog clamp applier. **K,** Lambert-Kay aorta clamp. **L,** Fogarty clamp-applying forceps, angled. **M,** Semb ligature-carrying forceps, close-up of tip. **N,** Bulldog clamp applier. *(From Tighe SM: Instrumentation for the operating room, ed 6, St Louis, 2003, Mosby.)*

Vessel and Patch Grafts

Prosthetic grafts are used to replace abnormal, diseased, or injured segments of an artery or a vein. Many types of grafts are available in assorted sizes (Figure 34-8). The two most common types of grafts are knitted and woven grafts. Knitted grafts are soft and porous. They are preferred for small artery anastomosis or for very fragile vessels. Woven grafts are used for large artery replacement, because their tight weave prevents loss of blood through the graft.

Preclotting is a method of preparing a graft to prevent leakage. In this process, the graft is flushed with blood, which

provides a seal between the fibers of the graft. In the past, all synthetic grafts required preclotting. However, the procedure now is seldom required, because woven and knitted grafts are impregnated with collagen. If preclotting is required, 30 to 50 mL of blood is withdrawn from the patient before heparinization. The surgeon or technologist flushes the graft with blood. The graft then is placed in a small basin until the surgeon needs it.

Grafts are available as straight or bifurcated tubes made of Teflon, Dacron, or polytetrafluoroethylene (PTFE). To prevent waste and expense, only the appropriate size of graft,

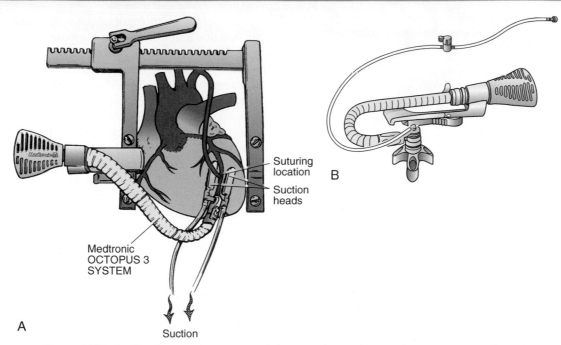

Suturing
location

Suction
heads

Medtronic
OCTOPUS 3
SYSTEM

A

Suction

B

Figure 34-7 A, The Octopus 3 coronary stabilizer attaches to the sternal retractor proximally and immobilizes the coronary artery. The device uses suction pads to minimize tissue motion at the anastomosis site. **B,** The Starfish left ventricular suction device holds the left ventricle apex and allows it to be retracted for access to lateral and posterior coronary arteries. *(From Seifert PC: Cardiac surgery: perioperative patient care, St Louis, 2002, Mosby.)*

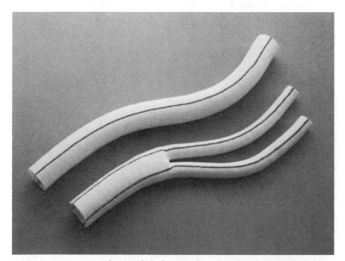

Figure 34-8 Straight and bifurcated arterial tube grafts. *(From Rothrock JC: Alexander's care of the patient in surgery, ed 12, St Louis, 2003, Mosby.)*

as determined by using graft sizers during the procedure, should be opened. As with all implants, the type, size, and serial number of the graft are recorded on the patient's operative record by the circulating nurse.

Patch grafts, also made of Teflon (PTFE), are used to strengthen a suture line or to close a defect (an abnormal opening in the tissue). Patches are cut to size as needed. Teflon felt material in the form of small pledgets is used along the suture line to reinforce the anastomosis. To prepare these, the scrub should place a mosquito clamp in the middle of the pledget and pass a suture through the pledget, or the clamp and pledget are passed to the surgeon for suture attachment.

Prosthetic Valves

A full set of prosthetic heart valves and their sizers, handles, and holders are required for valve replacement. The technologist should be familiar with the different types of valves and accessory equipment. Valves are extremely expensive and should be handled as little as possible. The scrub and the circulator must verify the type, size, and identification number of the valve. The circulator records the valve identification information on the patient's operative record. Two commonly used valves are the St. Jude Medical (mechanical) valve (Figure 34-9) and the Hancock porcine (biological) valve. Biological valves are stored in a glutaraldehyde solution, which must be removed by rinsing the valve in three separate basins of normal saline for 2 minutes in each basin (for a total of 6 minutes).

Pacemaker

A **pacemaker** is a device that produces electrical impulses that stimulate the heart muscle. This process is called *pacing the heart.* Pacing batteries may be temporary (external) or permanent (internal). Temporary electrodes are implanted on the surface of the heart at the time of cardiac surgery. Two types of permanent electrodes are used, endocardial (transvenous) electrodes and epicardial electrodes. An endocardial electrode is inserted into a vein and advanced into the right ventricle under fluoroscopy (Figure 34-10). An epicardial electrode is sutured directly to the heart on the atrium, the ventricle, or both. Endocardial transvenous insertion is more common. The electrode or electrodes are connected to a generator, and an alligator cable is used to connect them to the external battery for temporary pacing during heart surgery.

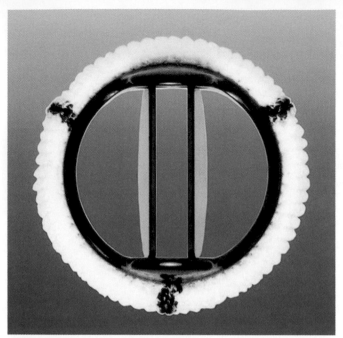

Figure 34-9 St. Jude Medical bileaflet valve prosthesis. *(From Rothrock JC: Alexander's care of the patient in surgery, ed 12, St Louis, 2003, Mosby.)*

Defibrillator

Defibrillator paddles are required to convert **fibrillation** (ineffectual quivering of the ventricles) into a functional rhythm. The two paddles are kept readily available on the sterile field. When needed, such as during ventricular fibrillation, the surgeon places a paddle on each side of the heart and instructs the circulator to set the charge on the defibrillator. The application of electricity to the heart shocks the cells, converting the rhythm back to normal. When the defibrillator is in use, all personnel must stand clear of the patient to avoid receiving an electric shock.

Disposable, adhesive defibrillator patches may be used during repeat sternotomy or minimally invasive procedures.

Fibrillator

The temporary pacing wires attached to the alligator cables (used for temporary pacing) may also be used with a fibrillator to create fine fibrillation of the heart. The wires are connected to the fibrillator power source and the heart is fibrillated (causing it to quiver) during repair of a leaking anastomosis. After the air is removed or the repair is completed, the heart is defibrillated.

Cardiopulmonary Bypass

The **heart-lung machine** takes the place of the heart and lungs by pumping and perfusing blood, which has been shunted outside the body. The heart-lung pump collects the blood, removes excess carbon dioxide, oxygenates the blood, and returns it to the body (Figure 34-11). The tubing and oxygenator for the heart-lung machine are assembled and primed by a perfusionist (pump technician). Sterile cannulas, which **shunt** the blood away from the heart, are delivered to the scrub, who prepares them for surgical insertion into the heart.

The surgical technologist should be familiar with the basic function and operation of the pump. This includes the size of the pump lines and how they connect to the patient. The scrub should also know which lines infuse blood and which remove blood, as well as the types of cannulas and catheters.

- *Venous cannula:* Straight-ended with multiple holes in the distal tip. This type of cannula is used to shunt blood from the heart. A two-stage venous cannula also has openings in the midportion of the catheter.
- *Aortic cannula:* May have a straight or an angled tip to direct the blood toward the descending thoracic aorta. This cannula carries oxygenated (arterial) blood.
- *Femoral arterial cannula:* Also carries oxygenated (arterial) blood, is tapered to match the size of the artery, and has a beveled end to allow easier insertion.
- *Coronary antegrade perfusion cannula:* Has a cuff near its tip to prevent the cannula from being inserted too far into the coronary arteries. It is used to infuse cardioplegic solution directly into the heart; a retrograde cannula is placed in the great cardiac vein.
- *Left ventricular sump (vent) catheter:* Drains air and blood within the heart and prevents the accumulation of blood, which can cause distention of the ventricle and injure the heart muscle.
- *Right superior pulmonary vent catheter:* Also used to decompress the left ventricle and remove intracardiac air.

DRUGS

Heparin

Heparin sodium is an anticoagulant that prevents the conversion of fibrinogen to fibrin, an essential part of the body's clotting mechanism. The drug does not dissolve blood clots, but only prevents them from forming. It is administered through a large vein or the right atrium before cannulation for cardiopulmonary bypass or before a blood vessel is occluded. It prevents clot formation in the bypass circuit while the patient is on the heart-lung machine. The drug dosage is calculated according to body weight. Heparin also is distributed to the surgical technologist for local use on the field.

Protamine Sulfate

Protamine sulfate is administered to reverse the anticoagulant effects of heparin. Intravenous protamine is administered after bypass has been completed and the cannulas have been removed. Some patients have a reaction to protamine, and the surgeon may elect to allow heparin reversal to proceed without it.

Lidocaine

Lidocaine (Xylocaine) 1% is commonly used in the treatment of ventricular **arrhythmia**. This drug controls particular rhythmic patterns, including premature ventricular contractions and ventricular **tachycardia**. These arrhythmias can develop into ventricular fibrillation in which the heart stops beating and instead quivers without coordination, effectively stopping circulation.

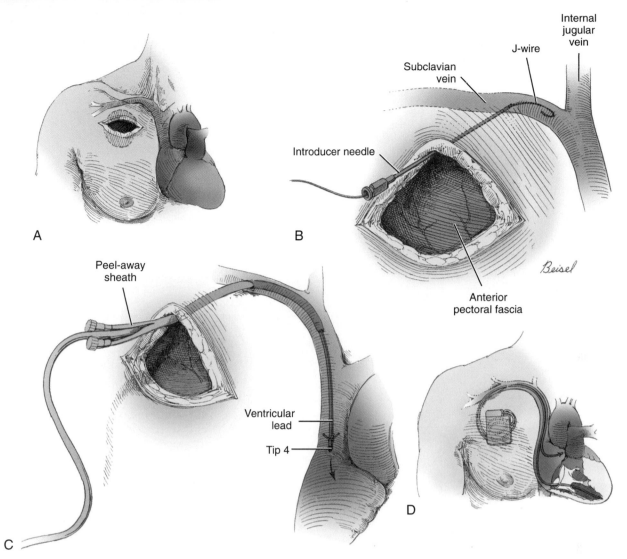

Figure 34-10 **Insertion of a pacemaker. A,** A transverse incision is made for the skin pocket. **B,** Needle insertion into the subclavian vein is performed to introduce the J-tip guidewire. **C,** The pacing electrode is introduced and advanced into the right ventricle. **D,** Completion of the pacemaker procedure, with the pulse generator placed in the pocket. *(Modified from Waldhausen JA, Pierce WS, Campbell DB: Surgery of the chest, ed 6, St Louis, 1996, Mosby.)*

Epinephrine

Epinephrine has many actions, including cardiac stimulation. Under normal circumstances, it cannot start a heart that has stopped beating, but it can stimulate the adrenergic receptors in the heart.

Cardioplegic Solution

Cardioplegia is the intentional interruption of the heart's pumping action. A cardioplegic solution may contain a mixture of potassium chloride, lidocaine, dextrose, insulin, albumin, tromethamine, and Plasmanate. The exact type and amount of the drugs in the solution vary. The solution may be cooled or warmed for administration.

A cardioplegic solution is administered by two methods. In antegrade cardioplegic infusion (after the aortic **cross clamp** has been applied), a needle is placed in the aorta (proximal to the aortic clamp) where it exits the left ventricle (the aortic "root"). The cardioplegic solution is infused into the aorta. It then flows into the right and left coronary openings and into the coronary circulation. In retrograde cardioplegic infusion, a catheter is placed in the coronary sinus of the right atrium and into the great cardiac vein. The cardioplegic solution is then infused into the coronary venous system.

SURGICAL PROCEDURES

MEDIAN STERNOTOMY

Surgical Goal

A median sternotomy is a midline incision used for surgical procedures of the heart and great vessels in the thoracic cavity.

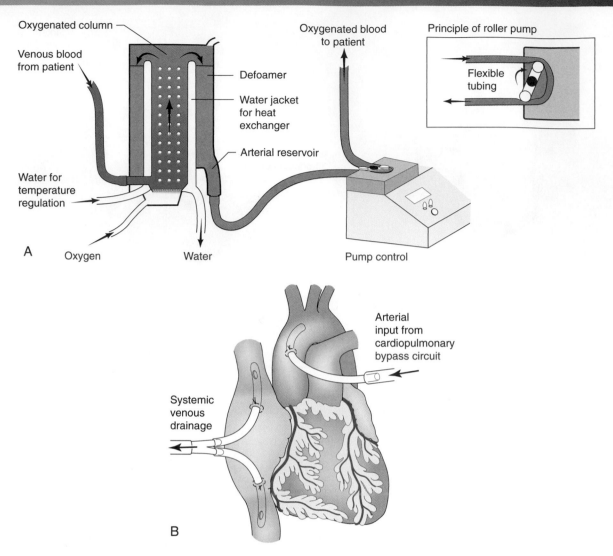

Figure 34-11   **A,** Schematic of cardiac bypass (heart-lung machine). **B,** Cannulation of the heart. *(From Garden O, Bradbury A, Forsythe J, Parks R: Principles and practice of surgery, ed 5, Edinburgh, 2007, Elsevier/Churchill Livingstone.)*

TECHNIQUE

Sternotomy

1 The surgeon makes a midline thoracic incision.
2 The xiphoid is divided.
3 The sternum is divided.

Discussion (Sternotomy)

The patient is placed in the supine position, prepped, and draped for a midline thoracic incision. The surgeon makes a midline incision from the sternal notch to 2 to 3 inches (5 to 7.5 cm) below the xiphoid. The subcutaneous tissue and linea alba (the fascial layer distal to the xiphoid) are divided with the knife or electrosurgical unit (ESU). The surgeon digitally separates the underlying tissue from the sternal notch and xiphoid. The xiphoid then is divided on the midline with heavy curved scissors. A sternal saw is placed in the center of the xiphoid or sternal notch, and the bone is divided.

The assistant elevates the raw edges of the sternum with handheld retractors (e.g., Army-Navy retractors) while the surgeon coagulates bleeders with the ESU. A small amount of bone wax may be applied to the bone edges.

Before placing a self-retaining retractor, the surgeon protects the edges of the incision with towels or moist laparotomy sponges. The retractor then is opened slowly. This exposes the pericardium, which is incised with the ESU or scissors.

The surgeon elevates the pericardium with vascular forceps or a clamp to prevent injury to the heart. The pericardium is incised to expose the heart and ascending aorta. Lateral incisions are made as needed.

If the procedure requires bypass, traction sutures may be placed through the edges of the pericardium and sewn to the periosteum. An umbilical tape or vessel loop is used to encircle and retract the aorta. The heart and aorta are then cannulated for cardiopulmonary bypass. If an **off-pump procedure** is to be performed (i.e., cardiopulmonary bypass is not needed), cannulation is not required. However, the scrub

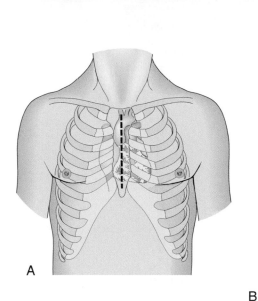

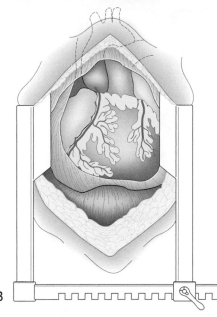

A

B

Figure 34-12 **Median sternotomy.** A, Incision. B, Right atrium and ascending aorta exposed with the retractor in place. *(From Garden O, Bradbury A, Forsythe J, Parks R: Principles and practice of surgery, ed 5, Edinburgh, 2007, Elsevier/Churchill Livingstone.)*

should be prepared to institute bypass if the patient's condition deteriorates. A median sternotomy is illustrated in Figure 34-12.

TECHNIQUE

Sternotomy Closure

1 Wires are placed through the sternum or a transverse plate system implanted.
2 The sternal edges are approximated.
3 The fascia and periosteum are approximated.
4 The subcutaneous tissue and skin are closed.

Discussion (Sternotomy Closure)

After the surgical procedure, drainage catheters are inserted to remove blood, fluid, and air from the pericardium and the pleural spaces (if they have been entered). Temporary pacing wires are placed on the epicardial surface of the heart. The surgeon places six to eight size 5 wire sutures through each sternal edge. When passing stainless steel sutures, the scrub holds the free ends of the wire to control the ends and protect them from contamination. The surgeon tightens the wires and twists each one to bring the sternal edges together. The surgeon uses a wire twister to make a final twist, burying the ends in the periosteum.

When Wolvek sternal approximation fixation instruments are used, the ends of the wires are threaded through small metal plates. The surgeon then tightens the ends and locks the wire into position by crimping the plate. The excess wire is cut with wire cutters and sharp tips are buried in the periosteum with the wire twister. Other approximation systems also are available. When a titanium transverse plate system is used, multiple thin plates and fine bone screws are used to approximate the sternum. This system has also been used in sternal dehiscence.

The surgeon approximates the fascia and periosteum with interrupted sutures, such as size 0 polyester sutures.

CARDIOPULMONARY BYPASS

Cardiopulmonary bypass diverts blood away from the heart and lungs so that surgery can be performed. An increasing number of cardiac procedures are performed without the use of cardiopulmonary bypass. However, many types of surgery, such as valve replacement and aneurysm repair, do require bypass.

The pump tubing is connected to cannulas that are inserted into the venae cavae and ascending aorta through a median sternotomy incision. The femoral artery and femoral vein occasionally are used when the great vessels are not accessible because of disease. Before cannulation, the anesthesia care provider administers heparin.

Cardiopulmonary bypass may be total or partial. The surgeon performs total bypass by tightening umbilical tapes around the venae cavae and cannulas. This forces all blood returning to the right side of the heart into the cannula and pump. It also prevents air from entering the venous line and obstructing the flow of blood to the pump when the right side of the heart is open. Total bypass also is used for procedures such as mitral valve replacement, repair of septal defects, and resection of a left ventricular aneurysm. In partial bypass, blood can escape around the cannula and enter the heart. Partial bypass often is used during aortic valve replacement. It also is used to support a patient in emergencies such as cardiac arrest or a ruptured aneurysm. Figure 34-13 illustrates a typical bypass circuit.

In both types of bypass, blood returns to the pump through the cannula by gravity drainage and is pumped back into the circulation by a roller head (or a centrifugal pump) on the bypass machine. When the right side of the heart is open and the patient is on bypass, the risk exists that air will enter the venous line. This can cause an "air lock" (a large amount of air in the venous line), which may obstruct the flow of blood to the pump. The vacuum created by the pump draws the air away from the heart and into the pump.

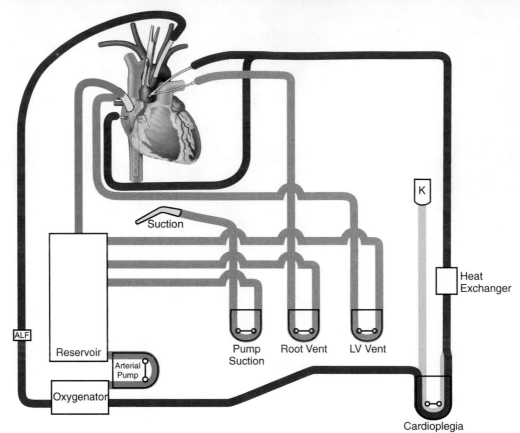

Figure 34-13 **Typical cardiac bypass circuit.** Bypass provides a bloodless surgical field and can be partial or total. In this drawing, venous blood is diverted through the venous line of the bypass circuit to a venous reservoir. The arterial pump then functions in the same way as the heart would by sending it through a heat exchanger, oxygenator, and arterial line filter. Blood is then returned through the arterial line to the patient's own system. *(From Miller R, Eriksson L, Fleisher L, et al: Miller's anesthesia, ed 7, Philadelphia, 2009, Churchill Livingstone.)*

The surgical technologist must always watch for the presence of air in the heart or pump lines and alert the surgeon immediately if air is noticed. Air must be removed to prevent an air embolus. The technologist should have a needle and syringe readily available for evacuating air. A 10-mL syringe with a 19-gauge needle can be used for both adult and pediatric patients.

Cannulation Techniques in Cardiopulmonary Bypass

AORTA   A purse-string suture is placed on the anterior portion of the ascending aorta and the ends are pulled through a Rumel tourniquet. A stab incision is made into the aorta and the incision is dilated with an aortic dilator or clamp. The surgeon controls bleeding by holding one finger over the hole as the cannula is inserted. The assistant controls the top end of the cannula, which is occluded by a tube-occluding clamp. The surgeon positions the cannula and the assistant tightens the suture to form a tourniquet. The tourniquet then is tied to the cannula with heavy silk suture. The surgeon clamps and unclamps the cannula to allow it to fill with blood and to remove the air. The cannula then is connected to the arterial perfusion line from the pump.

SUPERIOR AND INFERIOR VENAE CAVAE   If two cannulas are to be inserted, the surgeon uses vascular forceps to grasp the right atrial appendage (a small muscular pouch attached to the atrium) and places a curved partial occlusion vascular clamp (Beck or Glover clamp) across it. A purse-string suture of 2-0 polyester or polypropylene is placed through the occluded portion of the appendage. The assistant snares the ends of the suture through a piece of tubing and tags them with a hemostat.

The surgeon then excises the tip of the atrial appendage with scissors and applies clamps or forceps to the two edges of the atrial wall. The assistant controls the vascular clamp and retracts the atrial wall as the surgeon inserts the cannula. The technologist should control the end of the cannula during this procedure. The assistant removes the vascular clamp and controls the suture to prevent bleeding from the atrium.

The surgeon introduces the cannula into the superior vena cava. The assistant forms a tourniquet around the suture as previously described. The surgeon ties the cannula and tourniquet together with a heavy silk tie and then allows blood to fill the cannula by gravity or by lung inflation. The assistant places a tube-occluding clamp across the cannula. Care must be taken not to clamp the wire-reinforced portion of the cannula.

The inferior vena cava is cannulated through a similar technique. The major difference is that the cannula is inserted through the atrial wall instead of through the appendage. A knife blade and scissors may be used to open the atrium. The cannulas are connected to the venous return line from the pump.

TWO-STAGE CANNULATION Two-stage cannulation is similar to bicaval cannulation except that only one cannula is used. The cannula has holes both in the distal end (which is inserted into the inferior vena cava to drain the lower body) and in the midportion of the cannula (which lies in the atrium to drain blood from the superior vena cava).

FEMORAL ARTERY AND VEIN Cannulation of the femoral artery and vein is performed when partial bypass is needed to support the patient's circulation in an emergency or during surgical resection of the descending thoracic aorta and ascending aorta. The femoral artery also is cannulated whenever the ascending aorta cannot be cannulated and in some minimally invasive cardiac procedures.

After heparin has been given, the surgeon makes an incision in the groin over the femoral vessels with the knife. The subcutaneous tissue and fascial layers are divided with scissors. A self-retaining retractor is placed in the incision. The surgeon then isolates the common femoral artery with Metzenbaum scissors. The vessel is encircled with umbilical tape and secured in the jaw of a right-angle clamp. The assistant places a tube tourniquet over the ends of the tapes. The femoral vein is isolated using the same technique.

The surgeon occludes the femoral artery with small angled vascular clamps (e.g., a Glover or Cooley clamp). An arteriotomy is performed in the occluded segment with a #11 knife, and the incision is extended with Potts scissors. The opening may be dilated with a clamp. The surgeon inserts the cannula as the assistant removes the superior vascular clamp. The assistant tightens the umbilical tape to hold the cannula in place. The surgeon ties a heavy silk suture around the cannula and the tape and releases the tube-occluding clamp to allow blood to fill the cannula and evacuate air. The cannula then is connected to the arterial perfusion line.

In patients with pulmonary emboli, partial cardiopulmonary bypass using the femoral vein and the femoral artery can be used. Left heart bypass may be used to perfuse the lower body when the descending aorta is cross-clamped.

SUMP CATHETERIZATION

Surgical Goal

A sump catheter is inserted into the left ventricle soon after cardiopulmonary bypass has been established to suction blood and air and maintain cardiac decompression. By venting air, a sump catheter reduces the risk of air embolism in the systemic circulation.

Insertion of the Catheter: Left Ventricle

As soon as bypass is initiated, the surgeon elevates the **apex** of the left ventricle with a laparotomy sponge. A purse-string

suture is placed in the apex and snared through a tube tourniquet. The technologist connects the sump catheter to the pump line.

The surgeon makes a stab incision in the apex with a #11 knife blade and dilates the opening with a Schnidt clamp or similar clamp. The catheter is inserted and secured with the tourniquet. The surgeon ties the catheter and tourniquet together with heavy silk suture and lowers the apex into normal position.

Insertion of the Sump Catheter: Right Superior Pulmonary Vein

A right superior pulmonary vein catheter is used more often than a left ventricular apical catheter, which can damage the ventricular muscle.

The assistant retracts the right atrium to expose the right superior pulmonary vein as the surgeon places a purse-string suture. A tourniquet is placed over the suture ends. The surgeon makes a stab incision in the vein with a #11 knife blade, dilates the incision with a clamp, and inserts the catheter into the vein. The catheter is manipulated into the left atrium, across the mitral valve, and into the left ventricle. The tourniquet is then snugged down and a tube-occluding clamp is put in place across the catheter. The surgeon ties the catheter to the tourniquet with heavy silk suture and connects it to the pump suction line.

INFUSION OF A CARDIOPLEGIC SOLUTION

Surgical Goal

A cardioplegic solution is used to stop the heart; this reduces the energy required by the cardiac muscle by eliminating the energy requirements of contraction. The process of infusing a cardioplegic solution into the coronary arteries protects the cardiac muscle from damage while the aorta is occluded and the blood supply is interrupted. The solution may be infused directly into the coronary artery or transatrially into the coronary sinus. A cardioplegic solution can be infused indirectly into the aortic root just above the aortic valve.

TECHNIQUE

Direct Coronary Artery Infusion (Antegrade)

1 The ascending aorta is occluded and opened below the clamp.
2 The openings of the coronary arteries are identified and cannulated.
3 Solution is infused and the cannulas are removed immediately after each infusion.
4 The aorta is closed when the surgery has been completed.

Direct coronary artery infusion and the transatrial retrograde method (discussed later) are the methods most commonly used. The surgeon places a polypropylene purse-string suture in the aorta below the site of the cross-clamp. The ascending aorta is then occluded, and an indwelling catheter (e.g., a 14-gauge Angiocath) is inserted into the aorta below the clamp. The assistant connects the tubing from the cardioplegic solution to the catheter. A Y-connector can be inserted into the cardioplegic tubing and a suction line can be inserted to vent air from the aorta. Each line from the Y (cardioplegic solution and vent) can be occluded. When cardioplegic solution is being infused, the suction line is occluded; when the suction line is opened, the cardioplegic solution line is occluded.

The surgeon occludes the ascending aorta and opens it below the clamp. The coronary openings are located and the correct cannulas are determined. The technologist connects the cannulas to the tubing. The surgeon then gently inserts the cannulas into the opening of the coronary arteries and holds them in position until the pump perfusionist or anesthesia care provider completes the infusion. Solution is infused until the heart stops beating (Figure 34-14). The technologist should keep the cannulas and tubing secure in a towel until they are needed for subsequent infusions. The surgeon closes the aorta at the completion of surgery.

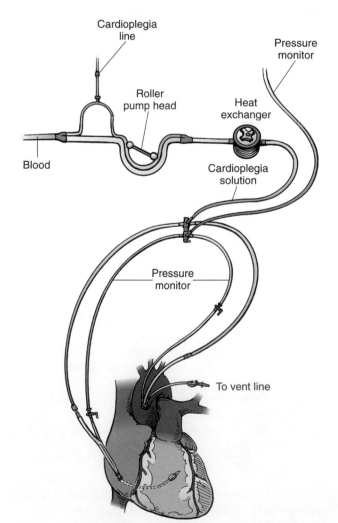

Figure 34-14 Infusion of a cardioplegic solution. *(Modified from Waldhausen JA, Pierce WS, Campbell DB: Surgery of the chest, ed 6, St Louis, 1996, Mosby.)*

TECHNIQUE

Indirect Coronary Artery Infusion (Antegrade)

1 The ascending aorta is occluded.
2 An indwelling catheter is inserted into the aortic root above the valve.
3 The catheter is connected to the tubing and filled with cardioplegic solution.
4 The solution is infused.
5 The indwelling catheter is removed immediately before the aorta is unclamped.
6 The defect made by the catheter is repaired with suture.

Cardioplegic solution is infused as often as necessary during the procedure. The surgeon withdraws the indwelling catheter and removes the clamp from the aorta. Air in the aorta is suctioned through the vent line. After removal of the catheter, the surgeon closes the defect with 5-0 polypropylene suture.

TECHNIQUE

Transatrial Cardioplegia via the Coronary Sinus (Retrograde)

1 A small purse-string suture is placed in the atrial wall and an incision is made in the center.
2 A retrograde cardioplegia catheter is passed through the atrial stab wound, inserted into the opening of the coronary sinus, and positioned in the coronary vein.
3 The proximal end of the catheter is connected to a line leading to the source of the cardioplegic solution.
4 The cardioplegic solution is infused to stop the heart.
5 When cardioplegia is no longer needed, the catheter is removed and the purse-string is tied to close the wound.
6 Cardioplegic solution often is infused by the retrograde route (into the coronary venous system) rather than by the arterial antegrade route. The cardioplegic solution flows from the coronary veins through the capillaries and into the coronary arteries, stopping the heart.
7 After placing a 5-0 polypropylene purse-string suture in the atrial wall, the surgeon incises the atrium with a #11 or #15 blade. The retrograde cardioplegia catheter is inserted into the atrium and guided to the entrance of the coronary sinus. Palpating the outer atrial wall, the surgeon positions the catheter in the sinus opening and advances it into the vein. The catheter is attached to tubing connected to the source of the cardioplegic solution in the bypass circuit.
8 When cardioplegia is no longer needed, the catheter is removed and the atrial incision is closed.

Decannulation

TECHNIQUE

Decannulation of the Ventricle, Venae Cavae, and Aorta

1 A tube-occluding clamp is placed across the catheter or cannula.
2 Suture ties are removed from the catheter.
3 The catheter is withdrawn and the suture is tied.

Discussion

The left ventricular catheter usually is removed from the ventricle before bypass is discontinued. The catheter is occluded with a tube-occluding clamp and the silk suture and tourniquet are removed. The catheter is withdrawn and the suture is tied securely to occlude the cannulation site. Additional sutures (often on pledgets) may be used for hemostasis. Decannulation of the venae cavae and aorta uses the same technique after bypass has been discontinued.

TECHNIQUE

Decannulation of the Femoral Artery and Vein
1 The cannula is occluded.
2 The umbilical tape is released.
3 The cannula is withdrawn and the femoral vein is occluded with a vascular clamp.
4 The venotomy is closed and all clamps and tapes are removed.
5 The artery is decannulated using the same technique.

At the conclusion of bypass, the surgeon occludes the femoral vein cannula. The assistant releases the cannula from the drapes and other attachments on the field. The surgeon then withdraws the cannula and occludes the vein with a vascular clamp. The venotomy is closed with continuous suture of 5-0 or 6-0 polypropylene. All clamps are removed and the artery is decannulated with the same technique.

Bleeding or hemorrhage can occur in the postoperative period if cannulation sites have not been closed securely, if heparin has not been adequately reversed with protamine, if dissection of the cannulated blood vessel occurs, or if surrounding tissue has been damaged. Atelectasis may persist because of lung deflation during bypass. Temporary cognitive, sensory, and perceptual changes may occur as a result of the effects of extracorporeal circulation.

CORONARY ARTERY BYPASS GRAFTING

Surgical Goal

Coronary artery bypass (CAB) of a narrow segment of one or more coronary arteries is performed to improve circulation to the heart. An autograft (tissue from the patient's own body) usually is used as the bypass graft. The procedure is commonly known by its acronym, CABG, for coronary artery bypass grafting.

Pathology

The inner and outer walls of the heart may be affected by coronary artery disease (CAD). CAD is caused by the buildup of cholesterol deposits in the arterial lining, a condition called **atherosclerosis**. This can affect any artery. A closely related disease is **arteriosclerosis**, which is loss of elasticity in and hardening of the arteries. Arteriosclerosis often is the result of diet and other environmental causes. When the flow of coronary blood is reduced, the myocardial cells are deprived of oxygen and other nutrients. This in turn can produce a weakening of the heart muscle or a myocardial **infarction**, resulting in tissue death.

TECHNIQUE

1 A median sternotomy incision is made.
2 A segment of the saphenous vein is removed. The internal mammary artery (IMA) is dissected from its retrosternal bed.
3 The heart is cannulated for cardiopulmonary bypass unless an off-pump procedure is planned.
4 The aorta is occluded and cardioplegic solution is administered into the aortic root.
5 The coronary artery is incised and the vein, IMA, or other graft conduit is anastomosed to the coronary arteriotomy.
6 The aorta is unclamped.
7 Venous and other free grafts are anastomosed to the ascending aorta. These may be anastomosed while the cross-clamp is applied.
8 Cardiopulmonary bypass is discontinued and decannulation is performed.
9 Pacing wires and chest tubes are inserted and the wound is closed.

Discussion

The surgeon performs a median sternotomy and cannulates for cardiopulmonary bypass. However, an increasing number of coronary bypass procedures are performed without the use of cardiopulmonary bypass. In patients with very complex, multivessel disease, bypass often is required. The assistant removes the greater saphenous vein from the leg, or the left or right radial artery may be harvested for use as a free graft. (This procedure is described and illustrated in Chapter 31.) Video-assisted endoscopic vein harvesting may be performed.

Preparation of the Internal Mammary Artery

The internal mammary artery (IMA) is dissected free from the retrosternal bed (Figure 34-15). The sternal edge may be elevated with a self-retaining retractor attached to the side from which the IMA is dissected. The left IMA commonly is used, although the right IMA also may be used.

After cardiopulmonary bypass has been instituted (if used), the surgeon identifies the segment of coronary artery to which the bypass graft will be anastomosed. Excess epicardial fat is removed from the arteriotomy site with a #64 Beaver blade or a #15 blade. The surgeon then occludes the ascending aorta and inserts the indwelling catheter for infusion of the cardioplegic solution and venting of air.

Next, the coronary artery is opened with a #11 knife blade (or Beaver blade), and the incision is extended with Diethrich or fine Potts coronary scissors. A Garrett dilator may be inserted into the lumen of the artery to assess its size. The technologist places the vein in a small basin with heparinized blood solution to keep the graft moist. The surgeon bevels the free end of the vein with Potts scissors. The vein then is sutured to the coronary artery with continuous or interrupted sutures (e.g., 6-0 or 7-0 polypropylene). When the anastomosis is complete, the assistant inflates the vein with a physiological solution to test for leaks and to determine the diameter and length of the graft when it is filled.

The surgeon performs all other anastomoses using the same technique. Size 8-0 polypropylene may be used for the

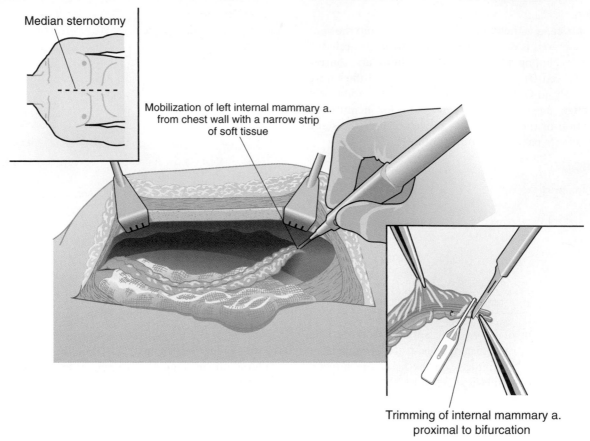

Median sternotomy

Mobilization of left internal mammary a.
from chest wall with a narrow strip
of soft tissue

Trimming of internal mammary a.
proximal to bifurcation

Figure 34-15 Harvesting of the internal mammary artery for coronary artery bypass. *(From Jones RH: Coronary artery bypass grafts. In Sabiston DC Jr, editor: Atlas of cardiothoracic surgery, Philadelphia, 1995, WB Saunders.)*

anastomosis (Figure 34-16). The aorta then is unclamped and the indwelling catheter is removed. A portion of the aorta is occluded with a vascular clamp (e.g., Lambert-Kay clamp). A #11 knife blade and aortic punch are used to create a hole in the occluded portion.

The surgeon inflates the vein to make sure it is not twisted and does not have any leaks and to determine the length needed to reach the aorta. The vein is then cut to the appropriate length and the end is beveled with Potts scissors. The anastomosis is performed between the vein and the hole in the aorta. The surgeon completes each anastomosis and removes the clamp from the aorta. When the procedures are performed off-pump, a small horseshoe retractor is positioned over the coronary arteriotomy to minimize cardiac movement during the distal anastomosis. The proximal aortic anastomosis is performed with partial occlusion of the aorta. In some patients, both distal and proximal anastomoses are created with the aorta cross-clamped.

Air is evacuated from the vein grafts with a 25- or 27-gauge needle. The surgeon inspects each anastomosis for leaks and any found are repaired before bypass is discontinued. The cannulas are removed and a pacemaker electrode may be sutured to the heart. Metal rings or radiopaque material may be placed around each vein graft on the aorta. These mark the veins in the event cardiac catheterization is performed in the postoperative period. The completed anastomosis is shown in Figure 34-17.

Off-Pump Coronary Artery Bypass

Off-pump coronary artery bypass (OPCAB) is performed through a median sternotomy. The Octopus retractor and left ventricular suction apparatus are commonly used to expose the coronary arteries.

A special rib retractor with endoscope is used to harvest the left IMA. The rib retractor is exchanged for another small thoracotomy retractor positioned to expose the anastomosis site. A stabilizing device is used to minimize cardiac movement during suturing. The anastomosis is performed in the traditional manner.

Complications include hemorrhage, atrial and/or ventricular arrhythmias, stroke, infection, **ischemia**, and death. Arterial grafts may spasm, producing changes in the electrocardiogram that can signal ischemia. A sufficiently normal blood pressure should be maintained for arterial grafts to function properly. CABG grafts may clot, causing a myocardial infarction.

TRANSMYOCARDIAL REVASCULARIZATION

Surgical Goal

In transmyocardial revascularization (TMR) a series of small-bore transmural channels are created with the carbon dioxide or holmium–yttrium-aluminum-garnet (holmium:YAG) laser to perfuse the myocardium. The goal is to increase blood flow to the heart in patients in whom bypass surgery or

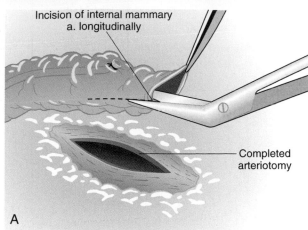

Incision of internal mammary
a. longitudinally

Completed
arteriotomy

A

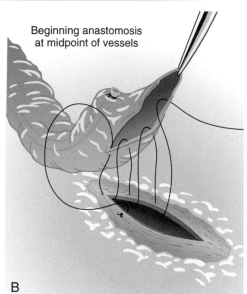

Beginning anastomosis
at midpoint of vessels

B

Figure 34-16 **Coronary artery bypass. A,** Potts scissors are used to open the vein graft. **B,** Anastomosis of the vein graft. *a.,* Artery. *(From Townsend CM: Sabiston textbook of surgery, ed 17, Philadelphia, 2001, WB Saunders.)*

medical management is not feasible. TMR may be used in conjunction with standard CAB.

TECHNIQUE

1 In patients not undergoing coronary artery bypass (CAB), a minithoracotomy is made on the side of the affected coronary artery.
2 The pericardium is opened to expose the heart.
3 The sterile laser probe is used to create channels into the heart muscle.
4 A chest tube may be inserted.
5 The incision is closed.

Discussion

If TMR is performed in conjunction with CAB, only laser-specific instruments and supplies should be used. If TMR is to be performed through a thoracotomy, chest instruments in addition to the laser supplies and equipment are used. External defibrillator patches are applied to all patients; pediatric internal defibrillator paddles may also be requested.

The surgeon uses a sterile laser probe to make the myocardial channels from the epicardium to the endocardium. Both the scrub and the circulating personnel keep track of the number of channels formed.

RESECTION OF A LEFT VENTRICULAR ANEURYSM

Surgical Goal

Resection of a left ventricular aneurysm reduces the risk of rupture and embolism.

Pathology

An aneurysm of the left ventricle most often is caused by a reduced blood supply from an infarcted coronary artery.

TECHNIQUE

1 A median sternotomy is performed.
2 Cannulation and total cardiopulmonary bypass are initiated.
3 A left ventriculotomy is performed and the aneurysm is resected.
4 The ventricle is closed.
5 The cannulas are removed.
6 Pacer electrodes are sutured to the heart, chest tubes are inserted, and the wound is closed.

Discussion

After a median sternotomy has been performed and bypass has been initiated, the surgeon cross-clamps the ascending aorta. The ventricle is incised with the long knife and the incision is extended with curved Mayo scissors. Allis clamps may be applied to the edges of the aneurysm for traction.

The surgeon assesses the mitral valve and removes any clots with forceps or suction. The technologist should keep the instruments clean to prevent clots from entering the bloodstream.

The aneurysm tissue is excised with curved Mayo scissors and a Dacron patch is inserted to repair the ventricle. An alternate technique is to resect the aneurysm tissue and then bring the edges of the ventricle together with suture of size 0 polypropylene or polyester. Strips of Teflon felt or pledgets are incorporated with the suture. A second or third row of sutures is placed through the ventricular edges for a more secure closure. The surgeon decompresses the ventricle using the sump catheter from the heart-lung machine. The catheter is removed before the final suture is placed. The apex of the ventricle may be aspirated with a 19-gauge needle. The wound then is prepared for closure as previously described, and the incision is closed. Resection of a left ventricular aneurysm is illustrated in Figure 34-18.

AORTIC VALVE REPLACEMENT

Surgical Goal

The aortic valve maintains one-way blood flow from the left ventricle to the aorta. Aortic valve replacement involves the replacement of a diseased valve.

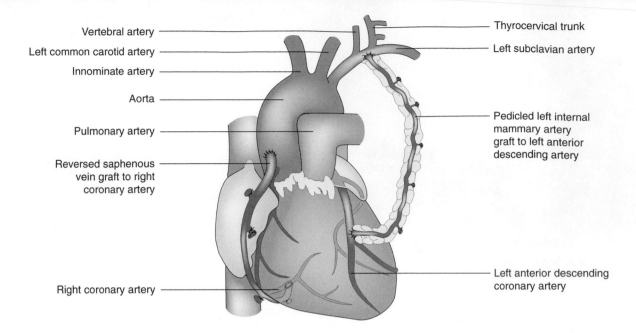

Figure 34-17 Completed coronary bypass with venous and left internal mammary artery grafts in place. *(From Garden O, Bradbury A, Forsythe J, Parks R: Principles and practice of surgery, ed 5, Edinburgh, 2007, Elsevier/Churchill Livingstone.)*

Pathology

Common causes of valve insufficiency are endocarditis, congenital anomalies, and calcification. A leaking valve allows blood to leak back into the left ventricle instead of going through the aorta. The left ventricle eventually fails as a result increased cardiac work.

Calcification of the valves also can occur. The valve leaflets may become stiff because of calcification or other thickening. This can reduce the opening of the valve to a small slit. The ventricle must work harder to pump a sufficient amount of blood through the narrowed orifice of the stenotic valve. This can lead to ventricular failure and insufficient blood flow to the brain, coronary arteries, and other organs.

TECHNIQUE

1 A median sternotomy and cardiopulmonary bypass usually are performed with a two-stage venous cannulation.
2 The ascending aorta is occluded and cardioplegic solution is infused through the aortic root or coronary sinus and into the coronary circulation.
3 A transverse incision is made in the anterior aortic wall.
4 A prosthetic valve is selected and sutured in place.
5 The aortotomy is closed and the aorta is unclamped.
6 Cardiopulmonary bypass is discontinued and the cannulas are removed.
7 Pacing wires and chest tubes are inserted and the wound is closed.

Discussion

The surgeon performs a median sternotomy and cannulates for cardiopulmonary bypass. A retrograde cardioplegic catheter is inserted into the coronary sinus. The ascending aorta is occluded and the cardioplegic solution is infused. The route through which the cardioplegic solution is delivered depends on the valve pathology. If aortic **stenosis** is present, the cardioplegic solution initially is infused through the aortic root. After the aorta is opened, subsequent cardioplegic infusions are given through the retrograde catheter. If aortic insufficiency is present, cardioplegic solution infused into the aortic root preferentially flows into the left ventricle. Fluid in the ventricular chamber distends and damages the ventricular wall. In these situations, retrograde cardioplegic solution is infused. Direct coronary perfusion rarely is required.

The surgeon opens the aorta with a transverse incision or, occasionally, a vertical incision. The valve cusps are incised with forceps and scissors or a long knife. If the valve leaflets are extensively calcified, the surgeon may debride the calcium with rongeurs. The technologist should keep the instruments clean with a damp sponge to prevent calcium particles and other materials from dropping back into the wound, where they might cause an embolus.

The annulus is measured with obturators. Different types of valve prostheses have their own unique sizing obturators. The scrub obtains the correct size of prosthesis from the circulating nurse. The surgeon places interrupted sutures through the annulus of the prosthetic sewing ring. Some surgeons prefer to use continuous suture of 2-0 or 3-0 polypropylene. Interrupted sutures in the aortic valve may be inserted in three series, corresponding to the three cusps of the valve. The distal suture ends are tagged with mosquito clamps or placed in a suture holder. When biological valves are used, they must be rinsed to remove the glutaraldehyde storage solution; the valve

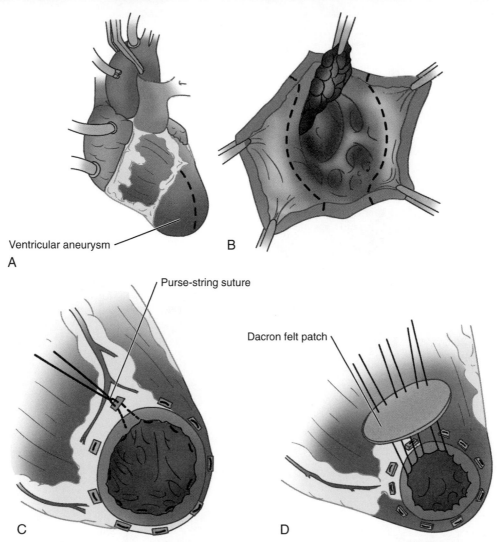

Ventricular aneurysm

A

B

Purse-string suture

C

Dacron felt patch

D

Figure 34-18 **Repair of a ventricular aneurysm. A,** Left ventricular apical aneurysm. **B,** The aneurysm is opened and clots are removed. **C,** A purse-string suture is used. **D,** A Dacron patch is sutured to the edge of the defect. *(Modified from Waldhausen JA, Pierce WS, Campbell DB: Surgery of the chest, ed 6, St Louis, 1996, Mosby.)*

must be kept moist with saline before it is implanted. If the leaflets become dry, the prosthesis can be damaged.

The surgeon seats the valve in position and ties all sutures. The aortotomy is closed with two 2-0 or 3-0 polypropylene sutures. One suture begins on the left side and the other suture begins on the right side. The sutures are tied in the middle portion of the aortotomy. Before tying the sutures, the surgeon allows air to escape from the suture line. The sutures are then tied securely. The surgeon may oversew the initial closure to enhance hemostasis. The aortic clamp is removed, and the aortic vent line is turned on to aspirate air. The surgeon also may elevate the left ventricular apex and insert a 19-gauge needle into the chamber to allow air to escape.

Bypass is discontinued, and the cannulas are removed. Temporary pacemaker electrodes may be sutured to the heart. Chest tubes are inserted, and the wound is closed in layers.

Complications include hemorrhage, atrial and/or ventricular arrhythmias, stroke, infection, ischemia, and death.

Additional complications include valve failure or malfunction. Aortic valve replacement is illustrated in Figure 34-19.

MITRAL VALVE REPAIR AND REPLACEMENT

Surgical Goal

In mitral valve repair and replacement, a diseased mitral valve is replaced to open a constricted valve (stenosis) or to prevent blood from regurgitating into the left atrium. The valve is repaired with an annuloplasty (or other reparative techniques). If the valve is severely damaged, it is replaced.

Pathology

The mitral valve is situated between the left atrium and left ventricle. Over time, a stenotic valve causes the left atrium to become dilated and can lead to arrhythmias, such as atrial fibrillation. Mitral valve disease may be caused by rheumatic heart disease, dilation of the annulus, ischemic heart disease, trauma, or changes in the tissue that produce regurgitation.

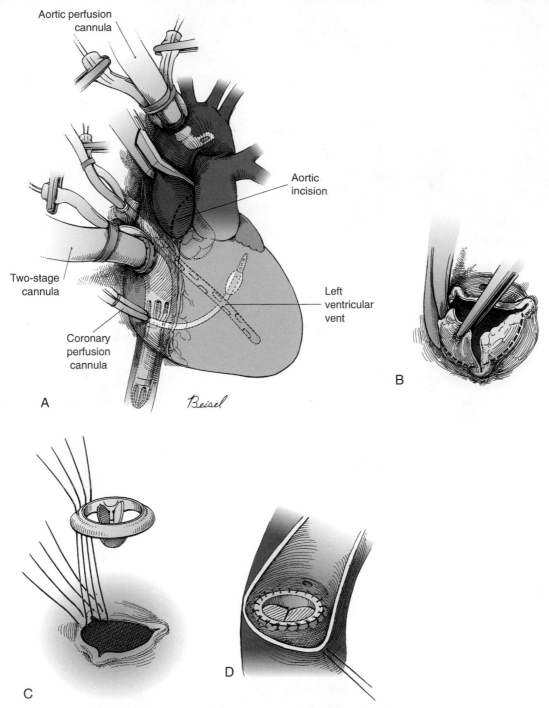

Aortic perfusion
cannula

Aortic
incision

Two-stage
cannula

Left
ventricular
vent

Coronary
perfusion
cannula

A

Beisel

B

C

D

Figure 34-19   **Aortic valve replacement. A,** Incision site and cannulation. **B,** Excision of the valve.
C, Valve replacement and placement of sutures. **D,** Completed suture line. *(Modified from Waldhausen
JA, Pierce WS, Campbell DB: Surgery of the chest, ed 6, St Louis, 1996, Mosby.)*

TECHNIQUE

1 A midline sternotomy is performed.

2 Cannulation of the superior and inferior venae cavae is performed for total cardiopulmonary bypass.

3 The ascending aorta is occluded and cardioplegic solution is infused through the aortic root and into the coronary arteries.

4 A left atriotomy is performed and the mitral valve is excised.

5 A prosthetic valve is sutured in place.

6 The atriotomy is closed and the aorta is unclamped.

7 Cardiopulmonary bypass is discontinued and the cannulas are removed.

8 Chest tubes and pacing wires are inserted and the wound is closed.

Discussion

MITRAL VALVE REPLACEMENT A median sternotomy is performed and both venae cavae are cannulated for total cardiopulmonary bypass. The ascending aorta is occluded and a cardioplegic solution is infused through the aortic root and into the coronary arteries.

The surgeon opens the left atrium with the long knife, extends the incision with scissors, and inserts an atrial retractor, which the assistant uses to expose the valve. The surgeon grasps the valve with a valve hook or long Allis clamp and excises the cusps with valve scissors or the knife. The chordae tendineae and papillary muscles of the anterior leaflet are cut; the posterior leaflet chordae often are left intact.

The annulus then is measured so that the technologist can obtain the correct size of prosthetic valve from the circulator. The surgeon places the sutures through the annulus and the prosthetic sewing ring using the same technique as described for aortic valve replacement. The valve is seated in position and the sutures are tied.

The atriotomy is closed with continuous 3-0 polypropylene suture. Before tying the sutures, the surgeon temporarily releases the vena cava tourniquets and allows the heart to fill with blood. The blood is allowed to spill out of the heart to remove air bubbles. The surgeon then ties the sutures securely. The aortic clamp is removed and the aorta is aspirated with a vent catheter to ensure that no air remains in the heart.

Cardiopulmonary bypass is discontinued and the cannulas are removed. A temporary pacemaker electrode may be sutured to the heart. Chest tubes are inserted and the wound is closed. Mitral valve replacement is illustrated in Figure 34-20.

MITRAL COMMISSUROTOMY Occasionally a mitral commissurotomy (opening of the commissures that bring the cusps of the valve together) is performed rather than valve replacement. This technique can be used to relieve stenosis when the valve leaflets are sufficiently flexible to allow it. The procedure is performed during bypass. The surgeon incises the commissures with a knife or breaks them apart with a mitral valve dilator (e.g., Gerbode or Tubbs dilator) to separate the cusps. The atrium then is closed as described for mitral valve replacement.

MITRAL RING ANNULOPLASTY A dilated mitral valve annulus can be repaired by placement of an annuloplasty ring in the annulus to allow the valve leaflets to come together more efficiently. Sutures are placed in the annulus and the annuloplasty ring and are tied. This procedure reduces the annular orifice, allowing the valve leaflets to close properly.

Related Procedure

TRICUSPID VALVE REPLACEMENT OR REPAIR In replacement procedures, the tricuspid valve is excised and replaced with a prosthetic valve through a right atriotomy. Total cardiopulmonary bypass is required. Tricuspid ring annuloplasty (similar to mitral valve annuloplasty) often is preferred over replacement.

RESECTION OF AN ANEURYSM OF THE ASCENDING AORTA

Surgical Goal

An aneurysm or dissection of the ascending aorta can rupture or prevent the aortic valve leaflets from closing properly. The goal of resection of an aneurysm of the ascending aorta is to repair the aneurysm and restore function to the valve.

Pathology

An aortic aneurysm is a potentially life-threatening condition in which the walls of the aorta (or any other vessel or heart chamber) balloon out because of cardiovascular disease (Figure 34-21). Aneurysms can be classified as saccular or fusiform. A **saccular aneurysm** is a ballooning out of a localized area in the artery. A **fusiform aneurysm** involves the entire circumference of the artery. Arteriosclerosis and atherosclerosis both contribute to these conditions. As the disease progress, the walls of the aorta become increasingly stiff and blocked by fatty deposits. The walls of the segment *distal to* the blockage (in the direction of blood flow) become weak and distended. Finally, the ballooning vessel begins to delaminate (the intimal layer separates) and blood is forced between the layers, resulting in rupture. This delamination is called *dissection* and the aneurysm then is referred to as a *dissecting aneurysm*. The condition requires immediate surgery to prevent rupture.

TECHNIQUE

1 A median sternotomy is performed.
2 The femoral artery is isolated and cannulated.
3 The venae cavae are cannulated.
4 Total cardiopulmonary bypass is initiated and a vent catheter of the right superior pulmonary vein is inserted.
5 The aorta is occluded distal to the aneurysm or dissection and the aortic wall is opened.
6 Retrograde cardioplegic solution is infused (the coronary arteries rarely are directly perfused).
7 A prosthetic graft is anastomosed to the proximal and distal aorta, and the aorta is unclamped.
8 Cardiopulmonary bypass is discontinued and the cannulas are removed.
9 Chest tubes are inserted and the wound is closed.

Discussion

A median sternotomy may be performed, after the femoral artery and vein have been isolated for cannulation, if the risk exists that the aorta may rupture when the chest is opened. After cannulation has been completed and the right superior pulmonary vein sump catheter has been inserted, the surgeon occludes the aorta distal to the aneurysm. The aneurysm is opened with scissors, and all clots and debris are removed. If the aorta is dissected, the location of the aortic tear is identified.

Retrograde cardioplegic solution is administered through the coronary sinus. The surgeon examines the aortic valve to determine the extent of injury and to replace it if necessary.

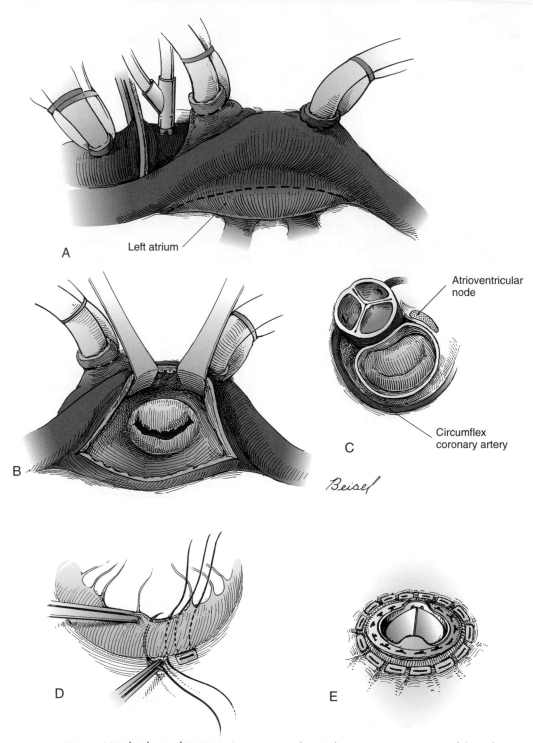

A, Left atrium

C, Atrioventricular node

Circumflex coronary artery

Beisel

Figure 34-20   Mitral valve replacement. A, Incision and cannulation sites. **B,** Exposure of the valve. **C,** Anatomical relationship between the mitral and aortic valves. **D,** Pledgets are placed with double-arm sutures. **E,** Completed valve replacement. *(Modified from Waldhausen JA, Pierce WS, Campbell DB: Surgery of the chest, ed 6, St Louis, 1996, Mosby.)*

The technologist should have valve instruments available on the setup tray to prevent delay. Valve suture should be ready for immediate opening if needed.

The surgeon obtains the appropriate size of graft from the technologist and performs the distal anastomosis with continuous suture of 3-0 polypropylene. When the anastomosis is complete, the surgeon occludes the graft with a vascular clamp and temporarily releases the aortic clamp to test the suture line. Additional sutures are placed as needed. Teflon felt pledgets are used to reinforce the suture line.

The surgeon cuts the graft to an appropriate length and performs the proximal anastomosis. Before tying the suture, the surgeon temporarily releases the aortic clamp to fill the graft and flush out air and clots. The right superior pulmonary vein sump catheter is then removed. After cardiopulmonary bypass has been discontinued, the cannulas are removed. The

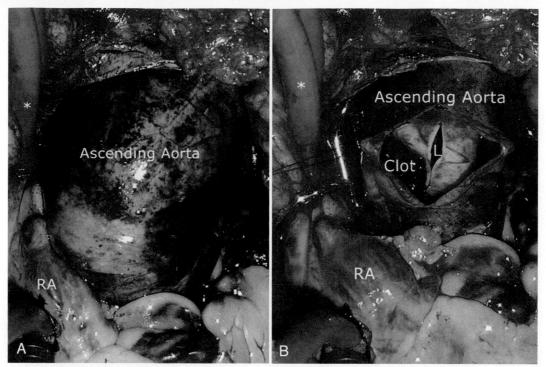

Figure 34-21 **Ascending aortic aneurysm. A,** Acute aortic dissection. **B,** The aorta has been opened, showing the true lumen. *RA,* right atrium. *(From Townsend CM: Sabiston textbook of surgery, ed 17, Philadelphia, 2001, WB Saunders.)*

surgeon may cover the graft with aneurysm tissue. The assistant closes the groin incision while the surgeon inserts chest tubes and closes the sternotomy.

The surgeon occasionally must replace both the aorta and the aortic valve. Special composite graft-valve prostheses are available for these procedures. If the coronary opening is obscured by the composite graft, the surgeon must reimplant the coronary opening or create bypass grafts that attach proximally to the aortic graft. Coronary bypass instruments should be available.

Postoperative complications include hemorrhage, stroke, infection, and death. Graft anastomoses may require repair if persistent bleeding arises. Neurological deficit or paralysis may be a complication of surgery on the descending thoracic aorta. Figure 34-22 illustrates the resection of an ascending aortic aneurysm.

RESECTION OF AN ANEURYSM OF THE AORTIC ARCH

Surgical Goal

An aneurysm or dissection of the aortic arch can impair blood flow to the brain and the upper body because of the frequent involvement of the aortic branches (i.e., the brachiocephalic artery, the left carotid artery, and the left subclavian artery). The goal of resection of an aortic arch aneurysm is to repair the aneurysm and restore adequate blood flow to the aorta and its branches.

Discussion

An aneurysm that extends or is limited to the aortic arch may require resection and anastomosis of both the aorta and its

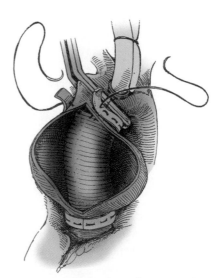

Figure 34-22 **Resection and repair of an ascending aneurysm.** *(From Rothrock J: Alexander's care of the patient in surgery, ed 17, Philadelphia, 2007, Mosby.)*

branching arch vessels using a graft. The femoral vein and artery are cannulated as for aneurysms of the ascending aorta. In some cases, the branch vessels cannot be clamped because of their location or because of their involvement in the aneurysm. In these cases, the surgeon may elect to turn off the pump for the period required to anastomose the arch vessels. Once the anastomoses are complete, the pump is started again and the remainder of the procedure is performed under bypass. Figure 34-23 illustrates the repair of an aortic arch aneurysm.

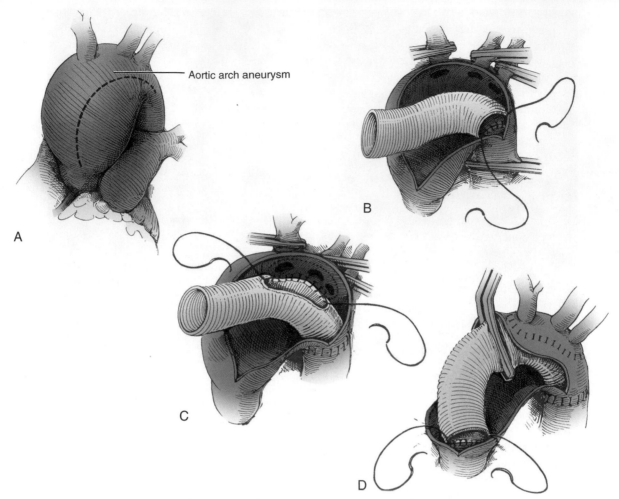

Aortic arch aneurysm

A

B

C

D

Figure 34-23   **Repair of an aortic arch aneurysm. A,** Incision. **B,** Distal anastomosis. **C,** Anastomosis of the graft below the arch vessels. **D,** Proximal anastomosis. *(Modified from Waldhausen JA, Pierce WS, Campbell DB: Surgery of the chest, ed 6, St Louis, 1996, Mosby.)*

RESECTION OF AN ANEURYSM OF THE DESCENDING THORACIC AORTA

Surgical Goal

The goal of surgical repair of an aneurysm of the descending thoracic aorta is to prevent rupture and life-threatening hemorrhage.

TECHNIQUE

1   A thoracotomy is performed.
2   The mediastinal pleura is incised.
3   The aneurysm or dissection is mobilized from the surrounding tissue.
4   Vascular occluding clamps are applied to the aorta and the aneurysm or dissection is resected.
5   The intercostal arteries are ligated.
6   A prosthetic graft is implanted.
7   The occluding clamps are removed from the aorta.
8   The graft may be enclosed by the remaining vascular wall.
9   The mediastinal pleura is closed.
10 Chest tubes are inserted and the wound is closed.

Discussion

The patient is placed in the lateral position, prepped, and draped for a thoracotomy. A thoracotomy incision is performed as described previously. After the chest has been opened and the retractors placed, the surgeon retracts the edges of the pleura with 2-0 silk sutures.

The surgeon begins to free the aneurysm from the surrounding tissue. Femoral vein–femoral artery cardiopulmonary bypass may be used to perfuse the kidneys and the rest of the lower body. If bypass is not used, speed is essential at this time because there is no flow to the lower body. The technologist must be alert and avoid unnecessary movements and loss of time while handling instruments.

The surgeon occludes the aorta proximal and distal to the aneurysm. The knife is then used to make a longitudinal incision into the aneurysm and the incision is extended with scissors. The outer layer of the aneurysm is preserved and retracted with 2-0 or 3-0 silk sutures. These flaps are used later in the procedure to cover the grafts and prevent them from adhering to the lung.

The surgeon removes all debris and blood clots inside the aneurysm using suction and tissue forceps. The technologist should have a small basin to receive loose debris and blood clots and a moist sponge to wipe debris from the instruments. The surgeon ligates the intercostal vessels along the posterior wall of the aneurysm with polyester sutures. Identifying the origin of these vessels may be difficult. To aid identification, the surgeon may irrigate the area with warm saline solution and look for bleeding points, indicating an open vessel. When hemostasis is secured, the graft is anastomosed to the aorta.

The surgeon transects the aorta immediately above and below the aneurysm and removes the middle segment. A graft then is implanted to replace the diseased segment.

ANASTOMOSING THE GRAFT The surgeon performs the proximal anastomosis with continuous suture of 3-0 or 4-0 polypropylene or polyester. A straight vascular clamp may be placed across the graft while the surgeon releases the proximal aortic clamp briefly to check for leaks. The surgeon reapplies the aortic clamp, removes the graft clamp, and places any additional sutures needed to control leakage. Teflon pledgets may be used to bolster the sutures.

After completing the proximal anastomosis, the surgeon trims the graft to the appropriate length and performs the distal anastomosis. Before the suture is tied, the graft is flushed to clear it of clots and debris. The suture is then tied and all clamps are removed, restoring blood flow to the lower body.

If cardiopulmonary bypass has been used, it is discontinued at this stage and the cannulas are removed. To complete the procedure, the surgeon covers the graft with remaining aneurysm tissue (if it has not been excised) using absorbable continuous or interrupted 2-0 or 3-0 suture. The mediastinal pleura is closed, chest tubes are inserted, and the wound is closed in layers.

ENDOVASCULAR REPAIR OF A THORACIC ANEURYSM

Endovascular repair of a descending thoracic aneurysm is now frequently used for the treatment of descending thoracic aortic aneurysm (DTAA). Devices currently used are the TAG Device (W.L. Gore & Associates, Flagstaff, Ariz). Others are under investigation at this time. A discussion on endovascular repair of abdominal aneurysm (EVAR) is found in Chapter 32 and clarifies the principles of endovascular repair.

Discussion

Endovascular repair of descending aortic aneurysms are performed on patients with fusiform-type aneurysms, which are at least double the normal size of the aorta. Computed tomography angiography is used to measure and evaluate the extent of disease to determine whether the patient is suitable for endovascular repair.

The surgical approach may be through an incision into the femoral artery or percutaneous insertion (without incision) may be possible. As in endovascular repair of abdominal aneurysm, a wire stent graft is deployed through the femoral artery and positioned at the level of the aneurysm. This is done under fluoroscopy and intraoperative angiography using the opposite groin for entry of angiocatheters.

For femoral surgery, a needle is inserted into the femoral artery and a guidewire is threaded into the thoracic portion of the aorta. The needle is removed. Because the guidewires may be over 6 feet long, the surgical technologist should take precautions to avoid contaminating the wire by anchoring the distal end of the wire with sterile towels or another weighted sterile object.

Dilators of increasing size are inserted over the guidewire; each dilator is inserted and removed in succession and replaced with a larger guidewire in order to enlarge the femoral artery.

An angiographic catheter is inserted into the patient's opposite femoral artery in order to visualize the interior of the aorta, to perform intraoperative angiograms, and to guide and verify the placement of the deployed stent. The surgeon uses fluoroscopy to identify the location of the arch vessels and to identify normal proximal and distal aortic tissue into which the endovascular stent graft will be secured. Intravascular ultrasound may be used to measure internal diameters and to note anatomic angles that can affect placement of the device(s). More than one device may be deployed when there is an extensive aneurysmal lesion.

When the target area is reached, the device is positioned and opened in the aorta. The surgeon confirms the proper placement of the endostent(s) and the absence of endoleaks. If hemostasis is not achieved, the surgeon may reposition the graft or replace the existing graft with another stent. If there is acute hemorrhage that cannot be repaired endoscopically, the technologist should be prepared for open surgery to complete the repair.

Recovery is considerably shorter after endovascular repair than after thoracotomy. Possible complications include bleeding and migration of the device, requiring adjustment and/or insertion of another device.

INSERTION OF AN ARTIFICIAL CARDIAC PACEMAKER

Surgical Goal

An artificial pacemaker is implanted in the body to correct cardiac arrhythmia caused by a disease of the conduction system. A pulse generator provides electrical impulses through the device's cardiac leads, which are implanted in the conductive tissue of the heart.

Pathology

Cardiac arrhythmia is an abnormal pattern of conductivity in the heart. Healthy individuals may have an arrhythmia. However, when the heart's conduction mechanism is affected by disease, certain arrhythmias can be life-threatening. Arrhythmias are named by type and origin. Some common arrhythmias are:

- *Ventricular tachycardia*: A heart rate over 120 beats per minute.
- *Atrial flutter*: A heart rate of 240 to 450 beats per minute.
- *Ventricular fibrillation*: Chaotic, disorganized stimulation of one or both ventricles that does not pump the blood.

- *Atrial fibrillation*: Chaotic, disorganized stimulation of one or both atria that prevents atrial contraction (which normally fills the ventricle with blood).
- **Bradycardia:** A heart rate below 40 to 60 beats per minute. Conduction disease can arise from ischemic heart disease, which can be caused by atherosclerosis, infection, or congenital defects.

TECHNIQUE

Temporary Pacemaker

1 An electrode is sutured to the right atrium and/or the right ventricle or can be inserted transvenously.
2 The free end of the electrode is brought through the skin and secured with a suture.
3 The electrode is connected to an alligator cable attached to a temporary external pacemaker generator.

Discussion

A pacemaker may be implanted in the cardiac catheterization suite or in the perioperative period. Postsurgically, a pacemaker can be implanted via the transvenous route (a temporary pacer is used until it is replaced by a permanent pacing system).

A pacemaker may be implanted temporarily, such as during cardiac procedures, or the implantation may be permanent. Three approaches are used for permanent implantation, the transvenous, epicardial, and subxiphoid approaches. The transvenous and subxiphoid procedures, which do not require a thoracotomy, are commonly performed with the patient under local anesthesia with monitored anesthesia care. When the transvenous approach is used, the electrodes are placed with the aid of fluoroscopy.

A right or left subclavian venotomy is performed and the electrode is advanced into the right atrium, through the tricuspid valve, and into the right ventricle, where it is placed in the right ventricular apex. The pulse generator then is placed within the superficial tissues of the chest wall. An atrial electrode also may be placed in the atrial appendage for dual-chamber (atrial and ventricular) pacing.

Implantation of both permanent and temporary pacemakers through a thoracotomy is less common than placement through the transvenous approach (the procedures are discussed in the next section).

Temporary pacemaker leads are implanted before cardiopulmonary bypass is discontinued, because the field is more accessible with the lungs deflated (as occurs on bypass). Another reason the leads are implanted before bypass is discontinued is that if touching the heart during lead attachment causes an arrhythmia, perfusion to the body is not compromised. The surgeon sutures the metal wire electrode to the heart with 5-0 silk. Only the tip of the electrode is exposed wire; the remaining section is insulated.

The technologist prepares the electrode on a needle holder before or after bypass is discontinued. The assistant cuts the needle off the electrode after the surgeon places it through the myocardium. The surgeon then secures the electrode with 5-0 silk sutures. The surgeon brings the opposite end of the electrode through the skin and secures it with 2-0 silk sutures. The electrode is connected to an alligator cable and pacemaker generator. The anesthesia care provider then can pace the heart as necessary. Insertion of a transvenous pacemaker is shown in Figure 34-10.

Epicardial Pacemaker

Although permanent epicardial pacemakers are inserted less frequently than transvenous pacers, the intravenous route is not feasible in some cases, such as with stenosis of the subclavian vein. A sternotomy for cardiac surgery is not necessarily an indication for epicardial lead attachment, because leads may be inserted transvenously after sternotomy when temporary pacing is sufficient to maintain an acceptable heart rate.

The techniques for implanting the permanent pacemaker through a thoracotomy or short transverse incision are similar. Using the skin knife, the surgeon makes a short transverse incision below the xiphoid and across the diaphragm. The subcutaneous, fascial, and muscle layers are divided with the scalpel or ESU. A self-retaining retractor (e.g., a small Finochietto or a large Weitlaner retractor) is placed in the wound.

The surgeon exposes the right ventricle by opening the pericardium with the knife or dissecting scissors. Size 2-0 silk sutures are placed on the edges of the pericardium so that the assistant can put traction on the tissue. The surgeon then places several sutures of 4-0 silk or polyester through the ventricle and into the electrode's Silastic casing. The coiled metal tip of the electrode is placed in the myocardium and the sutures are tied. Additional sutures may be needed to secure the electrode. The coiled (pigtail) lead usually is inserted into the ventricle; the harpoon-like lead generally is attached to the atrium.

To test the electrode, the surgeon connects it to an alligator cable attached to the temporary external pacemaker generator. The circulator or anesthesia care provider activates the battery. If the electrode functions normally, it is connected to the permanent battery. The surgeon makes a pocket for the battery beneath the fascia of the chest or, less often, the abdomen. The battery is inserted into the pocket, which is closed with interrupted size 0 or 2-0 nonabsorbable sutures. Size 0 or 2-0 absorbable sutures are used to approximate the subcutaneous tissue and the skin is closed with the surgeon's suture of choice.

REPLACEMENT OF A PACEMAKER BATTERY

Surgical Goal

A malfunctioning pacemaker generator is replaced to produce continuous pacing.

Pathology

Pacemaker batteries have a limited life span and must be replaced periodically. A warning system, built into the battery, and routine patient assessment are normally sufficient to provide a wide measure of safety to prevent complete and sudden battery failure. Besides normal wear due to age, a battery may become damaged by trauma (e.g., direct blow to the patient and battery) or a fault in the circuitry.

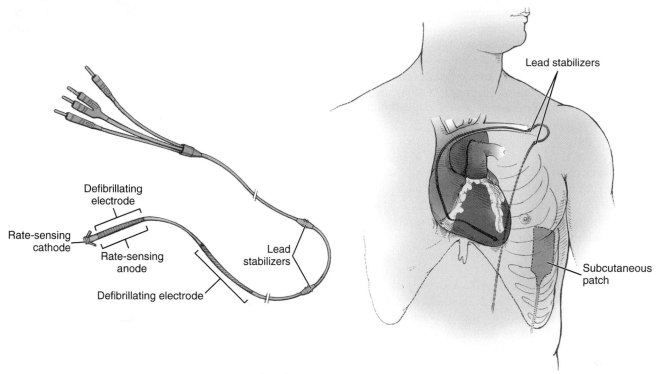

Figure 34-24 Internal cardioverter-defibrillator (ICD). *(From Rothrock J: Alexander's care of the patient in surgery, ed 17, Philadelphia, 2007, Mosby.)*

TECHNIQUE

1 Skin and subcutaneous tissue over the generator are incised.
2 The tissue layers are divided to expose the generator and electrode or electrodes.
3 The generator is removed from the tissue pocket.
4 The electrode is connected to an alligator cable and tested.
5 The electrode is inserted into the new generator.
6 The new generator is inserted into the tissue pocket and the wound is closed.

Discussion

The surgeon incises the skin over the generator. The underlying tissue layers are divided with sharp dissection to expose the electrodes and generator. The generator is removed from the tissue pocket and the electrodes are disconnected. The surgeon immediately connects the electrodes to the alligator cable of an external pacer generator so that the heart can be paced continually during the exchange of generators. The electrodes are then connected to the new generator. The surgeon places the new generator in the tissue pocket. Interrupted 3-0 absorbable suture are used to approximate the tissues over the generator. The skin is then closed with interrupted 4-0 sutures.

Complications include malfunction or failure of the device. Frequent shocking by an implanted defibrillator can wear out the battery; patients are monitored for excessive "shocks." Injury to blood vessels used for insertion of the device (e.g., the subclavian vein) is possible, as is infection of the generator pocket. Patients are observed for injury to the heart by assess-

ing electrocardiogram and blood pressure, and other hemodynamic parameters.

IMPLANTABLE CARDIOVERTER-DEFIBRILLATOR

The implantable cardioverter-defibrillator (ICD) (Figure 34-24) is an electronic cardiac defibrillating and monitoring device used in patients susceptible to ventricular fibrillation or ventricular tachycardia. Most ICDs also have pacing functions to treat bradycardia, which may occur after an episode of defibrillation. The device consists of a generator, sensing electrodes, and defibrillation/pacing electrodes. Newer transvenous ICD catheters have largely replaced the older models that used epicardial patch electrodes applied during open procedures.

The ICD may be implanted through a thoracotomy or a subxiphoid or median sternotomy incision, although most are inserted transvenously. The sensing leads are commonly placed in the right ventricle through a transvenous approach. The ventricular defibrillation leads are inserted into the heart transvenously and the generator is placed in the superficial tissue of the chest or abdominal wall. A subcutaneous thoracic patch occasionally is used to optimize defibrillation.

SURGERY FOR ATRIAL FIBRILLATION (CARDIAC ABLATION)

Surgical Goal

Cardiac ablation is the selective destruction of diseased conductive tissue to correct atrial fibrillation. Other conduction disorders include Wolff-Parkinson-White syndrome, which is characterized by multiple AV conduction pathways. By creating small areas of scar tissue in the cardiac muscle, electrical impulses are forced to follow an alternative conduction path or "maze." Ablation is commonly performed through a cardiac catheter, which delivers radiofrequency (RF) energy or cryoenergy. The procedure also may be performed through an open sternotomy.

Pathology

Atrial fibrillation is an abnormal heart rhythm. It may cause only minor discomfort or it may result in the pooling of blood in the atria. This can lead to insufficient cardiac output and thrombus (clotting), which in turn can lead to cerebrovascular accident or pulmonary embolism.

Discussion

INTERVENTIONAL CARDIAC ABLATION Depending on the anticipated origin of the problem, the electrophysiologist inserts a catheter percutaneously into the femoral vein or artery and threads the catheter retrograde to the right or left atrium and ventricle. The electrophysiologist tests various areas of the heart in an attempt to reproduce the dysrhythmia and then ablates the area of the heart where the rhythm disturbance originates. Postoperative considerations are similar to those for atrial fibrillation surgery.

TECHNIQUE

Sternotomy Approach

1 The surgeon performs a midline sternotomy. Cannulation of the superior and inferior venae cavae is performed for total cardiopulmonary bypass.
2 The ascending aorta is occluded and cardioplegic solution is infused through the aortic root and into the coronary arteries.
3 A right atriotomy is performed and the right atrial targets are ablated.
4 A left atriotomy is performed and the left atrial targets are ablated.
5 The atriotomies are closed and the aorta is unclamped.
6 Cardiopulmonary bypass is discontinued and the cannulas are removed.
7 Chest tubes and pacing wires are inserted and the wound is closed.

Postoperatively, patients are monitored for heart rhythm problems. In patients treated for atrial fibrillation, it may take up to 3 months for the heart to resume beating in the normal manner. Additional postoperative considerations include monitoring for bleeding, infection, and other potential complications related to heart surgery.

PERICARDIAL WINDOW

Surgical Goal

Accumulated blood or fluid in the pericardium can compress the heart and impede filling of the ventricles. This reduces the amount of blood ejected into the systemic circulation. Removal of the fluid, through the creation of a pericardial window, improves cardiac function.

Pathology

Pericardial effusion is caused by inflammation related to an infectious disease or a tumor. It may also be a result of a fluid shift related to homeostasis. Occasionally, a postoperative chest tube may become obstructed with clotted blood, causing drainage fluid to back up into the pericardium.

Discussion

The patient is placed in the supine position with a small roll under the left chest and the chest is prepped and draped. External defibrillator patches should be applied in case fibrillation occurs. A small incision is made in the fourth or fifth intercostal space and a retractor is inserted. The pericardium is exposed and a small portion (a "window") of the pericardial tissue is excised to allow fluid to leave the pericardium. The surgeon inserts a suction catheter and removes the excess fluid. One or more chest tubes are inserted, and the incision is closed.

PERICARDIECTOMY

Surgical Goal

Chronic inflammation of the pericardium can produce a fibrotic (and often calcified) coating over the heart that constricts the ventricles. Removal of the adherent scar tissue improves cardiac function.

Pathology

Constrictive pericarditis may develop because of viral infection, tuberculosis, or chronic pericarditis. The heart becomes encased within an adherent layer of scar tissue.

TECHNIQUE

1 A median or bilateral transverse sternotomy is performed.
2 Fibrous tissue is removed over the left ventricle between the parietal pericardium and the epicardium (visceral pericardium).
3 Both ventricles, atria, and venae cavae are decorticated.
4 Hemostasis is maintained.
5 Chest drainage tubes are inserted.
6 The sternum is approximated with wire.
7 The incision is closed.

Discussion

The patient is placed in the supine position and the anterior chest is prepped and draped. External defibrillator pads should be applied in case of ventricular fibrillation resulting from manipulation of the heart during dissection. A median sternotomy is performed with a sternal saw. Dissection of the dense adhesions can cause increased bleeding; suture ligatures of 4-0 or 5-0 polypropylene or silk, on pledgets if desired, may be used. Cardiopulmonary bypass often is available on a standby basis.

Basic sternotomy instruments are used in addition to lung retractors. An ultrasound debridement system occasionally is used for very dense calcification. Portions of adherent scar may be left in place if the risk of injury to underlying structures is great. Common examples are areas of the right and left coronary arteries. Bilateral dissection is performed to the phrenic nerves (which are identified and preserved).

HEART FAILURE

Surgical techniques to support a failing heart are available for temporary, long-term, or permanent support. When mechanical devices cannot reverse the decline of heart function, cardiac transplantation may be required.

INSERTION AND REMOVAL OF AN INTRAAORTIC BALLOON CATHETER

Surgical Goal

An intraaortic balloon catheter reduces the workload of the heart after myocardial infarction or in patients who cannot be taken off bypass. The intraaortic balloon catheter is inserted into the descending thoracic aorta in a retrograde direction via the femoral artery. The distal tip of the catheter is positioned just below the left subclavian artery. The balloon increases the supply of oxygen to the heart by increasing coronary blood flow during diastole and improves distal perfusion of the body's organs. When the ventricle contracts, the balloon deflates, creating a vacuum that lowers the pressure in the aorta. When the ventricle relaxes, the balloon inflates, increasing the volume of blood into the coronary arteries and distal organs (Figure 34-25). This produces additional blood flow to the brain, kidneys, and other organs. The size of the balloon is determined by the size of the femoral artery.

Pathology

Myocardial infarction, described earlier in the section on coronary artery bypass grafting, is caused by obstruction of the coronary artery and results in death of cardiac tissue. An intraaortic balloon catheter reduces the workload of a damaged heart following myocardial infarction. This also reduces the oxygen requirements of heart tissue and compensates for the loss of coronary artery function.

TECHNIQUE

Insertion

1 The femoral artery is exposed and isolated through a groin incision.
2 A heavy silk suture is tied around the proximal end of the balloon catheter to mark the level of insertion.
3 The femoral artery and branches are occluded and the artery is incised.
4 The catheter is inserted into the femoral artery and advanced into the descending thoracic aorta, almost to the left subclavian artery.

Removal

1 The groin is reopened and the femoral artery is isolated.
2 The balloon catheter is withdrawn and the artery is occluded.
3 The femoral artery is unclamped and the wound is closed.

Discussion

INSERTION The patient is placed in the supine position, prepped, and draped for a bilateral femoral incision. This is a precaution in case the first attempt to insert the balloon percutaneously is not successful because of aortoiliac stenosis. The procedure is performed with the patient under local anesthesia, or during cardiac surgery if the heart requires support.

The groin is incised and the incision is carried to the femoral artery and branches with sharp and blunt dissection. A small self-retaining retractor is placed in the wound. The common femoral artery and branches are mobilized with dissecting scissors and umbilical tapes or vessel loops are placed around the vessels for traction. Bolsters may be inserted over the loops and the ends tagged.

The surgeon measures the catheter against the distance between the patient's subclavian artery and the femoral artery and then marks this level by tying a suture around the proximal end of the catheter. The catheter is deflated with a syringe before insertion.

The femoral arteries are occluded with vascular clamps (e.g., Glover or DeBakey peripheral vascular clamps) or the umbilical tapes are used as tourniquets. The surgeon makes an incision in the common femoral artery with a #11 blade. Potts scissors are used to extend the incision as needed.

The scrub moistens the balloon with saline solution. The proximal clamp is removed from the artery and the surgeon inserts the catheter into the arteriotomy. The catheter is advanced to the level of the suture mark. The assistant controls bleeding while holding tension on the umbilical tape.

The pump technician evacuates the atmospheric air from the catheter with a 50-mL syringe and the pump is activated. The surgeon secures the catheter to the patient's leg with 2-0 silk suture. The wound may be irrigated with antibiotic solution.

The wound is closed in layers with absorbable and nonabsorbable sutures. A pressure dressing is applied to prevent the formation of a hematoma.

REMOVAL The previous wound is reopened, and the femoral artery is isolated. The balloon is deflated and the catheter is slowly withdrawn. The femoral artery is occluded and the incision is oversewn with continuous 5-0 polypropylene suture. Two sutures may be used. One suture is started at one side of the incision and the other suture is started on the opposite side; the two sutures are tied in the center of the femoral artery incision.

VENTRICULAR ASSIST DEVICE

Surgical Goal

A ventricular assist device (VAD) is used to wean patients from cardiopulmonary bypass when other means are ineffective. Patients awaiting heart transplantation also may be candidates for a VAD, which may consist of a polyurethane blood sac, flexible diaphragm, and pump assembly. The VAD maintains perfusion through cannulas placed in the chambers of

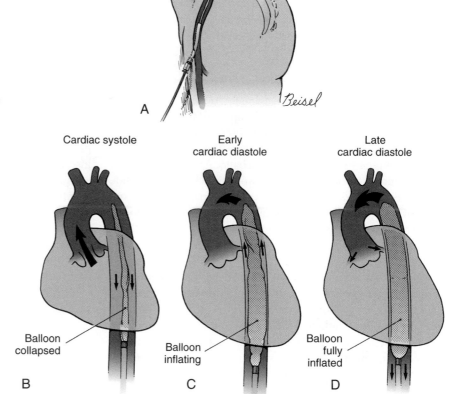

**Figure 34-25 Phases of balloon pumping.
A,** Placement of the balloon in the descending
aorta. **B,** Deflation of the balloon. **C,** Early inflation
of the balloon. **D,** Inflated balloon. *(Modified from
Waldhausen JA, Pierce WS, Campbell DB:
Surgery of the chest, ed 6, St Louis, 1996, Mosby.)*

Cardiac systole

Early
cardiac diastole

Late
cardiac diastole

Balloon
collapsed

Balloon
inflating

Balloon
fully
inflated

B

C

D

the heart and the great vessels according to the patient's need.
Power is provided by pneumatic, electrical, or battery-powered
pumps.

VADs may be use as a bridge to transplantation (supporting the heart until an organ donor becomes available). Some
newer left ventricular devices can be used as end-destination
therapy (the device remains permanently implanted).

Pathology

Patients may not regain sufficient cardiac capacity to sustain
full circulatory perfusion in spite of cardiac surgery with cardiopulmonary bypass. Blood must be pumped throughout the
circulatory system in order to sustain life. The ventricular

assist device is used when the heart is unable to fully perform
this function.

Discussion

In left ventricular assistance, blood is directed from the left
ventricle through the inflow cannula into the assist device and
returned to the ascending aorta through the outflow cannula
(Figure 34-26). Inflow and outflow are distinguished by the
direction of the blood flow relative to the VAD pump. Some
VAD pumps can be implanted in the chest cavity. Drivelines
from the pump exit through incisions in the chest.

In right ventricular assistance, blood is directed from the
right atrium into the pump and into the pulmonary artery. The

outflow cannula is sutured to the pulmonary artery. In biventricular assistance, left ventricular and right ventricular devices support the two ventricles simultaneously.

An extracorporeal VAD is used for temporary short-term assistance. The pump is connected to inflow and outflow cannulas, which are passed into the thoracic cavity through the chest wall. The pump itself is secured to the outer chest wall and covered with an occlusive dressing. An implantable VAD, which is used for long-term support, uses a pump that is surgically implanted in the chest or abdomen. If a battery pack is used, it is external and its cannulas are passed through the abdomen. VADs may be used as a bridge to transplantation, as an investigational tool, or as end-stage therapy.

Complications include malfunction of the device, infection, and stroke. Additional complications include hemorrhage and death. Graft anastomoses within the device may require repair if persistent bleeding develops.

HEART TRANSPLANTATION

Surgical Goal
The goal of heart transplantation is to replace a diseased heart with a healthy donor heart.

Pathology
Heart transplantation may be performed in suitable patients with end-stage cardiac disease. Patients suitable for heart transplantation include those with:

- Coronary artery disease
- Congenital heart disease

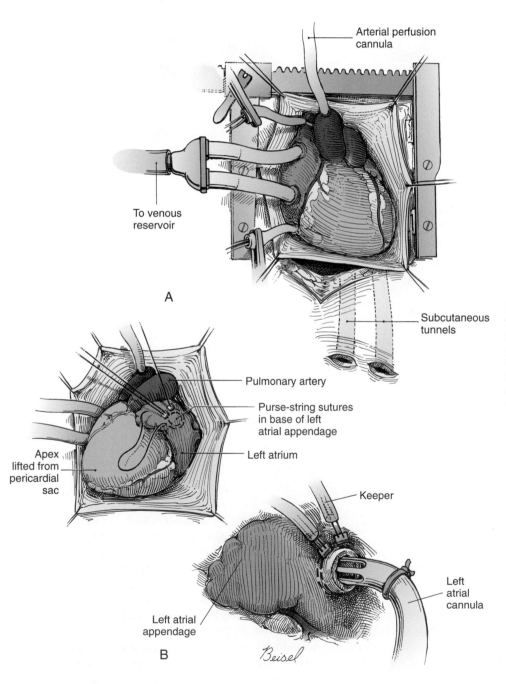

A

B

Beisel

Figure 34-26 Left ventricular assistance. A, Tunnels are developed from the pericardial space to the skin in preparation for placement of the arterial and atrial cannulas. **B,** Two purse-string sutures are placed at the neck of the left atrial appendage, the atrium is incised, and the atrial cannula is inserted.

Arterial perfusion cannula

To venous reservoir

Subcutaneous tunnels

Pulmonary artery

Purse-string sutures in base of left atrial appendage

Left atrium

Apex lifted from pericardial sac

Keeper

Left atrial cannula

Left atrial appendage

Continued

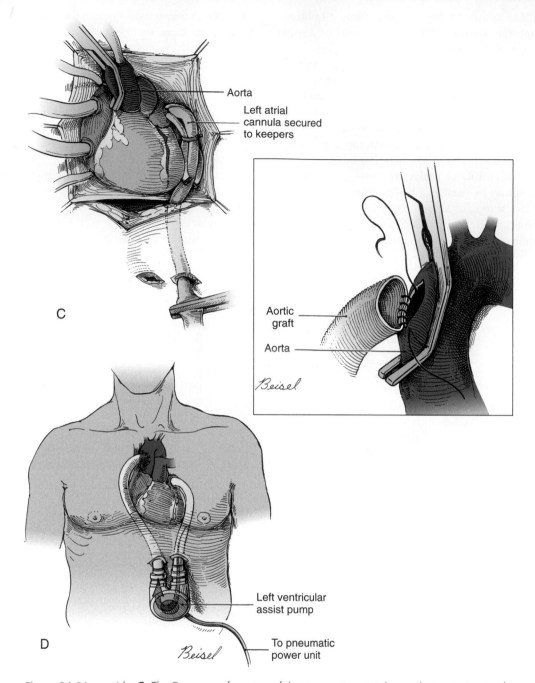

Aorta

Left atrial cannula secured to keepers

C

Aortic graft

Aorta

Beisel

D

Left ventricular assist pump

To pneumatic power unit

Beisel

Figure 34-26, cont'd   **C,** The Dacron graft portion of the composite arterial cannula is anastomosed to the side of the ascending aorta. The cannula is clamped and passed through the medial subcostal tunnel. **D,** Attachment of the pump. *(Modified from Waldhausen JA, Pierce WS, Campbell DB: Surgery of the chest, ed 6, St Louis, 1996, Mosby.)*

- Valve disease
- Rejection of previously transplanted heart

The native (recipient) heart is not removed until the donor procurement team has confirmed that the donor heart is acceptable. Tissue-matching protocols are scrupulously followed to prevent donor-recipient mismatch.

Two types of cardiac transplantation can be performed: orthotopic transplantation is performed more often and is the replacement of one heart with another (Figure 34-27); heterotopic ("piggyback") transplantation is the insertion of a second (donor) heart into the recipient patient's right pleural cavity.

The donor heart works in tandem with the recipient's native heart. This procedure occasionally is performed when a significant size mismatch exists between a small donor and a large recipient. Combined heart-lung procedures also may be performed.

As with other transplantation procedures, it is important to minimize any delay in removing the donor heart and transporting it to the recipient.

A modification of the orthotopic implantation technique has been developed that reduces some of the cardiac rhythm problems that can occur after transplantation. End-to-end

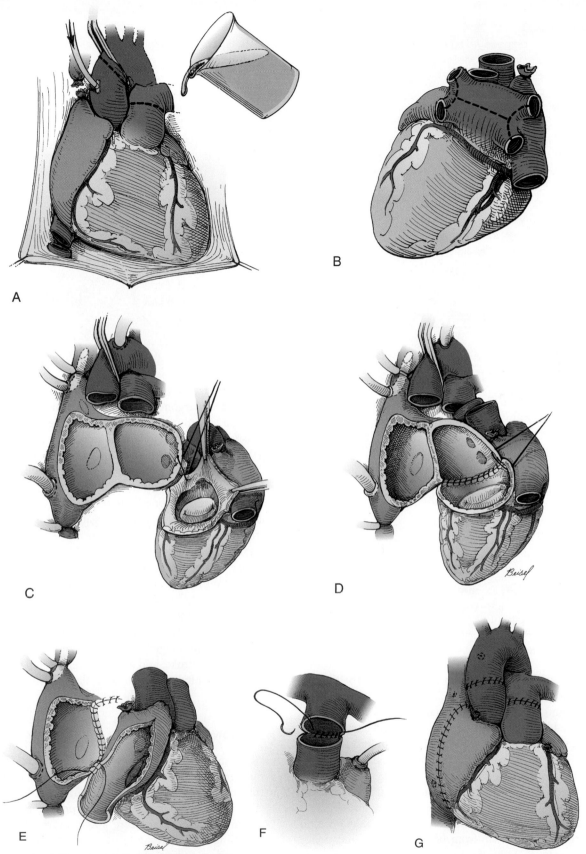

Figure 34-27 **Orthotopic heart transplantation. A,** Incision lines in the donor heart. **B,** Posterior portion of the heart incision lines connecting the pulmonary veins. **C** and **D,** Left atrial anastomosis. **E,** Right atrial anastomosis. **F,** Pulmonary artery anastomosis. **G,** Completed transplantation. *(Modified from Waldhausen JA, Pierce WS, Campbell DB: Surgery of the chest, ed 6, St Louis, 1996, Mosby.)*

TECHNIQUE

Heart Procurement

1 The donor is prepped from chin to knees.
2 A median sternotomy is performed.
3 A sternal retractor is inserted.
4 The pericardium is divided.
5 Umbilical tapes are placed around the aorta and the superior and inferior venae cavae.
6 Heparin is given.
7 The aorta, the superior and inferior venae cavae, and the main pulmonary artery are dissected.
8 The superior vena cava is ligated with heavy silk ties.
9 Cardioplegic solution is infused through the proximal aorta into the heart via the coronary arteries.
10 The venae cavae and the aorta are divided; the heart is lifted to expose the pulmonary veins. The veins are divided.
11 The pulmonary artery is divided just distal to the bifurcation.
12 The heart is removed and placed in a sterile bag containing cold preservative solution.

TECHNIQUE

Native Heart Excision

1 The patient is placed in the supine position and prepped from chin to knees.
2 A median sternotomy incision is made to expose the heart and great vessels.
3 Heparin is given.
4 Bicaval cannulation for cardiopulmonary bypass is performed.
5 Caval tapes are placed around each vena cava.
6 The patient is cooled, the aorta is cross-clamped, and the caval tapes are tightened around the venae cavae.
7 The pulmonary trunk and aorta are divided.
8 The atria are incised to leave intact the posterior portions of the right and left atrial walls and the interatrial septum.
9 The recipient's native heart is excised.

TECHNIQUE

Donor Heart Implantation

1 The donor heart is removed from the transport container and placed in a basin on the back table.
2 The surgeon inspects the heart and trims the atrial walls and great vessels in preparation for the anastomoses.
3 The donor heart is placed in the pericardial cavity and aligned with the remnant interatrial septum and the right and left atrial wall remnants of the recipient's heart.
4 The donor left atrial wall is anastomosed with running 3-0 polypropylene suture (suture size and type may vary according to the surgeon's preference).
5 The right atrial wall is anastomosed with running 3-0 polypropylene suture, followed by pulmonary artery anastomosis with 4-0 polypropylene suture.
6 The aorta is anastomosed with 3-0 running polypropylene suture.
7 Air is removed from the heart.
8 Chest drainage tubes and epicardial pacing wires are inserted.
9 The chest incision is closed.

anastomoses between the superior vena cava and the inferior vena cava are performed rather than the traditional atrial-to-atrial anastomoses. A cuff of the recipient left atrium is sewn to the donor left atrium; pulmonary artery and aorta anastomoses are performed in the usual manner. A pulmonary pressure monitoring line may be inserted before the patient leaves the operating room.

Complications of heart transplantation include rejection and infection. Transplant anastomoses may require repair if persistent bleeding develops. Rhythm changes may occur if retained conduction tissue from both the native and donor hearts is present.

Myocardial biopsies are required after surgery to detect possible rejection. Postoperatively, the transplant patient is placed on lifelong therapy with immunosuppressive medications to prevent rejection of the donor heart. Endomyocardial biopsies are taken regularly to monitor for rejection. Patients who have undergone cardiac surgery are commonly transported to a cardiovascular intensive care unit (CVICU) for intensive monitoring of blood pressure, heart rate, cardiac rhythm, chest tube drainage, and temperature.

Chest tube management is especially important to remove fluid from the pericardium; fluid buildup can compress the heart, causing tamponade. If the pleural cavities have been entered, chest tubes recreate a negative-pressure environment in the pleural cavity or cavities so that lung expansion (and gas exchange) can occur.

The endotracheal tube may be removed within a few hours after arrival in the CVICU, or it may remain in place until the patient is able to breathe independently. The patient's neurological, renal, pulmonary, and pain status are also closely observed and treated as necessary. Complications can include hemorrhage, prolonged ventilation, renal failure, infection, cardiac arrest, stroke, and death. Patients often are discharged from the hospital within 5 to 7 days unless complications develop.

KEY CONCEPTS

- Knowledge of the key anatomical structures of the heart and great vessels is necessary to a complete understanding of surgical procedures.
- Familiarity with diagnostic procedures of the heart is important for patient care and a more complete understanding of pathology.
- An understanding of cardiovascular pathology is important for patient care and case planning.
- Case planning in cardiac surgery requires specific understanding of the instruments, equipment, hemostatic materials and techniques, drugs, and sutures.

- In order to be effective in the scrub role, the surgical technologist must be knowledgeable about specific cardiac procedures and the steps involved in each procedure.

REVIEW QUESTIONS

1. What is the cause of endocarditis?
2. What is the difference between atherosclerosis and arteriosclerosis?
3. What is a cardioplegic solution?
4. What is the primary significance of coronary artery disease?
5. Define *dissecting aneurysm*.
6. Define *commissurotomy*.
7. What are the effects of ischemic heart disease on the heart's ability to conduct electrical impulses?
8. What is the purpose of atrial ablation?

BIBLIOGRAPHY

Carabello BA: Aortic stenosis: two steps forward, one step back, *Circulation* 115:2799, 2007.

Cohn LH, editor: *Cardiac surgery in the adult*, New York, 2008, McGraw-Hill.

Denholm B: Clinical issues: implant documentation, *AORN Journal* 87:433, 2008.

Fedak PWM, McCarthy PM, Bonow RO: Evolving concepts and technologies in mitral valve repair (review), *Circulation* 117:963, 2008.

Haywood PAR, Buxton BF: Contemporary graft patency: 5-year observational data from a randomized trial of conduits, *Annals of Thoracic Surgery* 84:795, 2007.

Kouchoukos NT, Blackstone EH, Doty DB, et al: *Kirklin/Barratt-Boyes cardiac surgery*, ed 3, vols 1 and 2, Philadelphia, 2003, Churchill Livingstone.

Levy MN, Pappano A: *Cardiovascular physiology*, ed 9, St Louis, 2007, Mosby.

Pelter MM: Electrocardiography: normal electrocardiogram. In Moser DK, Riegel B, editors: *Cardiac nursing: a companion to Braunwald's heart disease*, St Louis, 2008, Elsevier/Saunders.

Rubertone JA: Anatomy of the cardiovascular system. In Moser DK, Riegel B, editors: *Cardiac nursing: a companion to Braunwald's heart disease*, St Louis, 2008, Elsevier/Saunders.

Thompson J, Bertling G: Endovascular leaks: perioperative nursing implications, *AORN Journal* 89:839, 2009.

Wagner GS: *Marriott's practical electrocardiography*, ed 11, Philadelphia, 2008, Lippincott Williams & Wilkins.

35

Pediatric Surgery

CHAPTER OUTLINE

Introduction
Physiological and Anatomical
   Considerations

Pathology
Case Planning
Surgical Procedures

Neural Tube Defects

LEARNING OBJECTIVES

After studying this chapter the reader will be able to:

1. Identify key physiological and anatomical features in pediatric surgery
2. Discuss pediatric pathology as it relates to surgery

3. Discuss key elements of case planning for pediatric surgery
4. Describe psychosocial care of the pediatric patient
5. Discuss risk reduction techniques in pediatric surgery
6. List and describe common pediatric surgical procedures

TERMINOLOGY

Acquired abnormality: A physiological or anatomical defect that develops in fetal life as a result of environmental factors.

Atresia: The absence or blockage of a natural orifice or tubular structure.

Bolus: A compact substance (e.g., undigested food, fecal material) that occurs normally in the digestive tract.

Child life specialist: A trained professional who specializes in the psychosocial care of and communication with pediatric patients and their families.

Choanal: A term that describes the communicating passageways between the nasal fossae and the pharynx.

Coarctation: Narrowing of the passageway of a blood vessel, such as coarctation of the aorta, a congenital condition.

Congenital: A condition or an anomaly that develops during fetal life.

Ductus arteriosus: A normal fetal structure that allows blood to bypass circulation to the lungs. If this structure remains open after birth, it is called a *patent ductus arteriosus.*

Embryonic life: The first 8 weeks of gestational development.

Exstrophy: The eversion, or turning out, of an organ.

Fetus: Gestational life after 8 weeks.

Genetic abnormality: A birth anomaly that is inherited.

Homeostasis: The balance of physiological processes that maintain life.

Isolette: An infant-size "bed" and transport unit that is environmentally controlled and equipped with monitoring devices.

Magical thinking: A psychological process in which a person attributes intention and will to inanimate objects. Magical thinking may also describe a patient's belief that an event will happen because he or she wills it or wishes it. This is a normal developmental stage of toddlers.

Mutagenic substance: A chemical or other agent that causes permanent change in the cell's genetic material.

Nephroblastoma: Pediatric cancer of the kidney also known as Wilms tumor.

Neural tube defect: A congenital abnormality resulting from failure of the neural tube to close in embryonic development.

Omphalocele: A protrusion of abdominal contents through a congenital defect at the umbilicus.

Pyloric stenosis: A narrowing of the part of the stomach pylorus that leads to the small intestine.

Teratogen: A chemical or agent that can injure the fetus or cause birth defects.

INTRODUCTION

Pediatric surgery is a multidisciplinary field that encompasses many surgical specialties. Most procedures can be classified in one of three groups:

- Surgery for treatment of **congenital** anomalies
- Procedures for treatment of disease
- Trauma surgery

Innovative techniques in fetal surgery are also being developed and refined as a separate specialty of pediatric medicine.

Pediatrics includes the care of the child from neonate to late adolescence. Because many surgical procedures are an integral part of the child's growth and development, the patient often is followed into adulthood.

Pediatric surgery includes a variety of pathologies, which are not restricted to one body system. However, many pediatric surgeons specialize in a particular system or area of medicine, such as pediatric cardiology or maxillofacial or trauma surgery.

An important dynamic of pediatric surgery is the family's experience in the perioperative process. The family and patient cannot be separated in this specialty, and they require equal consideration in communication and psychosocial care.

The purpose of this chapter is to provide an overview of the physiological and psychological needs of the pediatric patient and to present *common* procedures. Procedures that are performed in both adult and pediatric patients are presented in that specialty chapter (e.g., hernia surgery is presented in Chapter 23 because it is performed on adults and children, whereas omphalocele, which is also an embryonic abdominal wall defect, is presented in this chapter). The procedures included in this chapter are performed most often in pediatric patients only.

The reader should refer to specialty chapters to review the surgical anatomy associated with each procedure presented in this chapter. Important physiological and psychosocial considerations are provided to highlight special needs of pediatric patients in the perioperative environment.

PHYSIOLOGICAL AND ANATOMICAL CONSIDERATIONS

The body's mechanisms for maintaining **homeostasis** (physiological balance) in a pediatric patient are different from those in an adult in many ways. Some of these differences create increased risks for the pediatric surgical patient.

THERMOREGULATION

All patients are at risk of hypothermia during surgery. However, pediatric patients, especially infants and neonates, are particularly vulnerable to hypothermia and hyperthermia. Important facts to remember are:

- Physiological mechanisms that normally regulate temperature in an adult are absent or undeveloped in the infant. Infants and children tend to lose more heat than they generate.
- Infants' relatively large skin surface area and low body weight can contribute to rapid lowering of the core temperature.
- Children and infants have extensive peripheral circulation, which contributes to relatively rapid cooling.
- Infants lack adequate insulation (fatty tissue) to maintain the core temperature in a cold environment.
- Infants and children show a wide range in temperature variation compared to adults.

Hypothermia

Environmental factors are an important cause of hypothermia in pediatric patients:

- Loss of body heat can occur through conduction when the patient's skin comes in contact with cold surfaces (e.g., a cold operating table or transport crib).
- Heat loss by radiation occurs as the patient's own body heat is given up to cold air in the operating room. Heat loss by radiation is intensified when body tissues are exposed during open procedures.
- Prep solutions contribute to hypothermia in two ways. Water absorbs heat from the body much more rapidly than

air. Consequently, cool prep solutions lower the body temperature by both conduction and evaporation.
- Wet linens, drapes, and bedclothes are a source of body cooling during the perioperative period.
- Anesthetics have a profound hypothermic effect in children. This is an added burden to the physiological stress of poor thermoregulation.

Hypothermia can result in a chain of physiological events that place the pediatric patient at risk for cardiac problems, apnea, and hypoglycemia. Pediatric patients, especially infants, have little metabolic tolerance for cold. They have little reserve fat and blood vessels are close to the skin, causing rapid heat loss. Approximately 60% to 75% of body heat is lost through radiation of body heat to the air. As the core temperature begins to drop, metabolism slows (approximately 50% at 82.4° F [28° C]). Heart rate and stroke volume decrease and systemic blood pressure falls. A drop in circulating blood and respiratory rate causes a decrease of up to 6% in normal oxygen intake. In the pediatric patient, this can be a critical level.

Shivering, a compensatory reaction to cold, normally occurs with hypothermia in adults. However, infants lack this mechanism. When an infant is cold, brown fat, found only in infants, is metabolized, using up oxygen and glucose. The result is hypoxemia and hypoglycemia. Electrolyte balance is disturbed, leading to loss of intravascular fluids into the skin. The effects of these physiological events can be rapid and severe. Cardiac arrhythmias leading to arrest may occur.

Hyperthermia

Environmental hyperthermia is less of a risk to pediatric surgical patients. However, elevated core temperatures can occur with misuse of warming devices. Warm light from the operating microscope may generate enough heat to raise an infant's core temperature, especially when the light is directed into a body cavity. Hyperthermia also can be induced in the perioperative period by too much covering. Waterproof drapes trap heat and may contribute to hyperthermia.

Physiological hyperthermia, such as malignant hyperthermia, is a greater risk in pediatric patients than in adults. (Chapter 14 presents a complete discussion of malignant hyperthermia, its causes, and the emergency response.)

PERIOPERATIVE INTERVENTIONS TO MAINTAIN NORMOTHERMIA

Steps to maintain the pediatric patient's temperature are implemented throughout the perioperative period. If the patient becomes chilled, it may be difficult to reestablish warmth, which must be done by using active warming methods.

Transport and Prewarming

Interventions to maintain the patient's temperature begin during transport to the surgical department. Infants and children may become chilled during transport; therefore personnel must make sure that adequate blankets are available before transport. Neonates may arrive in a heated **Isolette** (an infant-size transport unit that is environmentally controlled and equipped with monitoring devices). Infants and neonates should wear a head covering at all times. On arrival in the operating room, the patient is taken to a preheated holding area. A period of *prewarming* may be advisable in the holding area of the operating room. The patient is covered with a warm air blanket or placed on a warm air mattress for prewarming.

Intraoperative Warming

During surgery, a number of methods are used to maintain the core temperature.

- The operating room is prewarmed before the patient arrives. The anesthesia care provider and surgeon agree on the correct temperature for preparation of the patient.
- A warm air blanket may remain in use during the procedure. Upper and lower body mattresses are available for this purpose.
- A water-filled blanket may be used underneath the patient during surgery. Warm or cool water can be used to treat hyperthermia or to prevent hypothermia. Water blankets are programmable to maintain a constant temperature and have alarms in case flow is occluded.
- Overhead heating panels are used during the preoperative prep or whenever supplemental warming is needed. These are commonly used in neonatal and infant care in the surgical environment. A safe distance based on light aperture and intensity is established by the manufacturer. These parameters must be followed precisely, and the patient must be continuously monitored to prevent injury. Dehydration is a risk when overhead heating is used.
- A solution warmer is used during surgical procedures to maintain the correct temperature of irrigation solutions. Intravenous (IV) solutions are also prewarmed before administration.
- Surgical sponges are moistened with warm saline before use.

Monitoring

Pediatric biophysical monitoring uses many of the same techniques as in adult care. Esophageal and rectal probes assess the precise core body temperature. For short procedures, external measuring devices (axillary probes) are used.

FLUID BALANCE

Fluid balance (maintaining the correct amount and types of fluids in body spaces) is an important goal in the care of pediatric patients. Infants and children can become rapidly dehydrated. Before surgery begins, an IV line is inserted to maintain access to the circulatory system. Renal output is measured carefully and, if needed, tests can be done for specific electrolyte balance at any time. The high ratio of surface area to body volume in young children and infants contributes to an increased risk of acid-base imbalance in the blood. Arterial blood gas determinations can rapidly detect acid-base imbalance.

Certain surgical procedures, such as those of the gastrointestinal system, increase the risk of dehydration

and electrolyte shifts. The anesthesia care provider maintains constant monitoring to ensure that electrolyte imbalance is quickly brought under control.

Hemostasis is a critical element in pediatric surgery. Infants and children have little blood reserve and cannot tolerate persistent bleeding. All members of the surgical team are jointly responsible for monitoring blood loss as efficiently and accurately as possible. The scrubbed technologist must report the cumulative amount of irrigation fluid used during surgery so that this can be subtracted from the amount of fluid in each suction canister. Used sponges are maintained carefully, according to facility protocol, and weighed to determine blood loss.

The surgical technologist should have appropriate clamps, suture, and hemostatic materials and agents available according to the requirements of the procedure. The importance of the scrub's role during critical moments of hemorrhage cannot be overstated. The scrub should plan for such emergencies before surgery and mentally rehearse the steps needed to act quickly and correctly. Consulting with the surgeon on specific instruments and supplies *before surgery* reinforces learning.

RESPIRATORY SYSTEM AND AIRWAY

An important anatomical difference between the adult and pediatric respiratory systems is the structure of the airway. Failure to manage a pediatric patient's airway is among the leading causes of death in medical and traumatic emergency. The following are some of the important features of the pediatric airway:

- The tongue is large in proportion to the oral cavity.
- Infants less than 8 weeks of age are obligate nose breathers; this means that obstruction of the nasal passages may cause severe respiratory compromise.
- In infants and children, the trachea is much shorter and smaller than in adults.
- The airway is more delicate and less rigid than in an adult.
- The thoracic wall is weak and unstable in children. The costal and suprasternal muscles are prominent during airway obstruction or lung disease (e.g., pneumonia).
- Lung residual capacity is much lower in children than in adults. This contributes to much more rapid hypoxia if the airway is lost.

PATHOLOGY

During early **embryonic life,** organ systems develop from one of three cellular layers: the endoderm, the ectoderm, or the mesoderm (Figure 35-1). Each layer gives rise to a specific set of organs through a complex process. Figure 35-2 illustrates weekly developmental events as the embryo develops into a **fetus** in the first 10 weeks. Disturbances during the critical stages of germ cell differentiation and organ development can result in errors or defects in a structure or organ system.

Much of pediatric surgery is performed to correct structural defects that develop during fetal life; such a defect is called a *congenital or* **genetic abnormality.** The cause of the abnormality may be genetic (inherited) or acquired. An

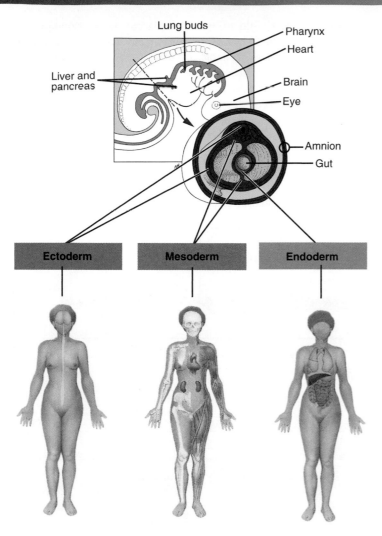

Lung buds
Pharynx
Heart
Liver and pancreas
Brain
Eye
Amnion
Gut

| Ectoderm | Mesoderm | Endoderm |

Figure 35-1 Embryonic membranes. In early embryonic life, three germ layers begin to develop into specific organ systems. (From Thibodeau G, Patton K: Anatomy and physiology, ed 6, Philadelphia, Mosby, 2007.)

acquired abnormality is the result of one or more *environmental agents* or conditions to which the fetus is exposed. The most vulnerable period in fetal life is the first 60 days. This is a period of rapid cellular and tissue differentiation.

An environmental agent (a chemical or drug) that injures the embryo or fetus is called a **teratogen.** Examples of teratogens are environmental mercury and alcohol. Certain drugs are also known to cause severe developmental defects. These include some recreational and prescription drugs.

A **mutagenic substance** causes gene mutation, a chemical change in the genetic structure. Mutation can cause retardation, skeletal deformity, or microcephaly (severely diminished brain development). Gamma radiation (x-rays) is both mutagenic and teratogenic.

The maternal diet is an important source of congenital birth defects. For example, lack of folic acid in the mother's diet causes specific spinal cord (neural tube) defects, such as spina bifida and anencephaly (absence of a cranial vault). A low-protein diet results in poor fetal development.

Certain *infectious agents* are also known be teratogenic. The following infectious microorganisms cause significant congenital abnormalities (listed in parentheses):

- *Toxoplasma gondii* (cerebral calcifications, microcephaly, heart defects)
- Rubella virus—the causative agent of measles (cataract, glaucoma, deafness, heart defects, retinal defects)
- Cytomegalovirus (hydrocephalus, deafness)
- Herpes virus (microcephaly, microphthalmia, retinal defect)
- Varicella-zoster virus—the causative agent of chickenpox (muscle atrophy, mental retardation)
- *Treponema pallidum*—the causative agent of syphilis (hydrocephalus, deafness, bone defects)

Table 35-1 presents important congenital and inherited abnormalities.

NOTE: Congenital defects of the skull and facial bones are presented in Chapters 29 and 30.

PSYCHOSOCIAL CARE OF THE PEDIATRIC PATIENT

Psychosocial care of the pediatric patient is a process that involves the child, parents or guardians, and perioperative staff. The goal of psychosocial care is to help patients and families develop strategies that can help them cope with the perioperative experience. The child's developmental stage, emotional state, and social support system are considered in planning for a safe, smooth surgical outcome. Planning for surgery usually includes a preoperative visit or counseling session involving the patient, family, and child life specialist. The **child life specialist,** who is trained in providing age-appropriate counseling to children about to undergo surgery, can explain the perioperative procedures. This helps reduce anxiety and allows both the patient and family to ask questions before surgery. One of the most important goals of preoperative planning is to provide patient and family education.

Allowing the child to ask questions in an informal setting demystifies the fearful aspects of surgery and engenders trust.

Pediatric patients tend to react to their environment in predictable ways according to their developmental age. This may or may not match the child's actual numerical age (Box 35-1), but it provides a basis on which to communicate and help orient the child to his or her surroundings in surgery.

It is important for all staff members to understand the basic developmental stages *and their significance in the perioperative*

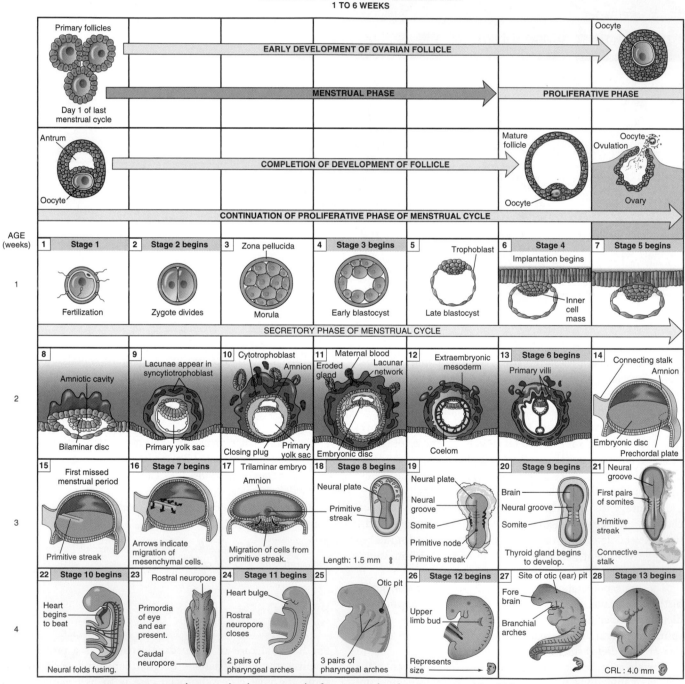

Figure 35-2   **Embryonic development in the first 10 weeks of embryonic and fetal life.** Disturbances during the critical stages of germ cell differentiation and organ development can result in errors or defects in a structure or organ system. *CRL,* Crown-rump length. *(From Thibodeau G, Patton K:* Anatomy and physiology, *ed 6, Philadelphia, Mosby, 2007.)*

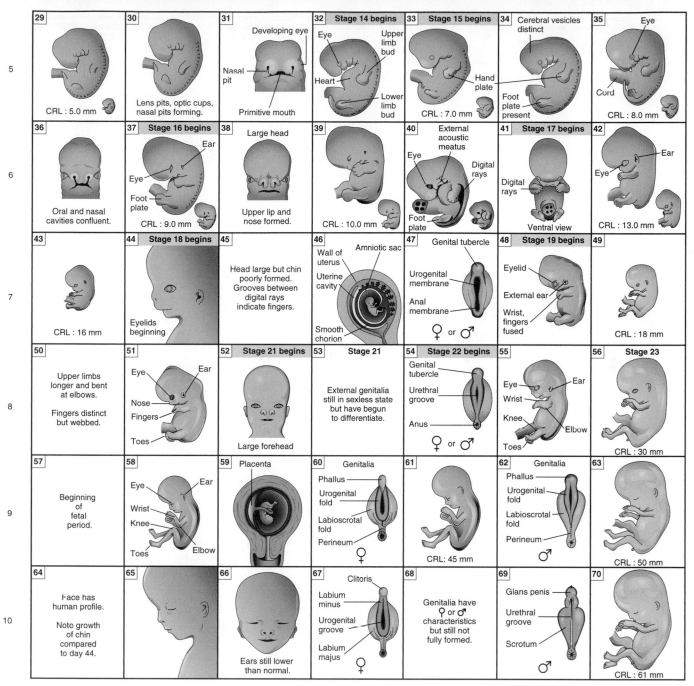

Figure 35-2, cont'd

setting. The greatest fears of young children undergoing surgery are:

1. Fear of the unknown
2. Fear of separation from the primary caregivers

Children appreciate supportive, positive statements about their perioperative experience. Trust in caregivers begins with honest but careful descriptions of what will happen to them. Certain words and phrases are avoided (Box 35-2) so that the patient does not develop a sense of fear or dread.

DEVELOPMENTAL STAGES OF THE CHILD

Childhood development traditionally is divided into age categories in which children display distinct social and cognitive characteristics (Erikson's stages of psychosocial development).

Infants (Birth to 18 Months)

Between birth and 18 months of age, children begin to develop trust in others. They require tactile comfort and are unable to tolerate sudden environmental changes. Loud noises may cause anxiety and fear. Between 7 months and 1 year, the child begins to fear separation from the parent or caregiver and usually has a strong mistrust of strangers. Transitional objects, such as a soft toy or blanket, are very comforting at this stage of development, and some facilities allow these to be brought into the surgical environment (they are labeled and returned to the parent or guardian for safekeeping). Parents may be

Table **35-1**	**Congenital and Genetic Abnormalities**	
Condition	**Description**	**Considerations**
Anencephaly	Congenital anomaly in which large parts of the brain fail to develop; occurs in 3 of 10,000 births.	Neonates with this lethal neural tube defect do not survive.
Atrial septal defect	Congenital cardiac defect in which a hole in the interatrial septum allows blood from the left atrium to flow into the right atrium.	Surgical repair is necessary to close the defect. See *Closure of an Atrial Septal Defect.*
Branchial cleft cysts and clefts	These are embryonic remnants or slits in the neck region that persist as cysts or fistulas after birth. They may not be diagnosed unless they interfere with structural function or become infected.	Surgical removal may be necessary.
Chest wall deformities	Two common chest wall deformities are *pectus excavatum* (PE) and *pectus carinatum* (PC). In PE the sternum is concave and may impinge on thoracic structures. In PC the sternum protrudes.	Surgical reconstruction is performed for cosmetic purposes or to relieve pressure on thoracic structures. See *Repair of Pectus Excavatum.*
Choanal atresia	Choanal atresia is a congenital anomaly characterized by a stricture or blockage of the passage between the nasal sinus and the pharyngonasal airways. Bilateral choanal atresia (both sides of the nasal passage are blocked) is a neonatal emergency; immediate treatment is required to maintain oxygen perfusion in the newborn.	Surgical repair is performed at birth in emergency cases. Endoscopic surgery and splinting of airways may be performed in nonemergency cases.
Cleft lip or palate	Partial or complete division of the lip or palate prevents the infant from suckling effectively. The defect occurs in about 1 in 700 live births.	Surgical reconstruction is performed in stages beginning at about 12 weeks of age. See *Repair of a Cleft Lip* and *Repair of a Cleft Palate.*
Coarctation of the aorta	Congenital narrowing of the thoracic aorta that restricts blood flow to the lower body.	Surgical treatment is necessary to restore circulation. See *Correction of Coarctation of the Aorta.*
Esophageal atresia	Complete or partial absence of the esophagus. The defect is associated with tracheoesophageal fistula (see below).	Surgical reconstruction of the esophagus is necessary for nutritional intake. See *Correction of Esophageal Atresia and Tracheoesophageal Fistula.*
Gastroschisis	An abdominal wall defect in which the viscera form outside the body. In this defect there is no sac surrounding the viscera. The cause is unknown.	Immediate surgical repair is required to preserve the viscera. See *Abdominal Wall Defects.*
Hirschsprung disease (megacolon)	Congenital absence of ganglion cells, which control the relaxation and contraction that occur in peristalsis of the bowel. This causes chronic bowel obstruction.	Surgery is performed to remove the disease bowel. See *Resection and Pull-Through for Hirschsprung Disease.*
Infantile hypertrophic pyloric stenosis (IHPS)	Also called *pyloric stenosis;* a congenital anomaly in which the longitudinal and circular muscles of the gastric pylorus are thickened. This results in obstruction at the pylorus.	Surgical treatment is performed to release the thickened bands of muscle and release the stricture. See *Pyloromyotomy.*
Omphalocele	A type of abdominal wall deformity in which the viscera develop outside the body, contained within a peritoneal sac.	Surgery is performed as soon as possible after birth to conserve the tissues involved. See *Repair of an Omphalocele.*
Patent ductus arteriosus	The ductus arteriosus is a fetal heart structure that shunts blood from the right ventricle into the systemic circulation. The ductus normally closes shortly after birth. A persistent or patent ductus arteriosus may result in heart failure	Surgical repair is necessary to close a patient ductus arteriosus. See *Closure of a Patent Ductus Arteriosus.*
Pulmonary valve stenosis	Congenital cardiac defect in which the pulmonary valve leaflets are fused, restricting circulation of blood from the right ventricle to the lungs.	Surgical repair is necessary to restore circulation. See *Correction of Pulmonary Valve Stenosis.*
Spina bifida	A congenital anomaly that includes several types of neural tube defects including incomplete closure of the bony spinal column around the spinal cord. The deformity often causes lower extremity paralysis and loss of bladder and bowel function. Spina bifida is associated with folic acid deficiency during pregnancy.	Surgical repair to close the superficial tissue layers is possible. However, nerve damage is not reversible. See *Repair of Myelomeningocele.*

Table 35-1	Congenital and Genetic Abnormalities—cont'd	
Condition	**Description**	**Considerations**
Syndactyly	Webbing of the fingers or toes as a result of incomplete separation of the digits in embryonic life.	See *Correction of Syndactyly*
Tetralogy of Fallot	A combination of congenital defects. The anomalies include pulmonary stenosis, ventricular septal defect, right ventricular hypertrophy, and transposition of the aorta.	Treatment is surgical repair of the defects. See *Repair of Tetralogy of Fallot.*
Tracheoesophageal fistula	A fistula connecting the esophagus with the trachea. The defect results in aspiration of liquid and food particles into the trachea.	The defect is surgically closed to prevent aspiration. See *Correction of Esophageal Atresia and Tracheoesophageal Fistula.*
Ventricular septal defect	Congenital cardiac defect in which blood from the left ventricle flows into the right ventricle and lungs, leading to congestive heart failure.	Surgical repair is necessary to close the defect. See *Closure of a Ventricular Septal Defect.*
Wilms tumor (nephroblastoma)	The most common primary renal malignancy of children. The tumor can become very large and spread from the abdomen to the lungs.	Surgical en bloc resection is performed when possible. The kidney, ureter, and adrenal gland are removed. More extensive dissection and resection may be required.

Box 35-1	Pediatric Age Groups

Neonate: Birth to 1 month
Infant: 1 month to 1 year
Toddler: 1 to 3 years
Preschooler: 3 to 6 years
School age: 6 to 10 years
Adolescent: 11 to 18 years

Box 35-2	Terms to Avoid (and Substitutes) in Caring for Pediatric Patients

Avoid	**Substitute**
Bad, no good	Good, good job!
Gas	Breeze, air
Stick, poke	Pinch
Strap in	Put on the safety belt
Stink	Smells funny
Feels strange	Feels funny
Cold water	Feels cool
Put to sleep	Nap

allowed into the operating room during induction and may be present in the postanesthesia care unit (PACU), depending on the facility's policy.

Toddlers and Preschoolers (3 to 6 Years)

Toddlers and preschoolers understand their environment in very literal terms and believe that they are personally responsible for events. A 3- or 4-year old may believe that surgery is a form of punishment or that the illness is the result of something the child did. Children in this age group have a strong fear of the unknown and show **magical thinking**, in which ordinary or inanimate objects have intentions (harmful or

benevolent). When communicating with the toddler or preschooler, health care professionals should give simple explanations and should avoid words that imply harm or injury. Children in this age group usually respond well to distraction as a means of soothing and calming.

Early and Middle School Age (6 to 12 Years)

Children in the early and middle school years use concrete reasoning (immediate experience) rather than complex abstract thinking; they are curious about objects and events in their environment. Children in this group fear harm and pain but are able to comprehend simple explanations of cause and effect. Patients in this age group can be comforted by knowing what to expect. All children have a need for privacy; however, children in this age group may have a heightened sense of invasion when exposed.

Adolescence (12 to 18 Years)

Patients between 12 and 18 years are able to project the significance of current events into the future. They understand the consequences of their illness but often focus on the social rather than the physical aspects. Among their greatest concerns are separation from their peers (including rejection by peers) and loss of mobility. A change in body image caused by a perceived disfigurement can be very disturbing. Disruption of their normal routines, especially those that contribute to socialization, is also upsetting. Fear of exposure and loss of privacy are extremely important in this age group, especially in middle adolescence.

Adolescents often reject or are mistrustful of care by strangers and need to demonstrate personal independence. This aspect of development increases their stoicism and they may refuse to take pain medication or to report pain, even when it is severe. Patients in this age group often find it difficult to admit fear, but they usually are grateful for straightforward, "no-nonsense" explanations of what is happening in their environment and why.

CASE PLANNING

ANESTHESIA

Many procedures that otherwise could be carried out using regional anesthesia or monitored sedation are performed in the pediatric patient using general anesthesia. This is partly because general anesthesia allows the anesthesia care provider to secure the airway and maintain full respiratory control during the procedure. General anesthesia is also necessary because children are unable to cooperate during regional anesthesia.

The differences between adult and pediatric anesthesia are primarily related to physiological and anatomical variations between the two populations. Important considerations in learning about pediatric anesthesia are:

1. Anesthesia (and surgery) involves the entire family, not just the patient.
2. Children are much more sensitive to small variations in drug doses than are adults.
3. IV fluids are commonly administered with microdrip tubing and a burette chamber. This provides accurate measurement of fluids.
4. Pediatric patients often are induced and maintained with inhalation anesthesia by mask or by laryngeal or endotracheal tube. Inhalation anesthetics are taken up quickly by the brain, allowing rapid induction.
5. IV access is usually obtained after induction to avoid patient struggling and anxiety.
6. Oral intake is restricted preoperatively in pediatric patients to reduce the risk of aspiration during anesthesia. As a general rule, clear liquids are withheld for 2 hours before surgery and breast milk for 4 hours. Solid food is withheld for 6 hours before surgery.[1]
7. Children are unable to cooperate fully during procedures that could otherwise be performed under regional anesthesia and therefore require a general anesthetic more often.

Preparation for Anesthesia

Pediatric patients are assessed and prepared for anesthesia using methods similar to those for adults. However, the psychological preparation must take into consideration the child's more extreme fears, especially the trauma of separation and fear of not waking up. Whenever possible, the family is prepared for the experience of anesthesia at least 4 days before surgery. Age-appropriate preparation may include familiarizing the child with anesthesia devices, surgical attire, and other objects that can cause anxiety. A brief review of preoperative preparation as it applies to pediatric patients is presented here:

1. A preoperative history is taken, including current health status, chronic and acute conditions, history of past diseases, and previous surgery.
2. The patient's current medications, anesthesia history, and allergies are recorded.
3. A review of systems is performed (i.e., routine physical assessment of each system).
4. The results of routine laboratory tests are reviewed.
5. Additional tests are requested as needed.
6. The preoperative medication and induction method are discussed with the family.
7. Special considerations for children are taken into account (e.g., loose or missing teeth, cardiac defects, croup, history of apnea, recent respiratory infection).

Preoperative Medication and Induction

Pediatric patients may be given an anxiolytic (anxiety-reducing) medication before surgery. However, this practice varies from institution to institution and among anesthesia care providers. Preoperative sedation may delay recovery from anesthesia and the method of administration (injection or a bitter-tasting oral medication) may increase anxiety in the child. Other drawbacks include an increased risk of falls and adverse physiological events, such as respiratory depression. If preoperative medication is required, a number of drugs are available (Table 35-2).

Table **35-2** Common Preoperative Medications Used in Pediatric Surgery		
Agent/Drug	**Route**	**Comments**
H$_2$ blocker (ranitidine, famotidine)	Oral, intravenous (IV)	Prevents gastrin-stimulated acid secretion
Ketamine	Intramuscular injection	Produces anesthesia within 3 minutes
	Oral	May be combined with midazolam for mask induction
Lidocaine 2.5% and prilocaine 2.5% (EMLA cream)	Topical	Applied to the skin before insertion of an IV cannula to reduce the pain of insertion
Methohexital (Brevital)	Rectal	Produces sleep within about 10 minutes
Metoclopramide (Reglan)	Oral or IV	Antiemetic
Midazolam (Versed)	Oral	May be administered by the parent
	Intranasal	Produces peak effect in 30 minutes
	Sublingual	May prolong anesthesia recovery
	Rectal	Causes antegrade amnesia after 10 minutes
Oral transmucosal fentanyl citrate	Oral transmucosal	May be used in lollipop form for pain relief in short procedures

INDUCTION Allowing one or both parents to be present during induction now is an accepted practice in many health care facilities. This has proved to reduce the need for preoperative medication in many pediatric patients. Parents who are not fearful themselves may stay with the patient from the time of arrival in the surgical department through the entire induction process. Patients older than 4 years are the best candidates for parental presence during induction. Infants and young children may be induced in the parent's or nurse's arms. The method of induction depends on the following conditions:

- The child's age
- Whether there is IV access
- The presence of a parent
- The preference and skill of the anesthesia care provider
- The American Society of Anesthesiologists (ASA) case classification (see Chapter 14)

Anesthesia may be induced by a combination of methods or by a single method:

- Mask inhalation
- Intramuscular injection
- Rectal administration
- Oral administration
- IV administration

If the child already has an IV line, intravenous induction with thiopental or propofol (Diprivan) is often administered for rapid, safe induction. Inhalation induction is easily performed with a cooperative child. The child can be asked to try on a mask and is praised for compliance. Even if the child refuses the mask, it can be held below the face. As soon as the child becomes sleepy, the mask can be fitted over the face. A child who arrives asleep may be administered an anesthetic through this "blow-by" method and quickly induced during sleep.

ANESTHESIA MAINTENANCE After induction or just before, the precordial stethoscope, pulse oximeter, and cardiac electrodes are placed. IV access is secured when the child is unconscious. Inhalation anesthesia is maintained through an endotracheal tube. Continuous inhalation anesthesia by mask can be used for short procedures (lasting less than 1 hour). Intraoperative monitoring is carried out as in adults and includes a minimum of electrocardiography, pulse oximetry, respiratory function, and blood pressure.

EMERGENCE AND RECOVERY When anesthetic agents are withdrawn or reversed, the patient experiences increased physiological stress from pain and other strong stimuli. The child's response during emergence from anesthesia depends on whether opioids, sedatives, or benzodiazepines were given. These can prolong emergence but also contribute to a smoother recovery. Patients who have had a routine surgical procedure without complications may remain in the operating room until the airway reflexes are intact and the endotracheal tube is removed. If the patient is to be transported to the intensive care unit, the endotracheal tube may be left in place and the patient maintained on ventilation. After the patient is admitted to the PACU, parents usually are permitted to remain with the child for comfort and reassurance.

The most common postanesthesia complications in pediatric patients are postoperative nausea and vomiting, which occur in 40% to 50% of children. Other, less common events include respiratory depression and delirium during emergence. (Chapter 14 presents a complete discussion of postanesthesia complications.)

SAFETY OF THE PEDIATRIC PATIENT

Pediatric specialization involves the same domains of safety required in surgery of the adult. The surgical technologist maintains a safe environment in collaboration with other members of the perioperative team. Pediatric patients *are particularly vulnerable* to risks related to their age, size, and stage of development. The student should review environmental risks that apply to all patients, which are covered in previous chapters. Specific risks and concerns are described in Table 35-3.

SAFE HANDLING OF DRUGS

Because of their small size and undeveloped organ systems, pediatric patients are at high risk of adverse events from overdosing. The surgical technologist participates in the medication process while in the scrubbed role. Pediatric medications are prescribed according to the child's weight in kilograms and the correct dose must be verified by the surgeon, circulating registered nurse, and technologist. Cumulative amounts of drugs, such as local anesthetics and vasoconstriction agents, given throughout the procedure must be recorded and tracked *in real time* to prevent an overdose. All safety precautions discussed in Chapter 13 apply to the pediatric patient, with special emphasis on the potential risks of errors made in measuring, dispensing, and documentation.

TRANSPORT OF THE PEDIATRIC PATIENT

Neonates and infants usually are transported to the operating room in a heated Isolette. Occasionally, a neonate may be carried to the operating room by a parent. Young children may walk to the surgical department (for outpatient cases) and are placed on a stretcher in the holding area for transportation to the operating suite. Transporting an inpatient toddler can present challenges because of this age group's innate curiosity and agility. The hospital crib is equipped with side and bottom pads and a flexible top may be used over the crib. During transport, a child may attempt to climb over the crib or stretcher rails. Also, it is critical to ensure that the child does not extend a limb through the rails.

POSITIONING THE PATIENT

The principles of safe patient positioning apply to pediatric patients as well as adults. Although the principles are the same

Table 35-3	Risks in the Perioperative Care of Pediatric Patients		
Domain of Care	**Specific Risk**	**Precautions/Prevention**	**Rationale**
Electrosurgery	Burns	• Use a pediatric-size patient return electrode (PRE) according to the manufacturer's specifications. • Never cut a PRE.	A PRE must be the correct size to properly disperse electricity flowing from the active electrode through the patient's body.
Patient transport	Falls	• Never turn your attention away from the patient during transport. • Do not abandon the patient *for any reason*. • Make sure that crib rails are secure.	Children (especially toddlers) are curious and extremely active. A child can quickly climb over the top of a crib or over stretcher rails.
Skin prep	Chemical burn Hypothermia	• Prep solutions may be diluted to prevent skin burns. • Follow the surgeon's orders for solution strength. • Use warmed solutions to prevent loss of body heat.	Infants and toddlers have very delicate skin. About 60% to 75% of body heat is lost through radiation. Additional cooling by evaporation can rapidly cause hypothermia.
Positioning	Skeletal injury	• Follow all the usual precautions for positioning the patient. • Pay careful attention to moving the patient's body within the normal range of motion. • Provide ample padding over skin, nerves, and blood vessels.	Children's joints are very flexible but fragile. Limbs and joints may be overstretched, causing injury because of the patient's small stature and apparent flexibility.
Surgical technique	Injury to body tissue	• Do not put any pressure on the patient's body (e.g., from heavy instruments, tension from power cords, or leaning over the patient during surgery).	Bruising and other injury can result from weight or pressure, not directly observed because drapes hide the patient's body. Pressure on the thorax may result in respiratory compromise.

for adults and children, it is important to use appropriate-size padding to fit the pediatric patient. Gel and foam pads are appropriate for infants and children, whose delicate skin must be protected from shearing pressure injury at all times. When creating a surgical position, the surgical technologist must keep in mind that a child's joints are extremely flexible. Care must be taken to move the patient's body within the normal range of motion and to consider anatomical restrictions related to injury or congenital defect. Adhesive tape should not be used when positioning children, because it can cause severe skin injury. Instead, soft Velcro straps designed for use with foam pads and supports should be used.

ELECTROSURGERY

All types of electrosurgical units (ESUs) are used in pediatric procedures, including monopolar and bipolar (high-frequency or radiofrequency) units. The safety principles for adult electrosurgery are the same for pediatric patients. The primary differences are the size of the active electrodes and the patient return electrodes (PREs). Active electrodes are selected according to the tissue and location in the body. Special pediatric-size PREs are used on children according to the child's weight. The parameters for size are established by the manufacturer of the electrode and must be followed. A PRE must *never* be cut or trimmed, because this can result in patient injury. (Chapter 18 presents a complete discussion of electrosurgery hazards for adults and pediatric patients.)

INSTRUMENTS

Pediatric instrument sets are assembled for a specialty such as cardiac, genitourinary, or gastrointestinal surgery. The instruments themselves may be smaller in all dimensions, or only the tips (working ends) may be smaller. For example, adult microsurgical instruments and those used in eye surgery often are used in pediatric plastic and genitourinary procedures. Fine scissors, needle holders, forceps, and calipers are found across these specialties. Pediatric instruments used in general surgery include a greater number of mosquito forceps (to replace Kelly and Crile clamps) and short Babcock and Allis clamps. Plastic shods (short lengths of plastic or silastic tubing) should be available to place over the tips of fine hemostats and should be available for all tag clamps. Smaller retractors (e.g., narrow Deaver, small Richardson, and "baby Balfour" retractors) are suited to children older than toddlers. Smaller self-retaining retractors are useful in pediatric general surgery, such as the small Weitlaner and various small spring retractors from thyroid and vascular surgery.

Minimally invasive techniques use very small trocars and endoscopes, which are designed in proportion to an infant or a child's body size. The instruments themselves are shorter and have finer tips than the adult-size versions.

SPONGES

Sponges used in open pediatric procedures usually (but not always) are smaller than those used in adult procedures. Radiopaque 4×4 sponges and 4×18 lap sponges are commonly used in pediatric procedures. Dissecting sponges must be mounted on a clamp, as in adult surgery; however, smaller, shorter clamps are used. For example, short ring forceps (sponge clamps) are used for 4 × 4 sponges. Mayo clamps, rather than long Péan clamps, are used for sponge dissectors. The guidelines and protocols for using only radiopaque sponges in the body cavity apply in pediatric surgery, just as in adult surgery.

SUTURES

Pediatric sutures naturally are smaller to meet the needs of more delicate tissues. In general, suture materials more often are absorbable than synthetic, except in cardiac, orthopedic, and reconstructive surgery. Nylon, Prolene, and other monofilament sutures are commonly used for skin and other connective tissues because they are the least reactive and rarely tear when pulled through tissue. The size of sutures depends on the patient's age and the tissue involved. Skin most often is closed with subcuticular sutures and colloidal skin adhesive.

SURGICAL PROCEDURES

REPAIR OF A CLEFT LIP

Surgical Goal

Repair of a cleft lip involves the closure of a cleft defect in the lip.

Pathology

The *philtrum* (the groove that extends from the upper lip to the nose) is formed during embryonic development by the joining of the median nasal processes. The lateral portions of the upper lip are formed by the maxillary processes. These formations occur during the first 8 weeks of development. Interruption of normal development and closure of these structures may result in a cleft lip. The cleft may be complete or incomplete and unilateral or bilateral. Bilateral cleft lip often is associated with clefts of the soft palate. An infant with a cleft lip is referred to a surgeon immediately after birth. The cleft is repaired in stages and the initial repair is performed at 10 to 12 weeks of age (Figure 35-3).

TECHNIQUE

1 The incision and anatomical landmarks are marked.
2 Incisions are made along the marked incision lines.
3 Dissection is performed.
4 The defect is closed.
5 Splints or dressings are applied.

Discussion

Pediatric plastic instruments are used to repair facial abnormalities. The patient is placed in the supine position with the head on a doughnut headrest and the arms at the sides. Before the prep, the surgeon draws the anatomical landmarks and the planned incisions on the skin with a skin scribe. If local anesthetic is to be used, it is injected at this time. The patient is prepped with povidone-iodine solution and then draped for a head and neck procedure.

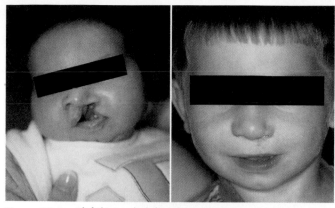

Figure 35-3 Cleft lip and cleft palate. This anomaly occurs in the first 8 weeks of embryonic life as a result of incomplete closure of the maxilla. *Left,* Three-month-old patient. *Right,* Patient at 5 years. *(From Townsend CM, Beauchamp DR, Evers MB, Mattox KL: Sabiston textbook of surgery, ed 18, Philadelphia, 2007, WB Saunders.)*

The incision is made with a #11 blade along the vermilion border toward the cleft-side midline. Double- or single-prong skin hooks are used for retraction, and the mucosa is separated off the orbicularis oris muscle with a #11 knife or tenotomy scissors. The surgeon then detaches the medial lip from the maxilla by incising the cleft at the top of the labial sulcus. This releases the medial lip.

A Z-plasty incision is made through the skin, muscle, and mucosa with a #11 or #15 blade. Hemostasis is maintained with the ESU. The procedure is repeated on the lateral portion of the cleft. When the dissection has been completed and the Z-plasty flaps have been created, the wound is ready to be closed. The mucosa is closed with interrupted absorbable sutures. The muscle then is closed with subcuticular absorbable sutures through the tips of the Z-plasty flaps. The vermilion border is closed with a subcuticular suture. The skin then is closed with absorbable suture (Figure 35-4).

REPAIR OF A CLEFT PALATE

Surgical Goal

Repair of a cleft palate involves closure of the palate to restore normal function.

Pathology

In the development of the midface, the palate arises from the joining of the medial nasal prominences on each side of the oral cavity to the maxillary prominence. Failure of these structures to meet results in a cleft palate. The degree of clefting can be complete or incomplete, depending on the level of fusion that occurred during embryonic development. Although cleft palate sometimes is seen in conjunction with cleft lip, they are separate malformations and are rarely related to one another. Infants with this condition are referred to a surgeon shortly after birth. However, the defects usually are not repaired until the infant is 11 to 12 months old to avoid interference with facial growth.

Before surgical repair of the palate, the infant may require myringotomy with tube placement, because cleft palate often is associated with chronic ear infection and partial deafness. The infant also may be fitted with a palatal prosthesis to allow for easier feeding until the time of repair.

TECHNIQUE

1 The incision is injected with a local anesthetic.
2 Incisions are made in the palate and the muscle.
3 The flaps are prepared.
4 The palatal incisions are closed.
5 The flaps are closed.
6 Dressings are applied.

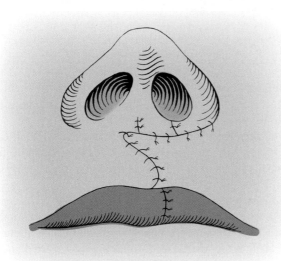

Figure 35-4   Repair of cleft lip.—rotation-advancement technique. *(From Cummings C, Flint P, Haughey B, Robbins K, Thomas J, et al: Otolaryngology: head and neck surgery, ed 4, Philadelphia, 2005, Mosby.)*

Discussion

The patient is placed in the supine position with the head on a doughnut headrest and with a shoulder roll to hyperextend the head. The surgeon may insert the cleft palate mouth gag, or Dingman mouth gag, before the prep. The palate is injected with a local anesthetic with epinephrine. This injection is given before the prep so that the hemostatic effects of the epinephrine have time to begin working before the initial incision. The patient then is prepped with povidone-iodine scrub and paint. If the mouth gag is already in place, it also must be prepped.

The surgeon first suspends the mouth gag from the Mayo stand. Once the gag is attached, the scrub must avoid jarring the Mayo stand because this can severely injure the patient.

The surgeon makes the initial incisions along the borders of the mucosa with a #15 blade. The incisions are extended through the oral mucosa, muscle, and nasal mucosa with a cleft palate blade (#6910 Beaver blade). After making the incisions, the surgeon elevates the nasal mucosa off the underlying muscle with the cleft palate blade and a Freer or Cottle elevator. This step is performed on both sides of the cleft. Figure 35-5 shows a rotation flap approach.

Next, the surgeon separates the oral mucosa from the overlying muscle. This step is performed in the same fashion as in the nasal mucosa. This creates three layers for closure.

After the mucosa has been elevated to the most lateral edges, the incisions are closed. The nasal mucosa is closed first with 4-0 absorbable suture on a 6-inch (15 cm) Crile-Wood needle holder and DeBakey forceps. The muscle is closed with 4-0 absorbable suture. The oral mucosa is closed with 4-0 or 5-0 absorbable suture. After closing the palate, the surgeon examines the wound and releases any areas under tension. The wound then is irrigated, and the mouth gag is removed.

Infants can begin to take liquids by sippy cup shortly after surgery. Any feeding method that involves sucking (bottles,

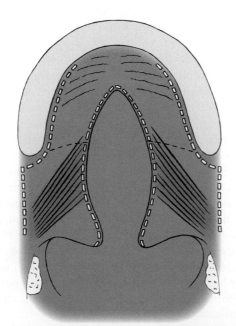
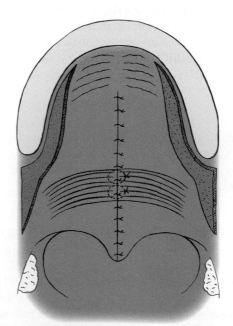

Figure 35-5   Repair of cleft palate using rotation closure. *Dotted lines* show lines of incision. *(From Cummings C, Flint P, Haughey B, Robbins K, Thomas J, et al: Otolaryngology: head and neck surgery, ed 4, Philadelphia, 2005, Mosby.)*

straws, cups with valves) is not used because this can disrupt the repair. Some surgeons require their postoperative patients to wear arm restraints for several weeks. This prevents the infant from putting anything in the mouth, which might disturb the repair.

OTOPLASTY

Surgical Goal

Otoplasty is performed to reconstruct the external ear after a traumatic injury or to correct protruding ears.

Pathology

Otoplasty can be performed in children or adults. In children, it usually is performed to reattach the ear closer to the head. This condition usually is the result of the absence or small size of the antihelical fold in the external ear (Figure 35-6). The repairs usually are performed before the patient starts school. The external ear may also be reconstructed after traumatic injury caused by fire, animal bites, or other accidents. Loss of the external ear or protruding ears can cause great anxiety and stress in children and can affect their social development and body image. A procedure for protruding ears is presented here; reconstruction of the ear is discussed later in the chapter.

TECHNIQUE

1 The antihelical fold is marked.
2 The posterior ear is injected with epinephrine and an ellipse of skin is excised.
3 Cartilage near the antihelical fold is incised and the anterior surface is scored.
4 Suture is placed in the cartilage.
5 The skin is closed.
6 Dressings are applied.

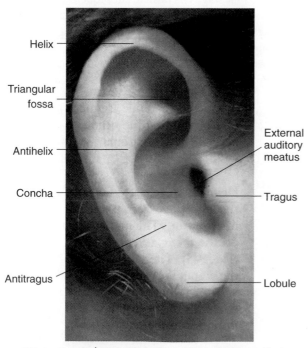

Figure 35-6 External ear. *(From Thibodeau G, Patton K: Anatomy and physiology, ed 6, Philadelphia, Mosby, 2007.)*

Labels on figure: Helix, Triangular fossa, Antihelix, Concha, Antitragus, External auditory meatus, Tragus, Lobule

Discussion

The patient is placed in the supine position with the affected ear up and the unaffected ear heavily padded to cushion pressure. The arms are tucked at the sides to give the surgeon full access to the head. The patient is prepped and a body and head drape is applied. If both ears are affected, a Mayfield headrest, which allows access to both ears, may be useful for positioning the head.

The antihelical fold is marked by the placement of 22-gauge needles that have been dipped in methylene blue. The surgeon performs this step by folding the external ear against the head and then inserting and withdrawing the needles from anterior to posterior. This procedure produces marks through all layers of the tissue. The scrub should have calipers available for this part of the procedure. The surgeon then injects the posterior ear with epinephrine, with or without a local anesthetic, and excises an ellipse of skin with a #15 blade and Adson toothed forceps or Brown-Adson forceps. Double-prong skin hooks are used to retract the skin flaps and the underlying tissue is elevated with a Freer elevator.

The cartilage can be scored with a #15 blade, making it more pliable, and then sutured in the postauricular area close to the head. An alternative technique is to excise the cartilage to create an antihelical fold, or it can be thinned with a power shaver to allow it to be molded. A 4-0 nonabsorbable suture (e.g., Mersilene, clear nylon, or polydioxanone surgical [PDS] suture) may be used to hold the cartilage in place.

The skin incision is closed with 3-0 absorbable suture. A bulky mastoid dressing consisting of Telfa, Kerlix fluffs, and Kerlix rolls is applied to the ear. This gives the newly formed ear adequate support and protection.

RECONSTRUCTION OF THE EAR

Surgical Goal

Congenital anomalies, which often accompany defects of the outer ear structure, require extensive surgical repair. In this procedure, only the cosmetic defect is addressed.

Pathology

Microtia is a congenital defect in which all or part of the external ear is missing. The deformity also affects the inner ear, resulting in deafness. Reconstructive surgery is performed in childhood before the patient reaches school age. Microtia may be present at birth or can be caused by accidents such as fire, dog bite, or other trauma.

Discussion

Reconstruction of the ear is performed in multiple stages with several operations. The technique varies, depending on the type and severity of the defect. A common method of reconstruction is to raise the skin where the ear normally would lie and insert a graft taken from the patient's costal cartilage. The tragus then is elevated in stages and the folds and ear lobe are created using grafts and skin flap techniques.

When an autograft is to be used, the patient is placed in the supine position. The surgeon creates a template (pattern) for the graft by placing a sheet of transparent material over the unaffected ear and tracing its outline on the material. The

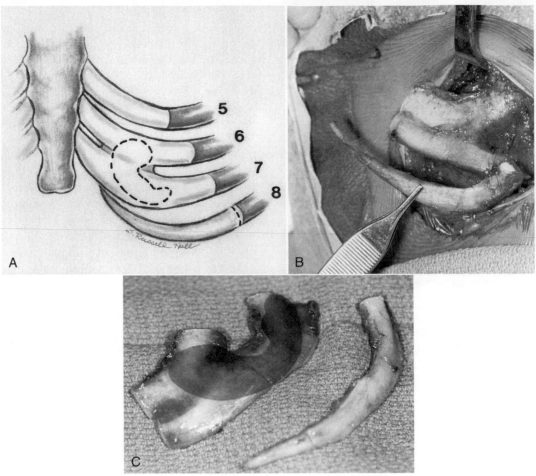

Figure 35-7 Reconstruction of the ear for microtia. **A,** A template is placed over the costal cartilage, and an autograft is removed from the tissue. **B** and **C,** Two separate graft components are required, for the pinna and the helix. *(From Cummings C, Flint P, Haughey B, Robbins K, Thomas J, et al: Otolaryngology: head and neck surgery, ed 4, Philadelphia, 2005, Mosby.)*

template then is placed over the affected ear and the ear remnants are traced on the template.

The surgeon makes an incision over the seventh, eighth, or ninth intercostal space. The template is placed over the costal cartilage and the tissue is excised, following the outline of the template. The incision is closed in layers in routine fashion.

The graft is shaped to form the basis of the pinna and helix. This is done with a power drill and small burr attachment. The surgeon may choose to work at the back table or at a separate draped table. The technologist should make sure that carving instruments, burrs, and elevators are neatly assembled for the surgeon's use. Clear nylon or fine stainless steel sutures are used to assemble the graft components. After the graft has been prepared, it is preserved in a safe location on the back table.

To prepare the implant site for the graft, the surgeon outlines the postauricular area where the graft will be inserted. The skin is incised and small bleeders are controlled with a needle-tip ESU. The skin is undermined and the graft is inserted into the skin pocket. The surgeon pulls the skin over the graft and sutures it in place. The lobe is transferred from the existing ear remnant. This completes the first stage of the reconstruction.

When the first stage has healed, subsequent operations are done to raise the frame of the ear and to construct the folds and recesses of the outer ear. These steps are performed by incising flaps of adjacent skin and rotating them into position. Fine sutures of nylon, Prolene, or other synthetic material are used to suture the flaps in place. Bulky dressings are used after ear repair to protect the reconstructed tissues from injury during healing. Figures 35-7 and 35-8 illustrate the techniques involved in ear reconstruction.

CORRECTION OF ESOPHAGEAL ATRESIA AND TRACHEOESOPHAGEAL FISTULA

Surgical Goal

The goal of surgical repair of esophageal atresia (EA) is to restore continuity of the esophagus. In repair of a tracheoesophageal fistula (TEF), an abnormal opening between the trachea and the esophagus is closed to prevent the flow of food and saliva from the esophagus to the lungs.

Pathology

Esophageal **atresia** (the absence or closure of a normal anatomical orifice) is a nongenetic defect in which the esophagus

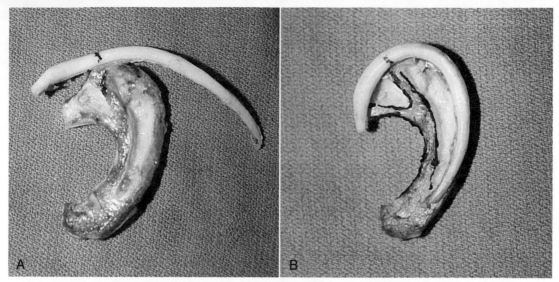

Figure 35-8 Construction of the implant taken from the costal cartilage. A, The framework is shaped with cutting burrs and carving instruments. B, The components are assembled using clear nylon or fine stainless steel sutures. (From Cummings C, Flint P, Haughey B, Robbins K, Thomas J, et al: Otolaryngology: head and neck surgery, ed 4, Philadelphia, 2005, Mosby.)

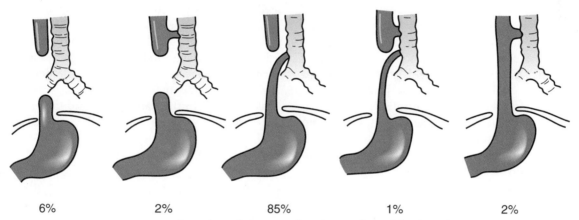

| 6% | 2% | 85% | 1% | 2% |

Figure 35-9 Variations of esophageal atresia and tracheoesophageal fistula, with the percentage of such defects represented by each variation. (From Townsend CM, Beauchamp DR, Evers MB, Mattox KL: Sabiston textbook of surgery, ed 18, Philadelphia, 2007, WB Saunders.)

is interrupted. The upper or proximal portion terminates in a blind pouch that does not communicate with the distal esophagus. Numerous variations of the anomaly can be seen, often including a tracheoesophageal fistula (Figure 35-9). A TEF is a direct passageway or duct between either esophageal section (distal or proximal) and the trachea.

Esophageal atresia prevents the normal passage of food and saliva to the stomach. A TEF between the proximal esophageal segment and the trachea causes aspiration of saliva and milk into the trachea and lungs; a TEF in the distal esophageal segment causes gastric secretions to flow into the lungs. EA may exist as a single anomaly or, more commonly, with TEF.

EA/TEF is associated with a number of other birth defects, some of which are lethal. These include:

- Imperforate anus
- Ventricular and atrial septal defect
- Tetralogy of Fallot
- Limb deformities
- Neural tube defect

In addition to these and other anomalies, the fetus with EA/TEF is prevented from swallowing amniotic fluid, a source of nutrition in fetal life. This results in low neonatal birth weight and size.

Surgical options for the correction of EA/TEF depend on the type and severity of the defect. Staged or delayed repair may be necessary if other life-threatening conditions (e.g., cardiac defects) take precedence or to allow normal growth and elongation of the esophagus. A colon graft may be used to elongate the esophagus, although primary closure is preferred when possible. Primary repair (anastomosis of the two esophageal segments) is performed when the two segments can be brought together and the infant's general physiological condition is good. An isolated TEF without EA can be repaired through a cervical approach. Primary closure of EA is described here.

TECHNIQUE

1 A right posterolateral thoracotomy is performed.
2 The tracheoesophageal fistula (TEF) is identified and retracted.
3 The TEF is divided and closed.
4 The proximal and distal esophageal pouches are mobilized.
5 The esophageal ends are excised and trimmed.
6 An end-to-end or end-to-side anastomosis is performed.
7 A chest tube may be placed.
8 The wound is closed.

Discussion

The technologist should have pediatric general surgical and thoracic instruments available. Silastic vessel loops and sponge dissectors should also be available. A pediatric Finochietto retractor is commonly used for retraction. The infant is placed in thoracotomy position with the head of the operating table slightly elevated. The prep extends from the neck to the iliac crest and includes the anterior and posterior chest.

The knife is used to make a transverse, posterolateral thoracotomy incision and the ESU is used to extend it into the latissimus muscles. Rake retractors can be used to retract the skin and subcutaneous layers while the muscle and fascia are divided. The scapula is retracted and the chest cavity is entered by incising the intercostal muscles. The ESU is used to divide the muscles. This exposes the pleura, which is dissected from the chest wall with small sponge dissectors. A Finochietto retractor is placed in the wound and pleural dissection continues to expose the azygos vein. This is clamped, ligated with 4-0 silk suture, and divided.

The esophageal defect is assessed. The anesthesia care provider advances the preplaced Replogle tube (nasogastric decompression tube). This demonstrates the blind proximal esophageal pouch. The TEF is located and encircled with a Silastic vessel loop. The fistula then is excised with fine dissecting scissors. The tracheal opening is closed with interrupted sutures of 4-0 or 5-0 absorbable synthetic suture. The surgeon tests the closure with warm saline irrigation solution. Bleeders are controlled with the ESU.

The proximal and distal esophageal segments are grasped with Babcock clamps, and the anastomosis site is examined. The surgeon excises the proximal pouch with fine dissecting scissors and smooth forceps. The distal portion, which is larger, is also excised to fit the proximal segment. An end-to-end anastomosis may be planned, or the proximal segment may be implanted in a circular incision made in the distal portion of the esophagus. The Replogle tube is advanced across the anastomosis site and traction sutures are placed through the esophageal segments. Absorbable 5-0 or 6-0 synthetic suture is used to create a single-layer anastomosis. Surgical alternatives include a double-layer closure and variations in the anastomosis to prevent tension on the esophagus. The Replogle tube may be left in place or withdrawn.

The wound is irrigated with warm saline, and bleeders are controlled with the ESU. A small chest tube maybe placed in the extrapleural space. The wound then is closed in layers with absorbable synthetic sutures.

Care of the infant immediately after surgery focuses mainly on the airway. Pharyngeal secretions are suctioned frequently for the first few days until the infant is able to swallow. The chest tubes are securely maintained and the incision sites are monitored for leakage or blockage. Oral feeding begins 2 to 6 days after surgery, after contrast studies have shown that the anastomosis is secure. Complications include infection, recurrent TEF, and leakage of the anastomosis.

PYLOROMYOTOMY

Surgical Goal

Pyloromyotomy is surgery to correct infantile hypertrophic pyloric stenosis, or simply **pyloric stenosis,** a thickening of the pylorus that results in stricture at the gastric outlet. The goal of surgery is to release the pyloric muscle fibers by incising them. This relaxes the gastric opening and allows food to pass normally out of the stomach into the intestine.

Pathology

Pyloric stenosis is a congenital anomaly involving the longitudinal and circular muscle fibers of the gastric outlet. The pylorus (or gastric outlet) of the stomach is enlarged and edematous, causing food to be regurgitated almost immediately after intake. This leads to dehydration and failure to thrive. The condition is about four times more common in male children. In the Ramstedt procedure, the muscle of the hypertrophic pylorus is split, and the mucosa is left intact.

TECHNIQUE

1 A right upper (subcostal) transverse incision is made.
2 The greater curvature of the stomach (near the pylorus) is grasped with a noncrushing clamp and brought out through the incision.
3 The anterior pylorus is incised.
4 A blunt instrument is used to split the muscle fibers.
5 The wound is closed.
6 The skin is closed with subcuticular suture.

Discussion

Ramstedt pyloromyotomy is commonly performed to treat pyloric stenosis. Either an open or a minimally invasive technique may be used. The open procedure is described here.

The infant is placed in the supine position. The chest and abdomen are prepped with an iodophor-povidone solution and draped for a laparotomy.

A 1- to 1.2-inch (2.5- to 3-cm) transverse incision is made in the right upper quadrant over the right rectus muscle. The fascial layers are divided transversely, but the rectus muscle is either retracted laterally or split in the middle. The edge of the liver is retracted superiorly, exposing the greater curvature of the stomach (near the pylorus), which is grasped with a noncrushing clamp and brought out through the incision. A damp gauze sponge is used to grasp the stomach, and with traction inferiorly and laterally, the pylorus is delivered from the

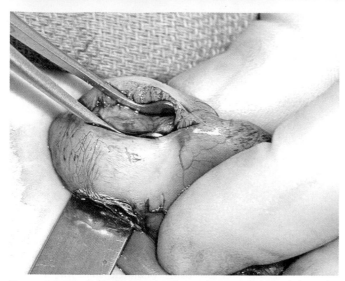

Figure 35-10   Pyloromyotomy. The pylorus is delivered from the wound and a short incision is made through the muscle layers. Here a pyloric spreader is used to release the muscle tissue. *(From Townsend CM, Beauchamp DR, Evers MB, Mattox KL: Sabiston textbook of surgery, ed 18, Philadelphia, 2007, WB Saunders.)*

incision. The ESU or knife is used to incise the serosa on the anterior wall of the pylorus to the level of the submucosa. A curved hemostat or pyloric spreader may be used to open out the muscle fibers and enlarge the pylorus (Figure 35-10). The pylorus is returned to the abdomen, and the abdominal incision is closed with 3-0 and 4-0 absorbable sutures. A flat dressing is placed over the wound.

RESECTION AND PULL-THROUGH FOR HIRSCHSPRUNG DISEASE

Surgical Goal

The goal of pull-through surgery for Hirschsprung disease (megacolon) is resection and reconstruction of the distal colon to restore functional peristalsis and prevent bowel obstruction.

Pathology

The normal intestine provides absorption, motility, secretion, and blood flow through a set of complex nerve plexuses that are nearly independent of the central nervous system. Reflexes for stool motility are located in the distal rectum. A **bolus** in this region causes the bowel to contract above the bolus and relax below it, moving stool through the sphincter. Hirschsprung disease is characterized by a congenital absence of ganglion cells, which control the relaxation and contraction that occur in peristalsis. The affected tissue begins at the anus and may extend proximally, causing functional obstruction in both the aganglionic and normal portions of the bowel. Severe distention, or megacolon, occurs in the bowel and abdomen.

Diagnosis of Hirschsprung disease is confirmed by rectal biopsy. The problem should be recognized soon after birth in neonates who have not passed meconium within the first 24 to 48 hours. Delayed diagnosis may result in necrotizing enterocolitis, which often is fatal if not treated promptly.

A colostomy may be performed soon after birth and intestinal correction delayed, or a single-stage procedure (without colostomy) may be performed in the first 48 hours of life. Many variations are possible for the procedure, which involves resection of the diseased bowel, endorectal pull-through of the distal colon, and anastomosis to the rectal musculature. This technique is similar to reconstruction after abdominoperineal resection (see Chapter 23).

TECHNIQUE

1. A left paramedian incision is made and if a colostomy is present, it is excised.
2. The sigmoid colon is mobilized and the superior hemorrhoidal vessels are divided.
3. Frozen section specimens may be taken to determine the presence of ganglia.
4. The pelvis is entered, the lateral rectal ligaments are divided, and the rectum is further mobilized
5. A long clamp (e.g., Babcock or ring forceps) is inserted transanally and a segment of the dissected colon is grasped.
6. Using counterpressure from the pelvis, the colon is everted and "pulled through" the anus.
7. The layers of the everted bowel are circumferentially incised and absorbable suture is used to anchor the rim of the retained portion of the colon to the rectum.
8. The diseased portion of bowel is divided and the anastomosis is performed with absorbable synthetic suture.
9. At the completion of this portion of the procedure, gowns, gloves, and setup are changed in preparation for the abdominal portion of the procedure.
10. The proximal edge of the muscular cuff is approximated to the seromuscular layer of the colon, completing the abdominal anastomosis.
11. The abdomen is irrigated and closed.

BOWEL RECONSTRUCTION FOR IMPERFORATE ANUS

Surgical Goal

Repair of an imperforate anus provides continuity of the lower intestinal tract to the outside of the body.

Pathology

An imperforate anus is a congenital malformation of the anorectal system in which the rectum and anus do not communicate with the outside of the body. This is one of many types of anorectal malformations that can occur during embryonic development. An imperforate anus may occur alone or in association with other anomalies of the genitourinary system. The defect may present in a variety of forms and is graded as high or low, depending on the severity and the location of rectal tissue in the distal gut. In the low form, which is the easier type to repair, the rectum has descended through the sphincter system. In more complex presentations, the rectum does not descend through the sphincter mechanism, and the malformation can include rectovaginal and rectourethral fistulas. A colostomy is performed on the neonate for diversion of feces until surgical repair is complete and the rectum and anus are functional.

TECHNIQUE

The techniques used to repair these anomalies depend on the type and severity of the defect. A low defect can be corrected with a pull-through procedure similar to that described previously. Combined laparoscopic-perineal surgery now is performed in many pediatric surgery centers. The technique described here is for a simple pull-through procedure.
1 The anus is located through a fistulous tract or by imaging studies.
2 The fistula is incised circumferentially.
3 The rectum is pulled through the anal structure and sutured to the skin.

Discussion

A Foley catheter is inserted during or before the skin prep. The prone position is used for a posterior approach. The hips are elevated on a soft pad. A change in position may be necessary during the procedure. A pediatric gastrointestinal set is required. A fine nerve stimulator is used throughout dissection to locate the anal structures.

A low imperforate anus is located through a fistulous tract that develops during embryonic life between the rectum and the anal structure. This fistula may or may not penetrate the perineal skin. If it is not visible, it can be approached through combined transverse and midline perineal incisions. The nerve stimulator is used to identify the exact location of the anus on the midline and to preserve the nerves necessary for continence. The tract is mobilized proximally with dissecting scissors and fine-toothed forceps. This dissection frees the rectum. Silk traction sutures may be placed through the edge of the distal fistula to aid mobilization of the tissue.

The mobilized rectum is grasped with Babcock forceps and delivered at the true rectum through a midline perineal incision. The edges of the rectum are carefully trimmed with fine dissecting scissors. The edges then are sutured to the skin at the site of the true anus. Multiple interrupted 4-0 or 5-0 synthetic absorbable sutures are used to create the anus.

REDUCTION OF AN INTUSSUSCEPTION

Surgical Goal

Intussusception, or the telescoping of one portion of the intestine into another, can be reduced with hydrostatic pressure (usually a barium enema) or by manual manipulation through a laparotomy incision. Nonoperative reduction is successful in about 50% of cases when performed within 24 to 48 hours.

Pathology

Intussusception is the most common cause of intestinal obstruction in children 3 months to 6 years of age and therefore among the most common surgical emergencies in this age group. A gangrenous bowel may rupture, leading to peritonitis.

TECHNIQUE

1 A transverse or low right paramedian incision is made and the peritoneum is entered.
2 The entire bowel is carefully inspected to determine whether the bowel wall at the intussusception is viable.
3 Manual manipulation is attempted to reduce the intussusception.
4 The bowel may require fixation after reduction to prevent recurrence.
5 Alternatively, if the viability of the bowel is in question, a resection with a possible colostomy is performed.
6 The abdomen is closed.

Discussion

In this procedure a routine laparotomy is performed as described in Chapter 23, using pediatric instruments. The surgeon locates the area of intussusception and reduces the obstruction by manually easing the bowel tissue into normal position. In cases when manual reduction is not possible, or if the bowel has perforated, a resection with end-to-end anastomosis is performed as described in Chapter 23. The wound is closed in routine manner.

REDUCTION OF A VOLVULUS

Surgical Goal

Reduction of a volvulus is performed to relieve intestinal obstruction by untwisting (counterclockwise detorsion) of the affected bowel. Depending on the viability of the affected bowel, a resection with anastomosis, ileostomy, or colostomy may be required.

Pathology

Volvulus is rotation of the intestine around itself or the attached mesentery. This can lead to strangulation of the blood vessels, ischemia in the bowel, and eventual gangrene of the affected portion. Volvulus is a rare condition; it affects children most often but can occur at any age. The developmental anomaly that causes volvulus is called *malrotation*. The central part of the intestine normally rotates into its final position in about week 10 of pregnancy. Occasionally this part of the intestine does not rotate fully, leaving the bowel predisposed to later twisting. Volvulus requires emergency surgery to prevent bowel perforation and peritonitis.

TECHNIQUE

1 The patient is placed in the supine position and the abdomen is prepped and draped.
2 A supraumbilical right transverse incision is made, extending from the midline laterally.
3 The bowel is thoroughly assessed.
4 The volvulus is reduced and any restrictive tissue bands are divided.
5 A resection and anastomosis, colostomy, or ileostomy may be performed.
6 The wound is closed.

Discussion

A routine laparotomy is performed as described in Chapter 23, and the volvulus is manually "untwisted." A bowel resection may be required if necrosis or perforation has occurred (refer to Chapter 23).

REPAIR OF AN OMPHALOCELE

Surgical Goal

An **omphalocele** is a congenital anomaly in which the abdominal viscera develop outside the body, contained within a peritoneal sac. The goal of surgery is to replace the contents of the abdomen in phases until the abdominal wall can be closed.

Pathology

An omphalocele is covered by a clear sac or membrane composed of peritoneum and amnion (Figure 35-11, *A*). The size of the omphalocele can range from very small, containing only a small portion of the intestine, to extremely large (*giant omphalocele*), including the intestine and other abdominal viscera such as the liver and spleen (Figure 35-12). The anomaly is associated with genetic defects, including trisomies 13, 18, and 21 in 30% of cases. Cardiac, musculoskeletal, and genitourinary defects are also associated with omphalocele.

Discussion

Surgical options for repair of an omphalocele depend on the size of the defect. Small defects (less than 0.8 inch [2 cm]) can be reduced in one step. In such cases, a primary abdominal closure is performed soon after birth.

Larger defects require multiple-stage procedures in which portions of the viscera are replaced in the abdominal cavity over a period of days or weeks. To prevent hypothermia, infection, and dehydration, a Silastic, Dacron-reinforced silo is sutured to the abdominal wall. The silo is reduced gradually, over a period of days, while the infant is in intensive care. When the omphalocele has been sufficiently reduced, the infant is taken to the operating room for complete closure of the abdominal wall. If the contents cannot be reduced completely, skin closure alone is performed. This results in a large abdominal wall hernia, which may be repaired later in childhood.

In some cases, the skin cannot be closed over the defect. In these patients, the abdominal contents are covered with a scarification agent, such as silver sulfadiazine. Granulation tissue leading to epithelialization (growth of skin tissue) occurs over a period of months, and repair is delayed for 1 to 2 years.

Shortly after birth, the omphalocele is protected with moist sponges and the infant prepared for surgery. General anesthesia is induced and the abdomen, umbilical cord, and sac are prepped and draped. A Foley catheter is inserted. A small defect is closed with 3-0 nonabsorbable suture.

Phased reduction of the omphalocele takes placed in the neonatal intensive care unit. Final closure is performed as for a laparotomy.

Gastroschisis

Gastroschisis is similar to an omphalocele defined previously, except that no peritoneal sac or membrane covers the

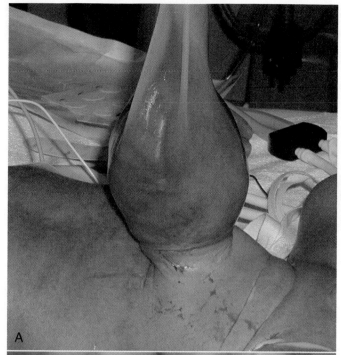

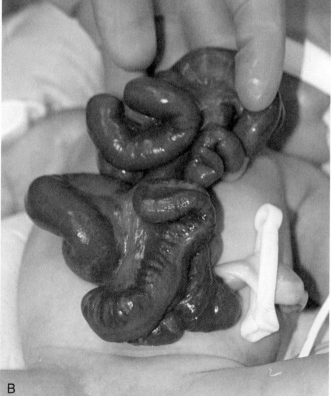

Figure 35-11 Defects of the abdominal wall. **A,** *Omphalocele:* The infant is born with the abdominal viscera outside the body; the organs are encased in a membrane. **B,** *Gastroschisis:* The abdominal viscera are not covered by a membrane. *(From Townsend CM, Beauchamp DR, Evers MB, Mattox KL: Sabiston textbook of surgery, ed 18, Philadelphia, 2007, WB Saunders.)*

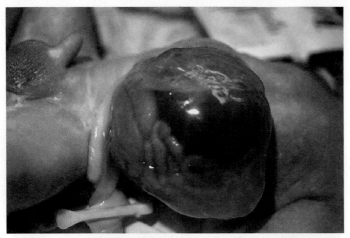

Figure 35-12   Giant omphalocele, with organs clearly visible. *(From Clark DA, Thompson JE, Barnemeyer BM: Atlas of neonatology, ed 7, Philadelphia, 2000, WB Saunders.)*

abdominal viscera (see Figure 35-11, *B*). Unlike with an omphalocele, associated anomalies are rare. Intestinal atresia (narrowing of the lumen) may be present. The exposed bowel often is thickened and edematous and may be abnormally short. This may be related to exposure to amniotic fluid or during fetal life. The cause of gastroschisis is not known.

Surgical treatment for gastroschisis is similar to that for an omphalocele, involving the use of a Silastic silo and phased reduction. However, repair is more urgent because of the absence of a protective peritoneum.

The primary risks of an omphalocele and gastroschisis are infection and bowel necrosis. A silo is closed as soon as possible after birth to prevent infection. Fluid loss from the exposed bowel can be significant; therefore the tissue is kept covered and moist during staged closure. Increased intra-abdominal pressure, which occurs after repair, may result in difficult ventilation and decreased urinary output. Adequate pain relief is provided by continuous infusion of morphine.

REPAIR OF BLADDER EXSTROPHY/ EPISPADIAS

Surgical Goal

The surgical goal of reconstruction is to restore the normal functions of the lower urinary tract.

Pathology

Bladder **exstrophy**/epispadias is a complex set of congenital anomalies involving the lower genitourinary tract and skeletal system. The anomalies arise from the same developmental defect, which occurs in the first trimester of fetal life. The anomalies associated with the defect are:

- Bladder exstrophy (the anterior bladder wall is exposed on the outside of the body through an abdominal wall defect)
- Epispadias (the urethra is fully exposed or terminates on the dorsum of the penis)
- Shortening of the penis, which also demonstrates chordee (bands of tissue that cause an upward curvature)

- Opening out of the glans and absence of the dorsal foreskin
- Anterior displacement of the vagina and anus
- Exposure of the bladder neck
- Possible presence of an omphalocele
- Divergence of the rectus muscles and widening of the pubic symphysis

Discussion

Reconstruction usually is performed in three stages, although this varies with the individual patient and with the surgical strategy chosen by the surgeon:

- *First stage:* Closure of the bladder and abdomen (24 to 48 hours of life)
- *Second stage:* Repair of epispadias (2 to 3 years old)
- *Third stage:* Achieving urinary continence (4 to 5 years old)
  Repair of an exstrophic bladder in the male is described here.

TECHNIQUE

1 The patient is placed in the supine position. A wide area is prepped, including the entire body anteriorly and posteriorly below the level of the nipple so that turning is possible, and the area is draped.

2 Traction sutures of 5-0 Prolene are placed in the glans penis and ureteral catheters are secured in each ureteral orifice.

3 The surgeon incises and completely dissects around the periphery of the bladder and urethral plate.

4 The incision is extended distally to the area where the ejaculatory ducts join the urethra, on both sides.

5 The umbilical cord is excised and an umbilicoplasty is performed during or after the initial procedure.

6 A paraexstrophy flap may be created if any question exists about the urethral length.

7 The bladder is completely mobilized, with preservation of its blood supply.

8 Inversion of the bladder plate and approximation of the corpora are the first stage of epispadias repair.

9 The corpora are approximated carefully in the midline to promote penile elongation.

10 The surgeon approximates the skin at the urethral plate inferiorly

11 The urethral plate is made tubular and ureteral catheters are placed bilaterally and brought out on each side of the bladder.

12 After two-layer closure of the bladder and urethral plate, the bladder is reduced into the pelvis and fixed with suture.

13 Sutures are placed to approximate the pubic halves. The drainage tubes are brought out superiorly and the fascia, subcutaneous tissue, and skin are approximated.

Figure 35-13 illustrates bladder exstrophy and epispadias and procedures for their repair.

ORCHIOPEXY FOR AN UNDESCENDED TESTICLE

Surgical Goal

The goal of surgery for congenital undescended testicle is to restore the testicle to its normal position in the scrotum. The procedure sometimes is called an *orchiopexy*; however, this term actually refers only to the surgical attachment of the testicle to the scrotal wall. Orchiopexy is performed for a variety of conditions, including surgical attachment for the prevention and treatment of testicular torsion.

Pathology

During normal fetal life, the testicles are retained within the abdomen. Just before birth, the testicles should descend into the scrotum. Occasionally one or both testicles fail to descend into the scrotum. This can result in sterility because of the testicles' exposure to the increased temperature in the abdominal cavity.

Discussion

The patient is placed in the supine position, prepped, and draped with the inguinal, groin, and scrotal areas on the affected side exposed. The surgeon makes an incision over the

TECHNIQUE

1. The surgeon enters and explores the inguinal region.
2. The testicle is identified.
3. The spermatic cord is mobilized.
4. The testicle is mobilized by sharp and blunt dissection.
5. A tunnel is made through the inguinal canal into the scrotum.
6. The testicle is brought through the tunnel and secured with sutures.
7. The inguinal layers are closed.

external ring, as for a hernia repair. The incision is carried into the deep inguinal tissues with sharp dissection.

Small bleeders are coagulated with the ESU or clamped with mosquito hemostats and ligated with fine absorbable sutures. The spermatic cord is identified and dissected with blunt and sharp dissection. The cord is dissected high in the internal ring to create sufficient slack to bring the testicle into the scrotum; the processus vaginalis is ligated.

The surgeon uses blunt dissection (e.g., Mayo or sponge forceps, or digital separation of the tissue) to create a tunnel for the testicle. A clamp is advanced through the external oblique fascia and the tissue is manually separated, forming a pocket in the scrotum.

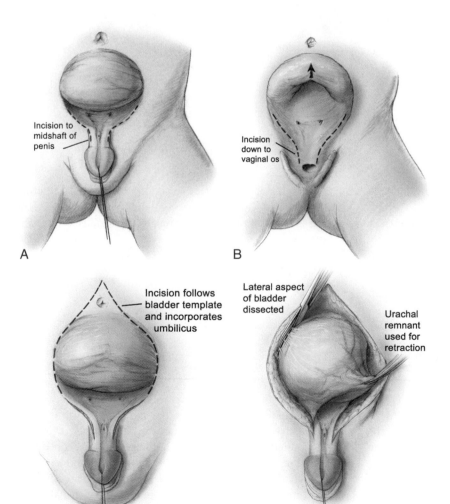

A — Incision to midshaft of penis

B — Incision down to vaginal os

C — Incision follows bladder template and incorporates umbilicus

D — Lateral aspect of bladder dissected — Urachal remnant used for retraction

Figure 35-13 Surgical reconstruction for bladder exstrophy and epispadias. **A,** The bladder plate is dissected from the abdominal wall. **B,** Incision in the female. **C** and **D,** Continuation of the incision.

Figure 35-13, cont'd **E**, Dissection of muscles from the symphysis pubis. **F**, Stents are placed in the bladder. **G**, A sound is placed in the urethra and closure begins. **H**, The symphysis, bladder, and rectus fascia are closed. *(From Wein AJ, editor: Campbell-Walsh urology, Philadelphia, 2007, WB Saunders.)*

The testicle is brought through the tunnel and the scrotum is incised to expose the scrotal septum. Several 3-0 or 4-0 absorbable sutures are placed through the septum and testicle, securing the testicle in place (Figure 35-14).

CLOSURE OF A PATENT DUCTUS ARTERIOSUS

Surgical Goal

Surgical closure of a **patent ductus arteriosus** (PDA) is performed to prevent arterial blood from recirculating through the pulmonary circulation. The ductus may be approached by an open incision or by the endoscopic route.

Pathology

The ductus arteriosus is a normal anatomical opening in the fetal heart. During fetal development, blood is pumped from the right ventricle into the systemic circulation by way of the ductus, which connects the pulmonary artery and descending thoracic aorta (Figure 35-15, *A*). At birth, the lungs expand and the ductus closes spontaneously within a short time (see Figure 35-15, *B*). If the ductus fails to close, arterial blood returns to the lungs, putting an added burden on the lungs and heart. The heart becomes enlarged and may fail. The ductus is closed surgically to correct this defect, usually during infancy.

TECHNIQUE

1 A left thoracotomy is performed.
2 The mediastinal pleura is incised.
3 The ductus is isolated.
4 The ductus is closed.
5 A chest tube is inserted and the chest is closed.

Discussion

Surgical repair of a PDA may be performed by minimally invasive surgery. An open procedure is described here.

The patient is placed in the supine position, prepped, and draped for a thoracotomy. A thoracotomy is performed as previously described. To begin the repair, the surgeon places a traction suture through the edges of the pleura (usually with 3-0 silk suture). The ends are tagged with a hemostat. The assistant retracts the pleura with the suture. The surgeon then carefully dissects the aorta and pulmonary artery with fine dissecting scissors to expose the ductus (Figure 35-16, *A*). A heavy silk suture may be passed around the ductus.

The surgeon continues the dissection until the ductus is fully isolated. Straight or angled vascular clamps are placed across the ductus, one close to the aorta and the other close to the pulmonary artery (Figure 35-16, *B*). In a newborn or a small infant, the surgeon may simply tie the ductus with size 0 silk, because the ductus is small and may not allow placement of the vascular clamps. Vascular clips also may be used.

In other situations, the surgeon may divide and oversew the cut edges. The surgeon cuts halfway through the ductus with Potts scissors or a knife. A 5-0 or 6-0 polypropylene suture is used to begin the closure of the ductus on the aortic side. The surgeon continues to incise the ductus and continues the suture to close the defect on the aortic side. The vascular clamp then is slowly released. Additional sutures are placed if needed. The end of the ductus closest to the pulmonary artery is sutured in the same manner. A topical hemostatic agent can be used to control bleeding at the anastomosis.

The mediastinal pleura is closed with a continuous suture of 3-0 or 4-0 silk or chromic gut. An appropriate-size chest tube is inserted and the wound is closed in layers (Figure 35-16, *C*).

CORRECTION OF A COARCTATION OF THE THORACIC AORTA

Surgical Goal
Correction of a coarctation of the thoracic aorta is performed to restore blood flow to the lower body and reduce cardiac workload.

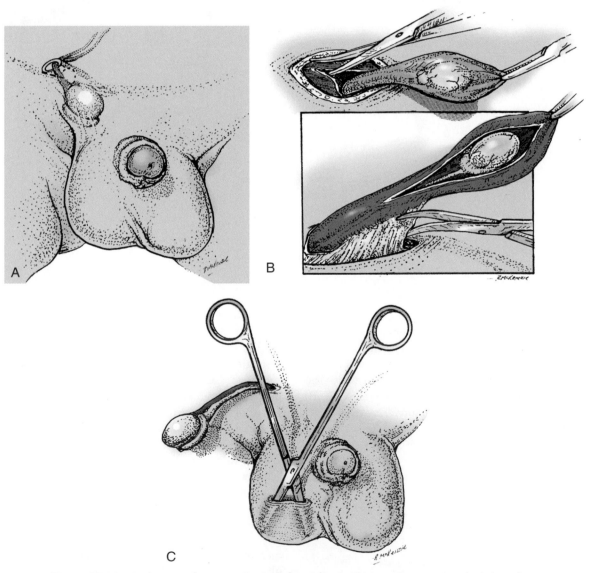

Figure 35-14 Orchiopexy for an undescended testicle. A, The testicle is approached through a transverse inguinal incision. **B,** The external ring is opened and the cremaster fibers are mobilized from the cord. **C,** Formation of the pouch.

Continued

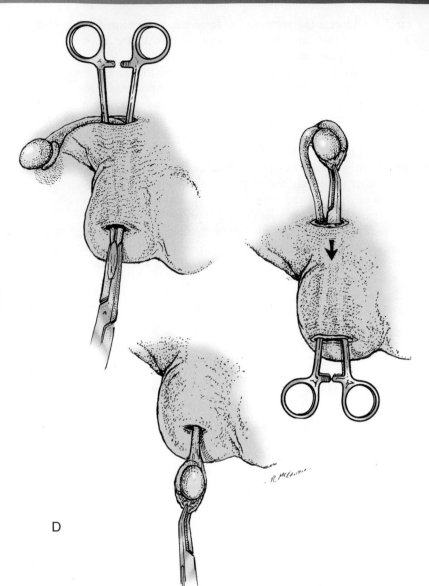

Figure 35-14, cont'd **D,** The testicle is brought through the tunnel. *(From Wein AJ, editor: Campbell-Walsh urology, Philadelphia, 2007, WB Saunders.)*

D

Pathology

Coarctation of the thoracic aorta is a congenital stenosis that usually occurs near the junction of the fetal ductus arteriosus and the aorta. Severe narrowing obstructs the normal flow of blood through the thoracic aorta and to the lower body. The heart becomes enlarged as a result of the increased work required to pump blood through a stricture. The lower body may be underdeveloped as a result of the defect.

TECHNIQUE

1 A thoracotomy is performed.
2 The mediastinal pleura is incised.
3 The ligamentum arteriosum is ligated and divided.
4 The aorta is occluded proximal and distal to the coarctation.
5 The aorta is transected and anastomosed, or a prosthetic graft is inserted.
6 The aorta is unclamped.
7 The wound is closed.

Discussion

The patient is placed in the lateral position, prepped, and draped for a thoracotomy. The thoracic cavity is entered through a posterolateral thoracotomy. A moist laparotomy sponge is placed over the lung, which is retracted by the assistant. The surgeon incises the mediastinal pleura and places 3-0 or 4-0 silk traction sutures in the edges. This exposes the aorta. Moist umbilical tape is placed around the aorta for mobilization and retraction.

The intercostal arteries are mobilized. Fine dissecting scissors are used to dissect the aorta in the area of the coarctation.

The surgeon ligates and divides the ductus (a ductus that has closed naturally is called the *ligamentum arteriosum*) to free the aorta and prevent bleeding from the ductus or ligamentum if it is still patent. Additional sutures of 4-0 silk are placed in the ductus if needed.

The surgeon occludes the aorta proximal and distal to the coarctation with straight or angled vascular clamps. The arteries that supply the coarctated segment also are ligated, and bulldog clamps may be placed on other vessels that lie between the coarctated segment and the cross clamps of the aorta. The aorta then is transected, and the stricture is removed.

The two ends of the aorta are anastomosed with 5-0 or 6-0 continuous suture. Interrupted sutures often are used in pediatric patients to allow growth. (In adults, 3-0 or 4-0 polypropylene suture is used.) If the two limbs of the aorta cannot be brought together easily (often the case in adults), a synthetic tube graft may be inserted, or a proximal portion of the left subclavian artery may be used to form a patch. In this technique, a part of the artery wall is swung around and anastomosed to the resected coarctation. The distal artery then is ligated.

All clamps are removed from the aorta and intercostal arteries. Blood flow to the lower body is restored. The surgeon inspects all suture lines for hemostasis and additional sutures are placed as needed. A topical hemostatic agent may be applied to control bleeding.

The mediastinal pleura is closed with 3-0 or 4-0 suture. A chest tube is inserted, and the wound is closed in layers. Figure 35-17 illustrates the repair of a coarctation of the thoracic aorta.

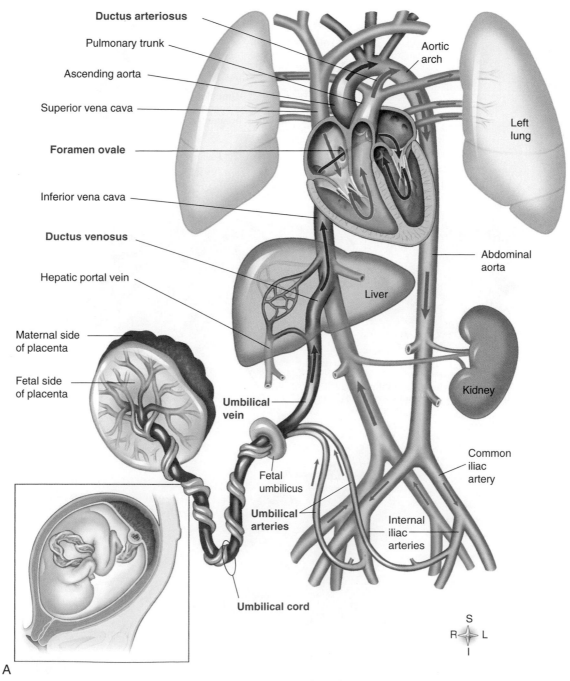

Figure 35-15 A, Fetal circulation.

Continued

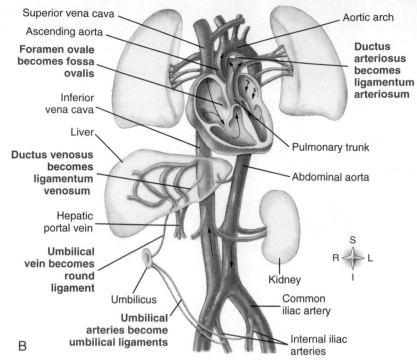

Superior vena cava

Ascending aorta

Foramen ovale becomes fossa ovalis

Inferior vena cava

Liver

Ductus venosus becomes ligamentum venosum

Hepatic portal vein

Umbilical vein becomes round ligament

Umbilicus

Umbilical arteries become umbilical ligaments

Aortic arch

Ductus arteriosus becomes ligamentum arteriosum

Pulmonary trunk

Abdominal aorta

Kidney

Common iliac artery

Internal iliac arteries

S
R · L
I

Figure 35-15, cont'd   B, Changes in fetal circulation at birth. *(From Thibodeau G, Patton K:* Anatomy and physiology, *ed 6, Philadelphia, Mosby, 2007.)*

B

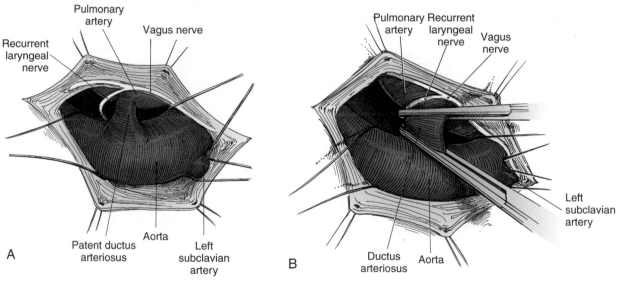

Pulmonary artery

Recurrent laryngeal nerve

Vagus nerve

Patent ductus arteriosus

Aorta

Left subclavian artery

A

Pulmonary artery

Recurrent laryngeal nerve

Vagus nerve

Ductus arteriosus

Aorta

Left subclavian artery

B

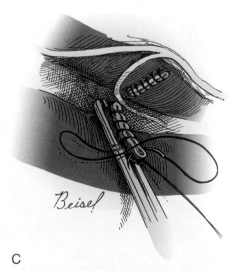

Beisel

C

Figure 35-16   Surgery for patent ductus arteriosus. A, Exposure of the patent ductus. **B,** Vascular clamps are placed across the ductus. **C,** Continuous suture closure. *(Modified from Waldhausen JA, Pierce WS, Campbell DB:* Surgery of the chest, *ed 6, St Louis, 1996, Mosby.)*

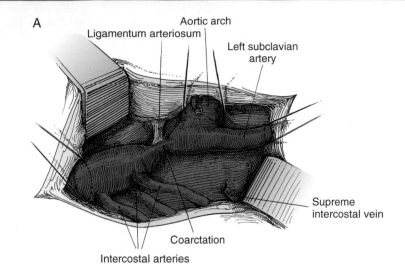

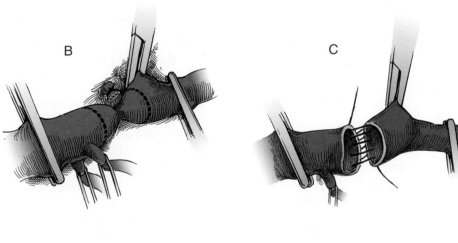

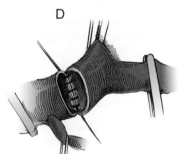

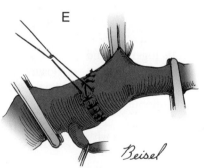

Beisel

Figure 35-17 **A,** Coarctation of the aorta. **B,** Arterial clamps are applied above and below the constriction, and the vessel is resected. **C** and **D,** Continuous absorbable suture is used in closure. **E,** Closure of the anterior wall is completed with interrupted or continuous sutures. *(Modified from Waldhausen JA, Pierce WS, Campbell DB: Surgery of the chest, ed 6, St Louis, 1996, Mosby.)*

CORRECTION OF PULMONARY VALVE STENOSIS

Surgical Goal

Valvulotomy is performed to release fused valve leaflets and restore circulation from the right ventricle to the lungs. Most cases are treated by balloon catheterization.

Pathology

Pulmonary valve stenosis usually is a congenital anomaly in which the pulmonary valve is narrowed. Severe stenosis may require emergency treatment.

TECHNIQUE

1 Cardiopulmonary bypass is initiated through a median sternotomy.
2 The venae cavae are encircled with umbilical tapes.
3 The pulmonary artery is opened and the fused leaflets are separated.
4 The pulmonary artery is closed.
5 Cardiopulmonary bypass is discontinued and the wound is prepared for closure.
6 The wound is closed.

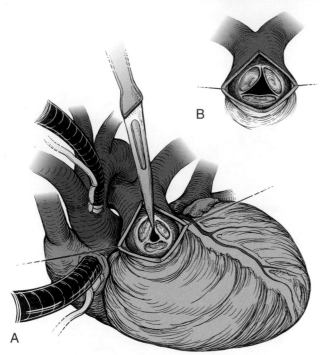

Figure 35-18 **Pulmonary valvulotomy. A,** The fused valve is incised. **B,** Completed valvulotomy. *(Modified from Mavroudis C, Backer DL: Pediatric cardiac surgery, ed 3, St Louis, 2003, Mosby.)*

Discussion

The surgeon enters the chest through a median sternotomy. The pericardial sac is incised with scissors, and the incision is extended downward to the diaphragm and upward to the innominate vein. Cannulas of the correct size are obtained and bypass is initiated.

An umbilical tape is placed on the aorta and a purse-string suture of 4-0 polypropylene or polyester is placed. The assistant brings the ends of the suture through a bolster (a short vinyl or Silastic tube that holds the suture ends together) and holds the suture with a hemostat. Heparin is administered to the patient. Bicaval venous cannulation and aortic cannulation are performed as described previously. Cardiopulmonary bypass is started.

To begin the repair, the surgeon isolates the vena cava with umbilical tape and a tourniquet is placed as previously described. The pulmonary artery above the valve is opened with scissors. The aorta may be occluded temporarily to create a drier field. The fused leaflets are separated with a knife, Metzenbaum scissors, or Potts scissors (Figure 35-18). The surgeon closes the pulmonary artery with 5-0 continuous suture. If the pulmonary artery is stenotic, a patch graft may be inserted to enlarge the artery.

CLOSURE OF AN ATRIAL SEPTAL DEFECT

Surgical Goal

An atrial septal defect is a congenital anomaly in which a hole in the interatrial septum allows blood from the left atrium to flow into the right atrium. The goal of surgery is to close the defect and reduce excessive blood flow to the pulmonary system.

Pathology

Blood normally flows from the left atrium into the left ventricle before entering the systemic circulation. An atrial septal defect causes the blood to shunt from the left atrium to the right atrium. This creates increased pressure on the right ventricle and lungs, causing the heart to enlarge and eventually fail. An atrial septal defect usually is closed during childhood. However, some patients reach adulthood before developing symptoms that require surgical repair.

TECHNIQUE

1 Cardiopulmonary bypass is initiated through a median sternotomy.
2 The aorta is occluded.
3 A right atriotomy is performed, the defect is closed, and the atriotomy is closed.
4 Cardiopulmonary bypass is discontinued and the wound is prepared for closure.
5 The wound is closed.

Discussion

The patient is prepped and draped for a median sternotomy. The sternotomy is performed and bypass is initiated. The surgeon may fibrillate the heart and occlude the aorta before performing a right atriotomy. A Richardson (pediatric) retractor is placed in the wound and the surgeon examines the defect. Additional supplies may be needed, depending on this assessment.

The surgeon may repair the defect with a primary closure or by inserting a patch or pericardial graft. Large defects require a patch graft, which is cut to size and sutured in place with polypropylene or nylon sutures. Air is removed from the left side of the heart before the final sutures are placed and tied. Bypass is discontinued, and the wound is prepared for closure. The incision is closed in layers. Figure 35-19 illustrates the procedure for closure of an atrial septal defect.

CLOSURE OF A VENTRICULAR SEPTAL DEFECT

Surgical Goal

A ventricular septal defect is incomplete closure of the septum between the right and left ventricle, which normally occurs during fetal life. This causes increased pulmonary pressure by allowing blood from the left ventricle to flow into the right ventricle and to the lungs, leading to congestive heart failure after birth. The septal defect is repaired to restore normal cardiac circulation.

Pathology

A ventricular septal defect is a hole in the intraventricular septum. It can occur in a variety of locations. Increased pressure in the left ventricle causes blood to flow through the defect into the area of lower pressure, the right ventricle.

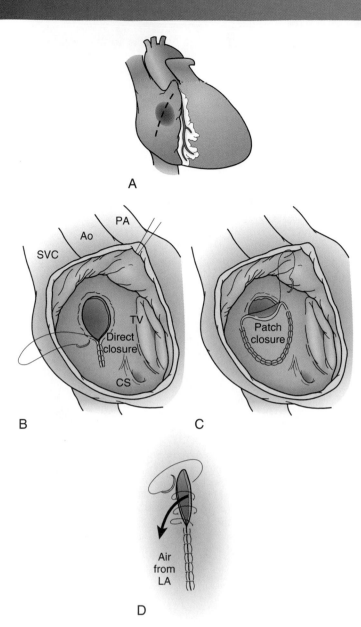

Figure 35-19 **Repair of an atrial septal defect.** **A,** The atrium is incised. **B,** Direct closure of the defect. *Ao,* Aorta; *CS,* coronary sinus; *PA,* pulmonary artery; *SVC,* superior vena cava; *TV,* tricuspid valve. **C,** Patch closure. **D,** Air is removed from the left atrium (*LA*). *(From Nichols DG, Ungerleider RM, Spevak PJ, et al, editors: Critical heart disease in infants and children, Philadelphia, 2006, Mosby.)*

TECHNIQUE

1 Cardiopulmonary bypass is initiated through a median sternotomy.
2 The aorta is occluded and a cardioplegic solution is infused into the coronary arteries.
3 A ventriculotomy is performed and the defect is closed.
4 The aorta is unclamped and the ventricle is closed.
5 Bypass is discontinued and the cannulas are removed.
6 A temporary pacemaker electrode is sutured to the heart.
7 Chest tubes are inserted and the wound is closed.

Discussion

The surgeon performs a median sternotomy and cannulates for total cardiopulmonary bypass as described in Chapter 34. The surgeon occludes the aorta with a pediatric vascular clamp and infuses a retrograde cardioplegic solution through the coronary sinus. A right ventriculotomy is performed with the knife or Mayo scissors. The surgeon may place sutures through the edges of the ventricle for traction.

The defect is assessed and a patch graft is sutured into place. Teflon pledgets may be used to reinforce the suture line. Air is removed from the left ventricle before final closure.

After removing the aortic clamp, the surgeon closes the ventricle with continuous suture. Bypass is discontinued and the cannulas are removed. A temporary pacemaker lead may be sutured to the right ventricle and right atrium. Chest tubes are inserted and the wound is closed.

TOTAL CORRECTION OF TETRALOGY OF FALLOT

Surgical Goal

Tetralogy of Fallot is a combination of congenital defects that includes pulmonary stenosis, ventricular septal defect, right ventricular hypertrophy, and dextroposition (displacement) of the aorta. Surgical repair is performed to correct cyanosis and restore normal blood flow.

Pathology

Tetralogy of Fallot causes reduced pulmonary blood flow and right-to-left shunting (from the right ventricle to the left ventricle) of blood. This shunting mixes deoxygenated blood with oxygenated blood and the mixture is pumped into the systemic circulation. The right ventricle becomes hypertrophied (enlarged) because of the work needed to pump the blood through the obstructed pulmonary system. The patient is cyanotic and increased oxygen demand results in reduced pulmonary blood flow. If delayed repair is necessary, a systemic-pulmonary shunt may be performed to increase blood flow to the lungs. This shunt improves oxygenation and allows the baby to develop to a stage at which total correction is possible.

TECHNIQUE

1 A median sternotomy is performed and bypass is initiated.
2 Cardioplegia is performed.
3 A right ventriculotomy is performed, the infundibular muscle is resected, and a pulmonary valvulotomy is performed.
4 The ventricular septal defect is closed and the right ventricle is closed with a patch.
5 Bypass is discontinued.
6 A temporary pacemaker lead is inserted.
7 Chest tubes are inserted and the wound is closed.

Discussion

The incision used for this procedure depends on whether a palliative shunt previously was performed. Total correction in the absence of a previous shunt is performed through a median sternotomy. After the chest has been opened, bypass is initiated. Cardioplegia then is performed as described previously.

The surgeon performs the right ventriculotomy with a knife and curved Mayo scissors. Retractors are inserted, and a portion of the infundibular muscle is excised. The technologist should wipe all instruments clean after use to prevent emboli from forming.

A pulmonary valvulotomy then is performed, and the ventricular septal defect is closed as previously described. After air is evacuated from the left ventricle, the clamp is removed from the aorta.

The surgeon closes the ventricle with continuous suture of 4-0 polypropylene. A patch of woven Dacron or Teflon is used to enlarge the right ventricular outflow tract (the area beneath the pulmonary valve). The pulmonary artery also may be enlarged with a patch, using a smaller size suture.

The pulmonary artery pressure and right ventricular pressure are measured to determine whether the surgery was successful. If the results indicate that additional surgery is required, additional surgical supplies are needed.

If the surgery is successful, bypass is discontinued and the wound is prepared for closure as described previously. Chest tubes are inserted, and the wound is closed. Complete repair of tetralogy of Fallot is illustrated in Figure 35-20.

REPAIR OF PECTUS EXCAVATUM

Surgical Goal

Pectus excavatum, or funnel chest, is a nongenetic defect of the chest wall marked by overgrowth of the costal cartilages, a sunken appearance in the anterior chest, and a restricted sternum. The goal of surgery is to reconstruct the chest wall to restore normal inspiratory function and improve body image.

Pathology

Pectus excavatum does not have a genetic component, but it may be associated with Marfan syndrome. Children born with the acquired defect may have mild to moderate paradoxical movement of the sternum with inhalation. Children have a typical slouching appearance, and older children may experience shortness of breath. Surgery is performed in adolescence or preadolescence.

In the Nuss procedure, a metal bar is placed under the sternum to lift the chest wall. The bar is left in place for 2 years or longer until growth is complete. The bar then is removed, a procedure for which local anesthesia is used.

As the child emerges from anesthesia, the PACU team ensures that the patient remains in the supine position to prevent the bar from being dislodged. Patients are kept in the hospital for at least 3 to 4 days for pain control and to ensure that the bar is stable. Epidural catheterization for continuous pain control is used in selected patients. Limited activity may be resumed 6 weeks after surgery.

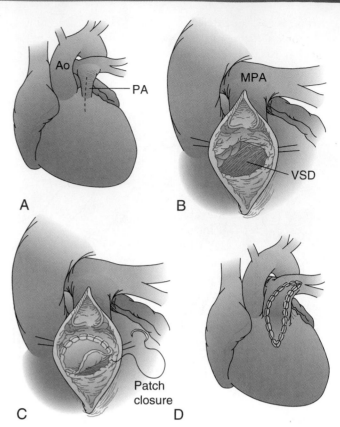

Figure 35-20   Repair of tetralogy of Fallot. A, Enlargement of the right ventricle; main pulmonary artery (*MPA*) connection. *Ao,* Aorta; *PA,* pulmonary artery. **B,** Resection of muscle from the ventricular septal defect (*VSD*). **C,** Closure of the VSD. **D,** Patch graft. *(From Townsend CM, Beauchamp DR, Evers MB, Mattox KL: Sabiston textbook of surgery, ed 18, Philadelphia, 2007, WB Saunders.)*

TECHNIQUE

1. The defect is measured and the skin is marked for insertion of the pectus bar.
2. The pectus bar is prepared using a plate bender.
3. Two 0.8-inch (2-cm) incisions are made in the midaxillary line following the skin marks.
4. Under thoracoscopic visualization, a curved introducer is inserted through one of the incisions and a tunnel is made.
5. The bar is inserted in inverted position and advanced to the opposite incision.
6. When the bar is in place, it is inverted to evert the sternum, creating a convex chest wall.
7. The bar may be stabilized with #3 steel wire and stabilizers.
8. The ends of the bar are buried in the subcutaneous tissue.
9. The wound is checked for bleeding and to ensure that the bar is stabilized.
10. The wounds are closed with synthetic absorbable sutures and flat dressings or Steri-Strips.

NEURAL TUBE DEFECTS

The neural tube is an embryonic structure that gives rise to the central nervous system (i.e., the spinal cord and the brain). During embryonic development, a variety of environmental conditions can cause defects in the neural tube. Normally, the embryonic spinal cord develops from a flat area, which then rolls into a tubal structure at about 28 days after conception. A **neural tube defect** occurs when the tube fails to close completely. The most common defects are spina bifida, anencephaly, and encephalocele. These are called *open defects* because the neural tissue is exposed at birth and leakage of cerebrospinal fluid (CSF) occurs.

- *Spina bifida* is an anomaly that includes several types of defects. The most common is a myelomeningocele. A myelomeningocele is an exposed portion of the spinal cord and nerves that is contained within a membranous sac, which may rupture at birth. Hydrocephalus, paralysis, bowel and bladder incontinence, and severe mental retardation are associated with a myelomeningocele. The defect can be closed, but nerve damage is permanent.
- *Anencephaly* is the absence of a cranial vault. The defect is incompatible with life and the neonate dies soon after birth. The defect can be diagnosed during routine prenatal ultrasound.
- *Encephalocele* is an anomaly in which meninges, CSF, and sometimes brain tissue are contained within a herniated sac. The incidence is 1 to 4 in 10,000 births, with a 50% survival rate.

Repair of a myelomeningocele is described later.

NEPHRECTOMY IN WILMS TUMOR

Surgical Goal

The goal of surgical treatment of Wilms tumor is excision of the kidney without trauma to the specimen, which might result in seeding cancerous cells in the retroperitoneal space. In some cases a partial nephrectomy may be performed; however, most cases are advanced at the time of diagnosis, requiring a more aggressive surgical approach. An open approach is usually preferred because it allows exploration of the perirenal tissues.

Pathology

Wilms tumor (**nephroblastoma**) is the most common malignancy of the kidney in children. However, the disease itself is rare. The tumor is responsible for 6% to 7% of all childhood cancers. Most cases are identified in children younger than 5 years. The disease can present in one or both kidneys and is more frequently encountered in females. Early diagnosis and absence of bilateral disease are indications of a successful outcome.

TECHNIQUE

1 The abdomen is entered and the peritoneal reflection mobilized.
2 The Gerota fascia is entered.
3 The regional anatomy is examined for signs of metastasis.
4 The renal pedicle is mobilized.
5 The renal vessels are identified, clamped, and ligated serially.
6 The ureter is identified and mobilized
7 The kidney and capsule are excised.
8 Lymph nodes may be excised before the wound is closed.

Discussion

The patient presenting for nephrectomy is usually between the ages of 2 and 5 years. A period of illness may have preceded the surgery, or a nonpainful mass diagnosed without other medical consequences. Cancer surgery in all families is emotionally difficult for the patient and family, but often intensified in the pediatric population. Support to the family is necessary throughout the perioperative period.

In case planning for the surgery, the surgical technologist should have pediatric laparotomy instruments, pediatric kidney pedicle clamps, and basic pediatric vascular instruments. These should include vascular forceps, fine dissecting scissors, handheld retractors, and a small assortment of vascular clamps. The procedure requires careful mobilization of the colon and kidney pedicle structures (renal vein, renal artery, and ureter) and dissection of the specimen from the retroperitoneal space. These techniques require small dissecting sponges, Silastic vessel loops (or a small Penrose drain) for traction on the ureter, and a number of short fine hemostats to tag and hold vessel loops and sutures. Plastic shods to insert over the tips of fine hemostats should be available for all tag clamps.

The surgeon's choice of a pediatric self-retaining retractor and ample sponges for cushioning the tissue edges should be available soon after opening. The surgical technologist must be careful to keep instruments not in use off the field to prevent injury.

Hemostatic materials including absorbable gelatin sponge, topical thrombin glue, and Gelfoam may be needed. Titanium or stainless steel vessel clips should be available in two sizes for clamping the renal vessels, and also for identification of residual tumor edges.

The patient is placed in supine position with a small gel pad under the operative flank for elevation and improved exposure. Prepping is performed using warm solution, and the patient is draped as soon as it is safe in order to prevent hyperthermia.

An abdominal incision (lateral or subcostal) is made to enter the abdominal cavity. (Normally a flank incision is not advised for this procedure.) After extending the incision as necessary, a self-retaining retractor may be positioned. The surgeon may gently explore the abdomen, including the liver, inferior vena cava, and periaortic area, for any signs of metastasis. (A full preoperative workup including magnetic resonance imaging should have ruled out bilateral disease; however, some exploration is necessary.) The technologist should have sponge sticks and a small Deaver retractor available. The surgeon will palpate the renal vein as it emerges from the vena cava to establish a landmark and also to check for any thrombosis related to the tumor.

In order to obtain access to the retroperitoneum, the peritoneal reflection of the colon is identified and mobilized. The ureter is identified and mobilized with a wide Silastic vessel loop or narrow Penrose drain. This allows the ureter to be retracted during dissection.

The perirenal fascia is dissected and the renal artery, vein, and accessory vessels are dissected, clamped, and ligated or clipped. The ureter can then be ligated using fine absorbable sutures (including one or more suture ligatures) and divided. The kidney and adrenal gland are carefully extracted to prevent seeding of cancer cells, with the Gerota fascia intact. Note that ligatures on pedicle structures may be left long and tagged with mosquito forceps until closure, to ensure that hemostasis is secure.

Before closing the wound, several lymph nodes may be removed for pathological analysis. However, extensive nodal dissection is not usually performed. Ligatures are now checked to ensure there is no leakage, and any bleeding is controlled using the ESU. The wound may then be gently irrigated with warm saline and closed in layers. A flat gauze dressing or subcuticular skin closure with Dermabond is used.

Immediate postsurgical complications include small bowel obstruction, hemorrhage, vascular complications, and wound infection. In the postoperative period, patients undergo radiation and chemotherapy according to the postoperative findings (staging). Lifelong care is necessary because Wilms tumor can recur after several years.

REPAIR OF A MYELOMENINGOCELE

Surgical Goal

The surgical goal of repair of a myelomeningocele is to close a dural and cutaneous defect and preserve neural function.

Immediate surgical repair is essential if the defect is leaking CSF; otherwise, the procedure is performed within 48 hours of birth to prevent infection.

Pathology

Spina bifida is a birth defect associated with incomplete closure of a section of the vertebral column. Spina bifida may occur at any point in the vertebral column but is most common in the lumbar and sacral spine. The defect may be small (spina bifida occulta) and not cause any neurological deficit for the infant, or it may cause herniation of the meninges and leakage of CSF (meningocele). The most significant form of spina bifida causes the spinal cord, meninges, and nerve roots to herniate through the skin (Figure 35-21). The structures generally are contained within a cyst or saclike enclosure. The neural tissue in the myelomeningocele is abnormal and even with repair, the patient still has some degree of neurological deficit, such as paralysis or loss of sensation below the level of the defect. A myelomeningocele often is accompanied by birth defects such as heart and urinary system problems, which may complicate the infant's care.

Hydrocephalus (excessive accumulation of cerebrospinal fluid within the ventricles of the brain) is discussed in Chapter 36. It often is associated with a myelomeningocele. If the hydrocephalus is significant, the surgeon may elect to place a

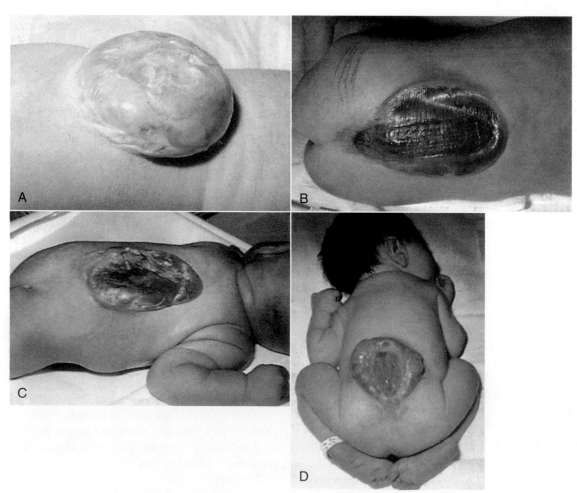

Figure 35-21   **Myelomeningocele. A,** A lesion covered by membrane. **B,** A flat lesion. **C,** A thoracolumbar lesion. **D,** Exposed spinal cord. *(From Rothrock J: Alexander's care of the patient in surgery, ed 17, Philadelphia, 2007, Mosby.)*

ventricular shunt at the time of myelomeningocele repair. If the hydrocephalus is less of a concern, the surgeon may postpone the shunt placement to allow the infant to recover from the primary surgery.

TECHNIQUE

1 The infant is positioned prone on small chest and hip rolls.
2 Fluid is aspirated from the sac and submitted for culture.
3 An incision is made around the circumference of the defect.
4 The tissue around the defect is explored and dissected free.
5 The dura is separated from the fascia and closed.
6 The fascia is separated from the muscle and closed.
7 The muscle and skin are closed.

Discussion

Infants with a myelomeningocele often undergo many surgical procedures to address the primary defect and associated birth defects. Consequently, latex sensitization often develops in these patients. Many institutions that routinely treat infants with a myelomeningocele use a latex-free protocol to minimize exposure and reduce sensitization. The surgical technologist should be familiar with the facility's policies and procedures for latex allergy to ensure that a safe environment is maintained for the patient.

Infants with a myelomeningocele are more vulnerable to hypothermia because of the exposure of their skin and neural structures to the ambient room temperature. The technician must ensure that the solutions used during the procedure are warm. Because of the delicate nature of this procedure and the patient's size, small, fine instruments are used.

The patient is placed in the prone position using small chest and hip rolls. If the neural sac is intact, the surgeon decompresses it with a 20-gauge needle attached to a syringe. The fluid is sent for culture and analysis.

The surgeon begins the procedure by making a circumferential incision around the defect with a #15 blade on a #3 knife handle. The technician should be prepared with bipolar ESU and 4 × 4 sponges to assist the surgeon with hemostasis. The incision is carried through the subcutaneous tissue until the fascia or dura is visualized.

The surgeon uses Metzenbaum scissors to remove the tissue over the exposed spinal cord and dissects along the side of the cord to reach the dura. The technician should be prepared with the bipolar ESU and moistened cottonoids, as necessary, for hemostasis during the dissection. Metzenbaum scissors are used to separate the dura from the fascia, and the dura is closed over the spinal cord with 4-0 braided nylon or silk suture.

The fascia is dissected from the muscle layer with Metzenbaum scissors and a #11 blade as necessary. The fascial layer is closed over the dura with nonabsorbable suture. The wound is irrigated with warm saline. The muscle layer is closed with absorbable synthetic sutures. If the defect is small, the surgeon may be able to reapproximate the skin edges easily; larger defects may require Z-plasty or flap closure with interrupted sutures of synthetic nonabsorbable material.

CORRECTION OF SYNDACTYLY

Surgical Goal
Surgery is performed to separate the fingers, which are joined at birth.

Pathology
During weeks 6 and 8 of gestation, the paddle-shaped hands and feet normally differentiate into separate fingers and toes. Syndactyly results when this separation fails to occur. It is the most common malformation of the limbs and is associated with at least 28 other specific syndromes, occurring in 1 per 2,000 births. The cause is unknown. The condition is classified as incomplete or complete, depending on whether the fingers are joined from the base (web) to the tip. In complex syndactyly, bone and soft tissue are shared by two fingers, whereas in simple syndactyly, only superficial tissues and skin are involved. Surgery is performed before school age. Simple syndactyly is shown in Figure 35-22.

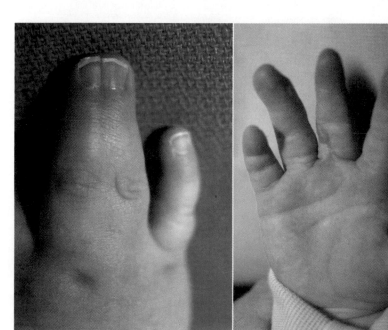

Figure 35-22 Syndactyly before and after surgical correction. (From Canale S, Beaty J: Campbell's operative orthopaedics, ed 11, Philadelphia, 2008, WB Saunders.)

TECHNIQUE

1 The skin incisions are marked.
2 A graft site is prepared and an inguinal graft is removed.
3 Skin flaps are raised.
4 The web space is reconstructed using a primary Z-closure on one side.
5 A skin graft is sutured in place.
6 Dressings are applied.

Discussion

The patient is placed in the supine position with the operative arm on a hand board. General anesthesia is induced. A tourniquet is applied, and the arm is prepped from the elbow to the hand. If a skin graft is required, the groin is prepped and draped separately.

To begin the procedure, the surgeon plans the incisions and draws them on the hand. If a graft is to be taken, this is done first. A small amount of skin is removed from the groin crease using the free-hand method and scalpel. The skin is handed to the surgical technologist to be kept moist until needed. The site is covered with a towel to protect it from contamination.

The skin incisions are made with a #15 knife and plastic surgery forceps. A Z-shaped or modified Z-incision is used. The tourniquet is released momentarily, and bleeders are controlled with a needle point bipolar ESU. The tourniquet can then be reinflated. The triangular flaps are closed on one finger with anchor sutures of 5-0 nylon and interrupted sutures to complete the repair.

The graft is positioned over the denuded area of the other finger and trimmed as needed. Tenotomy scissors or iris scissors may be used for this. The graft is sutured in placed with 4-0 or 5-0 interrupted nylon or absorbable synthetic sutures.

A Xeroform dressing can be placed over the graft site, and a stent dressing can be used to maintain close contact between the graft and finger. (Stent dressings are described in detail in Chapter 22.) The opposite finger is dressed with Xeroform and gauze. Webril is applied around each site while the fingers are widely separated. Many surgeons apply a hard cast to maintain the repair during healing. A simple syndactyly repair is shown in Figure 35-23.

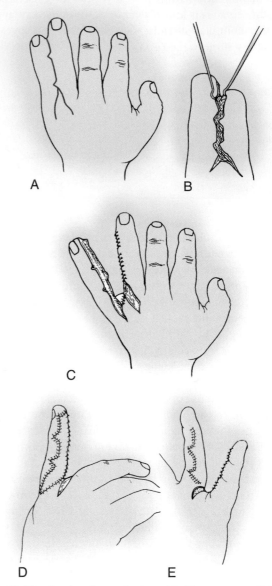

Figure 35-23   Syndactyly repair. **A** and **B**, Skin incisions. **C**, Reconstruction of the ring finger. **D** and **E**, Closure of the little finger and web space graft. *(From Canale S, Beaty J: Campbell's operative orthopaedics, ed 11, Philadelphia, 2008, WB Saunders.)*

KEY CONCEPTS

- Participation in pediatric surgery requires knowledge of specific surgical anatomy and pathology of numerous body systems.
- Case planning for pediatric surgery requires careful attention to patient care in the operative period, and attention to the size and age of the patient in order to select the correct instruments and equipment.
- Psychosocial care of the pediatric patient requires skill and understanding of the developmental age of the patient and an appreciation for the child's concerns.
- Special risk reduction procedures are used in pediatric surgery related to hemostasis and homeostasis.
- In order to be effective in the scrub role, the surgical technologist must be knowledgeable about specific pediatric procedures and the steps involved in each procedure.

REVIEW QUESTIONS

1. What are the disadvantages of administering a preoperative anxiolytic to a pediatric patient?
2. List at least five reasons infants are at risk for hypothermia.
3. Explain magical thinking and how this affects a toddler's view of the perioperative environment.
4. Explain the difference between an omphalocele and gastroschisis.

5. List at least six reasons pediatric patients should not be considered "small adults." Give examples from your knowledge of pediatric physiology.

6. What are the specific risks associated with transporting a pediatric patient?

7. What are the risks to tissue that is left exposed to the environment in conditions such as omphalocele and spina bifida?

8. Why might the presence of a parent upset a child during induction?

9. Explain the anatomical aspects of tetralogy of Fallot.

REFERENCE

1. American Society of Anesthesiologists: Practice guidelines for preoperative fasting and the use of pharmacologic agents to reduce the risk of pulmonary aspiration: application to healthy patients undergoing elective procedures—a report by the American Society of Anesthesiologists Task Force on Preoperative Fasting, *Anesthesiology* 90:3, 1999.

BIBLIOGRAPHY

Association of periOperative Registered Nurses (AORN): Pediatric medication safety, *AORN Journal* 83:1, 2006.

Busen N: Perioperative preparation of the adolescent surgical patient, *AORN Journal* 73:2, 2001.

Cartwright CC, Jimenez DF, Barone CM, et al: Endoscopic strip craniectomy: a minimally invasive treatment for early correction of craniosynostosis, *Journal of Neuroscience Nursing* 35:3, 2003.

Dreger V, Tremback T: Management of preoperative anxiety in children, *AORN Journal* 84:5, 2006.

Golden L, Pagala M, Sukhavasi S, et al: Giving toys to children reduces their anxiety about receiving premedication for surgery, *Anesthesia and Analgesia* 102:1070, 2006.

Hommertzheim R, Steinke E: Malignant hyperthermia: the perioperative nurse's role, *AORN Journal* 83:1, 2006.

Ingoe R, Lange P: The Ladd's procedure for correction of intestinal malrotation with volvulus in children, *AORN Journal* 85:2, 2007.

Phippen ML, Papanier Wells M: *Patient care during operative and invasive procedures*, Philadelphia, 2000, WB Saunders.

Swoveland B, Medvick C, Thompson G: The Nuss procedure for pectus excavatum correction, *AORN Journal* 74:6, 2001.

Touloukian RJ, Smith EI: Disorders of rotation and fixation. In O'Neill JA, Rowe MI, editors: *Pediatric surgery*, ed 5, vol 2, St Louis, 1998, Mosby.

Viitanen H, Paivi A, Viitanen M, Tarkkila P: Premedication with midazolam delays recovery after ambulatory sevoflurane anesthesia in children, *Anesthesia and Analgesia* 90:498, 2000.

CHAPTER OUTLINE

LEARNING OBJECTIVES

After studying this chapter the reader will be able to:

1. Identify key anatomical features of the nervous system
2. Describe basic physiology of the autonomic nervous system
3. Describe basic diagnostic procedures of the nervous system

4. Discuss key elements of case planning for pediatric surgery
5. List and describe common surgical procedures of the nervous system

TERMINOLOGY

Acoustic neuroma: A benign tumor of the eighth cranial nerve; more accurately referred to as a *schwannoma,* because it is composed of Schwann cells, which produce myelin.

Aneurysm: Dilation or ballooning of an artery wall as a result of injury, disease, or a congenital condition.

Arteriovenous malformation (AVM): A collection of blood vessels with abnormal communication between the arteries and veins. It may be the result of injury, infection, or a congenital condition.

Astrocytes: Cells that support the nerve cells (neurons) of the brain and spinal cord by providing nutrients and insulation.

Bone flap: A section of bone removed from the skull during craniotomy procedures.

Embolization: A technique used to occlude a blood vessel. A variety of materials, including platinum coils and microscopic plastic particles, are injected into the vessel under fluoroscopy control to stop active bleeding or prevent bleeding.

Intracranial pressure (ICP): The pressure within the skull exerted by the brain tissue, blood, and cerebrospinal fluid.

Stereotactic: A computerized method of locating a point in space or in tissue, using coordinates in three-dimensions. During stereotactic surgery, the precise location of a tumor or other tissue can be identified from outside the body. The tissue can then be targeted for destruction. The term originates from the Greek words *stereo,* meaning "three dimensional," and *tactos,* meaning "touched."

INTRODUCTION

Neurosurgery is a specialization of the brain, spine, and peripheral nerves. Access to the brain and spinal anatomy often requires penetration or removal of bony tissue. Therefore many procedures require both soft tissue and orthopedic instruments. Unlike most other tissues of the body, nervous tissue does not regenerate after trauma or disease. Many neurosurgical procedures are performed to restore function to other systems and alleviate pain, for tumor removal, and for the treatment of trauma or disease that is life threatening or that greatly reduces quality of life. Like other specialties, neurosurgical technology has advanced quickly in the past decade. Digital technology has created new techniques in neuroendoscopy, microsurgery, biomodeling, and navigation of the nervous system. This chapter is an introduction to neurosurgical techniques that are the basis of more advanced practice for the surgical technologist.

SURGICAL ANATOMY

The nervous system is a communication center for the body. It receives, processes, and interprets information from the environment. It then coordinates appropriate sensory and motor responses. The nervous system is divided structurally into two parts: the *central nervous system (CNS),* which includes the brain and spinal cord, and the peripheral nervous system (PNS), which includes the cranial and spinal nerves and their branches.

CELLS OF THE NERVOUS SYSTEM

Neurons

The neuron is the primary cell type of the nervous system located throughout the body. It transmits information to other neurons, muscle, and glandular tissue. The neuron has three main parts: the body (or soma), the axon, and the dendrites (Figure 36-1).

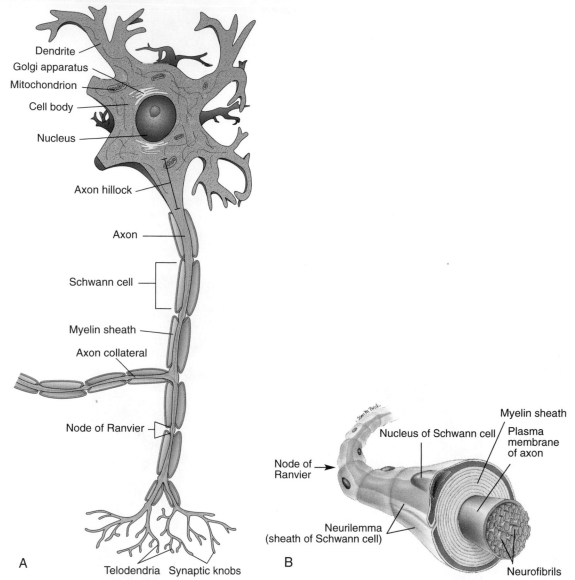

Figure 36-1 A, Structure of the neuron. Note the three main sections: the cell body, dendrites, and axon. **B,** Structure of the axon. The myelinated sheath of some neurons affects the speed of nerve transmission. *(A from Thibodeau G, Patton K: Anatomy and physiology, ed 6, St Louis, Mosby, 2007; B courtesy Brenda Russell, PhD, University of Illinois at Chicago.)*

- The *soma* acts as the sending and receiving area for nerve impulses and is the energy center for the cell.
- The *axon* carries nerve impulses away (efferent) from the cell.
- The *dendrites* carry nerve impulses toward (afferent) the cell.

Neuroglia and Schwann Cells

Neuroglia and Schwann cells provide support to the neurons. Brain and spinal cord tissue is composed primarily of neuroglia. **Astrocytes**, the most common type of neuroglia, fill the spaces between the neurons. Oligodendrocytes form myelin, the fatty sheath that provides insulation for the dendrites. Microglia are specialized immune cells that remove cellular debris. Ependymal cells line the brain ventricles and are involved in the production of cerebrospinal fluid (CSF).

Schwann cells are found in the peripheral nervous system. Their main functions are the production of myelin and the removal of cellular debris.

CENTRAL NERVOUS SYSTEM

Skull (Cranium)

The skull covers and protects the brain. It is composed of bony plates that are connected by a thin membrane called a *suture*. The major bones of the skull (Figure 36-2) are as follows:

- One *frontal bone*, which provides structure for the forehead and orbits.
- Two *parietal* bones on either side of the skull, which provide structure for the sides and roof of the cranium.
- Two *temporal* bones on either side of the skull, which contribute to the structure for the sides of the cranium.

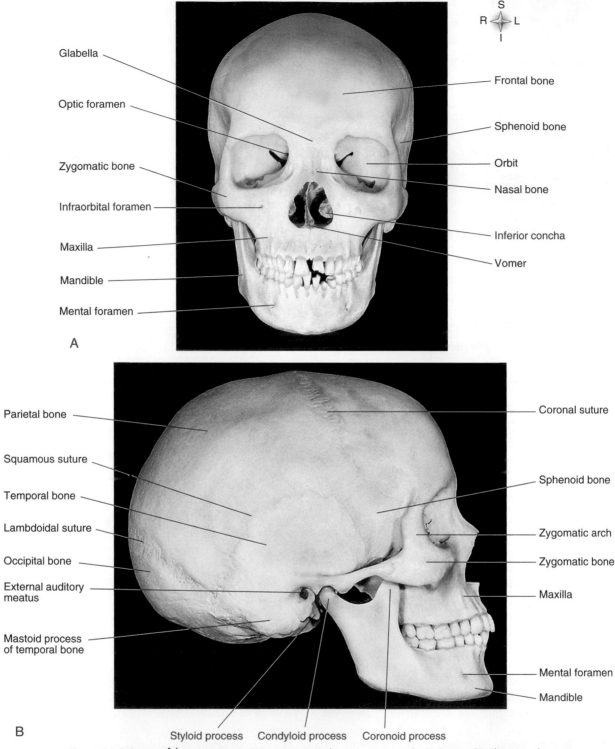

Figure 36-2 **Bones of the cranium. A,** Front view. **B,** Side view. *(From Vidic B, Suarez FR: Photographic atlas of the human body, St Louis, 1984, Mosby.)*

- One occipital bone, which provides structure to the back of the skull and a portion of the floor of the cranium.

The skull is covered by the multilayered scalp, which is composed of skin and highly vascular subcutaneous tissue. The *pericranium* is the periosteal layer of the skull bones. The pericranium is covered by muscle and the galea, a tough, fibrous tissue sheet. The skin of the scalp is very thick and highly vascular and contains numerous hair follicles.

Meninges

Directly beneath the skull lie the three protective coverings of the brain, the meninges. The outermost layer, the dura mater, is composed of very dense, fibrous tissue. The middle layer is the arachnoid mater. The arachnoid mater is a very delicate, serous membrane that has the appearance of a spiderweb. Beneath the arachnoid mater is the subarachnoid space, which is filled with CSF. The pia mater is the layer closest to the brain. This is a vascular membrane that contains portions of areolar

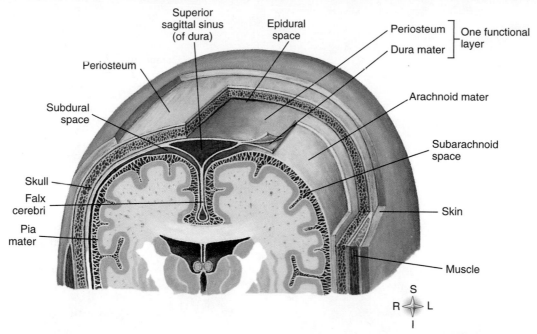

Figure 36-3 Surgical layers of the scalp, galea, meninges, and brain. *(From Abrahams P, Hutchings RT, Marks SC: McKinn's color atlas of human anatomy, ed 4, St Louis, 1999, Mosby.)*

connective tissue. This membrane dips down into the various crevices and convolutions of the brain. The layers of the scalp, superficial brain, and associated structures are illustrated in Figure 36-3.

Brain

The brain itself is divided into three main sections: the cerebrum, cerebellum, and brainstem. Each of these sections is further subdivided (Figure 36-4).

CEREBRUM The cerebrum, or forebrain, controls all motor activity and sensory impulses. It is divided into halves, the right and left cerebral hemispheres. Each hemisphere is subdivided into four lobes:

- The *frontal lobe* is responsible for thought and behavior.
- The *temporal lobe* controls memory, the senses, language, and emotions.
- The *parietal lobe* primarily controls language.
- The *occipital lobe* controls vision.

The cerebrum is the largest part of the brain, accounting for almost 88% of the total weight of the organ. The surface of the cerebrum is convoluted, having small bulges that occur throughout. These bulges are called *gyri* (sing., gyrus). Between the bulges are shallow indentations, called *sulci* (sing., sulcus). Larger deeper furrows in this area are known as *fissures*.

The outer tissue layer of the cerebrum is known as the *cerebral cortex*. This layer is composed of gray matter and is divided into lobes, which are named for the bones that lie over them. The gray matter is composed of nerve cells and blood vessels. The lobes and functional areas of the cerebrum are illustrated in Figure 36-5.

CEREBELLUM The cerebellum, or hindbrain, lies under the posterior cerebrum and is the second largest area of the brain

(Figure 36-6). Like the cerebrum, it is covered by a cortex composed of gray matter and is divided into lobes by fissures. The cerebellar lobes are the anterior, posterior, and flocculonodular lobes. The anterior and posterior lobes help control coordination and movement. The flocculonodular lobe helps control equilibrium. Coordination between the cerebrum and cerebellum is necessary for the "planning" and execution of movement. The sensory information provided by the cerebrum guides the coordinated movement of muscles and balance.

BRAINSTEM The brainstem is composed of three sections: the medulla oblongata, midbrain, and pons (Figure 36-7). The medulla oblongata is a continuous connection between the spinal cord and the pons. It is made up primarily of gray matter and closely resembles the spinal cord in internal structure except that it is much thicker. Lines of white matter are interspersed within the gray matter, and all impulses into and out of the spinal cord are located here. The medulla is responsible for vital functions such as control of the circulatory system, respiration, and heart rate.

The midbrain is situated between the forebrain and the hindbrain. The major structures of the midbrain are the thalamus, hypothalamus, pituitary gland, and pineal gland. The pituitary gland is composed of two sections, anterior and posterior, which coordinate with the hypothalamus to synthesize and secrete many vital hormones that are responsible for cell activity and physiological processes in the body. These essential hormones that are targeted include the growth hormone, thyroid stimulating hormone, adrenocorticotropic hormone, prolactin, luteinizing hormone, antidurectic hormone, oxytocin, and antidiuretic hormone. The pineal gland lies posterior to the pituitary and secretes melatonin which regulates periods of wakefulness and sleep (circadian rhythm) through a feedback mechanism from the retina. On the ventral side of the

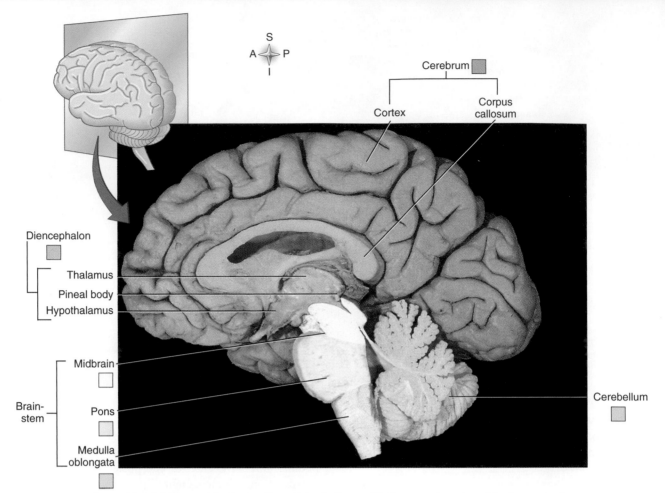

Figure 36-4 **Divisions of the brain.** *(From Vidic B, Suarez FR: Photographic atlas of the human body, St Louis, 1984, Mosby.)*

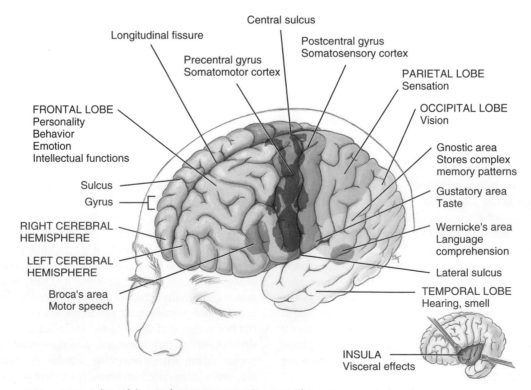

Figure 36-5 **Lobes of the cerebrum.** *(From Applegate E: The anatomy and physiology learning system, ed 2, St Louis, 2000, WB Saunders.)*

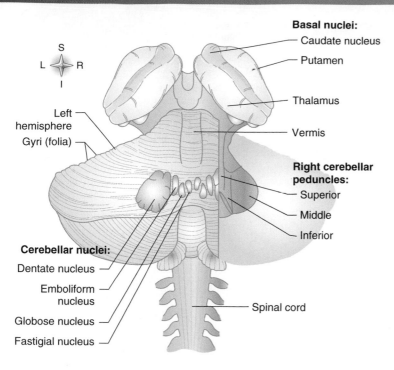

Figure 36-6 Posterior view of the cerebellum. *(From Abrahams P, Hutchings RT, Marks SC: McKinn's color atlas of human anatomy, ed 4, St Louis, 1999, Mosby.)*

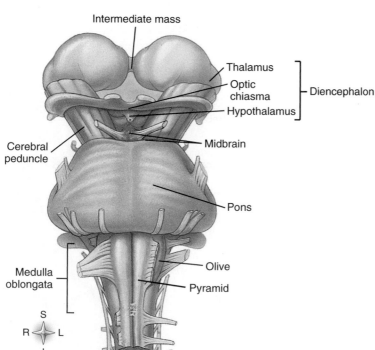

Figure 36-7 Brainstem and diencephalon. *(From Thibodeau G, Patton K: Anatomy and physiology, ed 6, St Louis, 2007, Mosby.)*

midbrain are two masses of white matter called the *cerebral peduncles.* White matter contains millions of myelinated nerve fibers that carry impulses between the neurons. On the dorsal side are four rounded tissue masses called the *corpora quadrigemina.* This section is responsible for relaying auditory and visual impulses.

The pons lies between the midbrain and the medulla, in front of the cerebellum. It consists mainly of white matter and serves as a relay between the medulla and the cerebral peduncles. The fifth, sixth, seventh, and eighth cranial nerves originate in this portion of the hindbrain.

VENTRICULAR SYSTEM

The ventricles are four cavities that are found between the various sections within the brain. They are filled with CSF, which bathes and nourishes the brain. Two lateral ventricles occupy the two halves of the cerebrum. These are connected by the interventricular foramen, which leads to the third ventricle. This ventricle opens into a narrow path, called the *cerebral aqueduct,* which leads directly into the fourth ventricle, lying near the base of the brain. The CSF leaves the fourth ventricle through three openings and then circulates around

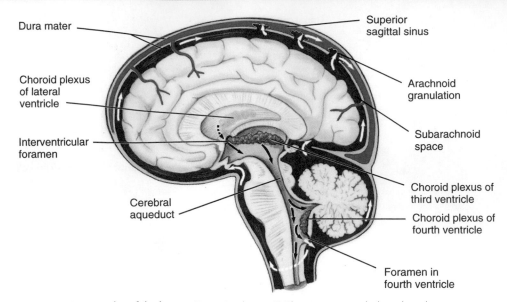

Figure 36-8 **Ventricles of the brain.** *(From Applegate E: The anatomy and physiology learning system, ed 2, St Louis, 2000, WB Saunders.)*

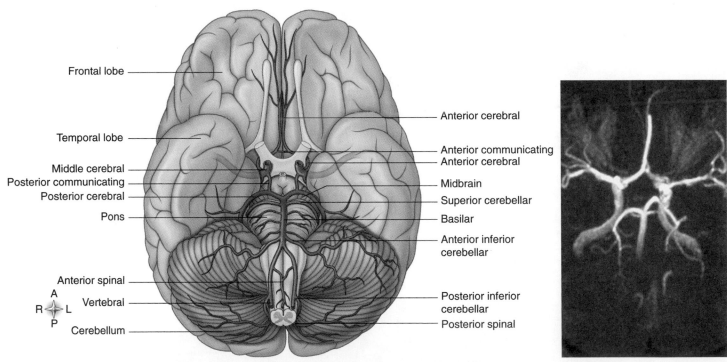

Figure 36-9 **Arteries of the brain.** *(From Drake R, Vogl AW, Mitchell AWM: Gray's anatomy for students, Edinburgh, 2005, Elsevier; and Abrahams P, Hutchings RT, Marks SC: McKinn's color atlas of human anatomy, ed 5, St Louis, 2003, Mosby.)*

the brainstem and cord. The ventricles are illustrated in Figure 36-8.

BLOOD SUPPLY TO THE BRAIN

The brain requires 20% more oxygen than the other organs in the body to function adequately. It receives arterial blood from two systems, the internal carotid arteries and the vertebral arteries. These systems communicate through a structure called the *circle of Willis*, which is located at the base of the brain (Figure 36-9). The circle of Willis gives rise to the other arteries that supply blood to the cerebral hemispheres and ensures continuity of the blood supply to the brain if any of the arteries are compromised. Blood is carried away from the brain by the cerebral veins that drain into the dural sinuses and internal jugular veins.

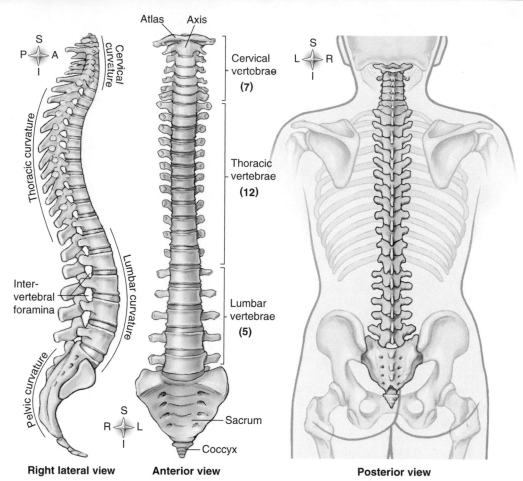

Figure 36-10 Spinal column. *(From Thibodeau G, Patton K: Anatomy and physiology, ed 6, St Louis, Mosby, 2007; and Standring S: Gray's anatomy, ed 38, Edinburgh, Churchill Livingstone, 2004.)*

VERTEBRAL COLUMN

The vertebral column provides structure and protects the spinal cord. The vertebral column is composed of 24 bones, or vertebrae, in addition to the sacrum and coccyx, which are separate in childhood but become fused in adulthood (Figure 36-10):

- 7 cervical vertebrae
- 12 thoracic vertebrae
- 5 lumbar vertebrae
- 5 sacral vertebrae (fused as one)
- 1 coccygeal vertebra, which also is a fused structure containing 1 to 3 separate vertebrae

The vertebrae are referred to by a numerical designation preceded by the first letter of the region where they are located (e.g., the first cervical vertebra is C-1; the first thoracic vertebra is T-1).

The atlas, or first cervical vertebra (C-1), supports the skull and is fused with the second vertebra, the axis (C-2), to provide rotational movement of the neck. The remaining vertebrae are similar in structure and appearance. Each vertebra has a body with a circular opening through which the spinal cord passes. Two pedicles extend backward from the body and form the transverse processes. The transverse processes project laterally and support the articulating surfaces, known as the *facets*.

Each vertebra has openings (intervertebral foramina) for the passage of spinal nerves. Muscles and ligaments hold the vertebral column together.

The vertebrae are separated by cartilaginous cushions called *intervertebral discs*. The tough outer layer of the disc is the annulus fibrosis and the jelly-like center layer is the nucleus pulposus (Figure 36-11).

SPINAL CORD

The spinal cord is located within the vertebral canal and is continuous with the medulla oblongata of the hindbrain. The cord originates at the foramen magnum, a large opening at the base of the skull, and terminates in the cauda equina at the first and second lumbar vertebrae. The spinal cord has 31 segments—8 cervical, 12 thoracic, 5 lumbar, 5 sacral, and 1 coccygeal.

Structurally, the spinal cord is somewhat flat on the dorsoventral side. It has an outer layer of white matter and an inner body of gray matter. A cross section of the cord reveals that the gray matter forms a rough H shape. The two dorsal portions of the H are called the *dorsal horns* and the two ventral portions are called the *ventral horns*. The cross portion of the H is called the *gray commissure,* and this portion encompasses a canal that traverses the length of the cord (Figure 36-12).

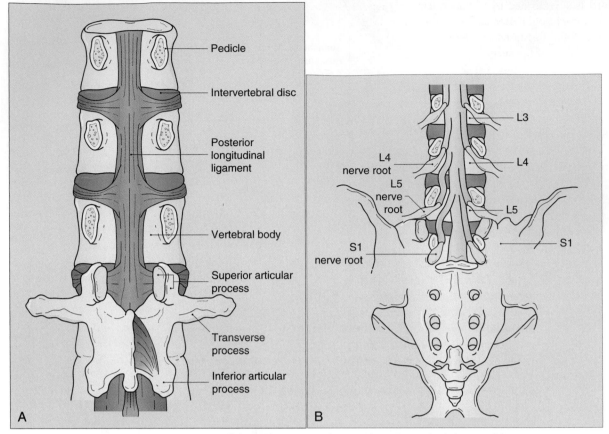

Figure 36-11 A, Posterior view of the lumbar spine, showing the intervertebral discs and bony processes. Note that the upper processes have been cut away to show the deeper structures. **B,** Lumbar spine, illustrating the nerve roots. *(From Rengachary S, Ellenbogen R: Principles of neurosurgery, ed 2, St Louis, 2005, Mosby.)*

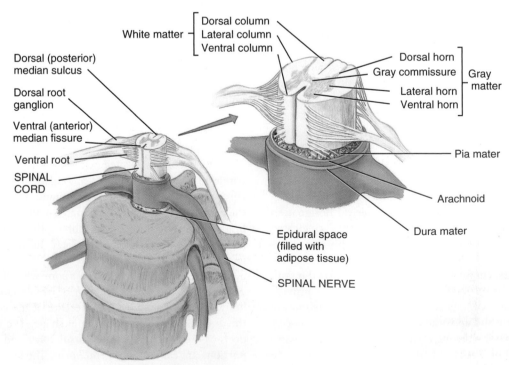

Figure 36-12 Cross section of the spinal cord. *(From Applegate E: The anatomy and physiology learning system, ed 2, St Louis, 2000, WB Saunders.)*

The cord is surrounded by the meninges—the outside dura mater, the arachnoid mater, and the inner pia mater. These are contiguous with the brainstem and continue beyond the spinal cord to the level of the second or third sacral vertebra.

Blood Supply to the Spinal Cord

Blood is supplied to the spinal cord via the branches of the vertebral artery, posterior spinal arteries, posterior inferior cerebral arteries, and various regions of the aorta. The anterior and posterior spinal veins are responsible for venous drainage from the cord.

CRANIAL NERVES

The cranial nerves are 12 pairs of nerves that originate in the brain and are responsible for the sensory and motor functions of the body. Each of the 12 pairs is designated by a Roman numeral, and each has a particular function:

- *I (olfactory):* Responsible for the sense of smell.
- *II (optic):* Conveys impulses for sight.
- *III (oculomotor):* Controls muscles that move the eye and iris.
- *IV (trochlear):* Controls the oblique muscle of the eye.
- *V (trigeminal):* A sensory nerve that controls the sensations of the face, forehead, mouth, nose, and top of the head.
- *VI (abducens):* Controls lateral movement of the eye.
- *VII (facial):* A motor nerve that controls the muscles in the face and scalp, as well as tears and salivation.
- *VIII (vestibulocochlear [acoustic]):* Controls hearing and equilibrium.
- *IX (glossopharyngeal):* Controls the sense of taste and pharyngeal movement, as well as the parotid gland and salivation.
- *X (vagus):* Innervates the pharyngeal and laryngeal muscles, heart, pancreas, lungs, and digestive systems; also controls the sensory paths of the abdominal viscera, the pleura, and the thoracic viscera.
- *XI (accessory):* Has two parts, a cranial portion and a spinal portion. The cranial portion joins the vagus nerve to help control the pharyngeal and laryngeal muscles. The spinal portion controls the trapezius and sternocleidomastoid muscles.
- *XII (hypoglossal):* Innervates the muscles of the tongue.

SPINAL NERVES

The spinal nerves occur in pairs and originate from the spinal cord near their corresponding vertebra. Each spinal nerve has two roots, a dorsal root and a ventral root. The dorsal root has an area of enlargement called the *dorsal root ganglion.* Each spinal nerve forms two branches, which are called *rami* (sing., *ramus*).

The cervical and thoracic nerves exit the spinal column through the vertebral foramina in a lateral direction. The lumbar, sacral, and coccygeal nerve roots exit from the distal spinal cord at the first lumbar vertebra. These particular nerve roots descend below the terminal point of the spinal cord and are referred to collectively as the *cauda equina* (horse's tail).

AUTONOMIC NERVOUS SYSTEM

The autonomic nervous system (ANS) is an involuntary system that transmits signals for vital functions such as the heart rate, respiration, and digestion. It connects the CNS to the visceral organs via the cranial and spinal nerves. The ANS can be further subdivided into complementary, sympathetic, and parasympathetic components. The sympathetic component is responsible for the "fight-or-flight" mechanism the body uses in response to a threat. The sympathetic response results in the diversion of blood (via vasoconstriction) from nonessential organs and systems (e.g., the gastrointestinal system and skin) to the brain, heart, lungs, and muscles. The parasympathetic component is responsible for the resting functions that promote energy conservation through the dilation of blood vessels and relaxation of muscle groups, as is seen with increased blood flow to the gastrointestinal tract to promote the digestion of food. The ANS and the CNS work together to maintain homeostasis.

SOMATIC NERVOUS SYSTEM

The somatic nervous system (SNS) connects the CNS to the skin and skeletal muscles via the cranial and spinal nerves. It is described as a voluntary system because many of its actions (e.g., blinking the eyelids) can be controlled. The SNS keeps the body in touch with its surroundings by processing sensory activity and controlling muscles.

PERIPHERAL NERVES

Peripheral nerves are composed of small bundles of nerve fibers, called *fascicles,* which are surrounded by a sheath called the *endoneurium.* The perineurium, which is composed of fibers of connective tissue, extends within the spaces between the nerve fibers and binds them together. The nerve unit is bound together by the epineurium.

DIAGNOSTIC PROCEDURES

HISTORY AND PHYSICAL EXAMINATION

The history and physical examination are done to determine past and present symptoms, trauma, and neurological illness or pathological abnormalities. Many neurological problems are not visible; therefore specialized techniques are used during the physical examination to evaluate the CNS and PNS. Baseline tests are listed in Table 36-1. In examining the patient, the neurosurgeon focuses on gait, speech, and mental status. Assessment of the patient's motor tone, strength, reflex response, and flexibility also is a critical element of the examination.

The patient's cerebellar function is evaluated by testing balance and coordination. Sensory function generally is evaluated during the cranial nerve examination.

Table **36-1**	**Cranial Nerve Evaluation**
Cranial Nerve (CN)	**Method of Testing**
I (olfactory)	Patient is asked to identify a smell.
II (optic)	Patient is asked to describe an object. Neurosurgeon evaluates visual field by asking when the patient first sees an object (e.g., the surgeon's finger) moving into the line of vision.
III (oculomotor)	Surgeon examines the patient's pupils for size, shape, equality, and reaction to light.
IV (trochlear)	Tested in conjunction with CN III.
V (trigeminal)	Patient is asked to identify sensations of hot and cold, pinpricks. Also asked to clench teeth and move jaw from side to side.
VI (abducens)	Surgeon has patient follow an object visually from side to side and up and down.
VII (facial)	Patient is asked to close eyes, smile, and frown.
VIII (vestibulocochlear)	Patient's response to verbal questions indicates that the nerve is grossly intact. Surgeon may also use a tuning fork to check bone and air conduction.
IX (glossopharyngeal)	Surgeon tests the patient's gag reflex with a tongue blade and asks the patient to swallow.
X (vagus)	Tested in conjunction with CN IX.
XI (spinal accessory)	Patient is asked to rotate the head and shrug the shoulders against resistance.
XII (hypoglossal)	Patient is asked to stick out the tongue.

IMAGING STUDIES

A variety of imaging studies may be performed before neurosurgery as part of the patient's diagnostic workup. Relevant studies must be available in the operating room or uploaded to the computer before the surgery begins.

Computed Tomography

Computed tomography (CT) is the gold standard for evaluating many cranial vascular disorders (e.g., **aneurysm**, acute hemorrhage). (Chapter 7 includes a discussion of the technical aspects of CT.)

Magnetic Resonance Imaging

Magnetic resonance imaging (MRI) is used extensively in neurosurgery to diagnose tumors, abscesses, ligament damage, and disc herniation. It provides clear visualization of these structures. In some facilities, MRI is done intraoperatively, either with a portable unit or in a dedicated operating suite. (Chapter 7 includes a description of the technology used in MRI.)

Functional Magnetic Resonance Imaging

Functional MRI (fMRI) is used for preoperative brain mapping. Preoperative brain mapping allows the neurosurgeon to localize areas of the brain responsible for certain motor skills, language, and sensory functions. Preoperative mapping also can determine the need for intraoperative mapping. Images of the brain are captured while the patient is asked to do certain tasks (e.g., name a list of objects). These images are processed by the MRI computer software, which generates three-dimensional images showing the active areas of the brain.

Stereotactic Magnetic Resonance Imaging

Stereotactic MRI combines standard MRI technology with a head frame or magnetic markers, called *fiducials,* to pinpoint a particular location in the brain and provide precise coordinates for surgery. This procedure greatly enhances surgical precision for a variety of interventions.

Magnetic Resonance Angiography

Using MRI technology, magnetic resonance angiography (MRA) produces very detailed images of vascular structures. It is useful for visualizing the cerebral circulation.

Angiography (Arteriography)

In angiography, an arterial catheter is used to inject a contrast medium into the patient's arterial system. The contrast medium outlines the structure of the vessels. Angiography often is used in the diagnosis of cerebral aneurysms and arteriovenous malformations. The principles of angiography are discussed in Chapters 7 and 32.

Digital Subtraction Angiography

Digital subtraction angiography (DSA) is an imaging technique used with standard angiography to selectively isolate vascular structures. Images are obtained before and after injection of the contrast medium. The precontrast image is "subtracted" from the data, revealing the vascular structure only. This technology is used less routinely since the advent of three-dimensional CT angiography.

Three-Dimensional CT Angiography

In three-dimensional CT angiography, a contrast medium is used to provide images of the intracranial vasculature, which later are reconstructed in a three-dimensional view by the CT program software. This technology is less invasive than DSA.

Myelography

Although myelography largely has been replaced by MRI, some surgeons use x-rays to visualize the spinal cord. For these imaging studies, a contrast medium is injected into the subarachnoid space of the cervical or lumbar spine. Plain x-rays are then taken to record the images produced by the contrast medium.

Discography

Discography is an imaging technique used to evaluate pathology of an intervertebral disc (e.g., herniation). In this procedure, a small amount of contrast dye is injected directly into the disc, and the patient's response is monitored in terms of the intensity and location of the pain resulting from the injection. Fluoroscopy is used for real-time assessment of the disc during the test. A CT scan may be performed afterward for a more detailed anatomical view of the disc.

Ultrasound

Ultrasound technology often is used before neurosurgery to assess the blood flow in the cerebral blood vessels. It is used intraoperatively for real-time imaging of cysts, tumors, and other structures in the brain or spinal cord.

Electroencephalogram

An electroencephalogram (EEG) measures the electrical activity of the brain. It typically is obtained to evaluate seizure disorders, head injuries, dementia, and metabolic conditions affecting the brain. In the perioperative setting, it can be used during a procedure to monitor the depth of anesthesia or to monitor brain activity in procedures that require occlusion of the carotid artery.

Electromyography

Electromyography (EMG) measures the conduction rate of motor nerves. During this test, needle electrodes are placed in the muscle and a low-voltage current is delivered. The period between stimulus and muscle contraction is measured. This test often is used to evaluate loss of nerve conduction caused by a herniated disc, spondylosis, or other types of impingement disorders.

Somatosensory Evoked Potentials

The somatosensory evoked potentials (SSEP) test measures sensory impulses from the body to the brain. This test may be performed preoperatively to assess nerve damage, or it may be performed intraoperatively to monitor changes in the nerves in spinal, carotid artery, or cerebral aneurysm surgery. Electrodes or fine needles are used to stimulate selected nerves, and function is determined by the elapsed time between stimulus and response.

CASE PLANNING

PSYCHOLOGICAL CONSIDERATIONS

All patients undergoing surgery arrive in the operating room with concerns about their safety and the surgical outcome. Because of the delicate nature of neurosurgery and the risk of impaired function after the surgery, neurosurgical patients often are very fearful or anxious. Patients facing cranial surgery may fear they will not awaken after the surgery or that they will lose their sight, hearing, or mobility. The fear of losing cognitive ability is very strong in many patients.

Patients who appear to be unaware or even unconscious often are highly aware of their surroundings. Although voluntary movement may be impaired, their sensory perception may be fully intact. The perioperative team can provide important emotional and psychological support to the patient.

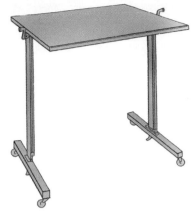

Figure 36-13 Mayfield instrument table. *(From Rothrock J: Alexander's care of the patient in surgery, ed 12, St Louis, 2003, Mosby.)*

ROOM SETUP AND EQUIPMENT

Because of the highly technical nature of neurosurgery procedures, a great deal of specialized equipment and accessories may be required. The surgical technologist shares responsibility for ensuring that all needed equipment and supplies are available and ready for use.

Standard Equipment

Standard furniture and equipment for the neurosurgery operating room include the following:

- Operating table with specialized head stabilizers
- Monopolar electrosurgical unit (ESU), bipolar ESU, or combined unit
- Nitrogen (inline or tank)
- Two suction units
- Surgeons' sitting stools
- Imaging equipment
- Operating microscope

A special overhead table (Mayfield table) may be used in place of the Mayo stand during neurosurgical procedures (Figure 36-13). The Mayfield table can be positioned over the patient during cranial surgery so that instruments and equipment can be passed to the surgeons, who stand at the patient's head. During spinal surgery, the table can be placed over the patient's lower body. The table is large enough to accommodate the many supplies and solutions needed during a neurosurgical procedure. In many cases, the Mayfield table is draped continuously with the patient to produce one large sterile field. If an overhead table is not used, the surgical technologist stands at the surgeon's dominant side so that instruments can be passed without any obstruction.

INSTRUMENTS

Hand Instruments

Neurosurgical instrumentation is often daunting to team members who are new to the specialty. Hundreds of different instruments are available, each having a particular shape and use. General surgery instruments are used for soft tissue access to neurological structures. Once exposure is accomplished,

| Box **36-1** | **Basic Neurosurgical Instruments** |

- Assorted bone rongeurs
- Assorted pituitary rongeurs
- Penfield dissectors
- Self-retaining retractors (e.g., Weitlaner, Adson-Beckman, Gelpi)
- Cranial self-retaining retractor systems (e.g., Greenburg, Budde, Leyla-Yasargil)
- Handheld retractors (e.g., Army-Navy, Richardson, Meyerding, Cushing, malleable, Senn; skin hooks)
- Toothed and untoothed forceps (e.g., bayonet, Cushing, Adson, Gerald, dural)
- Periosteal elevators
- Osteotomes and gouges
- Dural hooks, nerve hooks
- Scalp clip appliers or clip applier gun
- Bone curettes
- Bipolar forceps
- Frazier suction tips (assorted sizes)
- Microsurgical instruments as requested

specialty instruments are used to provide retraction and exposure, remove bone, extract disc fragments, and manipulate the delicate tissue of the brain and spinal cord.

Basic neurosurgical instruments are listed in Box 36-1. Instrumentation specific to the neurosurgical procedure is discussed in the surgical techniques section. Commonly used instruments are illustrated in Figures 36-14 through 36-17.

Microsurgical instruments are used in cranial surgery, spinal surgery, and some peripheral nerve procedures. These instruments are delicate and must be handled with care. When the surgeon is using an instrument under the microscope, the surgical technologist must remember that the surgeon is working within a very limited visual field. The scrub must anticipate which instrument will be needed next and pass it correctly so that the surgeon does not have to look away from the field to receive it. (Chapter 27 contains illustrations demonstrating this technique.)

Decontamination and sterilization processing for neurosurgical instruments generally is identical to processing for other hand instruments. However, special processing is required for instruments used in known or suspected cases of Creutzfeldt-Jakob disease (CJD). CJD is a fatal disease of the nervous system that is caused by a prion, which cannot be destroyed by normal disinfection and sterilization methods. Although guidelines for decontamination vary by institution, recommendations include the use of disposable instruments, which are isolated and incinerated upon disposal. (A discussion of prion disease can be found in Chapter 9.)

Further information on isolation and sterilization measures is available on the websites for the Centers for Disease Control and Prevention (CDC, at http://www.cdc.gov) and the Association of periOperative Registered Nurses (AORN, at http://www.aorn.org).

Power Instruments

Power instruments are used to remove and shape bone. Power drills and saws are used for cutting and remolding bone. Neurosurgical power equipment can be pneumatic (air-powered) or battery or electrically powered. The surgical technologist is responsible for the safe handling of power instruments on the surgical field. Switches must always be in the safety position, except during use, to prevent injury in the event of inadvertent activation. The surgical technologist also is responsible for irrigating the tip of the drill when it is in use to prevent overheating of tissue. Commonly used power systems are the Midas Rex system, the Hall perforator, and the Codman craniotome (a craniotomy saw) (Figure 36-18). A complete discussion of the care and use of power drills, including craniotomies, is covered in Chapter 31.

During a craniotomy, a perforator bit is used to drill holes in the cranial bones. The perforator is used with a power drill, called a craniotome, which is equipped with a safety clutch that stops the drill bit before it touches the dura.

IMPLANTS

A variety of materials are implanted in the course of many neurosurgical procedures. Implants include tissue, bone, plates, screws, rods, clips, shunts, coils, chemotherapeutic wafers, and generators. Specific devices are discussed as applicable in the Surgical Procedures section. In general, surgical technologists must take care in handling any implantable device to ensure its sterility and integrity. The scrub must also document the manufacturer's serial and lot numbers and any other information contained in the sterile packaging. When multiple devices are implanted, the scrub must communicate clearly with the circulator to ensure that the devices' correct locations are noted in the patient record.

The U.S. Food and Drug Administration (FDA) regulates the tracking of certain implantable devices and requires that manufacturers have processes in place to locate devices in the event of a recall. The FDA regulations govern devices for which failure would result in serious, adverse health consequences; those that are intended to be left in the human body for at least 1 year; and any implantable device that is life sustaining or life supporting and is used outside of a health care facility. Facilities may develop policies and procedures for tracking any implantable device, but at minimum they must track the devices identified by the FDA. Typical information used in tracking includes the following:

- Device identification (e.g., lot number, serial number, model or batch number)
- Date of manufacture and shipping
- Name, address, telephone number, and social security number of the patient in whom the device was implanted
- Location where the device was implanted
- Name, address, and telephone number of the physician who implanted the device

On occasion, a previously implanted device is removed during a procedure. This process is known as *explantation*. Surgical technologists should be familiar with their facility's policies regarding explanted devices; all explanted devices

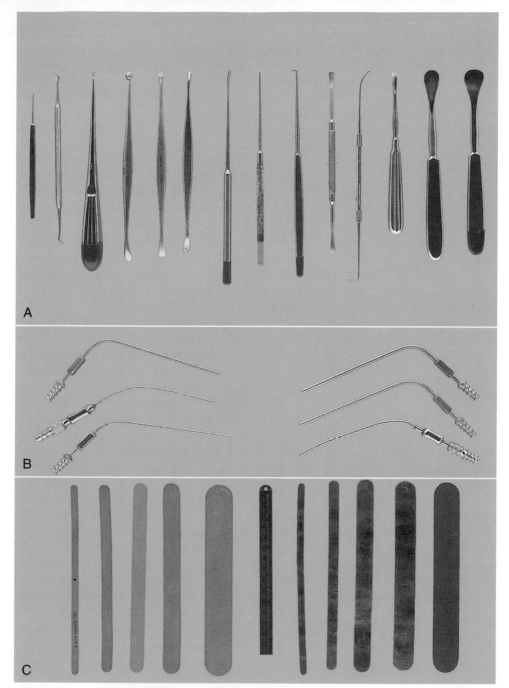

Figure 36-14 Neurosurgical instruments. A, *Left to right,* 1 dura hook; 1 Woodson dura separator; 1 Brun curette; 4 Penfield dissectors; 1 Adson dura hook, 1 nerve hook; 1 Freer elevator; 1 Kistner probe; 1 joker elevator; 2 Hoen periosteal elevators. **B,** Frazier suction tips. **C,** Brain retractors and spatulas. *(From Tighe SM: Instrumentation for the operating room, ed 6, St Louis, 2003, Mosby.)*

are sent for pathological examination before their final disposition.

WOUND MANAGEMENT

Sponges

Radiopaque 4 × 4 sponges are used in neurosurgical procedures to absorb blood and fluid and control bleeding. In addition to these, the neurosurgeon uses small, square, felted sponges made of cotton or rayon to control bleeding on neural and vascular tissue. These are commonly referred to as "patties" or "cottonoids" (see Chapter 22). Radiopaque threads are sewn into the body of each sponge, which also has a strong string, colored green, for visibility in the wound. Patties are supplied in a variety of sizes. The felted consistency allows the surgeon to use the sponge as a filter when suction is applied to the neural tissue. The suction tip is kept in contact with the patty so that the tissue underneath is not damaged.

Small cotton balls with radiopaque markers and strings also are used in neurosurgery. Cottonoids and cotton balls are always offered moist. The surgeon may place a cottonoid or cotton ball on top of the tissue and suction through it to avoid damaging the tissue. All sponges are counted on all neurosurgical procedures.

Drugs and Irrigation

Drugs used intraoperatively during neurosurgery include:
- Hemostatic agents
- Irrigation fluid
- Antibiotics in solution with injectable saline

The temperature of the irrigation solution is very important. To prevent tissue damage, the temperature should be below 120° F (48.9° C). Fluid that is too cold may contribute to hypothermia. A piston syringe is used to irrigate the tissue. A catheter or needle-tip irrigator similar to that used in eye surgery may also be used during microsurgery or nerve repair.

Among the more important drugs administered during cranial procedures is the osmotic diuretic, which removes fluid from tissue and prevents swelling as a result of surgical trauma. Drugs commonly used in neurosurgery are listed in Table 36-2.

Drains

A variety of drains are used in neurosurgery to evacuate blood, serum, and fluid and to eliminate dead space in the surgical wound. A lumbar drain may be placed in the subarachnoid space before a surgical procedure to remove CSF from the spinal canal or brain; this decompresses the tissue. A lumbar drain also can be used to monitor **intracranial pressure (ICP).** As an alternative, a ventricular drain may be placed for the same purpose. The surgical technologist must make sure strict sterility is maintained during the placement of this type of drain, because the drain acts as a direct conduit to the CNS, providing a portal of entry for infection. A separate surgical setup should be created for placement of the lumbar or ventricular drain.

Suture

Silk and nylon sutures are commonly used on neural tissue for dural retraction, closure, and repair. Peripheral nerve anastomosis usually is performed with fine nylon or Prolene suture. Wire is used to suture the cranial bones in place following craniotomy. Staples generally are used for skin closure in the scalp and back.

Cements and Adhesives

Bone cements and adhesives are used in neurosurgical procedures. Methylmethacrylate (see Chapter 31) is used in cranioplasty procedures and to construct antibiotic beads, which are used in cases of vertebral column infection. (The cranioplasty section, later in the chapter, presents more information on techniques used to prepare methylmethacrylate in cranial surgery.) Octylcyanoacrylate, an adhesive, may be used to close the skin edges of incisions that are not under pressure.

Dressings

Wound dressings are applied at the end of a neurosurgical procedure to protect the incision and provide an environment for wound healing. Spinal incisions are dressed with nonadherent Telfa and absorbent gauze pads secured with tape. Cranial dressings tend to be more complex and more difficult to secure. A single nonadherent strip (Telfa or mesh) is placed over the incision. Square gauze and bulky fluff gauze are added, followed by soft rolled gauze, which is wrapped around the head to secure the dressings. If an external brace is required, it is applied over the dressing.

ANESTHESIA

Neurosurgery of the cranium and spine usually is performed using general (inhalation) anesthesia. Selected procedures, such as the placement of brain electrodes, can be performed with the patient awake or under light sedation. Depending on the patient's condition, an "awake" intubation may be required for safety in some procedures of the cervical spine.

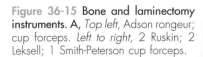

Figure 36-15 **Bone and laminectomy instruments. A,** *Top left,* Adson rongeur; cup forceps. *Left to right,* 2 Ruskin; 2 Leksell; 1 Smith-Peterson cup forceps.

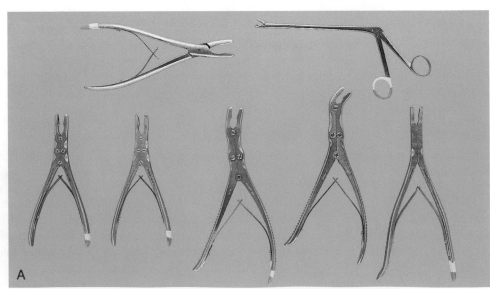

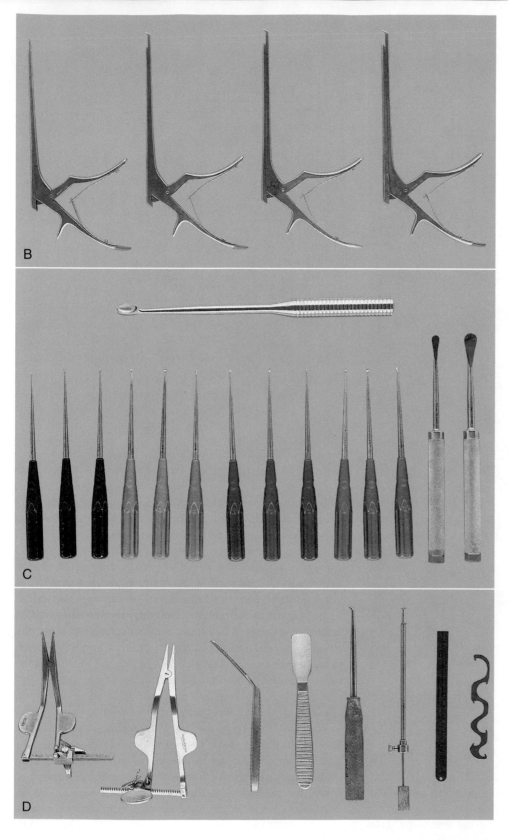

Figure 36-15, cont'd **B,** Kerrison rongeurs (up-biting). **C,** Curettes (colored handles) and Cobb elevators. **D,** *Left to right,* 2 Cloward vertebra spreaders; 2 Cloward blade retractors; 1 osteophyte elevator; 1 depth gauge; 1 ruler; 1 spanner wrench. *(From Tighe SM: Instrumentation for the operating room, ed 6, St Louis, 2003, Mosby.)*

Regional anesthesia can be used in peripheral nerve repair. The Bier block (see Chapter 14) is commonly used for nerve repair or transposition in the arm. The scalp incision site routinely is injected with a vasoconstrictive drug in a local anesthetic carrier (lidocaine) to maintain local vasoconstriction and a drier surgical field.

Extensive physiological monitoring is carried out during cranial procedures.

Thermoregulation is an important consideration for neurosurgical patients undergoing general anesthesia because most procedures are lengthy. Hypothermia can interfere with clotting, alter the metabolism of drugs, and impair wound

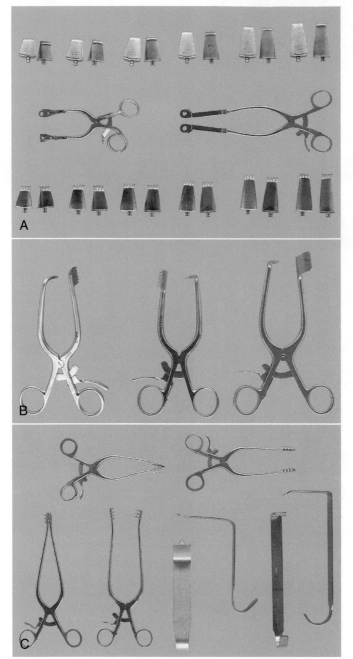

Figure 36-16 **Laminectomy retractors.** **A,** Cloward retractor with blunt and sharp blades. **B,** Williams retractors. **C,** *Top,* Adson retractors. *Bottom, left to right,* 2 Weitlaner retractors; 2 Taylor retractors; 2 Hibbs retractors. *(From Tighe SM: Instrumentation for the operating room, ed 6, St Louis, 2003, Mosby.)*

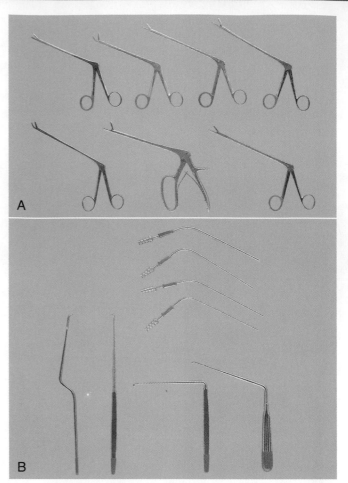

Figure 36-17 **Discectomy instruments.** **A,** Cushing pituitary rongeurs, straight and angled. **B,** Frazier suction tips *(top)* and nerve root retractors. *(From Tighe SM: Instrumentation for the operating room, ed 6, St Louis, 2003, Mosby.)*

healing. The anesthesia care provider implements a variety of measures to minimize the patient's risk of developing intraoperative hyperthermia, such as warming the anesthetic gases and fluids and using warm blankets and forced air warming blankets. Infants undergoing neurosurgical procedures are very vulnerable to the effects of hypothermia. An infrared light system often is used to keep the infant warm and reduce the risk.

In addition to standard anesthetic goals, specific areas of monitoring and care are required during neurosurgery. The patient's blood pressure is maintained within a normal or below-normal range to prevent bleeding and increases in ICP. Smooth emergence from anesthesia is extremely important to minimize the risk of laryngospasm and struggling. Often the surgical dressing is applied before the reversal agents are given to avoid overstimulating the patient, which might increase the blood pressure.

PATIENT POSITIONING

The long duration of neurosurgical procedures increases the risk of injury related to positioning. The surgeons and anesthesia care provider check any possible pressure points and make sure the areas are adequately padded. Because cranial procedures often use the prone position, respiratory clearance for expansion of the thorax is very important. (These points and others are covered in Chapter 19.)

Specialized Positioning Aids

HEADRESTS During cranial surgery, a variety of specialized positioning devices are used, including headrests and fixation devices that attach to the operating bed. Many different types of headrest are available, some designed with disposable or

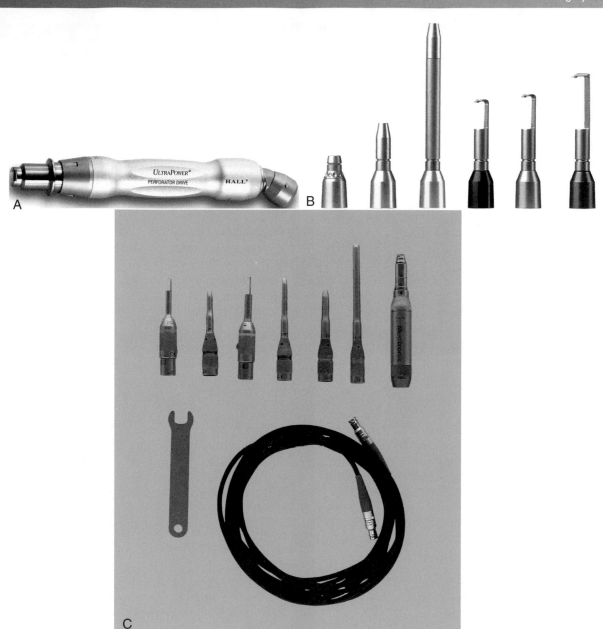

Figure 36-18 **Neurosurgical power instruments. A,** Hall perforator drill. **B,** Burr guards. L-shaped guards prevent the drill tip from penetrating the cranial meninges. **C,** Midas Rex drill and guards (Medtronic, Minneapolis, Minn). *(From Tighe SM: Instrumentation for the operating room, ed 6, St Louis, 2003, Mosby.)*

reusable detachable pins that are inserted into the patient's skull. The patient first is positioned with the headrest in place, and the pins then are reattached to the headrest to immobilize the head completely.

Two types of headrests commonly used are the Mayfield headrest and the three-pin fixation headrest (Figure 36-19). Skull tongs (e.g., Gardner-Wells tongs) may also be used to secure the patient's head in a particular position and as a means for attaching traction devices. The surgical technologist establishes a small sterile field on a prep table for the neurosurgeon to use when inserting the fixation pins or tongs (Figure 36-20). The scrub may also assist the surgeon with insertion or removal of the device.

When assisting the surgeon during patient positioning, the surgical technologist must take care to prevent injury to the patient's spine, shoulders, and head. Make sure the head is cradled securely and in anatomical position at all times to prevent hyperextension of the neck or sudden movement.

Operating Table

A specialty operating table is used in neurosurgery, especially for spinal and cranial procedures. These beds come with many accessories to optimize safe positioning. The Andrews bed and the Jackson spinal table are two examples of specialized operating beds. These specialized tables allow a wide variety of customized positions with clearance for C-arm fluoroscopy. An

Table 36-2 Medications Used in Neurosurgery

Agent	Form	Mechanism of Action	Special Considerations
Lidocaine with epinephrine	Injectable	Inhibits the conduction of nerve impulses and constricts blood vessels.	Must be clearly labeled when used on the sterile field to avoid confusion with other medications. Surgical technician must track the amount administered by the surgeon.
Mannitol	Injectable	Acts on the kidneys to move fluid from the tissues.	Given by the anesthesia care provider to prevent increased intracranial pressure and reduce cerebral or spinal cord edema.
Papaverine	Injectable/topical	Relaxes the blood vessel wall.	May be applied topically to the vessels feeding a cerebral aneurysm to prevent spasm.
Topical thrombin	Powder for reconstitution; packaged with diluent and spray pump, or diluent and spray tip syringe with diluent only	Catalyzes the conversion of fibrinogen to fibrin.	For external use only; must be refrigerated.
Gelatin matrix (FloSeal)	Gelatin matrix granules and topical thrombin packaged as a kit with syringes and mixing bowl	Matrix particles form a composite clot that seals the bleeding site; thrombin component converts the fibrinogen in the patient's blood to fibrin.	Product reaches maximum expansion at approximately 10 minutes. Excess product should be removed with gentle irrigation.
Absorbable gelatin sponge (Gelfoam)	Film, powder, and topical forms	Absorbs and holds blood and fluid within its interstices; exerts physical hemostatic effect.	Should not be used in the closure of skin incisions, because it may interfere with healing of skin edges. Often moistened with saline or topical thrombin before use.
Collagen hemostat (Avitene, Helistat, Instat)	Pads, powder, sheets, sponges	When in contact with a bleeding surface, attracts platelets, which aggregate into thrombi, initiating the formation of a physiological platelet plug.	Applied dry; excess material should be removed from the wound before closure.
Oxidized regenerated cellulose (Surgicel)	Fibrous, knitted, or sheer weave fabric	Allows platelets and aggregates of thrombin and particulate blood elements to cling and form a coagulum that can act as a patch.	Store at room temperature.

Modified from Ferrera D: Neurosurgery. In Rothrock JC, editor: *Alexander's care of the patient in surgery*, ed 14, St Louis, 2007, Mosby.

alternative to a dedicated spinal table is a laminectomy frame (e.g., the Wilson frame), which is positioned on the operating table and adjusted to elevate the thorax (see Chapter 19).

Cranial Surgery

Accurate positioning of the patient's head is crucial in cranial surgery. The location of the lesion determines the exact position and whether fixation is needed. Venous drainage and maintaining a low ICP are other important considerations when positioning patients for cranial procedures.

Risks Associated with Fowler Position

A significant risk of air embolisms is associated with sitting positions (e.g., Fowler or beach chair position). Air embolism can occur when air enters the vascular system through an open blood vessel, the exposed occipital muscles, or the sinuses of the brain. Air embolism is a surgical emergency for which all team members must be prepared. If an embolism occurs through the wound, the surgeon needs copious irrigation and sponges to cover the open vessels. This prevents any more air from entering the wound while attempts are made to locate the source of air entry. Another action the surgeon may take is to reposition the patient in a left lateral position. This prevents air that might have entered the heart from forming an air lock. The scrubbed surgical technologist should protect the sterile field and quickly move sterile equipment out of the way so that the patient can be positioned. When the patient is secured, the equipment is again moved into place.

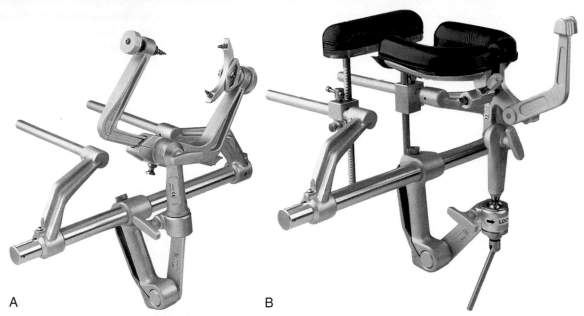

A   B

Figure 36-19 **Cranial headrests. A,** Three-pin suspension skull clamps. **B,** Mayfield headrest. *(From Rothrock J: Alexander's care of the patient in surgery, ed 12, St Louis, 2003, Mosby.)*

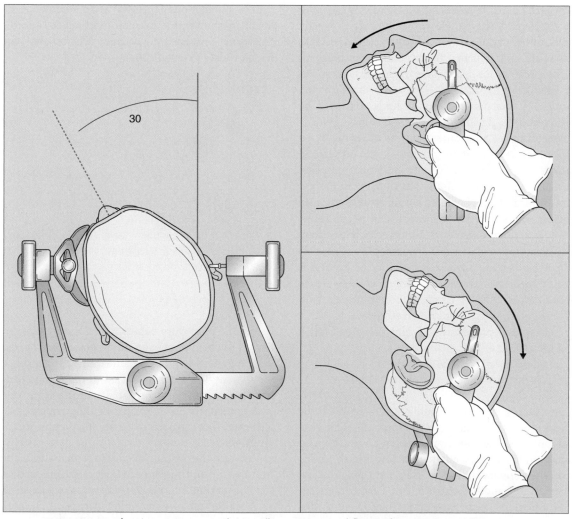

Figure 36-20 **Three-pin suspension clamps allow rotation and flexion for secure positioning.** *(From Rengachary S, Ellenbogen R: Principles of neurosurgery, ed 2, St Louis, 2005, Mosby.)*

Spinal Surgery

Procedures of the anterior cervical spine are performed with the patient in the supine position, often with the patient's head in a three-pin skull fixation device to maintain stability. Traction also may be used, with a chin harness attached to a weight to open the spaces between the cervical vertebrae. Procedures of the posterior cervical spine are performed with the patient in either the prone or sitting position.

Procedures of the thoracic spine may use the supine, lateral, or prone position or even a combination of positions, which may require an intraoperative position change. The prone position with spinal flexion is used for surgery on the lumbar spine. This spreads the lamina, decompresses the epidural veins, minimizes wound depth, and allows the great vessels of the abdomen to drop away from the spine

PREPPING AND DRAPING

Once the patient has been positioned, the skin prep is performed. When necessary, hair removal should be done as close to the time of surgery as possible. Head hair is only removed when it would interfere with the surgery. If the surgeon has ordered hair clipping, it is performed outside the operating room. Generally, hair removal is limited to the amount necessary to facilitate the incision and ensure a clean surgical field; rarely is the entire head shaved. However, the hair is usually held back with rubber bands and water-based gel. The patient's hair may be saved and returned to the patient as personal property. In preparation for procedures of the cervical spine, the surgeon may order the patient's nape to be shaved to the level of the ears. If the patient's hair is long, it should be secured to the top of the head with an elastic band.

Certain neurosurgical procedures, such as those involving harvesting of a bone or fat graft, may require a second surgical prep. A separate prep setup is used for the second prep site. (See Chapter 20 for a complete discussion of the skin prep.)

Because most surgeries involving the brain require complex draping routines, the surgeons may direct and complete the draping themselves. Drapes may be sewn directly to the scalp with silk sutures, adhesive drapes may be used, or surgical skin staple clips may be used. In any case involving the head, it is wise to have extra drapes available to secure a large sterile field. A specialized craniotomy drape with an attached fluid collection system often is used for cranial surgery.

Draping for spinal procedures is the same as for a laparotomy.

TEAM POSITIONING

For cranial procedures, the surgeon and assistant stand at the patient's head and the scrub stands to the surgeon's right or at the overhead table. During spinal procedures, a right-handed surgeon usually stands at the patient's left side and the assistant stands on the patient's right side. The scrub should stand to the patient's left unless otherwise directed. Peripheral nerve procedures on a patient's upper extremities may be performed with the surgical team seated around a hand table. Team positioning during procedures with the patient in the high Fowler position may need to be altered to accommodate standing platforms for scrubbed personnel to ensure safe access to the surgical field. Other considerations for team positioning include the presence of equipment such as the C-arm, surgical microscopes, Cavitron Ultrasonic Surgical Aspirator (CUSA) console, and other equipment.

CRANIAL PROCEDURES

BURR HOLES

Surgical Goal

In cranial surgery, holes are drilled in the cranium with a neurosurgical drill (craniotome). The procedure is performed most often to relieve pressure on the brain caused by the accumulation of fluid beneath the dura mater. Burr holes are also used when the skull is opened for a craniotomy.

Pathology

Traumatic head injury often causes blood to accumulate under the dura. The resulting hematoma causes pressure on the brain tissue, causing injury and alterations in consciousness or motor function. A skull fracture may or may not have occurred during the injury. Trauma usually is the result of a motor vehicle accident, sports injury, or intentional violence. Suspicion of a hematoma is treated as an emergency. CT scans are obtained quickly and a craniotomy often is performed as an emergency procedure to evacuate accumulated blood or infectious exudate from a brain abscess.

TECHNIQUE

1 The patient is placed in the supine position and the head is stabilized.
2 The incision line is marked and injected with lidocaine with epinephrine.
3 The scalp is incised and the pericranium elevated.
4 A craniotome with a perforating bit is used to drill a hole through the skull.
5 The dura is incised.
6 The clot, tissue debris, and fluid are evacuated.
7 Drains may be placed.
8 The wound is closed in layers.

Discussion

Before the procedure begins, the CT scans showing the location of the hematoma should be placed on the view boxes.

The patient is prepped and draped for a routine craniotomy. A surgical marker is used to mark the position of each burr hole. Some surgeons infiltrate the scalp with lidocaine with epinephrine to control bleeding, which usually is brisk. However, if the procedure is an emergency, this step may be omitted.

To begin the procedure, the surgeon makes a linear incision over the site of the proposed burr hole. The scrub should have the ESU and numerous 4 × 4 sponges available.

After the scalp is incised, a periosteal elevator is used to separate the pericranium from the skull.

A craniotome with a perforator bit is used to create the burr holes. The scrub must irrigate the perforator bit during drilling

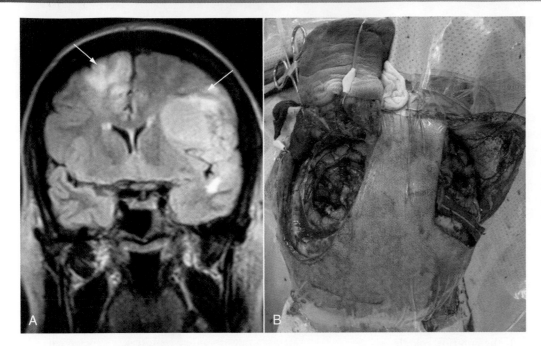

Figure 36-21 A, MRI showing a metastatic brain tumor. **B,** Simultaneous craniotomies for resection of tumors. *(From Townsend CM: Sabiston textbook of surgery, ed 17, Philadelphia, 2001, WB Saunders.)*

to prevent friction and thermal injury to the underlying tissue. Suction is applied adjacent to the irrigation stream to remove any bone particles from the field. The surgical technologist should have bone putty prepared in case of bleeding from the bone edges. Two or more burr holes may be drilled to evacuate the hematoma or fluid collection. The number of holes placed and their location depend on the size of the hematoma and its orientation. Typically, the first burr hole is placed in the temporal region immediately above the zygomatic arch and subsequent holes are placed in the parietal or frontal regions.

The surgeon uses a dura hook to elevate the dura and then incises it with a knife with a #15 blade. Metzenbaum scissors are used to create a larger opening.

Irrigation fluid is used to evacuate the clot. The scrub provides copious amounts of warm irrigation fluid. Several bulb syringes can be used simultaneously. Irrigation continues until the clot is evacuated and the irrigation return is clear.

Hemostasis is maintained with the ESU. In some cases, a drain may be inserted into the subdural or epidural space to promote complete evacuation of the hematoma. The dura is closed with braided nylon or silk. The galea is closed with absorbable suture and the skin is closed with staples or nylon suture.

CRANIOTOMY: TUMOR REMOVAL

Surgical Goal

A craniotomy is an incision into the cranium to permit access to the brain and intracranial structures. Intracranial access is achieved by creating a **bone flap** (a removable section of the cranium). Tumor removal is an indication for a craniotomy.

Pathology

A craniotomy may be required to provide access for treatment of a variety of intracranial conditions, such as a neoplasm,

cerebral aneurysm, arteriovenous malformation, or hemorrhage. Implantation of electrodes and stimulators also is performed through a craniotomy.

The presence of any type of tumor presents a risk, because the skull is a fixed space, and any tumor can impinge on surrounding tissue (Figure 36-21). Tumors that require resection are listed in Table 36-3.

TECHNIQUE

1. The patient is positioned using the horseshoe headrest or pin fixation.
2. The incision line is marked and injected with lidocaine with epinephrine to promote vasoconstriction of the wound edges.
3. The incision is carried through the galea.
4. Scalp clips are applied to the scalp edges with a clip applier or clip gun to provide hemostasis.
5. The scalp flap is retracted and the pericranium is stripped off the skull with periosteal elevators.
6. Burr holes are placed and extended with rongeurs and curettes.
7. A Penfield or Woodson dissector is used to release the dura from the bone.
8. The burr holes are connected; a craniotome with a dura guard and cutting blade is used to produce the bone flap.
9. The bone flap is elevated from the dura and removed or retracted.
10. Retraction sutures are placed in the dura, which is opened.
11. The resection site is irrigated and hemostasis is achieved.
12. The dura is closed to form a watertight seal.
13. The bone flap is replaced and secured with wire or miniplates and miniscrews.
14. The muscle is approximated and the galea is closed.
15. The skin is closed with staples or suture.

Table **36-3**	**Common Brain Tumors Resected During a Craniotomy**
Tumor Type	**Special Considerations**
Ependymoma: A cancerous tumor composed of the ependymal cells that line the brain ventricles and spinal cord.	Commonly located in the fourth ventricle of the brain. Often slower growing than other brain tumors. More common in children.
Astrocytoma: A cancerous tumor composed of astrocytes, the most prominent glial cell.	A four-tiered grading system, established by the World Health Organization (WHO), is used to rank the severity of the tumor and prognosis. Grade I tumors have a more favorable outcome than grade IV tumors. Glioblastoma multiforme (GBM), a type of grade IV tumor, is extremely aggressive and commonly occurs in the sixth and seventh decades of life.
Oligodendroglioma: A cancerous tumor composed of oligodendrocytes (cells that produce myelin).	Occurs primarily in adults and usually is located in the cerebral hemispheres.
Meningioma: A benign tumor composed of cells from the arachnoid.	More common in females than in males.

Discussion

The craniotomy approach depends on the location of the pathology; it may be made through the anterior, middle, or posterior fossa. In addition, a craniotomy may be classified as frontal, parietal, temporal, or occipital, depending on the planned location of the incision. The patient is placed in the supine, prone, or sitting position. During a craniotomy, a section of the cranium (i.e., a bone flap) is removed. The size of the flap is determined by the size and location of the tumor. A superficial tumor is easier to access and requires a smaller flap than a deep, large tumor. The bone flap is created by drilling multiple burr holes in the skull and then "connecting" them with a protected saw blade (Figure 36-22). This provides a safe method of making an incision into the cranium. The bone flap can be folded back and secured during the procedure or removed completely (a free flap). In either case, the bone is reattached at the close of the procedure.

After infiltrating the incision site with local anesthetic for hemostasis, the surgeon makes a curved incision in the scalp. The surgical assistant applies digital pressure to the wound edges; therefore the scrub should make sure that numerous folded 4 × 4 sponges are available. The monopolar ESU is used for hemostasis.

The surgeon uses scalp clips to secure the edges of the scalp and provide continuous hemostasis during the procedure. Scalp clips are supplied in a disposable preloaded applier, or the scrub may be required to load them onto a manual applier. If manual loading is performed, two appliers should be used for rapid delivery. One is used while the other is loaded.

Blunt and sharp dissection are used to free the galea from the skull. The scalp flap, with the scalp clips in place, is secured to the drapes with silk suture, towel clips, hemostats, or scalp hooks attached to rubber bands tethered by a hemostat. A self-retaining retractor (e.g., a Weitlaner retractor) may also be used to hold the scalp back. A moistened 4 × 4 sponge may be placed over the flap to prevent the tissue from drying.

A periosteal elevator is used to remove the periosteum from the bone and prepare it for drilling the burr holes. To create a bone flap, the surgeon "connects" the burr holes by dividing the bone between each hole with a saw. This frees the

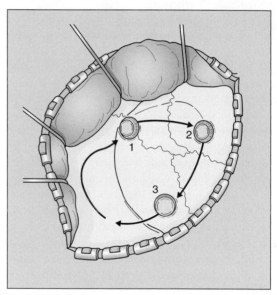

Figure 36-22 Craniotomy. An incision is made to the cranial bone, and scalp clips are applied. Three burr holes are drilled, and the bone is cut between the holes. *(From Rengachary S, Ellenbogen R: Principles of neurosurgery, ed 2, St Louis, 2005, Mosby.)*

cranial segment, which is removed to provide access to the brain tissue below. The flap is turned back or removed.

During the procedure to create a bone flap, the scrub should provide a continuous stream of irrigation fluid over the drill tip or saw during drilling. This prevents the bone tissue from heating as a result of friction. After each burr hole is made, the surgeon removes the bone debris and dust with a curette and enlarges the holes. A Kerrison or a small, double-action rongeur can be used to excise more bone if necessary. The scrub should have bone putty available at this time to aid hemostasis.

The surgeon uses a #3 Penfield or Sachs dura separator to loosen the dura from the skull before connecting the burr holes with the craniotome. The surgeon then wedges two periosteal elevators under the flap to lift it from the dura. If any dura remains attached to the skull flap, a joker elevator may be used to release it.

If the flap is to be turned back (left partly attached), the surgeon places moistened 4 × 4 sponges around it to prevent drying. The flap then is turned back and secured with a towel clip or nylon suture. If a free flap is created, the scrubbed surgical technologist must maintain a firm grip on the bone flap as it is transferred from the surgeon to avoid dropping it. The scrub is responsible for the safety of the flap until it is reattached. The flap must stay hydrated and must be clearly identified in the surgical field. It should be placed in a dedicated basin and covered with antibiotic solution or normal saline. The basin is placed in a protected area of the back table to prevent contamination or contact with instruments and supplies. The flap must be clearly identified to anyone scrubbing in during the case.

After the flap is created, Gelfoam and cottonoid sponges are placed at the periphery of the open dura. A self-retaining retractor system may be placed at this time. In preparation for entry into the brain tissue, the scrub should have a bipolar ESU and a #5 or #6 Frazier suction tip available. The surgeon uses a dura hook to lift the dura away from the brain and incises it with a #15 knife blade mounted on a #7 handle. The incision is extended with Frazier dura scissors or Lahey-Metzenbaum scissors and toothed Adson or Cushing tissue forceps. The technologist should prepare traction sutures of 4-0 silk on a fine controlled-release needle. These are used to secure the dura away from the wound. The brain then is exposed.

A surgical microscope may be used to magnify the tumor bed. The surgeon uses brain spoons, curettes, and delicate rongeurs to remove the tumor. The CUSA also can be used to fragment and debulk neurological tumors.

The scrub should have irrigation fluid available at all times during the procedure. A 30- or 50-mL syringe or bulb syringe is used. A variety of cottonoid sponges and topical hemostatic material also should be available throughout the dissection of the brain tissue. A tissue specimen may be submitted for frozen section during the procedure. All specimens are identified as soon as they are received and passed off the sterile field.

Whenever possible, the entire tumor is removed. If the size or location of the tumor prevents complete removal (e.g., if the tumor is too close to a vital speech or vision center), the surgeon debulks it. In debulking, the surgeon removes as much of the tumor as possible while preserving function in the adjacent areas. Debulking relieves pressure on remaining brain tissue and may make any postoperative radiation or chemotherapy more effective.

After removing the tumor, the surgeon irrigates the wound with antibiotic solution. The dura then may be closed with fine silk sutures or left unsutured.

If the tumor is identified as a high-grade astrocytoma (e.g., glioblastoma multiforme), the surgeon may implant Gliadel wafers in the tumor bed before closing the dura. The Gliadel wafer is impregnated with an antineoplastic agent that delivers chemotherapy directly to the tumor site. The surgical technologist and surgeons must double-glove when handling the wafers for protection from the chemicals. The surgeon places up to eight wafers in the tumor bed and secures them in place with ½-inch (1.25-cm) strips of Surgicel before closing the dura. The scrub should ensure that any instruments used in

placing the wafers are passed off the sterile field so that they do not come in contact with healthy cranial tissue. Any opened but unused wafers should be disposed of according to the facility's policy and procedure for disposal of chemotherapeutic agents. The team regloves before proceeding with cranial closure.

The surgeon then prepares the bone flap for reattachment to the cranium. When transferring the free flap back to the surgeon at the end of the procedure, the scrub should verify that the surgeon has a firm grip on the flap before releasing it. The surgeon reattaches the flap with wire sutures. A craniotome drill is used to place small holes in the bone flap and the edges of the skull. Short lengths of #28 steel wires are passed through the holes to attach the flap. A wire twister is used to secure the suture ends to the bone.

Alternately, the surgeon may attach the bone flap with cranial plates and screws. The loose pericranium and galea are attached over the burr holes and bone flap with absorbable synthetic or silk sutures. The scalp clips then are removed and the muscle and subcutaneous layers are approximated with 3-0 absorbable or silk sutures. The skin is closed with 4-0 nylon suture or staples.

Postoperative Considerations

Any surgical manipulation of the brain raises the possibility of postoperative seizures, swelling, and increased ICP. Intraoperative swelling may necessitate leaving the bone flap off and loosely closing only the skin to give the brain space to expand. Should this occur, the bone flap may be packaged in a sterile condition according to the facility's policy and procedure and frozen for later reimplantation (see the Cranioplasty section). Because of the risk of increased ICP and seizure activity, patients undergoing a craniotomy are monitored in the intensive care unit postoperatively. Increased ICP usually is manifested by changes in the patient's neurological status, such as a decreased level of consciousness, changes in pupil size and reaction, and changes in the ability to move the extremities on command. The surgeon assesses the patient's pupil size and neurological status after transfer from the operating bed to the transport device. Any change from the patient's baseline may necessitate immediate removal of the bone flap or reexploration of the wound. The scrub must therefore maintain the integrity of the sterile field and instrumentation until the patient is transferred from the operating suite.

Longer term complications from a craniotomy include infection of the bone flap or brain tissue, persistent seizure activity (e.g., epilepsy), and unresolved neurological deficits.

CRANIECTOMY

Surgical Goal

A craniectomy is the removal of cranial bone to access the structures below it. This procedure differs from a craniotomy, because the bone that is removed is not replaced.

Pathology

A craniectomy may be done to remove bone from any region of the skull for decompression of the brain or evacuation of epidural or subdural hematomas. More commonly, a craniectomy is performed to remove tumors in the posterior fossa. Tumors in this region may occur in the cerebellum, fourth ventricle, or brainstem. A posterior fossa craniectomy is described in this section.

TECHNIQUE

1 The patient is placed in the sitting position.
2 An occipital burr hole is made for placement of a ventricular catheter.
3 The incision line is marked and injected with lidocaine with epinephrine to promote vasoconstriction of the wound edges.
4 The incision is made.
5 Hemostasis is maintained.
6 A skin flap is created and retracted.
7 One or more burr holes are placed.
8 A Penfield or Woodson dissector is used to release the dura from the bone.
9 Rongeurs are used to enlarge the burr holes and remove an adequate amount of bone for exposure.
10 The dura is opened.
11 The brain is explored for tumor or other pathology and resected if necessary.
12 The dura is closed.
13 The muscle is reapproximated and the skin is closed.
14 The patient is placed in the supine position. The skull fixation is removed before the individual emerges from anesthesia.

Discussion

The patient is placed in a sitting or beach chair position with the head stabilized at the forehead with pin fixation or tongs. A tall Mayfield table is used and standing platforms are required so that the surgical technologist is accessible to the surgeons without compromise to the sterile field. The procedure may also be performed with the patient prone. A routine prep is performed.

To lower the ICP and provide an additional means of decompression, the surgeon may place a ventricular drain through a burr hole before beginning the craniectomy. If this is done before the main procedure, the technologist prepares a separate surgical field and assists as necessary. The burr hole is made as previously described. The burr hole may also be made concurrently with the procedure.

After infiltrating the incision site with a local anesthetic for hemostasis, the surgeon makes a midline or upwardly curved incision between the mastoid tips. The surgical assistant applies digital pressure to the wound edges. A folded 4 × 4 sponge should be available to place over the wound edge for added pressure. The monopolar and bipolar ESUs are used for hemostasis.

The skin flap is retracted with Weitlaner retractors. A Key periosteal elevator is used to free the muscles, which are then divided with the monopolar ESU.

One or more holes are drilled into the occipital bone, and the holes are extended with a large rongeur or a craniotome

burr. The dura mater is stripped from the underside of the bone, and a double-action rongeur (e.g., Kerrison or Leksell rongeur) is used to enlarge the craniectomy to the desired size and to smooth the bone edges. The scrub should anticipate that bone bleeding may occur and be prepared to supply the surgeon with bone putty to help control the bleeding. Moistened cottonoid strips and Gelfoam are also placed to prevent air embolism.

The surgeon tents the dura with a dura hook and opens it with a #15 blade in a #7 knife handle. A cottonoid strip may be placed on the brain tissue to protect the brain as the dural incision is extended with Metzenbaum scissors.

The extent to which the posterior fossa is explored depends on the nature of the disease. The exploration may include opening of the cisterna magna, draining of the spinal fluid, and inspection of the cerebellar hemispheres.

When the brain has been exposed, brain retractors are placed over cottonoid strips to increase exposure. The surgical technologist must keep the handles of the handheld retractors dry to prevent them from slipping in the surgeon's hand; however, the inserted edge should be kept wet to prevent damage to the brain. During the procedure, cranial nerves may be identified with a nerve stimulator.

After removal of the lesion, the surgeon must check for adequate hemostasis because of the increased venous pressure in the cranium. The dura mater may be partly or fully closed, and the muscle, fascia, and skin are closed as for a craniotomy. The patient must remain anesthetized until being returned to a supine position with the pin fixation or tongs removed.

The formation of an intracerebral hematoma is a risk after craniectomy. A hematoma can contribute to increased ICP and damage the cerebral tissue. Longer term complications that may occur include those previously discussed in the craniotomy section and CSF leakage.

CEREBRAL ANEURYSM SURGERY

Surgical Goal

Aneurysm surgery is performed to isolate a cerebral aneurysm from the normal circulation while preserving flow to the nearby vessels.

Pathology

An intracranial aneurysm is the bulging of an artery within the cerebral circulation. Aneurysms can take many forms and shapes. They are caused by a weakening of the arterial wall, which occurs as a congenital defect or as a result of trauma or infection. As blood flows through the vessel, the weakened aneurysm wall becomes thin (Figure 36-23). This creates a high risk of sudden rupture and hemorrhage, which can be quickly fatal. Types of cerebral aneurysms are listed in Table 36-4.

Discussion

Aneurysms vary in size, shape, and location and the surgical treatment is adjusted to each individual case. The goal is to prevent rupture. This may require application of a surgical clip (small clamp), wrapping, or a combination of techniques. In

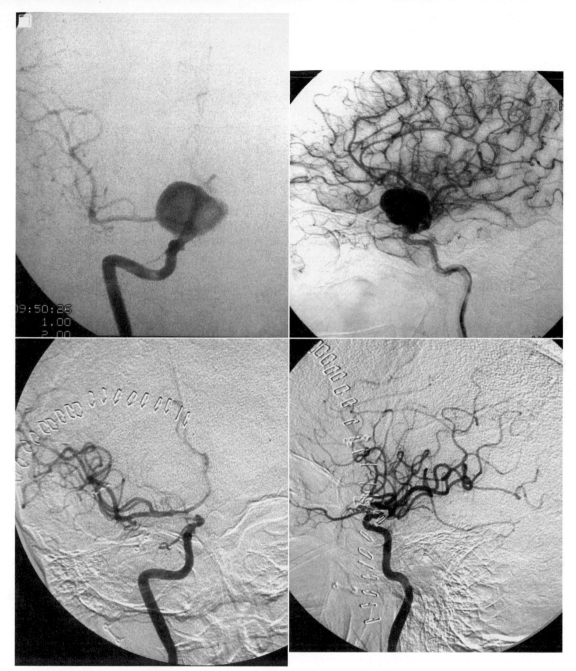

Figure 36-23 **Cerebral aneurysm.** *(From Le Roux P, Winn H, Newell D: Management of cerebral aneurysms, Philadelphia, 2004, WB Saunders.)*

TECHNIQUE

1 A lumbar drain may be placed before the patient is positioned.

2 The patient's head is placed in a three-point pin fixation device and the patient is positioned according to the anatomical location of the aneurysm.

3 The incision line is marked and injected with lidocaine with epinephrine to promote vasoconstriction of the wound edges.

4 A craniotomy is performed to expose the dura.

5 The operating microscope is brought to the field and adjusted.

6 The arachnoid webs and other tissue are dissected away as necessary to allow visualization of key intracranial structures.

7 The arteries supplying the aneurysm are identified.

8 One or more clips are applied to the base of the aneurysm.

9 A needle is used to aspirate the aneurysm sac after the clip is placed.

10 Hemostasis is achieved

11 The dura is closed.

12 The muscle is reapproximated and the skin is closed.

Table **36-4**	Types of Cerebral Aneurysms	
Type	**Description**	**Special Considerations**
Saccular	Any aneurysm with a saclike outpouching that comes off a stem or neck. Many saccular aneurysms are referred to as *berry aneurysms* because they resemble a berry.	This is the most common type of aneurysm. It appears at a branch in the arterial system, usually in the circle of Willis or the middle cerebral artery. Multiple aneurysms may be present.
Fusiform	An aneurysm that does not have a stem or neck; also known as an *atherosclerotic aneurysm*.	Typically occurs in older patients. Most commonly located in the vertebrobasilar system.
Giant	Any saccular or fusiform aneurysm larger than 25 mm.	Commonly located on the internal carotid artery.

selected cases, an endovascular coil can be placed inside the vessel under fluoroscopic guidance. This procedure can be performed as an interventional radiology procedure using a minimally invasive approach. The coil occludes the vessel and may be inserted before open surgery to prevent rupture until surgery can be safely performed.

A lumbar drain, connected to a drainage bag with a stopcock, may be placed by the neurosurgeon before the patient is prepped or positioned. The drain is used to control the volume of CSF in the ventricles, if needed, during the procedure. The anesthesia care provider opens the stopcock and releases CSF into the drainage bag to promote brain relaxation and reduce the ICP. The surgical technologist should ensure that the lumbar drain is prepared and isolated in a separate sterile field. Drains are supplied in a prepackaged kit with all the necessary components for insertion. The scrub may be responsible for assisting the surgeon in the insertion of the drain.

The patient is always placed in a three-point pin cranial fixation system to ensure absolute head stability and immobility. After the pins are placed and attached to the fixation device, the patient is positioned. The approach for most cerebral aneurysms is a frontal, bifrontal, or frontotemporal (i.e., pterional) craniotomy. The craniotomy is performed as previously described.

A self-retaining brain retractor system is placed after the dura is opened and tacked back from the surgical field. Moistened cottonoids or Gelfoam strips are placed beneath the retractor blades for cushioning and hydration. The retractors are essential for gentle, consistent retraction of the cerebral tissue. The system allows for placement of retractors in almost any direction. Each system is configured differently, but all are designed to be secured to the patient's head, to the skull pin fixation device, or to a post and coupling attached to the operating bed. The surgeon may periodically adjust the retractor blades to ensure that the tissue beneath remains perfused and the brain is not bruised.

The draped operating microscope is brought to the field and positioned. At this point, the surgeon may request a draped sitting stool with an arm rest. The arachnoid is opened with microscissors, hooks, dissectors, and a microbipolar ESU. As the arachnoid is opened, CSF is released, which further relaxes the brain.

Dissection continues until the surgeon visualizes the aneurysm. Dissection is meticulous to avoid undue manipulation of the aneurysm. The surgeon needs a large supply of moistened cottonoids and suction during this phase of the procedure. The microscopic suction tips can easily become occluded with blood and debris. The scrub should have several suction tips available on the field so that the tips can be changed out quickly with minimal interruption to the flow of the procedure.

The aneurysm is occluded at its base with one or more aneurysm clips. Aneurysm clips are available from a variety of manufacturers but share common characteristics (Figure 36-24). The clip is composed of a body, a pivot point, and two blades. The blades of the clip come in different lengths and are configured in a variety of ways, including straight, curved, and angled up, down, or sideways, to allow for anatomical variation.

The scrub must be familiar with the basic aneurysm clips and clip appliers available for use. Clips are supplied as permanent or temporary devices. Temporary clips have blades that open wider than permanent clips and they also have lower closing force. They are used to occlude the arterial source to the aneurysm temporarily or to test-occlude the base of the aneurysm before the permanent clip is applied. Temporary clips generally are gold colored, for easy identification, and should be discarded after use.

Permanent clips have a greater closing force and are designed to remain in place as a permanent implant. Fenestrated clips have an open blade. These clips may be used for indirect access to the aneurysm. A Sundt-type clip has a Teflon-lined lumen and is used to encircle the vessel completely when bleeding is encountered. Clip appliers may have a spring-loaded configuration or a pistol grip. They may have a hinged shaft to improve visualization. The scrub must make sure that at least two clip appliers are available for each type of clip used.

When handling aneurysm clips, the scrub must not compress the clips or manipulate them in any way while loading them in the applier. The clip should be compressed only by the surgeon immediately before placement, because opening and closing the clip alters its closing force and the clip may not seat securely.

The surgeon prepares the aneurysm for occlusion by continuing to isolate and identify the proximal and distal vasculature. This phase of the surgery requires careful handling of tissues, because of the risk for it to rupture. Rupture can occur at any time during the procedure but is more likely to happen during dissection. The scrub should always be prepared for the possibility of rupture by having a temporary clip loaded on a clip applier. If rupture occurs, suction and moistened cottonoids are needed immediately.

The surgeon places the clip across the neck of the aneurysm (Figure 36-25). Additional clips are used as necessary to ensure that the aneurysm and its feeder vessels are occluded.

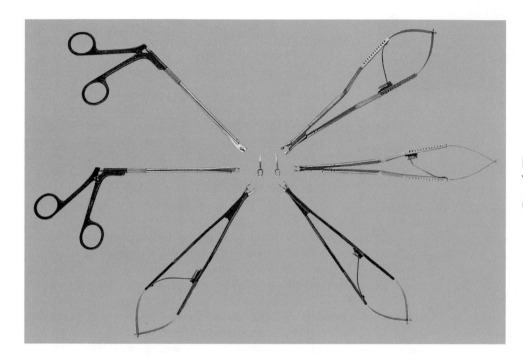

Figure 36-24 **Yasargil aneurysm clips with assorted appliers.** *(From Tighe SM:* Instrumentation for the operating room, *ed 6, St Louis, 2003, Mosby.)*

Once the aneurysm is occluded, the surgeon requires a 30-gauge needle attached to the syringe to aspirate the aneurysm sac. This maneuver removes any blood in the aneurysm and allows the surgeon to establish that there is no filling of the aneurysm and the clip is secure. In cases of giant aneurysms, the surgeon may open the dome of the aneurysm (aneurysmectomy) after the clips are placed to evacuate blood, clots, or tissue debris. If a clip cannot be applied to occlude the aneurysm, the surgeon may attempt to occlude it by wrapping or coating the vessel with a piece of the galea, methylmethacrylate, or cyanoacrylate.

After clip placement, the surgeon may request a cottonoid moistened with papaverine to apply to the vessels surrounding the aneurysm to prevent vessel spasm. Wound closure follows as outlined for a craniotomy. The pin fixation device is removed before the patient emerges from anesthesia.

ARTERIOVENOUS MALFORMATION RESECTION

Surgical Goal

Arteriovenous malformation (AVM) resection is performed to correct the fistula that occurs when an abnormal communication exists between the cerebral arteries and veins.

Pathology

An AVM is an abnormal communication or fistula between the arteries and veins. AVMs are commonly diagnosed in adults between 20 and 40 years of age. As the connection becomes larger under pressure, blood is diverted from surrounding brain tissue. When this occurs, multiple hemorrhages from the dilated blood vessels can cause seizures and subarachnoid hemorrhage.

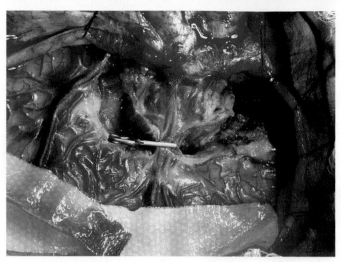

Figure 36-25 Aneurysm clip applied over a defect. *(From Rengachary S, Ellenbogen R: Principles of neurosurgery, ed 2, St Louis, 2005, Mosby.)*

TECHNIQUE

1 The patient's head is placed in a three-point pin fixation device and positioned according to the anatomical location of the arteriovenous malformation (AVM).

2 The incision line is marked and injected with lidocaine with epinephrine to promote vasoconstriction of the wound edges.

3 A craniotomy is performed.

4 Using techniques discussed in the section on aneurysm surgery, the surgeon isolates the AVM and applies aneurysm clips to the feeder vessels.

5 The AVM is dissected further and resected.

6 Closure is as described for a craniotomy.

Discussion

Some AVMs may be very complex and involve many vessels, making surgical resection risky. A multidisciplinary approach often is used in treating these patients. An interventional radiologist may be involved in the patient's care before surgery to embolize the AVM and reduce its size. During **embolization**, platinum coils, glue, or microscopic plastic particles are placed in the vessels feeding the AVM. The materials close off the feeder vessels, reducing the vascularity of the AVM to reduce the chance of rupture. Embolization may also be used after craniotomy for AVM resection, if required, to secure additional vessels not accessible during open surgery. Radiosurgery with the gamma knife is another option that may be used as an adjunct to surgery.

The procedure to resect an AVM is similar to the procedure for clipping a cerebral aneurysm. A craniotomy approach is used and the AVM is exposed using the same techniques described in the previous section. Because of the complexity of the vascular structure of most AVMs, microscopic dissection to identify the feeder vessels can be prolonged. A microtipped bipolar ESU is used extensively during this dissection. The scrub must have several microbipolar forceps available to allow for rapid exchange when the tips become coated with eschar. The scrub should observe the dissection on the video monitor to anticipate when the bipolar instrument will need to be exchanged and to make sure that the flow of instruments, sponges, and other materials is seamless and that the surgeon does not have to look away from the microscope.

Once the AVM is exposed, the surgeon uses the bipolar ESU to occlude smaller vessels. Multiple aneurysm clips are placed on the larger feeder vessels. The AVM then is resected with the bipolar ESU. The scrub should be prepared with strips of Surgicel and Gelfoam to line the AVM cavity. The wound is closed as described for cerebral aneurysm clipping. Figure 36-26 illustrates the techniques used in the treatment of an AVM.

CORRECTION OF CRANIOSYNOSTOSIS

Surgical Goal

A linear strip craniectomy is performed to correct the premature closure of an infant's cranial suture lines by separating the involved bones and treating the bones to prevent resealing until the brain has completed most of its growth.

Pathology

Craniosynostosis is a congenital deformity of the skull that results from premature closure of one or more of the cranial sutures of the skull. Fusion of each of the major cranial vault sutures can have different effects on the skull, generally causing growth restriction perpendicular to the suture (Figure 36-27). Fusion of multiple sutures can lead to increased ICP as the brain grows. Surgery usually is performed when the infant is 6 weeks to 6 months of age, because the skull bones are more malleable and a better cosmetic result can be achieved. The following procedure is used to treat sagittal hypostasis, the most common form of craniosynostosis.

TECHNIQUE

1 The patient is positioned supine with the head in a headrest.

2 The incision line is marked and injected with lidocaine with epinephrine to promote vasoconstriction of the wound edges.

3 An incision is made at the midpoint between the anterior and posterior fontanels and is extended from ear to ear.

4 The scalp is separated from the skull with blunt dissection, leaving the pericranium intact. Scalp clips are applied to the wound edges.

5 Burr holes are made in the cranium.

6 The burr holes are connected to form strips of bone.

7 The dura is dissected from the bone strips.

8 Hemostasis is maintained.

9 The bone strips are reshaped and replaced to correct the defect.

10 Absorbable plates and screws are placed to anchor the strips in their new configuration.

11 Closure proceeds as described for a craniotomy.

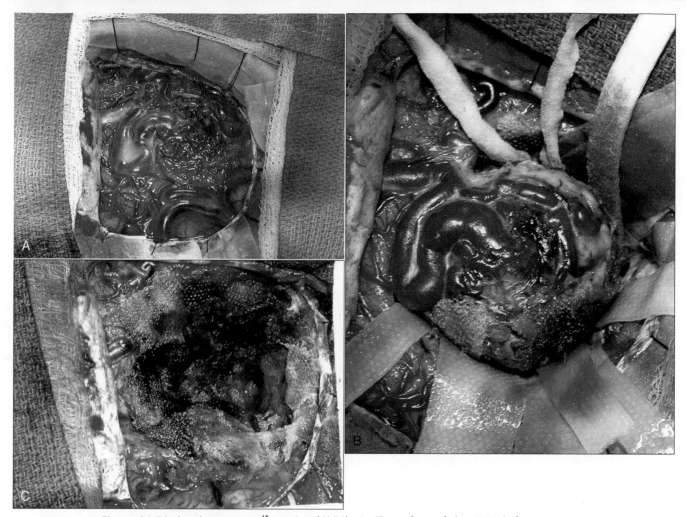

Figure 36-26 Arteriovenous malformation (AVM). **A,** The surface of the AVM before resection. **B,** The AVM has been separated from the surrounding area of the brain. **C,** Appearance of the resection cavity after resection. *(From Rengachary S, Ellenbogen R: Principles of neurosurgery, ed 2, St Louis, 2005, Mosby.)*

Discussion

Preoperative preparation of a pediatric patient includes protection against hypothermia. The operating room temperature is increased and extra draping layers or warm air mattress may be used. The scrub must ensure that irrigation solutions are warm to prevent the loss of heat through exposed tissues.

The scalp is incised over the area where the premature closure of the suture line has caused the deformity. The surgical assistant applies digital pressure to the wound edges; therefore the scrub should ensure that an ample supply of folded 4 × 4 sponges is available. A zigzag incision may be made to provide a more cosmetic result.

Scalp clips are applied (see the craniotomy procedure for special considerations when using scalp clips), and the scalp is secured away from the field with a towel clip, suture, or hooks attached to rubber bands. The scrub should have moistened 4 × 4 sponges available to place over the scalp surface to prevent it from drying during the procedure.

The periosteum is lifted from the bone with a small Key elevator. A small round burr on a drill is used to place a series

of burr holes, which are connected with a bone saw to form bone strips. The number of strips cut depends on how extensive the correction needs to be. The calvarial bone is soft and cuts easily but is still vulnerable to heat damage from the burrs and cutting blades; the scrub therefore must be ready to provide gentle irrigation during cutting to prevent heat buildup.

The dura mater is stripped from the underside of the skull using blunt dissection with a nerve hook. The bone strips are then removed with a heavy scissors, a craniotome, or a small Kerrison rongeur. Bone putty should be available for hemostasis of the bone edges.

The surgeon reshapes the bone strips by bending them or shaving them with a fine burr. After the pieces have been reshaped, the surgeon places them back on the head, usually in an altered configuration, and secures them in place with absorbable suture, plates, and screws (Figure 36-28). Hemostasis is achieved using the bipolar and monopolar ESUs, Gelfoam strips, and Surgicel as needed. The scalp clips are removed and closure proceeds as described for a craniotomy.

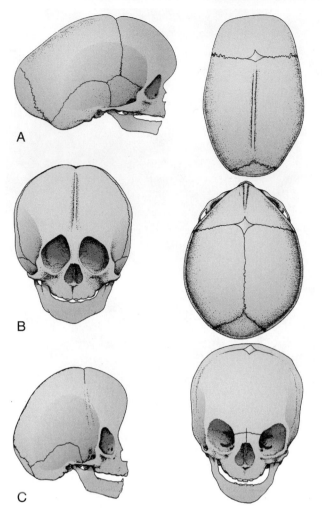

Figure 36-27 Craniosynostosis. Effects on the skull resulting from fusion of major vault sutures. **A,** Sagittal sutures. **B,** Metopic sutures. **C,** Coronal sutures. *(From Choux M, DiRocco C, Hockley A, et al: Pediatric neurosurgery, London, 1999, Churchill Livingstone.)*

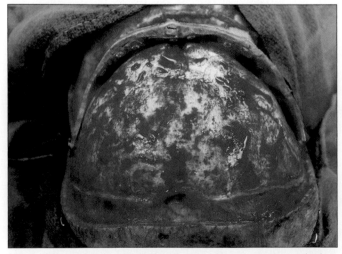

Figure 36-28 Craniosynostosis. Absorbable plates are applied to cranial strips after repair. *(From Rengachary S, Ellenbogen R: Principles of neurosurgery, ed 2, St Louis, 2005, Mosby.)*

CRANIOPLASTY

Surgical Goal

In this procedure, an area of bone in the skull is replaced with a bone graft or prosthetic material to restore the continuity of the skull, protect the brain, and improve the patient's cosmetic appearance.

Pathology

Deformities of the skull resulting from trauma or disease may leave a portion of the brain and dura mater exposed. More commonly, cranial defects may occur as a result of an infection of the bone flap after elective craniotomy.

If the cranial defect is clean (e.g., in closed trauma), the repair may be performed immediately. If the wound is contaminated (e.g., bone flap infection, open trauma), repair is delayed. The bone flap created by craniotomy may have been removed and stored under sterile conditions to allow the brain to expand and to reduce the ICP. In other circumstances, calvarial bone strips are used to cover the exposed area, protect it from injury, and improve the patient's appearance. Methylmethacrylate most often is used for prosthetic replacement. However, some surgeons use an acrylic prosthesis that is customized for the patient with three-dimensional imaging and computer-aided design (CAD). The following description is for the process of methylmethacrylate cranioplasty.

TECHNIQUE

1. The patient is positioned according to the location of the defect.
2. The incision line is marked and injected with lidocaine with epinephrine to promote vasoconstriction at the wound edges.
3. An incision is made through the existing scar.
4. Scalp clips are applied.
5. Blunt dissection is used to separate the scalp from the skull.
6. The bone edges are trimmed and a bony ledge is created.
7. The methylmethacrylate is prepared, allowed to cure to the desired consistency, and placed in the bag provided by the manufacturer.
8. The bag containing the methylmethacrylate is molded to the defect.
9. The bag is removed from the wound and allowed to cool.
10. The cooled prosthesis is placed back in the wound and trimmed and smoothed as necessary to fit.
11. The prosthesis is secured in place with wire.
12. Closure proceeds as previously described for a craniotomy.

Discussion

The patient is positioned, prepped, and draped for access to a particular area of the skull. The scalp is incised over the defect as for a craniotomy. The surgeon may excise the scar overlying the defect.

Depending on the nature of the previous injury or disease, remnants of bone may be present in the affected area. If bone fragments are present, the surgeon uses a rongeur to reduce them. If the affected area is completely devoid of bone, the surgeon trims the periphery of the area with rongeurs to form a saucer-like ledge. This prevents the prosthesis from slipping below the level of the skull and helps seat it in place. The scrub should retain all the bits of trimmed bone as specimens.

When the surgeon has completed this procedure, the wound is irrigated with warm saline solution. An antibiotic irrigant also may be used at this time.

The scrub uses a commercially prepared cranioplasty kit containing a premeasured amount of powder and solvent to form the methylmethacrylate prosthesis. Methylmethacrylate is flammable and must be mixed in a well-ventilated area. A vacuum system specifically designed for methylmethacrylate mixing may be used to minimize the fumes released as part of the chemical reaction. A single dose is supplied in each cranioplasty kit. If additional material is needed, it should be mixed separately. The entire package of powder is emptied into a stainless steel mixing bowl or a disposable sterile bowl supplied by the manufacturer. The entire volume of solvent is then added. A spatula is used to mix the substances for approximately 30 seconds. The scrub should cover the bowl after the initial mixing to prevent evaporation and should test the consistency of the cement periodically. The cement becomes doughy and pulls away from the walls of the mixing bowl within 5 minutes.

While the cement is still doughy, the scrub places it in the plastic bag provided in the kit and passes it to the surgeon. The surgeon then flattens and molds the bag over the cranial defect until it fits. This step must be performed quickly, because the cement gives off heat as it hardens and can damage the underlying tissue. The surgeon removes the molded cement from the defect to allow the cement to cure. While the cement is curing (usually 15 to 20 minutes), the surgeon may assess the wound for any small bleeders. During this time, the scrub should prepare a dental drill or similar drill and a fine drill point.

When the cement plate has hardened, the surgeon drills several holes in its edge. Similar holes are drilled at the periphery of the skull defect. Any rough spots in the cement plate are smoothed with a large burr attached to a power drill or craniotome. The surgeon then fits the cement plate into the defect and secures it by passing fine stainless steel wires through the holes. The wound is irrigated and closed in routine fashion.

Because cranioplasty does not involve the manipulation of brain tissue, neurological complications are rare. Infection involving the scalp or replanted bone may occur, and resorption of the bone may occur if calvarial bone strips are used.

VENTRICULOPERITONEAL/VENTRICULAR SHUNT

Surgical Goal

Ventricular shunting is used to divert the cerebrospinal fluid away from the ventricles of the brain to another location in the body, such as the peritoneal cavity, pleural space, or atrium of the heart, where the CSF can be absorbed. This reduces intracranial pressure.

Pathology

Hydrocephalus is a condition involving an inappropriate amount of CSF in the intracranial space at an inappropriate pressure. CSF is produced by the epidermal cells in the lateral third and fourth ventricles. CSF circulates through the foramen of Monro into the third ventricle, through the cerebral aqueduct (aqueduct of Sylvius), and into the fourth ventricle. From the fourth ventricle, it flows through the cerebromedullary cistern down the spinal cord and over the cerebral hemispheres (Figure 36-29). Hydrocephalus can occur as a result of an overproduction of CSF, or it may be the result of a condition that interferes with the normal absorption of fluid. Hydrocephalus can develop in children and adults. Persistent hydrocephalus can interfere with cerebral blood flow and cause enlargement of the skull in infants. In selected cases, surgical intervention is aimed at removing the excess fluid to relieve pressure on the brain. A ventriculoperitoneal shunt most often is used to divert CSF.

TECHNIQUE

1 The patient is positioned supine with the head slightly rotated opposite the side of the shunt and the neck extended in a straight line to the abdomen.

2 A scalp incision is made and hemostasis is achieved.

3 A small scalp flap is created and retracted.

4 A burr hole is made.

5 The ventricular catheter is placed through the burr hole into the lateral ventricle.

6 The reservoir and valve are connected to the ventricular catheter.

7 A subcutaneous tunnel is created from the burr hole to the neck. The end of the tunnel is marked and the neck incision is made at that site.

8 The peritoneal catheter is connected to the reservoir and valve.

9 An abdominal incision is made.

10 A second subcutaneous tunnel is created from the neck incision to the abdomen.

11 The peritoneal catheter is threaded through the abdominal incision.

12 Flow of cerebrospinal fluid through the end of the peritoneal catheter is verified.

13 The peritoneal catheter is placed in the peritoneal cavity and secured with a purse-string suture.

14 The incisions are closed.

Discussion

Shunt systems vary by manufacturer, but common components include a ventricular catheter, a CSF reservoir, a valve, and a peritoneal catheter (Figure 36-30). Valves are designed for one-way flow and are supplied with a variety of pressure and flow settings. The scrub should read the manufacturer's specifications and instructions before the procedure is performed. As with all Silastic or other implant materials, the shunt should be handled carefully and protected from contamination by lint, dust, or glove powder. The shunt components should be soaked in antibiotic solution before they are

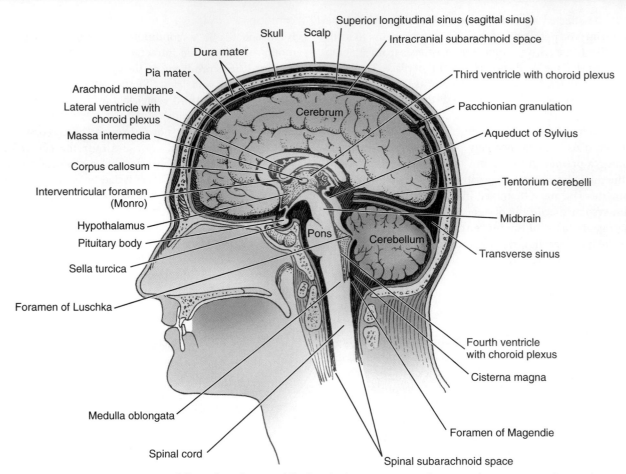

Figure 36-29 **Normal flow of cerebrospinal fluid in the brain.** *(From Applegate E: The anatomy and physiology learning system, ed 2, St Louis, 2000, WB Saunders.)*

implanted. The scrub is responsible for priming the assembly with saline and ensuring that no air is present in the system. Because ventricular shunting may be performed on adults or children, the scrub should ensure that the instruments and sutures selected are appropriate for the age and size of the patient.

The surgeon may choose a frontal, parietal, or occipital approach to place the ventricular catheter. The patient is positioned in a flat plane, according to the approach chosen, to facilitate insertion of the tunneling device from the neck to the abdomen.

After the patient is prepped and draped, the surgeon makes a curved incision in the scalp over the area where the burr hole will be drilled. The burr hole is placed as previously described, and the dura is incised.

A bipolar ESU is used to open the pia. Intraoperative ultrasound may be used to confirm the location of the ventricle before catheter insertion is attempted. The scrub loads the ventricular catheter on an introducer, and the surgeon inserts it through the burr hole into the lateral ventricle. The introducer is removed and CSF flow through the catheter is confirmed. If no CSF flow is present, the catheter is removed, the introducer is replaced, and the procedure is attempted again. When CSF flow is confirmed, the reservoir and valve are attached to the ventricular catheter and secured with 2-0 silk sutures.

A tendon passer is used to create a subcutaneous tunnel from the burr hole to the neck. The surgeon makes a small neck incision and completes any dissection using the Metzenbaum scissors. The catheter is brought through the tunnel and the surgeon confirms that CSF is still flowing through the valve before connecting the peritoneal catheter.

The surgeon makes a small abdominal incision and dissects through the subcutaneous tissue and fascia to reach the peritoneum. The scrub should be prepared for this step with Senn retractors, monopolar ESU, and Metzenbaum scissors. A tunneling device is used to create space in the soft tissues from the abdominal incision to the neck incision.

The peritoneal catheter is brought through the tunnel and CSF flow is confirmed. The catheter may be flushed with normal saline to ensure that it has not become occluded with blood or debris. The upper valve can also be pumped to confirm that the shunt is working. After confirming patency, the surgeon uses 3-0 absorbable synthetic sutures to secure the catheter to the peritoneum.

The incisions are closed with absorbable synthetic suture. The scalp and abdominal skin incisions are closed with staples or with interrupted 4-0 nylon suture. The neck incision can be closed with a running subcuticular stitch or interrupted sutures.

The most common complication after ventricular shunt placement is shunt malfunction as a result of blockage of the

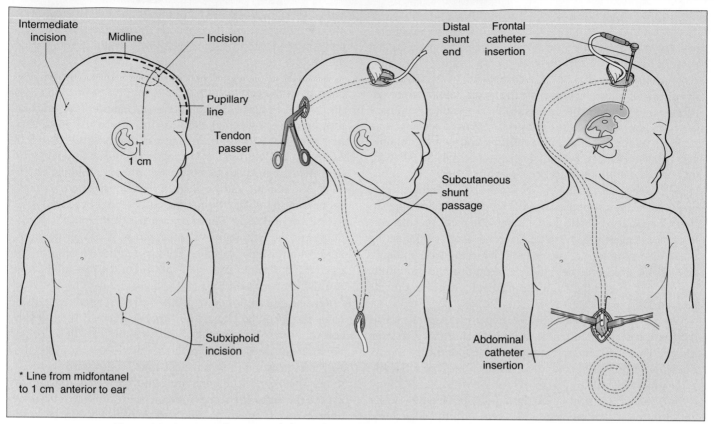

Figure 36-30 Ventriculoperitoneal shunt. The patient is positioned and exact positions are marked. A subcutaneous tunnel is created for the shunt and the catheter is inserted. *(From Rengachary S, Ellenbogen R: Principles of neurosurgery, ed 2, St Louis, 2005, Mosby.)*

valve or catheter. This complication can occur shortly after placement or at any time after the shunt is in place. Overdrainage or underdrainage also can occur and can cause patients to exhibit a variety of symptoms ranging from headache to neurological deficits. Shunts placed in infants and children need to be replaced periodically to accommodate their growth.

TRANSSPHENOIDAL HYPOPHYSECTOMY

Surgical Goal

The goal of hypophysectomy is to remove all or a part of the pituitary gland. This procedure may be performed to slow the growth and spread of endocrine-dependent malignant tumors or to excise a pituitary tumor. The surgical approach is through the sphenoid.

Pathology

The pituitary gland is responsible for the storage, release, and secretion of a variety of hormones. The gland is attached by a stalk to the hypothalamus and rests in the sella turcica. It is adjacent to critical structures such as the optic chiasma and cavernous sinuses. The cavernous sinuses contain several cranial nerves and the internal carotid arteries. Because the gland is uniquely located, symptoms from a tumor often are noticed as visual field anomalies or may be related to pressure on cranial nerves III through VI. Tumors may damage the adjacent brain tissue through mass effect by displacing structures, blocking CSF flow, or creating pressure.

TECHNIQUE

1 The patient is positioned in a semisitting position with the head secured with three-point pin fixation.
2 Preoperative fluoroscopy is used to confirm the correct position.
3 Topical and infiltration anesthetics are applied to the nasal mucosa.
4 The patient's face, mouth, nasal cavity, and a small abdominal area are prepped and draped.
5 The gingiva and nasal mucosa are incised and lifted from the septum.
6 Bone and nasal cartilage are resected and preserved.
7 The sphenoid sinus is examined.
8 The sinus is opened and the floor of the sella turcica is identified.
9 The sella turcica is opened with a pneumatic drill.
10 The microscope is used to visualize the pituitary tumor.
11 The tumor and gland are resected.
12 The sella turcica is packed with fatty tissue and the floor is reconstructed with cartilage from the nasal septum.
13 The nasal mucosa is sutured and the gingival incision is closed.
14 Nasal packing and splints are inserted.

Discussion

Transsphenoidal hypophysectomy requires an interdisciplinary approach. An otorhinolaryngologist participates in the surgery during access to the sella turcica. An open or endoscopic approach may be used (see Chapter 28 for a discussion of endoscopic sinus techniques). The scrub should have combined sinus instrumentation available. Specialized pituitary instrumentation, which includes self-retaining specula, long pituitary spoons and scoops, rongeurs, and curettes, should also be available. The operating microscope may be prepared and draped before the start of surgery.

Before the start of surgery, the scrub should prepare a side table that includes supplies needed for injection and application of a local anesthetic. Supplies include nasal specula, cottonoids, syringes, and several 25-gauge needles. The circulating nurse dispenses topical cocaine and lidocaine with epinephrine to this nonsterile field. Before beginning the procedure, the surgeon injects the nasal and gingival mucosa to provide hemostasis.

The scrub also is responsible for preparing a separate sterile field with a few basic instruments for obtaining a fat graft from the abdomen. The fat graft is harvested before the transsphenoidal procedure begins to maintain the flow from a clean to a contaminated area.

The patient is placed in the three-point pin fixation device and positioned in a semisitting position with the neck flexed toward the left and the head rotated to the right. The surgical approach is from the patient's right side. After the patient has been positioned, the C-arm is used to confirm that the positioning is accurate for access to the sella. Often the floor is marked with a piece of tape where the C-arm's wheels are placed so that it can be repositioned in the same location during the procedure. Because the patient is in a semisitting position, the risk of air embolism exists. Refer to the posterior fossa craniectomy procedure for information about intraoperative air embolism.

To secure hemostasis before the incision, the otorhinolaryngologist injects the nasal submucosa and gingival mucosa with lidocaine with epinephrine. Cottonoids saturated with cocaine solution are used to pack the nose. The anesthesia care provider may insert a throat pack so that any blood or fluid from the procedure does not enter the patient's stomach.

The scrub should note the number of cottonoids placed in the nose for reconciliation during the sponge count. Although a counted sponge is not typically used for the throat pack, the scrub should note its presence and remind the anesthesia care provider to remove it at the end of the procedure.

The procedure begins with the harvesting of the fat graft from the abdomen. The surgeon makes a small incision below the belt line. A small amount of subcutaneous fat is removed with the monopolar ESU and Metzenbaum scissors. The fat may be harvested from any location in the abdomen, but the site usually is chosen for a cosmetic result. Alternately, muscle may be removed from the patient's thigh for use as packing material. The surgical technologist should keep the tissue graft in a basin filled with saline or wrapped in a moistened Telfa strip on the back table until it is needed. The surgeon uses 2-0 polyglactin suture to close the subcutaneous tissue. The skin can be closed with staples or running subcuticular stitches of 3-0 or 4-0 nylon or polypropylene suture. The scrub should protect the incision with a sterile towel for the remainder of the procedure.

Next, the otolaryngologist exposes the sella. This may be done endoscopically (see Chapter 28 for details) or by incising the septal cartilage with a #15 blade and elevating the mucous membrane with a septal elevator. The otorhinolaryngologist removes nasal bone and cartilage until the sella is exposed. If necessary, the otorhinolaryngologist may open a window in the patient's gingiva to gain exposure. The scrub should retain any pieces of bone and cartilage in a small basin on the surgical field for reimplantation at the end of the procedure.

The surgical technologist drapes the C-arm with a sterile drape and the radiology technician moves it into place, aligning it with the tape placed on the floor earlier. Fluoroscopy is used at this stage to confirm exposure of the sphenoid sinus and the floor of the sella.

Once exposure is confirmed, a drill or rongeur is used to enter the sphenoid sinus. The surgeon removes the mucosa covering the sphenoid with a pituitary rongeur. The surgical microscope is positioned. With the microscope in place, the surgeon opens the roof of the sphenoid with a narrow osteotome. Small pieces of bone are removed with a rongeur to expose the dura. The surgeon uses a #11 blade with a bayonet knife handle to open the dura and then dissects the dura off the pituitary gland with a dura hook. Angled microscissors are used to further open the dura and separate it from the gland. The microbipolar ESU is used to control any bleeding.

Before tumor resection begins, the tumor mass is biopsied and sent for frozen section identification to confirm the presence of pituitary tissue. After positive identification, the surgeon uses microblunt ring curettes, enucleators, suction, and microdissectors to remove the tumor mass. Bleeding is controlled with the ESU, cottonoids, and Gelfoam packing.

Using the fat graft or muscle tissue obtained at the start of the procedure, the surgeon packs the floor of the sella and reinforces the graft with pieces of nasal cartilage and bone to prevent a CSF leak. The otorhinolaryngologist closes the gingival incision (if used) with polyglactin suture, reapproximates the nasal mucosa, and places flexible polyethylene splints in the patient's nose to maintain septal alignment. The splints are secured anteriorly with nylon or polypropylene suture. Gauze, Telfa strips, or nasal tampons coated with antibiotic ointment may be packed into the nasal cavity after the splints are placed. The patient is returned to a supine position and the pin fixation device is removed before the patient emerges from anesthesia.

Patients who have undergone transsphenoidal hypophysectomy are monitored in the intensive care unit postoperatively for changes in neurological status and CSF leakage. Leakage of CSF indicates that the sella is not sealed and the patient is at risk for infection. Because the pituitary gland has been manipulated or partly resected, patients may experience symptoms related to underproduction or overproduction of the various hormones controlled by the gland. These symptoms may be present immediately postoperatively or may manifest in the weeks or months after the procedure.

Some patients require lifelong hormonal replacement after hypophysectomy.

RESECTION OF A VESTIBULAR SCHWANNOMA (ACOUSTIC NEUROMA)

Surgical Goal

Resection of a vestibular schwannoma is performed to remove tumors from the vestibular branch of cranial nerve VIII while preserving the function of the nerve. A suboccipital, translabyrinth, or middle fossa approach can be used. Vestibular schwannomas may also be treated with radiosurgery. Each approach is associated with particular advantages and disadvantages. The choice of one approach over another is based on the surgeon's preference and the size and location of the tumor. The translabyrinth approach is discussed here.

Pathology

A schwannoma, also called an **acoustic neuroma,** is a benign, slow-growing tumor composed of Schwann cells. As the tumor grows, it impinges on cranial nerve VIII, causing one-sided hearing loss, ringing in the ears, dizziness, and problems with balance. The tumor also can cause pressure on the nearby seventh cranial nerve, causing facial numbness and pain. If the tumor is left untreated and continues to grow, it eventually may cause deafness.

TECHNIQUE

1 The patient is positioned supine with the head turned.
2 The postauricular incision line is marked and injected with lidocaine with epinephrine.
3 A tissue graft is obtained.
4 The incision is made and hemostasis is achieved.
5 The periosteum is stripped from the mastoid bone.
6 A cutting burr is used to open the mastoid.
7 The operating microscope is used to visualize the inner ear.
8 Select structures of the inner ear are removed.
9 Bone is removed from the structures around the inner ear.
10 The dura is opened.
11 The tumor is removed.
12 The mastoid cavity is packed.
13 The wound is closed.

Discussion

Resection of a vestibular schwannoma involves a multidisciplinary team approach. The neurosurgeon partners with an otologic surgeon to ensure that the patient receives optimum care.

The patient is positioned supine with the head at the foot of the table so that the surgeon can be seated for the procedure. A facial nerve monitor may be used to assess the functioning of the facial nerve during the procedure. The surgeon injects the postauricular incision line and continues the injection into the internal auditory canal.

A tissue graft is obtained from the patient's abdominal fat or postauricular fascia. This tissue graft is placed in saline by the scrub and retained on the back table until the end of the procedure.

The surgeon makes the initial incision behind the patient's ear and carries it through the fascia. The scrub should be prepared with 4 × 4 sponges and the monopolar ESU for hemostasis. A Lempert elevator is used to strip the periosteum off the mastoid bone and bone wax is used to control any bleeding from the bone.

Self-retaining retractors are placed and the surgeon opens the mastoid cavity with a large cutting burr on a high-speed drill handpiece. The scrub should irrigate the drill tip in the usual manner during drilling. Gelfoam strips and cottonoids may be used for hemostasis after the mastoid is opened.

The operating microscope is brought to the field . The drill is used to remove the semicircular canals, utricle, and saccule. Fine microsurgical instrumentation (e.g., alligator forceps, cup forceps, picks, and dissectors) is used during this phase of the procedure to remove any remaining bone covering the dura of the posterior and middle fossa.

Microscissors or a microknife is used to open the dura and access the tumor. Any bleeding that is encountered is managed with the bipolar ESU or a vessel clip. If necessary, the surgeon dissects the tumor away from the facial nerve before proceeding with removal. The surgeon uses micropituitary rongeurs, alligator forceps, and micropicks to remove the tumor. In some cases, the surgeon may use the CUSA to fragment the tumor. Hemostasis is maintained with Gelfoam strips, Surgicel, cottonoids, and the bipolar ESU. The Surgicel and Gelfoam must be removed before the tissue graft is placed, because these materials will swell and can exert pressure on the surrounding vessels and the brainstem.

The surgeon closes the dura with 4-0 silk sutures and packs the tumor bed and cavity with the tissue graft. The skin is closed with interrupted subcuticular absorbable sutures.

STEREOTACTIC SURGERY

Surgical Goal

Stereotactic surgery uses computer-based technology to identify specific structures or lesions in the brain for diagnosis or treatment. Precise identification of lesions on a coordinate system results in minimal damage to surrounding tissue. A three-dimensional frame-based or frameless guidance system is used for accuracy.

Pathology

The stereotactic approach may be used for tumor biopsy or removal, resection of AVMs, brain mapping, implantation of electrodes, catheter placement, ventriculostomy, and the treatment of movement disorders and intractable pain. It is used in conjunction with minimally invasive radiosurgical techniques to ablate tumors and AVMs and to treat functional disorders such as trigeminal neuralgia, Parkinson disease, and essential tremor.

Discussion

The patient undergoes a preoperative MRI or CT scan. The films must be available during the procedure for the surgeon to use in planning the placement of the stereotactic head

TECHNIQUE

1 A stereotactic head frame is placed on the patient's head and secured with skull pins (framed system); alternatively, fiducials (i.e., adhesive radiographic markers) are placed on the skin (frameless system).

2 An MRI or a CT scan is performed to locate the target and determine the coordinates to be used.

3 The patient returns to the operating room and the coordinates are loaded into the system's computer.

4 A burr hole is placed.

5 Instrumentation is introduced through the burr hole as needed for the procedure.

6 Closure is as described for a burr hole procedure.

7 The frame or fiducials are removed.

frame or fiducials. If a framed system is used, the skin is infiltrated with local anesthetic at the skull pin insertion points.

With the frame (or fiducials) in place, the patient is sent to CT or MRI, where predetermined anatomical landmarks are used as guides and the coordinates are determined (Figure 36-31). The computer determines the target trajectory. For many surgical approaches, the use of stereotaxis allows the surgeon to plan the best line of sight with the least amount of tissue damage.

The patient is transferred to the operating room with the frame or fiducials in place. General anesthesia is used if the procedure will be extensive. The surgeon places burr holes as previously described. After making the burr holes, the surgeon uses hollow cannulas, coagulating electrodes, cryosurgical probes, wire loops, and other biopsy instruments to access and treat target areas in the brain.

DEEP BRAIN STIMULATION

Surgical Goal

The goal of deep brain stimulation (DBS) is to change the electrical activity of the brain in a controlled manner using electrodes and a pulse generator.

Pathology

DBS has been used to treat movement disorders such as Parkinson disease and some pain disorders. It has been used experimentally to treat depression and Tourette syndrome, a neurological disorder characterized by uncontrollable motor movements (tics) and vocalizations.

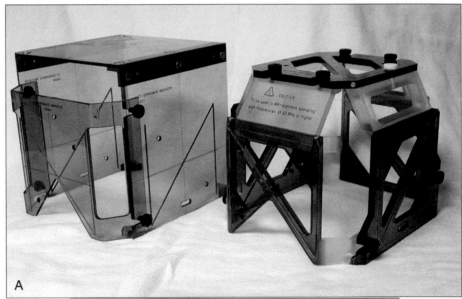

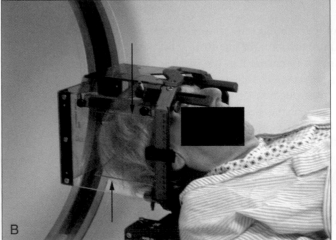

Figure 36-31 A, Frame reference plate array for Leksell stereotactic system. **B,** Reference plates attached to the patient. *(From Rengachary S, Ellenbogen R: Principles of neurosurgery, ed 2, St Louis, 2005, Mosby.)*

TECHNIQUE

1 A stereotactic approach is used to prepare the patient for implantation of the electrodes.
2 The lead is inserted through the burr hole to the target area and connected to a generator.
3 The generator is activated and the response of the symptom to the stimulus is evaluated.
4 The lead is repositioned and retested as necessary to alleviate the patient's symptom.
5 An extension is connected to the lead and tunneled subcutaneously from the head to the area where the generator is implanted.
6 A pocket is created for the generator below the clavicle or in the abdominal fat.
7 The burr hole is closed as previously described. The generator pocket is closed.

Discussion

The patient undergoing DBS implantation is awake so that correct placement of the electrode can be confirmed. The brain does not have any pain receptors. Local anesthesia is used for placement of the stereotactic frame and burr holes in the cranium.

The patient is placed in the sitting position. The procedure begins as described for stereotactic surgery. The DBS system consists of three components: the lead, the extension, and the generator. Using the stereotactic coordinates, the surgeon passes the lead through the brain tissue until the tip is in contact with the target tissue. The patient is asked to perform certain tasks during placement of the lead. Any abnormalities, such as an alteration in speech or inability to perform cognitive tasks, may indicate that the electrode is not placed correctly.

After placement is confirmed, the surgeon connects the lead to a test generator and activates the generator to determine the effect on the patient's symptoms. The generator is adjusted as necessary to achieve optimum control of the symptoms. An extension is connected to the lead.

The surgeon uses a tunneling device to create a subcutaneous tunnel from the head to the area where the generator will be implanted. Depending on the surgeon's preference and the patient's anatomy, the generator pocket is created beneath the clavicle or in the subcutaneous abdominal fat. Hemostasis is maintained with the monopolar ESU as necessary. The extension is passed through the tunnel and connected to the generator. The surgeon irrigates both areas copiously with antibiotic solution and uses a subcuticular stitch with 3-0 absorbable suture or staples for closure. The generator is programmed with a remote device using the settings derived from the testing phase.

ENDOSCOPIC VENTRICULOSCOPY

Surgical Goal

The goals of endoscopic ventriculoscopy include relief of ventricular obstruction to restore CSF circulation, visualization of the third ventricle, decompression, or tissue removal. Stereotactic techniques may be used to improve accuracy.

Pathology

Conditions that may be treated with endoscopic ventriculostomy include intraventricular cysts and tumors and hydrocephalus. Cysts may develop in the third ventricle and attach to the roof or floor. A variety of malignant or benign tumors may form in the third ventricle or may metastasize from other sites. The presence of a cyst or tumor may cause hydrocephalus, or hydrocephalus may be the result of other conditions. The procedure described here is for correction of hydrocephalus.

TECHNIQUE

1 The patient is placed in the supine position.
2 The incision line is marked and injected with lidocaine with epinephrine to promote vasoconstriction of the wound edges.
3 An incision is made and a burr hole is placed.
4 The dura is opened and the operating sheath is placed.
5 The endoscope is passed through the sheath and the ventricle is visualized.
6 The floor of the ventricle is punctured and then dilated.
7 Closure proceeds as described for a burr hole procedure.

Discussion

If stereotaxis is used for ventriculoscopy, the stereotactic system is applied as described in the discussion of stereotactic surgery, and the patient is placed under general anesthesia. Patients undergoing ventriculoscopy without stereotaxis are positioned supine, with the head resting on a soft headrest and elevated 30 degrees to promote venous drainage, minimize CSF loss, and reduce the likelihood of air entering the patient's vasculature.

After marking the incision and injecting it with lidocaine and epinephrine, the surgeon incises the skin and places a burr hole over the right lateral ventricle. The dura is opened with scissors or a #11 blade attached to a #7 knife handle and the bipolar ESU is used for hemostasis.

The surgeon inserts a peel-away catheter through the burr hole into the lateral ventricle and removes the stylet to confirm the flow of CSF. The sides of the catheter are peeled downward and stapled or sutured to the drapes.

A cannula with an irrigation port is placed through the sheath tract. Sterile intravenous tubing is attached to the irrigation port and passed off the field to be attached to a bag of warmed Ringer lactate. A flexible or rigid endoscope is connected to the video camera and adjusted as necessary to ensure a clear image. The endoscope is passed through the cannula and the irrigation is started. The surgeon adjusts the flow of irrigation fluid as necessary using the stopcock on the port to ensure that any bleeding is cleared from the field and the ventricles remain distended. The scrub should be prepared with suction to keep the surgical field clear of irrigation fluid.

The surgeon passes the endoscope into the lateral ventricle and navigates the scope through the foramen of Monro to visualize the floor of the third ventricle. The floor of the third ventricle is opened with a blunt instrument, monopolar or bipolar ESU, or blunt wire, and a 3 or 4 French (Fr) Fogarty catheter is passed through the opening and inflated to enlarge it. The surgeon advances the endoscope into the third ventricle through the opening.

Any arachnoid bands or membranes that impede the flow of CSF are bluntly disrupted with the Fogarty catheter. The surgeon inspects the ventricle and observes the floor of the ventricle for movement to confirm communication of the CSF between the ventricles and subarachnoid space. The Fogarty balloon is deflated and the catheter is removed.

The surgeon removes the endoscope and sheath and places Gelfoam in the burr hole for hemostasis. A ventricular drain may be placed before closure. Closure proceeds as described for the burr hole procedure.

MICROVASCULAR DECOMPRESSION OF CRANIAL NERVES

Compression of cranial nerves by nearby blood vessels can result in a variety of painful conditions. The compression may injure the protective myelin sheath over the nerve, causing it to misfire or fire erratically if stimulated in any way. Compression also interferes with the nerve's ability to shut off the pain signals after the stimulation is removed. Common conditions related to cranial nerve compression include the following:

- *Trigeminal neuralgia (tic douloureux):* Associated with severe pain in the eyes, lips, nose, scalp, forehead, and jaw.
- *Glossopharyngeal neuralgia:* Characterized by pain in the tongue, throat, tonsils, and ear.
- *Hemifacial spasm:* Characterized by periodic muscular contractions over one side of the face.

Compression of the vestibular nerve may result in vertigo and ringing in the ears.

During microvascular decompression surgery, a retromastoid (behind the mastoid bone) incision is used. The operating microscope is used to identify the impinging vessel, which is released from the nerve. A small piece of synthetic material (e.g., Teflon or polyvinyl alcohol) is placed between the compressing vessel and the nerve.

CEREBRAL REVASCULARIZATION

Cerebral revascularization (also referred to as a *cerebral bypass*) is performed to improve the blood flow to an ischemic area of the brain. Indications for the procedure include chronic cerebral ischemia, moyamoya disease, a giant intracerebral aneurysm, or a skull base tumor. During the procedure, the surgeon creates an anastomosis between an extracranial artery and an intracranial artery to bypass a stricture or blockage below the bifurcation of the common carotid artery. Typically, an artery in the scalp is anastomosed to a branch of the middle cerebral artery. This bypass establishes increased blood flow to the cerebral circulation and may be used to prevent a major stroke.

SPINAL PROCEDURES

ANTERIOR CERVICAL DISCECTOMY AND FUSION (OPEN)

Surgical Goal

The goal of an anterior cervical discectomy is to excise one or more herniated cervical intervertebral discs. Spinal fusion restores continuity to the spine after the disc is removed.

Pathology

The most common indication for anterior cervical discectomy and fusion is a herniated cervical disc. A patient with a herniated cervical disc has pain in the neck, shoulders, or arms, accompanied by numbness and weakness in the hands and arms. Depending on the level of herniation, the patient may experience more severe symptoms, such as difficulty walking.

Cervical spondylosis is a degenerative condition generally attributed to age-related changes in the cervical discs. During the aging process, the discs lose fluid, fragment, and collapse. As the discs collapse, increased mechanical stress is placed on the bone, which may result in the formation of bony spurs along the spinal canal. Symptoms of cervical spondylosis include neck and shoulder pain, pain in the back of the head, and numbness and weakness in the arms. If spondylosis is severe, the spinal cord may be affected (myelopathy), and the patient may experience symptoms such as problems with walking and balance.

TECHNIQUE

1. The patient is positioned supine with the right or left hip elevated.
2. The incision lines on the neck and hip are marked and injected with lidocaine with epinephrine to promote vasoconstriction of the wound edges.
3. An incision is made along the border of the iliac crest.
4. A bone graft is obtained and placed in antibiotic solution.
5. The hip incision is closed in layers and covered with a sterile towel.
6. A transverse incision is made in the neck.
7. The trachea and esophagus are retracted.
8. Intraoperative radiographs are taken to confirm the anatomical location of the disc.
9. The cervical vertebrae are dissected out to identify the disc space.
10. Disc fragments are removed.
11. The previously removed bone graft is shaped and placed in the disc space.
12. Cervical plates and screws are used to secure the bone graft.
13. The wound is closed in layers.
14. A cervical collar is placed on the patient before the individual emerges from anesthesia.

Discussion

The patient is placed in the supine position. Cervical traction may be applied with Gardner-Wells tongs or a chin harness

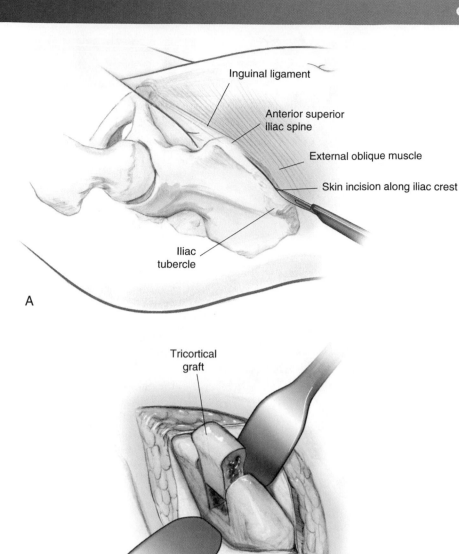

Inguinal ligament

Anterior superior
iliac spine

External oblique muscle

Skin incision along iliac crest

Iliac
tubercle

A

Tricortical
graft

B

Figure 36-32 Iliac crest bone graft. **A,** Incision over the iliac crest. **B,** Plug graft. *(From Miller MD, Chhabra AB, Hurwitz SR, Mihalko WM: Orthopaedic surgical approaches, Philadelphia, 2008, WB Saunders.)*

attached to a weight. Alternately, the arms may be pulled downward with soft gauze looped at the wrists and secured to the operating table frame to open the intervertebral spaces. The right or left hip is elevated on a sandbag or rolled bath blanket. This facilitates exposure of the iliac crest for removal of the bone graft. The surgeon marks both sites and infiltrates them with lidocaine with epinephrine. Both sites are prepped and draped in routine fashion. In some cases, the surgeon may elect to use cadaver bone instead of the patient's bone. If this is the case, prep of the iliac crest is unnecessary.

Two methods are used to take the bone graft. The Cloward method uses a special dowel cutter that creates a "plug" of bone from the iliac crest. Alternatively, an osteotome and a mallet can be used to shear the surface of the iliac crest and create short slivers of bone for the graft. Regardless of the method, the surgeon incises the iliac crest and deepens the incision with the monopolar ESU (Figure 36-32). When the bone has been exposed, a self-retaining retractor is placed

in the wound. The surgeon then uses a periosteal elevator to strip the crest of periosteum.

The graft is placed in a basin, where it may be moistened with saline solution. (Some evidence indicates that soaking the bone in saline destroys cells.) The decision is up to the surgeon. Bleeding vessels on the surface of the iliac crest are controlled with bone wax and the surface is smoothed with a rasp or rongeur. The wound is irrigated. The wound may or may not be closed at this time. Some surgeons pack the wound with sponges and delay closure until the neck procedure is completed, in case additional bone graft is needed. If the surgeon chooses to close the wound at this point, a count is taken. After verification of the count, the surgeon closes the wound in layers with size 0 or 1-0 absorbable synthetic suture on a cutting needle and closes the skin with subcuticular stitches or staples. A drain may be placed before closure. The wound should be covered with a sterile towel for the duration of the procedure.

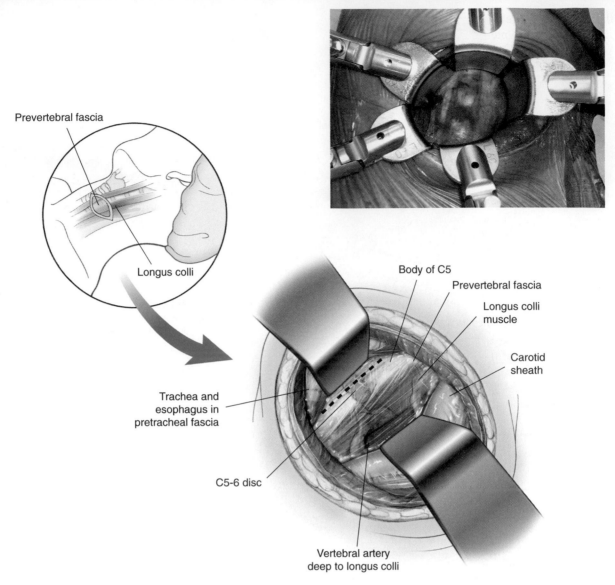

Prevertebral fascia

Longus colli

Trachea and
esophagus in
pretracheal fascia

C5-6 disc

Body of C5

Prevertebral fascia

Longus colli
muscle

Carotid
sheath

Vertebral artery
deep to longus colli

Figure 36-33 **Anterior cervical fusion and discectomy.** *(From Miller MD, Chhabra AB, Hurwitz SR, Mihalko WM: Orthopaedic surgical approaches, Philadelphia, 2008, WB Saunders.)*

The surgeon makes a transverse incision in the skin crease of the neck at the level of the cricoid cartilage. The incision is extended through the platysma muscle with Metzenbaum scissors or the monopolar ESU. Using the scissors for both blunt and sharp dissection, the surgeon defines the medial edge of the sternocleidomastoid muscle. This plane of dissection is carried laterally between the carotid artery and medially between the esophagus and trachea. A small self-retaining retractor is placed in the wound. Hemostasis is maintained with the monopolar and bipolar ESUs and cottonoid sponges.

The surgeon incises the muscle fibers to expose the vertebrae (Figure 36-33). A layer of fascia overlying the vertebra is incised with a #15 knife blade mounted on a #7 handle. A small handheld retractor may be needed by the assistant to help retract the muscle to expose the vertebra. Next, the surgeon incises and removes the anterior longitudinal ligament. With the disc then clearly visible, radiographs are taken

to verify the diseased disc. The surgeon may insert a hypodermic needle into the disc body for identification during the radiographic procedure. The scrub should be prepared for this and provide a sterile radiographic cassette cover if needed. In some cases, the C-arm may be used for real-time confirmation by fluoroscopy.

Once the anatomy has been confirmed, the surgeon places a self-retaining retractor (e.g., a Cloward or Caspar retractor) in the wound. Care is taken in placing these retractors to avoid damaging the carotid artery and esophagus. Usually a combination of sharp and dull blades is used. The retractor systems allow for customization with a variety of blade curvatures, lengths, and retraction surfaces.

With the retractors in place, the surgeon incises the disc with a #15 knife blade. Pituitary rongeurs and fine curettes are used to remove the disc. The disc is removed piece by piece, and the surgical technologist must retrieve the bits of disc from the rongeur or curette with a moistened 4 × 4 sponge. The surgeon may use an intervertebral spreader to expose the disc. A small drill bit or burr may be used to expose the dura within the interspace. The dura then is elevated with a sharp nerve hook or dura hook and incised with a #15 knife blade. When the interspace has been adequately enlarged and all traces of disc have been removed, the surgeon uses a depth gauge and calipers to measure the defect. These measurements are used to size the bone graft.

While the bone graft is being prepared, the neck wound should be covered with a saline-soaked 4 × 4 sponge to prevent tissue drying and with a sterile towel to protect it from contamination. The surgeon examines the graft and cuts it to the appropriate size to fit into the intervertebral space. Any extra bits of bone from the graft must be saved, because they may be used later to fill the interspace. The surgeon places the graft in the interspace and taps it with a mallet so that it fits snugly between the vertebrae. If the Cloward dowel cutter has been used, the Cloward impactor is used to place the graft. Cervical plates and screws may be used to secure the bone graft in place. In this instance, the surgeon drills pilot holes in the vertebrae on either side of the graft. The scrub must be prepared with irrigation to cool the drill bit while the holes are drilled. The surgeon places the plate in position and secures it with screws. An intraoperative radiograph may be taken to confirm the position of the bone graft, plate, and screws.

The wound then is irrigated with normal saline or antibiotic solution. Bleeding vessels are controlled with the monopolar and bipolar ESUs or a topical hemostatic agent. If it was not closed at the start of the procedure, the hip wound is closed at this time. The surgeon closes the cervical incision in layers with 3-0 polyglactin sutures and staples. Both wounds are dressed in routine fashion, and a rigid cervical collar is placed to help support the neck and maintain cervical alignment.

When the patient is moved from the operating table to the stretcher, particular care is taken to keep the head in alignment with the body to prevent dislodgment of the graft.

Postoperative hemorrhage, edema, and CSF leakage are possible after any surgery on the spine. Hemorrhage or edema can damage the spinal cord and cause the patient to exhibit neurological changes such as inability to move the extremities or numbness or weakness. The surgeon assesses the patient's neurological status immediately after transfer from the operating bed to the transfer device by testing the patient's ability to follow commands and move the extremities. The surgical technologist should maintain the integrity of the sterile field until the patient has been transferred from the operating room in case reexploration of the surgical site is necessary.

Longer term complications after spinal surgery include wound infection or meningitis, hardware failure (if used), and nonunion of the bone graft (if used).

POSTERIOR CERVICAL LAMINECTOMY

Surgical Goal

Posterior cervical laminectomy is performed to access the cervical spinal cord and to remove a portion of the cervical lamina.

Pathology

Posterior cervical laminectomy may be required to access neurological tumors. Tumors may occur in the cervical spinal cord or form in the vertebral elements of the cervical spine. Metastatic tumors are common in the bone. Patients with cervical spinal cord tumors typically experience neck pain and numbness and weakness in the upper extremities.

Cervical stenosis is a common condition in older adults that may affect the spinal cord. Cervical stenosis occurs when the discs degenerate and bone spurs form on or between the vertebral surfaces, or the ligaments in the spine buckle, causing pressure on the spinal cord. Symptoms vary, depending on the amount of compression and the location of the stenosis. Most often, symptoms include pain and numbness that radiate down the patient's arm. Cervical stenosis left untreated can seriously damage the spinal cord.

Traumatic injury may result in fracture of the cervical spine and damage to the spinal cord, resulting in a variety of neurological deficits, depending on the level of injury. Decompression laminectomy may be necessary to remove bone fragments and fuse or fixate the spine to prevent ongoing damage to the cord.

TECHNIQUE

1 The patient is positioned prone on a laminectomy frame with the head in pin fixation or in the sitting position with the head in pin fixation.

2 The incision is marked and infiltrated with lidocaine and epinephrine. If a bone graft is required, an additional site is marked and infiltrated. (The section on the procedure for anterior cervical discectomy provides details on obtaining the bone graft.)

3 A midline incision is made and the soft tissue and muscle are retracted.

4 Intraoperative radiographs are taken to confirm the correct vertebral level.

5 Bone is removed from the lamina to reduce pressure.

6 The disc is removed as necessary.

7 If indicated, a fusion or fixation is performed to stabilize the neck.

8 The wound is closed in layers.

9 Bupivacaine may be injected into the soft tissue and musculature to reduce postoperative pain.

10 A rigid cervical collar or external cervical brace system (e.g., halo brace) is placed before the patient emerges from anesthesia.

Discussion

The patient may be positioned in the sitting position or prone on chest rolls or a laminectomy frame for this procedure (Figure 36-34). The position used depends on the surgeon's preference and the pathological condition. The sitting position may provide better exposure for the higher vertebrae. A three-point pin fixation clamp is used in both positions to ensure that the patient's head and cervical spine remain as immobile as possible during the procedure. Immobilization is especially critical in traumatic injuries to the spine.

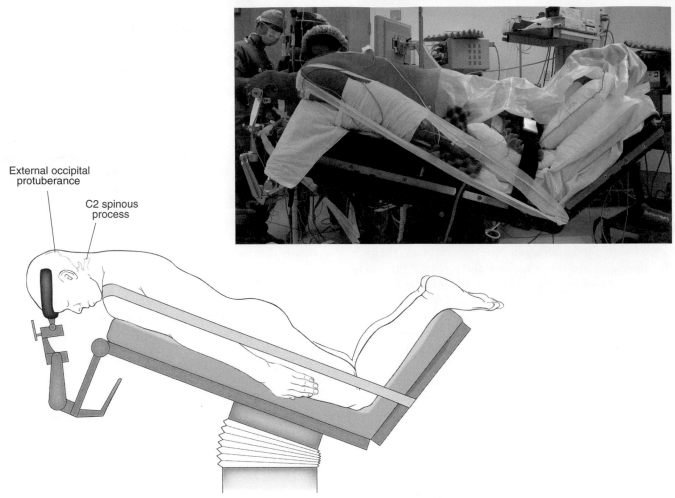

External occipital
protuberance

C2 spinous
process

Figure 36-34 **Posterior cervical laminectomy.** The patient is placed in the prone position. *(From Miller MD, Chhabra AB, Hurwitz SR, Mihalko WM: Orthopaedic surgical approaches, Philadelphia, 2008, WB Saunders.)*

The surgeon marks the incision site and infiltrates it with lidocaine with epinephrine. If a fusion is planned, an additional site on the patient's hip is marked and infiltrated. Both sites are prepped and draped in routine fashion.

If necessary, a bone graft is harvested from the patient's hip. Alternatively, cadaver bone may be used. The surgeon's preference and the patient's condition determine which method is used. Harvesting of the bone graft may be done at the start of the procedure or after the laminectomy is performed. The scrub should always be prepared for the possibility that a bone graft may be needed and ensure that the proper draping material and instrumentation are available.

After palpating the cervical spinous processes to determine the location of the incision, the surgeon makes a midline incision and begins to expose the musculature of the neck. A monopolar ESU is used for hemostasis, along with 4 × 4 sponges. The surgeon uses sharp dissection with Metzenbaum scissors and blunt finger dissection to separate the muscle layers. A self-retaining retractor (e.g., Weitlaner or Beckman-Adson retractor) is placed to help maintain exposure. Dissection continues until the spinous processes are visualized. The surgeon uses a variety of periosteal elevators (e.g., Cobb or

Key elevator) to clean the periosteum off the bone and gain exposure. Moistened cottonoids and Gelfoam may be used to aid hemostasis.

An intraoperative radiograph is obtained after exposure is completed. The surgeon places a towel clip on the vertebral process or inserts a spinal needle into the disc space to provide a marker, and the radiograph is taken. The scrub should provide a sterile cassette cover or sterile draping over the radiograph cassette holder. Depending on the patient's position, C-arm fluoroscopy may be used for real-time imaging.

The term *laminectomy* refers to the removal of the bony roof of the spinal canal. In a laminectomy, additional bone may also be removed from one or both sides of the vertebra to open up the spinal canal as needed. The surgeon begins the laminectomy with a Leksell rongeur to remove the spinous process and then uses Kerrison rongeurs in a variety of sizes to remove smaller pieces of bone (Figure 36-35). The scrub should be prepared to assist in removing the pieces of bone from the instrument with a moistened 4 × 4 sponge. Any bone fragments retrieved should be placed in a small bowl filled with saline. The surgeon may also use a high-speed drill (e.g., the Midas Rex) to perform the laminectomy. A variety of

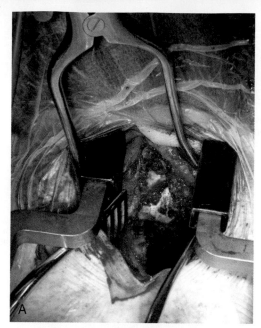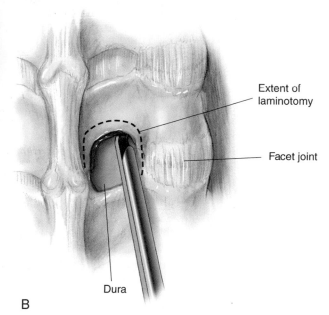

Figure 36-35 Posterior cervical laminectomy. A, With self-retaining retractors in place, the lamina is exposed. **B,** A Kerrison up-biting rongeur is used to remove bone. *(From Miller MD, Chhabra AB, Hurwitz SR, Mihalko WM:* Orthopaedic surgical approaches, *Philadelphia, 2008, WB Saunders.)*

cutting and shaping burrs are available. If necessary, the disc is removed with pituitary rongeurs and curettes, as described for an anterior discectomy.

In cases of cervical fracture, the surgeon may fuse the vertebra with a bone graft or with a variety of internal fixation methods, including plates, screws, and cables. The method of fixation varies, depending on the level of fracture and the severity of injury. (Chapter 31 presents a discussion of techniques of internal fixation.)

When the laminectomy and discectomy are completed, the surgeon irrigates the wound with antibiotic solution and secures hemostasis with the ESU. The wound is closed in layers with size 0 or 1-0 polyglactin suture on a cutting needle. The skin usually is closed with staples.

The wound is dressed with a simple gauze dressing. A rigid cervical collar is applied before the patient emerges from anesthesia. The collar provides stabilization while the laminectomy heals. Patients who have undergone fusion and instrumentation may require additional stabilization with a halo brace.

APPLICATION OF A HALO BRACE

Surgical Goal
A halo brace is used to provide traction and restore spinal alignment to the cervical spine. It may also be used to provide initial decompression of the spinal cord after injury.

Pathology
Fracture of the cervical spine requires immobilization to prevent displacement of the bone and impingement on the spinal cord. A halo traction brace is applied to maintain alignment during healing after traumatic injury and select cervical spine procedures.

TECHNIQUE

1 The patient is placed in the supine position.
2 A local anesthetic is injected into the pin sites.
3 Four to six people log-roll the patient and the back panel of the vest is placed.
4 The posterior bars are attached to the back panel of the vest.
5 The halo pins are placed and tightened.
6 The halo ring is attached to the posterior bars.
7 The front panel of the vest is placed and the anterior bars are secured to the vest.
8 The halo ring is attached to the anterior bars.
9 The pins are adjusted as needed for optimum immobilization.

Discussion
Cervical halo systems may vary by manufacturer but commonly consist of a halo ring that surrounds the head and is held in place by pins, a frame made of four upright bars and connectors to attach the bars to the halo, and a vest, which is a plastic structure that covers the chest and acts as a foundation for the brace.

The patient is positioned supine with the head extending over the edge of the bed and manually stabilized by the surgical assistant. The surgeon injects the pin sites with local anesthetic for hemostasis. Most systems use a four-pin configuration. The surgeon injects two sites on either side of the patient's eyes over the orbital ridge and two sites just behind the ears.

The patient is log-rolled onto the side and the surgeon slides the back panel of the halo vest into place. The posterior bars are secured to the back panel of the vest by sliding them through the connectors and tightening the connectors with an Allen wrench.

An appropriate-size ring is selected, and the pins are placed through the pin sockets in the ring. The surgeon positions the ring over the patient's head until the tips of the pins just touch the skin. Each pin is tightened by hand, starting with a front pin, and then the diagonally opposite back pin, until all the pins pierce the skin and are secure in the outer layer of the skull bone. The front panel of the vest is placed over the chest, and the anterior bars are placed through the connectors and tightened. The halo ring is attached to the bars with connectors in the front and back. A torque wrench is used to tighten the pins to 6 to 8 pounds (2.7 to 3.6 kg) of tightness. Once the ring and bars are secured, the straps on the side of the vest are buckled. The scrub must ensure that the wrenches that come with the vest are sent with the patient after the procedure, in case the halo device must be removed in an emergency. Often the wrenches are taped to the front of the vest for easy access.

LUMBAR LAMINECTOMY AND DISCECTOMY

Surgical Goal

Lumbar laminectomy is performed to access the lumbar spinal cord and remove a portion of the lumbar lamina. Discectomy is performed to excise and remove a portion of the intervertebral disc.

Pathology

Lumbar laminectomy as a stand-alone procedure most often is performed to decompress the spinal column in cases of spinal stenosis, to gain access to a spinal cord tumor, or as a step in a more extensive surgery to correct a spinal deformity.

Discectomy is used to treat a herniation of the intervertebral disc. Disc herniation refers to a tear in the outer ring (annulus fibrosis) that allows the softer middle portion of the disc (nucleus pulposus) to bulge out (Figure 36-36). Disc herniation occurs most frequently between the fourth and fifth lumbar vertebrae or between the fifth lumbar vertebra and the sacrum. Disc herniation may be the result of general wear and tear or of a traumatic event, such as lifting while bent at the waist.

TECHNIQUE

1 The patient is positioned prone on a laminectomy frame or in the knee-chest position on a spinal table.
2 The incision is marked and infiltrated with lidocaine and epinephrine.
3 A midline incision is made and hemostasis is maintained as the tissue is dissected to the level of the fascia.
4 The fascia is incised and the spinous processes are exposed.
5 Intraoperative radiographs are taken to confirm the correct vertebral level.
6 Bone is removed from the lamina.
7 Disc is removed as necessary.
8 The wound is closed in layers.
9 Bupivacaine may be injected into the soft tissue and musculature to reduce postoperative pain.

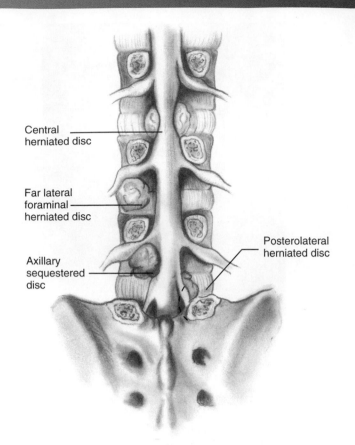

Figure 36-36 **Lumbar laminectomy.** Locations of possible disc hernias. (From Vaccaro AR, Betz RR, Zeidman SM: Principles and practice of spine surgery, St Louis, 2003, Mosby.)

Discussion

After induction and placement of an endotracheal tube, the patient is placed in the prone position on a laminectomy frame (e.g., Wilson or Jackson frame) or a specialized spinal operating bed.

To begin the procedure, the surgeon may inject the incisional site with a small amount of local anesthetic with epinephrine to aid hemostasis. A midline vertical incision is made over the spine with a #20 knife blade. The surgeon deepens the wound with the knife or monopolar ESU to the level of the fascia and incises the fascia with toothed forceps and the monopolar ESU. Two angled Weitlaner retractors are inserted into the wound for better exposure.

The scrub should have a large number of unfolded 4 × 4 sponges available at this time. The surgeon packs the sponges along the vertebra with periosteal elevators. This is done both to aid hemostasis and to expose the vertebrae by retracting the larger back muscles. Because the wound is now deep, the surgeon may replace the Weitlaner retractors with Beckman-Adson, Meyerding, or Taylor retractors (Figure 36-37). If Taylor retractors are used, the surgical technologist should have roller gauze available. The surgeon wraps the gauze around the tail of the retractor and drops the opposite end to the circulating nurse, who secures it to the table frame or a sandbag to keep the retractor in place.

Intraoperative radiographs are obtained to confirm the correct vertebral level. The surgeon may request a spinal

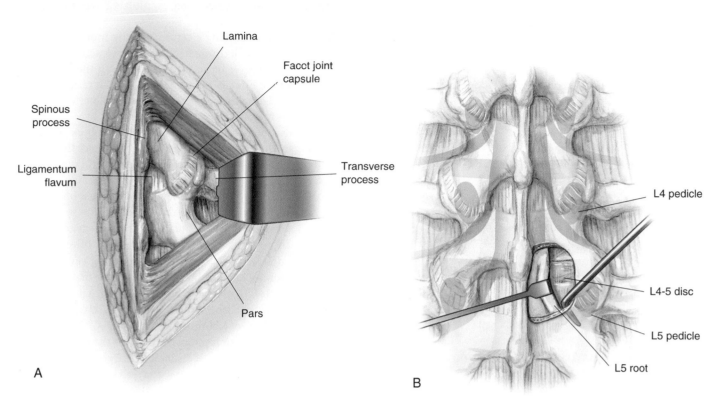

Figure 36-37 A, Lumbar laminectomy—exposure of the vertebrae with a Hibbs retractor in place. **B,** A Kerrison rongeur is used to decompress the lamina. *(From Miller MD, Chhabra AB, Hurwitz SR, Mihalko WM: Orthopaedic surgical approaches, Philadelphia, 2008, WB Saunders.)*

needle to mark the level or may clamp a towel clip through the spinous process. Generally, the radiographic cassette is loaded into a portable radiograph stand draped by the scrub. C-arm fluoroscopy may also be used.

The surgeon uses a large rongeur to remove small pieces of the spinous process and expose the lamina. Up-biting and down-biting Kerrison rongeurs then are used to excise the lamina and create access to the disc. The surgeon may also use a high-speed drill with a cutting burr to remove the bone. Any bone chips removed must be retained as specimens. After the lamina has been removed, cottonoid sponges are used instead of 4 × 4 sponges. To prevent the dura from tearing, the surgeon uses a dental probe or Freer-type elevator to loosen any dura attached to the lamina. The surgical technologist should be prepared with a small piece of bone wax on the end of a Penfield elevator or on the edge of a small medicine glass to aid hemostasis.

The surgeon identifies the yellowish ligamentum flavum (the ligament that connects each vertebra to the next) and incises it with a #15 knife blade mounted on a #7 handle. Down-biting Kerrison rongeurs are used to remove any ligament that obstructs the surgeon's view of the disc. The disc is now approachable.

The assistant retracts the vertebral nerve with a Love retractor or similar nerve root retractor as the surgeon snips off pieces of the bulging disc with a Takahashi or pituitary rongeur. As the disc is removed, the surgeon may use a curette for further

evacuation. The scrub must clean the tips of the instrument with each bite and keep the fragments as specimens. These specimens should be kept separate from the bone fragments previously retrieved. The scrub must remain alert during this maneuver, because the surgeon cannot turn away from the wound (because the risk of spinal cord damage is great).

After the herniated disc has been removed, the surgeon closes the wound. The fascial layer usually is closed with size 0 absorbable synthetic sutures and a large cutting needle. Before closing the muscle layer, the surgeon may inject a local anesthetic to control postoperative pain. The muscle and subcutaneous layers are closed with 2-0 sutures. The skin is closed according to the surgeon's preference (a variety of materials may be used), and the wound is dressed in routine fashion.

FORAMINOTOMY

Foraminotomy is performed to relieve pressure on the spinal nerves. The spinal nerves pass through the intervertebral foramina as they branch off the spinal cord. When the nerves are compressed by bone, herniated disc, scarring, or ligament hypertrophy, the patient may experience symptoms of pain, numbness, or weakness in the area served by that particular nerve.

Foraminotomy often is an adjunct procedure to laminectomy, but it may also be performed as a minimally invasive, stand-alone procedure through a small incision. The surgeon widens the foramen with a high-speed drill or fine-tip rongeurs.

MICRODISCECTOMY

Surgical Goal

During microdiscectomy, a small window is made in the lamina for access to an intervertebral disc. This is a minimally invasive approach to lumbar laminectomy and discectomy.

Pathology

See Lumbar Laminectomy and Discectomy.

TECHNIQUE

1   The patient is positioned prone on a laminectomy frame or in the knee-chest position on a spinal operating bed.
2   The incision is marked and infiltrated with lidocaine and epinephrine.
3   A guide needle is inserted through the skin under fluoroscopic visualization.
4   A guidewire is placed through the needle to confirm the correct vertebral level fluoroscopically.
5   Dilators in progressively larger sizes are placed over the guidewire to separate the muscles and expose the intralaminar space.
6   A tubular retractor is placed and the dilating tubes are removed.
7   The operating microscope (or an endoscopic telescope) is used to visualize the spinal anatomy.
8   Bone is removed and the nerve root is retracted.
9   The disc is removed.
10 The incision is closed if necessary.
11 A small dressing is applied.

Discussion

Microdiscectomy may be performed using general anesthesia, local anesthesia, or local anesthesia with sedation. The patient may be positioned in the lateral decubitus position, the prone position on a laminectomy frame, or in the knee-chest position on an Andrews table. If general anesthesia is used, induction and intubation take place before positioning. Some surgeons prefer using local anesthesia, because they believe that they can better monitor the patient's responses to pain.

The surgeon injects the incision line with lidocaine with epinephrine to promote hemostasis. The C-arm is used to confirm placement of a guide needle through the skin to the level of the affected lamina. The surgeon passes a guidewire through the needle and removes the needle, leaving the guidewire in place. The scrub should be prepared with a Crile clamp to secure the guidewire while the needle is removed.

A dilating tube is placed over the guidewire to separate the soft tissue and muscle. The surgeon removes the guidewire and leaves the dilating tube in place. A sequence of progressively larger tubes is placed over the existing tube to further dilate the space.

A tubular retractor is placed over the dilating tubes and docked on the lamina. The retractor is secured to a post that clamps onto the operating bed for stability. The dilating tubes are removed, leaving the retractor in place. The operating microscope is positioned and adjusted. Alternately, an endoscope attached to a camera and monitoring system may be used.

The scrub places a long electrode on the monopolar ESU, and the surgeon uses it through the tubular retractor to remove any remaining muscle or soft tissue overlying the lamina. A small window of bone is removed through the retractor with a Kerrison or Leksell rongeur. Some surgeons prefer to use a high-speed powered drill with a long cutting burr for removing the bone. The surgeon removes a window of bone, preserving the ligamentum flavum underneath to protect the dura.

A nerve root retractor is passed through the tubular retractor and the nerve root is gently retracted. The epidural veins are coagulated with the bipolar ESU and dissected off the disc space. A special endoscopic knife is used to incise the disc surface. The surgeon uses standard disc rongeurs to remove any extruded portions of the disc. The nerve root retractor is removed and the area is inspected visually. The surgeon irrigates the wound with normal saline to ensure that all debris is cleared and to visualize any bleeding areas. Any necessary hemostasis is accomplished with the bipolar ESU and Gelfoam pledgets soaked in topical thrombin.

The tubular retractor is removed. Because the wound is very small, minimal closure is necessary. The surgeon may use size 0 and 3-0 polyglactin sutures for a layered closure and then 4-0 polyglactin sutures for subcuticular closure. The wound edges are approximated with Steri-Strips or Dermabond glue.

LUMBAR FUSION

Surgical Goal

Lumbar fusion is performed to stabilize the spine using a bone graft or metal implant. The graft stimulates the growth of new bone between the vertebral elements, causing the area to fuse. If necessary, metal implants are used to further stabilize the spine and offer greater support.

Pathology

A fusion may be required after laminectomy or as a means to stabilize traumatic or pathological fractures. Fusion may also be indicated after removal of a tumor or as a corrective procedure for spinal deformities. The technique described here details the procedure for a posterior lumbar interbody fusion with pedicle screws and rods.

Discussion

Two types of fusion are commonly used in the lumbar spine, posterolateral fusion and interbody fusion. Both types may be used independently or in conjunction with one another. In posterolateral fusion, the bone graft is placed between the transverse processes and fixed in place with screws (or wire) placed through the vertebral pedicles and attached to metal rods. In interbody fusion, the surgeon places the bone graft between the vertebrae in the area normally occupied by the intervertebral disc. The graft may or may not be secured with instrumentation.

The surgeon performs a laminectomy to prepare the area for fusion (refer to the discussion of lumbar laminectomy for the procedural steps). Using external landmarks and

TECHNIQUE

1. A lumbar laminectomy is performed and a bone graft is obtained.
2. The area where the screws will be placed is identified.
3. A high-speed drill with a cutting burr is used to remove the cortical surface of the bone.
4. The screw entrance hole is identified.
5. The screw hole is tapped and widened.
6. The pedicle screws are placed on either side of the vertebra and guide pins are attached to the screw heads.
7. The bone graft is placed between the vertebrae.
8. An appropriate-size rod is selected and connectors are placed over the rod.
9. The rod-connector assembly is threaded over the guide pins and secured.
10. Hemostasis is maintained and a drain is placed.
11. The wound is closed in layers.
12. An external brace may be placed before the patient emerges from anesthesia.

radiographic confirmation, the surgeon identifies the pedicle canal entry site and removes the cortical layer over the bone with a high-speed cutting burr. The scrub should be prepared with irrigation and suction while the surgeon is using the drill. Next, the surgeon places a bone probe through the entry site to determine its depth.

Pedicle markers are placed in the canal, and the proposed screw path is confirmed with real-time fluoroscopy with the C-arm or a lateral radiograph. After confirming the path, the surgeon taps the hole and widens it as appropriate for the screw configuration. The screw is placed in the pedicle until the base of the screw head makes contact with the bone. The process is repeated until the desired number of pedicle screws has been placed on either side of the spine.

A guide pin guide is positioned over the screw head and a guide pin is threaded through it. The guide pin is tightened onto the screw and the guide pin guide is removed. The process is repeated for each screw. When the screws are in place, the surgeon places the bone graft between the vertebrae.

The surgeon selects the rod to be used. Rods are available in a variety of diameters and lengths and can be customized for the patient with a rod bender and rod cutter. The surgeon places lateral connectors onto the rods and tightens the connector screws to secure the connectors to the rods. The connector-rod assembly is slid over the guide pins down to the pedicle screws. A lock nut is placed over the guide pin and secured over the connector. The guide pin is removed and the process is repeated until all the connectors are secured to the pedicle screws. A screwdriver is used to tighten the lock nuts into place.

Hemostasis is maintained with the ESU and the wound is irrigated with antibiotic solution. Gelfoam strips and Surgicel may also be used to aid hemostasis. The surgeon closes the wound in layers with size 0 or 1-0 absorbable synthetic suture and skin staples. To further immobilize the spine and promote patient comfort, the surgeon may place an external lumbar brace or jacket on the patient before he or she emerges from anesthesia.

CORRECTION OF SCOLIOSIS

Surgical Goal

Surgical correction of scoliosis is performed to restore anatomical alignment to the spine, prevent further curvature, and provide stability.

Pathology

Scoliosis is a three-dimensional spinal deformity. Typically, the spine is curved from side to side in an S or C concave-convex configuration. It also may have a degree of rotation. Scoliosis may occur in patients with muscular dystrophy or cerebral palsy, but in most cases the cause is unknown. The condition is familial and occurs more frequently in females than in males. Scoliosis usually is diagnosed during childhood or adolescence. Patients with scoliosis can have varying degrees of cosmetic deformity and may experience back pain and difficulty breathing as a result of rib cage compression. Many surgical procedures are available to provide correction and stabilization. Surgery involves the implantation of metal rods or other implants through an anterior or posterior approach and fusion with bone grafting. The hardware is designed to distract the spine and realign it to a more normal curvature, and fusion is used to maintain the new alignment. A basic posterior segmental rodding technique with hooks is described here.

TECHNIQUE

1. The patient is positioned prone on a spinal operating bed. A bone graft will be obtained; therefore the position may be altered to provide access to the iliac crest.
2. The incisions are marked and infiltrated with lidocaine and epinephrine.
3. The bone graft is obtained.
4. A midline lumbar incision is made and hemostasis is maintained.
5. The spinous processes are exposed and the anatomical level is confirmed by radiographs.
6. Curettes and elevators are used to clear the soft tissue and ligament attachments over the vertebrae.
7. A facetectomy is performed and a bone graft is placed.
8. The hook sites are prepared and the hooks are placed.
9. The rods are prepared and attached to the hooks with connectors.
10. Distraction of the curves is achieved by bending the rods and securing them in the new position with the connectors and cross-links.
11. The bone graft is placed.
12. The wound is closed in layers; staples are used for skin closure.

Discussion

The patient is positioned prone on a spinal operating bed, and the surgeon marks the incision lines for a midline lumbar incision and an iliac crest bone graft. A bone graft is obtained and prepared as described in the procedure for an anterior cervical discectomy.

The surgeon performs a midline lumbar incision and maintains hemostasis with the monopolar ESU and digital pressure with 4 × 4 sponges. The incision is extended into deep tissue, and Weitlaner retractors are placed for exposure. A Cobb elevator is used to strip the periosteum off the spinous processes. The scrub should be prepared to provide a spinal needle or towel clamp to the surgeon for radiographic localization of the anatomical levels after the spinous processes have been prepared.

Once the anatomical levels have been confirmed, the surgeon uses curettes and pituitary rongeurs to clean the surface of the vertebrae. Larger self-retaining retractors are placed as needed to maintain exposure and aid visualization. The surgeon may use a high-speed drill with a cutting burr to decorticate the bone further in preparation for the fusion and instrumentation.

A thoracic facetectomy is performed by placing a cut through the facet at the base of the lamina and carrying it along the transverse processes, leaving the fragment hinged. An additional cut is made in the upper articular facet with a Cobb gouge to produce another hinged fragment. The surgeon places cancellous bone chips in the defects.

Next, the surgeon prepares the hook sites. Two types of hooks are used, *pedicle* and *laminar*. Pedicle hooks are used in the thoracic spine and laminar hooks are used in other areas of the spine. The surgeon introduces a pedicle finder into the facet joint and enlarges the space as necessary with a drill. The pedicle hook is inserted and secured. The laminar hooks are temporarily placed on either the superior or inferior edge of the lamina, depending on the direction of distraction needed for correction of the curvature. The surgeon removes the laminar hooks and performs a lumbar facetectomy as previously described. The laminar hooks are replaced and the surgeon prepares the rods.

The rods are available in a variety of lengths and curvatures. The surgeon can also customize the curvature using rod benders if necessary. After choosing and modifying the rods, if necessary, the surgeon places the rods into the hooks. The hooks are top loading. The surgeon places a set screw into the first hook where the rod is securely seated. If necessary, a rod cam or ratcheted rod reducer is used to manipulate the rods into place over the hooks. Once the rods are in place, the surgeon uses set screws to secure them to the hooks. At this point, the surgeon evaluates the distraction and compression by attaching cross-links to the rods and tightening the connectors.

A high-speed drill or Cobb elevator is used to decorticate the vertebral surfaces to prepare them for the bone graft. The bone graft is placed and the wound is closed in layers as previously described for other spinal procedures. An external brace may be placed before the patient emerges from anesthesia to help maintain alignment and provide comfort.

SPINAL TUMORS

Surgical Goal
A spinal tumor is removed surgically to restore circulation of spinal fluid and increase patient mobility and also for pain management.

Pathology
Tumors of the spinal cord may be primary (the tumor is composed of cells derived from the nervous system) or secondary (arising from a distant or metastatic location). Primary tumors may be malignant or benign. Secondary tumors are always malignant.

Spinal tumors are differentiated according to their location; they are either extradural (outside the dura mater) or intradural (inside the dura mater). Intradural tumors can be further identified by their proximity to the spinal cord. Intramedullary tumors are found within the spinal cord and extramedullary tumors are found inside the dura mater but outside the spinal cord.

Extradural tumors include sarcomas, carcinomas from a metastasis, lipomas, neurofibromas, chondromas, angiomas, granulomas, and abscesses. Intradural extramedullary tumors usually are benign tumors that originate either from the dura mater or from the arachnoid space around the spinal cord. Gliomas are the most common intramedullary tumors; they have a very poor prognosis because of their ability to infiltrate the cord, making them difficult to remove.

TECHNIQUE

1 A laminectomy is performed and the dura is exposed (see the lumbar laminectomy procedure for details).
2 The dura is incised and retracted with sutures.
3 The tumor is excised.
4 The dura is closed.
5 Wound closure proceeds as described for a laminectomy.

Discussion
During spinal surgery for tumor removal, a variety of materials or a dural graft may be needed to restore continuity of the dura. This is necessary for large invasive tumors. Graft materials include a portion of the patient's pericranium, bovine pericardium, or biosynthetic dura substitutes. Handling techniques for the dural replacement materials vary, depending on the material and amount used. The scrub should anticipate the possibility of dural replacement in this procedure and ensure that the surgeon's preferred material is available, along with any items needed to prepare it.

The surgeon performs a laminectomy and then removes the ligamentum flavum with scissors, scalpel, or Kerrison or Cloward rongeur. The epidural fat is removed and the dura mater is exposed. The dura mater is elevated with a nerve hook and the surgeon uses a #15 blade to nick it. Using a groove director, the surgeon extends the dural incision. The dural edges are retracted with 4-0 silk and dural needles. The cord then is exposed.

The tumor is identified, gently dissected free, and removed. Dissection can be performed with suction, bipolar ESU forceps, pituitary scoops, curettes, rongeurs, or the CUSA. Hemostasis is maintained with the bipolar ESU, cottonoids, hemostatic clips, Gelfoam, and topical hemostatic agents. The wound is irrigated, and the dura is tightly closed or a duraplasty is performed to ensure a watertight seal. Once the dura has been closed, wound closure progresses as described for a laminectomy.

NEUROSURGICAL PAIN MANAGEMENT

CORDOTOMY

Surgical Goal

The goal of cordotomy (or chordotomy) is to disable pain-conducting tracts in the spinal cord.

Pathology

A variety of conditions may cause severe or intractable pain. In these conditions, the nerve fibers may be damaged or injured, resulting in incorrect neural transmission and pain. Cordotomy is performed primarily on patients with somatic or visceral pain related to cancer. Somatic pain arises from pressure on ligaments, tendons, fascia, muscles, bone, and blood vessels. Patients with tumors in the legs, hips, chest, or abdominal space may report somatic pain. Visceral pain in cancer patients is characterized by cramping and aching and generally is related to extensive involvement of the pancreas, colon, or reproductive organs. Somatic cancer pain may be treated with an anterolateral cordotomy, whereas visceral pain requires a bilateral cordotomy.

Other conditions less commonly treated with a cordotomy include phantom limb pain (pain perceived to be located in an amputated limb), severe spinal cord injury, and pain associated with peripheral nerve injury.

A percutaneous cordotomy may be performed as a minimally invasive technique using stereotactic guidance to locate the tracts associated with enervated tissue and destruction of the nerve bundle with a thermoregulated cordotomy electrode. Open cordotomy is used if percutaneous cordotomy is not feasible or was previously unsuccessful. Regardless of the method used, cordotomy may require repeat surgery, because the effect of surgery diminishes over the first 6 months after the procedure.

TECHNIQUE

1 A laminectomy is performed and the dura is exposed.
2 The dura is incised and retracted with sutures.
3 The operating microscope is used to locate the nerve tract.
4 A specialized ball electrode is placed against the nerve tract and radiofrequency current is applied.
5 The dura is closed.
6 The wound is closed.

Discussion

Electrophysiological nerve monitoring may be used in the procedure to monitor the spinal nerve responses to manipulation. The surgical technologist should be aware of the location of any electrodes placed in the patient before surgery to avoid dislodging them during the draping procedure. The operating microscope should be draped before the start of surgery.

The surgeon performs a laminectomy and opens the dura as previously described. The operating microscope is used to visualize the nerve tract and determine the depth for the electrode placement. Using careful blunt dissection with microsurgical instruments, the surgeon frees the dorsal root branches from the cord. The spinal cord must be slightly rotated to provide safe access to the nerve tracts. The surgeon places a silk suture through a clip and attaches the clip to the dentate ligament of the cord. The suture is used to gently put traction on the cord and rotate it approximately 45 degrees. A dental mirror is used to visualize the anterior spinal artery and other vascular structures. Blunt dissection continues until the correct spinal tract is identified.

A specialized ball electrode is inserted at the cordotomy site, and a grounding needle electrode is placed in the nearby paraspinal muscle. A radiofrequency signal is generated, causing a lesion in the area in direct contact with the ball electrode. The lesion prevents the transmission of pain signals to the area beyond it. If bilateral cordotomies are required, the procedure is repeated on the opposite side. When the procedure has been completed, the wound is closed as described in the procedure for a spinal cord tumor.

RHIZOTOMY

Surgical Goal

Rhizotomy is performed to selectively sever nerve roots in the spinal cord to relieve severe pain or symptoms related to neuromuscular conditions, such as multiple sclerosis, or spasticity arising from cerebral palsy or spinal cord injury.

Pathology

(Refer to the Pathology section in the cordotomy procedure for a discussion of pain syndromes that may be amenable to rhizotomy.) Spasticity refers to a form of increased tone or tension in the muscles that occurs as a result of damage to the motor pathways from the CNS. Spasticity may occur in patients with cerebral palsy, multiple sclerosis, spinal cord injuries, and other disorders.

TECHNIQUE

1 A laminectomy is performed and the dura is exposed.
2 Ultrasound is used to locate the tip of the spinal cord where the separation of sensory and motor nerves occurs.
3 The dura is incised and retracted with sutures.
4 The operating microscope is used to expose and isolate the sensory nerves.
5 The nerves are tested with electromyography (EMG) for the degree of spasticity.
6 Selective nerves are severed.
7 The dura is closed
8 The wound is closed.

Discussion

The patient is positioned for a lumbar laminectomy. EMG electrodes are placed and tested before the skin prep is performed. The surgeon performs a multilevel lumbar laminectomy, as described earlier in this chapter, and exposes the spinal cord and spinal nerves.

Intraoperative ultrasound is used to identify the area where the sensory and motor nerves arise from the spinal cord. Only the sensory nerves are severed in a rhizotomy. The operating microscope is brought to the field, and the surgeon carefully identifies and isolates the sensory nerves using blunt dissection with microsurgical probes. The surgeon uses a Silastic pad to separate the sensory nerves from the motor nerves. It is important that the spinal cord and nerve roots stay moist. The scrub should be prepared with moistened cottonoids and periodic irrigation.

After the sensory nerves have been exposed, the surgeon divides the nerve root into three to five rootlets and tests each one with EMG. EMG helps the surgeon identify which rootlets are responsible for the pain or spasticity response, because these rootlets show increased activity on the EMG recording. The surgeon uses microscissors to sever the nerve roots that show abnormal activity. The dura is closed and the wound is irrigated with saline. Wound closure proceeds as described for lumbar laminectomy.

DORSAL COLUMN STIMULATOR

Surgical Goal

Implanted dorsal column stimulators are used to manage chronic pain. The device generates an electrical impulse that causes a tingling sensation, which alters the perception of pain by the patient.

Pathology

Dorsal column stimulators may be used to treat a variety of chronic pain conditions, such as intractable back pain, complex regional pain syndrome, phantom limb pain, and postherpetic neuralgia (severe localized pain that occurs after an attack of shingles).

TECHNIQUE

1 A needle is placed into the epidural space and the electrode is threaded through the needle and connected to a stimulator.

2 The patient is awakened and the trial stimulator is activated.

3 The electrode is repositioned as necessary and the stimulator is adjusted according to the patient's responses.

4 The stimulator is disconnected and additional local anesthetic is infiltrated into the surrounding area.

5 The electrode is anchored and tunneled through the skin.

6 Any incisions are closed and the electrode is reconnected to the trial stimulator.

7 The patient is discharged to home for 4 to 7 days to use the stimulator and determine whether the treatment will be effective.

8 The patient returns for phase 2 and is positioned and sedated as previously described.

9 The stimulator site is infiltrated with lidocaine and epinephrine.

10 A subcutaneous pocket is created and the stimulator is placed in the pocket.

11 A tunneling tool is used to create a pathway from the stimulator to the previously implanted electrode.

12 The electrode is connected to the stimulator and the incision is closed in layers.

Discussion

The dorsal column stimulator procedure is performed in two phases to allow for a trial period in which to determine whether the device will be effective at relieving the patient's pain. The procedure frequently is performed with the patient sedated, because the surgeon must be able to awaken the patient and ask questions during placement of the electrode.

During both phases, the patient is positioned prone on a fluoroscopic table and sedated. The procedure can be lengthy; therefore the patient is made as comfortable as possible and sedated. The surgeon infiltrates the patient's back with lidocaine with epinephrine. A 3-mL syringe filled with saline is attached to a 15-gauge Tuohy needle, and the needle is inserted through the skin and ligaments and maneuvered into the epidural space. During the placement, the surgeon gently presses the plunger of the syringe and notes the resistance of the saline solution to the pressure. Loss of resistance is considered an indication of entry into the epidural space.

The surgeon threads the electrode through the needle under fluoroscopic guidance. A stylet is included in the electrode to assist the surgeon in placement. Once the electrode is placed at the anatomical target, it is anchored and attached to a temporary cable, which is passed off the sterile field and attached to a trial stimulator. The patient is awakened and the stimulator is activated. The patient is questioned about the presence or absence of sensations and their locations as the stimulator settings are adjusted.

After confirming the functioning of the device, the surgeon disconnects the electrode from the cable and makes a small vertical incision over the site of the Tuohy needle. The monopolar ESU is used for hemostasis, and Metzenbaum scissors are used to undermine the subcutaneous tissue. The surgeon removes the Tuohy needle and electrode stylet, leaving the electrode in place. Next, the electrode is anchored to prevent it from migrating with an anchoring device supplied by the manufacturer.

The surgeon attaches the electrode to a percutaneous extension lead and tunnels it under the skin. The electrode remains under the skin, and a portion of the extension lead is brought out through the skin. The subcutaneous layers and skin are closed with polyglactin sutures and staples. The externalized lead is attached to a temporary stimulator for a trial period of 4 to 7 days.

At the end of the trial period, the patient is questioned about the success of pain reduction. A 50% reduction of pain is considered an indicator of success and qualifies the patient to move to phase 2. If the trial was not successful, the electrode and extension lead are removed.

For the phase 2 procedure, the patient is positioned prone and sedated. The surgeon opens the previous midline incision and disconnects the extension lead from the electrode. Next, the site for stimulator placement is chosen. A variety of anatomical locations are suitable for the implantation, including the buttocks, abdomen, lateral chest, or subaxillary space.

The surgeon makes a horizontal incision over the proposed stimulator site and, using blunt and sharp dissection, creates a pocket large enough to house the stimulator. The monopolar ESU and 4 × 4 sponges are used for hemostasis. The pocket is purposely made shallow so that the stimulator can be easily programmed through a device held over the skin.

A small tunneler is used to connect the midline incision to the pocket. A new extension lead is attached to the electrode and passed through the tunneler to the pocket. The stimulator is placed in the pocket and connected to the extension lead. The surgeon closes the wound in layers with 3-0 polyglactin sutures and staples. The device is activated after the procedure has been completed and the wound dressing applied.

PERIPHERAL NERVE PROCEDURES

ULNAR NERVE TRANSPOSITION

Surgical Goal

The surgical goal of an ulnar nerve transposition is to free the ulnar nerve from a groove on the medial epicondyle, thereby restoring function and eliminating desensitization of the affected arm.

Pathology

The ulnar nerve is a peripheral nerve that travels through the groove of the medial epicondyle from the upper to the lower arm. The ulnar nerve can be injured by trauma, elbow fractures and dislocations, and repeated bending of the elbow as part of occupational or recreational activities. Symptoms generally include reduced sensation in the affected arm, hand atrophy or, in severe cases, a claw hand deformity.

TECHNIQUE

1 A long incision is made over the lateral elbow.
2 The muscles are divided.
3 The ulnar nerve is freed from the surrounding soft tissues.
4 The nerve is repositioned.
5 Hemostasis is maintained.
6 The wound is closed.

Discussion

The patient is placed in the supine position with the operative arm on an arm table, suspended over the patient, or laid across the patient's body, depending on the surgeon's preference. A pneumatic tourniquet is applied to the upper arm, and the procedure for exsanguination performed.

The surgeon makes the skin incision over the median epicondyle. Using blunt and sharp dissection with Metzenbaum scissors, the surgeon mobilizes the ulnar nerve. Delicate scissors are used to free a section of the nerve, and moist umbilical tapes, vessel loops, or a Penrose drain is looped around the nerve to aid manipulation.

The surgeon continues the dissection around the nerve to free a portion extending from above the elbow to below the elbow. A flap of fascia over the medial epicondyle is created with scissors. The nerve then is transposed (moved) from the groove at the back of the medial epicondyle of the humerus to the front of the epicondyle and positioned under the fascial flap. The fascial flap is loosely reapproximated with 2-0 Dexon sutures to protect the nerve. The tourniquet pressure is released, and the wound is checked for bleeders. The bipolar

ESU is used for hemostasis as needed. The wound is irrigated with sterile saline or an antibiotic solution and closed in layers with Dexon suture and dressed with gauze. A splint or cast is applied to the arm.

PERIPHERAL NERVE RESECTION AND REPAIR

Surgical Goal

In peripheral nerve repair, a severed nerve, usually in the hand or forearm, is anastomosed to restore function.

Pathology

Peripheral nerve injuries are commonly caused by industrial or home accidents involving tools or machinery. Successful repair depends on the patient's age, the extent of injury to adjacent tissue, and the type of injury to the nerve. An injury may be a clean-cut type (e.g., caused by a sharp object such as a knife or glass shard) or an injury that causes the nerve to shatter. If the nerve is severely damaged, it may be replaced with a nerve graft taken from another location in the body. The procedure described here is an upper extremity nerve repair.

TECHNIQUE

1 The patient is prepared for routine hand or forearm surgery.
2 The wound is debrided if necessary.
3 The nerve is anastomosed.
4 The wound is closed and dressed with supportive material.

Discussion

The procedure to repair a severed peripheral nerve usually is performed as an emergency. If nerve repair is delayed, the risk of a poor outcome increases. Several common methods of peripheral nerve repair are the funicular suture technique and the epineural suture technique. In the funicular technique, the funiculi (the fibers that make up the nerve) are joined individually. In the epineural technique, the epineurium (the component of connective tissue that surrounds the nerve) is anastomosed and the individual funiculi are not sutured together. An alternative to direct anastomosis of the severed ends or transplanted autograft, is the use of a biograft *nerve conduit*. This is a commercially available biograft that can be used to bridge nerve gaps of less than 3 mm.

In preparation for peripheral nerve repair, the scrub should have microinstruments or eye instruments available, as well as an operating microscope or surgical loupes, bipolar ESU, nerve stimulator, and a physiological saline solution, such as that used in eye surgery. Fine 6-0, 7-0, and 10-0 sutures swaged to small cutting needles also are needed. The choice of suture material and size depend on the surgeon's preference, but monofilament nylon usually is used.

The patient is positioned supine with the affected arm or hand resting on a hand table. A pneumatic tourniquet is used as previously described. The procedure may be performed using general or regional anesthesia.

If the limb has been extensively damaged, the surgeon may want to debride (excise any devitalized or ragged tissue) before

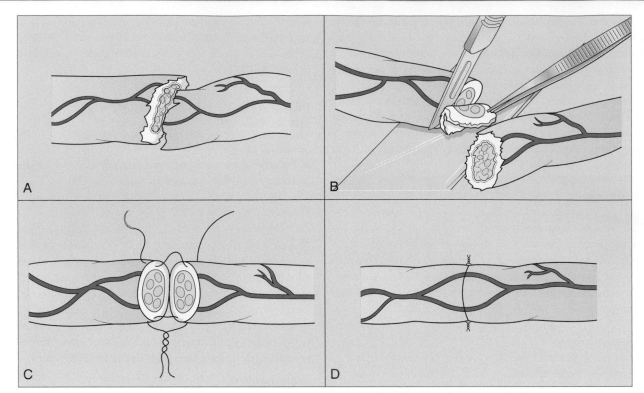

Figure 36-38 **End-to-end nerve anastomosis. A,** Tear injury. **B,** Debriding of the nerve. **C,** Placement of sutures through the epineurium. **D,** Completed repair. *(From Rengachary S, Ellenbogen R: Principles of neurosurgery, ed 2, St Louis, 2005, Mosby.)*

beginning the nerve repair. Debridement usually takes place in conjunction with the skin prep or immediately after it. If the surgeon wants to perform the skin prep and debridement, the scrub or circulator should supply the surgeon with copious amounts of sterile saline solution, sponges, antiseptic soap, a fine scalpel, tissue forceps, and dissecting scissors.

When debridement has been completed, the limb is draped in routine fashion and the tourniquet is inflated. Some surgeons drape the limb first and then perform the debridement. The first step of the actual procedure is the mobilization of the injured nerve. The surgeon uses fine dissecting scissors and thumb forceps to gently free the severed nerve from its surrounding tissue.

Before the anastomosis is started, the jagged ends of the nerve must be severed. Two fine traction sutures are placed through each end of the nerve and are used to bring the nerve ends into approximation. The surgeon incises the ends of the nerve with a #15 blade to ensure that the damaged fibers are removed and clean edges are available for the anastomosis. A moistened wooden tongue blade may be used as a firm surface on which to place the nerve. The nerve ends are cut serially in 1-mm slices under the operating microscope until the ends appear satisfactory for anastomosis (Figure 36-38).

In the epineural technique, the surgeon places several 6-0 or 7-0 nylon sutures, one through each quadrant of the nerve. For funicular repair, each individual funiculus is joined with interrupted sutures of 10-0 nylon. During the anastomosis, the scrub should irrigate the nerve frequently with balanced saline solution, such as that used in eye surgery, to prevent the nerve from drying out.

If a nerve conduit is used, the surgical technologist places the appropriate size collagen graft in sterile saline for 5 minutes, or according to the manufacturer's directions. After soaking the graft will assume a hydrated appearance and is ready for use. Size 8-0 or 9-0 nylon sutures are used to attach the graft. The severed ends of the nerve are threaded inside the graft, and four mattress sutures are used to tack the graft in place at each end. The wound is then irrigated with normal saline or lactated ringer's solution before wound closure.

After the repair, the tourniquet is released and the wound bed is inspected for bleeders. Hemostasis is maintained with the bipolar ESU, Gelfoam strips, and topical thrombin as necessary. The tissue layers are approximated with 3-0 and 4-0 polyglactin interrupted sutures. A dressing of cotton gauze and plaster splints or other casting material is used to immobilize the limb until healing is complete.

KEY CONCEPTS

- Knowledge of the key anatomical structures of the central and peripheral nervous systems is necessary to a complete understanding of surgical procedures.
- Familiarity with diagnostic procedures of the nervous system is important for patient care and a more complete understanding of pathology.
- A basic understanding of neuropathology is important for patient care and case planning.
- Case planning in neurosurgery requires specific understanding of the instruments, hemostatic materials and techniques, drugs, and patient positioning.

- In order to be effective in the scrub role, the surgical technologist must be knowledgeable about specific neurosurgical procedures and the steps involved in each procedure.

REVIEW QUESTIONS

1. Why is hemostasis particularly important during cranial surgery?
2. How is excess cerebrospinal fluid surgically shunted out of the brain?
3. What precautions should be taken to prevent loss of or damage to the bone flap during craniotomy?
4. Why are burr holes required to remove a bone flap?
5. Name several specialty instrument sets that might be needed during neurosurgery (e.g., orthopedic set).
6. Neurosurgical procedures can be quite lengthy. What safety and environmental precautions are particularly important to protect the patient from injury during a long procedure?
7. The Fowler position carries a high risk of embolism. Explain why.
8. Why is a subdural hematoma an emergency condition?
9. What methods of hemostasis are used during cranial surgery?
10. During laminectomy, small bits of bone are removed from the lamina in rapid succession. What is the role of the scrub during this part of the procedure?
11. In what cranial procedures might a fat graft be needed?
12. Describe the supplies that might be needed for debridement of a hand after an industrial accident.

BIBLIOGRAPHY

Asthagiri A, Pouratian N, Sherman J, et al: Advances in brain tumor surgery, *Neurologic Clinics* 25:975, 2007.

Baron EM: *Cervical spondylosis: diagnosis and management.* Accessed July 13, 2008, at http://www.emedicine.com/neuro/topic564.htm.

Brackmann DE, Green JD: Translabyrinth approach for acoustic tumor removal, *Neurosurgery Clinics of North America* 19:251, 2008.

Brown JA: Principles of pain management. In Rengachary SS, Ellenbogen RG, editors: *Principles of neurosurgery*, ed 2, St Louis, 2005, Mosby.

Drake JM, Iantosca MR: Cerebrospinal fluid shunting and management of pediatric hydrocephalus. In Schmidek HH, Roberts DW, editors: *Operative neurosurgical techniques: indications, methods and results*, ed 5, Philadelphia, 2006, WB Saunders.

Drummond JC, Patel PM: Neurosurgical anesthesia. In Miller RD, editors: *Miller's anesthesia*, ed 6, Philadelphia, 2005, Churchill Livingstone.

Fanciullo GJ, Ball PA: Spinal cord stimulation and intraspinal infusions for pain. In Schmidek HH, Roberts DW, editors: *Operative neurosurgical techniques: indications, methods and results*, ed 5, Philadelphia, 2006, WB Saunders.

Freeman BL: Scoliosis and kyphosis. In Canale ST, Beaty JH, editors: *Campbell's operative orthopaedics*, ed 11, Philadelphia, 2008, Mosby.

Harrop JH: *Spinal cord tumors: management of intradural intramedullary neoplasms.* Accessed July 18, 2008, at http://www.emedicine.com/Med/topic2905.htm.

Jobe MT, Martinez SF: Peripheral nerve injuries. In Canale ST, Beaty JH, editors: *Campbell's operative orthopaedics*, ed 11, Philadelphia, 2008, Mosby.

Kolaski K: *Myelomeningocele.* Accessed June 28, 2008, at http://www.emedicine.com/pmr/TOPIC83.HTM.

Lonser RR, Apfelbaum RI: Neurovascular decompression in surgical disorders of cranial nerves V, VII, IX, and X. In Schmidek HH, Roberts DW, editors: *Operative neurosurgical techniques: indications, methods and results*, ed 5, Philadelphia, 2006, WB Saunders.

MGI Pharma: *How to use Gliadel wafers.* Accessed July 4, 2008, at http://www.gliadel.com/hcp/about/how.aspx.

Polletti CE: Open cordotomy and medullary tractotomy. In Schmidek HH, Roberts DW, editors: *Operative neurosurgical techniques: indications, methods and results*, ed 5, Philadelphia, 2006, WB Saunders.

Qureshi NH, Harsh G: *Skull fracture.* Accessed June 28, 2008, at http://www.emedicine.com/med/TOPIC2894.HTM.

Roberts GA, Dacey RG: General techniques of aneurysm surgery. In LeRoux PD, Winn HR, Newell DW, editors: *Management of cerebral aneurysms*, Philadelphia, 2004, WB Saunders.

Schmidek HH, Roberts DW: *Schmidek and Sweet's operative neurosurgical techniques: indications, methods and results*, ed 5, Philadelphia, 2006, WB Saunders.

Seidel HM, Ball JW, Dains JE, Benedict GW, editors: *Mosby's guide to physical examination*, ed 6, St Louis, 2007, Mosby.

Shen FH, Samartzis D, Khanna AJ, Anderson DG: Minimally invasive techniques for lumbar interbody fusions, *Orthopedic Clinics of North America* 38:373, 2007.

St-Arnaud D, Paquin M: Safe positioning for neurosurgical patients, *AORN Journal* 87:1156, 2008.

Sugarman RA: Structure and function of the neurologic system. In McCance KL, Huether SE, editors: *Pathophysiology: the biologic basis for disease in adults and children*, ed 5, St Louis, 2006, Mosby.

Sutton LN: Spinal dysraphism. In Rengachary SS, Ellenbogen RG, editors: *Principles of neurosurgery*, ed 2, St Louis, 2005, Mosby.

Tarlov EC, Magge SN: Microsurgery of ruptured lumbar intervertebral disc. In Schmidek HH, Roberts DW, editors: *Operative neurosurgical techniques: indications, methods and results*, ed 5, Philadelphia, 2006, WB Saunders.

U.S. Food and Drug Administration: *Medical device reporting.* Accessed June 29, 2008, at http://www.fda.gov/cdrh/devadvice/.

Wang PP, Avellino AA: Hydrocephalus in children. In Rengachary SS, Ellenbogen RG, editors: *Principles of neurosurgery*, ed 2, St Louis, 2005, Mosby.

Wright PE: Carpal tunnel, ulnar tunnel, and stenosing tenosynovitis. In Canale ST, Beaty JH, editors: *Campbell's operative orthopaedics*, ed 11, Philadelphia, 2008, Mosby.

Yaremchuk MJ: Surgical repair of major defects of the scalp and skull. In Schmidek HH, Roberts DW, editors: *Operative neurosurgical techniques: indications, methods and results*, ed 5, Philadelphia, 2006, WB Saunders.

Yeung AT, Yeung CA: Minimally invasive techniques for the management of lumbar disc herniation, *Orthopedic Clinics of North America* 38:363, 2007.

37

Emergency Trauma Surgery

CHAPTER OUTLINE

LEARNING OBJECTIVES

After studying this chapter the reader will be able to:

1. Explain the trauma system used in the United States
2. Describe the lethal triangle of trauma physiology
3. Discuss compartment syndrome
4. Describe the principles of Advanced Trauma Life Support (ATLS) trauma management
5. Explain what is meant by *damage control surgery*
6. Discuss the elements of case planning for common trauma surgeries

TERMINOLOGY

Advanced Trauma Life Support (ATLS): A program established by the American College of Surgeons for protocols and training in trauma medicine.

Algorithms: Treatment pathways established to allow systematic and consistent methods of medical and surgical management.

Blunt injury: Trauma that results in deep tissue injury without rupture of the skin.

Cardiac rupture: Tearing of the atria or ventricles as a result of trauma.

Cardiac tamponade: Pressure on the heart causing restriction and damage to the conduction system.

Coagulopathy: Condition in which the body's normal blood clotting mechanism ceases to function, characteristic in severe multitrauma.

Compartment syndrome: Increased pressure in any compartment of the body such as the cranium, abdominal cavity, or a limb caused by trauma.

Contusions: Bruising.

Damage control surgery: Surgery whose objective is to stop hemorrhage and prevent sepsis without attempting reconstruction or anatomical continuity.

Definitive diagnosis: Evidence-based diagnosis of a medical problem using normal investigative procedures such as imaging studies.

Definitive procedure: A planned surgical procedure, usually with specific objectives for reconstruction or restoring continuity of anatomical structures.

Exsanguinating: Hemorrhage with the potential to deplete the patient's total blood volume.

Flail chest: Rib fracture in at least three adjacent ribs in two locations each. This condition requires immediate surgery.

Focused assessment with ultrasound for trauma (FAST): A protocol of ATLS in which ultrasound is used in a focused area to diagnose severe trauma.

Hemorrhagic shock: A type of shock characterized by vascular failure due to severe bleeding.

Hemothorax: Bleeding into the pleural space.

Metabolic acidosis: A potentially lethal physiological condition occurring in shock, characterized by abnormally low blood pH.

Occult injury: An injury that is not detected in normal assessment procedures.

Penetrating injury: Tissue damage that occurs when an object enters the body through the skin, or the body is propelled against an object, breaking the skin.

Pneumothorax: Injury that results in air in the pleural space causing displacement or collapse of the respiratory structures.

Resuscitation: In trauma medicine, the process of restoring physiological balance following severe trauma.

INTRODUCTION

Trauma is the leading cause of death between the ages of 1 and 45 and the third leading cause of death in all age groups.[1] The World Health Organization predicts that injury will be the leading cause of death and disability in all age groups by 2020. Most civilian trauma patients arrive at the emergency department after normal working hours and on weekends, when fewer staff members are available. A systems approach is used to focus all available resources on the most effective patient care.

The current principles of trauma medicine and surgery have been heavily influenced by the work of U.S. armed forces in Iraq and Afghanistan. As a result of these experiences, new trauma techniques have been developed, especially in the areas of resuscitation and staged surgical repair. At the same time, older procedures that were thought to be lifesaving in the civilian environment have been refined or discarded. For example, in the 1970s and 1980s, pneumatic antishock garments were routinely used to control exsanguinating injuries. The device—a tubular pneumatic body suit—was placed on the victim and then inflated as a tamponade against severe hypotension in the trunk area. Although the results did raise the victim's blood pressure, many patients inevitably died as a result of blood loss related to hypertension caused by the device. Some blood-clotting products that were developed for battle situations caused severe burns, and some increased the hemorrhage on removal. These products, however, led to the development of more sophisticated resuscitation techniques and chemical hemostatics that are used in both civilian and military medicine.

This chapter is an introduction to the fundamentals of trauma surgery. The material in this discussion assumes that the surgical technologist has already acquired more than minimal training in all aspects of the nonemergency role and is ready to approach the more intense study of trauma surgery. The new vocabulary and concepts introduced here serve as a basis for increased learning by practice. Naturally, there will be variations on these practices and specific methodologies. However, the principles of trauma care are fairly constant.

Preparation of the surgical technologist in an emergency role involves several important domains of practice. Most of the skills acquired in routine surgical procedures contribute to advanced practice in emergency situations. Although some additional techniques are necessary, the focus is more on *how* these familiar skills are applied, and above all, *prioritization* of tasks.

During a true surgical emergency, more so than in any other scenario, teamwork is key to a successful outcome for the patient. In all types of emergencies, urgency and *timing* require that one person (the surgeon in this case) be the decision maker. In a true emergency, there is little or no time for discussion or dispute. A sudden change in the patient's condition can result in a swift reordering of priorities and actions. This might mean a change of instrumentation from one system to another, such as orthopedic to vascular instruments, or sudden need for autotransfusion equipment. The role of the surgical technologist is therefore critical to the pace and flow of a procedure.

Although the ability to respond quickly to the demands of the surgery is important, so is *accuracy*. Accuracy in emergency terms means "getting it right the first time." Rapid response is ineffective or harmful if the response is incorrect. An instrument or suture passed in the wrong position, passing an inappropriate type or size of retractor for the needed exposure, incorrectly identified medications, and garbled communication are examples of errors that cost time and increase patient risk.

Clear communication is the pivot point of team efforts in an emergency. There may be many people attending the patient at one time during the emergency. These can include several circulators, more than one scrub person and even scrub team, surgical specialists (scrubbed or not), and other medical personnel present in the operating room during the setup and operative procedure. This is an opportunity for shared expertise, but also for miscommunication. The atmosphere may be distracting and noisy with multiple activities and requests to the circulators for medications, instruments, and assessment results. The surgical technologist must therefore be attentive not only to the tasks at hand, but also to the responsibility of clear communication, which should be deliberate, clearly spoken, and precise. Timing in communication is also very important. During the procedure, the scrub is dependent on the circulator to distribute needed items on the sterile field. The circulator must meet the requirements of the whole team while maintaining communication with other professionals outside the department such as the laboratory, blood bank, and intensive care unit (ICU). The basic tasks of the surgical technologist in the assistant circulator role are listed in Box 37-1.

TRAUMA SYSTEMS

The current trauma system in the United States provides for the designation of the health care facilities that are capable of treating emergency trauma, and specific training for all physicians who might be asked to treat trauma victims in their facilities. The system involves coordinated resources in the hospital and the community. Trauma centers are designated by a numerical system, levels I through V, with level I having the greatest capacity to handle all types of trauma. These designations are based criteria established by the Committee on Trauma of the American College of Surgeons and by individual state laws. The criteria are extensive and include such things as the number and type of trauma specialists (e.g., neurology, orthopedics, pediatrics), equipment available, and ability to transport victims quickly. Assessment capacity, community education in trauma prevention, and ability to perform a variety of specialty trauma procedures are also considered in the classification system. Communication between the field and facility is also of primary importance. Level I trauma centers must have state-of-the-art equipment that enables rescue and transport teams to communicate with facility trauma specialists in real time.

Penetrating injury is most commonly caused by gunshot and knife wounds.

Table 37-1 shows blunt trauma mechanisms and their associated injuries.

Box **37-1**	Tasks of the Surgical Technologist in the Assistant Circulator Role in Trauma Surgery

1. Gather and distribute sterile supplies in a logical manner (first to be used, first opened).
2. Handle the patient meticulously during transport and positioning.
3. Ensure that adequate amounts of irrigation solutions are prewarmed.
4. Assistance in maintaining patient normothermia using warm air blankets as directed by the anesthesia care provider.
5. Participate in sponge management and counting.
6. Set up and monitor the use of nonsterile equipment and attachments.
7. Maintain a safe operative environment by managing blood and fluid spillage on floors and other nonsterile surfaces.
8. Participate in communication between the sterile team and others involved in the multidisciplinary care team outside the surgical department (e.g., laboratory, x-ray, blood bank, central supply).
9. Assist in arranging for immediate postoperative patient transport and destination (ICU, trauma ICU, pediatric ICU).
10. Obtain the results of imaging or other investigations performed in the preoperative period.
11. Maintain documentation in real time, as events occur, if possible.
12. Obtain whole blood or blood products from the blood bank, according to facility policy.

ICU, Intensive care unit.

Physician certification in trauma care is achieved through the American College of Surgeon's **Advanced Trauma Life Support (ATLS)** course, which is globally recognized (see http://www.facs.org/trauma/atls/index.html). The course focuses on ATLS treatment guidelines and protocols for trauma management. Nonphysician health personnel may audit the course in some regions, but certification is reserved for licensed physicians only.

TRAUMA INJURIES

Unintentional trauma, such as automobile accidents (including pedestrian versus automobile), falls, bicycle accidents, and industrial accidents, leading to serious and lethal injury, has yielded injury patterns that are somewhat predictable. Intentional injuries such as those caused by firearms and other weapons have also been studied extensively in the past decade. To become familiar with the type of surgical interventions that are used to treat injuries, it is helpful to classify injuries by type. In **blunt injury**, the skin is unbroken, and the injuries are internal. In civilian populations, blunt injuries occur most commonly from motor vehicle accidents, falls, and interpersonal violence. In **penetrating injury,** the object that causes the injury creates an open wound and deeper injuries.

TRAUMA PATHOPHYSIOLOGY

The decision to perform emergency trauma surgery and the extent of the surgery are based on a unique set of criteria. A complex chain of physiological events occurs in severe trauma cases, especially in multiple trauma patients. These events often require a deviation from nontrauma **algorithms** (treatment pathways) that usually guide the surgeon and other attending consultants toward a course of action. The mechanisms are complex, and many are not completely understood even by specialists. However, an understanding of very basic trauma physiology is important to appreciate the decisions that must be made during all phases of trauma management.

THE LETHAL TRIANGLE

Three physiological conditions are a primary focus of assessment and decision making in severely injured patients. Together, the three conditions are called the "triangle of death," lethal triangle, or lethal triad. The three conditions are:

- *Hypothermia:* Subnormal core body temperature for an extended period of time
- *Metabolic acidosis:* Lower than normal blood pH
- *Coagulopathy:* Potentially lethal disorder of the normal blood-clotting system

Patients who survive the first hour after injury are at risk for these conditions, which are related to hemorrhage, shock, and the body's immune response to trauma.

Hemorrhagic Shock

In Chapter 14 it was stated that there are a number of different kinds of shock, caused by different pathologies. In this discussion, the focus is on **hemorrhagic shock**. This is vascular failure caused by prolonged, severe blood loss, the most common cause of mortality in trauma.

The body's compensatory mechanisms that are triggered by hemorrhage occur at the microcirculatory level. In the healthy body, blood delivers oxygen to the cells and also carries metabolic waste out the cells. The microcirculatory pathway responsible for these functions is called the *nutrient pathway.* The *nonnutrient pathway* provides warmth to the entire body, from core to extremities, necessary to sustain life. During severe hemorrhage and a drop in blood pressure, vasoconstriction occurs in the peripheral circulation. This mechanism preserves blood flow to the heart, kidneys, and brain. However, the diversion of blood to these vital structures causes the extremities, abdominal organs, and muscles to become deprived of normal circulation. In response to the loss of peripheral circulation, the cells begin to take on interstitial fluid from the vascular system. This further decreases blood pressure. At the same time, certain inflammatory chemicals are released in the body, and these are ultimately toxic to the nonvital organs in the absence of a normal circulatory system.

Table 37-1 Mechanisms of Blunt Injury

Mechanism of Injury	Additional Considerations	Potential Associated Injuries
Motor Vehicle Collisions		
Head-on collision		Facial injuries Lower extremity injuries Aortic injuries
Rear-end collision		Hyperextension injuries of cervical spine Cervical spine fractures Central cord syndrome
Lateral (T-bone) collision		Thoracic injuries Abdominal injuries—spleen, liver Pelvic injuries Clavicle, humerus, rib fractures
Rollover	Greater chance of ejection Significant mechanism of injury	Crush injuries Compression fractures of spine
Ejection from vehicle	Likely unrestrained Significant mortality	Spinal and pelvic injuries
Windshield damage	Likely unrestrained	Closed head injuries, coup and contrecoup injuries Facial fractures Skull fractures Cervical spine fractures
Steering wheel damage	Likely unrestrained	Thoracic injuries Sternal and rib fractures, flail chest Cardiac contusion Aortic injuries Hemo-/pneumothorax
Dashboard and front panel damage		Pelvic and acetabular injuries Dislocated hip
Restraint/Seat Belt Use		
Proper three-point restraint	Decreased morbidity	Sternal and rib fractures, pulmonary contusions
Lap belt only		Chance fractures, abdominal injuries, head and facial injuries/fractures
Shoulder belt only		Cervical spine injuries/fractures, "submarine" out of restraint devices (possible ejection)
Airbag deployment	Front-end collisions Less severe head/upper torso injuries Not effective for lateral impacts More severe injuries in children (improper front seat placement)	Upper extremity soft tissue injuries/fractures Lower extremity injuries/fractures
Pedestrian Versus Automobile		
Low speed (braking automobile)		Tibia and fibula fractures, knee injuries
High speed		Waddle triad—tibia/fibula or femur fractures, truncal injuries, craniofacial injuries "Thrown" pedestrians at risk for multisystem injuries
Bicycle and Motorcycle Accidents		
Automobile versus bicycle		Closed head injuries "Handlebar" injuries Spleen/liver lacerations Additional intraabdominal injuries Consider penetrating injuries
Non–automobile related		Extremity injuries "Handlebar" injuries

Continued

Table **37-1**	**Mechanisms of Blunt Injury—cont'd**	
Mechanism of Injury	**Additional Considerations**	**Potential Associated Injuries**
Falls from A Great Height Vertical impact		**Mortality 50% at 36-60 Feet** Calcaneal and lower extremity fractures Pelvic fractures Closed head injuries Cervical spine fractures Renal and renal vascular injuries
Horizontal impact		Craniofacial fractures Hand and wrist fractures Abdominal and thoracic visceral injuries Aortic injuries

Modified from Martin R, Meredith J: Management of acute trauma. In Townsend CM Jr, Beauchamp RD, Evers BM, Mattox KL, editors: *Sabiston textbook of surgery*, ed 19, Philadelphia, 2012, WB Saunders.

Inflammatory factors cause swelling in the peripheral tissues and organs, resulting in further ischemia and blood stasis, microclotting, and tissue death.

Hypothermia

In the initial stages of hypovolemic shock, the blood vessels constrict, causing increased vascular resistance. If shock deepens, further compensation occurs in the body as described previously. In the healthy individual, body heat is produced by the consumption of oxygen in the cells through aerobic metabolism. This is especially pronounced in the muscles and abdominal organs. During shock, these tissues are deprived of adequate blood flow, stalling aerobic metabolism. This in turn causes the life-threatening hypothermia. Nearly all critical trauma patients are hypothermic by the time medical care is available. The hypothermic state can be made more severe through skin exposure during the initial assessment when clothing is removed, as well as lack of warmth during transport to the medical facility and even during treatment. Therefore, steps to restore and maintain the patient's core temperature are a critical component of patient care before, during, and after emergency surgery. Persistent hypothermia quickly leads to other life-threatening physiological changes, described next.

Coagulopathy

During hemorrhage, the autonomic nervous system triggers the release of angiotensin, vasopressin, antidiuretic hormone, glucagon, cortisol, epinephrine, and norepinephrine. In the *early* stages of hemorrhagic shock, these hormones and the biochemical changes they cause are beneficial. They increase cardiac output and peripheral vasoconstriction, protecting the heart and brain from oxygen starvation. It is even common for blood pressure to remain within normal limits during the early compensatory stage of shock, even in the presence of severe hemorrhage. However, in the next stage of shock, further constriction of capillaries results in cellular death of those tissues deprived of blood and oxygen.

One of the primary consequences of the mechanisms just described is **coagulopathy** (dysfunction of the normal blood clotting process). Continued hypothermia and capillary constriction lead to fluid shifts that dilute the circulating blood. Total platelet supply and coagulation factors necessary for clotting also become diluted or lost completely with the addition of intravenous crystalloid fluids given as a strategy of treatment. In compensation for blood loss, the body releases additional thrombin. However, at this stage, circulation is sluggish, and this causes thrombin to be withdrawn from the vascular system and deposited in organs, leading to thrombin depletion, cellular destruction, and eventual failure. This constellation of events is called *disseminated intravascular coagulation (DIC)*. Even if major hemorrhage is halted through surgery or other mechanical means, *microhemorrhage* remains unchecked in DIC because the circulating platelets, thrombin, and coagulation factors have been deposited in the viscera and are ineffectual. DIC may be prevented by replacing the lost coagulation factors *early* in the crisis. However, the spiral of events can occur very rapidly, and once past a certain point, the process is irreversible.

NOTE: DIC can occur in all forms of shock.

Metabolic Acidosis

During shock, lack of oxygen supply to muscles and abdominal organs causes another phenomenon called **metabolic acidosis** (abnormally low blood pH). As tissue perfusion decreases during hemorrhage and shock, cells are not oxygenated. The shift from aerobic to anaerobic metabolism at the cellular level creates the waste product lactic acid. Without a circulatory system or other normal physiological process to rid the body of metabolic waste, serum lactate levels rise, resulting in life-threatening metabolic acidosis.

COMPARTMENT SYNDROME

The compensatory mechanisms in acute injury can lead to the condition called **compartment syndrome**. In simple terms, this is tissue swelling within a closed area such as muscle bundles (surrounded by sheets of fascia and encased by superficial tissues) or the abdomen. When the tissue swelling reaches a critical point, circulation to the area is blocked and the oxygen deprived tissues become necrotic. Acute compartment syndrome (ACS) requires emergency surgery to relieve the pressure. Compartment syndrome can occur anywhere in the body but is seen most commonly in the abdomen, in limbs, and in brain injury. Surgical management of ACS is discussed later in the chapter.

NOTE: *Acute compartment syndrome, or ACS, which can affect any closed compartment of the body, unfortunately has the same acronym as abdominal compartment syndrome (ACS), which refers only to the abdominal cavity. Acute abdominal compartment syndrome (AACS) is another term that refers to abdominal compartment syndrome that arises suddenly.*

ATLS PRINCIPLES OF TRAUMA MANAGEMENT

Lifesaving trauma management under the ATLS guidelines is based on specific objectives:

1. The clinical problem that is the most lethal (the greatest threat to life) is treated first.
2. Treatment is initiated even when a **definitive diagnosis** (a diagnosis confirmed by assessment or investigation) is not established.
3. Treatment may be initiated even when there is no detailed history.

ATLS trauma assessment is performed in two stages, the primary survey and the secondary survey.

PREHOSPITAL CARE AND THE GOLDEN HOUR

Prehospital care takes place before the patient arrives at the trauma center. First responders such as emergency medical technologists, trauma nurses, and rescue personnel arriving on the scene of the trauma are involved in prehospital care in the field and in transit. The principles of care in the first hour are based on a concept known as the *Golden Hour*. This refers to the first critical hour following injury. Trauma-related morbidity and mortality are partially related to the time elapsed between the trauma event and resuscitation attempts. About 50% of victims with injury to the aorta, heart, spinal cord, or brainstem die from their injuries within minutes of the trauma. A further 30% of victims die in the first few hours. Of these, half will have died from hemorrhage and the remaining from damage to the central nervous system. Overall, hemorrhage is the primary cause of death in traumatic injury.

Field Care: The Primary Survey

The primary survey is the initial patient assessment, performed by first responders. Elements of the survey follow the ABCDE sequence:

1. *Airway and cervical spine control*: The patient's own or an artificial airway is secured and the cervical spine stabilized with a rigid collar to prevent further injury and to maintain the airway.
2. *Breathing and oxygenation*: The patient is assessed for thoracic injury such as pneumothorax, flail chest, or hemothorax (discussed later) that might compromise breathing. In the case of an open thorax, immediate artificial ventilation is established. Broken ribs or a crushed sternum may also prevent adequate ventilation.

3. *Circulation and hemorrhage*: Blood loss due to hemorrhage must be controlled in the early phase of the emergency to prevent coagulopathy and eventual exsanguination. Multiple intravenous lines are established for blood testing and administration of fluids and drugs. **Occult injury** (such as hidden hemorrhage) is a significant clinical problem in the prehospital and emergency department phases.
4. *Dysfunction and disability of the central nervous system*: Traumatic brain injury (TBI) may result in cessation of vital functions, including respiration. A rapid neurological assessment is performed to ascertain whether TBI has occurred.
5. *Exposure of injuries and environmental control (thermoregulation)*: Once vital functions are restored, the full extent of the victim's injuries is assessed. This requires removal of clothing and steps to prevent or treat hypothermia.

The primary survey may determine the need for immediate emergency surgery, or if the patient is stable enough, the secondary survey is started right away. Resuscitation begins immediately in the early assessment stages of trauma and continues as long as necessary.

Resuscitation

Resuscitation is the process of restoring physiological balance in injury. In the context of trauma, resuscitation refers to restoration from hemorrhagic shock, including establishment of normal circulating blood volume (hemodynamics), tissue perfusion, and vascular tone. Resuscitation is initiated as soon as medical help is available and continues through out the prehospital, emergency department, preoperative, surgical, and ICU phases of recovery.

The process of trauma resuscitation is not a straightforward case of replacing blood or restoring normal fluid balance. This is because increased intravascular fluids such as colloids and crystalloids can dilute the circulating blood, platelet, and coagulation factors and can result in decreased oxygen supply to vital organs. As blood pressure is increased, the rate of blood loss also increases. Increasing the blood pressure can also disrupt or dislodge clots that have already formed. Resuscitation is therefore a critical part of trauma response that requires careful monitoring and reevaluation throughout the emergency. The primary objectives of resuscitation in hemorrhagic shock are to achieve and maintain normothermia and to maintain the patient's intravascular volume in a balanced state of sufficient oxygen-carrying capacity, adequate levels of coagulation factors, and fluid pressure without increasing hemorrhage. Resuscitation involves placing at least two large-bore venous cannulas for mechanical pump infusion of blood products, plasma, colloids, crystalloid, and washed salvaged blood. The pump maintains fluids between 38° and 40° C.

Hospital Care: The Secondary Survey

The secondary survey is performed once the patient is stable enough to be moved. However, a patient requiring *immediate, lifesaving surgery* may be transported directly to the operating room after the primary assessment. The secondary assessment includes a head-to-toe examination to look for less obvious injuries that may also be critical. In this phase, the patient is able to undergo investigations including ultrasound, radiology, and magnetic resonance imaging (MRI). Further interventions such as placing additional intravenous lines, a urinary catheter, or a nasogastric tube are performed at this time. An important aspect of the secondary survey is the verbal history obtained from the patient or witnesses who can provide details of the trauma. This can assist with the diagnosis obtained through imaging studies and other tests. If time does not allow complex investigations, the attending physician attempts to find out about the patient's general health, allergies, and other information that might affect the treatment plan. This is done by interviewing the victim's family, if they are available.

NOTE: All multiple-trauma patients recover in the ICU for continued resuscitation and monitoring.

RECORDS AND CONSENT

Consent for invasive procedures, including emergency surgery, is obtained from the patient if he or she is able, or from responsible individuals according to hospital policy. Documentation of all care is vital so that subsequent care providers have accurate information on what was done and when throughout the assessment and treatment plan. The collection of forensic evidence and related documentation is also mandatory. This normally takes place in the emergency department but may be continued in the operating room.

MANAGEMENT OF FORENSIC EVIDENCE

Forensic medicine is a complex topic in which the methods and means of interpersonal violence are studied. The surgical technologist working in an urban trauma facility is likely to have some contact with forensic evidence. Although an extended discussion of forensics is beyond the scope of this textbook, the surgical technologist should be familiar with some aspects of evidence management.

The concepts of forensics was introduced in Chapter 3, and some guidelines were presented in that discussion. However, it is worth reviewing these with regard to trauma surgery.

Death from firearms is the second leading cause of mortality in the United States, and approximately 115,000 cases of firearm injury are treated each year. The most common firearm used in personal violence is the handgun. However, other weapons are also used, and many of these fire-jacketed or exploding bullets. The manner in which these weapons are handled on the surgical field may determine whether they can be used as legal evidence. Therefore, it is very important for the surgical technologist to use technique that is consistent with maintaining specimens correctly:

- When passing any instrument that will come in contact with a bullet, fragment, shrapnel, or other ballistic item, also ensure that the tips of the instrument are protected with rubber shods or completely covered with sponge. Markings on the fragment or bullet may not be visible without magnification but are nevertheless present on all weapons.

- Avoid any contact between the bullet or fragment and other metal, such as a metal container or other bullets retrieved. Do not toss a projectile into a basin. Pad the basin and set the projectile into it. Careless handling can easily scratch the item and obscure evidential marks.
- Do contain ballistic fragments or whole bullets in separate containers and label them according to exact location, as identified by the surgeon.
- Do use plastic containers to avoid damage to the projectile.
- Projectiles should be sent in a dry container unless directed otherwise by the laboratory. Do not wash the item before submitting it to pathology.
- Fragments of cloth or other nonprojectile items removed from a wound must be preserved as specimens and the exact location documented.
- When labeling specimens, do not speculate on the type of projectile.

DAMAGE CONTROL SURGERY

The decision to perform emergency surgery even in the absence of a definitive diagnosis is highly influenced by the physiological events described earlier. Once the decision is made, the extent of surgical repair may be limited to **damage control surgery**. This is a specific surgical strategy whose exact technique depends on the body systems involved and the likelihood of improving the prognosis using surgical intervention. The goal of damage control surgery is to focus solely on lifesaving maneuvers:

- Control of hemorrhage
- Control of fecal spillage (abdominal and pelvic injury)
- Packing a body cavity
- Delayed or phased closure of the wound
- Relief of compartment syndrome
- Splinting or external fixation to prevent extension of injuries

Damage control surgery is based on the concept that the severely wounded patient is physiologically unstable and may quickly succumb to exsanguinating hemorrhage leading to deepening shock, hypothermia, inadequate organ perfusion, and coagulopathy. A secondary but immediate concern is sepsis caused by wound contamination. Damage control surgery stops the immediate cause of potential harm without extensive or elaborate reconstruction to restore anatomical form or continuity of tissues. It focuses on the immediate dangers so that the patient can be quickly moved to the ICU for resuscitation. Damage control surgery can be performed on any area of the body. The most common types are thoracic, abdominal, retroperitoneal, cranial, and orthopedic. Each system requires slightly different surgical techniques and equipment. These are discussed later in the chapter. If the patient is stabilized in 12 to 48 hours, he or she can then be returned to surgery for a **definitive procedure** (surgical treatment using a planned method and techniques intended to provide a lasting repair). The procedure often involves extensive wound repair in one or multiple (staged) procedures. If during the resuscitation the patient shows no improvement or there is evidence of continuing hemorrhage, damage control surgery can be repeated to find and correct the source of the bleeding. Staged or phased procedures after damage control surgery are therefore performed for more extensive reconstruction, or as a lifesaving measure in the presence of further hemorrhage or to treat compartment syndrome.

CASE PLANNING FOR TRAUMA SURGERY

All health care facility surgical departments prepare emergency case carts in preparation for specific emergencies likely to arrive for treatment. These include basic setups for craniotomy, cesarean section, and abdominal aneurysm. Emergency carts may be adapted for other types of emergencies, or a general emergency cart may be prepared and placed on standby. This contains linens drapes, towels, Mayo covers, extra table drapes, and general surgery instruments and supplies. Even when emergency carts are prepared ahead of time, case planning according to the body system (e.g., orthopedic, cranial, abdominal, thoracic), and anatomical location will help the surgical team quickly assemble other equipment needed to start an emergency procedure.

INSTRUMENTS

Planning for instrumentation should start with basic instruments and be modified according to the systems involved, with specialty instruments distributed on the sterile field during the case setup or as needed. The multiple injury patient may require multiple system instruments. To avoid having instruments sets opened but not used, specialty instruments can be placed unopened on a cart outside the operating room in the sterile core. In this way they are easily and quickly available without adding more equipment to the setup. On the other hand, if it is known that the patient has both thoracic and abdominal injuries, it is wise to have both sets open so the scrub can prepare both as time allows.

SOLUTIONS AND DRUGS

Copious amounts of irrigation solution are often needed during trauma surgery. These are used to flush and clean the wound of tissue debris and foreign objects. If major debridement is required and has not been performed in the emergency department, additional warm fluids will be needed. The scrubbed surgical technologists should have two separate suction systems including separate tubing, suction tips, and irrigation devices. All solutions must be distributed warm and maintained warm during the surgery in order to combat hypothermia, which is an important element of the lethal triangle described earlier. Antibiotic irrigation is likely to be used in open trauma cases and can be distributed as needed at the close of surgery. In order to track blood loss, the circulator may place empty solution bottles in a designated area of the room for counting when time permits.

SUTURE AND HEMOSTATIC DEVICES

Hemostasis is a priority in all trauma surgery. The choice of suture therefore depends on the systems involved. Suture ligatures and free ties should be available throughout the surgery. Initially, 2-0 and 3-0 nonabsorbent ligatures should be immediately available. A general rule to follow is that nonabsorbent suture material will be favored in open trauma or possible bowel contamination of the wound because of the risk of infection, which would quickly dissolve absorbent materials. Size 0 would be needed in the event of major blood vessel damage, whereas 2-0 and 3-0 are adequate for smaller branching and peripheral vessels. It is best to have two sizes of tapered curved needles available for suture ligatures, because these can be used on blood vessels and also on vascular bundles that might be encountered in deep tissue layers. Two electrosurgical unit (ESU) systems (handpieces and power units) should be available. One can be held in reserve until called for by the surgeons.

Thrombin-based tissue sealants are used only if there is no coagulopathy present because these depend on an intact coagulation response. Dry hemostats such as gelatin, collagen, and oxidized cellulose may also be ineffective in the presence of coagulopathy. However, in the absence of this condition, the scrub should anticipate the need for topical hemostatic agents including thrombin-based materials.

The choice of skin closure materials is usually deferred until the close of surgery. In the case of damage control surgery, the wound may be left open without sutures, or a single-layer closure in heavy nonabsorbent material might be used. The type of closure may not be known until the extent of the trauma is determined and the condition of the patient is assessed at the end of surgery. Wound drains will be secured using nonabsorbent suture, size 2-0 or 3-0, on a $\frac{3}{8}$ cutting needle.

It may be safe to assume, for planning purposes, that autotransfusion might be used in cases of severe hemorrhage. The unit and accessories should be placed on standby but not opened during case preparation unless requested by the surgeon.

DRAINS AND DRESSINGS

The physiological changes brought about by trauma cause severe edema in the regional tissues, including those not directly injured. Postoperative serosanguinous pooling is controlled with wound drains, whereas fluid and electrolyte imbalance is managed through systemic resuscitative measures. Thoracic wounds require a closed chest drainage system (Pleur-Evac type), which is discussed in Chapter 33. Abdominal, pelvic, and other soft tissue trauma may require suction drainage by one or more drain systems such as a Hemovac, Jackson-Pratt, or negative-pressure wound therapy (NPWT) system (e.g., Wound V.A.C.).

Dressings and packing used in trauma surgery vary according to the type of wound and its classification, the tissues involved, and whether the wound will be packed and left without any primary closure until the next stage of repair. The clinical information needed to make this decision is often not known until the full extent of the injuries has been assessed during the surgical procedure.

SPONGES

The nature of trauma surgery and the objectives of damage control procedures require all possible methods of hemostasis, including the use of many surgical sponges. A large surgical wound may require 100 or more laparotomy sponges that must be immediately available on the sterile field, with many packs held in reserve for immediate distribution as needed. Whereas a normal abdominal or thoracic case might require 10 to 20 lap sponges to start the case, in trauma surgery at least 40 should be available as soon as the procedure begins. The 4 ×4 sponge mounted on sponge forceps is usually only required for deep swabbing in a relatively dry wound.

Tracking sponges during emergency trauma surgery can be problematic. An initial (baseline) count may not have been possible because of the urgency of the procedure, and depending on the course of events during surgery, additional sponges may be provided without a proper count. At a minimum the number of sponge packs (groups of 5 or 10) can be recorded as they are distributed on the field. This does not guarantee a correct count but can serve as a basis for estimation. The scrub and circulator must use practical judgment about the need to count sponges during the procedure. As time allows, the circulator retrieves bloodied sponges discarded off the sterile field and places them in a sponge holder as usual, to be counted when an opportunity arises. Wound packing is a technique of damage control surgery and is described later in the chapter. Although it is not ideal, the surgeon may use laparotomy sponges for packing the abdominal cavity, and these remain in place until the next procedure (usually within 24 hours).

Special closure and dressing techniques such as planned nonclosure of an abdominal wound require items that can be gathered toward the end of the procedure. These include plastic viscera bags (Bogota bag), Velcro sheets, plastic draping sheets, and Silastic mesh.

PREOPERATIVE CARE OF THE PATIENT

MOVING AND HANDLING

Positioning the trauma patient requires precise coordination among members of the surgical team. The real potential for extending the patient's injuries exists during moving and handling. Although splints and spinal support may have been applied at the scene of the accident or in the emergency department, *occult injuries* (those not detected during the assessment) may exist. For example, fractured bone ends can easily tear through adjacent blood vessels, nerves, and other soft tissue. Sudden movement of the body may shift blood clots. Particular attention is given to maintaining stability of the spine. In order to minimize this risk, basic precautions are exercised:

- All moves are directed by one person—the anesthesia care provider or surgeon. It is necessary to have a lead person in charge of coordinating the moves to avoid further injury to the patient.

- Patients often arrive in the operating room with stabilization devices in place. These include vacuum or rigid splints for extremities, torso splints, and the cervical collar for maintaining alignment of the cervical spine. No support devices are removed until the anesthesia care provider and surgeon state that it is safe to do so.
- Sudden shifts in fluid balance can occur during moving and handling. Active bleeding and shock can cause shifts in fluid spacing, which can become more severe with sudden postural changes. Postural changes such as raising and lowering the lower extremities must be made slowly with physiological monitoring in place.
- When moving and handling the pregnant patient, care is taken to avoid compression of the vena cava, which can compromise fetal circulation. The patient should always be maintained in left lateral position.

MAINTAINING PATIENT NORMOTHERMIA

Maintaining the patient's core temperature as close to normal as possible is a major goal of emergency treatment. This means that exposure is kept to an absolute minimum and that warmed blankets are available all times during preoperative preparations. A warm-air heating blanket can be used intermittently between investigations in different locations of the facility. All intravenous infusion and irrigation solutions are prewarmed. The room temperature is prewarmed higher than 29.4° C (85°F) and maintained until active warming devices achieve normothermia.[2]

AIRWAY

Maintaining the patient's airway is a priority of the anesthesia care provider. An emergency airway such as a tracheostomy or cricothyroidotomy may have been performed in the emergency department. This may be converted to a different type when the patient arrives in the operating room. In this case the anesthesia care provider may require surgical assistance and instruments to perform the procedure.

CONTINUING PHYSIOLOGICAL EVALUATION

The unstable trauma patient is continually evaluated for physiological changes from the time he or she arrives at the health care facility. Baseline tests that are performed in the emergency department are repeated at regular intervals. These include tests for blood gases, electrolyte levels, oxygen saturation, platelet and other blood components, and renal function, as well as many others. Some of the tests are urgent and the results are needed to detect life-threatening metabolic changes. In these cases, the laboratory is notified when the patient arrives so that time can be dedicated to the emergency. A runner may be identified in the surgical department or among the circulating team to transport blood samples quickly and also to communicate with laboratory staff. In many facilities, reports can be read out over the communication system directly from departments within the hospital to the operating room where the patient is being treated.

Imaging procedures that were performed during the secondary assessment can be uploaded to the operating room's dedicated computer almost immediately. However, not all hospitals have such capabilities, and the physical output of any imaging studies will need to be retrieved from where they were taken back to the operating room.

EMOTIONAL SUPPORT

The conscious trauma patient may arrive at the emergency department disoriented and frightened. Powerful emotional reactions to the trauma can affect the body's physiological mechanisms through the same chemicals that induce and prolong metabolic shock. Health care personnel can and should offer reassurance to the patient and provide orientation as to where the patient is and what is happening. In a severe emergency, all activity is focused on lifesaving measures. However, whenever possible, it is important to provide some measure of emotional comfort.

The family of the patient is likely to arrive during the most urgent phases of assessment. The operating room supervisor or person in a similar role is often responsible for seeing that family members have a quiet place to wait. This person should also provide intermittent updates on the patient's condition.

OPENING A CASE AND STERILE SETUP

Teams that work together on a regular basis are able to plan the amount of time needed to open a case for a particular procedure fairly accurately. However, emergency trauma surgery presents challenges that are not conducive to preplanning. Often the extent of the injuries is not known to the team until the patient arrives in the department. The patient's condition may fluctuate, requiring nursing personnel to divide their time between direct patient care and distributing sterile items to the sterile team. On occasion there may be very little time between the patient's arrival in the operating room and the start of surgery. This means that the scrub might be donning gown and gloves at the same time the surgeons arrive. In this situation, assistant circulators can be very valuable to help get the case opened and underway.

In emergency circumstances, some of the usual routines are abbreviated. This includes sponge and instrument counts. Although this is not an ideal situation, the American College of Surgeons has stated that standardized counting procedures may be suspended in life-threatening situations.[3] AORN has also stated in their recommended practices that surgical counts may be waived to in circumstances in which the time required presents an unacceptable delay in patient care.[4]

There is a tendency in opening up an emergency case to bring in many more instruments and supplies than will be needed. Although it is wise to have items immediately available, it is also important to consider which supplies and instruments are certainly needed and which can be held in reserve. Another consideration is not to overload the back table with so many instruments and supplies that they cannot be located quickly as needed. Professional judgment and experience determine which items should be immediately available and which should be held in reserve. If there is a high probability that extra instrument sets are needed, these can be opened onto smaller instrument tables at the periphery of the sterile field.

A general rule that most surgical technologists follow when setting up for an emergency is to prepare items in order of their immediate use on the field. The term *up* means "up on the Mayo, ready to use." The following is a suggested order:
1. Gowns, gloves, drapes arranged in order of use.
2. Draping completed.
3. ESU, suction up.
4. Light handles in place.
5. Knife mounted and up.
6. Four laparotomy sponges on the field, four in warm saline for immediate use.
7. Superficial and self-retaining retractors up.
8. Hemostats up.
9. Once the wound is opened, preparation for evacuation of free blood and wound packing.

Trauma patients who arrive with an open thorax as a result of emergency department thoracotomy require a modification of the suggested sequence. Retraction and exposure may be the first surgical objective, followed by rapid control of bleeding.

NOTE: It is wise to keep in mind at all times during an emergency that if the problem cannot be visualized, it cannot be managed.

SKIN PREP AND DRAPING

The decision to modify the skin prep for emergency technique lies with the medical and nursing team. A minimum skin prep may be to simply pour prep solution over the operative area including a wide or "whole body" coverage of prep solution. The area of the prep is usually not clearly delineated unless the patient workup (assessment, history, diagnostic and assessment procedures) indicates that the patient is stable and normal protocols can be followed. However, damage control surgery is performed in many trauma cases, and by definition, these procedures are carried out because of severe hemorrhage that precludes "normal" patient prep.

As with the surgical prep, draping may be performed with fewer drapes, possibly excluding all but the top drape. In any event, discussion on this should be avoided once the patient is in the room. The surgical technologist takes direction from the surgeon, who will normally relate this information while the patient is being transferred to the operating table. Sometimes it is necessary to simply have all drapes on hand and allow the surgeon to select the type she or he wants as the drapes are applied.

MANAGING THE STERILE FIELD IN EMERGENCY TRAUMA

Management of the sterile field during emergency trauma surgery requires a high level of attention to the wound itself and the immediate needs for instruments and supplies. Unlike other types of surgery, in which there are known steps and procedures, trauma surgery is performed according to a succession of priorities that can change rapidly. It can be helpful to remember that the surgical priorities are to control and prevent hemorrhage and minimize contamination (in the case of bowel spillage and large penetrating wounds that may contain fragments). These objectives are the basis of surgical management and apply to all types of trauma surgery.

The role of the scrubbed surgical technologist is to provide the most efficient and safest means of expediting the procedure. This means carrying out most of the usual tasks of the scrub role while predicting immediate needs. For example, as stated earlier, retraction must precede hemostasis in most cases. However, if the bleeding is **exsanguinating** (capable of depleting the patient's total blood volume), the area is first packed to slow the flow. Hemostasis can be achieved using suture ligatures or rapid anastomosis (of a lacerated blood vessel). The process of hemostasis is predictable even if the steps of the entire procedure are not clear at the start.

Infection is the second leading cause of mortality in trauma patients. Containment methods are used during surgery to limit tissue exposure to bowel contents or foreign objects. Bowel technique, which is described in Chapter 23, is used to the extent possible within the limits of time. Debridement, described later, and irrigation are other methods used to prevent sepsis. As with hemostasis, the techniques used to mitigate wound contamination are predictable, and the surgical technologist can plan for them ahead of time.

Elements of the surgery that are not so predictable are sudden changes in the course of the surgery, such as occur when occult injury is discovered or the patient's physiological status suddenly deteriorates, requiring a change in surgical strategy. These examples demonstrate the need to watch the wound even while performing other tasks such as clearing away instruments from the top drape or preparing supplies.

LAPAROTOMY WITH STAGED CLOSURE

Abdominal injury is the leading cause of trauma morbidity and mortality in all age groups. Blunt trauma is caused by motor vehicle accidents, including motorcycles, pedestrian versus vehicle encounters, falls, and assault. Penetrating wounds are most commonly caused by knife or gunshot. Difficulty in rapid and accurate diagnosis may lead to a high rate of occult abdominal injuries to vital organs and vascular structures of the abdomen. Most commonly injured are the spleen, liver, pancreas, small bowel, and retroperitoneal structures, with accompanying injuries to the omentum and mesentery.

Damage control laparotomy with staged closure is an exploratory process in which the sources of hemorrhage are found and controlled. No reconstruction is attempted unless absolutely necessary. The abdomen is packed using sponges, left unsutured, and covered with mesh or a transparent wound cover.

In the stable patient, diagnosis of abdominal injury is performed mainly by computed tomography (CT) or **focused assessment with ultrasound for trauma (FAST)**. In some cases diagnostic peritoneal lavage (DPL) may be performed using a peritoneal catheter set (Figures 37-1 and 37-2). This can be done in the emergency department or in surgery. Unstable patients who are hypotensive, indicating hemorrhage, may be taken to surgery before a definitive diagnosis is made. This means that the need to immediately address obvious exsanguinating hemorrhage outweighs the time

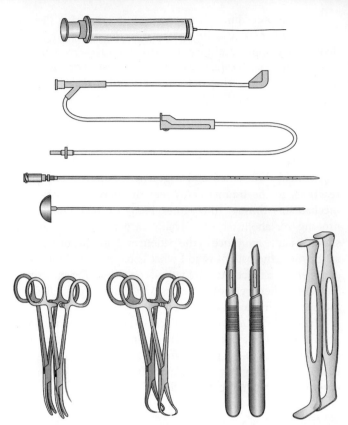

Figure 37-1 Standard instruments for open diagnostic peritoneal lavage. *Top to bottom:* 20-mL syringe, diagnostic peritoneal lavage catheter with slide closure, trocar, obturator. Right to left bottom: Army Navy retractors, # 15 knife, # 11 knife, towel clips to elevate the peritoneum, Kelly or Crile hemostats. *(From Roberts J, Hedges J, editors:* Clinical procedures in emergency medicine, *ed 5, Philadelphia, 2010, WB Saunders.)*

required to pinpoint the exact location of the hemorrhage in the abdomen in the assessment phase. The surgical objective in all damage control surgery is to secure hemostasis and prevent sepsis as quickly as possible in order to return the patient to the ICU for complete resuscitation.

CASE PLANNING FOR ABDOMINAL TRAUMA

Following the general recommendations for case planning discussed earlier, the surgical technologist should have a general surgery or laparotomy instrument set. He or she should also be prepared for subphrenic, retroperitoneal, and pelvic exploration. In this case extra-long instruments should be on hand.

Box 37-2 lists suggested instruments and materials to *supplement* a major laparotomy set for a total abdominal exploration. These may be opened immediately at the start of surgery or held in reserve for distribution as needed to the field.

DAMAGE CONTROL TECHNIQUES

Damage control technique for abdominal trauma consists of the following steps:
1. Pack the wound in a systematic manner.
2. Evaluate for active bleeding and repair.

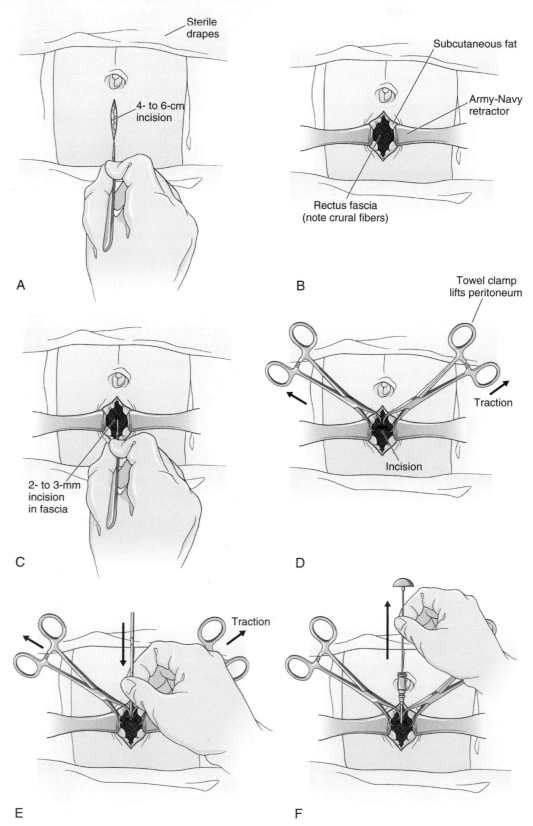

Figure 37-2 Procedure for diagnostic peritoneal lavage (DPL). A, After bladder decompression with Foley catheter, an infraumbilical incision is made with a #11 scalpel. **B,** Blunt dissection using Army-Navy retractors to fascia. **C,** A 2- to 3-mm incision is made through the fascia with a #15 knife. **D,** Each side of the rectus fascia is grasped with towel clips and lifted for insertion of the trocar and DPL catheter. **E,** Trocar with DPL catheter is inserted into the fascial opening and through the peritoneum. **F,** After the peritoneum has been entered, the catheter is gently advanced into the peritoneal cavity while withdrawing the trocar. If aspiration is negative, the catheter is attached to an infusion bag of normal saline or lactated Ringer solution for irrigation. *(From Roberts J, Hedges J, editors: Clinical procedures in emergency medicine, ed 5, Philadelphia, 2010, WB Saunders.)*

3. Evaluate for bowel spillage and repair.
4. Perform minimal or no primary closure.
5. Apply abdominal coverings.

As soon as the skin incision is made, the surgical technologist should have at least eight laparotomy sponges moistened with warm saline and wrung dry. Two suction systems and an ESU should also be immediately available. Once the incision has been extended with the knife and ESU, the abdomen is evacuated for blood, clots, and fluid. Packing may begin as

soon as the abdomen has been evacuated, or it may be only partially packed during exploration. If possible, the scrub should take note of how many sponges have been positioned in each quadrant. If the patient has an intact coagulation process, packing all four quadrants using laparotomy sponges absorbs free abdominal blood and fluid, slows the bleeding, and allows the surgeon to identify the origin of the hemorrhage. In contrast to nonemergency surgery, meticulous repair is avoided.

The most common abdominal injuries are to the liver, spleen, pancreas, small intestine, and mesentery. The injuries may extend into the pelvic cavity and also include these structures. Injury to the solid organs (such as in liver or pancreatic injury) may require partial resection or total removal (such as splenectomy) in order to control hemorrhage. Refer to Chapter 23 for details on these procedures.

The methods used for creating a temporary closure vary according to the surgeon's training and experience with certain materials. Table 37-2 lists a variety of temporary abdominal closure systems. Before the wound is covered, the cavities are thoroughly irrigated and checked again for hemorrhage. The four quadrants of the abdomen are repacked and drainage tubes put in place. One method of covering the wound is to enclose the bowel in a plastic bowel bag and sponges. Silastic mesh may be placed over these. A self-adhesive plastic drape impregnated with iodophor is used in the final layer. If continuous vacuum suction is used, this includes a foam covering that is cut to fit the size of the wound, which is then covered with an adherent drape (Figure 37-3).

In a staged closure, the dressings are taken down in phases, according to the patient's progress toward full resuscitation in

---

Box 37-2 Suggested List of Special Instruments and Materials for Emergency Damage Control Laparotomy

Retractors
Omni self-retaining, with specialty blades
Deaver set, wide
Harrington

Clamps
Long right-angle (Mixter type), delicate tip
Kidney pedicle
Vascular clamps: Satinsky, DeBakey straight, curved, tangential occlusion

Forceps
Vascular forceps, standard and long, straight atraumatic
DeBakey type, single-tooth delicate

Supplies and Materials
One or two bowel bags
Elastic vessel loops
Shods for hemostats

Table 37-2 Techniques for Temporary Abdominal Closure

Technique	Description	Mechanism
Vacuum-assisted closure (VAC)	A perforated plastic sheet covers the viscera, and a sponge is placed between the fascial edges. The wound is covered by an airtight seal, which is pierced by a suction drain connected to a suction pump and fluid collection system.	The (active and adjustable) negative pressure supplied by the pump keeps constant tension on the fascial edges while it collects excess abdominal fluid and helps resolve edema.
Vacuum pack	A perforated plastic sheet covers the viscera, damp surgical towels are placed in the wound, and a surgical drain is placed on the towels. An airtight seal covers the wound, and negative pressure is applied through the drain.	The negative pressure keeps constant tension on the fascial edges, and excess fluid is collected.
Artificial burr (Wittmann patch)	Two opposite Velcro sheets (hooks and loops, one on each side) are sutured to the fascial edges. The Velcro sheets connect in the middle.	This technique allows for easy access and stepwise reapproximation of the fascial edges.
Dynamic retention sutures	The viscera are covered with a sheet (e.g., ISODrape, Microtek [Microban], Huntersville, NC). Horizontal sutures are placed through a large-diameter catheter and through the entire abdominal wall on both sides.	The sutures keep tension on the fascia and may be tightened to allow staged reapproximation of the fascial edges. This may be combined with a vacuum system.
Plastic silo (Bogota bag)	A sterile x-ray film cassette bag or sterile 3-liter urology irrigation bag is sutured between the fascial edges or the skin and opened in the middle.	This is an easy technique that allows for easy access. The bag may be reduced in size to approximate the fascial edges.
Mesh, sheet	An absorbable or nonabsorbable mesh or sheet is sutured between the fascial edges. Examples are Dexon, Marlex, or Vicryl mesh. Examples of sheets are Silastic or silicone sheets.	The mesh or sheet may be reduced in size to allow for reapproximation. Nonresorbable meshes may be removed or left in place at the end of the open abdominal period.

Modified from Diaz J, Duton W, Miller R: The difficult abdominal wall. In Townsend CM Jr, Beauchamp RD, Evers BM, Mattox KL, editors: *Sabiston textbook of surgery*, ed 19, Philadelphia, 2012, WB Saunders.

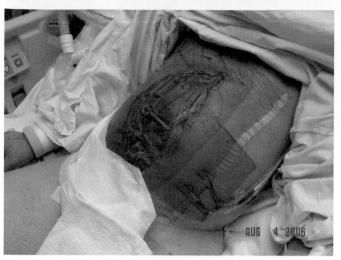

Figure 37-3 Vacuum-assisted closure. This system uses a foam sheet with vacuum suction that distributes the pull of fluid over a large area, preventing tissue damage. In this image, a surgical towel has been placed between two adhesive drapes, and then placed in the wound. Suction drainage tubes are placed at the wound periphery and brought out through the skin. These are attached to wall suction for continuous drainage. (*Modified from Martin R, Meredith J: Management of acute trauma. In Townsend CM Jr, Beauchamp RD, Evers BM, Mattox KL, editors: Sabiston textbook of surgery, ed 19, Philadelphia, 2012, WB Saunders.*)

the ICU. Or, the abdomen may be reentered emergently if the patient's condition is deteriorating and there is strong suspicion of continuing hemorrhage or abdominal compartment syndrome.

ABDOMINAL COMPARTMENT SYNDROME

Acute abdominal compartment syndrome (ACS) is a postoperative complication requiring emergency response. A combination of immune response to tissue trauma, and resuscitative procedures leads to severe edema of the abdominal viscera and severe ascites. In the closed abdomen (one that has been primarily closed at surgery) the intraabdominal pressure is greater than can be tolerated by the vascular system. This results in tissue death from ischemia and can also cause mechanical obstruction to the patient's ability to ventilate. Elevated central venous pressures also leads to increased intracranial pressure, rupture of the retinal capillaries, and decreased cardiac output due to tamponade.

The treatment for ACS is immediate surgical opening of the abdominal cavity. Temporary abdominal closure as described earlier prevents ACS.

ORTHOPEDIC TRAUMA

Among the indications for urgent damage control surgery of the skeletal system are near amputation, crushing injury, potentially septic trauma, and pelvic fracture. The objective of early intervention in these cases is to prevent further injury related to vascular and soft tissue damage, decrease the risk of sepsis, prevent or treat compartment syndrome, and decrease blood loss. Stabilization of the bones is therefore often the surgical priority for fractures. In selected cases,

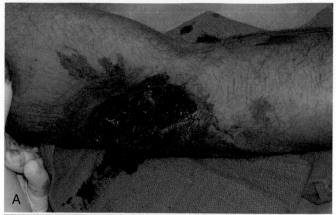
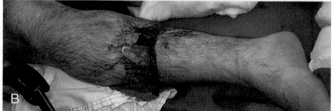
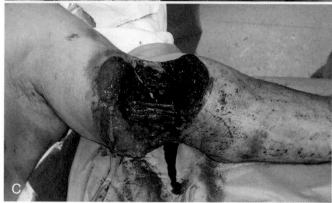

Figure 37-4 Fractures requiring emergency surgery. A, This open fracture of the tibial shaft shows severe soft tissue damage. **B,** Tibial fracture without gross contamination. **C,** Near-amputation of the forearm. This type of injury requires extensive vascular repair in order to salvage the limb. (*From Canale S, Beaty J: Campbell's operative orthopaedics, ed 11, Philadelphia, 2009, Mosby.*)

conversion to definitive intramedullary nailing of long bones may be attempted. In near amputation such as that shown in Figure 37-4, repair of major vascular structures may require emergency reconstruction. However, the decision to proceed with a definitive vascular procedure is weighed against causing further immune system reaction by a prolonged surgical procedure. Pelvic fracture is associated with high mortality after a motor vehicle accident due to instability of the pelvic ring and multiple injuries to the venous system that are difficult to access surgically. Repair of soft tissue in orthopedic trauma usually takes place over several days and includes phased debridement to assess tissue viability.

PREOPERATIVE CARE OF THE ORTHOPEDIC PATIENT

Potential complications in the multiple orthopedic trauma patient are:

- *Life-threatening hemorrhage:* Hemorrhage may be addressed with direct pressure on the wound. Early stabilization is critical.
- *Infection from open fractures:* Antibiotic therapy is started early in treatment. Further contamination is avoided by keeping the wounds covered with sterile barriers (e.g., loose dressings, drapes) and exposing only when necessary in the preoperative period.
- *Neurological injury:* Care is taken during wound assessment to avoid causing or extending nerve damage.
- *Vascular damage, compartment syndrome, and limb loss:* Transporting, moving, and handling the patient can result in extension of injuries including vascular damage. Compartment syndrome may occur early and must be treated quickly.
- *Loss of limb function:* Full debridement and identification of nerves, tendons, and blood vessels for reconstruction take place once the patient is stabilized. Debridement may be repeated within 24 hours.

Preoperative care of the patient is directed toward prevention or treatment of these complications. The surgical technologist in an assistant circulator role may be directly or indirectly involved in presurgical care of the patient. Good communication is essential, because there may be many people in the circulator role and the environment may be noisy.

Preoperative care of the patient may include debridement in the emergency department. If the primary assessment reveals exsanguinating hemorrhage, emergency surgery takes precedence over debridement. In this case the patient may arrive in the operating room very quickly after transport to the health care facility. If there is a pelvic fracture, the patient may have a pelvic binder in place, and this is only released with direction from the surgeon and anesthesia care provider. Limb traction may have been applied in the emergency department. If so, the anesthesia care provider and surgeon direct all transfers in order to maintain traction. Anesthesia is started as soon as clinically safe, and the patient can then be carefully positioned, prepped, and draped.

CASE PLANNING

Instruments and Equipment

Instrumentation required for damage control surgery includes a major orthopedic set and general surgery instruments. Soft tissue repair may be delayed for phased procedures; however, one set of soft tissue instruments and equipment is needed for debridement and another for the surgical repair. Open fracture of the long bones is most often stabilized with an external fixation system. Intramedullary nailing may also be performed in selected cases. If the method is preplanned before the patient arrives, naturally this equipment and hardware is included in the setup. However, if the stabilization methodology is not known, the surgical technologist should have certain equipment available to open on immediate request. A suggested list is shown in Box 37-3.

A high-impact pelvic fracture with open fracture of the leg is initially stabilized using a pin and frame external fixation system. This allows exploration of the wound. Severe pelvic

---

| Box **37-3** | Suggested Repair Equipment to Be Available for Damage Control |

- Low- and high-speed drills (low speed usually preferred) with extra drill bits
- Hand drill
- Kirschner wires
- Threaded Steinman pins
- Heavy pin cutters
- Pin or clamp and frame fixation system (surgeon's preference) and olive wires
- Self-tapping screw fixation system
- Intramedullary nailing system, dynamic or static locking (surgeon's preference)

---

fracture is associated with a high rate of tissue damage to the pelvic structures and severe hemorrhage arising from the venous system. Wound exploration requires right angle clamps, fine long curved hemostats, and narrow retractors such as a Deaver set. If there is involvement of the lower intestinal or genitourinary tract, these instruments sets must also be available. An ample supply of Silastic vessel loops with bolsters and clamp covers should also be available.

Drapes

Emergency orthopedic surgery can require large amounts of solutions both for debridement and for normal surgical wound irrigation. Impermeable drapes, gowns, and cover sheets are therefore used whenever possible. Runoff from irrigation solutions must be controlled using pocket drapes. Sterile team members should have leggings available to prevent soaking through the scrub suit.

Intraoperative Imaging

Operative fluoroscopy may be used for external fixation pins or nail placement. Intraoperative imaging is especially beneficial in trauma where there is significant tissue displacement.

Intraoperative Debridement

If debridement takes place in the operating room, special supplies are needed. Tissue dissection is straightforward and performed with basic soft tissue instruments plus fine dissecting scissors such as pediatric-size Metzenbaum, tenotomy, or plastic surgery type scissors. Dissection around blood vessels and ducts may require vascular forceps. Bone and other connective tissue debridement can be performed using a knife or fine rongeur. However, bone is spared whenever possible. An ample supply of fresh (new) knife blades, #10 and #15, should be available throughout the procedure as they can quickly become dull and inaccurate when used for debridement.

DAMAGE CONTROL ORTHOPEDIC SURGERY

The primary goals of damage control orthopedic surgery are control of hemorrhage, stabilization of the fractures, and prevention of sepsis.

The surgical technologist in the scrub role maintains a high level of wound management as described in detail in Chapter 22. Particular highlights of wound management in the multiple trauma orthopedic patient are to:

- Assist in maintaining hemostasis using all appropriate technologies available.
- Use and have available appropriate-size instruments for the tissues.
- Clear the sterile field of all instruments not in use; maintain a clean, orderly field.
- Keep tissues moist; tendons are particularly vulnerable.
- Protect the sterile field and maintain strict aseptic technique.

Debridement

Wound debridement is removal of nonviable or dead tissue and nontissue debris from a traumatic or infected wound. Patients with open traumatic wounds, without or without fracture, are at high risk of morbidity and mortality from infection. Therefore debridement is a necessary part of treatment. The procedure may be performed in the emergency department before an emergent surgical procedure or as a part of the procedure itself. However, if immediate life-saving surgery is required, debridement may be performed at the patient's beside after both patient and fracture are stabilized.

Open fractures are by definition contaminated and require some level of debridement, which may include excision of skin edges and deeper tissues that have been crushed or macerated in the trauma. As a rule, bone tissue is not removed, and tendon is removed only if it is obviously nonviable. In preparation for debridement, the wound is draped with an extra-wide margin exposed beyond the periphery of the wound. The area is prepped as usual but extended to include a large anatomical region such as the entire limb. Debridement is performed using the surgical knife, Metzenbaum or fine scissors such as tenotomy or pediatric-size Metzenbaum, toothed tissue forceps, and the appropriate retractors for the tissue involved. Hemostasis is maintained as usual with ligation or ESU. The wound may be enlarged to encompass muscle, fascia, and in some cases devitalized medullary canal tissue. Tissue and debris may be collected in basins placed on the field. The surgeon will reduce or cut back the tissue margins until bleeding on the margins signals viability. All tissue and nontissue fragments are saved as specimens. Viable bone fragments recovered during debridement must be kept moistened with saline, because they may be used during repair.

Following surgical debridement, the wound must be copiously irrigated. Routine low-pressure irrigation using a bulb or Asepto syringe may be used, or the surgeon may use a pulsating lavage system. In either case, warm normal saline is used. Topical bacitracin may be used as an additive to the irrigation solution. Regardless of the mechanics of irrigation, the surgical technologist should prepare the surgical field for large quantities of fluid. Debridement may be repeated within 6 to 8 hours.

EMERGENCY TREATMENT OF FRACTURES

External fixation is currently the most common method of damage control orthopedic surgery. This strategy plays a significant role in stabilization to prevent further tissue damage, pain control, and maintaining limb length. All attempts will be made to resuscitate the multiple trauma patient to the point where damage control surgery can be attempted. This is because further insult to the body increases the immune responses, which lead to deterioration of the patient's condition.

Control of hemorrhage takes priority in damage control orthopedic surgery. If the source of the bleeding has been identified and is accessible, the area may be packed with lap sponges and the packs systematically removed to secure hemostasis. In the case of unstable pelvic fracture, abdominal, retroperitoneal, or pelvic structures may be severely injured. A focused assessment with ultrasound performed preoperatively aids in the identification of free blood. In the case of abdominal or pelvic bleeding, a laparotomy may be required to secure hemostasis. Bleeding in the retroperitoneal cavity is more difficult to identify and stop because it often arises from the venous plexus, which is difficult to access. Also, an unstable pelvic ring may extend the injuries. Because of these difficulties, a pelvic stabilizer may be applied at the start of surgery or in the emergency department. The C-clamp stabilizer is a temporary bar device held in place with pins (Figure 37-5). A more complex external or internal fixation system replaces the C clamp during the first or later phased surgeries.

Long bone fractures are initially stabilized using an external fixation system such as the Ilizarov system, cage, or lateral fixator. These are held in place with pins or wires and once the fractures are stabilized allow the limb to be moved without risk of further tissue damage (Figure 37-6). Application of the device is straightforward. The scrub should have the surgeon's preferred system, including the bar and wire components and tools needed to assemble and adjust the framework. Figure 37-7 illustrates a cage system implanted under the image intensifier.

A second option that may be used in damage control surgery of the long bones is intramedullary nailing. However, this method is used only on patients who are hemodynamically stable enough to undergo the procedure in the early phases of the emergency. The current practice favors external fixation for severe open fracture of the long bones in the multiple-injury patient. Procedures for intramedullary nailing are described in Chapter 31.

THORACIC INJURY

Blunt thoracic injury accounts for at least 20% of all trauma mortality and contributes to 50% of all trauma mortality in the United States. The main cause of all thoracic injury is a motor vehicle accident. Life-threatening injuries to the thoracic structures and chest wall include those that cause mechanical impingement on respiratory and cardiac function, injury to the heart and great vessels, pulmonary injuries, and other soft tissue injuries such as esophageal and diaphragmatic trauma.

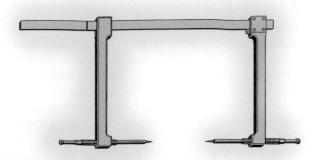

Figure 37-5   Pelvic stabilizer. This **C**-clamp device is used to provide temporary stabilization of the fractured pelvis intraoperatively or until a more permanent device can be implanted. The device can be inserted in the emergency department and is held in place by two lateral pins. (*From Canale S, Beaty J:* Campbell's operative orthopaedics, *ed 11, Philadelphia, 2009, Mosby.*)

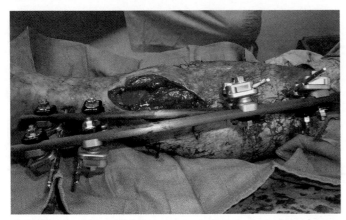

Figure 37-6 External fixation using a unilateral pin and bar fixation device. (*From Canale S, Beaty J:* Campbell's operative orthopaedics, *ed 11, Philadelphia, 2009, Mosby.*)

Open thoracotomy may be performed in the emergency department to evacuate a **cardiac tamponade** (hemorrhage into the pericardial sac sufficient to prevent the heart from contracting effectively) or to control hemorrhage of the heart, lung, or large vessels, including the aorta. Once the immediate emergency has been addressed, the patient is then transferred rapidly to the operating room for further surgery. Indications for immediate surgical intervention include tension pneumothorax, open pneumothorax, flail chest, massive hemothorax, and pericardial tamponade. These conditions are described later.

CASE PLANNING

Case planning for thoracic emergency should include instrumentation and supplies for three systems:

- Cardiovascular
- Respiratory
- Orthopedic

The most urgent (lethal) injury is of course treated first, but total damage control surgery often involves at least two of the three systems. Priorities of the cardiovascular system are focused on management of hemorrhage and cardiac function. The respiratory system is restored by repair of the injured structures including the chest wall. Fractures of the ribs can be life threatening when the fractured end punctures or lacerates vital soft tissues, or in the case of multiple rib fracture that impinges on the lung (flail chest) described later in this section.

Rapid setup and delivery of instruments for damage control thoracotomy should be prioritized by the following:

1. *Determining the location of potentially lethal injury requires good exposure.* This translates to suction (at least two suction systems immediately available), sponges, and appropriate retractors. A Finochietto self-retaining and Deaver set should be available from the start of surgery.

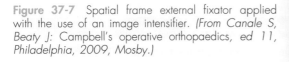

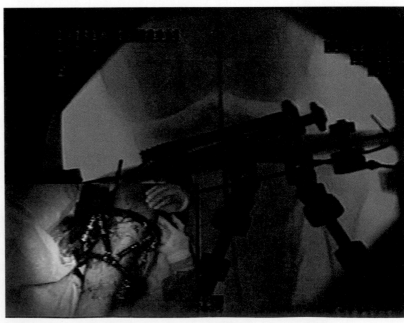

Figure 37-7 Spatial frame external fixator applied with the use of an image intensifier. (*From Canale S, Beaty J:* Campbell's operative orthopaedics, *ed 11, Philadelphia, 2009, Mosby.*)

2. *The thoracic cavity may be packed as soon as free blood is removed.* Prepare a large basin to receive clots. Have at least 10 to 15 lap sponges dipped in warm saline and wrung dry. Always have at least 30 sponges in reserve for immediate use.

3. If the surgeon's preference for suture on myocardium and great vessels is not known, have available 2-0 and 3-0 Prolene. Fibrin glue may also be used to seal wounds in damage control surgery.

4. The strategy for chest wall closure is usually deferred until the end of the case. The wound may be closed in one layer. Chest tubes and underwater seal drainage are required.

INJURIES OF THE CHEST WALL

The chest wall must be intact for normal respiration. Disruption in the rib and sternal structures that protect the heart, lungs, and great vessels can have serious consequences for the respiratory and cardiac systems. Open injury of the chest wall in which negative pressure is lost requires immediate lifesaving measures to restore respiratory function. This can be done in the field or in the emergency department. A common method for sealing the chest wall is application of petrolatum gauze over the wound, which is an effective temporary sealant. Evacuation of air is performed using needle thoracostomy or immediate insertion of chest tubes. Extensive open chest wounds require mechanical ventilation.

CARDIOVASCULAR TRAUMA

Blunt Cardiac Rupture

Cardiac rupture is the tearing of the ventricles or atria, pericardium, chordae, valves, or other associated structures. It is among the most lethal of thoracic injuries and may include "explosive" rupture of the ascending aorta and shearing of the descending aorta, which occurs as the first rib and clavicle strike the vertebral column in high-speed, high-energy impact accidents. Diagnosis is made by investigating the mechanism of the injury from witnesses and through echocardiogram. Cardiovascular trauma is usually accompanied by other serious injuries including pulmonary, abdominal, and head injury. Diagnosis of these is generally based on focused sonogram and radiography, and survival is often based on an intact pericardium and ability to control hemorrhage from other sites. The most common cause of blunt cardiovascular trauma is a motor vehicle accident in which the driver impacts the steering wheel. Other causes are falls, blast injury, and crushing injury. Cardiac injury can be complicated by conduction disorder, dysrhythmia, and intraventricular thrombi. Treatment for cardiac rupture may be performed in the emergency department initially by pericardiocentesis, emergency thoracotomy, and pericardiotomy. The patient is then immediately transported to the operating room. The patient who has had thoracotomy in the emergency department may arrive with an inflated Foley catheter controlling a small hole in the heart or direct manual compression on larger wounds. Only about 10% require bypass for repair in the operating room. The surgical treatment is immediate control of hemostasis and repair of the ruptured myocardium and other damaged structures. Damage control surgery of the heart includes packing the chest cavity and rapid repair of the structures using abbreviated traditional means and temporary closure of the thoracic cavity. A definitive procedure follows when the patient has been resuscitated.

Penetrating Cardiac Wound

Penetrating wounds of the heart caused by civilian gunshot or knife are now common in urban areas. Emergency department treatment includes fluid and blood resuscitation and tube thoracostomy (insertion of a chest tube) to treat pneumothorax, which usually occurs with penetrating wounds. Echocardiography is performed quickly and the patient transferred to the operating room. The most lethal complications in penetrating cardiac injury are exsanguinating hemorrhage into the pleural cavity or cardiac tamponade. The patient with increasing cardiac tamponade must be treated quickly, and this may require immediate emergency department thoracotomy. Gunshot wounds to the thorax are associated with high mortality, especially with high-velocity bullets. Knife wounds result in laceration of structures that can often be repaired, if the patient is treated quickly to avoid fatal hemorrhage. Other less frequent causes of penetrating wounds to the heart and vessels are various types of impalement injuries related to industrial and home accidents.

Surgical treatment includes evacuation of free blood, restoring heart function, and repair of damaged tissues. This requires a complete cardiovascular setup with repair sutures or the surgeon's choice. The repair may be definitive but somewhat abbreviated. For example, suturing over pledgets may be too time consuming. Patch grafts are preferred over tube grafts.

Aortic Injury

Injury to the aorta is most often the result of a high-speed, head-on collision (unrestrained passenger or driver) or high-impact lateral blow to the chest. Car versus pedestrian accidents, a fall from a great height, and ejection from a motor vehicle also contribute to the incidence of aortic trauma. Mortality is high, especially with complete rupture of the aorta. Of patients with blunt aorta injury, 60% to 90% die at the scene of the accident or shortly after arrival in the trauma center. Diagnosis may be difficult, especially in the multiple-trauma patient. Echocardiography, FAST, and radiography are used in the assessment, along with analysis of the mechanism of injury and presenting symptoms.

Surgical repair of the aorta is definitive and may require cardiopulmonary bypass to prevent postoperative paraplegia related to cross-clamping the aorta. Synthetic grafts or direct anastomosis are techniques used in repair. Although most procedures require open surgery for assessment and repair of associated injuries, some cases of aortic trauma can be managed using endovascular stenting via the femoral or iliac artery.

PULMONARY TRAUMA

Pulmonary trauma occurs most frequently in motor vehicle accidents as described earlier for cardiovascular injury. An additional cause is a blast injury, which occurs in intentional violence and occasionally in industrial accidents. Pulmonary injury ranges from severe lung and bronchial tears to a variety of conditions in which respiration is compromised because of loss of the lungs' mechanical ability to expand. Thirty percent to 75% of pulmonary **contusions** (bruising of the lung parenchyma leading to hemorrhage into the alveolar spaces) occur with blunt chest trauma. It is the most common thoracic injury in children. Any pulmonary injury that compromises ventilation and gas exchange must be treated emergently. Treatment begins in the emergency department with thoracostomy or possible thoracotomy and is continued in the operating room. Emergency surgery requires a basic emergency setup including major thoracic and vascular instruments. An autotransfusion system should also be available.

Flail Chest

Flail chest is a critical condition in which three or more *adjacent* ribs are broken in two locations (Figure 37-8). This allows the ribs, still attached to each other by connective tissue, to move freely over the thoracic structures. More importantly, the segment moves *paradoxically*: inward with inspiration, and outward on expiration. The goal of treatment is to restore ventilation and treat underlying injuries. Intubation and assisted ventilation are performed in extreme cases so that surgery can be initiated on injuries to the internal structures, which are almost always present and account for the 8% to 35% mortality with flail chest.

Pneumothorax

Pneumothorax is the presence of air in the pleural space that prevents lung expansion. This condition is always found in penetrating pleural injury. Three types of pneumothorax include *simple*, *communicating*, and *tension*. **Pneumothorax** is the presence of air in the potential space between the lung and pleura that prevents full expansion of the lung. A simple pneumothorax is defined as one in which there is no communication with atmospheric air and no thoracic structures are displaced (Figure 37-9). This can be caused by a fractured rib end entering the pleural space on impact, or from a gunshot or stab wound. *Communicating pneumothorax* occurs when the pleural wound communicates with the outside atmosphere. This results in collapse of the lung on the affected side with complete loss of ventilation (Figure 37-10). This type of pneumothorax is sometimes referred to as a "sucking" chest wound because of the sound made as air is forced in and out of the wound during attempted respiration. *Tension pneumothorax* occurs when air in the pleural space increases to a point where the mediastinum, lung, and great vessels are pushed and eventually compressed into the opposite side of the chest cavity. This is a critical injury resulting in rapid hypoxia, shock, and acidosis.

Pneumothorax is detected using CT scan and FAST. Treatment can be initiated in the field or in the emergency department by needle thoracostomy or by insertion of chest tube in the case of tension pneumothorax. The presence of underlying injuries may require rapid transfer to the operating room.

Hemothorax

Hemothorax is free blood in the pleural cavity, reducing lung capacity by the same mechanisms as pneumothorax. A common cause is laceration of lung tissue, including the parenchyma (lung covering). Emergency thoracotomy is performed when blood reaches or exceeds 1500 mL. The patient can quickly become hypovolemic with complications related to failed gas exchange. The surgical goal in this case is to repair the lacerations, restore respiratory function, and replace the blood loss. A thoracostomy is performed in the emergency department for initial treatment. In this case a size 36 to 40 Fr chest tube is inserted under local anesthetic and connected to an underwater sealed drainage system. The patient is then transferred to the operating room.

Laceration of the Lung

Pulmonary laceration or deep pulmonary laceration is associated with hemothorax and multiple rib fractures. A severe laceration can arise from the bronchi or from the lung tissue

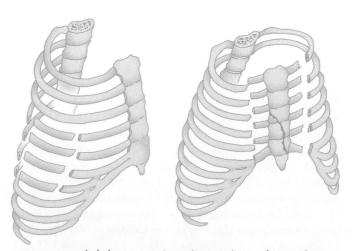

Figure 37-8   Flail chest. Note that adjacent ribs are fractured in two sections, creating a lateral or central section that is free floating. Flail chest is an indication for immediate emergency surgery. (*From Marx J, Hockberger R, Walls R: Rosen's emergency medicine: concepts and clinical practice, ed 7, Philadelphia, 2010, WB Saunders.*)

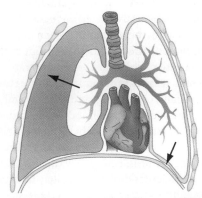

Figure 37-9   Closed pneumothorax. This is a simple pneumothorax in the right lung with air in the pleural cavity and collapse of the lung. (*From Marx J, Hockberger R, Walls R: Rosen's emergency medicine: concepts and clinical practice, ed 7, Philadelphia, 2010, WB Saunders.*)

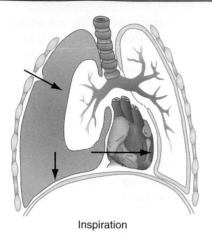
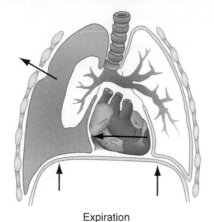

Inspiration   Expiration

Figure 37-10 **Communicating pneumothorax.** The right lung is collapsed, and there is a defect in the chest wall that communicates to the outside. (From Marx J, Hockberger R, Walls R: Rosen's emergency medicine: concepts and clinical practice, ed 7, Philadelphia, 2010, WB Saunders.)

itself. In these cases the patient may undergo emergency department thoracotomy to clamp the tissue and then may be moved quickly to the operating room for complete repair. Damage control surgery may include lobectomy in selected cases. However, initially the bleeding is controlled with rapid suturing. Some surgeons prefer to use staples for a temporary repair (refer to Chapter 33).

Diaphragm Injury

Diaphragmatic injury occurs most frequently with motor vehicle accidents and falls from a great height. This injury involves the herniation of abdominal contents into the thoracic cavity through a defect in the diaphragm. This presents a risk of strangulation of abdominal structures that is made worse as the negative intrathoracic pressure pulls the organs into the thoracic cavity. Rupture of the diaphragm caused by blunt or penetrating trauma can be life threatening and requires emergency surgery. Surgery can be performed laparoscopically, but full evaluation of all injuries often requires open surgery. The method of repair is definitive unless additional injuries indicate damage control laparotomy. Routine diaphragmatic surgery is described in Chapter 23. These techniques are also used to repair the ruptured diaphragm.

MAJOR PERIPHERAL VASCULAR TRAUMA

Trauma of the major arteries may threaten limb viability or vital structures and is therefore considered extremely urgent. In the United States, 70% to 90% of peripheral vascular injuries occur as a result of penetrating trauma related to violence. Gunshot wounds remain the leading cause of death in 15- to 34-year-olds. Ninety percent of victims are males and are usually under the age of 40.[5]

The method of assessment in vascular trauma depends on the severity of the wounds and the patient's condition at the time of arrival at the health care facility. Patients with severe, pulsating hemorrhage from an open wound and other obvious indications of limb-threatening injury are often taken directly to the operating room without preoperative diagnostic workup. Intraoperative angiography may be performed after bleeding is under control and the patient is hemodynamically stable. Other less serious but nonetheless urgent cases are diagnosed using color flow Doppler, CT scan, and MRI. The value of diagnostic procedures must be weighed against the time required to produce the results.

Specific areas of vascular injury are often associated with another trauma. For example, the most common vascular injury is to the femoral artery and vein caused by hip fracture. Trauma to the iliac artery is almost always accompanied by involvement of the intestine, bladder, and pelvis. In this case, damage control laparotomy is performed. The most common arterial injury of the arm is the brachial artery, seen mostly with penetrating trauma, fracture of the humerus, and animal bites.

Vascular injury is divided into two major categories according to cause—penetrating and blunt trauma.

PENETRATING TRAUMA

In civilian medicine, penetrating trauma to blood vessels is most frequently caused by gunshot and knife wounds. The trajectory, perimeters of wound damage, and path of bullets have been expertly studied in the field of ballistics. Data gathered by civilian, military, and human rights organizations have greatly benefited the surgeon's ability to predict the extent of trauma and therefore more effective exploratory surgery and treatment. There is a wide variation in penetrating ability, lateral tissue damage, and shape of bullet wounds, according to the type of weapon and bullet involved. Surgeons are challenged to learn about new or modified weapons that are introduced for civilian interpersonal violence. All bullets produce a typically elongated track. Jacketed or semijacketed types also expand (explode) early in impact or late in the path. This means that tissue damage and vascular injury may occur distant from the entry wound. Shotgun or pellet wounds present a larger scope of impact that may result in migration of fragments into distant tissues.

Knife trauma results in partial or total severing of vascular structures. Small wounds may be easily explored and treated, whereas larger, deeper penetrating wounds can be fatal and require emergency surgery.

BLUNT TRAUMA

Blunt vascular trauma occurs as a result of crushing injuries such as those that occur in motor vehicle or industrial accidents.

A fractured long bone may also impinge on vascular bundles, causing blunt trauma, occlusion, and limb ischemia. Loss of blood supply to the lower limb forces the tissue into anaerobic metabolism, accumulation of lactic acid, and tissue death.

CASE PLANNING

Urgent vascular trauma surgery commonly includes other systems. A vascular setup and general surgery instruments should be prepared, along with all supplies needed for a major vascular case including drugs, solutions, hemostatics, Silastic vessel loops, and other vascular supplies, such as Fogarty catheters for removing thrombi in damaged vessels. Orthopedic and amputation instruments should also be available for limb surgery.

Sutures and supplies should include basic peripheral vascular sutures such as Mersilene, Prolene, or Pronova on vascular needles. Grafting is usually not performed in emergency surgery. Instead, direct repair and anastomosis techniques are used. As soon as the technologist is able to identify (or is informed) of the vessels to be repaired, the appropriate-size sutures should be quickly prepared. It is better to have made an intelligent guess than to have no repair sutures available. Both single-arm and double-arm (for anastomosis) sutures should be immediately available. Unless the surgeon identifies which suture materials are needed for ties, silk, size 2-0 and 0, should be prepared on right angle passers to start the case.

In cases where the limb is in danger of ischemia and compartment syndrome, the anesthesia care provider and surgeon may implement a forced cooling protocol to slow the metabolism in the limb. In this case, sterile ice slush and cold irrigation may be required on the field.

SURGICAL TREATMENT

Preoperative treatment in the emergency department includes resuscitative measures and attempts to stanch the hemorrhage, if the source can be accessed. A Foley catheter may be inserted at the wound site and used as a tamponade. In some cases, vascular repair may not take precedence over other life-threatening injuries, which are addressed first while arterial or venous injuries are treated by direct compression. The patient is transferred to the operating room as soon as possible in the presence of exsanguinating vascular trauma complicated with other injuries.

If the vascular injury involves a major neurovascular bundle or the limb has been severely mangled, amputation may be performed. A generalized list of priorities of the surgery will be:

- Exposure to the site of injury
- Gaining access to the injured vessels by evacuation, retraction, and careful dissection
- Hemorrhage control by clamping or direct pressure followed by direct repair or temporary graft
- Blood and fluid replacement (continued resuscitation)
- Repair or removal of bone or foreign body fragments to prevent further injury

The type of repair performed on the vessels depends on the patient's condition. Damage control surgery for major injury favors direct repair of the vessel including anastomosis. However, a temporary synthetic graft may be implanted for a short period (usually no more than 24 hours) in order to perfuse a limb in an unstable patient.

INJURIES OF THE BRAIN AND SPINAL CORD

Traumatic brain injury accounts for approximately one third of all deaths from trauma, representing about 52,000 deaths each year. The main causes of TBI are falls and motor vehicle accidents. TBI is the leading cause of death in patients younger than 25 years. Two thirds of total deaths due to brain injury in the 0- to 4-year-old group are due to child abuse. The objective of emergency medical and surgical intervention is to avert secondary injuries related to increased cranial pressure and the physiological changes that occur with severe head trauma. Figure 37-11 shows the events contributing to secondary brain injury.

BLUNT TRAUMA

Because brain injury is irreversible, all attempts are made to prevent secondary events that accompany the initial trauma. These include management of hemorrhage and intracranial pressure due to bleeding and cerebral edema. These can occur with blunt trauma to the head or when the head in motion (such as in a fast-moving vehicle) is suddenly stopped. This has two effects: the shearing injury of neural tissue and blood vessels, and the physical impact of the brain against the cranium. These can result in rupture of blood vessels, laceration of tissue, and *avulsion* (separation or tearing away of one tissue layer from another).

Assessment for head injury relies on laboratory findings and imaging studies using CT neuroimaging and MRI. The decision for emergency neurosurgery depends on the presence of other life-threatening injuries and the patient's hemodynamic status. Damage control surgery includes drilling burr holes in the cranium and ventriculostomy (placement of a drainage catheter in a ventricular space to relieve pressure). Definitive surgery to relieve intracranial pressure related to hemorrhage is craniotomy with evacuation of blood and clots and securing hemostasis.

PENETRATING BRAIN INJURY

The most common cause of penetrating brain injury in the United States is gunshot. Gunshot wounds account for approximately 21,000 deaths per year. As with injury to other systems by gunshot, the type of weapon, speed and type of bullet, and exact path in the tissue determine the lethality of the injury. Patients who survive the initial impact are evaluated for location of the injured tissue, extent of hemorrhage, and secondary effects—mainly hypoxia, ischemia, and hypotension. Emergency surgical management is usually craniotomy for control of intracranial pressure.

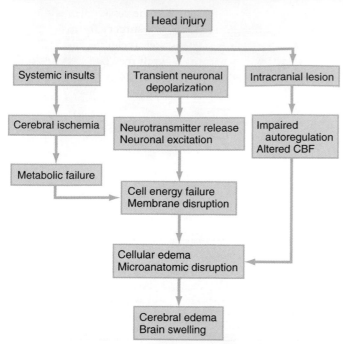

Figure 37-11 Factors contributing to traumatic brain injury. *CBF,* Cerebral blood flow. *(From Marx J, Hockberger R, Walls R: Rosen's emergency medicine: concepts and clinical practice, ed 7, Philadelphia, 2010, WB Saunders.)*

CASE PLANNING

Planning for craniotomy is detailed and requires many specialty instruments and supplies. Therefore, an emergency craniotomy cart is available on standby in health care facilities that receive trauma patients. The cart contains essential items including but not limited to standard linens, suction tubing, ESU equipment, hemostatic materials, scalp clips, surgical sponges, and neurosurgical instrument sets, including craniotomes, power saws, and drills.

Preparing for multiple-injury cases that include an emergency neurosurgical procedure plus additional setups can be difficult because of the amount of neurosurgical equipment required. A sequential setup may be possible if the surgeon knows ahead of time the priority of multiple repairs. Two or more setups can be confined to separate back tables that are brought forward in order of need. Damage control neurosurgery (see later discussion) requires few instruments, and the equipment can be quickly separated from the emergency cart. The scrub can then switch back tables as needed. An alternative strategy is that more than one scrubbed team operates simultaneously on different injuries. In this case, each team has a dedicated setup.

Positioning the patient requires care to maintain the spine in a neutral position. Cervical spine injury is not ruled out until a conclusive (often time-consuming) assessment has been completed. The urgency of surgery may override full evaluation. The patient usually arrives with a stabilizing cervical collar, and transfer to the operating table requires logrolling with a lateral transfer device. The supine position can be used if cervical injury has been completely ruled out. In this case, the head is turned with the affected side up. A prone or beach chair position may also be used if it does not interfere with surgery of other systems.

Draping for emergency craniotomy with multiple injury sites must accommodate these sites. In such cases the top drape can be extended only as far as the periphery of the other site, and a second procedure drape is used to overlap the craniotomy drape. A penetrating brain injury is considered contaminated because the penetrating object is not sterile and scalp tissue including hair is often dragged into the wound.

POSSIBLE EMERGENCY NEUROSURGICAL PROCEDURES

Depending on the location of the injury and source of hemorrhage, a number of different approaches are used in emergency neurosurgery. These are described here.

- *Subdural hematoma:* Hematoma between the dura and brain. These are often associated with acceleration-deceleration trauma.
- *Epidural hematoma:* Hematoma arising between the dura and deepest layer of the cranium. These are usually associated with fracture and can be rapidly fatal.
- *Traumatic subarachnoid hemorrhage:* This type of injury may be associated with tearing of subarachnoid vessels.
- *Intracerebral hematoma:* A traumatic intracerebral hematoma occurs as a shearing injury that ruptures small arteries deep within the brain. They occur as a result of impact of the brain against the cranial vault rather than as a direct injury. Traumatic (direct) intracerebral injury carries a high mortality rate.

NOTE: The procedures for craniotomy and cranioplasty are detailed in Chapter 36.

SPINAL TRAUMA

Approximately 50% of spinal injuries are caused by motor vehicle accidents in patients who were unrestrained at the time of the accident. Most of the remaining 50% are caused by falls, gunshot wounds, or sport injuries.

These data are kept by the National Spinal Cord Injury Association (http://www.spinalcord.org/).

Spinal cord injury occurs when the supporting ligaments, intravertebral discs, and bony structures are disrupted, causing the spine to move in opposing directions. The protective structures that hold the spine in alignment occur as two separate columns. If one column remains intact, it acts as a brace against injury. However, if both the posterior and anterior columns are disrupted, the likelihood of spinal cord injury is greatly increased. Primary injury to the spinal cord can worsen at any time during transport and treatment as long as the spinal column is unsupported. Therefore stability of the spine is a primary consideration in emergency response. Emergency personnel in the field now apply cervical and full-body stabilization devices to accident victims, sometime before they are extricated from the accident debris. Stabilization devices are not removed until there is definitive evidence that no spinal injury exists.

Many different types of spinal fractures have been identified. Injury to the spinal cord depends on the direction of impact and penetration of the spinal cord by bone or other connective tissues, such as the ligaments that extend along the spinal column. Diagnostic imaging (CT, MRI) and laboratory tests are used to confirm a diagnosis.

Spinal cord injuries are divided into two main types, primary and secondary. Primary injury occurs when blunt or penetrating trauma severs neural tissue in the spinal column. Primary injury also occurs when a dural hematoma impinges on the cord. Secondary injury occurs as a result of a cascade of physiological changes that occur with trauma, including the lethal triad discussed previously, and injury related to moving and handling the patient after admission to the health care facility.

A further classification of spinal cord lesions is the complete and incomplete lesion. *Complete* lesions cause complete loss of motor and sensory function distal to the injury. *Incomplete* lesions result in varying degrees of combined motor and sensory loss depending on the nature of the lesion, its location, and the extent of injury. Emergency surgery is usually not performed on patients with complete lesions. However, an incomplete lesion can benefit from exploratory surgery that includes removal of foreign bodies, bone fragments, or other tissue impinging on the spinal cord, removal of hematomas, and mechanical stabilization using a spinal orthopedic system or by application of a halo brace. These procedures are described in Chapter 36 and are performed on stabilized patients.

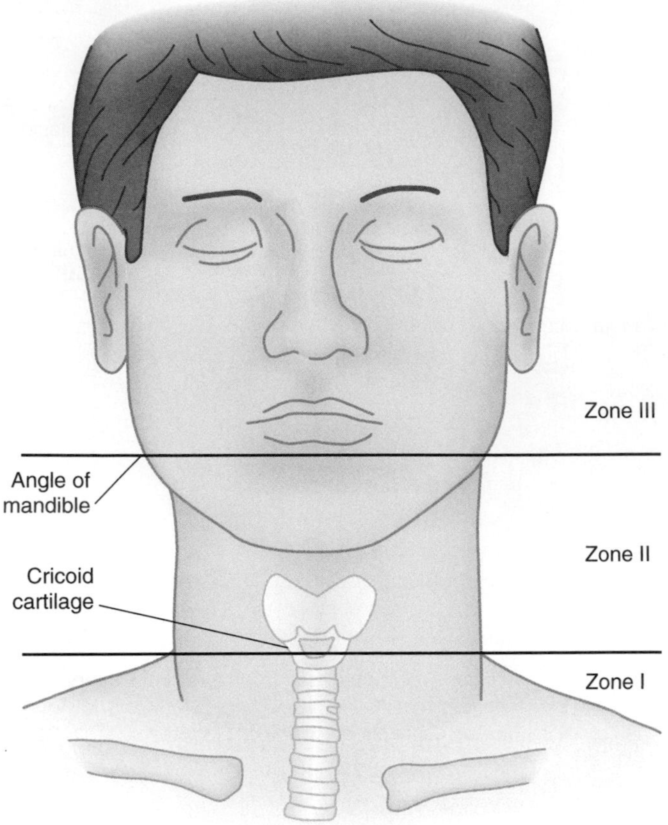

NECK TRAUMA

Life-threatening neck trauma of the soft tissues may involve the airway, blood vessels, and laryngeal structures. Severe hemorrhage from any of the vital structures can result in shock or obstructed airway. Three classifications of neck trauma are blunt, penetrating, and strangulating (also called near hanging), and these account for up to 5% of all traumatic injuries. Blunt trauma is rare compared with other mechanisms of injury.

A penetrating injury is most commonly related to gunshot and knife wounds and shrapnel from home-made explosives.

Emergency response for injuries of the neck depends on the structures suspected of injury and the anatomical regions shown in Figure 37-12. Diagnosis employs a combination of physical assessment for signs of hemorrhage, airway obstruction, and neurological damage, in addition to imaging studies—CT scan and MRI.

PREOPERATIVE CARE OF THE PATIENT

Cervical spine injury is not ruled out in the patient with severe neck trauma, and field response includes placement of a cervical collar. Intubation may be required, and in this case rapid sequence intubation (RSI) is performed. In this technique, a fast-acting, short-duration sedative is administered and

Figure 37-12 Divisions of the neck. Critical injury to the neck is divided according to specific regions, referred to as zones. *(From Marx J, Hockberger R, Walls R: Rosen's emergency medicine: concepts and clinical practice, ed 7, Philadelphia, 2010, WB Saunders.)*

orotracheal intubation performed unless there is massive facial trauma. If RSI is not possible, a surgical airway such as cricothyrotomy is performed in the emergency department or in the field. Care of the patient in the immediate preoperative phase is the same as for all trauma patients, with attention to preventing hypothermia, spinal protection, and monitoring vital signs while in transit. Although many neck injuries can be treated conservatively, those involving major blood vessels or the airway may require immediate surgery. A gunshot wound may contain pellets that can migrate into an open blood vessel and into the heart or brain. Severe hemorrhage of the carotid, subclavian, or jugular vein may impinge on the airway.

CASE PLANNING

Case planning for neck trauma must include vascular instruments, sutures, and supplies such as those used in carotid surgery (refer to Chapter 32). Fine dissecting instruments should also be available for exploration of the upper respiratory structures. This will require a variety of retractors, such as those used in thyroid procedures and for carotid endarterectomy. Drugs and hemostatic agents should be distributed as for carotid procedures.

Patients are normally positioned supine with prep and draping as for wide thyroidectomy. In the event of cervical fracture, stabilization devices will be managed by the anesthesia care provider, and positioning is carried out with care to maintain a neutral spine.

SURGICAL MANAGEMENT OF NECK INJURY

Surgical management of vascular injuries in the neck is usually definitive unless there are other, more urgent concurrent injuries that require immediate attention. Direct anastomosis or patch graft techniques are used to control vascular hemorrhage. Airway trauma may also be treated by direct repair with tracheostomy. Combined laryngotracheal trauma usually occurs in blunt trauma in motor vehicle accidents and also in near-hanging incidents. A fractured cricoid cartilage leads to airway obstruction. Immediate control of hemorrhage and removal of airway obstruction are the surgical objectives in these cases.

KEY CONCEPTS

- The Committee on Trauma of the American College of Surgeons has developed extensive criteria for the designation of trauma facilities. These facilities are graded according to their capacity to attend trauma patients and other criteria involving community trauma response.
- The physiological consequences of multiple or severe trauma can develop into an irreversible cascade of events initiated by the immune system. These are often called the "lethal triad" and include severe hypotension, metabolic acidosis, and coagulopathy.
- Treatment protocols for the lethal triad are initiated as soon as medical help is available to trauma victims. Actions taken in the first hour often determine whether the injuries are fatal.
- Compartment syndrome is severe compression of tissues within a compartment of the body, including the cranium, abdomen, or limb. Unless relieved, compartment syndrome can lead to ischemia and necrosis of the tissue involved.
- ATLS trauma management defines specific protocols and objectives. The main objectives are to treat life-threatening clinical problems such as severe hemorrhage immediately and then transport the patient to the ICU for resuscitation. Phased surgical procedures then follow when the patient is stable.
- Damage control surgery is defined as surgery that only addresses hemorrhage and the threat of sepsis. Reconstructive and other types of prolonged procedures are delayed until the patient is stable.
- Case planning for emergency trauma surgery includes a multisystem approach based on possible surgical interventions. The surgical technologist can develop expertise in trauma surgery by building on the principles and techniques of nonemergency surgery.

REVIEW QUESTIONS

1. The trauma system used in the United States involves assigning numeric levels to health care facilities. Explain this system.
2. Explain what is meant by the "golden hour" as it applies to emergency trauma.
3. Explain compartment syndrome.
4. Define "lethal triangle" as it applies to emergency trauma. Briefly describe the elements of the triangle.
5. Compare and contrast *damage control surgery* with surgery performed for nonemergency.
6. How does case planning for emergency trauma surgery differ from case planning of nonemergency cases?
7. Why is it no longer recommended to perform extensive repair and reconstruction surgery in the initial stages of emergency trauma?
8. Explain the *primary survey* which is performed by first responders in the field.
9. Describe the appropriate care of forensic specimens during surgery and the rationale for using this protocol.
10. Why are displaced pelvic fractures life-threatening?
11. Distinguish between flail chest, pneumothorax, and hemothorax.

REFERENCES

1. Townsend CM, Beauchamp DR, Evers M, Mattox KL, editors: *Sabiston textbook of surgery*, ed 19, Philadelphia, 2012, WB Saunders.
2. Association of periOperative Registered Nurses (AORN): Unplanned perioperative hypothermia. In *Standards, recommended practices and guidelines, 2011 edition*, Denver, 2011, AORN.
3. American College of Surgeons: *Statement on the prevention of retained foreign bodies after surgery*. Accessed April 20, 2012, at http://www.facs.org/fellows_info/statements/st-51.html.
4. AORN: Recommended practices for prevention of retained surgical items. In *Perioperative standards and recommended practices, 2011 edition*, Denver, 2011, AORN.
5. Modrall J, Weaver F, Yellin A: Diagnosis and management of penetrating vascular trauma and the injured extremity, *Emergency Medicine Clinics of North America* 16:129, 1998.

BIBLIOGRAPHY

Borden Institute and the U.S. Department of Defense: *Emergency war surgery, third United States revision*, Washington, DC, 2004, U.S. Government Printing Office.
Canale S, Beaty J: *Campbell's operative orthopaedics*, ed 11, Philadelphia, 2009, Mosby.
Martin R, Meredith J: Management of acute trauma. In Townsend CM Jr, Beauchamp RD, Evers BM, Mattox KL, editors: *Sabiston textbook of surgery*, ed 19, Philadelphia, 2012, WB Saunders.
Marx J, Hockberger R, Walls R: *Rosen's emergency medicine: concepts and clinical practice*, ed 7, Philadelphia, 2010, WB Saunders.
Miller R, Eriksson L, Fleisher L, Weiner-Kronish J, Young W: *Miller's anesthesia*, ed 7, Philadelphia, 2009, Churchill Livingstone.
Roberts J, Hedges J, editors: *Clinical procedures in emergency medicine*, ed 5, Philadelphia, 2010, WB Saunders.

American Hospital Association Guideline for Patient Rights

THE PATIENT CARE PARTNERSHIP: UNDERSTANDING EXPECTATIONS, RIGHTS, AND RESPONSIBILITIES

When you need hospital care, your doctor and the nurses and other professionals at our hospital are committed to working with you and your family to meet your health care needs. Our dedicated doctors and staff members serve the community in all its ethnic, religious, and economic diversity. Our goal is for you and your family to have the same care and attention we would want for our families and ourselves.

The following sections explain how you can expect to be treated during your hospital stay. They also cover what we will need from you to care for you better. If you have questions at any time, please ask them. Unasked or unanswered questions can add to the stress of being in the hospital. Your comfort and confidence in your care are very important to us.

WHAT TO EXPECT DURING YOUR HOSPITAL STAY

- *High-quality hospital care.* Our first priority is to give you the care you need, when you need it, with skill, compassion, and respect. Tell your caregivers if you have concerns about your care or if you have pain. You have the right to know the identity of doctors, nurses, and others involved in your care, and you have the right to know when they are students, residents, or other trainees.
- *A clean and safe environment.* Our hospital works hard to keep you safe. We use special policies and procedures to avoid mistakes in your care and keep you free from abuse or neglect. If anything unexpected and significant happens during your hospital stay, you will be told what happened, and any resulting changes in your care will be discussed with you.
- *Involvement in your care.* You and your doctor often make decisions about your care before you go to the hospital. Other times, especially in emergencies, those decisions are made during your hospital stay. When decision making takes place, it should include discussing your medical condition and information about medically appropriate treatment choices. To make informed decisions with your doctor, you need to understand:
  - The benefits and risks of each treatment
  - Whether your treatment is experimental or part of a research study

- What you can reasonably expect from your treatment and any long-term effects it might have on your quality of life
- What you and your family will need to do after you leave the hospital
- The financial consequences of using uncovered services or out of network providers

Please tell your caregivers if you need more information about treatment choices.

- *Discussing your treatment plan.* When you enter the hospital, you sign a general consent to treatment. In some cases, such as surgery or experimental treatment, you may be asked to confirm in writing that you understand what is planned and agree to it. This process protects your right to consent to or refuse a treatment. Your doctor will explain the medical consequences of refusing recommended treatment. It also protects your right to decide whether you want to participate in a research study.
- *Getting information from you.* Your caregivers need complete and correct information about your health and coverage so that they can make good decisions about your care. That information includes:
  - Past illnesses, surgeries, or hospital stays
  - Past allergic reactions
  - Any medicines or dietary supplements (e.g., vitamins and herbs) you are taking
  - Any network or admission requirements under your health plan
- *Understanding your health care goals and values.* You may have health care goals and values or spiritual beliefs that are important to your well-being. They will be taken into account as much as possible throughout your hospital stay. Make sure your doctor, your family, and your care team know your wishes.
- *Understanding who should make decisions when you cannot.* If you have signed a health care power of attorney stating who should speak for you if you become unable to make health care decisions for yourself, or a "living will" or "advance directive" that states your wishes about end of life care, give copies to your doctor, your family, and your care team. If you or your family need help making difficult decisions, counselors, chaplains, and others are available to help.
- *Protecting your privacy.* We respect the confidentiality of your relationship with your doctor and other caregivers, and the sensitive information about your health and health

care that are part of that relationship. State and federal laws and hospital operating policies protect the privacy of your medical information. You will receive a Notice of Privacy Practices that describes the ways that we use, disclose, and safeguard patient information and explains how you can obtain a copy of information about your care from our records about your care.

- *Preparing you and your family for your departure from the hospital.* Your doctor works with hospital staff and professionals in your community. You and your family also play an important role in your care. The success of your treatment often depends on your efforts to follow medication, diet, and therapy plans. Your family may need to help care for you at home.

- *Helping you to identify sources of follow-up care and letting you know whether our hospital has a financial interest in any referrals.* As long as you agree that we can share information about your care with them, we will coordinate our activities with your caregivers outside the hospital. You can also expect to receive information and, where possible, training about the self-care you will need when you go home.

- *Helping you with your bill and filing insurance claims.* Our staff will file claims for you with health care insurers or other programs, such as Medicare and Medicaid. They also will help your doctor with needed documentation. Hospital bills and insurance coverage often are confusing. If you have questions about your bill, contact our business office. If you need help understanding your insurance coverage or health plan, start with your insurance company or health benefits manager. If you do not have health coverage, we will try to help you and your family find financial help or make other arrangements. We need your help with collecting needed information and other requirements to obtain coverage or assistance.

While you are here, you will receive more detailed notices about some of the rights you have as a hospital patient and how to exercise them. We are always interested in improving. If you have questions, comments, or concerns, please contact _____.

Common Surgical Medications

Category	Type	Examples
Antiinfectives		
Antibiotics	Aminoglycosides	Amikacin Gentamicin Neomycin Tobramycin
	Antiretrovirals	Didanosine Efavirenz Lamivudine Stavudine Zidovudine
	Cephalosporins	Cefotaxime Cefoxitin Ceftriaxone Cefuroxime
	Fluoroquinolones	Ciprofloxacin Gemifloxacin Levofloxacin
	Lincosamines, vancomycin, ketolides	Clindamycin Vancomycin Telithromycin
	Macrolides	Azithromycin Clarithromycin Erythromycin
	Penicillins	Amoxicillin Ampicillin Penicillin G Penicillin V Piperacillin Ticarcillin
	Sulfonamides	Sulfadiazine Sulfamethoxazole and trimethoprim Sulfisoxazole
	Tetracyclines	Doxycycline Minocycline Tetracycline Tigecycline
Antiviral	Antiretroviral	Didanosine Efavirenz Lamivudine Stavudine Zidovudine
Antifungal	Systemic	Amphotericin Anidulafungin Caspofungin Micafungin

Category	Type	Examples
Blood		
Blood Derivatives	—	Whole blood
		Packed red cells
		Leukoreduced red blood cells
		Frozen-thawed red cells
		Platelet concentrate
		Fresh frozen plasma
		Cryoprecipitate
		Factor IX prothrombin concentrate
		Granulocyte concentrate
Anticoagulants	Heparins	Unfractionated heparin
		Low-molecular-weight heparin
		Warfarin (Coumadin)
	Thrombolytics	Recombinant tissue plasminogen activator
		Urokinase
Coagulants		Topical thrombin
Central Nervous System Agents		
General Anesthetics	Inhalation	Nitrous oxide
		Isoflurane
		Sevoflurane
		Desflurane
		Enflurane
	Dissociative	Ketamine
Analgesics	Opiates	Morphine
		Codeine
		Hydromorphone
		Hydrocodone
		Oxycodone
		Oxymorphone
	Nonopiates	Ibuprofen (antiinflammatory)
		Diclofenac (antiinflammatory)
		Acetaminophen
Sedatives/Hypnotics	Intravenous	Propofol
		Etomidate
		Dexmedetomidine
	Barbiturates	Thiopental
		Methohexital
	Benzodiazepines	Midazolam
		Lorazepam
		Alprazolam
		Diazepam
Neuromuscular Blocking	Depolarizing	Succinylcholine
	Nondepolarizing	Atracurium
		Cisatracurium
		Pancuronium
		Rocuronium
		Vecuronium
Diagnostic Agents		
Contrast Media	Iodinated	Diatrizoate
		Metrizoate
	Paramagnetic	Gadoxetate disodium
		Gadopentetate dimeglumine
		Gadobenate dimeglumine

Continued

Category	Type	Examples
Electrolyte and Fluid Balance		
Crystalloids	Normal saline—0.9% sodium chloride	
	Lactated Ringer solution	
	PlasmaLyte (balanced crystalloid)	
	Dextrose 0.5% in water (D5W)	
Electrolytes/Solutes	Sodium	
	Potassium	
	Calcium	
	Magnesium	
	Chloride	
	Lactate	
	Bicarbonate	
	Gluconate	
Colloids	Albumin	
	Hydroxyethyl starches	
	Gelatins	
	Dextran	
Diuretics	Acetazolamide	
	Bumetanide	
	Furosemide	
	Hydrochlorothiazide	
	Indapamide hemihydrate	
	Amiloride HCl (potassium-sparing)	
	Spironolactone (potassium-sparing)	
Local Anesthetics		
Injectable	Procaine	
	Chloroprocaine	
	Lidocaine	
	Mepivacaine	
	Prilocaine	
	Bupivacaine	
	Ropivacaine	
Topical	Benzocaine	
	Cocaine	
	Dibucaine	
	Lidocaine	
	Tetracaine	
Gastrointestinal Drugs		
Histamine-2 Receptor	Cimetidine	
	Famotidine	
	Ranitidine	
Gastric Proton Pump Inhibitors	Lansoprazole	
	Omeprazole	
	Rabeprazole	
	Pantoprazole	
	Esomeprazole	
Antiemetics	Dolasetron	
	Droperidol	
	Granisetron	
	Metoclopramide	
	Ondansetron	
Obstetrical Drugs		
Oxytocics	Carboprost	
	Dinoprostone	
	Oxytocin	
	Syntometrine	
	Ergometrine	

Category	Type	Examples
Corticosteroids		
Corticosteroids	Dexamethasone	
	Prednisone	
	Betamethasone	
Cardiac Drugs		
Antianginals	Amlodipine	
	Atenolol	
	Diltiazem	
	Isosorbide	
	Nifedipine	
	Nitroglycerin	
	Propranolol	
	Verapamil	
Antiarrhythmics	Adenosine	
	Amiodarone	
	Atropine	
	Digoxin	
	Esmolol	
	Isoproterenol	
	Lidocaine	
	Procainamide	
	Quinidine	
	Verapamil	
Antihypertensives	Amlodipine	
	Candesartan	
	Captopril	
	Doxazosin	
	Felodipine	
	Lisinopril	
	Losartan	
	Nitroprusside	
Inotropics	Dobutamine	
	Dopamine	
	Digoxin	
	Epinephrine	
	Milrinone	
Vasodilators	Ambrisentan	
	Bosentan	
	Iloprost	
	Nesiritide	
	Nimodipine	
	Sildenafil	
Hemostatic Devices (Hemostasis)		
Gelatin Sponge	Gelfoam	
	Surgifoam	
Collagen Powder	Avitene	
	EndoAvetine	
	Instat MCH	
Oxidized Cellulose	Surgicel gauze or sponge tuft	
Fibrin Combination Sealant	Tisseel	
	Floseal	
	Surgiflow	
	CrossSeal	
	Omnex	
	CoSeal	
	Dermabond	

Continued

Category	Type	Examples
Other	Platelet gel	
	Ostene bone putty	
	BioGlue	
Dyes and Stains		
	Gentian violet	
	Methylene blue	
	Indigo carmine	
	Lugol solution	
Chemotherapeutic Agents		
Intravesical	Doxorubicin	
	Epirubicin	
	Thiotepa	
	Mitomycin	
	Interferon	
	Gemcitabine	

Medications Used During Ophthalmic Surgery

Drug/Brand Name	Description/Uses
Mydriatics (Drugs that dilate the pupil but permit focusing)	
Phenylephrine (Neo-Synephrine, Mydfrin), 2.5%, 10%	Objective examination of the retina, testing of refraction, and easier removal of lenses; mydriatics may be used alone or with a cycloplegic drug.
Cycloplegics (Drugs that paralyze accommodation and inhibit focusing)	
Tropicamide (Mydriacyl), 1%	Anticholinergic, dilation of the pupil, examination of the fundus, and refraction.
Atropine, 1%	Dilates the pupil, inhibits focusing; anticholinergic, potent, and has a long duration of action (7 to 14 days).
Cyclopentolate (Cyclogyl), 1%, 2%	Anticholinergic; dilates the pupil, inhibits focusing.
Scopolamine hydrobromide (Isopto Hyoscine), 0.25%	Anticholinergic; dilates the pupil, inhibits focusing.
Homatropine hydrobromide (Isopto Homatropine), 2%, 5%	Anticholinergic; dilates the pupil, inhibits focusing.
Epinephrine (1:1,000) preservative free (PF)	Dilates the pupil; added to bottles of balanced salt solution (BSS) for irrigation to maintain pupil dilation during cataract surgery or vitrectomy.
Miotics	
Carbachol (Miostat), 0.01%	Potent cholinergic; constricts the pupil, used intraocularly during anterior segment surgery.
Carbachol (Isopto Carbachol), 0.75%, 1.5%, 2.25%, 3%	Potent cholinergic; constricts the pupil, used topically to reduce intraocular pressure (IOP) in glaucoma.
Acetylcholine chloride (Miochol-E), 1%	Cholinergic; rapidly constricts the pupil, used intraocularly during anterior segment surgery; reconstitute immediately before using.
Pilocarpine hydrochloride, 1%, 4%	Cholinergic; constricts the pupil, used topically to lower IOP in glaucoma.
Topical Anesthetics	
Tetracaine hydrochloride (Pontocaine), 0.05%	*Onset:* 5-20 s *Duration of action:* 10-20 min
Proparacaine hydrochloride (Ophthaine), 0.05%	*Onset:* 5-20 s *Duration of action:* 10-20 min
Injectable Anesthetics	
Lidocaine (Xylocaine), 1%, 2%, 4%	*Onset:* 4-6 min *Duration of action:* 40-60 min, 120 min with epinephrine
Methylparaben free (MPF)	Preservative free; adjunct to topical anesthetic.

Medications Used During Ophthalmic Surgery—cont'd

Drug/Brand Name	Description/Uses
Bupivacaine (Marcaine, Sensorcaine), 0.25%, 0.50%, 0.75%	*Onset:* 5-11 min *Duration of action:* 8-12 hr with epinephrine; often used in 0.75% strength in combination with lidocaine for blocks
Mepivacaine (Carbocaine), 1%, 2%	*Onset:* 3-5 min *Duration of action:* 2 hr (longer with epinephrine)
Etidocaine (Duranest), 1%	*Onset:* 3 min *Duration of action:* 5-10 hr

Additives to Local Anesthetics

Epinephrine, 1:50,000 to 1:200,000	Combined with injectable local anesthetics to prolong anesthesia and reduce bleeding.
Hyaluronidase	Enzyme mixed with anesthetics (75 units per 10 mL) to increase diffusion of anesthetic through tissue, improving the effectiveness of the block; contraindicated if skin inflammation or malignancy is present.

Viscoelastics

Sodium hyaluronate (Healon, Amvisc, Provisc, Vitrax) in a sterile syringe assembly with blunt-tip cannula	Lubricant and support; maintains separation between tissues to protect the endothelium and maintain the anterior chamber intraocularly; removed from anterior chamber to prevent postoperative increase in pressure; should be refrigerated (except Vitrax); allow 30 min to warm to room temperature.
Sodium chondroitin–sodium hyaluronate (Viscoat) in a sterile syringe assembly with blunt-tip cannula	Maintains deep chamber for anterior segment procedures, protects epithelium of cornea, and improves visualization; may be used to coat intraocular lens before implantation; should be refrigerated.
Duovisc	Packages of separate syringes of Provisc and Viscoat in the same box.

Viscoadherents

Hydroxypropyl methylcellulose 2% (Ocucoat) in a sterile syringe assembly with blunt-tip cannula	Maintains a deep chamber for anterior segment procedures, protects epithelium of cornea, and may be used to coat intraocular lens before implantation; removed from anterior chamber at end of procedure; stored at room temperature.
Hydroxyethylcellulose (Gonioscopic Prism Solution)	Bonds gonioscopic prisms to the eye; stored at room temperature.
Hydroxypropyl methylcellulose 2.5% (Goniosol)	Bonds gonioscopic prisms to the eye; stored at room temperature.

Irrigants

Balanced salt solution (BSS, Endosol)	Used to keep the cornea moist during surgery; also used as an internal irrigant in the anterior or posterior segment.
BSS enriched with bicarbonate, dextrose, and glutathione (BSS Plus, Endosol Extra)	Used as an internal irrigant in the anterior or posterior segment; must be reconstituted immediately before use by adding part I to part II with the transfer device.

Hyperosmotic Agents

Mannitol (Osmitrol)	Intravenous (IV) osmotic diuretic; increases the osmolarity of the plasma, causing the osmotic pressure gradient to pull free fluid from the eye into the plasma, thereby reducing the IOP.
Glycerin (Osmoglyn, Glyrol)	Oral osmotic diuretic given in chilled juice or cola; increases the osmolarity of the plasma, causing the osmotic pressure gradient to pull free fluid from the eye into the plasma, thereby reducing the IOP.

Antiinflammatory Agents

Betamethasone sodium phosphate and betamethasone acetate suspension (Celestone)	Glucocorticoid; injected subconjunctivally after surgery for prophylaxis; also used to treat severe allergic and inflammatory conditions.
Dexamethasone (Decadron)	Adrenocorticosteroid; injected subconjunctivally after surgery for prophylaxis; also used to treat severe allergic and inflammatory conditions and intraocularly for endophthalmitis.
Methylprednisolone acetate suspension (Depo-Medrol)	Glucocorticoid; injected subconjunctivally after surgery for prophylaxis; also used to treat severe allergic and inflammatory conditions.

Continued

Medications Used During Ophthalmic Surgery—cont'd

Drug/Brand Name	Description/Uses
Antiinfective Drugs	
Polymyxin B/bacitracin (Polysporin ointment)	Topical treatment of superficial ocular infections of the conjunctiva or cornea; also used prophylactically after surgery.
Polymyxin B/neomycin/bacitracin (Neosporin ointment)	Topical treatment of superficial infections of the external eye; used prophylactically after surgery; hypersensitivity to neomycin is possible.
Neomycin and polymyxin B sulfates and dexamethasone (Maxitrol ointment or suspension)	Topical treatment of steroid-responsive inflammatory ocular conditions or bacterial infections of the external eye; hypersensitivity to neomycin is possible.
Tobramycin/dexamethasone (TobraDex)	Topical treatment or prevention of superficial infections of the external part of the eye; also has antiinflammatory properties.
Cefazolin (Ancef, Kefzol)	Injected subconjunctivally for prophylaxis after eye procedures; also used topically, intraocularly, and systematically for endophthalmitis.
Gentamicin sulfate (Garamycin)	Injected subconjunctivally for prophylaxis after eye procedures; also used topically, subconjunctivally, and intraocularly for endophthalmitis.
Ceftazidime (Fortaz, Tazicef, Tazidime)	Injected subconjunctivally and intraocularly for the treatment of endophthalmitis.
Other Drugs	
Cocaine, 1% to 4%	Used topically only, never injected; used on cornea to loosen epithelium before debridement and on nasal packing to reduce congestion of mucosa.
5-Fluorouracil (5-FU)	Antimetabolite used topically to inhibit scar formation in glaucoma-filtering procedures; handle and discard in compliance with the regulations of the Occupational Safety and Health Administration (OSHA) and health care facility's policies for safe use of antineoplastics.
Mitomycin (Mutamycin)	Antimetabolite used topically to inhibit scar formation in glaucoma-filtering procedures and pterygium excision; handle and discard in compliance with OSHA's and health care facility's policies for safe use of antineoplastics.
Tissue plasminogen activator (TPA) (Activase)	Thrombolytic agent; used for the treatment of fibrin formation in patients who have had vitrectomy and for the lysis of clots on the retina.
Fluorescein	*IV diagnostic aid:* Used in fluorescein angiography to diagnose retinal disorders. *Topical stain:* Fluorescein strip temporarily stains the cornea yellow-green in areas of denuded corneal epithelium.
Timolol maleate (Timoptic)	Beta-adrenergic receptor blocking agent; used in the treatment of elevated IOP in ocular hypertension or open angle glaucoma.
Acetazolamide sodium (Diamox)	Carbonic anhydrase inhibitor; given IV to reduce the secretion of aqueous humor, resulting in a drop in IOP; also has a diuretic effect.
Dextrose, 50%	Added to BSS, Endosol, BSS Plus, or Endosol Extra for diabetic patients during intraocular procedures.

From Rothrock JC: *Alexander's care of the patient in surgery,* ed 13, St Louis, 2007, Mosby.

Contents of Crash Cart

Gloves
Cutdown tray
Kerlix
Syringes
Povidone-iodine solution and swabs
Intravenous (IV) tubing
Cardiac monitor/defibrillator
Sharps container
Ambu bag with mask
Cardiac board (backboard)
Oxygen compressed cylinder with gauge
Nasopharyngeal airways
Oropharyngeal airways
Endotracheal tubes with stylet
Laryngoscope handle and McGill forceps
Assortment of laryngoscope blades
CO_2 detector
50% dextrose injection USP 25 g (0.5 g/mL)
98.4% sodium bicarbonate injection
USEP 50 mEq (1 mEq/mL)

Sodium bicarbonate 10-mEq syringe (pediatrics)
Atropine 0.5 mg/5 mL-syringe
Lidocaine 50 mg/5 mL-syringe
2 g lidocaine (8 mg/mL)
2% lidocaine HCl injection USP 100 mg/5 mL
Epinephrine injection 1:10,000, 1 mg (0.1 mg/mL)
400 mg dopamine
0.9% sodium chloride injection 10 mL
Pressure cuff
Blood pressure cuff
Suction catheter kit
Tourniquet
Butterfly catheter
Spinal needles
Small dressings
IV catheters
Tape
Three-way stopcock
Assorted needles

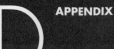

NOTE: Infectious disease organisms are discussed in Chapter 9. Pathology associated with surgical treatment is discussed by system in their respective chapters.

Skin and Superficial Tissues

Basal cell carcinoma	Slow-growing neoplasm of the skin related to excessive exposure to ultraviolet light.
Cellulitis	Bacterial infection of superficial tissues, especially in immunocompromised patients.
Chemical injury	Burn caused by strong alkaline or acidic chemicals; results in tissue necrosis and liquefaction.
Cold thermal injury	Tissue necrosis related to prolonged exposure to freezing temperature.
Electrical injury	Trauma related to electrical systems, lightning, or electrical devices. May result in paralysis, cardiopulmonary arrest, and burns.
Keratosis	Hornlike skin lesion related to excessive exposure to ultraviolet light.
Melanoma	Rapidly growing, potentially metastatic neoplasm originating in the melanocyte of the skin.
Nevus	Circumscribed pigmented lesion of the skin or connective tissue, usually congenital. May be a cancerous precursor lesion.
Squamous cell carcinoma	Neoplasm of the squamous cells.

Skeletal System and Connective Tissues

Ankylosing spondylitis	Inflammatory arthritic condition associated with other inflammatory diseases such as inflammatory bowel disease, psoriasis, and rheumatoid disease.
Avascular necrosis	Infarction of bone and marrow tissue resulting in ischemia and necrosis; may be idiopathic or related to trauma.
Bursitis	Inflammation of the joint capsule related to disease or injury.
Carpal tunnel syndrome	Inflammation of the medial tendon sheath related to overuse or repetitive use.
Cyst	Fluid-filled sac encapsulated by a membrane.
Fibromyalgia	Condition of widespread pain located in "tender points" that can be elicited by digital compression.
Gout	A disease caused by deposition of monosodium urate in the tissue related to hyperuricemia. The disease results in arthritis and soft tissue inflammation.
Infectious arthritis	Acute bacterial infection of a joint space. Most commonly affects the knee; usually caused by *Staphylococcus aureus* infection.
Marfan syndrome	Inherited connective tissue disease that may affect numerous body systems. Manifestation depends on which system is affected.
Myasthenia gravis	Autoimmune disorder resulting in extreme muscle weakness. May affect any muscle of the body.
Muscular dystrophy	Genetic disorder resulting in progressive muscle weakness and degeneration.
Osteomalacia	Extreme softening of the bones resulting in deformity. May be due to vitamin D deficiency or other disease process.
Paget disease	Inherited chronic disease of the axial skeleton that results in bone destruction and disorders of the osteoblast cells. The cause is unknown.
Degenerative disc	Condition in which fibrocartilage or softer nucleus of the intervertebral disc is damaged through the aging process, injury, or disease, resulting in degeneration of the tissues and instability of the spine.
Pectus carinatum	Congenital deformity of the chest wall most commonly resulting in protrusion of the upper sternum and depression of the lower anterolateral chest wall.

Pectus excavatum	Congenital deformity of the chest wall resulting in depression of the sternum that may restrict breathing.
Radial dysplasia	Historical term for *radial longitudinal deficiency*. The condition results in a shortened forearm with radial deviation and is associated with other systemic diseases.
Rheumatoid arthritis	Inflammatory autoimmune disorder affecting the joints. The disease tends to be progressive and affects other body systems.
Rickets	Nutritional disease related to deficiency of calcium phosphate, or vitamin D.
Talipes equinovarus	Congenital deformity involving the calcaneotalar-navicular complex of the foot.

Diseases of the Nervous System

Astrocytoma	Tumor of the astrocyte cells occurring in the brain or spinal cord; may become rapidly malignant.
Arteriovenous malformation	In the nervous system, refers to abnormal connection between arteries and veins without capillaries. The cause is unknown.
Cerebral palsy	Term used to describe a large group of disorders caused by disturbances in fetal development. May present as problems of development, orthopedic deformity, perception, and cognition.
Glioma	Tumor of the neuroglial cells arising from the brain or spinal cord.
Meningioma	Slow-growing tumor arising from the arachnoid cells of the arachnoid villi; most are benign.
Parkinson disease	Degenerative disease of the extrapyramidal dopaminergic system. The disease is characterized by four main signs: tremor, rigidity, akinesia (loss of muscle movement), and postural problems.
Seizure disorder (epilepsy)	Electrical disturbance in brain activity resulting in unprovoked seizures. There are many causes.
Encephalitis	General term meaning inflammation of the brain.

Ear, Nose, and Throat

Choanal atresia	Congenital stricture of the choana.
Infection	The most common infections are otitis externa (swimmer's ear) and atopic dermatitis. Other causes can be viruses and fungi.
Infection/inflammation	Infections of the nose may be caused by bacteria or fungi. The most common causes of inflammation of the nose are allergies and nasal polyps.
Polyp	Lobular growth on mucous membrane tissue of the same tissue origin.
Laryngitis	Inflammation of the larynx; a symptom of many different diseases affecting the throat.
Mastoiditis	Infection of the mastoid cavity; may be associated with severe otitis media. With the introduction of modern antibiotics, the condition is rarely seen in developed countries.
Meniere disease	The cause of Meniere disease is unknown. It is characterized by recurrent vertigo (dizziness) that lasts several hours, sensorineural hearing loss at low frequency, and ringing in the ears (tinnitus).
Nonmalignant tumor	Nonmalignant tumors include juvenile nasal angiofibroma and inverting papilloma. Although these are not cancerous, they can cause nasal obstruction.
Otitis externa	Superficial infection of the outer ear.
Otitis media	Infection of the middle ear. May be acute or chronic. It is more common in childhood, especially when children are exposed to cigarette smoke and other air pollutants.
Ruptured tympanic membrane	Tear or puncture of the tympanic membrane usually associated with infection of the middle ear.
Sinusitis	Inflammation or infection of the air cavities of the nose and face.
Vertigo	A sensation of dizziness.
Tinnitus	Ringing or other sounds in the ear; may be idiopathic or symptomatic of a number of ear diseases.
Trauma	Injury to the external ear can result in avulsion of the ear or hematoma.

The Eye

Conjunctivitis	Inflammation of the conjunctiva related to infection or allergy.
Glaucoma	A group of diseases related to increased intraocular pressure and damage to the optic nerve. Increased pressure may be due to blockage of aqueous humor circulation or drainage.
Cataract	Opacity of the lens of the eye usually related to aging process.
Macular degeneration	Age-related complex degeneration of the photoreceptors, retinal pigment epithelium, and choriocapillaris of the eye, leading to blindness.

Continued

Cardiovascular

Aneurysm	Outpocketing or ballooning of an artery or heart chamber in an area weakened by disease or congenital defect. The aneurysm may continue to progress, growing larger until it ruptures.
Angina	Chest pain associated with blockage of the coronary artery, most commonly due to arteriosclerosis. Blockage results in ischemia of the heart muscle and pain. Occurs most commonly on exertion.
Arteriosclerosis	A group of vascular diseases characterized by hardening and stiffening of the arteries caused by calcium deposits and fatty substances in the arterial wall. The disease is related to age, smoking, diabetes, and hypertension.
Atherosclerosis	The most common form of arteriosclerosis; an obstructive disease of the arteries in which the vessels are infiltrated with calcium and fatty fibrous deposits, causing reduced elasticity as well as obstruction and ischemia. Risk factors include smoking, a high-fat diet, obesity, and inactivity.
Cardiac fibrillation	Ineffective quivering or uncoordinated movement of the heart muscle rather than normal regular contraction of the atria and ventricles.
Congestive heart failure	Failure of the heart to pump related to cardiac tissue damage or disease. Right heart failure results in inability to pump blood into the pulmonary circulation, causing peripheral edema and congestion of the abdominal viscera. Left heart failure causes blood to back up into the pulmonary circulation with overload.
Coronary artery disease	Arteriosclerosis of the coronary arteries leading to cardiac ischemia.
Embolus	A moving vascular obstruction—usually a blood clot, but may also be a fat globule, plaque, air, or foreign body.
Endocarditis	Inflammation or infection of the endocardium lining the heart chambers.
Gangrene	Tissue necrosis as a result of ischemia and loss of oxygen to the tissue. Dry gangrene is not related to bacterial infection.
Heart block	Damage or disease of the conduction cells of the heart resulting in inability to initiate or sustain electrical activity necessary for contraction of the muscle. Heart block may be partial or complete.
Intermittent claudication	Not a disease, but a symptom—intermittent muscle pain on exertion related to arteriosclerosis. The pain is relieved with rest.
Mitral stenosis	Hardening and malfunction of the mitral valve.
Murmur	Not a disease, but a sign of valvular disorder that can be detected on auscultation.
Myocardial infarction	Necrosis of heart muscle due to ischemia (lack of blood supply and therefore oxygen); often associated with coronary artery disease.
Myocarditis	Inflammation or infection of the heart muscle.
Pericarditis	Inflammation or infection of the pericardium surrounding the heart.
Raynaud syndrome	Spasm of the blood vessels of the fingers and toes in a cold environment or during stress, resulting in blanching of the skin. The condition is often idiopathic (no known cause).
Rheumatic heart disease	An acute manifestation of the streptococcal disease rheumatic fever that becomes chronic over time. Rheumatic heart disease usually affects the heart valves, causing deformities and malfunction.
Thrombophlebitis	The presence of a thrombus in a superficial or deep vein with accompanying inflammation.
Thrombus	A stationary blood clot or other obstruction in the vascular system.
Atelectasis	Condition in which the lung alveoli remain collapsed because of hypoxia related to trauma or because of disease.

Blood and Lymph

Anemia	Deficiency of red cells or hemoglobin related to excessive blood loss or destruction (hemolytic anemia).
Aplastic anemia	Bone marrow depression related to stem cell disease and loss of blood cells, white blood cells, and platelets.
Polycythemia	Abnormally high total red blood cell mass with hematocrit greater than 55%.
Leukemia	Cancer of the hematopoietic stem cells.
Hodgkin disease	Malignant lymphoma; cancer of the lymph system and structures.

Respiratory System

Chronic obstructive pulmonary disease	Inflammatory disease of the respiratory system caused by exposure to cigarette smoke. Main features of the disease are airflow limitation, chronic airway irritation, mucus production, and airway scarring.
Cystic fibrosis	Genetic disorder affecting multiple systems, including dehydrated secretions in the pulmonary system, pancreas, liver, and intestinal tract requiring long-term care.
Atelectasis	Collapse of all or part of the lung.
Aspiration	Inhalation of an object, particle, or liquid into the airway.
Pulmonary embolus	An embolus that has entered the respiratory circulation with potential to cause death due to ischemia and necrosis of lung tissue.
Bronchitis	Inflammation of the bronchi.
Empyema	Suppurative infection in the lung; lung abscess.
Pneumothorax	Positive pressure in the pleural cavity due to presence of air.
Pleuritis	Inflammation or infection of the pleural sac.
Pulmonary effusion	Not a disease but a symptom—accumulation of fluid in the pleural space. There are multiple causes related to disease or trauma.

Gastrointestinal System

Salivary gland disorders	These include salivary gland stones, infection, and neoplasms of the glands.
Sjögren syndrome	Inflammatory disease that may affect the functioning of the salivary glands.
Esophageal atresia	Narrowing or stricture of the esophagus due to congenital defect or disease.
Esophageal varices	Engorged veins of the esophagus as a result of blood that has backed up from the hepatic circulation.
Fistula	A tract, usually congenital in origin, that penetrates the esophagus and emerges outside the organ.
Hiatal hernia	Herniation of a portion of the stomach at the juncture with the diaphragm, allowing the stomach to slide partially into the thoracic cavity.
Pyloric stenosis	Congenital defect involving thickened bands of muscle tissue at the pyloric sphincter that prevent nutritional intake.
Peptic ulcer disease	Ulceration of the stomach or duodenum is mainly caused by *Helicobacter pylori* bacteria and ingestion of noxious substances.
Diverticular disease	Abnormal outpockets within the intestinal lining that trap material and become infected.
Inflammatory bowel disease	Multiple inflammatory pathologies arising from the large and small intestines. Many are related to autoimmunity.
Intussusception	Telescoping of bowel tissue, usually in a child, leading to obstruction. If undetected, can cause ischemia and necrosis.
Obstruction	Any condition of the bowel that creates a physical obstruction of bowel contents or causes bowel tissue to lose peristaltic tone.
Volvulus	Twisted or looped section of bowel leading to obstruction and necrosis.
Nutritional/psychiatric diseases	Anorexia and bulimia nervosa are two disorders found only in Western society in which the individual refuses food and purges the body of nutrition to the point of death.
Celiac disease	Inflammatory condition of the small intestine related to ingestion of wheat, rye, and barley, associated with genetic factors.
Crohn disease	Inflammatory and ulcerative condition of the small intestine related to genetic predisposition.

Liver, Pancreas, and Spleen

Cholecystitis	Inflammation or infection of the gallbladder.
Cholelithiasis	Presence of gallstones in the bile ducts or gallbladder.
Cirrhosis	Disease of the liver in which the tissue becomes sclerotic and inflamed and ceases to function normally.
Cirrhosis and portal hypertension	End-stage alcoholic liver disease is characterized by fibrosis of the liver, which prevents the flow of blood and bile. Blood backs up into the portal vein, causing congestion and rupture of the esophageal venous plexus.

Continued

Diabetes type 1	Autoimmune disease resulting in destruction of insulin-producing cells in the pancreas and alterations in normal carbohydrate metabolism.
Diabetes type 2	Acquired disease in which there is relative resistance to insulin and dysfunction of the beta cells in the pancreas.
Pancreatitis	Inflammatory disease of the pancreas and peripancreatic fat that often results in tissue fibrosis and necrosis. Chronic pancreatitis is most commonly associated with alcohol abuse or biliary disease.
Portal hypertension	Impaired hepatic circulation due to sclerosis of the liver sinusoids, causing blood to back up in to the digestive tract.

Endocrine Disorders

Hyperadrenalism (Cushing disease)	Disorder in which excessive glucocorticoid is produced, related to pituitary adenoma secreting adrenocorticotropic hormone.
Hypoadrenalism (Addison disease)	Disease of adrenal insufficiency as a result of bilateral destruction of the adrenal cortex, usually as a result of autoimmune causes.
Hyperparathyroidism	Abnormally high production of parathyroid hormone, which regulates calcium and phosphorus in the body.
Thyroid nodule	Usually benign. May be related to iodine deficiency or cystic condition of the thyroid.
Hyperthyroidism (Graves disease)	Autoimmune disease resulting in multinodular thyroid gland and excessive production of thyroid hormone.
Hypothyroidism (Hashimoto disease)	Hypothyroidism may be congenital or acquired. Thyroid hormone is essential for brain development in the fetus. In adults, hypothyroidism is caused by thyroidectomy or radiation of the thyroid for cancer treatment.

Female Reproductive System

Abnormal uterine bleeding	Uterine bleeding that occurs at irregular intervals. Note: The term *dysfunctional uterine bleeding* is no longer used.
Cystocele	Herniation of the bladder into the anterior vaginal wall, usually related to multiple childbirths and weakening of the vaginal tissue.
Endometriosis	Presence of endometrial tissue in locations of the body other than the uterine lining. The tissue remains under hormonal control and may bleed and become painful.
Fibrocystic disease	Usually refers to the breast, in which one or more cysts can develop within the connective tissue. Polycystic disease refers to ovarian cysts.
Leiomyoma	Benign tumor of the myometrium.
Menorrhagia	Regular menstrual bleeding but excessive flow.
Pelvic inflammatory disease	Refers to an infectious process. Usually related to *Chlamydia* but may also be caused by any other sexually transmitted disease.
Rectocele	Herniation of the rectal wall into the posterior vaginal wall. Usually related to multiple childbirths and weakening of the vaginal tissue.

Obstetrical Complications

Abruptio placentae	Premature separation of the placenta from the uterine wall, often related to high blood pressure during pregnancy.
Breech presentation	Occurs when the baby's feet, knees, or buttocks are delivered ahead of the rest of the body.
Cephalopelvic disproportion	Occurs when the mother's birth canal is too small or the baby is too large for delivery.
Ectopic pregnancy	Implantation of the fertilized ovum occurring outside the uterus, usually in the fallopian tube.
Nuchal cord	Condition in which the umbilical cord is wrapped one or more times around the baby's neck, with risk of compression of the cord against the birth canal.
Spontaneous abortion	Loss of pregnancy before the 20th week of gestation.
Preeclampsia	Hypertension during pregnancy that contributes to high risk for the woman and fetus.

Male Reproductive System

Balanitis and balanoposthitis	Inflammation of the glans or foreskin; may be related to infection.
Benign prostatic hypertrophy	Enlargement of the prostate gland, usually with age. Although benign, may cause voiding problems.
Cryptorchidism	Undescended testicle in the child or adult usually related to congenital defect. May result in sterility if left untreated.

Epispadias	Rare congenital defect in which the anterior urethra is incompletely developed, resulting in a meatus located on the ventral side of the penis or in other locations depending on the extent of the defect.
Hypospadias	Congenital defect in which the external urethral meatus is located on the ventral side of the penis; accompanied by stricture.
Erectile dysfunction	Inability to achieve or maintain erectile function of the penis. May be related to many different causes, including functional, medical, and emotional origins.
Hydrocele	Fluid-filled sac arising in the layers of the tunica vaginalis of the testicle, often related to inguinal hernia or other inguinal defect.
Orchitis	Inflammation or infection of the testicle.
Phimosis, paraphimosis	Tightness in the prepuce preventing retraction over the glans or return to its normal position. May be related to infection or scarring.
Prostatitis	Inflammation or infection of the prostate gland.
Spermatocele	Fluid-filled cyst at the spermatic cord.
Testicular torsion	Twisting of the testicle on itself resulting in ischemia and necrosis. The condition usually occurs as a sports injury but may have underlying structural causes.
Varicocele	Abnormal dilation of the testicular blood vessels.

Urogenital System

Calculi (stones)	Stones are formed by crystalline minerals and salts precipitated from filtrate produced in the kidney.
Cancer of the kidney	Primary cancer of the kidney arises from the cortex and renal pelvis. The greatest risk factor is smoking.
Cystic kidney disease	Renal cysts originate in the nephron as a result of obstruction. Fluid-filled cysts impinge on vascular structures, causing loss of kidney function. Cystic disease may be acquired or congenital. Polycystic disease is hereditary and has no treatment.
Cystitis	Infection of the urinary bladder.
Urinary reflux	Backward flow of urine or filtrate in the renal system.
End-stage renal disease	Renal failure that cannot be reversed. It has many causes, including diabetes, hypertension, systemic lupus erythematosus, nephrotic syndrome, and infection (ingestion of *Escherichia coli* is a common cause of renal failure).
Polycystic disease	Inherited disease in which fluid-filled cysts replace normal kidney tissue.
Glomerulonephritis	Kidney infection and autoimmune disorders may affect any part of the nephron and glomerulus. Glomerulonephritis is a general term rather than a specific disease.
Hydronephrosis	Distention and loss of function of the ureter or renal pelvis related to urinary reflux (backward movement of urine) caused by obstruction such as a stricture, stone, or tumor.
Trauma to the kidney	Injury to the kidney is usually caused by a blow to the flank or back. Most commonly occurs during contact sports or as a result of intentional violence.
Wilms tumor (nephroblastoma)	The most common tumors in children—arising in the kidney.
Addison disease	Adrenal insufficiency. A rare disorder with many different causes, including autoimmune disease and certain tumors.
Cushing syndrome	Overproduction of glucocorticoid, which is secreted by the adrenal glands; the condition can be related to several pathological conditions of the pituitary gland, an adrenal tumor, or other tumors.
Cancer of the bladder	The most common form of urinary tract cancer; tumors are derived from the bladder lining.
Neurogenic bladder disorder	General term that refers to pathogenic loss of bladder function related to neurological damage. Common causes are spinal cord injury, cerebrovascular accident, brain lesion, peripheral nerve disease, and infection.
Trauma to the bladder	Traumatic injury to the bladder occurs most often in motor vehicle accidents and is related to pelvic fracture.
Urinary incontinence	The most common cause of urinary incontinence is loss of sphincter control at the bladder neck. This may be related to multiple childbirths or advancing age. Hypertrophy of the prostate also causes involuntary loss of urine.

Continued

Urinary retention	Retention of urine related to medical or psychological problem.
Urinary tract infection (UTI)	Infection of the lower urinary tract. It is commonly caused by *E. coli* contamination of the distal urethra or by a sexually transmitted disease. Chronic UTIs may result in scarring of the urethra that requires surgery.

Genetic Disorders

Achondroplasia	Deficiency of growth hormone resulting in short stature but normal body proportions.
Marfan syndrome	See Skeletal System and Connective Tissues.
Albinism	Inherited condition of melanin production resulting in little or no pigment in the skin, eyes, or hair.
Phenylketonuria	Inherited metabolic defect in which a baby is born without the ability to break down phenylalanine, an essential amino acid.
Sickle cell disorder	Inherited disorder of the blood cells in which healthy red blood cells are replaced with more fragile sickle-shaped cells, which carry less oxygen and may cause vessel blockages.
Tay-Sachs disease	A congenital defect of chromosome 15 that results in inability to produce hexosaminidase A, which helps break down gangliosides in nerve cells. The condition is usually fatal.
Down syndrome	Genetic condition in which a person has 47 rather than the normal 46 chromosomes. The condition is accompanied by many defects including developmental delay, structural deformity, and delayed mental and social development.
Developmental disorder	Any physical or mental condition that results in delay or arrest of normal physical, social, or mental development.

Glossary

Abandonment: A health professional's failure to stay with a patient and provide care, especially when there is an implied contract to do so.

Abdominal peritoneum: The serous membrane lining the walls of the abdominal cavity. The retroperitoneum is the posterior aspect. In surgical discussions, abdominal usually refers to the anterior aspect.

Abduction: Movement of a joint or body part away from the body.

ABHES: Accrediting Bureau of Health Education Schools. Organization that offers accreditation to higher education institutions.

Ablate: To remove or destroy tissue.

Ablation: The complete destruction of tissue.

ABO blood group: Inherited antigens are found on the surface of an individual's red blood cells. These antigens identify the blood group (i.e., type A blood has type A antigens). Also known as blood type.

Absorbable suture: Suture material that is broken down and metabolized by the body.

Accommodation: A process in which the lens continually changes shape to maintain the focus of an image on the retina.

Accountability: Accepting responsibility for one's actions. In a professional context, this means that roles and actions accepted by an individual within the context of their occupation require the person to accept responsibility for the consequences of carrying out those tasks.

Accreditation (of a health care facility): The process by which a hospital or other health care facility is evaluated by an independent organization. Accredited facilities are those that meet the standards of the accreditation agency.

Acoustic neuroma: A benign tumor of the eighth cranial nerve; more accurately referred to as a *schwannoma*, because it is composed of Schwann cells, which produce myelin.

Acquired abnormality: A physiological or anatomical defect that develops in fetal life as a result of environmental factors.

ACS: American College of Surgeons. A professional organization that establishes educational standards for surgeons and surgical residency programs.

Active electrode monitoring (AEM): A method of reducing the risk of patient burns during monopolar electrosurgery. AEM systems stop the electrical current whenever resistance is high anywhere in the circuit.

Active electrode: In electrosurgery, the point of the electrosurgical instrument that delivers current to tissue.

Activities of daily living (ADLs): Basic activities and tasks necessary for day-to-day care, such as dressing, bathing, toileting, and meal preparation.

Acute illness: Sudden onset of disease or trauma or disease of short duration, usually 3 weeks or less.

Adhesion: Scar formation of the abdominal viscera.

Administration: Individuals who manage an institution, plan its activities, and provide oversight for day-to-day operations and employees. The administration is also a liaison between the facility and the community, government, and media.

Administrative laws: Laws created by an agency or a department of the U.S. government.

Adnexa: A collective term for the ovaries, fallopian tubes, and their connective and vascular attachments.

Advance directive: A document in which a person gives instructions about his or her medical care in the event that the individual cannot speak for himself or herself. Examples are a living will and a medical power of attorney.

Advance health care directive: A written document stating an individual's specific wishes regarding his or her health care to be enacted in the event the person is unable to make decisions.

Advanced Trauma Life Support (ATLS): A program established by the American College of Surgeons for protocols and training in trauma medicine.

Adverse reaction: An unexpected harmful reaction to a drug.

Aerobes: Organisms that favor an environment with oxygen. Strict aerobes cannot live without oxygen.

Aerosol droplets: Droplets of moisture small enough to remain suspended in the air; such a droplet can carry microorganisms within it.

Aesthetic surgery: Surgery that is performed to improve appearance but not function; also called *cosmetic surgery*.

Agency for Healthcare Research and Quality (AHRQ): Agency that provides disaster-related research, resources, training, and recommendations for health care facilities, communities, and individuals.

Aggression: The exertion of power over others through intimidation, sarcasm, or bullying.

Agonist: A drug that produces a response in the body by binding to a receptor.

Air exchange: The exchange of air between areas separated by a physical boundary. Standards for air exchange are regulated by health and safety organizations.

Airborne transmission precautions: Precautions that prevent airborne transfer of disease organisms in the environment.

Airway: The anatomical passageway or artificial tube through which the patient breathes.

Algorithms: Treatment pathways established to allow systematic and consistent methods of medical and surgical management.

Allergy: Hypersensitivity to a substance, a response produced by the immune system.

All-hazards approach: An integrated strategy for disaster management that focuses on the common features of all disasters, regardless of the cause or origin.

Allied health profession: A profession that follows the principles of medicine and nursing but that focuses on an expertise set apart from those practices.

Allograft: A tissue graft in which the donor and recipient are of the same species.

Alloy: A combination of several different kinds of metals. Alloys are used in the manufacture of stainless steel.

Alloys: Substances that are mixtures of pure metals.

Alternating current (AC): A type of electrical current in which electricity changes direction to complete its circuit and transmits high-voltage electricity.

AMA: American Medical Association. An association founded in 1847 made up of medical doctors whose mission is to promote healthy lifestyles across all patient populations.

American Red Cross: National organization that provides humanitarian assistance and technical support during disasters and emergencies.

Amnesia: The loss of recall of events or sensations.

Amniotic fluid: Water around the fetus in the uterus.

Amniotic membranes: Two membranes that encase the fetus, amniotic fluid, and placenta during pregnancy.

Ampere: A unit measuring the amount of energy passing a given point in a stated period of time.

Amplification: In wave science, the phenomenon of increasing wave height by lining up the peaks and troughs of individual waves.

Amplitude: In electromagnetic wave energy, the height of a wave.

Anaerobes: Organisms that prefer an oxygen-poor environment. Strict anaerobes cannot survive in the presence of oxygen.

Analgesia: The absence of pain, produced by specific drugs.

Anastomosis: The surgical creation of an opening between two blood vessels, hollow organs, or ducts.

Anesthesia: The absence of sensory awareness or medically induced unconsciousness.

Anesthesia care provider (ACP): A professional who is licensed to administer anesthetic agents and manage the patient throughout the period of anesthesia.

Anesthesia machine: A biotechnical device used to deliver anesthetic gases or volatile liquids and provide physiological monitoring.

Anesthesia technologist: An allied health professional trained to assist the anesthesia care provider.

Anesthesiologist: A physician specialist in the administration of anesthetics and pain management.

Anesthetic: A drug that reduces or blocks sensation or induces unconsciousness.

Aneurysm: A weakness in the arterial wall resulting in ballooning of the artery and possible rupture. It could be a result of injury, disease, or a congenital condition.

Angioplasty: Dilation of an artery using endovascular techniques (i.e., an arterial catheter); may include insertion of a supportive stent inside the artery to maintain blood flow.

ANSI: American National Standards Institute. Organization that creates business and health standards to serve as a baseline for assessment.

Antagonist: A drug or chemical that blocks a receptor-mediated response.

Anterograde amnesia: In anesthesia, the patient's inability to recall events that occur after the administration of specific drugs. After the drug is metabolized and cleared from the body, normal recall returns.

Antibiotics: Drugs that inhibit the growth of or kill bacteria.

Antisepsis: A process that greatly reduces the number of microorganisms on skin or other tissue.

Antiseptic: Chemical agent approved for use on the skin that inhibits the growth and reproduction of microorganisms.

Anxiolytic: A drug that reduces anxiety.

AORN: Association of periOperative Registered Nurses. The professional organization for surgical nurses; originally known as the Association of Operating Room Nurses.

Apex: The lower left tip of the left ventricle of the heart; also, the rounded upper portion of each lung.

APGAR score: Method of assessing a neonate according to respiratory rate, color, reflex response, heart rate, and body tone.

Apnea: Absence of breathing.

Aponeurosis: A tendinous sheet that separates muscles or attaches a muscle to bone.

Approximate: To bring tissue together by sutures or other means.

ARC/STSA: Accreditation Review Council on Education in Surgical Technology and Surgical Assisting. The ARC/STSA establishes, maintains, and promotes quality standards for education programs in surgical technology and surgical first assisting.

Arch bars: Metal plates wired to the teeth to occlude the jaw during maxillofacial surgery or during healing. Arch bars maintain the patient's normal bite (occlusion).

Argon: An inert gas used in electrosurgery to direct and shroud the electrical current.

Arrhythmia: An abnormal heartbeat (also called *dysrhythmia*).

Arterial blood gas test (ABGs): A blood test that determines carbon dioxide and oxygen saturation, pH, and other important parameters of respiration and oxygen perfusion.

Arteriosclerosis: A disease characterized by thickening, hardening, and loss of elasticity of the arterial wall.

Arteriosclerosis: Disease of the arteries characterized by loss of elasticity and hardening of the arterial walls.

Arteriotomy: An incision made in an artery, usually to perform an anastomosis with a graft or another artery or to remove plaque or a thrombus.

Arteriovenous fistula (or AV shunt): Surgically created vascular access for patients undergoing hemodialysis.

Arteriovenous malformation (AVM): A collection of blood vessels with abnormal communication between the arteries and veins. It may be the result of injury, infection, or congenital condition.

Arthrodesis: Surgical fusion of a joint.

Arthroscopy: Endoscopic surgery of a joint.

Asepsis: The absence of pathogenic microorganisms on an animate surface or on body tissue. Literally, *asepsis* means "without infection." In surgery, asepsis is a state of minimal or zero pathogens. Asepsis is the goal of many surgical practices.

Aseptic technique: Methods or practices in health care that reduce infection.

Aspiration: Inhalation of fluid or solid matter.

Assertiveness: Communicating one's personal and professional needs to others; protecting one's own rights while respecting those of others.

Assistant circulator: The surgical technologist in the nonsterile role of the surgical team responsible for monitoring conditions in the operating room as related to patient care, safety, documentation, distribution of sterile supplies and counts. A registered perioperative nurse in this role would be considered a circulator and will have additional responsibilities.

Association for the Advancement of Medical Instrumentation (AAMI): The AAMI is an authoritative source of standards for sterilization and disinfection.

AST: Association of Surgical Technologists. The professional association for surgical technologists (website: http://www.ast.org).

Astrocytes: Cells that support the nerve cells (neurons) of the brain and spinal cord by providing nutrients and insulation.

Atherosclerosis: A disease characterized by the buildup of cholesterol deposits in the arterial lining.

Atom: A discrete unit made of matter consisting of charged particles.

Atresia: The absence or blockage of a natural orifice or tubular structure.

Auscultation: Listening to the lungs, heart, or abdomen through the stethoscope.

Autograft: The surgical transplantation of tissue from one part of the body to another in the same individual.

Autotransfusion: Also called *blood salvaging*. A method of retrieving blood lost at the operative site, reprocessing it, and infusing it back to the patient.

Auxiliary water channel: A channel in the flexible endoscope used to deliver irrigation fluid at the tip.

Back table: A large stainless steel table on which most of the sterile surgical supplies and instruments are placed for use during surgery. Before surgery, the back table is covered with a sterile drape and sterile instruments and other equipment are opened onto its surface. Supplies needed for immediate use are transferred to the Mayo stand.

Bactericidal: Able to kill bacteria.

Bacteriostatic: Chemical agent capable of inhibiting the growth of bacteria.

Benign: A term used to characterize a tumor that does not have the capability to spread to other parts of the body and usually is composed of tissue similar to its tissue of origin.

Bicoronal incision: An incision made between the frontal and the parietal bones bilaterally.

Bicortical screws: Screws that penetrate both cortical layers and the intervening spongy layer of the bone.

Bier block: Regional anesthesia in which the anesthetic agent is injected into a vein.

Bifurcation: The Y-shape of an artery or graft.

Billroth I procedure: A gastroduodenostomy, or surgical anastomosis, of the stomach and the duodenum.

Billroth II procedure: A gastroduodenostomy, or surgical anastomosis, of the stomach and the jejunum.

Bioactive implant: An orthopedic implant that releases calcium to enhance healing.

Bioavailability: The extent and rate at which a drug or its metabolites (products of breakdown) enter the systemic circulation and reach the site of action.

Bioburden: A measure of the number of bacterial colonies on a surface.

Biocompatibility: A term that describes a material that is compatible with tissue (i.e., causes no toxic or inflammatory effect).

Biofilms: Dense colonies of bacteria that adhere tightly to surfaces. Biofilms, which are resistant to chemical disinfectants and scrubbing, are a matrix of extracellular polymers produced by microorganisms. These substances bind the microorganisms tightly to a living or nonliving surface, making them highly resistant to antimicrobial action. Biofilm increases the risk of disease transmission on internal medicine devices such as catheters and endoscopic instruments.

Biological grafts: Grafts derived from live tissue, whether human or animal.

Biological indicator: A quality control mechanism used in the process of sterilization. It consists of a closed system containing harmless, spore-forming bacteria that can be rapidly cultured after the sterilization process.

Biomechanics: The relationship between movement and biological or anatomical structures.

Biomedical engineering technician: Professional who specializes in the maintenance, repair, maintenance, and safe operation of devices used in medicine, including surgical equipment.

Biopsy channel: A channel that extends the full length of a flexible endoscope and is used to retrieve biopsy tissue.

Biopsy: Removal of a sample of tissue for pathological analysis.

Biosynthetic: A type of graft or implant material made of synthetic absorbable material.

Bioterrorism: The intentional release of biological agents (e.g., bacteria, viruses, mycotoxins) to create illness and death in humans, animals, and the environment. Modes of transmission include air, water, and food.

Bipolar circuit: An electrosurgical circuit in which current travels from the power unit through an instrument containing two opposite poles in contact with the tissue and then returns directly to the energy source.

Birth canal: The maternal pelvis and soft structures through which the baby passes during birth.

Bispectral index system (BIS): A monitoring method used to determine the patient's level of consciousness and prevent intraoperative awareness.

Blebs: Areas of overdistention in lung tissue.

Blended mode: In electrosurgery, a combination of intermediate frequency and intermediate wave intervals to produce a specific effect on tissue.

Blood-borne pathogens: Harmful microorganisms that may be present in and transmitted through human blood and body fluids.

Blowout fracture: A severe fracture of the orbital cavity in which a portion of the globe may extrude outside the cavity.

Blunt dissection: The technique of separating tissue layers by teasing them apart with a rough sponge dissector.

Blunt injury: Trauma that results in deep tissue injury without rupture of the skin.

Body image: In psychology, the way a person sees himself or herself through the eyes of others. A negative body image can severely affect a patient's sense of identity and social and personal interactions.

Body language: Communication through facial expressions, posture, and gestures.

Boiling point: The temperature of a substance when its state changes from a liquid to a gas.

Bolus: A compact substance (e.g., undigested food, fecal material) that occurs normally in the digestive tract.

Bone flap: A section of bone removed from the skull during craniotomy procedures.

Bowel technique: A method of preventing cross-contamination between the bowel contents and the abdominal cavity.

Box lock: The hinge point of many surgical instruments.

Bradycardia: A slow heart rate (usually a heart rate less than 60 beats per minute in an adult).

Breathing bag: The reservoir breathing apparatus of the anesthesia machine. Gases are titrated and shunted into the breathing bag, which is connected to the patient's airway.

Breech presentation: Presentation of the baby in which the buttocks or feet deliver first.

Bridle suture: In ophthalmic surgery, a temporary traction suture placed through the sclera and used to pull the globe laterally for exposure of the posterolateral surface. It is called a *bridle suture* because of its resemblance to the reins of a horse's bridle.

Broaches: Fin-shaped rasps used to enlarge the medullary canal for insertion of an implant. The broach is the same shape as the implant.

Bronchospasm: Partial or complete closure of the bronchial tubes.

CAAHEP: Commission on Accreditation of Allied Health Education Programs. Accredits health science programs, including those for surgical technology.

Calculi: Stones caused by the precipitation of minerals, such as calcium, and other substances from the urine or kidney filtrate.

Camera control unit (CCU): The main control source for the video camera. The unit captures video signals from the camera head and processes them for display on the image system.

Cannula: In minimally invasive surgery, a cannula is a slender tube inserted through the body wall that is used to receive and stabilize telescopic instruments.

Cannulated: A device having a hollow core; for example, an instrument with a central channel that can be fitted over a guidewire or pin.

Capacitative coupling: In minimally invasive surgery, the unintended transmission of electricity from the active electrode to an adjacent conductive pathway, sometimes resulting in a patient burn.

Capacitive coupling: A specific burn hazard of monopolar endoscopic surgery. It occurs when current passes unintentionally through instrument insulation and adjacent conductive material into tissue.

Capillary action: The ability of suture material to absorb fluid.

Carbon dioxide: An inert gas used as a lasing medium during laser surgery.

Cardiac cycle: The pumping action of the heart from one beat to the next.

Cardiac rupture: Tearing of the atria or ventricles as a result of trauma.

Cardiac tamponade: Pressure on the heart causing restriction and damage to the conduction system.

Cardioplegia: Intentional stopping of the heart during cardiac surgery. This is achieved with a cardioplegic solution, which often contains a mixture of potassium chloride, lidocaine, dextrose, insulin, albumin, tromethamine, and Plasmanate.

Case cart system: A method of transporting clean and sterile equipment. Equipment is prepared by the central services or supply department and sent to the operating room. All equipment is contained within a covered movable storage cart.

Case planning: The process of organizing and implementing the tasks and equipment required for a surgical procedure.

Casting: A method of immobilizing a limb by the application of rigid or semirigid material along the length of the limb. A cast can be fully or partially circumferential.

Cataract: Clouding of the eye, caused by a disease in which the crystalline lens of the eye, its capsule, or both become opaque. This prevents light from focusing on the retina, resulting in visual distortion. Cataracts may develop as a result of disease or injury.

Cauterization: The use of a hot object to burn tissue to achieve coagulation.

Cavitation: A process in which air bubbles are imploded (burst inward), releasing particles of soil or tissue debris.

Cavitron Ultrasonic Surgical Aspirator (CUSA): This instrument destroys tumors through the use of high-frequency sound waves (ultrasound).

Central core: The restricted area of the operating room, where sterile supplies and flash sterilizers are located.

Central nervous system depression: This refers to a decrease in sensory awareness caused by drugs or pathologic condition.

Central Processing (CP) department: The area of the hospital where medical devices and equipment are processed; also called Central Surgical Supply or the Surgical Processing department.

Central processing technicians: Skilled professionals who specialize in processing and maintaining medical devices used in the health care facility.

Central processing unit (CPU): The component of a computer that contains the circuitry, memory, and power controls.

Cerclage: A procedure in which a suture ligature is placed around the cervix to prevent spontaneous abortion.

Certification: Acknowledgment by a private agency that a person has achieved a minimum level of knowledge and skill. Certification usually is established by graduation from an accredited institution and passing a written examination. Certification does not confer legal status.

Cerumen: A substance produced by the cerumen glands of the ear (i.e., ear wax).

Chain of command: A hierarchy of personnel positions that establishes both vertical and horizontal relationships between positions.

Chemical barrier: The barrier formed by the action of an antiseptic; it not only reduces the number of microorganisms on a surface, but also prevents recolonization (regrowth) for a limited period.

Chemical indicator: A method of testing a sterilization parameter. Chemical strips sensitive to physical conditions, such as temperature, are placed with the item being sterilized and change color when the parameter is reached; sometimes called a chemical monitor.

Chemical name: The name of a drug that reflects its molecular structure.

Chemical sterilization: A process that uses chemical agents to achieve sterilization.

Child life specialist: A trained professional who specializes in the psychosocial care of and communication with pediatric patients and their families.

Chisel: An orthopedic instrument used to slice bone; one side is straight and the other is beveled.

Choanal: A term that describes the communicating passageways between the nasal fossae and the pharynx.

Cholesteatoma: A benign tumor of the middle ear caused by shedding of keratin in chronic otitis media.

Chronic illness: An illness that has continued for months, weeks, or years.

-cidal: A suffix indicating death. For example, *bactericidal* means "able to kill bacteria."

Circuit: The path of free electrons as they move through conductive material. In a *closed circuit*, the electrons proceed unhindered and electrical energy is maintained; in an *open circuit*, the path of the electrons is interrupted, which stops the flow of current.

Cirrhosis: A disease of the liver in which the tissue hardens and the venous drainage becomes blocked. It usually is caused by chronic alcoholism but may result from other disease conditions.

Cleaning: A process that removes organic or inorganic soil or debris using detergent and mechanical or hand washing.

Closed chest drainage: A system of removing air or fluid from the thoracic cavity and restoring negative pressure so that the lungs can expand properly after thoracic surgery or trauma to the chest wall.

Closed reduction: Alignment of bone fragments into anatomical position by manipulation or traction.

Coagulopathy: Condition in which the body's normal blood-clotting mechanism ceases to function, characteristic in severe multitrauma.

Coagulum: A sticky semiliquid substance that forms when tissue is altered by electrical or ultrasonic energy.

Coarctation: Narrowing of the passageway of a blood vessel, such as coarctation of the aorta, a congenital condition.

Cobalt-60 radiation: A method of institutional bulk sterilization used by manufacturers to sterilize prepackaged equipment using ionizing radiation.

Coherency: A quality of laser light in which all light waves are lined up with troughs and peaks matching.

Coherent light waves: Light waves that are lined up so that the troughs and peaks are matched.

Coitus: Sexual intercourse.

Colposcopy: Microscopic examination of the cervix.

Coma: The deepest state of unconsciousness, in which most brain activity ceases.

Comminuted: A fracture in which there are multiple bone fragments.

Compartment syndrome: Extreme tissue swelling within a closed compartment of the body or closed external device such as a cast. Edematous tissue can exceed the capacity of the space it is held in, causing sufficient pressure to cause tissue necrosis.

Compartment syndrome: Severe swelling and tissue injury caused by constriction of the blood and lymph. Compartment syndrome can progress to tissue necrosis.

Complete blood count (CBC): A blood test that measures specific components, including the hemoglobin, hematocrit, red blood cells, and white blood cells.

Composite graft: A biological graft composed of different types of tissues such as skin and muscle.

Compression injury: Tissue injury caused by continuous pressure over an area.

Compression: Mechanical force in which a structure is compacted or pressed together. Compression is used to repair tissue. A compression injury (e.g., compression fracture) results when bone or other tissue is compacted.

Computed tomography (CT): An imaging technique that allows physicians to obtain cross-sectional x-ray views of the patient. The result is a CT scan.

Concentration: A measure of the quantity of a substance per unit of volume or weight.

Conduction: The transfer of heat from one substance to another by the natural movement of molecules, which sets other molecules in motion.

Conductive: The quality of a material to give up electrons easily and thus transmit electrical current.

Conductivity: The relative ability of a substance to transmit free electrons or electricity.

Congenital: A condition or an anomaly that develops during fetal life and is present at birth.

Consciousness: Neurological status in which a patient is able to sense environmental stimuli such as sight, sound, touch, pressure, pain, heat, and cold.

Consensus: Agreement among members of a group.

Containment and confinement: A foundation concept of aseptic technique in which sterile and nonsterile surfaces are separated by physical barriers or distance (space).

Contaminated: Rendered nonsterile and unacceptable for use in critical areas of the body.

Contamination: The consequence of physical contact between a sterile surface and a nonsterile surface in surgery. Contamination also can result from airborne dust, moisture droplets, or fluids that act as a vehicle for transporting contaminants from a nonsterile surface to a sterile one.

Continuing education: More formally called *professional development*. It demonstrates an ongoing learning process in an individual's profession. Continuing education (CE) credits are provided by a professional organization. Credits are earned by attending lectures and in-service presentations or by study and examination. Usually only peer-reviewed professional literature qualifies for CE credits.

Continuous wave lasers: Lasers that emit laser light continuously rather that in pulses.

Contracture: Tissue that heals without scar formation, causing limited mobility.

Contraindications: Contraindications to a protocol, drug, or procedure are circumstances that make its use medically inadvisable because it increases the risk of injury or harm.

Contrast media: Radiopaque solutions (i.e., not penetrated by x-rays) that are introduced into body cavities and vessels to outline their inside surfaces.

Control head: The proximal section of a flexible endoscope where the controls are located.

Controlled substances: Drugs that have the potential for abuse. Controlled substances are rated according to their risk potential; these ratings are called *schedules*.

Contusion: Bruising.

Convection: The displacement of cool air by warm air. Convection usually creates currents as the warm air rises and the cool air falls.

Cord prolapse: Complication of pregnancy in which the umbilical cord emerges from the uterus during labor and may be compressed against the maternal pelvis or the vagina. This can cause obstructed blood supply to the fetus.

Coroner's case: A patient death that requires investigation by the coroner, as well as an autopsy on the deceased.

Count: A systematic method of accounting for all sponges, needles, instruments, and other items that can be retained in the patient.

Cross-clamp: To place a clamp across a structure to occlude it.

Cross-contamination: The spread of infection from one person to another or from an object to a person.

Cruciate: Cross-shaped.

Cryoablation: A method of tissue destruction in which a probe is inserted into a tumor or tissue mass. High-pressure argon gas is injected into the probe, causing the surrounding tissue to freeze and eventually slough off.

Cryosurgery: The use of extremely low temperature to destroy diseased tissue.

Cryotherapy: A technique in which a cold probe is used to freeze tissue, such as the sclera, ciliary body (for glaucoma), or retinal layers, after detachment.

CST: Certified surgical technologist. A surgical technologist who has successfully passed the certified examination given by the National Board of Surgical Technology and Surgical Assisting.

CST-CFA: Certified surgical technologist–certified first assistant. A surgical technologist with advanced training who has successfully passed the certification examination for surgical first assistants and is credentialed by the National Board of Surgical Technology and Surgical Assisting.

Cultural competence: The ability to provide support and care to individuals of cultures and belief systems different from one's own.

Culture: The process of growing a microbe in a laboratory setting so that it can be studied and tested.

Curettage: The removal of tissue by scraping with a surgical curette.

Current: The flow of electricity.

Cutting mode: In electrosurgery, the use of high voltage and relatively low frequency to cut through tissue.

Cystocele: A herniation of the bladder into the vaginal wall.

Damage control surgery: Surgery whose objective is to stop hemorrhage and prevent sepsis without attempting reconstruction or anatomical continuity.

Damages: Money awarded in a civil lawsuit to compensate the injured party.

Database: In computer technology, a compilation of information, usually lists or numerical information, that can be manipulated or calculated.

Debridement: The removal of devitalized tissue, debris, and foreign objects from a wound. Debridement is performed on trauma injuries, burns, and infected wounds either before surgery or as part of the surgical procedure.

Declared state of emergency: A status conferred on a disaster by the state governor or the president (for a federal declaration). An official declaration of emergency entitles the state in which the disaster occurs to receive federal aid through the Federal Emergency Management Agency (FEMA).

Decontamination area: A room or department in which soiled instruments and equipment are cleaned of gross matter and decontaminated to remove microorganisms.

Decontamination: A process in which recently used and soiled medical devices, including instruments, are rendered safe for personnel to handle.

Defamation: A derogatory statement concerning another person's skill, character, or reputation.

Definitive diagnosis: Evidence-based diagnosis of a medical problem using normal investigative procedures such as imaging studies.

Definitive procedure: A planned surgical procedure, usually with specific objectives for reconstruction or restoration of continuity of anatomical structures.

Dehiscence: Separation of the layers of a surgical wound.

Delegation: The assignment of one's duties to another person. In medicine, the person who delegates a duty retains accountability for the action of the person to whom it is delegated.

Delirium: A state of confusion and disorientation. In the past delirium was defined as a distinct stage of induction and emergence from general anesthesia. However, this stage is rarely demonstrated in association with modern anesthetics.

Dentition: The number, type, and pattern of the teeth.

Dependent areas of the body: Areas of the body subject to pressure from gravity and weight. For example, the sacrum is a dependent area when a person is in the supine position.

Deposition: The testimony of a witness given under oath and transcribed by a court reporter during the pretrial phase of a civil lawsuit.

Dermatome: A medical device used for removing single-thickness skin grafts.

Dermoid cyst: A mass arising from the germ layers of the embryo that contains tissue remnants, including hair and teeth.

Desiccation: The removal of water from tissue, causing it to die.

Detergent: A chemical that breaks down organic debris by emulsification (separation into small particles) to aid in cleaning.

Determination of death: A formal medical process to determine brain death.

Diagnostic endoscopy: A diagnostic procedure in which a long, flexible, fiberoptic tube is inserted into a body cavity for viewing and diagnosis.

Diastole: That phase of the cardiac cycle when the ventricles contract.

Diastolic pressure: The pressure exerted on the walls of the blood vessels during the resting phase of cardiac contraction.

Diathermy: Low-power cautery used to mark the sclera over an area of retinal detachment.

Differential count: A test that determines the number of each type of white blood cells in a specimen of blood.

Diffusion (oxygen): The molecular passage of oxygen across the alveoli and into the bloodstream.

Diffusion: Uniform dispersal of particles in a solution or across a membrane.

Digital output recorder: During video-assisted surgery, digital signals are captured from the video camera and transmitted to an image system. The digital output recorder processes these signals.

Dilator: Graduated smooth instrument that is used to increase the diameter of an anatomical opening in tissue.

Dilemma: A situation or personal conflict that arises from a need to make a decision when none of the choices are acceptable.

Diluent: The liquid component of a drug that must be reconstituted from a powder to a solution for purposes of administration.

Direct coupling: In minimally invasive surgery, the transmission of electricity directly from one conductive path to another, such as from the active electrode to a conductive instrument.

Direct current (DC): A type of low-voltage electrical current in which electrons flow in one direction to complete a circuit. Battery power uses direct current.

Direct inguinal hernia: A hernia that results from an acquired weakness in the inguinal floor.

Direct transmission: The transfer of microbes by direct physical contact with the microbes.

Disaster recovery: A phase of the disaster cycle in which the community returns to a functional level after a disaster. Recovery has no defined interval and may take years.

Disaster: A catastrophic event that affects a large portion of the population and poses significant risk to human life and property. A disaster overwhelms local resources and requires outside assistance.

Discharge against medical advice (AMA): Self-discharge by a patient who has not necessarily met discharge criteria.

Discharge criteria: Objective criteria used to determine whether a patient is safe for discharge from the health care facility.

Disinfection: Destruction of microorganisms by heat or chemical means. Spores usually are not destroyed by disinfection.

Dislocation: Displacement of a joint from its normal position.

Dispersive electrode: A component of the electrosurgical circuit that spreads current at the point where it exits the body and thus prevents injury.

Dissecting sponge: A small compact sponge used to dissect soft tissue planes; also referred to as a sponge dissector. The dissecting sponge is always mounted on a clamp for use in the surgical wound.

Distraction: A mechanical process in which a structure is elongated. Distraction can be used to suspend a limb (and thereby stretch the soft tissue and bones) during surgery. A distraction injury is caused by the pulling apart or stretching of tissue (the opposite of a compression injury).

DNAR: "Do not attempt resuscitation." Emphasizes the patient's desire to refuse intervention to resuscitate.

DNR: "Do not resuscitate." An official request to refrain from certain types of resuscitation, usually cardiopulmonary resuscitation.

Docking: In robotic surgery, the process of positioning the robotic instruments in the exact location over the patient so that instruments can be safely attached to their ports in the body cavity.

Doppler duplex ultrasonography: A type of ultrasonography that amplifies sounds that pass through tissue and produces a visual image of blood flow.

Doppler effect: The effect perceived when the origin or receiver of sound waves moves. The perception is a change in the frequency of the waves and corresponding pitch.

Doppler studies: A technique that uses ultrasonic waves to measure blood flow in a vessel.

Doppler ultrasound: A medical device that uses the Doppler effect and ultrasonic waves to measure and record blood flow as well as tissue density and shape.

Dosage: The regulated administration of prescribed amounts of a drug. Dosage is expressed as a quantity of drug per unit of time.

Dose: The quantity of a drug to be taken at one time or the stated amount of drug per unit of distribution (e.g., 0.5 mg per milliliter of solution).

Double gloving: Wearing two pairs of gloves, one over the other, to reduce the risk of contamination as a result of glove failure or puncture.

Double-action rongeur: A bone-cutting instrument with two hinges in the middle. This increases leverage and strength of the instrument.

Droplet nuclei: Dried remnants of previously moist secretions containing microorganisms. Droplet nuclei are an important source of disease transmission.

Drug: A chemical substance that when taken into the body, changes one or more of the body's functions.

Drug administration: The giving of a drug to a person by any route.

Ductus arteriosus: A normal fetal structure that allows blood to bypass circulation to the lungs. If this structure remains open after birth, it is called a *patent ductus arteriosus.*

Duty cycle: In electrosurgery, the duration of current flow sometimes is referred to as the duty cycle. The duty cycle can intermittently be applied to produce the desired effect on tissue.

Dyspnea: Difficulty breathing.

Eclampsia: A seizure during pregnancy, usually as a result of pregnancy-induced hypertension.

Ectopic pregnancy: Implantation of the fertilized ovum outside the uterus.

Efficiency: The economic use of time and energy to prevent unnecessary expenditure of work, materials, and time.

Effusion: Fluid in the middle ear.

Electrocardiography: A noninvasive assessment of the heart's electrical activity displayed on a graph, the electrocardiogram. In the United States, *electrocardiogram* is abbreviated correctly as ECG. EKG is the European abbreviation.

Electrocution: Severe burns, cardiac disturbances, or death as a result of electrical current discharged into the body.

Electrolytic media: Fluids that contain electrolytes and therefore can transmit an electrical current.

Electromagnetic field: A three-dimensional pattern of force created by the attraction and repulsion of charged particles around a magnet.

Electromagnetic waves: The natural phenomenon of wave energy, such as electricity, light, and radio broadcasts. The type of energy is determined by the frequency of the waves.

Electron: A negatively charged particle that orbits the nucleus of an atom.

Electrostatic discharge: The sudden release of electrical energy from surfaces where charged particles have accumulated because of friction.

Electrosurgery: The direct use of electricity to cut and coagulate tissue.

Electrosurgical unit (ESU): Medical device commonly used in surgery to coagulate blood vessels and cut tissue.

Electrosurgical vessel sealing: A type of bipolar electrosurgery in which tissue is welded together using low voltage, low temperature, and a high-frequency current.

Electrosurgical waveforms: The transduced or actual waves generated when frequency, voltage, and power are delivered in different combinations during electrosurgery.

Element: A pure substance composed of atoms, each with the same number of protons (e.g., iron, copper, uranium).

Elevator channel: A channel that extends the full length of a flexible endoscope and receives biopsy forceps or other instruments.

Elevator: A straight instrument with a curved sharp or dull tip used to separate tissue layers such as periosteum from bone.

Elimination: The physiological process of removing cellular and chemical waste products from the body.

Embolism: A clot of blood, air, organic material, or a foreign body that moves freely in the vascular system. An embolus travels from larger to smaller vessels until it cannot pass through a vessel. At that level, it interrupts the flow of blood and may result in severe disease or death.

Embolization: A technique used to occlude a blood vessel. A variety of materials, including platinum coils and microscopic plastic particles, are injected into the vessel under fluoroscopy control to stop active bleeding or prevent bleeding.

Embolus: A moving substance in the vascular system. An embolus may consist of air, a blood clot, atherosclerotic plaque, or fat.

Embryonic life: The first 8 weeks of gestational development.

Emergence: The stage in general anesthesia in which the anesthetic agent is withdrawn and the patient regains consciousness.

Emergency: A more geographically isolated event than a disaster that can be handled by local emergency services, such as ambulances, the fire department, or paramedics.

Emoticons: Small images or acronyms used to convey emotion in email and SMS (text message) communication.

Empyema: A pus-filled area of the lung.

End of life: A period within which death is expected, usually days to months.

Endarterectomy: The surgical removal of plaque from inside an artery.

Endocoupler: A device that connects the endoscope to the camera.

Endoscopic procedure: Medical assessment of body cavities using a fiberoptic instrument (endoscope).

Endospore: The dormant stage of some bacteria that allows them to survive in extreme environmental conditions, including heat, cold, and exposure to many disinfectants. Endospores are commonly referred to as spores.

Endotracheal tube: An artificial airway (tube) that is inserted into the patient's trachea to maintain patency.

Endovascular repair: Endoscopic surgery of the vascular system.

Entry site: In microbial transmission, the sites where microorganisms enter the body.

Enucleation: Surgical removal of the globe and accessory attachments.

Enzymatic cleaner: A specific chemical used in detergents and cleaners to penetrate and break down biological debris, such as blood and tissue.

Epidural: A type of anesthesia in which the anesthetic is delivered through a small tube in the patient's back to relieve pain in labor. The patient usually is in bed and catheterized during labor in which this form of anesthesia is used.

Episiotomy: A perineal incision made during the second stage of labor to prevent the tearing of tissue.

Epispadias: A rare congenital abnormality in which the opening of the urethra is on the dorsum of the penis. This anomaly does not usually occur in isolation but is part of a more complex set of defects of the urogenital system.

Epistaxis: Bleeding arising from the nasal cavity.

Eschar: Burned tissue fragments that can accumulate on the electrosurgical tip during surgery; eschar can cause sparking and become a source of ignition.

Eschar: Charred and burned tissue created by a high-voltage current.

Eschar: Tissue that has been burned (second- and third-degree burns) but remains adherent to the wound. Eschar is nonelastic and may constrict underlying structures, impairing vital functions.

Escharotomy: Excision of eschar to release stricture in surrounding tissues.

Esmarch bandage: A rolled bandage made of rubber or latex that is used to exsanguinate blood from a limb.

Esophageal varices: Distended veins of the esophagus, caused by advanced liver disease. The condition occurs as a result of portal vein obstruction arising from fibrosis of the liver. Esophageal varices may bleed profusely.

Ethical dilemma: Situation in which ethical choices involve conflicting values.

Ethics: Core values that define one's relationship with others.

Ethylene oxide (EO): A highly flammable toxic gas that is capable of sterilizing an object.

Event related: An activity or process linked with an event.

Event-related sterility: A wrapped sterile item may become contaminated by environmental conditions or events, such as a puncture in the wrapper. Event-related sterility refers to sterility based on the absence of such events. The shelf life of a sterilized pack is event related, not time related.

Evert: To turn outward or inside out.

Evidence-based practice: Professional practices, methods and their standards based on established scientific research rather than opinion or tradition.

Evisceration: Protrusion of the viscera outside the body as a result of trauma or wound disruption.

Examination under anesthesia (EUA): Fracture and dislocation may be fully assessed when general anesthesia is used.

Excimer: A type of lasing energy that is created when electrons are removed from the lasing medium.

Excitation source: In laser technology, the energy that causes the atoms of a lasing medium (gas or solid) to vibrate.

Exenteration: Removal of the entire contents of the orbit.

Expiration: The act of breathing out (exhalation).

Exploratory laparotomy: A laparotomy performed to examine the abdominal cavity when less invasive measures fail to confirm a diagnosis.

Exposure time: This is the amount of time goods are held at a specific time, temperature, and pressure during a sterilization process. Exposure time varies with the size of the load, type of materials being sterilized, and type of sterilizer. Exposure time is sometimes called the hold time.

Exsanguinating: Hemorrhage with the potential to deplete the patient's total blood volume.

Exstrophy: The eversion, or turning out, of an organ.

External fixation: A method of stabilizing bone fragments in anatomical position from outside the body. A cast is an example of an external fixation device.

Extracorporeal shock wave lithotripsy (ESWL): A procedure in which ultrasonic sound waves are used to pulverize kidney or gallbladder stones.

Extracorporeal: A term meaning "outside the body." In minimally invasive surgery, it refers to a technique for placing sutures in which the knots are formed outside the body and then tightened after they have been introduced into the surgical wound.

Extravasation: The absorption of the fluid into the vascular system, leading to increased blood pressure and possible death related to fluid overload. This occurs during surgery when distention fluid used during endoscopic procedures is absorbed through large blood vessels in the bladder or uterus.

Extubation: Withdrawal of an artificial airway.

Facilitator: A group leader who coordinates the direction and flow of a group meeting without influencing the content of people's contributions. It is similar to an *enabling* position in which people are encouraged to express ideas without fear of judgment.

Fasciotomy: A surgical treatment for compartment syndrome in which the fascia is incised to release severe tissue swelling, which can result in necrosis.

Federal Emergency Management Agency (FEMA): Federal agency responsible for all aspects of coordination, management, and response for nationally declared disasters. It also provides extensive training programs in disaster preparedness management and response for professionals and members of the community.

Feedback: The response to a message; a component of effective communication.

Fenestrated drape: A sterile body sheet with a hole or "window" (*fenestration*) that exposes the incision site. The fenestrated drape is positioned after other drapes and towels have been placed in keeping with the procedure. Fenestrated drapes are differentiated by type (e.g., laparotomy, thyroid, kidney, eye, ear, and extremity drapes).

Fetal demise: Death of the fetus.

Fetus: Gestational life after 8 weeks.

Fibrillation: Uncoordinated muscular activity in the heart muscle, which results in "quivering" rather than pumping action.

Fibroid: See Leiomyoma.

Fistula: An abnormal tract or passage leading from one organ to another or from an organ to the skin; usually caused by infection.

Flail chest: Rib fracture in at least three adjacent ribs in two locations each. This condition requires immediate surgery.

Flammable: Capable of burning.

Fluoroscopy: A radiological technique that provides real-time images of an anatomical region.

Focal point: The exact location where light rays converge after passing through a convex lens.

Focused assessment with ultrasound for trauma (FAST): A protocol of ATLS in which ultrasound is used in a focused area to diagnose severe trauma.

Foley catheter: A retention catheter with an expandable balloon at the distal end.

Fomite: An intermediate inanimate source in the process of disease transmission. An object, such as a contaminated surgical instrument or medical device, can become a fomite in disease transmission.

Footboard: Operating table attachment that braces the patient's weight when the table is tilted toward the feet.

Frequency: In electricity, the periodicity of electromagnetic waves. In physics, the number of waves that pass a point in 1 second. The unit of measurement for frequency is the hertz (Hz).

Friable: A descriptive term for tissue that means fragile and easily torn, and may bleed profusely. Some disease states produce friable tissue. The liver and spleen normally are friable.

Frozen section: A procedure in which a tissue specimen is flash-frozen and sectioned for examination under the microscope. The procedure is used to verify suspected malignancy during surgery.

Fulguration: A process of tissue surface destruction used in electrosurgery.

Full-thickness skin graft (FTSG): A skin graft composed of the epidermis and dermis.

Fungicidal: Able to kill fungi.

Fusiform aneurysm: A type of aneurysm that involves the entire circumference of a blood vessel.

Gain: In electronics, the intensity of the signal.

Gas plasma sterilization: A process that uses the form of matter known as plasma (e.g., hydrogen peroxide plasma) to sterilize an item. Also referred to as plasma sterilization.

Gas scavenging: The capture and safe removal of extraneous anesthetic gases from the anesthesia machine.

Gastrostomy: A surgical opening through the stomach wall connecting to the outside of the body or another hollow anatomical structure.

General anesthesia: Anesthesia associated with a state of unconsciousness. General anesthesia is not a fixed state of unconsciousness, but rather ranges along a continuum from semiresponsiveness to profound unresponsiveness.

Generation: In pharmacology, refers to a drug group that was developed from a previous prototype (e.g., first-generation cephalosporin).

Generic name: The formulary name of a drug that is assigned by the U.S. Adopted Names Council.

Genetic abnormality: A birth anomaly that is inherited.

Germicidal: Able to kill germs.

Gestational age: The age of the fetus as measured in the number of weeks from conception.

Glasgow Coma Scale (GCS): A standardized method of measuring a patient's response to external stimuli.

Glaucoma: A group of diseases characterized by elevation of the intraocular pressure. Sustained pressure on the optic nerve and other structures may result in ischemia and blindness.

Glomerular filtration rate (GFR): An indication of kidney function in which the serum creatinine (normally filtered by the kidney) level is measured.

Gouge: A V-shaped bone chisel.

Graft: An implant used to replace or augment existing tissue. A graft may be obtained from the patient, another person, an animal source, or synthetic or biosynthetic materials.

Gravitational energy: The natural attractive force of masses in the universe.

Gravity displacement sterilizer: A type of sterilizer that removes air by gravity.

Gross contamination: Contamination of a large area of tissue by a highly infective source.

Grounding pad: An alternate name for the patient return electrode.

Grounding: A path for electrical current to flow unimpeded through a material and disperse back to the source or disperse into the ground.

Groupthink: In sociology and group behavior theory, the conformity of a group to one way of thinking and behaving. Groupthink creates two factions, those who agree (in group) and those who disagree (out group). This generates resentment and conflict in the workplace.

Half-life: The time required for half of a drug to be cleared from the body.

Hand washing: A specific technique used to remove debris and dead cells from the hands. Hand washing with an antiseptic also reduces the number of microorganisms on the skin.

Handover (hand-off): A verbal and written report from one nurse to another to provide updated patient information.

Haptic feedback: Tactile feedback conveyed from tissue to the hand when a hand instrument is used. Robotic instruments do not provide any tactile feedback.

Harmonics: The quality of sound related to the frequency of the sound waves.

Heart-beating cadaver: A cadaver maintained on cardiopulmonary support to provide tissue perfusion. This is done to maintain viability in organs for donation.

Heart-lung machine: Medical device used during cardiac bypass. Systemic blood is shunted out of the body via cannulas, which are implanted in the heart. The device collects the blood, removes excess carbon dioxide, oxygenates it, and returns it to the body through separate cannulas.

Hematocrit (Hct): The ratio of red blood cells to plasma.

Hematoma: A blood-filled space in tissue, the result of a bleeding vessel.

Hemodialysis: A process in which blood is shunted out of the body and passed through a complex set of filters for the treatment of end-stage renal disease (and in some cases, poisoning); also called *renal replacement therapy*.

Hemodynamic: A term referring to the pressure, flow, and resistance in the cardiovascular system.

Hemoglobin (Hgb): The oxygen-carrying molecule found in red blood cells.

Hemoptysis: Bloody sputum or bleeding arising from the respiratory tract.

Hemorrhage: Continuous bleeding from a pathological cause.

Hemorrhagic shock: A type of shock characterized by vascular failure due to severe bleeding.

Hemostat: A surgical clamp most often used to occlude a blood vessel.

Hemostatic agents: Substances applied to bleeding arising from the surface of tissue to enhance rapid coagulation (e.g., topical gelatin sponge applied on area of capillary bleeding on the spleen).

Hemothorax: The presence of blood in the thoracic cavity or between the pleural sac and lungs, usually caused by trauma.

Hernia: A protrusion of tissue under the skin through a weakened area of the body wall.

High definition (HD): A type of video format. The clarity of the image is based on the number of signals (pixels) emitted by the camera. HD format has a 16:9 aspect ratio, which is 7 times greater than standard definition.

High level disinfection (HLD): A process that reduces the bioburden to an absolute minimum.

High-efficiency particulate air (HEPA) filters: Filters installed in the operating room ventilation system that remove 99.97% of particles equal to or larger than 0.3 micrometers.

High-vacuum sterilizer: A type of steam sterilizer that removes air in the chamber by vacuum and refills the chapter with pressurized steam. Also known as a prevacuum sterilizer.

Holmium:YAG: A solid crystal lasing medium that penetrates a wide variety of substances, including renal and biliary stones and soft tissue.

Homeostasis: The balance of physiological processes that maintain life.

Hook wire: A device used to pinpoint the exact location of a nonpalpable mass detected during a mammogram. Also referred to as a hook needle. A fine wire is inserted into the mass during the examination, and the tissue around the needle is removed for pathological examination and definitive diagnosis.

Hospital policy: Rules or regulations that hospital employees are required to follow. They are created to protect patients and employees from harm and to ensure smooth operation of the hospital.

Hot wire: In electrical circuits, the hot wire is the one that carries the electrical current.

Hydrodressing: A dressing impregnated with a water-based gel. This type of dressing prevents the wound from drying.

Hyperextension: Extension of a joint beyond its normal anatomical range.

Hyperflexion: Flexion of a joint beyond its normal anatomical range.

Hyperlinks: In computer technology, electronic links between files and the electronic addresses for data associated with those links. Hyperlinks allow data to be obtained electronically and quickly from another computer through a computer network.

Hyperplasia: An excessive proliferation of tissue.

Hypersensitivity: Allergic immune response to a substance causing a range of symptoms from mild inflammation to anaphylactic shock and death.

Hypertrophic scar: A raised scar characterized by excess collagen.

Hypertrophy: Enlargement of an organ or tissue.

Hypotension: Decreased blood pressure.

Hypothermia: Body temperature that is below normal.

Hypoxia: Lack of oxygen in the tissue.

Imaging studies: Diagnostic tests that produce a picture or image.

Imaging system: The combined components of the endoscopic system, which create the image captured in the focal view of the endoscope.

Immediate-use sterilization: Items to be sterilized shortly before surgery must be processed so they are ready as close to the time of surgery as possible. This is referred to as immediate-use sterilization, previously called *flash sterilization.*

Impedance: The constriction of electrical current by a nonconductive material or an area of high density. This results in the transformation of electricity into thermal energy; the ability of a substance to stop or alter the flow of electrons through a conductive material (resistance).

Impervious: Waterproof.

Implant: Any medical device placed in the body with intention to be permanent or semipermanent. Examples include orthopedic hardware (e.g., plates, screws, rods), synthetic grafts, internal cardiac pacemakers, molded silicone used in plastic and reconstructive surgery, and intraocular implants used in cataract surgery.

Implanted electronic device (IED): An electronic device that monitors and corrects physiological conditions. Electrosurgery may interfere with the function of such devices, which include pacemakers, internal defibrillators, deep brain stimulators, and ventricular assist devices.

In situ: A term meaning "in the natural position or normal place, without disturbing or invading surrounding tissues."

Inactive electrode: An alternate term for the patient return electrode.

Inanimate: Nonliving.

Incarcerated hernia: Herniated tissue that is trapped in an abdominal wall defect. Incarcerated tissue requires emergency surgery to prevent ischemia and tissue necrosis.

Incident report: A written description of any event that caused harm or presented the risk of harm to a patient or staff member in the course of normal health care.

Incise drape: A plastic adhesive drape that is positioned over the incision site after the surgical skin prep. The incise drape creates a sterile surface over the skin.

Incisional hernia: The postoperative herniation of tissue into the tissue layers around an abdominal incision. This may occur in the immediate postoperative period or later, after the incision has healed.

Incompetent cervix: A condition in which previous cervical injury results in repeated spontaneous abortions.

Incomplete abortion: Expulsion of the fetus with retained placenta before 20 weeks of gestation.

Indirect inguinal hernia: A hernia that protrudes into the membranous sac of the spermatic cord. This condition usually is due to a congenital defect in the abdominal wall.

Induction: Initiation of general anesthesia with a drug that causes unconsciousness.

Indwelling catheter: A urethral or ureteral catheter that is left in place.

Inert: Causing little or no reaction in tissue or with other materials.

Infarction: Necrosis and death of tissue related to obstruction of blood flow.

Infection: The state or condition in which pathogenic microorganisms invade and colonize in the body or body tissues.

Inflammation: The body's nonspecific reaction to injury or infection that results in redness, heat, swelling, and pain.

Informed consent: A process and a legal document that states the patient's surgical procedure and the risks, consequences, and benefits of that procedure.

Insertion tube: The long narrow portion of the flexible endoscope that is inserted into the body.

Inspiration: The act of taking a breath (inhalation).

Instrument channel: A channel that extends the full length of a flexible endoscope and receives instruments during flexible endoscopy.

Insufflation: In minimally invasive surgery, inflation of the abdominal or thoracic cavity with carbon dioxide gas.

Insulate: To cover or surround a conductive substance with nonconductive material.

Insulator: A substance that does not conduct electrical current and is used to prevent electricity from seeking an alternate path.

Insurance policy: A contract in which the insurance company agrees to defend the policy holder if that individual is sued for acts covered by the policy.

Integrated operating room: A type of structural and engineering design in which digital and computerized components such as cameras, monitors, and environmental controls can be controlled from a central location in the room. Components such as endoscopic control units and monitors are built into the room structure rather than as separate portable units.

Internal drives: Data storage devices that are an integral part of the computer.

Internal fixation: A method of surgically repairing a fracture by implanting a device that holds the bone fragments in place. Metal plates, rods, pins, and screws are examples of internal fixation devices.

Internet: A worldwide public network of computers that are connected by wires, fiberoptic cables, or satellite signals. Computers connected to this system can receive and transmit data to other computers in the system.

Interrupted sutures: A technique of bringing tissue together by placing individual sutures close together.

Intracorporeal: A term meaning "inside the body." In minimally invasive surgery, it refers to a suture technique in which sutures are knotted and secured inside the patient.

Intracranial pressure (ICP): The pressure within the skull exerted by the brain tissue, blood, and cerebrospinal fluid.

Intranet: A computer network within a facility or organization that can be accessed only by those employed by or affiliated with the organization.

Intraoperative awareness (IOA): A rare condition in which a patient undergoing general anesthesia is able to feel pain and other noxious stimuli but unable to respond.

Intraosseous: Refers to administration of a drug directly into the bone marrow.

Intrathecal: Refers to administration of a drug into the spinal canal.

Intravasation: The unintended absorption of irrigation fluids into the vascular system, which causes fluid overload and can result in cardiac arrest.

Intravascular ultrasound: A diagnostic tool in which a transducer is introduced into an artery and ultrasound is used to translate the physical characteristics of the lumen into a visible image.

Intravascular volume: Fluid volume within the blood vessels.

Intubation: The process of inserting an invasive artificial airway.

Invasive procedure: A medical or nursing procedure in which the skin is broken or a body cavity is entered.

Ischemia: Loss of blood supply to a body part either by compression or as a result of a blockage in the blood vessels. Prolonged ischemia causes tissue death from lack of oxygen to the tissue.

Isolated circuit: An electrical circuit that has no ground reference or method of conducting current into the ground at the site of use. Current is directed from the energy source, through the patient, and back to the source.

Isolette: An infant-size "bed" and transport unit that is environmentally controlled and equipped with monitoring devices.

Isotope: An atom of a specific element with the correct number of electrons and protons but a different number of neutrons.

Job description: A document that specifies duties, responsibilities, location, pay, and management structure of a job.

Job title: The name of a job, such as "Certified Surgical Technologist" or "Chief of Surgery."

Keloid: A hypertrophic scar occurring in dark-skinned individuals. The scar may become bulbous and usually does not reduce over time.

Keratoplasty: Surgery of the cornea. The term *penetrating keratoplasty* refers to corneal transplantation.

Kinetic energy: The energy of motion; the kinetic energy of an object is mathematically related to its speed.

Knot pusher: A device used to secure suture knots during minimally invasive surgery.

Kübler-Ross, Elisabeth: A Swiss psychiatrist who proposed a theory of developmental or psychological stages of the dying experience.

Labor: The process of regular contraction of the uterine muscle that results in birth.

Laminar airflow (LAF) system: A ventilation system that moves a contained volume of air in layers at a continuous velocity, with 800 to 900 air exchanges per hour.

Laparotomy: A procedure in which the abdominal cavity is surgically opened. The techniques used for laparotomy are used for all open surgical procedures of the abdomen.

Laryngeal mask airway (LMA): An airway consisting of a tube and small mask that is fitted internally over the patient's larynx.

Laryngoscope: A lighted instrument used to assist endotracheal intubation.

Laryngospasm: Muscular spasm of the larynx, resulting in obstruction.

Laser: Acronym for *light amplification by stimulated emission of radiation.*

Laser classification: Industry and international system for grading laser energy according to its ability to cause injury.

Laser head: The component of the laser system that holds the lasing medium.

Laser medium: A solid or gas that is sensitive to atomic excitation by an energy source, which creates intense laser light and energy.

Lateral abuse: Verbal abuse or sabotage of people of equal job or professional ranking.

Lateral heat: The unintentional heating of tissue outside the direct area of electrosurgical application. Also called *thermal spread.*

Lateral transfer: Transferring the patient from one horizontal surface to another, such as from a bed to a stretcher.

Latex: A naturally occurring sap obtained from rubber trees that is used in the manufacture of medical devices, supplies, and patient care items.

Laws: Standards of conduct that apply to all people in a given society.

Le Fort I fracture: A horizontal fracture of the maxilla that causes the hard palate and alveolar process to become separated from the rest of the maxilla. The fracture extends into the lower nasal septum, lateral maxillary sinus, and palatine bones.

Le Fort II fracture: A fracture that extends from the nasal bone to the frontal processes of the maxilla, lacrimal bones, and inferior orbital floor. It may extend into the orbital foramen. Inferiorly, it extends into the anterior maxillary sinus and the pterygoid plates.

Le Fort III fracture: This fracture involves separation of all the facial bones from their cranial base. It includes fracture of the zygoma, maxilla, and nasal bones.

LEEP: Loop electrode excision procedure. In this technique, an electrosurgical loop is used to remove a core of tissue from the cervical canal.

Leiomyoma: A fibrous benign tumor of the uterus that usually arises from the myometrium.

Liable: Legally responsible and accountable.

Libel: Defamation in writing.

Licensure: Professional status, granted by state government, that defines the limits (scope) of practice and regulates those who hold a license.

Ligate: To place a loop or tie around a blood vessel or duct.

Ligation loop: A commercially prepared suture loop used to secure structures during minimally invasive surgery.

Light cable: The fiberoptic light cable that transmits light from the source to the endoscopic instrument. Sometimes called a *light guide.*

Light source: A device that controls and emits light for endoscopic procedures.

Linea alba: A strip of avascular tissue that follows the midline and extends from the pubis to the xiphoid process.

Living will: A legal document signed by the patient stating the conditions and limitations of medical assistance in the event of near death or a prognosis of death.

Lobectomy: Surgical removal of one or more anatomical sections of the liver.

Logistics supply chain: The event-related process of handling material goods from the point of procurement to the point of delivery to the end user.

Lumen: The inside of a hollow structure, such as a blood vessel.

Magical thinking: A psychological process in which a person attributes intention and will to inanimate objects. Magical thinking may also describe a patient's belief that an event will happen because he or she wills it or wishes it. This is a normal developmental stage of toddlers.

Magnetic field: A three-dimensional force pattern created by the positive and negative charges of a polar magnet.

Magnetic resonance imaging (MRI): A diagnostic technique that uses radiofrequency signals and magnetic energy to produce images.

Malignant: A term used to characterize tissue that shows disorganized, uncontrolled growth (cancer). Malignant tissue has the potential to spread locally or to distant areas of the body. It is then termed *metastatic*.

Malignant hyperthermia (MH): A potentially rare and fatal syndrome of hypermetabolism that occurs in association with inhalation anesthetics and neuromuscular blocking agents. It results in an extremely high body temperature, cardiac dysrhythmia, and respiratory distress.

Malpractice: Negligence (as defined by the law) committed by a professional. Malpractice may be committed if a person deliberately acts outside of his or her scope of practice or while impaired.

Maslow's hierarchy of human needs: A model of human achievement and self-actualization developed by psychologist Abraham Maslow.

Mass casualty event (MCE): An emergency in which the number of victims overwhelms the human and material capacity of available health care services. An MCE usually is associated with a geographically isolated event (e.g., transportation accident, industrial accident).

Mastectomy: A procedure in which breast tissue, including the skin, areola, and nipple, is removed, but the lymph nodes are not removed. Also called a simple mastectomy.

Master controllers: In robotic surgery, the nonsterile hand controls that manipulate surgical instruments.

Mastication: Chewing.

Material Safety Data Sheet (MSDS): A government-mandated requirement for all chemicals used in the workplace. The MSDS describes the formulation, safe use, precautions, and emergency response. The MSDS must be available for each chemical an employee is required to handle in his or her work.

Maxillomandibular fixation (MMF): See arch bars.

McBurney incision: An incision in which the oblique right muscle is manually split to allow removal of the appendix.

Mean arterial pressure (MAP): The average amount of pressure exerted throughout the cardiac cycle.

Meatotomy: A procedure in which a small incision is made in the urethral meatus to relieve a stricture. A topical anesthetic is used.

Meconium: A nearly sterile fecal waste that accumulates while the fetus is in the uterus. It is passed within the first few days after birth.

Medical device: Any equipment, instrument, implant, material, or apparatus used for the diagnosis, treatment, or monitoring of patients.

Medical ethics: A branch of ethics concerned with the practice of medicine.

Medical power of attorney: A legal document signed by a person who is giving another individual the power to make health care decisions for the first person if he or she becomes incompetent, unconscious, or unable to make decisions for himself or herself.

Medical Reserve Corps (MRC): Medical volunteer agency that is committed to supporting public health and emergency responses in the community.

Menarche: The onset of menstruation, menses.

Menorrhagia: Excessive bleeding during menses.

Message: An idea, concept, thought, or feeling expressed during communication.

Metabolic acidosis: A potentially lethal physiological condition occurring in shock, characterized by abnormally low blood pH.

Metastasis: The spread of malignant or cancerous cells to a local or distant area of the body.

Missed abortion: An abortion in which the products of conception are no longer viable but are retained in the uterus.

Mitigation: A process or intervention intended to reduce the level of injury or harm. For example, mitigation against the effects of a hurricane includes early warning systems that may predict the strength and location of the storm.

Mobility: The ability of an organism to move. As a protective mechanism, mobility allows an organism to move away from harmful stimuli.

Modified radical mastectomy: A procedure in which the entire breast, nipple, and areolar region are removed. The lymph nodes also are usually removed.

Mohs surgery: A procedure in which a malignant tissue mass is removed and cut into quadrants before frozen section. These quadrants are used to map the tumor and determine the exact location of malignant margins.

Molecule: A specific substance made up of elements that are bonded together.

Momentum: The mathematical relationship between the weight and velocity of a mass.

Monitored anesthesia care (MAC): Monitoring of vital functions during regional anesthesia to ensure the patient's safety and comfort.

Monochromatic: A characteristic of laser light in which the frequency of each wave is the same.

Monopolar circuit: In electrosurgery, a continuous path of electricity that flows from the electrosurgical unit to the active electrode, through the patient and the return electrode, and back to the electrosurgical unit.

Morbid obesity: A condition in which the patient's body mass index (BMI) is 40 or higher, and the individual is at least 100 pounds (45 kg) over the ideal weight despite aggressive attempts to lose weight.

Muscle recession: Surgery in which the eye muscle is moved back to release the globe.

Muscle resection: Surgical shortening of an eye muscle to pull the globe into correct position.

Mutagenic substance: A chemical or other agent that causes permanent change in the cell's genetic material.

Nasogastric (NG) tube: A flexible tube inserted through the nose and advanced into the stomach. The NG tube is used to decompress the stomach or to provide a means of feeding the patient liquid nutrients and medication.

Nasolaryngoscope: A flexible endoscope that is passed through the nose to visualize the larynx.

Nasopharyngeal airway: Artificial airway between the nostril and the nasopharynx; used in semiconscious patients or when an oral airway is contraindicated.

National Certifying Examination for Surgical Technologists: A comprehensive written examination required for official certification by the Association of Surgical Technologists, developed by the NBSTSA.

National Disaster Life Support Education Consortium (NDLSEC): Organization of health professionals committed to providing education, standards, and guidelines for volunteers so that the needs of the public are met during a disaster or emergency situation.

National Disaster Medical System (NDMS): Agency that maintains a database of trained on-call medical, paramedical, and allied health personnel for emergency deployment during a disaster.

National Fire Protection Association (NFPA): Organization that develops and distributes codes and standards that aim to lessen the threat of fire and hazards, as well as their potential impact in the community.

Natural disaster: Widespread damage and risk of injury caused by forces of nature, such as a hurricane, tornado, earthquake, floods, and extreme heat or cold.

NBSTSA: National Board of Surgical Technology and Surgical Assisting. The NBSTA (formerly the Liaison Council on Certification for the Surgical Technologist) is responsible for all decisions related to certification such as eligibility, renewal, and revocation, as well as developing the certification examination.

NCCT: National Center for Competency Testing. A nonprofit organization that provides a certification examination for nonaccredited programs and on the job training, and for other trained surgical technologists whose programs are not recognized by the Association of Surgical Technologists.

Negligence: Negligence as it applies to health professionals can occur in two ways: it can be a failure to do something that a reasonable person, guided by the ordinary professional considerations would do it can be the act of doing something that a reasonable and prudent person would not do.

Neodymium:YAG: A solid lasing medium known for its attraction to protein and deep penetration into tissue.

Neoplasm: A tumor, which may be benign or malignant.

Nephroblastoma: Wilms tumor.

Neural tube defect: A congenital abnormality resulting from failure of the neural tube to close in embryonic development.

Neuromuscular blocking agent: A drug that blocks nerve conduction in striated muscle tissue.

Neuropathy: Permanent or temporary nerve injury that results in numbness or loss of function of a part of the body.

Neutral electrode: An alternate term for the patient return electrode.

Neutral zone (no-hands) technique: A method of transferring sharp instruments on the surgical field without hand-to-hand contact. A neutral zone is identified, and sharps are exchanged in this zone.

Neutron: A subatomic particle located in the nucleus of the atom. It has no electrical charge.

Nonabsorbable suture: Suture material that resists breakdown in the body.

Nonconductive: The quality of a substance that resists the transfer of electrons and therefore electrical current.

Noncritical items: Items that are not required to be sterile because they do not penetrate intact tissues. Patient care items such as a blood pressure cuff and a stethoscope are noncritical.

Non–heart-beating cadaver: A cadaver in which perfusion at and after death was not possible. Only certain tissues may be procured for donation.

Nonelectrolytic: Nonconductive; nonelectrolytic solutions must be used for bladder distention or continuous irrigation whenever the electrosurgical unit (ESU) is used.

Nonsterile personnel: In surgery, team members who remain outside the boundary of the sterile field and do not come in direct contact with sterile equipment, sterile areas, or the surgical wound. The

circulator, anesthesia care provider, and radiographic technician are examples of nonsterile team members.

Nonsterile team members: Surgical team members who handle only nonsterile equipment, supplies, and instruments. The circulator is the primary nonsterile team member.

Nonwoven: A fabric or material that is bonded together as opposed to a process of interweaving individual threads.

Normal spontaneous vaginal delivery (NSVD): A normal delivery of the fetus, without the need for medical intervention. The normal birth process.

Norms: Behaviors that are accepted as part of the environment and culture of a group. Norms usually are established by custom and popular acceptance rather than by law, although the two may not be mutually exclusive.

Nosocomial infection: Another term for a hospital-acquired infection (HAI) or health care–acquired infection; an infection acquired as a result of being in a health care facility.

Nuchal cord: A complication of pregnancy in which the umbilical cord is wrapped around the neck of the fetus. This may lead to obstructed blood flow to the fetus.

Nuclear medicine: Medical procedures that use radioactive particles to track target tissues in the body.

Nucleus: The center of an atom.

Nutrition: Usually refers to the intake of food by an organism.

Obturator: A blunt-nosed instrument that is inserted through the sheath of a rigid endoscope or hysteroscope to protect the tissue as the instrument is advanced.

Occlusion: In maxillofacial surgery, this refers to the patient's bite pattern when the jaw is closed.

Occult injury: An injury that is not detected in normal assessment procedures.

Occupational exposure: Exposure to hazards in the workplace; for example, exposure to hazardous chemicals or contact with potentially infected blood and body fluids.

Odontectomy: Tooth extraction.

Off-pump procedure: A procedure performed without a cardiopulmonary bypass (i.e., "the pump").

Omphalocele: A protrusion of abdominal contents through a congenital defect at the navel.

Open reduction: Surgical access (through an incision) to bring bone fragments into anatomical alignment.

Opportunistic infection: Infection in a weakened individual, or as the of result specific drugs, usually by colonization of a bacterium that does not usually cause disease. The host may be debilitated by another disease or the immune system may be compromised.

Optical angle: The angle at which light is transmitted at the distal end of a fiberoptic or video endoscope.

Optical resonant cavity: The component of a laser system in which the lasing medium is contained and light is transformed.

Organizational chart (organigram): A graphic depiction of an organization's chain of command that shows the lines of vertical (higher and lower) and horizontal (equal) administrative authority.

Oromaxillofacial surgery: Surgery involving the bones of the face, primarily for repair of fractures and reconstruction of congenital anomalies.

Oropharyngeal airway (OPA): Artificial airway that is inserted over the tongue into the larynx; used in patients in whom endotracheal intubation is difficult or contraindicated.

ORT: Operating room technician; former name for surgical technologists (name changed to *surgical technologist* in the early 1970s).

Orthopedic system: A specific (usually patented) set of instruments and implants used for an orthopedic technique. For example, arthroplasty implants are marketed as systems that include the joint components and instruments that are designed for use with that implant.

Orthostatic (postural) blood pressure: Refers to a technique used to check the patient's blood pressure in the upright and recumbent positions.

Ossicles: The bones of the middle ear that conduct sound (i.e., the malleus, incus, and stapes).

-ostomy: A suffix that refers to an opening between two hollow organs; for example, gastroduodenostomy, a surgical procedure that joins the stomach and duodenum.

Ostomy: A technique in which a new opening is made between a tubular structure such as the intestine or ureter and the outside of the body or another hollow structure or organ.

Ototoxic: A substance that can injure the ear.

Oxidizers: Agents or substances capable of supporting fire.

Oxygen-enriched atmosphere (OEA): An environment that contains a high percentage of oxygen and therefore presents a high risk for fire.

Pacemaker: A device that stimulates the heart muscle to contract.

Packing: A method of applying a dressing to a body cavity. In nasal procedures, 0.25- or 0.49-inch (0.63- or 1.25-cm) gauze strips are inserted into the nasal cavity to absorb drainage, control bleeding, or expose the mucosa to topical medication. "Packing" a wound may refer to any dressing that is introduced into an anatomical space or cavity.

Palpating: Assessing a part of the body by feeling the outline, density, movement, or other attributes.

Pandemic: A public health emergency in which an infectious disease spreads throughout a large population, often across international boundaries.

Papanicolaou (Pap) test: A diagnostic test in which epithelial cells are taken from the endocervical canal and examined for abnormalities that can lead to cervical cancer.

Papilloma: A benign epithelial tumor characterized by a branching or lobular tumor. (Also called a *papillary tumor.*)

Paranasal sinuses: Air cells surrounding or on the periphery of the nasal cavities. These are the maxillary, ethmoid, sphenoid, and frontal sinuses.

Parenteral: Refers to administration of a drug by injection.

Paresis: Paralysis of a structure (e.g., vocal cord paresis).

Partial thromboplastin time (PTT): A test of blood coagulation used in patients receiving heparin to determine the correct level of anticoagulation.

Parturition: Birth.

Pathogen: A disease-causing (pathogenic) microorganism.

Patient return electrode (PRE): A critical component of the monopolar electrosurgical circuit. The PRE is a conductive pad that captures electricity and shunts it safely out of the body and back to the electrosurgical unit.

Patient-centered care: Therapeutic care, communication, and intervention provided according to the unique needs of the patient and centered on those needs.

Peak effect: The period of maximum effect of a drug.

Penetrating injury: Tissue damage that occurs when an object enters the body through the skin, or the body is propelled against an object, breaking the skin.

Peracetic acid: A chemical used in the sterilization of critical items.

Percutaneous: A term for a procedure that is performed "through the skin." For example, in percutaneous nephroscopy, the nephroscope is inserted into the kidney through a skin incision.

Perforation: A defect in the tympanic membrane caused by trauma or infection.

Perfusion (oxygen): The distribution of oxygen to tissues.

Perfusion: Circulation of blood to a specific tissue, organ, system, or the whole body is called perfusion. Perfusion is necessary to maintain life in the cells.

Perfusion: Flow of blood to tissue.

Perineum: The anatomical area between the posterior vestibule and the anus.

Periodic table: A standardized chart of all known elements.

Perjury: The crime of intentionally lying or falsifying information during court testimony after a person has sworn to tell the truth.

Personal protective equipment (PPE): Clothing or equipment that protects the wearer from direct contact with hazardous chemicals or potentially infectious body fluids.

Personnel policy: A policy that sets forth the health care facility's job descriptions, role delineations, requirements for employment, and rules of conduct for personnel.

Phacoemulsification: The destruction of cataracts using ultrasound technology.

Pharmacodynamics: The biochemical and physiological effects of drugs and their mechanisms of action in the body.

Pharmacokinetics: The movement of a drug through the tissues and cells of the body, including the processes of absorption, distribution, and localization in tissues; biotransformation; and excretion by mechanical and chemical means.

Pharmacology: The study of drugs and their action in the body.

Phonation: Vibration of the vocal cords during speaking or vocalization.

Photodamage: Damage to the skin caused by ultraviolet light.

Photon: In physics, the name given to a light particle.

Physical barrier: In surgery, a barrier that separates a sterile surface from a nonsterile surface. Examples are sterile surgical gloves, gowns, and drapes. A physical barrier, such as a clean surgical cap, also can prevent a bacteria-laden surface, such as the hair, from shedding microorganisms.

Physiological monitoring: Assessment of the patient's vital metabolic functions.

Physiological: Refers to the biochemical and metabolic processes of an organism.

PID: Pelvic inflammatory disease. PID is caused by a sexually transmitted disease or some other source of infection. It causes scarring of the fallopian tubes and adhesions in the abdominal and pelvic cavities.

Pixel: An element within each silicone chip contained within a device that produces electronic images such as those seen on a surgical image system used in minimally invasive surgery.

Placenta: The organ that transfers selected nutrients to the fetus during pregnancy.

Placenta previa: A complication of pregnancy in which the placenta implants completely or partly over the cervical os. In this position, the placenta begins to bleed as it separates from the cervix during labor.

Placental abruption: Premature separation of the placenta from the uterine wall after 20 weeks' gestation and before the fetus is delivered.

Plasma: A gaseous state in which the atom's nucleus becomes separated from the electrons.

Plication: Folding tissue and securing it in place surgically.

Pneumatic tourniquet: An air-filled tourniquet used to prevent blood flow to an extremity during surgery.

Pneumoperitoneum: An abdomen insufflated or distended with carbon dioxide gas during laparoscopy.

Pneumothorax: Injury that results in air in the pleural space causing displacement or collapse of the respiratory structures.

Polyp: Excessive proliferation of the mucosal epithelium.

Porcine: Derived from pig tissue.

Positron emission tomography (PET): A type of medical imaging that measures specific metabolic activity in the target tissue.

Postanesthesia care unit (PACU): The critical care area where patients are taken after surgery for monitoring and evaluation as they emerge from anesthesia.

Postexposure prophylaxis (PEP): Recommended procedures to help prevent the development of blood-borne diseases after an exposure incident such as a needlestick injury.

Postmortem care: Physical care of the body to prepare it for viewing by the family and for mortuary procedures.

Potassium-titanyl-phosphate (KTP): A low-power lasing medium that produces a very small diameter beam well suited to microsurgery.

Potential energy: Energy stored in the form of gravity, chemical bonds, nuclear particles, and mechanical springs.

Practice acts: State law that establish and regulate the conditions under which professionals may practice including licensure, registration, educational requirements, scope of duties, and functions.

Preclotting: The process of soaking a graft or patch of synthetic graft material in the patient's blood or plasma before insertion. Most grafts no longer need preclotting.

Prenatal: The period of pregnancy before birth.

Preoperative medication: One or more drugs administered before surgery to prevent complications related to the surgical procedure or anesthesia.

Prescription: An order for a drug written by a qualified medical staff member.

Presentation: A term that refers to the part of the baby that comes down the birth canal first.

Press-fit: To impact or press a joint implant into position. Press-fitted implants do not require bone cement.

Primary intention: The wound-healing process after a clean surgical repair.

Prion: An infectious protein substance that is resistant to common sterilization methods.

Process challenge monitoring: A sealed, harmless bacteriological sample is included in a load of goods to be sterilized. The sample is recovered following the sterilization process and cultured to test for viability. This process is also called biological monitoring.

Professional attributes: Positive behaviors and traits of a professional, highly regarded by the public and professional peers. They include such traits as honesty, reliability, tact, diplomacy, and commitment to the profession.

Professional ethics: Ethical behavior established by authoritative peers of a particular profession, such as medicine or law.

Prognosis: A prediction of the patient's medical outcome (e.g., poor prognosis, good prognosis).

Proprietary name: The patented name given to a drug by its manufacturer.

Proprietary school: Private, for-profit school.

Protective reflexes: Nervous system responses to harmful environmental stimuli, such as pain, obstruction of the airway, and extreme temperature. Coughing, blinking, shivering, and withdrawal (from pain) are protective reflexes.

Prothrombin time (PT): A measurement of the time required for blood to clot.

Pterygium: A triangular membrane that arises from the medial canthus; the tissue may extend over the cornea, causing blindness.

Ptosis: Drooping or sagging of any anatomical structure.

Pulmonary embolism (PE): An obstruction in a pulmonary vessel caused by a blood clot, air bubble, or foreign body. Causes sudden pain and possible pulmonary arrest.

Pulmonary function tests (PFTs): Tests performed to measure the function and strength of the pulmonary system.

Pulse oximeter: A monitoring device that measures the patient's hemoglobin oxygen saturation by means of spectrometry.

Pulse pressure: A measurement of the difference between the systolic pressure and diastolic pressure. This can be a significant sign of metabolic disturbance.

Pulsed wave lasers: Lasers that apply laser light intermittently to the target tissue.

Punitive: Actions intended to punish a person who has violated the law.

Pyloric stenosis: A narrowing of the part of the stomach (pylorus) that leads to the small intestine.

Q-switched lasers: An alternate name for pulsed wave lasers.

Radiant exposure: In laser technology, the combination of the concentration of laser energy and the length of time tissue is exposed to it.

Radioactive seeds: Small "seeds" of radioactive material implanted in tissue for cancer treatment.

Radiofrequency: Electromagnetic energy in which the frequency is in the area of radio transmission. In electrosurgery, radiofrequency electromagnetic waves are used to produce the desired surgical effect.

Radiofrequency ablation (RFA): The use of radiofrequency waves to destroy a tissue mass or surface.

Radionuclides or isotopes: In nuclear medicine, radioactive particles are directed at the nucleus of a selected element to create energy. These special elements are referred to as *radionuclides* or *isotopes.*

Radiopaque: A substance that is impenetrable by x-rays (gamma radiation).

Range of motion: The normal anatomical movement of an extremity.

Raytec: A surgical sponge folded to 4 by 4 inches. The Raytec derives its name from one of the companies that manufacture surgical sponges.

Ream: To enlarge a preexisting hole, depression, or channel, such as the medullary canal.

Receiver: The person to whom a message is communicated by a sender.

Receptacle: An outlet in an electrical circuit that receives a plug containing live current, completing the circuit.

Reduce: To replace or push herniated tissue back into its normal anatomical position.

Reduction: The process of manipulating a bone structure to restore anatomical position.

Reflection: Communication with the patient that helps the individual connect his or her current feelings with events in the environment. Also, the behavior of a wave when it reaches a nonabsorbent material. The wave reverses and is directed back toward the source.

Reflux: Flow of a body fluid in the direction opposite its normal path. Urinary reflux is backward flow of urine into the ureter or kidney.

Refraction: A phenomenon of physics in which light rays are bent as they pass through a transparent medium that is denser than air. In the eye, refraction occurs as light enters the front of the eye and passes through the cornea, lens, aqueous humor, and vitreous.

Regional block: Anesthesia in a specific area of the body, achieved by injection of an anesthetic around a major nerve or group of nerves.

Replantation: Surgical attachment of the hand, thumb, or fingers after traumatic amputation.

Reprocessing: Activities or tasks that prepare used medical devices for use on another patient; these activities include cleaning, disinfection, decontamination, and sterilization.

Required request law: A law requiring medical personnel to request organ recovery from a deceased person's family.

Resectoscope: A cutting instrument used to remove and coagulate tissue piece by piece. It is used in conjunction with endoscopic procedures to remove tumors or other tissue, such as the prostate or endometrium.

Resident flora: Microorganisms normally present in specific tissues. Resident flora are necessary to the regular function of these tissues or structures. Also called *normal flora.*

Resident microorganisms: The microorganisms that normally colonize certain tissues of the body, usually without harm to the host.

Residual activity: The antimicrobial action of an antiseptic or a disinfectant that continues after the solution has dried.

Resistance: In electricity, the measurement of a substance's ability to inhibit the flow of electricity.

Restricted area: The area of the operating room where only personnel wearing surgical attire, including masks, shoe coverings, and head coverings, are allowed. Doors are kept closed, and the air pressure is greater than that in areas outside the restricted area.

Resuscitation: In trauma medicine, the process of restoring physiological balance following severe trauma.

Retained foreign object: An item that is inadvertently left inside the patient during surgery.

Retention catheter: A type of urinary catheter that remains in place. Also called an *indwelling* or *Foley catheter.*

Retrograde pyelography: Imaging studies of the renal pelvis in which a contrast medium is instilled through a transurethral catheter. *Retrograde* refers to flow, which is opposite the normal direction.

Return electrode monitoring (REM): A safety system used in electrosurgery in which the PRE transmits continuous feedback on the quality of impedance in the electrode and stops the current when it becomes dangerously high.

Reusable: A designation used by manufacturers to indicate that a medical device can be reprocessed for use on more than one patient.

Rigor mortis: The natural stiffening of the body that starts approximately 15 minutes after death and lasts about 24 hours.

Risk management: The process of tracking, evaluating, and studying accidents and incidents to protect patients and employees. Risk management produces change in policy or enforcement of policy if the risk reaches an unacceptable level.

Risk: The statistical probability of a given event based on the number of such events that have already occurred in a defined population.

Robot: A mechanical device that can be programmed to perform tasks.

Role confusion: Lack of clarity about one's job duties and requirements.

Rongeur: A hinged instrument with sharp, cup-shaped tips that is used to extract pieces of bone or other connective tissue.

Running suture: A method of suturing that uses one continuous suture strand for tissue approximation.

Saccular aneurysm: A type of aneurysm in which a saclike formation with a narrow neck projects from the side of the artery.

Safe Medical Device Act: A federal regulation that requires the reporting of any incident causing death or injury that is suspected to be the result of a medical device.

Sanitation: A method that reduces the number of bacteria in the environment to a safe level.

Scrub: The scrubbed surgical technologist or nurse assisting in surgery. Also refers to the surgical hand scrub performed before surgery and if the hands are contaminated with body fluids.

Scrubbed personnel: In surgery, members of the surgical team who work within the sterile field. Also called *sterile personnel.*

Sedation: An arousable state in which an individual is unaware of sensory stimuli. Depression of the central nervous system.

Sedative: A drug that induces a range of unconscious states. The effects are dose dependent. At low doses, sedatives cause some drowsiness. Increasing the dose causes central nervous system depression, ending in loss of consciousness.

Segmental resection: Anatomical resection of the liver in which segments divided by specific blood vessels and biliary ducts are removed.

Selective absorption: The absorption of a lasing medium into tissue being lased according to its color and density.

Semirestricted area: A designated area in which only personnel wearing scrub suits and hair caps that enclose all facial hair are allowed.

Sender: The person who communicates a message to another.

Sensation: The ability to feel stimuli in the environment (e.g., pain, heat, touch, visual stimuli, sound).

Sensorineural hearing loss: Hearing impairment arising from the cochlea, auditory nerve, or central nervous system.

Sentinel event: An unexpected incident resulting in serious physical injury, psychological harm, or death. The *near miss* of injury or harm is also considered a sentinel event.

Sentinel lymph node biopsy (SLNB): A procedure in which one or more lymph nodes are removed to determine whether a tumor has metastasized. Other lymph nodes may be removed periodically to determine whether metastasis has occurred.

Serial lenses: An optical system in which several lenses are lined up to produce a clear, well-defined image. Surgical endoscopes use serial lenses.

Serosa: The delicate outer layer of tissue of most organs.

Serosanguineous fluid: Exudate or discharge containing serum and blood.

Sexual harassment: An extreme abuse of power in which an individual uses sexualized language, gestures, or unwanted touch to coerce or intimidate another person.

Shank: The area of a surgical instrument between the box lock and the finger ring.

Sharps: Any objects that can penetrate the skin and have the potential to cause injury and infection, including but not limited to needles, scalpels, broken glass, broken capillary tubes, and exposed ends of dental wires.

Sharps: Any objects used in health care that are capable of penetrating the skin, causing injury.

Shear injury: Tissue injury or necrosis that results when two tissue planes are forcefully pulled in opposite directions. Shearing usually occurs when the body is pulled or slides by gravity across a high-friction surface, such as a bed sheet. Shearing can lead to a decubitus ulcer.

Shelf life: The length of time a wrapped item remains sterile after it has been subjected to a sterilization process.

Shelter-in-place: During a disaster, individuals may be required (or may choose) to shelter-in-place rather than evacuate the hazardous areas. This means that people remain where they are until the environment is safe or until rescue workers can reach the site.

Shunt: To bypass a structure or carry fluid from one anatomical location to another.

Side effects: Anticipated effects of a drug other than those intended. Side effects may be uncomfortable for the patient or may have a positive outcome.

Single-action rongeur: A heavy cutting instrument that has one hinge.

Single-stage prep: Also called a *paint prep*. The skin prep is performed using only antiseptic solution, which is painted on the skin at the operative site.

Single-use items: Instruments and devices intended for use on one patient only; sometimes called disposable items.

Skeletal traction: Traction device in which bone fragments are connected by pins or rods that are surgically inserted into the bone.

Skin flap: A flap that is created by incising the skin and cutting it away from the underlying tissue to which it is attached. The flap can be increased in size or "raised" as it is enlarged by dissection.

Slander: Spoken defamation.

Smoke plume: Toxic smoke emitted by tissue during electrosurgery and laser surgery.

Solid: A state of matter in which the molecules are bonded very tightly. Characteristics of solids are hardness and the ability to break apart into other solid pieces.

Solution: Any liquid antiseptic combined with water.

Spatula needle: A flat-tip suture needle commonly used in ophthalmic surgery.

Spaulding system: A system used to determine the level of microbial destruction required for medical devices and supplies based on the risk of infection associated with the area of the body where the device is used. Categories include critical, semicritical, and noncritical.

Specific gravity: The ratio of the density of a fluid compared to water. The specific gravity of urine is an important diagnostic tool.

Sphygmomanometer: An instrument used to measure blood pressure.

Split-thickness (or partial-thickness) skin graft (STSG): A skin graft that consists of the epidermis and a portion of the papillary dermis.

Sponge stick: A 4- × 4-inch sponge folded and mounted on a sponge forceps for use deep in the body.

Sporicidal: Able to kill spores.

Spray coagulation: An alternate term for fulguration.

Staghorn stone: A large, jagged kidney stone that forms in the renal pelvis.

Staging: An international method of classifying tissue to determine the level of metastasis in cancer.

Standard definition (SD): A type of video format. The clarity of an image is based on the number of signals (pixels) emitted by the camera. A standard definition format displays 640 × 480 pixels in a rectangular image.

Standard Precautions: Guidelines issued by the Centers for Disease Control and Prevention (CDC) to reduce the risk of transmission of blood-borne and other pathogens.

Standards of conduct: A set of rules or guidelines an organization writes for its members. The rules pertain to how people behave and are based on the principles that the organization values, such as professionalism and personal integrity.

States of matter: The physical forms of matter. The four states of matter are gas, liquid, solid, and plasma.

Static electricity: The buildup of charged particles on a surface.

Statutes: Laws passed by state legislative bodies.

Stenosis: The narrowing of a hollow structure such as a blood vessel or duct.

Stent: A tubular device placed inside an artery for dilation, support, and prevention of stricture.

Stereoscopic viewer: In robotic surgery, the binocular lens system of the surgeon console.

Stereotactic: A computerized method of locating a point in space or in tissue, using coordinates in three dimensions. During stereotactic surgery, the precise location of a tumor or other tissue can be identified from outside the body. The tissue can then be targeted for destruction. The term originates from the Greek words *stereo*, meaning "three dimensional," and *tactos*, meaning "touched."

Sterile field: An area that includes the draped patient, all sterile tables, and sterile equipment in the immediate area of the patient. The patient is the center of the sterile field.

Sterile item: Any item or medical device that has been exposed to a process that destroys all microbes, including spores.

Sterile personnel: Members of the surgical team who have performed a surgical scrub or hand and arm antisepsis procedure. They don sterile gown and gloves and either perform the surgery or assist directly. Sterile personnel include the surgeon, assistant(s), and scrub. Other sterile personnel such as a scrub nurse, students, and preceptors may also be part of the sterile team.

Sterile setup: The process of organizing and arranging sterile supplies and equipment before surgery.

Sterile: Completely free of all microorganisms.

Sterility: A state in which an inanimate or animate substance harbors absolutely no viable microorganisms.

Sterilization: A process by which all microorganisms, including spores, are destroyed.

Sternotomy: An incision made into the sternum.

Stoma: An opening created in a hollow organ and sutured to the skin to drain the organ's contents (e.g., an intestinal or ureteral stoma). A stoma may be a temporary or permanent method of bypass.

Stoma appliance: A two- or three-piece medical device used to collect drainage from a stoma. The appliance is attached to the patient's skin and completely covers the stoma. This allows free drainage into a collection device or bag.

Strabismus: Inability to coordinate the extraocular muscles, which prevents binocular vision.

Straight catheter: A urinary catheter used for one-time drainage of the bladder. It may be called a "red Robinson" or simply a "Robinson" catheter.

Strangulated hernia: A hernia in which abdominal tissue has become trapped between the layers of an abdominal wall defect. The strangulated tissue usually becomes swollen as a result of venous congestion. Lack of blood supply can lead to tissue necrosis.

Strike-through contamination: An event in which fluid from a nonsterile surface or air penetrates the protective wrapper of a sterile item, causing it to become contaminated.

Subciliary incision: Skin incision made approximately 2 mm inferior to the lower eyelashes.

Subcutaneous mastectomy: A procedure in which the breast is removed, but the skin, nipple, and areola are left intact. Also called a lumpectomy.

Subpoena: A court order requiring its recipient to appear and testify at a trial or deposition. Medical records also can be the subject of subpoenas.

Suppurative: Having developed pus and fluid.

Suprapubic catheter: A bladder catheter inserted through the skin in the suprapubic area of the abdomen.

Suprapubic pressure: Pressure that is applied downward on the patient's abdomen just above the pubic bone.

Surge capacity: The number of patients a health care facility can manage in an emergency.

Surgeon's preference card: A database or card system listing the methods, materials, and techniques used by each surgeon for specific procedures.

Surgical conscience: In surgery, the ethical motivation to practice excellent aseptic technique to protect the patient from infection. Surgical conscience implies that the professional practices excellent technique regardless of whether others are observing.

Surgical hand scrub: A specific technique for washing the hands before donning a surgical gown and gloves before surgery. The scrub is performed with timed or counted strokes using detergent-based antiseptic. The surgical hand scrub is designed to remove dirt, oils, and transient microorganisms and reduce the number of resident microorganisms.

Surgical handrub: The systematic application of antiseptic foam or cream on the hands before gowning and gloving for a sterile procedure. The surgical handrub may be used as an alternative to the traditional hand scrub under certain conditions.

Surgical site infection (SSI): Postoperative infection of the surgical wound, most commonly caused by the normal bacteria found on the patient's skin or shed from the skin or hair of members of the surgical team.

Surgical wound: The superficial and deep tissue layers of the surgical incision. This is the center of the surgical field.

Swage: The area of an atraumatic suture where the suture strand is fused to the needle. Also called an atraumatic suture.

Synthetic grafts: Grafts derived from synthetic material compatible with body tissue. Synthetic grafts may be soft, semisolid, or liquid.

Systole: A phase of the cardiac cycle in which the ventricles contract.

Systolic pressure: The pressure exerted by blood on the walls of vessels during the contraction phase of the cardiac cycle.

Tachycardia: A fast heart rate (usually over 120 beats per minute in the adult).

Tamponade: An instrument or other device that puts pressure on tissue, usually to stop bleeding.

Tapered needle: A suture needle that has a round body that tapers to a sharp point. It punctures tissue, making an opening for the body of the needle to follow.

Technetium-99: A radioactive substance used to identify sentinel lymph nodes.

Telesurgery: A type of robotic surgery in which surgery is performed from a nearby location through computer-mediated instruments. In telesurgery, no direct physical contact with the instruments occurs.

Tenaculum: A grasping instrument with sharp pointed tips, generally used to manipulate or grasp tissue such as the thyroid or cervix.

Tensile strength: The amount of force or stress a suture can withstand without breaking.

Teratogen: A chemical or agent that can injure the fetus or cause birth defects.

Terminal decontamination: Thorough cleaning and disinfection of supplies or an environment such as the operating room suite after patient use. Specific protocols and procedures are used during terminal decontamination.

The Joint Commission: The accrediting organization for hospitals and other health care facilities in the United States.

Therapeutic communication: A purposeful method of communication in which the caregiver responds to explicit or implicit needs of the patient.

Therapeutic touch: The purposeful touching of another person to convey empathy, care, and tenderness.

Therapeutic window: Range of drug doses that can treat disease effectively while staying within the safety range.

Thermal conductivity: The ability of a substance to conduct heat. Different substances have different abilities to conduct or transmit heat.

Thermoregulation: A complex physiological process in which the body maintains a temperature that is optimal for survival.

Thoracic outlet syndrome: A group of disorders attributed to compression of the subclavian vessels and nerves. Such compression can cause permanent injury to the arm and shoulder.

Thoracotomy: An incision made into the thoracic cavity.

Thromboembolus (embolus): A blood clot that breaks loose and enters the systemic circulation, causing obstruction or occlusion of a blood vessel. (Also referred to as a *thrombus*.)

Thrombus: Any organic or nonorganic material blocking an artery; generally refers to a blood clot or atherosclerotic plaque but also includes fat or air.

Throw: A loop that forms a knot.

Tie on a passer: A strand of suture material attached to the tip of an instrument.

TIMEOUT: A procedure for verifying the patient's identity, correct surgical procedure, site, and side. TIMEOUT takes place after the patient has been positioned, prepped, and draped but before the first incision. The procedure is promoted by the Association of Surgical Technologists (AST) and described in detail by the Association of periOperative Registered Nurses (AORN) and the World Health Organization (WHO).

Tincture: Any liquid antiseptic combined with alcohol.

TM: The tympanic membrane.

TNM classification system: An international system in which *T* refers to the extent of the tumor, *N* refers to the lymph node involvement, and *M* is the extent of the metastasis. It determines the extent of metastasis and the level of cell differentiation, two important factors in the treatment and prognosis of cancer.

Topical: Refers to application of a drug to the skin or mucous membranes.

Topical anesthesia: Anesthesia of superficial nerves of the skin or mucous membranes.

Torsion: Twisting of an organ or a structure on itself. Torsion may cause local ischemia and necrosis.

Tort: Legal wrongdoing that results in injury to a person or property.

Traction: A mechanical method of applying pulling force to fractured bone in order to bring the fragments into alignment.

Traction injury: A nerve injury caused by stretching or compression of the nerve.

Trade name: The name given to a drug by the company that produces and sells it.

Traffic patterns: The movement of people and equipment into, out of, and within the operating room.

Transcervical: Literally, "through the cervix." In surgery, a transcervical approach means that surgery is performed by passing instruments through the cervix.

Transconjunctival incision: Incision made through the conjunctiva.

Transcutaneous: Literally, "through the skin"; it refers to a procedure in which a needle or other medical device is inserted from the outside of the body to the inside through the skin.

Transdermal: Refers to administration of a drug by absorption through the skin, such as with ointments or patches impregnated with the drug.

Transfer board: A thin Plexiglas, fiberglass, or roller board that is placed under the patient to move the person from the operating table to the stretcher or bed.

Transient flora: Microorganisms that do not normally reside in the tissue of an individual. Transient microorganisms are acquired through skin contact with an animate or inanimate source colonized by microbes. Transient flora may be removed by routine methods of skin cleaning.

Transitional area: An area in which surgical personnel or visitors prepare to enter the semirestricted and restricted areas. Transitional areas include the locker rooms and changing rooms.

Transmission-based precautions: Standards and precautions to prevent the spread of infectious disease by patients known to be infected.

Transosteal implants: Bone plates with retaining posts used in the procedure for dental implants.

Transsphenoidal: Literally, "across or through the sphenoid bone." Surgery of the pituitary gland may be performed by approaching it through the sphenoid bone.

Transurethral: Surgical access through the urethral orifice. The term also may describe an instrument that enters the bladder through the urethral meatus.

Trendelenburg position: The position in which a prone or supine patient is tilted with the head down.

Tumor marker: An antigen present on the tumor cell or a substance (protein, hormone, or other chemical) released by cancer cells into the blood.

Tunable dye laser: A type of laser formed by the combination of argon gas and specific dyes that alter tissue absorption of the lasing beam.

Tympanostomy tube: A tube that is placed in a myringotomy to produce aeration of the middle ear.

U.S. Pharmacopeia (USP): An organization that establishes standards for drugs approved by the U.S. Food and Drug Administration (FDA) for their labeled use. All approved drugs have been tested for consumer safety and written information is available about their pharmacological action, use, risks, and dosage.

Ultrasonic cleaner: Equipment that cleans instruments using ultrasonic waves.

Ultrasonic energy: High-frequency energy created by vibration or excitation of molecules. This type of energy destroys tissue by breaking molecular bonds.

Ultrasound: A technology that uses high-frequency wave energy to identify anatomical structures and anomalies. In ultrasound imaging, sound waves are transformed into visual images on a screen.

Umbilical tapes: Lengths of cotton mesh tape used to loop around a blood vessel for retraction. See *vessel loop.*

Unconsciousness: A neurological state in which the person is unable to respond to external stimuli. Unconsciousness can be induced with drugs or may be caused by trauma or disease.

Undermine: A surgical technique in which a plane of tissue is created or an existing tissue plane is lifted, such as skin from the fascia.

Underwriters Laboratories (UL): A nonprofit agency that tests and certifies electrical equipment in the United States.

Unrestricted area: An area that people dressed in street clothes may enter.

Unretrieved device fragment: A portion of a medical device that has broken off or come apart in the body and is not detected or removed. Examples are fragments of a broken surgical needle and a hinge pin of a surgical instrument.

Uterus: The muscular organ that holds the fetus and the placenta during pregnancy.

Vector: A living intermediate carrier of microorganisms from one host to another. An example is the transmission of the bubonic plague. The vector is a flea and the bacterium is transmitted to the human through a bite from an infected flea.

Venous stasis: Pooling of blood in the veins caused by inactivity or disease. Stasis can cause distention of the veins.

Ventilation: The process of inflating and deflating the lungs during breathing.

Ventral hernia: A weakness in the abdominal wall, usually resulting in protrusion of abdominal viscera against the peritoneum and abdominal fascia.

Verbal abuse: Deliberate attempts to devalue, intimidate, bully, or embarrass another person using loud, vulgar, sexualized, or intimidating language.

Veress needle: A spring-loaded needle used to deliver carbon dioxide gas during insufflation.

Vessel loop: A device used to retract a vessel during surgery. A length of thin Silastic tubing or cotton tape (umbilical tape) is passed around the vessel. The ends can be threaded through a bolster (a 0.12- to 0.24-inch [0.3- to 0.6-cm] length of rubber or Silastic tubing) to secure the loop against the blood vessel.

Video cable: In video-assisted endoscopy, the cable that transmits digital data from the camera head to the camera control unit and from the image system to the output recorder.

Video printer: A device that stores and prints output data viewed through the video endoscope.

Viricidal: Able to kill viruses.

Virion: A complete virus particle.

Virulence: The degree to which a microorganism is capable of causing disease.

Viscera: The organs or tissue of the abdominal cavity.

Vital signs: Cardinal signs of well-being: pain, temperature, pulse, respiration, and blood pressure. These are measured to assess a patient's basic metabolic status.

Volatile: A substance with a low boiling point such as alcohol that converts to a vapor at low temperature.

Voltage: The electrical force in a circuit, measured as the amount of force that passes a given point over a stated period. Voltage is measured in volts (V).

Vulnerability: Exposure to the risk of harm. In disaster management, vulnerable populations are those with a higher than normal risk. This may be related to their age, mobility, inaccessibility, or other condition that hinders or prevents aid.

Washer-sterilizer/disinfector: Equipment that washes and decontaminates instruments after an operative procedure.

Wave: In physics, a naturally occurring phenomenon in which energy is transmitted in the form of peaks (high points) and troughs (low points).

Wavelength: The distance between peaks in a complete wave cycle.

White balance: A procedure for adjusting the light color of the video camera to other components of the system.

Win-lose solution: In conflict resolution, a solution that leaves one party satisfied but the other party dissatisfied.

Win-win solution: In conflict resolution, a solution that allows both parties in a conflict to gain.

Wire localization: A biopsy procedure in which a hook wire is inserted under fluoroscopy into tissue suspected of being cancerous. The tissue surrounding the hook wire is removed.

World Wide Web: In computer technology, a network of links to data via an Internet system. It uses a special computer language protocol and is only one of many types of systems for transmitting data through a computer network.

Woven wrappers: Also called linen or cloth wrappers, these are fabric cloths used to wrap clean, disinfected supplies in preparation for a sterilization process.

Xenograft: A graft made up of tissue taken from one species and grafted into another species (e.g., a porcine graft implanted in human tissue).

A

Note: Page numbers followed by *b* indicated boxes; *f* figures; and *t* tables.